Diseases of the Liver and Biliary System in Children

EDITED BY

DEIRDRE KELLY
MD, FRCP, FRCPI, FRCPCH
Professor of Pediatric Hepatology, Liver Unit, Birmingham Children's Hospital, Birmingham, UK

THIRD EDITION

FOREWORD BY

DAME SHEILA SHERLOCK

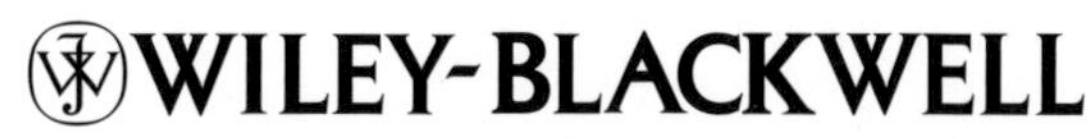

A John Wiley & Sons, Ltd., Publication

Blackwell Publishing was acquired by John Wiley & Sons in February 2007. Blackwell's publishing program has been merged with Wiley's global Scientific, Technical and Medical business to form Wiley-Blackwell.

Registered office: John Wiley & Sons Ltd, The Atrium, Southern Gate, Chichester, West Sussex, PO19 8SQ, UK

Editorial offices: 9600 Garsington Road, Oxford, OX4 2DQ, UK
The Atrium, Southern Gate, Chichester, West Sussex, PO19 8SQ, UK
111 River Street, Hoboken, NJ 07030-5774, USA

For details of our global editorial offices, for customer services and for information about how to apply for permission to reuse the copyright material in this book please see our website at www.wiley.com/wiley-blackwell

A catalogue record for this book is available from the British Library.

Library of Congress Cataloging-in-Publication Data

Diseases of the liver and biliary system in children / edited by Deirdre Kelly. — 3rd ed.
p. ; cm.
Includes bibliographical references and index.
ISBN 978-1-4051-6334-7 (alk. paper)
1. Liver—Diseases. 2. Biliary tract—Diseases. 3. Pediatric gastroenterology. I. Kelly, Deirdre A.
[DNLM: 1. Liver Diseases. 2. Child. 3. Infant. WS 310 D611 2008]
RJ456.L5D57 2008
618.92'362—dc22

2007037665

ISBN: 9781405163347

A catalogue record for this title is available from the British Library

Set in 9/12pt Meridien by Graphicraft Limited, Hong Kong
Printed and bound in Singapore by COS Printers Pte Ltd

First published 1999
Second edition 2004
Third edition 2008

1 2008

Contents

Contributors

Estella M. Alonso MD
Professor of Pediatrics, Northwestern University, Feinberg School of Medicine; Siragusa Transplant Center, Children's Memorial Hospital Chicago, IL, USA

Ulrich Baumann MD
Consultant Paediatric Hepatologist, The Liver Unit, Birmingham Children's Hospital, Birmingham, UK

Sue V. Beath BSc, MB BS, MRCP(UK), DTM, FRCPCH
Consultant Paediatric Hepatologist, The Liver Unit, Birmingham Children's Hospital, UK

Jacqueline Blyth BSc, MSc (Health Psychology), ClinPsyD, CSci, CPsychol, AFBPsS
Clinical Psychologist, Birmingham Children's Hospital, Birmingham, UK

Elizabeth Boxall PhD, FRCPath, FFPH
Consultant Clinical Scientist, Health Protection Agency, West Midlands Public Health Laboratory, Heart of England Foundation Trust, Birmingham, UK

Rachel M. Brown BSc MBChB FRCPath
Consultant Paediatric Hepatologist, Department of Histopathology, Birmingham Children's Hospital, Birmingham, UK

Anupam Chakrapani MD, DCH, FRCPCH
Consultant in Inherited Metabolic Disorders, Department of Inherited Metabolic Disorders, Birmingham Children's Hospital NHS Foundation Trust, Birmingham, UK

Mei-Hwei Chang MD
Professor, Department of Paediatrics, National Taiwan University Hospital, Taipei, Taiwan

Victoria Clark BChD, M Dent Sci, FDS (paeds)
Consultant in Paediatric Dentistry, Birmingham Children's Hospital, Birmingham, UK

Carla Colombo MD
Associate Professor of Pediatrics, University of Milan, Fondazione IRCCS "Ospedale Maggiore Policlinico, Mangiagalli e Regina, Elena", Cystic Fibrosis Centre, Milan, Italy

Suzanne Davison BSc, MRCP, MRCPCH
Paediatric Hepatologist, Children's Liver and GI Unit, St James's University Hospital, Leeds, UK

Elwyn Elias MD
Consultant Hepatologist, Liver Unit, University Birmingham Foundation Trust Hospital, Birmingham, UK

Jean de Ville de Goyet FRCS, MD, PhD
Professor of Paediatric Surgery, Tor Vergata University, Roma, Italy; Paediatric Liver and Transplant Surgery, Bambino Gesu Children's Hospital, Roma, Italy

Graham Gordon BSc, SRN, RSCN
Principle Specialist Nurse (Hepatology and Transplantation), The Liver Unit, Birmingham Children's Hospital, Birmingham, UK

Anne Green BSc, MSc, PhD, FRCPath, FRCPCH, FIBiol, FRSC
Consultant Paediatric Biochemistry and Professor of Paediatrics and Child Health, University of Birmingham, Birmingham, UK; Consultant Clinical Biochemist, Research and Development, Clinical Chemistry & Inherited Metabolic Disorders, The Birmingham Children's Hospital NHS Trust, Birmingham, UK

Jane Hartley MB.ChB, MRCPCH, M.Med.Sc
Department of Medical and Molecular Genetics, Birmingham University and Birmingham Children's Hospital, Birmingham, UK

Marie-Therese Hosey DDS, MSc (Med Sci), BDS, FDS, RCPS
Professor of Paediatric Dentistry, King's College Dental Institute, Denmark Hill, London, UK

Deirdre A. Kelly MD, FRCP, FRCPI, FRCPCH
Professor of Paediatric Hepatology, The Liver Unit, Birmingham Children's Hospital, Birmingham, UK

A. David Mayer MS, FRCS
Consultant Liver Transplant Surgeon, Queen Elizabeth Hospital and Birmingham Children's Hospital, UK

Janet E. McDonagh MD, FRCP(UK)
Clinical Senior Lecturer in Paediatric and Adolescent Rheumatology, Division of Reproductive and Child Health, University of Birmingham, Birmingham, UK

Patrick J. McKiernan BSc, MRCP, FRCPCH
Consultant Paediatric Hepatologist, The Liver Unit, Birmingham Children's Hospital, Birmingham, UK

Giorgina M. Mieli-Vergani MD, PhD
Director of Paediatric Liver Centre, Institute of Liver Studies, King's College London School of Medicine at King's College Hospital, Denmark Hill, London, UK

Alastair J.W. Millar MBChB, FRCS(Eng & Edin), FRACS (paed surg), FCS(SA), DCH
Charles F.M. Saint Professor of Paediatric Surgery, University of Cape Town and Red Cross War Memorial Children's Hospital Rondebosch, Cape Town, South Africa

Bruce Morland MBChB, MRCP, DM, FRCPCH
Consultant Oncologist, Birmingham Children's Hospital, Birmingham, UK

Karen F. Murray MD
Professor of Pediatrics; Director, Hepatobiliary Program, Division of Gastroenterology and Nutrition, Seattle Children's Hospital and Regional Medical Center, Seattle, WA, USA

Carolyn Patchell BSc, SRD
Head of Dietetic Services, Birmingham Children's Hospital, Birmingham, UK

Seng-Hock Quak MBBS, Mmed (Paed), FAMS, FRCP (Glas), FRCPCH, MD
Department of Paediatrics, National University Hospital, Singapore

Julie Reed BSc, MPhil, ClinPsyD
Consultant Clinical Psychologist, Birmingham Children's Hospital, Birmingham, UK

Jorge Reyes MD
Chief, Division of Transplant Surgery, University of Washington Medical Center, Chief, Transplantation Services, Children's Hospital and Regional Medical Center, Seattle, WA

Eve A. Roberts MD, FRCPC
Adjunct Professor of Paediatrics, Medicine and Pharmacology, University of Toronto, The Hospital for Sick Children, Toronto, Ontario, Canada

Kathleen B. Schwarz MD
Director, Pediatric Liver Center and Professor of Pediatrics, Johns Hopkin's University School of Medicine, Baltimore, MD, USA

Ross Shepherd MD, FRACP, FRCP
Professor of Pediatrics, Washington University School of Medicine, Medical Director, Liver Care Center, St Louis Children's Hospital, St Louis, MO, USA

Anupam Sibal MD
Group Medical Director, Senior Consultant Pediatric Gastroenterologist & Hepatologist, Indraprastha Apollo Hospitals, New Delhi, India

Robert H. Squires MD
Professor of Pediatrics, Clinical Director, Pediatric Gastroenterology, Hepatology and Nutrition, Children's Hospital of Pittsburgh, Pittsburgh, PA, USA

Stuart Tanner CBE, FRCP, FRCPH
Emeritus Professor of Paediatrics, University of Sheffield, UK

Michelle Thomson MRCP
Consultant Dermatologist, The Birmingham Skin Centre, City Hospital, Birmingham, UK

Indra D.M. van Mourik MD, MRCP, FRCPCH
Consultant Paediatric Hepatologist, The Liver Unit, Birmingham Children's Hospital, Birmingham, UK

Diego Vergani MD, PhD
Professor of Liver Immunopathology, Institute of Liver Studies, King's College London School of Medicine at King's College Hospital, Denmark Hill, London, UK

Peter F. Whitington MD
The Sally Burnett Searle Professor of Pediatrics and Transplantation, Northwestern University Feinberg Medicine School; Chief, Division of Gastroenterology, Hepatology and Nutrition, Director of the Siragusa Transplantation Center, Children's Memorial Hospital, Chicago, IL, USA

Jaime Liou Wolfe MD
Division of Pediatric Gastroenterology and Nutrition, Johns Hopkin's University School of Medicine, MD, USA

Foreword to the First Edition

Although the Ancient Egyptians believed that the liver had mystic powers of healing, and Hippocrates gave a full description of hepatic encephalopathy, modern hepatology has only taken off in the last 50 years. Accelerated progress has followed discovery of the hepatitis viruses, now a virtual alphabet from A to E and beyond. Hepatobiliary imaging and endoscopy have added to the progress. Developments have depended not only on specialist hepatologists, but on developments in other related disciplines of medicine—particularly virology, immunology, biochemistry, and now, molecular medicine. A huge literature is available describing liver disease in adults, but pediatrics has lagged behind.

This book covers all the essentials of pediatric hepatology and is therefore particularly timely. The material covered is wide, from such aspects as the psychology of parents of children on transplant waiting lists to the genetic disturbances of bilirubin and bile salt transport in the neonate. The chapter authors have been well chosen. They are international authorities, active both clinically and in research. They write lucidly from personal experience.

Many helpful algorithms and tables are included. The references at the end of each chapter have been carefully selected and are up-to-date . . . This book should be available in every pediatric department. It should be at hand at all times to offer practical advice on any childhood liver disease. General pediatricians will certainly benefit. It would be a suitable gift to reward a trainee.

This book fills a real gap in our knowledge of liver disease. It will be a well-deserved success.

PROFESSOR DAME SHEILA SHERLOCK
1918–2001

Preface

Pediatric liver disease is a significant cause of morbidity and mortality worldwide. Sophisticated molecular genetic techniques have not only identified new genes and categorized rare diseases, but have also given us an insight into pathophysiology and potential therapy. Research into genomics and proteomics has extended our understanding of the mechanisms involved in cellular regulation and regeneration. National and international collaboration through clinical databases has helped us refine our diagnosis and treatment of diseases such as biliary atresia and acute liver failure.

Advances in diagnosis and treatment—particularly the successful development of transplantation—have dramatically improved the outcome for infants and children with liver disease, so that many can now expect to grow into adult life. This success brings its own challenges, as adult specialists now need to learn to manage young people with a lifetime of chronic disease. They need to become familiar with pediatric diseases new to them in a population prone to teenage behavior and nonadherence.

The investigation and management of significant pediatric liver disease rightly remains within the remit of specialist or transplant units. Nevertheless, the recognition of the incidence of liver disease, the implications of new therapies, and the necessity for multidisciplinary working are as important for general pediatricians as for pediatric gastroenterologists, surgeons, and hepatologists. The gratifying survival of increasing numbers of young people with liver disease into adult life means that it is essential for adult practitioners to be cognisant of pediatric liver disease.

The third edition of this book summarizes the advances of the last 4 years and provides a practical approach to the diagnosis and management of pediatric liver diseases, highlighting the importance of multidisciplinary teamwork and holistic management of the child and family. The remit has been extended to include information on structure and function, with an emphasis on the basic mechanisms of disease. New chapters describe the effects of liver disease from pregnancy to adolescence, to reflect the increasing survival of young women with liver disease into adult reproductive life, and the importance of managing adolescent transition.

It should interest the adult gastroenterologist and hepatologist, the general pediatrician, and the pediatric trainee, as well as providing guidance for nurses and allied health professionals.

DEIRDRE A. KELLY
Birmingham, September 2007

Acknowledgments

The investigation and management of pediatric liver disease requires much skill and a dedicated multidisciplinary approach. I am indebted to my colleagues in the Liver Unit, in Birmingham Children's Hospital, and elsewhere across the globe for their knowledge and expertise.

I was fortunate that so many distinguished contributors worldwide agreed to share their own areas of expertise and learning, which have enhanced this book.

I particularly wish to thank the many colleagues who provided clinical slides and material—particularly Dr. Helen Alton, Dr. Kathryn Foster, and Dr. Rachel Brown.

Finally, I am grateful to Audrey Bergan for her help in editing and coordinating this book.

Dedications

First Edition

To my sons, Eoin and Lochlinn Parker
and my husband, Ian Byatt.

Second Edition

To the memory of my parents, Frank and Kathy Kelly, who started me on my medical career.

Third Edition

To all the children and families who have taught me so much.

1 Structure Function, and Repair

1 Structure Function and Repair of the Liver

Ulrich Baumann, Alastair J.W. Millar, and Rachel M. Brown

The liver is an organ that has fascinated mankind ever since medicine existed. Ancient medicine was aware of the liver's central role in nutrition, and for Galen it was a "principal instrument" of the body. In Greek mythology, Prometheus—the friend of mankind who was chained to a rock by the god Zeus as punishment for giving humans the use of fire—suffered daily as an eagle devoured his liver, only for it to restore itself overnight. This association with Prometheus and the capacity of the liver to regenerate has been quoted many times in textbooks, editorials, and reviews.

Most lay people understand the principal roles of the heart, brain, and kidney, but are unfamiliar with the liver. Patients and families find it difficult to understand the functions of the liver and the implications of liver failure, and this has to be taken into consideration when counseling children and their families. In order to gain an understanding of liver disease, it is necessary to study the basics of the development, anatomy, and function of the liver and its responses to injury.

Structure

Development

Overview

The development of the liver has been extensively studied.[1,2] Human liver development begins during the third week of gestation from the ventral foregut endoderm (the future duodenum), which gives rise to the liver bud or hepatic diverticulum. The liver bud grows into the septum transversum and the cardiac mesoderm. These structures provide connective tissues to the developing liver and appropriate gene expression, which is regulated in a time-specific manner by liver-enriched transcription factors such as hepatocyte nuclear factor 6 (HNF6),[3] required for normal development in the endoderm and is mesoderm. This process is termed "mesoderm inductive signaling."[4,5] In this environment, cells from the liver bud form thick plates of hepatoblasts surrounding sinusoids fed from vitelline vessels derived from the wall of the yolk sac. Sheets of liver cells are initially many layers thick, but by 5 months after birth, the plates are two cells thick. The adult pattern of plates one cell thick (Figure 1.1) is not seen until at least 5 years of age.[6] The liver reaches a peak of relative size at the ninth gestational week, accounting for 10% of fetal weight. In the healthy neonate, it represents up to about 5% of the body's weight; during adolescence, this decreases to the final adult proportion of 2% of body weight, or a weight of 1400 g in the female and 1800 g in the male.

Vascular development

The liver grows under the influence of its blood supply. Initially, blood is provided by the symmetrical vitelline veins, which ultimately join to form the portal vein. Later, blood is supplied by the left and right umbilical veins, rich in oxygen and nutrients, from the placenta. The right umbilical vein then disappears, leaving the left umbilical vein as the principal supplier. Blood in the left umbilical vein takes one of three routes—supplying sinusoids on the left side of liver; supplying sinusoids in the right half of the liver via retrograde flow through a connection with the left branch of the portal vein; or to the inferior vena cava via the ductus venosus. Ultrasound studies in fetuses near term have shown that the left lobe receives almost exclusively nutrient-rich umbilical vein blood, whilst the right lobe only receives 50% of its supply from the umbilical vein, with the remaining 50% coming from the nutrient-poor portal vein.[7] The left lobe is therefore significantly better perfused *in utero*, and as such is relatively larger than in adults and better able to withstand hypoxic insults. At birth, the left umbilical vein becomes the ligamentum teres, and the ductus venosus becomes the ligamentum venosum. Hepatic artery branches appear later in development, emerging in portal tracts (Figure 1.2) first near the hilum and then toward the periphery. This spatial and temporal sequence mirrors that seen in the developing bile ducts. The artery appears before the definitive bile duct and may be formed at least in part from portal constituents, specifically myofibroblasts, rather than growing into the portal tracts from the hilum.[8]

Diseases of the Liver and Biliary System in Children, 3rd edition. Edited by Deirdre Kelly. © 2008 Blackwell Publishing, ISBN: 978-1-4051-6334-7.

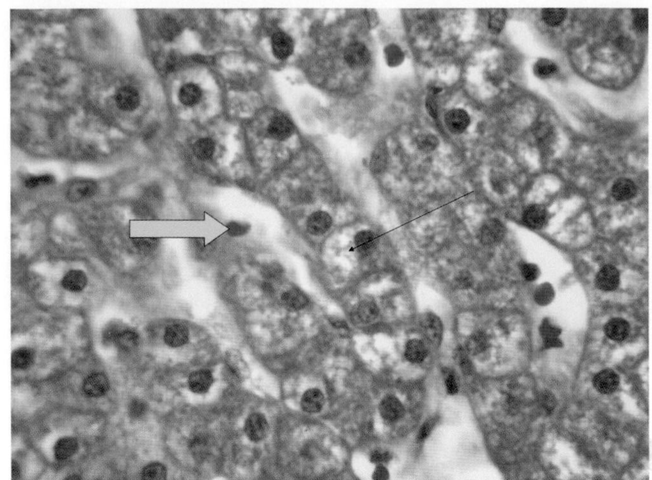

A

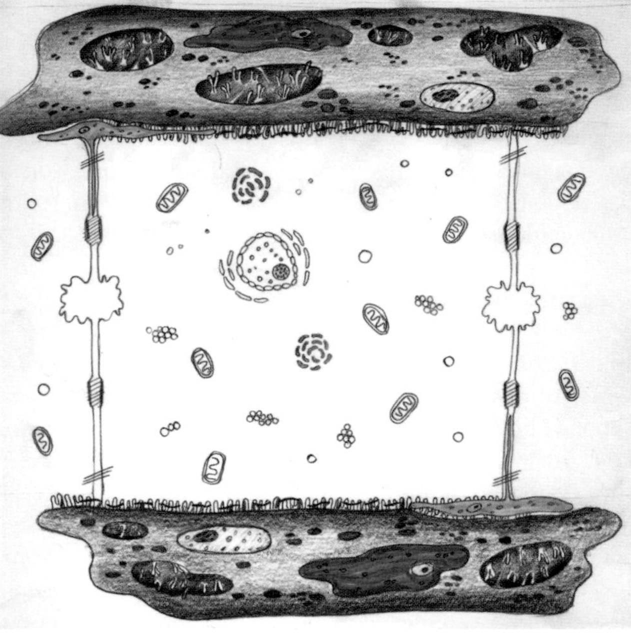

B

Figure 1.1 Mature hepatic plates and sinusoids. **A** Mature hepatic plates and sinusoids are easily identified on light microscopy. The small black arrow shows a hepatocyte in a plate one cell thick, while the large blue arrow shows an erythrocyte in a sinusoid. (Hematoxylin–eosin, original magnification × 400.) **B** Schematic view of the cellular arrangement of the hepatocyte in the hepatic plate, with stellate cells (yellow) located in the space of Disse and Kupffer cells (brown) in the sinusoidal lumen.

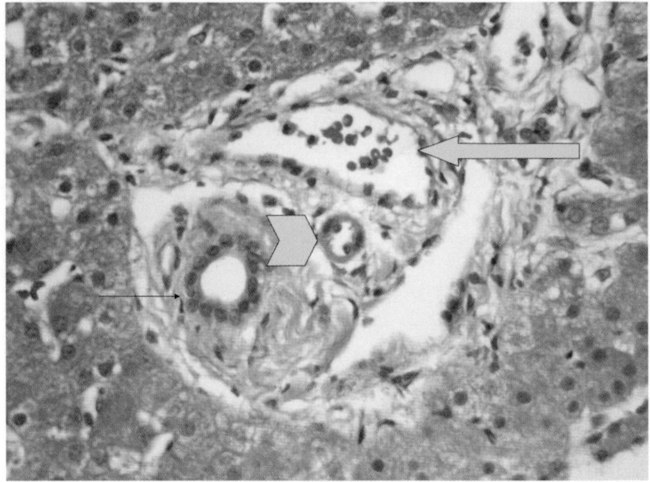

Figure 1.2 Normal portal tract. The normal portal tract consists of the hepatic artery (blue arrowhead), the portal vein branch (blue arrow), and bile duct (small black arrow). (Hematoxylin–eosin, original magnification × 200.)

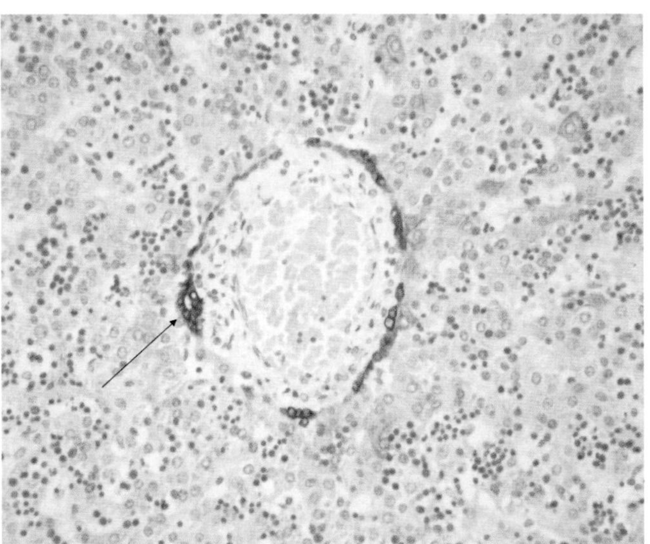

Figure 1.3 The ductal plate. The oval-shaped ductal plate highlighted in this 17-week fetus on cytokeratin immunohistochemistry (AE1/AE3) is undergoing the process of remodeling. A tubular structure has formed within the ductal plate (arrow), which will subsequently become incorporated into the developing portal tract to occupy a position as seen in Figure 1.2. (Original magnification × 200.)

Biliary development

The extrahepatic and intrahepatic biliary systems develop from the endoderm as two independent subunits, which merge at the end of the developmental process. The extrahepatic bile ducts and gallbladder develop from the elongated stalk of the hepatic diverticulum as the duodenum withdraws from the septum transversum. Formation of the intrahepatic bile duct system begins around the eighth week of gestation. The hepatoblasts around the margins of the mesenchyme of the portal tracts become smaller and strongly express cytokeratins (intermediate cytoskeletal components, of which there are many types). This sleeve of cells surrounding the portal vein branch, with its associated mesenchyme, is the *ductal plate* (Figure 1.3).

A discontinuous second layer of cells now forms around the first, resulting in a double layer around variable stretches of the portal perimeter. Within this double layer, slit-like lumens appear. The cells destined to form ducts express biliary-type cytokeratins, identifiable by immunohistochemistry; hepatoblasts not involved in the evolution of the ductal plate differentiate toward mature hepatocytes and express different cytokeratins. The early liver cells are bipotential, capable of differentiating into biliary epithelial cells or mature hepatocytes. Contact with the portal mesenchyme orchestrates the differentiation toward biliary epithelium; the portal myofibroblasts have been implicated specifically in this process.[8] Signals include bone morphogenic protein and transforming growth factor-β.[3] The unique nature of the portal mesenchyme in inducing this differentiation is evidenced by the fact that ductal plates do not form around the central veins. From 12 weeks' gestation onward, the ductal plate is *remodeled*.

Both ductal plate development and its subsequent remodeling begin in the largest portal areas near the hilum and proceed outward toward the smaller portal tracts.[9] The tubular structures that have formed in the double-layered ductal plate become surrounded by portal mesenchyme and separated from the parenchyma. Connections are retained between the newly forming duct in the portal tract and the ductal plate and hence to the canaliculi (canals of Hering). As only a single duct persists, remodeling requires the disappearance of unwanted elements of the ductal plate by apoptosis. Failure of the precise scheme of spatial and temporal remodeling leads to persistence of the ductal plate, known as "ductal plate malformation," which can affect any caliber of portal tract.[10] Periportal cells may retain the ability to differentiate toward bile duct epithelium, seen as the ductules that appear at the portal tract margins in biliary diseases. Speculation surrounds the origin of the ductules—either from metaplasia of mature hepatocytes or biliary epithelial cells, or from progenitor cells located in the canals of Hering, possibly of bone-marrow origin.[5,11] This topic is further considered in the section on regeneration below.

At term, the remodeling process has only just reached the smallest peripheral portal tracts, where a ductal plate may therefore persist. Canaliculi appear as intercellular spaces between hepatocytes before bile secretion begins,[12] from about 12 weeks, and the intrahepatic biliary system is in luminal continuity with the extrahepatic bile duct. However, the proliferation and development of the intrahepatic biliary system is not complete by 40 weeks of gestation, and bile duct genesis continues postpartum. The number of bile ducts per portal tract continues to increase and only reaches the adult 1 : 1 pairing of hepatic arteries and bile ducts per portal tract at about 15 years of age.[13–15]

Mature macroanatomy

The liver occupies most of the right upper quadrant of the abdomen. Physical examination demarcates the borders of a normal liver in the midclavicular line, from the fifth intercostal space to just below the costal margin. In infants, a liver palpable below the right costal margin is normal. A normal liver span on percussion and palpation can be estimated as:

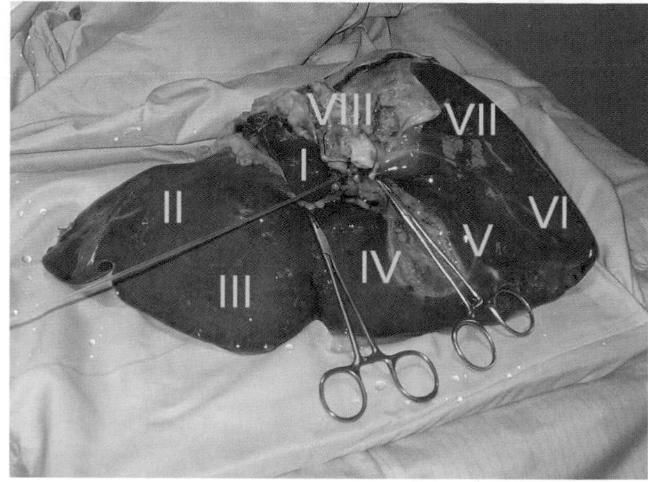

A

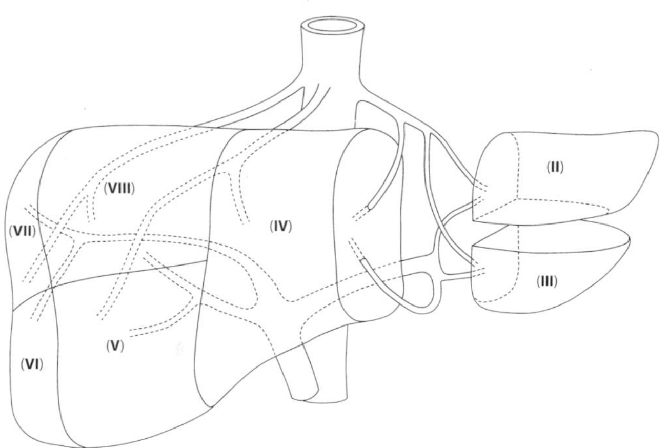

B

Figure 1.4 Segmental anatomy of the liver. **A** Dorsoposterior view of a normal adult liver. All segments can be seen only from this perspective. **B** Schematic view of the anterior aspect of a normal liver. The retrograde blood supply of segment IV is shown, which is of relevance in split-liver techniques in liver transplantation. Segments II and III are also used for reduction hepatectomies and living related donor transplantation.

- < 1 year: 4–5 cm
- 1–5 years: 6–7 cm
- 5–12 years: 8–9 cm

A prominent left lobe that is palpable in the epigastrium may be normal in infants, but in older children is suggestive of pathology.

The macroscopic division of the liver into the right, left, quadrate, and caudate lobes does not correspond to the segmental organization into eight segments (Figure 1.4). The right and left lobes of the liver are defined by the principal plane, or "Cantlie's line," from the gallbladder bed anteriorly to the left side of the inferior vena cava posteriorly and between the right and left branch of the portal vein, with the quadrate lobe and most of the caudate lobe functionally belonging to the left hemiliver.[16] The right and left halves of the liver are further subdivided into two sectors by the right and left fissures, which roughly correspond to the positions of the right and left hepatic veins. The shape of the left lateral segment (segments III and II) varies greatly between a thin, "flatfish" lobe and a short, thick lobe—particularly segment III—or "blowfish" shape. This has particular relevance in monosegmental liver transplantation.[17]

More important than the topographic description of macroscopically visible lobes is the segmental organization of the liver, which provides the basis for all major liver surgery, including liver transplantation.[18,19] The caudate lobe is segment I, and the remainder of the segments are labeled according to their clockwise position. Each segment has its own independent vascular and biliary supply, which is surrounded by a fibrous sheath, the extension of Glisson's capsule.[20] Partial hepatectomies for tumor surgery or liver transplantation follow these segmental borders and are different from the traditional lobar macroanatomy.[21,22]

Portal venous anatomy

The portal vein, a valveless vein, drains blood from the splanchnic area and commences behind the neck of the pancreas as a cranial continuation of confluence of the superior mesenteric vein and the splenic vein. It is interesting that in several animal species, the portal vein takes a helical or spiral shape. This has been less well documented in humans.[23] The significance of this helical structure and the implications for its effect on blood flow have yet to be defined, but the structure has been documented using color duplex Doppler ultrasonography.[24] The portal vein is also unique in that, instead of the normal pattern of solely circular smooth-muscle fibers, there are two distinct muscle layers: a relatively thin inner layer consisting of circular smooth-muscle cells, resembling the normal media of a vein, and an outer layer of longitudinal muscle with abundant vasa vasorum—architecture that closely resembles that of the gastrointestinal tract.[25] The portal vein branches in an extrahepatic position at the hilum into a right and left portal vein; the latter supplies the caudate and quadrate lobe before it enters the parenchyma. The venous return from the gallbladder drains into the right branch of the portal vein. Each segment of the liver is supplied by its own branch of the portal vein. Anomalies of the portal vein are rare, but those most frequently seen are an abnormal position anterior to the head of the pancreas, typically associated with the biliary atresia and splenic malformation syndrome (absent intrahepatic inferior vena cava, polysplenia, situs inversus, and malrotation) and an abnormal communication with the inferior vena cava, resulting in a congenital portocaval shunt (Abernethy syndrome).[26]

Hepatic artery anatomy

The arterial supply to the liver and biliary tree is notorious for the variation in its origin and course relative to the surrounding anatomy, due to the complex embryological development of the celiac and superior mesenteric arteries.[27] The usual arrangement of the hepatic artery, originating from the celiac axis and dividing into a right and left branch above the level of the gastroduodenal artery, is only present in about 60% of cases. In about 25% of individuals, the right hepatic artery arises from the superior mesenteric artery and may act as a fully replaced right hepatic artery or as an accessory artery. This artery runs through the head of the pancreas and lies posterior to the common bile duct and has particular relevance in its supply to the right liver bile ducts and gallbladder.

In a similar proportion of individuals, the left lobe of the liver may be partially or completely supplied by an artery arising from the left gastric artery, which runs in the gastrohepatic omentum and enters the hilar plate at the level of the umbilical fissure. Other less common anomalies are a very short common hepatic artery with long right and left arteries, with the gastroduodenal artery arising from the right hepatic artery or even arising separately from the celiac trunk.

The blood supply to the bile ducts is entirely arterial and may be divided anatomically into hilar, supraduodenal, and pancreatic sections. The blood supply to the mid-portion of the common duct is axial, with a 3-o'clock and a 9-o'clock artery running alongside the duct, receiving an average of eight contributions from all of the surrounding named vessels. There is a 60% contribution from the gastroduodenal artery and 40% from the right hepatic artery. An additional supply to the supraduodenal duct is a consistent retroportal artery, arising from the celiac axis or superior mesenteric artery close to their origin from the aorta.[28] These all form a plexus of vessels surrounding the bile ducts, which extend into the liver. The ducts at the hilum receive blood from the right and left hepatic arteries and multiple small vessels that enter the caudate lobe. These vessels may be arranged in an arcade pattern, suggesting good collateral supply, or in a tree-like fashion from either the left or right hepatic arteries. It is also important to note the frequency of segment IV arterial supply either from the right, proper, or left hepatic artery, which has important implications for split-liver transplantation. From corrosion-cast studies, it is obvious that a very important role for the hepatic arteries is the nourishment of the biliary system, and impairment of this blood supply will lead to ischemic consequences, with necrosis or stricture.[28,29]

Hepatic vein anatomy

The hepatic venous anatomy is relatively simple, as there are three main hepatic veins, which lie above the portal structures within the liver. They divide the liver into sectors along an oblique plane; thus, the right hepatic vein divides the right lobe of the liver into posterolateral and anteromedial sectors; the middle hepatic vein separates the liver into right and left, and the left hepatic vein also divides the liver into a posterolateral sector (segment II) and an anteromedial sector (segments IV and III). The caudate lobe also has bilateral drainage with a relatively clear median plane, with direct venous channels into the inferior vena cava—more on the left, as this part of the caudate lobe is the larger and more consistent.

The right hepatic vein may not be dominant, and much of the right posterior sector may drain into the inferior vena cava (IVC) as a large accessory, caudally placed vein. There is a short extrahepatic course, and in 60% of cases there are no branches just before joining the IVC, which lends itself to separate dissection and ligation.

There are multiple other "dorsal" hepatic veins that drain directly into the IVC, which are thin-walled and fragile and require delicate ligation during right hepatectomy. The middle hepatic vein drains into the left hepatic vein within the liver substance, resulting in a common confluence in most cases, and receives branches from the right and left liver to a variable extent—mainly segments V, IVb, and VIII. This venous drainage area becomes crucially important in living-donor right liver transplants, as adequate drainage must be ensured for the donor (segment IV) as well as the graft (segments V and VIII) (Figure 1.4).

Biliary anatomy

The interlobular or terminal bile ducts belong to the portal triad and have a diameter of < 100 μm. They are accompanied by arterial vessels, which supply oxygenated blood to the bile ducts and also play a role in the immediate reabsorption of organic compounds from primary bile into the general circulation. Bile is then drained into the septal, segmental, and right or left hepatic ducts. The left hepatic duct drains segments II, III, and IV, and the right hepatic duct drains segments V, VI, VII, and VIII. Segment I, the caudate lobe, has its own biliary drainage. Variations of this are common, and in 78% of individuals the caudate lobe drains into both the left and right hepatic duct.[30] The right and left hepatic ducts join to form the common hepatic duct. The left hepatic duct lies predominantly outside the liver parenchyma, and this can be used to advantage in dealing with more distal bile duct strictures.[31]

An important and common anomaly is for the right sectional (sectoral) duct to cross to the left and drain into the left hepatic duct. There is considerable variation in ductal anomalies, which are recorded in textbooks of anatomy and surgery. In about 70% of cases, there is a clear right–left confluence, and in 12% there is a trifurcation of the ducts at the porta hepatis,[32] but many patterns of drainage are discernible. The right hepatic posterior and anterior sectoral ducts may drain separately at different levels or may join the left duct, as mentioned. A right posterior sectoral duct may join the hepatic duct as low as the insertion of the cystic duct or may even drain into the gallbladder.

The cystic duct joins the hepatic duct in most cases at an acute angle on the right side. However, the level of insertion is variable and may be anterior or on the left, with a spiral or parallel configuration around the duct. The term "hepatocystic triangle" describes the inferolateral base, with the cystic duct and hepatic duct medially and the inferior surface of the liver superiorly. Calot's triangle is the inferior part of this, with the cystic artery as the base of the inverted triangle.[33] The cystic duct drains the gallbladder, which lies in the median plane between the two functioning halves of the liver on its anterior undersurface. The length and diameter of the cystic duct also vary greatly—from 4 mm to 65 mm in length and from 3 mm to 9 mm in diameter.

The gallbladder lies wrapped in the extension of Glisson's capsule and may be embedded within the liver substance to a variable degree, or may even have a mesentery of its own suspended from the undersurface of the liver.

The common bile duct, with a mean diameter of 6 mm in adults, passes distally behind the duodenum and sometimes through the pancreas to reach its destination in the mid-second part of the duodenum, surrounded by sphincter muscle. At its terminal portion, it is joined by the pancreatic duct, with a short common channel in most cases. However, not infrequently there may be pancreaticobiliary malunion with a long common channel, which is associated with choledochal dilation and cystic change due to pancreatic juice reflux (see the section on choledochal cysts in Chapter 19, pp. 441–444).

Lymphatics

Hepatic lymph is generated in the space of Disse, which is continuous with the lymph vessels. Lymphatic vessels originate in the connective-tissue spaces within the portal tracts and flow toward the hepatic hilum. Lymphatics in the hepatic capsule drain to vessels either at the hilum or around the hepatic veins and inferior vena cava and eventually into the thoracic duct.[1]

Microanatomy

Microanatomy is intimately related to function and is best considered by linking individual cellular constituents and their local relationships with function. Blood from the hepatic artery and portal vein needs to come into intimate contact with hepatocytes to allow the metabolism of dietary molecules and detoxification of compounds, and to distribute the diverse proteins synthesized by the liver. In order for the liver to fulfill its exocrine function, bile secreted into intercellular canaliculi has to find its way to the biliary duct system and ultimately to the intestine. These functions require a complex interaction between individual cells, as well as regulation of blood supply and innervation. The way in which groups of cells are organized into "functional units" has been the subject of much debate and is discussed further below.

Cellular constituents of the liver

The liver parenchyma consists of a number of different cell types. About 80% are hepatocytes; biliary epithelial cells account for 1%, sinusoidal endothelium 10%, Kupffer cells (hepatic macrophages) 4%, and lymphocytes 5%.

Hepatocytes, arranged in branched and anastomosing cords, are between 30 and 40 μm in size. In keeping with

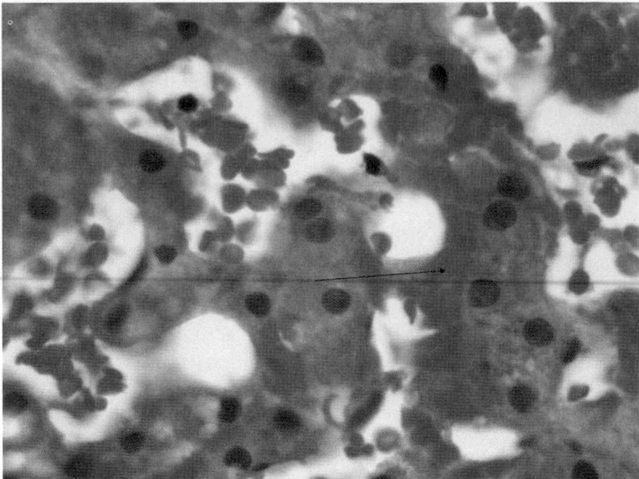

Figure 1.5 The space of Disse. Liver histology in a child with Budd–Chiari syndrome. The space of Disse is not normally visible, but in this image from a patient with Budd–Chiari syndrome, blood has been forced into the space of Disse and renders it visible. (Hematoxylin–eosin, original magnification × 400.)

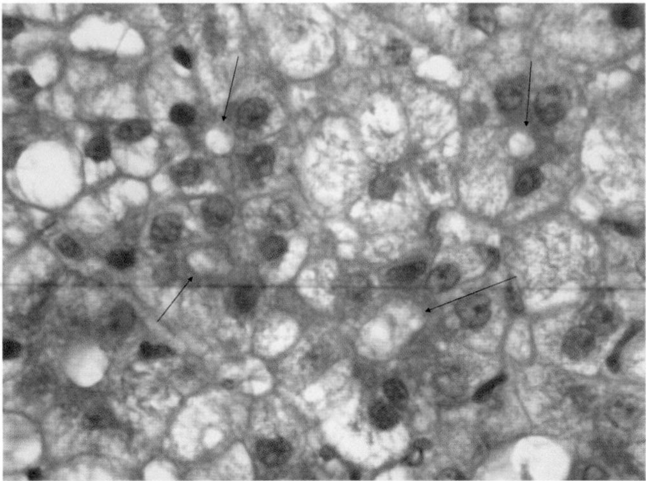

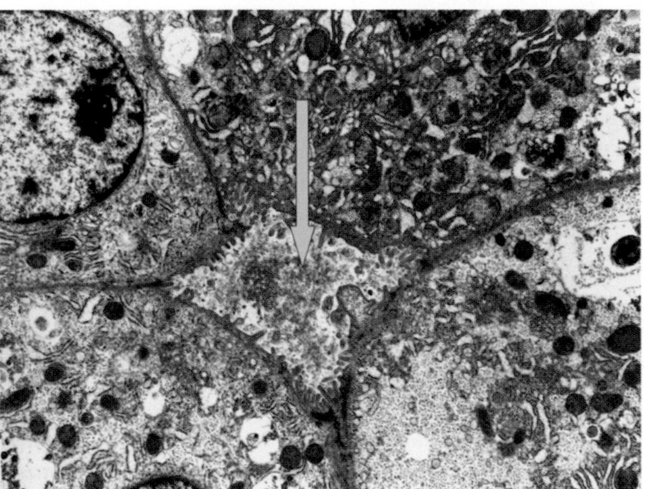

Figure 1.6 Bile canaliculi in cholestatic liver disease. **A** Canaliculi in a child with neonatal cholestasis. The canaliculi are not visible in the normal liver. In this child with neonatal hepatitis, they are distended by bile plugs, making them prominent (arrows). (Hematoxylin–eosin, original magnification × 400.) **B** Electron microscopy of a canaliculus. The arrow shows granular bile in a canaliculus in a child on parenteral nutrition. There are microvilli lining the edge of the canaliculus.

their diverse functions, they are rich in organelles, up to 1000 mitochondria can be seen in a single cell, and apparatus for protein production is also abundant (e.g., endoplasmic reticulum and Golgi complex).[6,32] Particulate glycogen forms much of the "background" of the cell. The hepatocytes have different surfaces or "domains," where they abut other hepatocytes, with which they communicate via gap junctions (lateral domain). The basal domain is where the hepatocyte contacts blood in the sinusoid, and the apical domain forms the canaliculus. The latter two domains are covered with microvilli, providing an enlarged surface area. The sinusoids are lined by a specialized endothelium, which has fenestrae (apertures) to facilitate the transfer of molecules and particles. The sinusoidal endothelium lacks a basement membrane, further facilitating exchange between blood and hepatocyte.

Between the endothelial cells and the basal aspect of the hepatocytes lies the space of Disse (Figure 1.5). This is not normally visible with light microscopy, but can be seen if there is hepatic venous obstruction. The space of Disse contains extracellular matrix components, including type IV collagen, laminin, and proteoglycans. This matrix is not merely an extracellular scaffold, but also interacts via adhesion molecules with the hepatocytes. The extracellular matrix can modulate the cell phenotype and serves as a reservoir for cell growth factors, cytokines, and albumin, which can be released by matrix degradation.

The apical domain constitutes 15% of the hepatocyte cell membrane and forms the bile canaliculus. Again, canaliculi are not normally visible on light microscopy, but become so in cholestatic disease (Figure 1.6). The canaliculus is delineated from the third (lateral) domain by tight junctions. The bile canaliculi constitute the outermost reaches of the biliary tree. They are spaces 1–2 μm wide, which are interconnected and form a network of intercellular channels, which receive the bile secreted from hepatocytes. Actin and myosin filaments of the hepatocyte propel the bile into the canals of Hering (ductules or cholangioles), which are lined with a mixture of biliary epithelium and hepatocytes.[34] They have a diameter of less than 15 μm and are located at the periphery of a portal triad. They are not visible with routine light microscopy.

Kupffer cells are located on the luminal side of the endothelial wall. They have a phagocytic function and are also an important source of cytokine secretion. Hepatic stellate cells (previously known as Ito cells) produce extracellular matrix, store vitamin A and lipid, and have fine extensions surrounding the sinusoids, possibly related to control of vascular tone. When activated, they transform into myofibroblasts and have an important role in fibrosis.

Functional anatomy/regulation of blood supply

The dual blood supply to the liver, by the hepatic artery and portal vein, is almost unique in the body. In resting conditions, the liver receives about a quarter of the cardiac output. About 30% of this hepatic inflow is oxygen-rich blood via the hepatic artery; the remaining 70% is nutrient-loaded blood from the intestine and spleen, supplied by the portal vein. Arterial and portal blood mixes freely at the level of the sinusoids. Total blood flow into the liver varies considerably and is reduced during sympathetic stimulation or sleep. In contrast, portal blood flow increases following a meal. It is most stimulated by a protein-rich feed and only moderately by carbohydrates, with little effect following lipids. The arterial blood supply is not determined by oxygen demand. In normal livers, only half of the oxygen supplied is extracted, and in situations in which metabolic rates increase, oxygen extraction rises without an increase in arterial flow. Portal and arterial flow are closely related, and an experimental reduction of portal flow in dogs resulted in arterial hyperemia. Clinically, this phenomenon becomes apparent in liver transplantation, when thrombosis of either the hepatic artery or the portal vein leads to compensatory flow rates in the other vessel.

About 20–25% of the normal liver consists of blood, which is situated in the large vessels. This is about 10–15% of the body's total blood volume, and the liver thus serves as a reservoir with capacitance function. Liver blood volume can increase by 4% for each 1-mmHg increase in hepatic venous pressure and may be tripled to about 60% in states of severe outflow obstruction. In hemorrhagic shock, in sympathetic stimulation, and in vascular dehydration, the liver can replace systemic volume rapidly. In animal studies, it has been observed that 7% of the total blood volume can be replaced from the liver, while in dogs a 60% decrease in liver blood content can be achieved within seconds by sympathetic stimulation.

Portal vein perfusion pressure is approximately 6–10 mmHg. Arterial perfusion pressures depend on systemic perfusion pressures. The sinusoidal perfusion pressure is determined by a number of factors in the afferent and efferent vessels, including muscular sphincter, autonomic nervous innervation, and paracrine function.

In the normal liver, the sinusoids consist of a fenestrated endothelial capillary that receives blood from arterioles and venules, with a perfusion pressure of 2–4 mmHg. The distribution of blood flow in the sinusoids is determined by variation in the size of the Kupffer and endothelial cells, which swell and shrink to control the patency of the sinusoidal lumen. The role of stellate cells, which are thought to be myofibroblasts, remains unclear, although their ability to induce fibrosis appears to be the dominant effect on sinusoidal perfusion in states of liver disease.

Functional versus anatomical units

In the absence of connective-tissue septa delineating structural units, different models have been used to define the smallest functional unit in the liver (Figure 1.7):

• The *classic lobule*, hexagonal in shape, was described in 1833.[35] It corresponds to the unit that is outlined by connective tissue in other species, such as the pig. It has a hepatic vein branch ("central vein") at its center. Blood arriving in the portal tracts at the periphery of the hexagon will feed sinusoids around the whole of their circumference, rather than all draining into the interior of the hexagon. It therefore has limited application as a true primary unit. The *primary lobule*, described by Matsumoto *et al.*,[36] uses the portal vein branches to act as the center of the functional unit, giving rise to tortuous and branching three-dimensional units surrounding portal vein branches, but it does include the *classic lobule* as a secondary structure.[6,32] This model is based on actual vascular reconstruction (rather than the gelatin infusions used in the acinar concept, below) and is gaining widespread acceptance.[37] Descriptive histology in the lobular models hence includes such terms as "centrilobular" hepatocytes (those around the central vein).

• The work of Rappaport *et al.* in 1954 defined the functional unit as an acinus.[38] The axis of the acinus is formed by the terminal branch of the portal vein, not visible in routine microscopy. The three zones of the acinar concept are illustrated in Figure 1.7. Descriptive histology in the acinar concept refers to these three acinar zones, and it should be noted that these do not equate to the regions described in the lobular concept. "Acinar zone 3" is not exclusively "perivenular," but rather extends in an arc-like fashion from one portal tract to another. The acinar concept proved popular for pathologists from an observational point of view. In severe liver damage, necrosis is presumed to occur in the least well oxygenated, most vulnerable hepatocytes first. In the lobular concept, the least well oxygenated hepatocytes would be centrilobular, and necrosis would therefore be seen in the perivenular region exclusively. In practice, however, necrosis occurs in a portal–central distribution, and this corresponds to the most peripheral acinar regions (zone 3; Figure 1.7). Many studies of functional heterogeneity within the liver do not support the acinar concept, however, and as mentioned above, the *primary lobule*, based on the actual branching of the portal vein, is gaining in popularity.

However the functional unit is defined, the function of the hepatocytes, sinusoidal endothelium, Kupffer cells, and

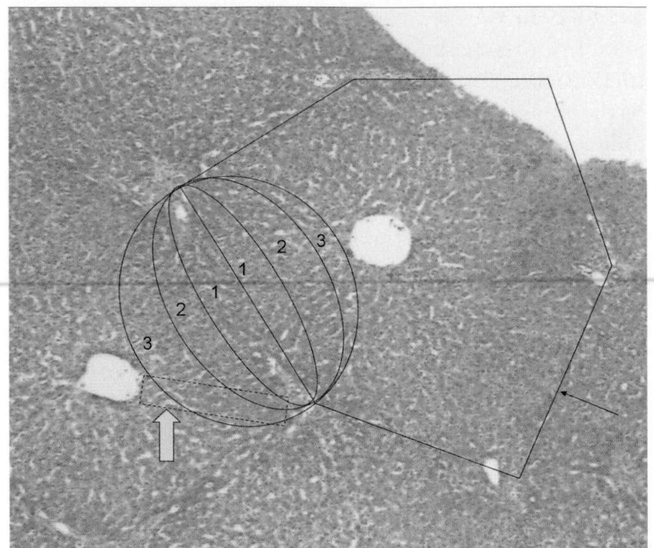

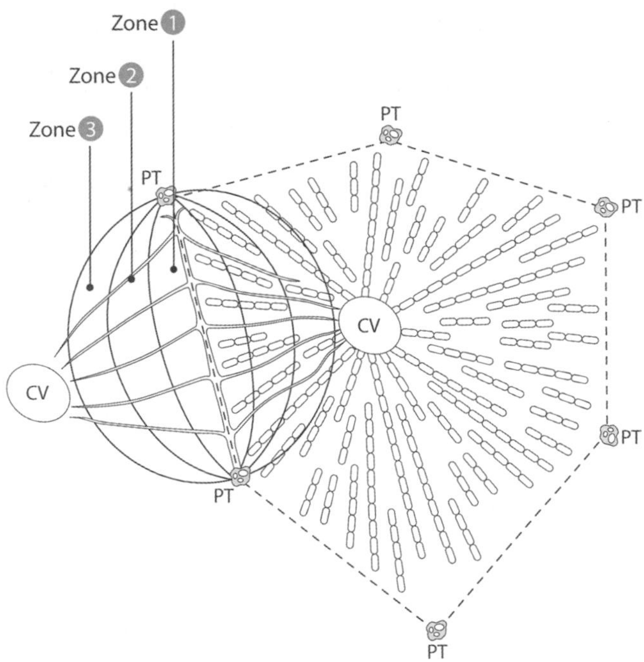

Figure 1.7 A Light microscopy of normal liver tissue. The small arrow points to the approximate outline of a classic hepatic lobule, centered around a central vein. In schematic diagrams, this is often illustrated as a regular hexagon, with portal tracts at four points and "nodal points of mall" at the other two. This is rarely reproducible in practice, leading to the slightly irregular hexagon shown. The elliptical structure denotes postulated acinar zones 1, 2, and 3, centered around a terminal portal venule (not visible). This occupies portions of two adjacent classic lobules. The dotted rectangle shows the location of portal central bridging necrosis, which is observed in the clinical situation and which made the acinar concept popular from a pathological point of view. (Hematoxylin–eosin, original magnification × 40). **B** Schematic view of the same anatomical and functional units of the liver.
CV, central vein; PT, portal tract.

extracellular matrix composition, varies between regions. "Periportal," "perivenular," and—although it does not correspond to a true acinar zone—"midzonal" serve as useful descriptors for considering functional differences or gradients. Gene expression also shows a functional gradient.[32] The phenotypic variation may be determined by the declining gradient in oxygen concentration, the decreasing glucagon–insulin ratio, or other autocrine signals. Periportal hepatocytes are responsible for oxidative energy metabolism, such as beta-oxidation and amino acid catabolism, bile formation, and cholesterol synthesis. Perivenous hepatocytes are involved in glucose uptake for glycogen synthesis, glycolysis, liponeogenesis, and ketogenesis.

Innervation

The liver is innervated by the autonomic nervous system, through sympathetic nerve fibers from the celiac ganglia and some parasympathetic input from the vagus nerve. Sympathetic nerves supply a dense perivascular plexus around the hilar blood vessels into the sinusoids, where nerves course in the space of Disse and surround isolated hepatocytes and stellate cells. Parasympathetic nerve fibers accompany the hepatic inflow system, forming a plexus around hepatic artery and portal vein, but there is little cholinergic innervation beyond the portal tract.[39]

It has been suggested that gap junctions may also provide direct electrical coupling between cells, bypassing the need for nervous innervation. Cholinergic stimuli increase metabolic activity, whereas adrenergic stimuli increase glucose mobilization into the blood. The realization that hepatic function is effective even in the denervated graft following liver transplantation has challenged long-standing views about the role of the autonomic nervous system in regulating metabolic activity in the liver. More recent studies have suggested that α-adrenergic innervation is involved in hepatocyte replication.

Function

The liver is the central organ for metabolic homeostasis. Its main functions are:

- Regulation of uptake and processing of nutrients from the intestinal tract
- Synthesis and biotransformation of proteins, carbohydrates, and lipids
- Excretion of bile and elimination of hydrophobic compounds
- Regulation of energy metabolism
- Endocrine functions and mediation of normal growth and development
- Immunological function
- Drug metabolism
- Regulation of fluid balance

Uptake and processing (synthesis, storage and degradation) of proteins, carbohydrates, and lipids

Proteins

The liver accounts for 15% of total body protein production, and the majority of these proteins are secreted as plasma proteins. Proteins are synthesized following the activation of genetic promoter sequences by transcription factors. Following translation and modification, proteins are secreted from the sinusoidal aspect of the hepatocytes into the circulation. Nutritional status and hormone secretion regulate the level of protein production. There is a surge of protein production in acute illnesses—the acute-phase response, in which C-reactive protein is the most commonly measured sign. The liver is responsible for synthesizing many proteins, such as albumin, transport proteins such as ceruloplasmin, coagulation and fibrinolytic proteins, complement, and protease inhibitors. Proteins are not stored in the liver, but amino acids are recycled to synthesize new molecules. The liver also plays a role in protein and glycoprotein degradation. Amino acid degradation takes place in the liver, generating the highly toxic metabolite ammonia, which is associated with hepatic encephalopathy (see Chapters 7 and 15). The urea cycle, which is active almost exclusively in the liver, is largely responsible for its removal, and urea cycle defects present with severe encephalopathy (see Chapters 5 and 13).

Carbohydrates

Glucose, fructose, and galactose are taken up by the hepatocytes from portal blood. Glucose is converted to glucose-6-phosphate and used to replenish glycogen stores, or else used in triglyceride production. The liver, under the influence of hormones—principally insulin (which reduces glucose output) and glucagon (which increases glucose output)—has a major role in maintaining blood glucose. Glucose is either released from glycogen (glycogenolysis) or synthesized from substrates such as lactate (gluconeogenesis). In conditions of stress or fasting, glucose uptake is reduced and glucose production is increased from glycogenolysis. Hypoglycemia is a sensitive test of liver function and is a sign of severe hepatic necrosis, indicating loss of liver function (see Chapter 7). For the same reason, many infants with severe liver disease are unable to maintain their blood sugar levels during prolonged fasts.

Lipids

The liver is essential for cholesterol and lipoprotein metabolism. Cholesterol is a component of all cell membranes and is essential for the production of steroid hormones and bile acids. Cholesterol homeostasis is controlled by uptake from lipoproteins and chylomicrons, which increase hepatic cholesterol, and by the enzyme 3-hydroxy-3-methylglutaryl coenzyme A (HMG CoA), which synthesizes cholesterol *de novo.* The amount synthesized in the liver is twice that absorbed from the diet. In the liver, cholesterol is either "free" or stored as cholesterol ester. The degradation of cholesterol takes place through the synthesis of bile acids and biliary excretion of cholesterol (see below). A number of cholestatic liver diseases (e.g., biliary atresia or Alagille's syndrome) lead to elevated plasma cholesterol due to deficient biliary excretion and catabolism.

Chylomicrons, which transport water-insoluble lipids, carry dietary fat from the intestine to the circulation. They deliver triglycerides to peripheral tissues, and the resulting cholesterol-rich chylomicron remnant is taken up by the liver. The liver also synthesizes fatty acids from glucose in times of dietary excess, and these are subsequently stored as triglycerides, which are the principal source of energy. Fatty acids that are not converted to triglycerides or used in the synthesis of other molecules are oxidized, following modification, to ketone bodies in the mitochondria, or in the case of very-long-chain fatty acids in the peroxisomes. Microvesicular steatosis in hepatocytes is a sign of mitochondrial or peroxisomal disease or drug toxicity (see Chapters 5, 9, and 13).

Very-low-density lipoproteins (VLDLs) are the main lipoproteins secreted by the liver and carry triglyceride and cholesterol to other tissues, where they are converted to low-density lipoproteins (LDLs). High-density lipoproteins (HDLs) carry cholesterol from the peripheral tissues back to the liver. Fatty liver occurs when the synthesis of triglycerides exceeds the liver's capacity for export or internal metabolism.

Bile and bile acids

Bile is produced in hepatocytes and is modified in the bile ducts. In adults, about 600 mL of isotonic watery bile with a pH of 7.8 is produced daily in order to facilitate the excretion of many compounds, including drugs, toxins, and waste products, and to provide bile salts to the intestine for the emulsification and absorption of dietary lipids. Bile formation is an osmotic process and is traditionally classified as "bile salt–dependent" (the relationship of canalicular bile flow to bile salt excretion) and "bile salt–independent" (the active secretion of electrolytes and other solutes).

The main components of bile are bile acids (12%), phospholipids (4%), cholesterol (0.7%), and conjugated bilirubin (0.1%). Lecithin increases the solubility of cholesterol in bile by micelle formation exponentially to allow a 10-fold concentration of bile acids and cholesterol in the gallbladder. Of the electrolytes in bile, only sodium is concentrated to about 280 mmol/L; other electrolytes and bicarbonate are less concentrated, or unchanged. The primary bile acids—cholic acid and chenodeoxycholic acid—are synthesized from cholesterol by 7α-hydroxylase and subsequently conjugated with taurine and glycine to enhance affinity to both acids and bases ("amphophilia").

Primary bile salts are transformed by intestinal bacteria into secondary bile salts—cholic acid into deoxycholic acid and chenodeoxycholic acid into lithocholic acid and subsequently to ursodeoxycholic acid (UDCA). They are reabsorbed in the ileum and returned to the liver via the portal vein. In normal conditions, UDCA represents only 3% of the bile salt pool. It is more hydrophilic than the other bile salts and is used therapeutically to stimulate bile secretion; it may prevent the hepatocytes from damage caused by hydrophobic bile salts. Only lithocholic acid is poorly reabsorbed and excreted, so that the gallbladder bile consists of the four bile salts at a ratio of 10 : 10 : 5 : 1. In chronic liver disease, this balance is shifted to a predominant production of chenodeoxycholic acid, which lowers the bile pH.

Hepatic bile formation and the biliary excretory function are closely related. The rate of bile flow is determined by the enterohepatic circulation of bile salts and by the rate of secretion of bile salts, cholesterol, phospholipids, and glutathione, which means that if bile excretion is impaired in liver disease, there is reduced excretion of both endogenous and exogenous compounds. Bile salts are the main organic solutes in bile, and their active transport against a 1000-fold concentration gradient into the bile canaliculus is the driving force for hepatic bile formation. In adults, the enterohepatic circulation of bile salts occurs more than six to eight times in 24 h, enabling the body to retain most of the 5–6 g in the body bile salt pool. Neonates have about half the bile salt pool of an adult, and ileal bile salt reabsorption is lower. Their intestinal bile acid concentration may be low, leading to poor micelle formation and reduced uptake of fat-soluble vitamins and dietary lipid in comparison with older children and adults. Although this is rarely a cause of malnutrition and/or steatorrhea, it needs to be considered in cholestatic conditions when early supplementation of fat-soluble vitamins is indicated. Bile acid uptake from portal blood is physiologically lower in neonates in comparison with older children, and elevated levels of bile acids may be mistaken for cholestatic liver disease.

Intrahepatic and extrahepatic bile salt transport

The transport processes for bile salts are complex, and—despite the recent discovery of different membrane-bound bile salt transporters—they are still not fully understood. Hepatocytes are polarized cells that absorb substrates from the blood in the sinusoids, such as bile salts, phospholipids, and metabolites of toxic substances, and transport them across the cell to the canalicular membrane to secrete into bile. The sinusoidal uptake of conjugated bile salts (e.g., taurocholate) by hepatocytes at the basolateral plasma membrane is mediated by an active transport process driven by a sodium gradient via the sodium-dependent transporter for the uptake of bile salts, sodium taurocholate cotransporting polypeptide. The uptake of unconjugated bile salts at the sinusoidal membrane is sodium-independent and mediated by the organic anion transporting polypeptide. This transporter also transports steroids such as progesterone and cyclosporine. After uptake into hepatocytes, the intracellular transport across the cell is thought to be mediated by binding to cytosolic proteins, ligandins, and Y9 proteins or fatty acid–binding proteins. Some free intracellular bile salts reach the canalicular plasma membrane by diffusion.

Excretion of bile salts across the canalicular plasma membrane is the rate-limiting step in the transport of bile salts from blood into bile. Canalicular secretion of monovalent bile salts is facilitated by the adenosine triphosphate–dependent "bile salt excreting pump" (BSEP).[40] A defect in this transporter is responsible for the genetic condition known as progressive familial intrahepatic cholestasis (PFIC). In contrast to monoanionic bile salts, divalent sulfated and glucuronidated bile salts are excreted into bile by the multidrug resistance–associated protein 2 (Mrp2), also known as canalicular multispecific organic anion transporter (cMOAT). Failure to express Mrp2 at the canalicular membrane results in conjugated hyperbilirubinemia and forms the basis of the hereditary Dubin–Johnson syndrome. Canalicular phospholipid secretion is mediated by a different transporter protein, multidrug resistance protein type 3 (Mdr3), which is important in preventing bile salt–induced toxic damage to the biliary epithelium. Failure to express this transporter results in progressive familial intrahepatic cholestasis type 3 and biliary cirrhosis[41] (see Chapter 4). FIC-1 is an aminophospholipid translocator in the canalicular membrane of hepatocytes that is also found on the apical membrane of enterocytes. It is responsible for the transport of phosphatidylserine and phosphatidylethanolamine. A genetic defect in the expression or function of this transporter causes progressive familial intrahepatic cholestasis type 1 (PFIC-1) and benign recurrent intrahepatic cholestasis type 1 (BRIC-1; see Chapters 3 and 4).

Excretion of bilirubin

As well as its role in facilitating bile salt homeostasis, the biliary system also serves as the primary pathway for eliminating bilirubin, excess cholesterol, and hydrophobic xenobiotics. About 80% of bilirubin is derived from the breakdown of erythrocytes; the remainder stems from heme-containing myoglobin, cytochromes, and other enzymes. Mononuclear phagocytic cells oxidize heme to form biliverdin, which is then reduced to bilirubin. This unconjugated bilirubin is albumin-bound, transported to the hepatic sinusoids, and actively transported into the hepatocytes via the basolateral membrane. If the unconjugated bilirubin is displaced from albumin, it may diffuse across the blood–brain barrier and cause kernicterus in neonates.

Bilirubin uridine diphosphate (UDP) glucuronyltransferase (UGT1A1) conjugation with one or two molecules of glucuronic acid in the endoplasmic reticulum converts bilirubin (conjugated bilirubin), which is excreted as hydrophilic bilirubin glucuronides via the canalicular membrane. Following intestinal excretion, bacterial beta-glucuronidases degrade most of these bilirubin glucuronides to colorless urobilinogen. About 20% of urobilinogen is reabsorbed in the ileum and colon and returned to the liver via the portal vein. Some of this urobilinogen is excreted into the urinary tract.

UGT1A1 belongs to the UGT family of conjugating enzymes, which catalyze glucuronidation of various substrates, including steroid hormones, carcinogens, and drugs, and which are expressed in a wide range of tissues. Splicing variation of the original transcripts of the *UGT1A1* gene on chromosome 2q37 leads to different mRNAs of the enzyme. Of several isoforms, only UGT1A1 is physiologically active. Decreased activity of the enzyme in the newborn period contributes to the physiological jaundice common in the neonate. Mutations in the *UGT1A1* gene either reduce the affinity of UGT1A1 toward bilirubin or reduce enzyme activity. Complete absence of UGT1A1 activity causes Crigler–Najjar syndrome type 1, and a significant reduction of activity causes Crigler–Najjar syndrome type 2. Only a very mild reduction of UGT1A1 activity by missense mutation or reduced expression of the enzyme is present in 6% of the general population, causing Gilbert's syndrome, in which there is a mild elevation of unconjugated bilirubin (see Chapter 4).

Regulation of energy metabolism

The energy metabolism of the body is integrated by the liver through glucose metabolism and fatty acid oxidation. The liver has a central role in maintaining blood glucose homeostasis at constant levels between 3.3 and 6.1 mmol/L in order to supply glucose as an energy substrate for the brain, renal medulla, or blood cells. This glucostat function of the liver is primarily achieved by controlling the storage and release of glucose from glycogen, followed by glycolysis and gluconeogenesis. The glycogen content of a liver of a 10-kg child is around 20–25 g, increasing to about 70–80 g in an adult. As the normal resting glucose requirement is between 4 and 6 mg/kg/min, the glycogen stores last for less than a day of fasting, after which gluconeogenesis is activated. In prolonged fasting, total body glucose requirements decrease from 160 g/glucose/day to 40 g/glucose/day after 5–6 weeks of starvation in the adult. The healthy body can tolerate this, because fatty acid oxidation becomes the main source of fuel for respiration. Soskin postulated as early as 1940 that the blood glucose concentration is the primary stimulus to control glucose uptake or output.[42] Glucose uptake into the hepatocyte is insulin-independent and has a direct regulatory effect on glycogen synthesis. Conversion of excess glucose to fatty acids only takes place when hepatic glycogen stores are complete. Such fatty acids are esterified to triglycerides and exported from the liver as very-low-density lipoproteins (VLDLs). Triglycerides in VLDLs from the liver and from the intestinal absorption of lipids are hydrolyzed by lipoprotein lipase and taken up in the peripheral tissues, where fatty acids are metabolized for energy or stored.

Endocrine function

The liver plays an active role in endocrine regulation. In response to growth hormone activation, the liver produces the majority of the circulating mitosis-inducing (mitogenic) polypeptides insulin-like growth factor 1 and 2 (IGF-1 and IGF-2), which have anabolic and metabolic effects and regulate the proliferation of various cells. The specific endocrine effect of the IGFs and other hormones, such as steroid hormones, is modulated by different binding proteins (IGF-binding proteins 1–6, sex hormone–binding globulin, or thyroid-binding globulin) that are synthesized in the liver. These binding proteins transport the hormones, regulate their metabolic clearance, and directly modulate hormone interactions with specific receptors.[43,44] Thyroxine (T_4) is converted into the metabolically active form of T_3 in the liver, which accounts for the low T_3 syndrome in patients with decompensated cirrhosis. Hormonal dysfunction in liver disease may develop from reduced clearance of hormones (e.g., gynecomastia in men), from portosystemic shunting, dysregulated synthesis of binding proteins, or impaired end-organ sensitivity to the hormone—i.e., insulin resistance in cirrhosis.

Immunological function

The liver contains many lymphocytes, both of the adaptive immune system, which require previous exposure to antigen for efficacy, and also cells of the innate immune system—natural killer (NK) cells (Pit cells).[45] The liver also contains a population of cells that express both T-cell and NK-cell markers,[46] which play a role in the clearance function of the liver in filtering gut-derived endotoxins and microorganisms. Kupffer cells are macrophages that are important in the phagocytosis of particulate material and cellular debris (they are conspicuous in acute hepatitis), but also play a role in cytokine release and antigen presentation. Following liver transplantation, donor Kupffer cells are rapidly (within days) replaced by recipient Kupffer cells infiltrating the liver.

Drug metabolism

The liver is the prime site for drug metabolism in the body, which occurs in two phases. The first is an oxidation reaction, mediated by the cytochrome P450 enzymes. Reactive oxygen species that are toxic to the cell are generated during this process and require a range of antioxidant mechanisms (molecules—e.g., glutathione and vitamin E; and enzymes—e.g., superoxide dismutase) to render them inert. The metabolized drug, which may itself be toxic, enters the second phase of metabolism, which involves conjugation with hydrophilic compounds—e.g., glucuronic acid or glutathione. Once rendered hydrophilic, the drug metabolite is excreted via the kidneys or the bile. The enzymes responsible for drug metabolism may be either induced or inhibited by other drugs or chemicals, and there can also be idiosyncratic differences between individuals in drug metabolism. Severe liver failure reduces the ability to metabolize drugs, so that drug effects are prolonged (e.g., sedatives or anesthetic agents), or there may be an accumulation of toxic metabolites, which complicates hepatic encephalopathy.

Liver function and fluid balance

As described above (functional anatomy/regulation of blood supply), the liver can retain and release a significant volume of whole blood and/or plasma and hence influence the circulating blood volume. Although the direct interaction between the liver and kidney is not fully understood, impaired liver function leads to a reduced ability to excrete sodium and water. A number of factors are involved, which include: hyperaldosteronism and/or increased tubular sensitivity to aldosteronism; increased renal sympathetic nerve activity; and reduced renal perfusion. Splanchnic vasodilation is probably an initial adverse event that leads to renal vasoconstriction, followed by a reduction of renal blood flow and of the glomerular filtration rate. Sodium retention is the first sign of renal dysfunction, followed by water retention, leading to dilutional hyponatremia in plasma. Plasma volume expansion due to sodium and water retention, together with sinusoidal hypertension (portal pressure gradient of > 12%), is a key factor in the pathogenesis of cirrhotic ascites, which indicates the progression from compensated to decompensated cirrhosis.

Growth and repair

Functional development of the liver and physiological adaptations at birth

At birth, the change from placental to enteral nutrition stimulates bile acid secretion and the enterohepatic circulation. The switch from umbilical venous to portal blood supply means that new molecules and bacteria are carried to the immature neonatal liver by the portal vein. This is best demonstrated by the immaturity of bile formation and the development of physiological jaundice in neonates (see above). The liver is vulnerable in the presence of prematurity, hypoxia, sepsis, drug administration, or total parenteral nutrition.[47–49] α-Fetoprotein, one of the main fetal serum proteins, is synthesized by fetal hepatocytes 25–30 days after conception, and by the yolk sac and intestinal epithelium. Levels peak by the end of the first trimester and exponentially fall until normal adult levels are reached approximately at the end of the first year of life. Albumin levels are close to adult levels at birth, but coagulation proteins are low, increasing the risk of bleeding and hence the need for vitamin K administration at birth. Bile acids are synthesized from 5 to 9 weeks' gestation and bile secretion begins at 12 weeks, but canalicular transport mechanisms and the distal bile ducts, where the bile is extensively modified, are still under development for 4 weeks after birth.[6,49] γ-Glutamyltransferase, located at the canalicular surface of the hepatocytes, is slightly elevated in the serum in the first few months of life.

In utero, the placenta carries out most of the metabolic and detoxifying functions that normally take place in the liver. To cope with this change, hepatic enzymes are rapidly induced at birth. Many conjugation reactions are mature by 2 weeks, but some UDP-glucuronyltransferase genes are not fully expressed for 2 years.[50] The cytochrome P450 group and peroxisomal enzymes also show early functionality. The first feed stimulates insulin production and storage of glycogen. Term newborns have hepatic glycogen stores, but these are quickly depleted, making the infants prone to hypoglycemia unless fed frequently. If the infant is unwell, acute-phase proteins may have a long half-life, because the immature liver is unable to clear them.[48]

At 12 weeks' gestation, the liver is the main site of hemopoiesis, but the bone marrow becomes active from 5 months of gestation. It is normal to see evidence of residual hemopoiesis in the neonatal liver for up to 6 weeks after birth,[48] but it is particularly prominent in neonatal hepatitis. Hemosiderin (as hemopoiesis decreases) and copper-associated protein accumulate in the liver and are deposited in periportal hepatocytes. Both are normal constituents of the neonatal liver and are not indicative of disease.

Liver growth and regeneration

The expected life span of a hepatocyte is about 200–500 days. In normal children and adults, hepatic regeneration occurs by replication of mature cells. This process can be up-regulated—for instance, following trauma or partial hepatectomy, the liver can be reconstituted by proliferation of mature hepatocytes within days and weeks. The liver cell mass is highly flexible and varies throughout life, depending on metabolic demands such as disease or pregnancy. It is likely that liver is also regenerated from progenitor cells in the liver, bone marrow–derived stem cells, and mechanisms of cell fusion, but it is still not clear how this is controlled. Initial studies were based on the search for a growth factor that would stimulate hepatocyte regeneration and control of human hepatocyte replication. Studies of rodents suggested the presence of alternative pathways, including a putative progenitor cell compartment. Animal models in which the growth stimulus from partial hepatectomy was combined with growth arrest of fast-replicating mature hepatocytes using toxins such as 2-acetylaminofluorene or 5-aminouracil led to the proliferation of pluripotent so-called "oval cells" in the canals of Hering.[51,52] The phenotype of these putative hepatic progenitor cells, the oval cell, and the existence of a stem cell compartment was accepted for animals. The presence of similar oval cells in humans was more difficult to demonstrate, partly because of the inability to transfer the experimental model into an acceptable human study and partly because of phenotypic differences between humans and mice. The finding of the hemopoietic stem cell marker and proto-oncogene c-*kit* in certain biliary cells from diseased pediatric liver was one of the first steps in demonstrating the presence of this type of stem cell compartment in humans.[53] An understanding of the physiology of liver regeneration was improved by animal studies conducted by Petersen *et al.*,[54] which were confirmed in humans by Theise *et al.*[55] They demonstrated the presence of Y chromosome–positive hepatocytes and biliary epithelium in female recipients of a therapeutic bone-marrow transplant from male donors, confirming the ability of human bone marrow–derived stem cells to differentiate into the hepatic cell lineages. However, clinically, bone marrow–derived cells are only marginally involved in physiological repair, since in acute liver failure regeneration occurs via proliferation of hepatic progenitor cells, whereas following partial hepatectomy it is restored by replication of normally quiescent hepatocytes.

Liver regeneration is now known to vary in accordance with circadian rhythms and metabolic requirements. Increased metabolic demands and proinflammatory cytokines are likely to be essential. Effects of cytokines (tumor necrosis factor-α, interleukin-6) and growth factors (hepatocyte growth factor) are probably linked by the effect of the tissue-bound metalloproteinases. Experiments with hepatocytes and cocultured biliary epithelium have shown that the degradation of extracellular matrix by metalloproteinases to release growth factors is an essential step in hepatocyte proliferation.

The limitations of understanding of hepatic regeneration have led to persistent problems in clinical hepatocyte transplantation. Therapeutic liver repopulation is an attractive option in a number of metabolic conditions and has been successfully performed in a small number of patients. It remains problematic to achieve persistent engraftment of adequate numbers of cells, because it has not been possible to create an environment that allows preferential replication of transplanted cells. It is possible that significant medical and surgical hepatic preconditioning, similar to myeloablation in bone-marrow transplantation, will be necessary to provide an appropriate environment for persistent engraftment.[56] Clinical studies in this field are limited by the need to match the long-term outcome with orthotopic liver transplantation, at around 90%.

Liver fibrosis

The outcome of most disease processes in the liver is fibrosis. In hepatic fibrogenesis, stellate cells produce an excess of type I and III collagen, which replaces the normal extracellular matrix. Activation of these cells by injured hepatocytes, biliary cells, or inflammatory stimuli leads to the conversion of quiescent vitamin A–storing cells into proliferative, contractile, and fibrogenic myofibroblasts. The dogma that hepatic fibrosis is irreversible is increasingly being challenged, and an understanding of stellate-cell activation is an essential step forward here.[57] Different metalloproteinases that cleave collagens are mainly involved in matrix degradation of the liver, although neutrophils, macrophages, and stellate cells also contribute to this process. Tissue inhibitors of matrix metalloproteinases (TIMPs) are the key regulators in determining the reversal of fibrosis. Sustained TIMP-1 expression inhibits protease activity for matrix degradation and blocks apoptosis of activated stellate cells. A number of phase I clinical trials are being planned to investigate the use of these drugs to prevent or reverse fibrosis.[58]

References

1 Saxena R, Zucker SD, Crawford JM. Anatomy and physiology of the liver. In: Zakim D, Boyer TD, eds. *Hepatology: a Textbook of Liver Disease*, 4th ed. Philadelphia: Saunders, 2003: 3–30.

2 Lemaigre F, Zaret KS. Liver development update: new embryo models, cell lineage control, and morphogenesis. *Curr Opin Genet Dev* 2004;**14**:582–90.

3 Beaudry JB, Pierreux CE, Hayhurst GP, *et al.* Threshold levels of hepatocyte nuclear factor 6 (HNF-6) acting in synergy with HNF-4 and PGC-1alpha are required for time-specific gene expression during liver development. *Mol Cell Biol* 2006;**26**:6037–46.

4 Costa RH, Kalinichenko VV, Holterman AX, Wang X. Transcription factors in liver development, differentiation, and regeneration. *Hepatology* 2003;**38**:1331–47.

5 Crosby HA, Nijjar SS, de Ville de Goyet J, Kelly DA, Strain AJ. Progenitor cells of the biliary epithelial cell lineage. *Semin Cell Dev Biol* 2002;**13**:397–403.

6 Roskams T, Desmet V, Verslype C. Development, structure and function of the liver. In: Burt AD, Portmann BC, Ferrell LD, eds. *Macsween's Pathology of the Liver.* Edinburgh: Churchill Livingstone, 2007: 1–74.

7 Haugen G, Kiserud T, Godfrey K, Crozier S, Hanson M. Portal and umbilical venous blood supply to the liver in the human fetus near term. *Ultrasound Obstet Gynecol* 2004;**24**:599–605.

8 Libbrecht L, Cassiman D, Desmet V, Roskams T. The correlation between portal myofibroblasts and development of intrahepatic bile ducts and arterial branches in human liver. *Liver* 2002;**22**:252–8.

9 Vijayan V, Tan CE. Developing human biliary system in three dimensions. *Anat Rec* 1997;**249**:389–98.

10 Desmet VJ. Ludwig symposium on biliary disorders, part I. Pathogenesis of ductal plate abnormalities. *Mayo Clin Proc* 1998;**73**:80–9.

11 Theise ND, Saxena R, Portmann BC, *et al.* The canals of Hering and hepatic stem cells in humans. *Hepatology* 1999;**30**:1425–33.

12 Tan CE, Vijayan V. New clues for the developing human biliary system at the porta hepatis. *J Hepatobiliary Pancreat Surg* 2001;**8**: 295–302.

13 Van Eyken P, Sciot R, Callea F, Van der Steen K, Moerman P, Desmet VJ. The development of the intrahepatic bile ducts in man: a keratin-immunohistochemical study. *Hepatology* 1988;**8**: 1586–95.

14 Nakanuma Y, Hoso M, Sanzen T, Sasaki M. Microstructure and development of the normal and pathologic biliary tract in humans, including blood supply. *Microsc Res Tech* 1997;**38**:552–70.

15 Crawford JM. Development of the intrahepatic biliary tree. *Semin Liver Dis* 2002;**22**:213–26.

16 Cantlie J. On a new arrangement of the right and left lobes of the liver. *J Anat Physiol (London) (Section Proc Anat Soc Great Britain & Ireland)* 1898;**32**:4–9.

17 Kasahara M, Kaihara S, Oike F, *et al.* Living-donor liver transplantation with monosegments. *Transplantation* 2003;**76**:694–6.

18 Bismuth H, Houssin D, Castaing D. Major and minor segmentectomies "réglées" in liver surgery. *World J Surg* 1982;**6**:10–24.

19 Bismuth H. Surgical anatomy and anatomical surgery of the liver. *World J Surg* 1982;**6**:3–9.

20 Launois B, Jamieson GG. The importance of Glisson's capsule and its sheaths in the intrahepatic approach to resection of the liver. *Surg Gynecol Obstet* 1992;**174**:7–10.

21 Clavien PA, Petrowsky H, DeOliveira ML, Graf R. Strategies for safer liver surgery and partial liver transplantation. *N Engl J Med* 2007;**356**:1545–59.

22 Crawford JM. Liver and biliary tract. In: Kumar V, Abbas A, Faustto N, eds. *Robins and Cotran Pathologic Basis of Disease*. Philadelphia: Saunders, 2004: 877–939.

23 Van As AB, Hickman R, Engelbrecht GH, Makan P, Duminy F, Kahn D. Significance of the portal vein helix. *S Afr J Surg* 2001;**39**:50–2.

24 Rosenthal SJ, Harrison LA, Baxter KG, Wetzel LH, Cox GG, Batnitzky S. Doppler US of helical flow in the portal vein. *RadioGraphics* 1995;**15**:1103–11.

25 Attardi G. Demonstration in vivo and in vitro of peristaltic contractions in the portal vein of adult mammals (rodents). *Nature* 1955;**176**:76–7.

26 Howard ER, Davenport M. Congenital extrahepatic portocaval shunts—the Abernethy malformation. *J Pediatr Surg* 1997;**32**: 494–7.

27 Daly JM, Kemeny N, Oderman P, Botet J. Long-term hepatic arterial infusion chemotherapy. Anatomic considerations, operative technique, and treatment morbidity. *Arch Surg* 1984;**119**: 936–41.

28 Northover JM, Terblanche J. A new look at the arterial supply of the bile duct in man and its surgical implications. *Br J Surg* 1979;**66**:379–84.

29 Stapleton GN, Hickman R, Terblanche J. Blood supply of the right and left hepatic ducts. *Br J Surg* 1998;**85**:202–7.

30 Healey JE Jr, Schroy PC. Anatomy of the biliary ducts within the human liver; analysis of the prevailing pattern of branchings and the major variations of the biliary ducts. *AMA Arch Surg* 1953;**66**:599–616.

31 Hepp J, Couinaud C. [Approach to and use of the left hepatic duct in reparation of the common bile duct; in French.] *Presse Med* 1956;**64**:947–48.

32 Couinaud C. Liver anatomy: portal (and suprahepatic) or biliary segmentation. *Dig Surg* 1999;**16**:459–67.

33 Rocko JM, Di Gioia JM. Calot's triangle revisited. *Surg Gynecol Obstet* 1981;**153**:410–4.

34 Roskams TA, Theise ND, Balabaud C, *et al.* Nomenclature of the finer branches of the biliary tree: canals, ductules, and ductular reactions in human livers. *Hepatology* 2004;**39**:1739–45.

35 Kiernan F. The anatomy and physiology of the Liver. *Philos Trans R Soc London* 1833;**123**:711–70.

36 Matsumoto T, Komori R, Magara T, *et al.* A study on the normal structure of human liver, with special reference to its angioarchitecture. *Jikeikai Med J* 1979;**26**:1–40.

37 Malarkey DE, Johnson K, Ryan L, Boorman G, Maronpot RR. New insights into functional aspects of liver morphology. *Toxicol Pathol* 2005;**33**:27–34.

38 Rappaport AM, Borowy ZJ, Lougheed WM, Lotto WN. Subdivision of hexagonal liver lobules into a structural and functional unit; role in hepatic physiology and pathology. *Anat Rec* 1954;**119**:11–33.

39 McCuskey R, Robert S. Anatomy of efferent hepatic nerves. *Anat Rec* 2004;**280**:821–6.

40 Jansen PL, Strautnieks SS, Jacquemin E, *et al.* Hepatocanalicular bile salt export pump deficiency in patients with progressive familial intrahepatic cholestasis. *Gastroenterology* 1999;**117**:1370–9.

41 Jacquemin E. Progressive familial intrahepatic cholestasis. Genetic basis and treatment. *Clin Liver Dis* 2000;**4**:753–63.

42 Soskin S. The liver and carbohydrate metabolism. *Endocrinology* 1940;**26**:297–308.

43 Holt RI, Crossey PA, Jones JS, Baker AJ, Portmann B, Miell JP. Hepatic growth hormone receptor, insulin-like growth factor I, and insulin-like growth factor-binding protein messenger RNA expression in pediatric liver disease. *Hepatology* 1997;**26**: 1600–6.

44 Holt RI, Miell JP, Jones JS, Mieli-Vergani G, Baker AJ. Nasogastric feeding enhances nutritional status in paediatric liver disease but does not alter circulating levels of IGF-I and IGF binding proteins. *Clin Endocrinol (Oxf)* 2000;**52**:217–24.

45 Lang KS, Georgiev P, Recher M, *et al.* Immunoprivileged status of the liver is controlled by Toll-like receptor 3 signaling. *J Clin Invest* 2006;**116**:2456–63.

46 Doherty DG, Norris S, Madrigal-Estebas L, *et al.* The human liver contains multiple populations of NK cells, T cells, and CD3+CD56+ natural T cells with distinct cytotoxic activities and Th1, Th2, and Th0 cytokine secretion patterns. *J Immunol* 1999;**163**:2314–21.

47 Suchy F, Narkewicz MR. Development of the liver and bile ducts. *J Pediatr Gastroenterol Nutr* 2002;**35**(Suppl 1):S4–6.

48 Beath SV. Hepatic function and physiology in the newborn. *Semin Neonatol* 2003;**8**:337–46.

49 Knisely AS. Biliary tract malformations. *Am J Med Genet A* 2003;**122**:343–50.

50 Strassburg CP, Strassburg A, Kneip S, *et al.* Developmental aspects of human hepatic drug glucuronidation in young children and adults. *Gut* 2002;**50**:259–65.

51 Oh SH, Witek RP, Bae SH, *et al.* Bone marrow-derived hepatic oval cells differentiate into hepatocytes in 2-acetylaminofluorene/partial hepatectomy-induced liver regeneration. *Gastroenterology* 2007;**132**:1077–87.

52 Golding M, Sarraf CE, Lalani EN, *et al.* Oval cell differentiation into hepatocytes in the acetylaminofluorene-treated regenerating rat liver. *Hepatology* 1995;**22**:1243–53.

53 Baumann U, Crosby HA, Ramani P, Kelly DA, Strain AJ. Expression of the stem cell factor receptor c-*kit* in normal and diseased pediatric liver: identification of a human hepatic progenitor cell? *Hepatology* 1999;**30**:112–7.

54 Petersen BE, Bowen WC, Patrene KD, *et al.* Bone marrow as a potential source of hepatic oval cells. *Science* 1999;**284**:1168–70.
55 Theise ND, Nimmakayalu M, Gardner R, *et al.* Liver from bone marrow in humans. *Hepatology* 2000;**32**:11–6.
56 Grompe M. Principles of therapeutic liver repopulation. *J Inherit Metab Dis* 2006;**29**:421–5.
57 Friedman SL, Bansal MB. Reversal of hepatic fibrosis—fact or fantasy? *Hepatology* 2006;**43**:S82–8.
58 Hemmann S, Graf J, Roderfeld M, Roeb E. Expression of MMPs and TIMPs in liver fibrosis—a systematic review with special emphasis on anti-fibrotic strategies. *J Hepatol* 2007;**46**:955–75.

2 Investigating the Liver

2 The Approach to the Child with Liver Disease: Differential Diagnosis and Useful Investigations

Deirdre A. Kelly

The approach to the child with liver disease should be systematic and based on an accurate clinical history and a thorough physical examination. This chapter will outline the main diagnostic categories and summarize key investigations. Further detail will be provided in individual chapters. Investigating the liver relies on a multidisciplinary approach involving clinical chemistry, hematology, radiology, histopathology, and microbiology. It is essential to understand the many functions of the liver and to recognize the effects of hepatic dysfunction on other body systems (Table 2.1; see also Chapter 1).

Neonatal liver disease

Almost two-thirds of children who have liver disease present in the neonatal period with persistent jaundice. Although physiologic jaundice is common in neonates, infants who develop severe or persistent jaundice should be investigated to exclude hemolysis, sepsis, or underlying liver disease. Neonatal jaundice that persists beyond 14 or 21 days should always be investigated, even in breast-fed babies (see Chapter 4). It is essential to establish whether the jaundice is due to an increase in conjugated or unconjugated hyperbilirubinemia. The common causes of unconjugated hyperbilirubinemia are rhesus incompatibility, breast-milk jaundice, and Crigler–Najjar syndrome type I or II (see Chapter 4). Liver disease is associated with a rise in conjugated hyperbilirubinemia.

The clinical history should include:

- Details about the mother's pregnancy (drugs, alcohol, smoking, intercurrent illnesses, pruritus of pregnancy, hepatitis status, risk factors—e.g., drug abuse)
- Birth weight and gestational age
- Vitamin K administration
- Family history
- Consanguinity
- The history of the present illness should include:
  —Date of jaundice
  —Color of stools and urine
  —Drug history, particularly parenteral nutrition
  —Bleeding, petechiae, or bruising
  —Feeding history and weight gain
  —Diarrhea and vomiting
  —Immunizations, if relevant

The differential diagnosis can be guided by the birth weight and gestational age (Figure 2.1) and is between extrahepatic biliary disease, the neonatal hepatitis syndrome, and metabolic liver disease (see Chapters 4, 5, and 13).

Clinical features suggesting liver disease include:

- Family history, consanguinity, or dysmorphic features suggesting metabolic or inherited liver disease (Figure 2.2).
- Pale stools and dark urine, suggesting cholestasis or obstruction (Figure 2.3).
- Bruising, petechiae, or bleeding, suggesting vitamin K deficiency from malabsorption or inadequate administration at birth.
- Hypoglycemia could be secondary to metabolic disease, hypopituitarism, or acute liver failure.
- Hepatomegaly is a nonspecific sign, as is slow weight gain or failure to thrive.
- Splenomegaly suggests an intrauterine infection, metabolic liver disease, or advanced liver disease with hepatic fibrosis and early portal hypertension.
- Ascites is rare and suggests an intrauterine infection, inborn error of metabolism, rhesus hemolytic disease, or advanced liver disease.

If the infant is acutely ill, then sepsis, metabolic disease, or acute liver failure should be considered (see Chapters 5 and 7).

Liver disease in older children

Liver disease in children older than 6 months may be acute or chronic (Figure 2.4). As in infancy, there is a predominance

Diseases of the Liver and Biliary System in Children, 3rd edition. Edited by Deirdre Kelly. © 2008 Blackwell Publishing, ISBN: 978-1-4051-6334-7.

Table 2.1 Functions of the liver.

Function	Effect of dysfunction	Assessment
Metabolism/storage		
Carbohydrate/glycogen	Loss of glucose homeostasis	Hypoglycemia on fasting/stress
Lipid	Lipid accumulation in hepatocytes	High/low cholesterol
	↓ Oxidation of fatty acids	↑ Lactate
		↑ FFA : BOH ratio
		↑ Acylcarnitine
		Organic aciduria
Protein	↑ Catabolism	Low BCAA, urea
		↑ Ammonia
		↑ Tyr, –Phe, –Met
Synthesis		
Albumin	Loss of muscle mass	Low albumin
		Protein energy malnutrition
Factors II, VII, IX, X	Coagulopathy	Prolonged PT/PTT
Degradation		
Drugs	Prolonged drug effect—e.g., sedation	Clinical
Estrogens	Telangiectasia	Clinical
	Gynecomastia	
Toxic products	Encephalopathy	Abnormal EEG/clinical signs
Bile synthesis and excretion	Cholestasis	↑ Conjugated bilirubin
	Fat malabsorption	↑ GGT
		↑ ALP
		↑ Cholesterol
	Fat-soluble vitamin deficiency	Anthropometry
	Pruritus	
	Malnutrition	

ALP, alkaline phosphatase; BOH, β-hydroxybutyrate; BCAA, branched-chain amino acids; EEG, electroencephalogram; FFA, free fatty acids; GGT, γ-glutamyl transpeptidase; Met, methionine; Phe, phenylalanine; PT, prothrombin time; PTT, partial thromboplastin time; Tyr, tyrosine.

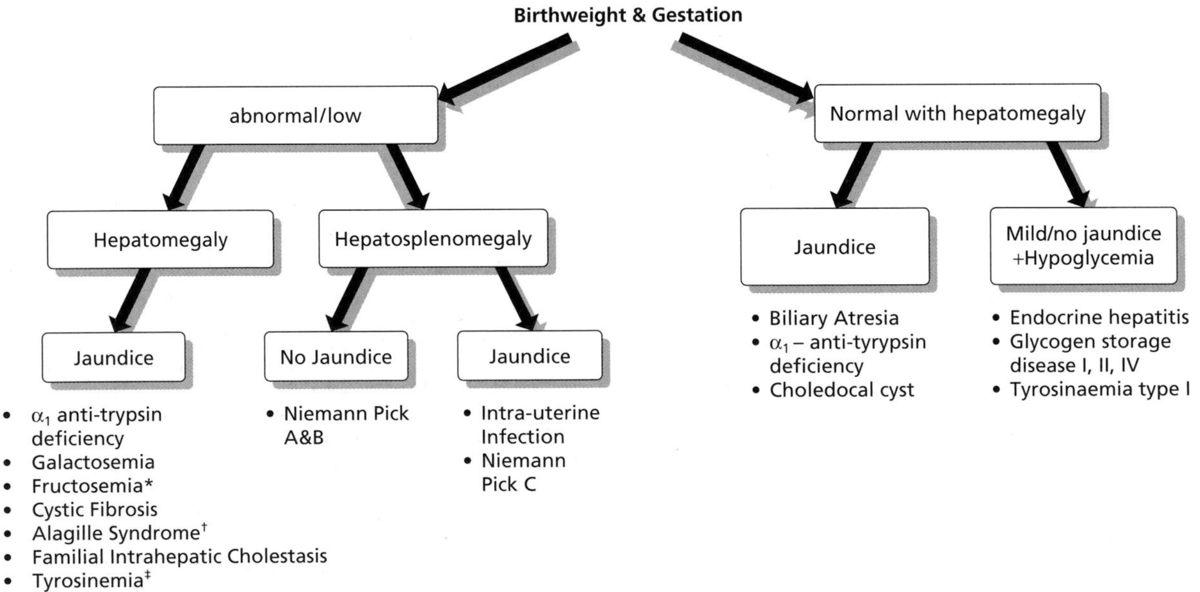

Figure 2.1 The approach to the diagnosis of neonatal liver disease. * Presents on weaning; † dysmorphic; ‡ jaundice may be mild.

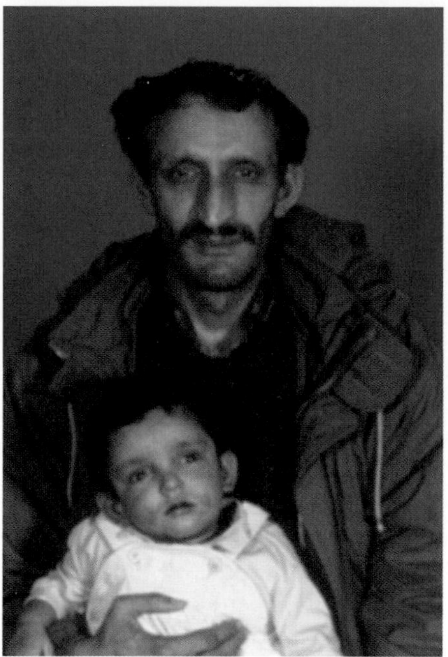

Figure 2.2 Dysmorphic features suggest inherited metabolic disease. In Alagille's syndrome, which is an autosomal-dominant disorder. The characteristic facies consists of a broad forehead, deep-set eyes, mild hypertelorism, and a pointed chin. It can be difficult to diagnose in an infant, but the diagnosis may be obvious in the parent.

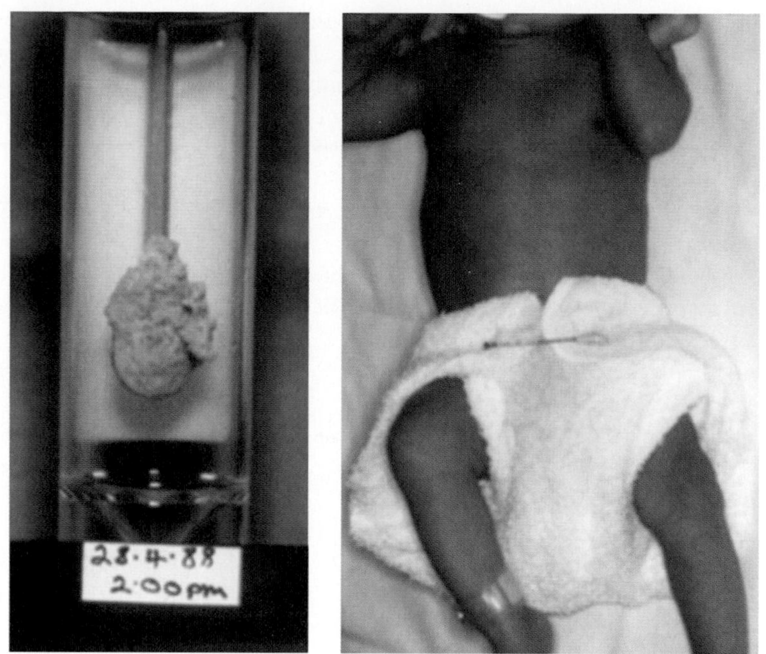

Figure 2.3 A, B Cholestasis with pale stools and dark urine is characteristic of biliary obstruction, usually due to biliary atresia.

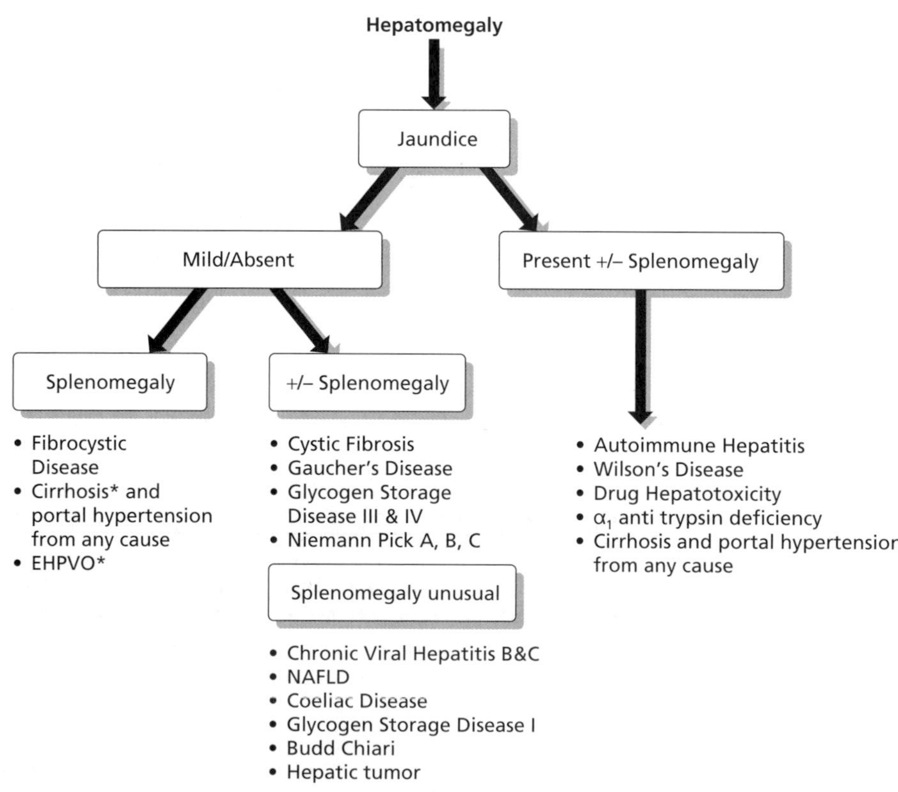

Figure 2.4 The approach to the older child with liver disease. * Liver may be small. EHPVO, extrahepatic vein obstruction; NAFLD, nonalcoholic fatty liver disease.

of inherited disorders and multisystem involvement. Jaundice may not be a prominent feature. Acute or chronic liver disease may be due to infection, autoimmune disease, drug-induced hepatitis, or metabolic disease, or may be secondary to disease elsewhere (Figure 2.4; see also Sections 6 and 7, Chapters 8–14).

The clinical history for either acute or chronic liver disease should include:

- Previous history, particularly of neonatal jaundice (α_1-antitrypsin deficiency and Niemann–Pick C disease may be associated with transient jaundice)
- Evidence of hypoglycemia
- Weight gain or loss
- Diarrhea or inflammatory bowel disease
- Pruritus
- Bleeding, bruising, epistaxis
- Hematemesis or melena
- Skin rashes or joint pains
- Drug history, especially transfusions
- Ear piercing, tattooing, previous surgery
- Immunizations
- Family history and consanguinity
- Symptoms of extrahepatic disease/autoimmune disease
- Allergies
- Developmental history
- Deterioration in school performance (Wilson's disease or Niemann–Pick C)
- Foreign travel
- Household contacts
- Local epidemics
- Recreational activity
- Intravenous drug abuse
- Pets

Acute liver disease

The clinical presentation varies depending on the etiology, but the following clinical features are common:

- A prodrome of malaise, lethargy, and anorexia
- Nausea, vomiting, or diarrhea
- Weight loss
- Abdominal discomfort or tender hepatomegaly
- Hepatomegaly
- Splenomegaly
- Ascites (rarely, except for acute Budd–Chiari syndrome)
- Rash or joint pains
- Jaundice may or may not be present

The differential diagnosis of acute hepatitis includes:

- Viral hepatitis A or B, seronegative hepatitis
- Autoimmune hepatitis
- Drug hepatoxicity
- Metabolic liver disease, especially Wilson's disease (see Chapters 6, 8, 9, and 14)

Acute liver failure is the development of massive hepatic necrosis with subsequent loss of liver function, with coagulopathy and with or without hepatic encephalopathy. The disease is uncommon, but has a high mortality. The child may present within hours or weeks with jaundice, encephalopathy, coagulopathy, hypoglycemia, and electrolyte disturbance. The main causes are infection (seronegative hepatitis), autoimmune hepatitis, drug toxicity (acetaminophen) and metabolic disease (see Chapter 7).

Chronic liver disease

Chronic liver disease may affect every organ in the body (Figure 2.5). It may be asymptomatic, and the diagnosis may be made:

- After incidental detection of abnormal liver enzymes or hepatomegaly
- After family screening for hepatitis B/C or metabolic disorders
- In a transfusion recipient following diagnosis of donor infection
- In coexistent disease—e.g., inflammatory bowel disease, celiac disease
- In a recipient of a known toxic agent—e.g., methotrexate

The clinical presentation varies from acute hepatitis to the insidious development of hepatosplenomegaly, cirrhosis, and portal hypertension with lethargy and malnutrition. Common symptoms include:

- Intermittent fatigue, anorexia, and weight loss
- Abdominal discomfort
- Variable or fluctuating jaundice with pruritus and pale stools
- Hematemesis or melena from variceal bleeding. This may be the presenting symptom, especially in cirrhosis with portal hypertension or extrahepatic portal hypertension.

The differential diagnosis of chronic liver disease is illustrated in Figure 2.4. Common physical features are:

- Palmar erythema, or "liver palms," is a nonspecific red discoloration of the palms and fingertips, indicative of a hyperdynamic circulation, which is associated with chronic liver disease and cirrhosis (Figure 2.6).
- Spider nevi, or spider angiomas, are telangectasia consisting of a central arteriole with superficially radiating small vessels, resembling spiders' legs. The lesion will blanch when pressure is applied to the center. Although spider nevi do occur in healthy children at puberty, the presence of more than five is suggestive of chronic liver disease. Superficial distended veins (telangectasia) are common on the face (Figure 2.7).
- Abdominal distension may be due to hepatosplenomegaly or ascites. Distended abdominal veins are a sign of portal hypertension (Figure 2.8).
- Fat malabsorption leads to malnutrition and rickets, often with pathological fractures (Figure 2.9).

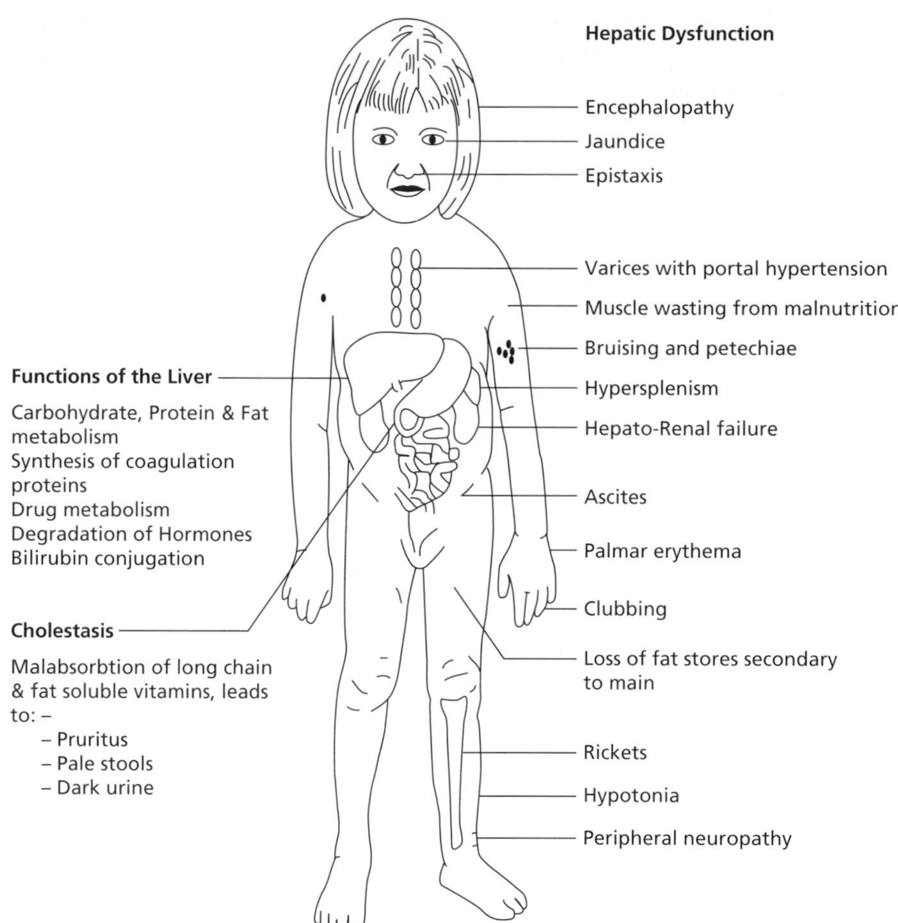

Figure 2.5 Multiorgan involvement in chronic liver disease.

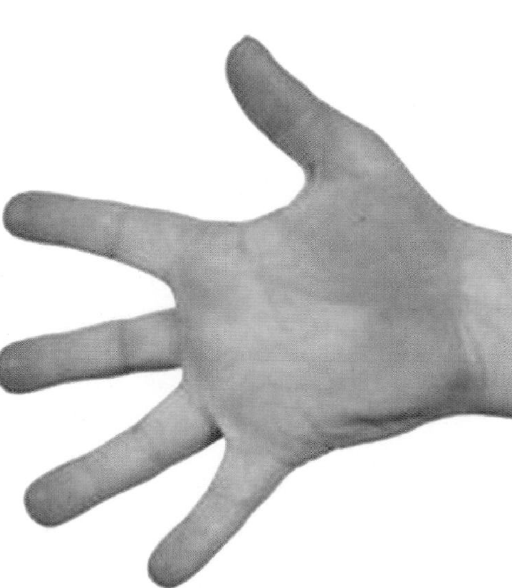

Figure 2.6 Palmar erythema is a sign of liver disease.

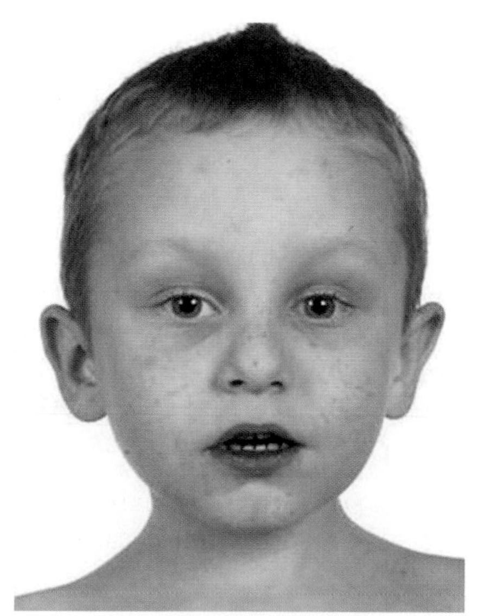

Figure 2.7 Facial telangiectasia is a sign of cirrhosis or hepatic decompensation.

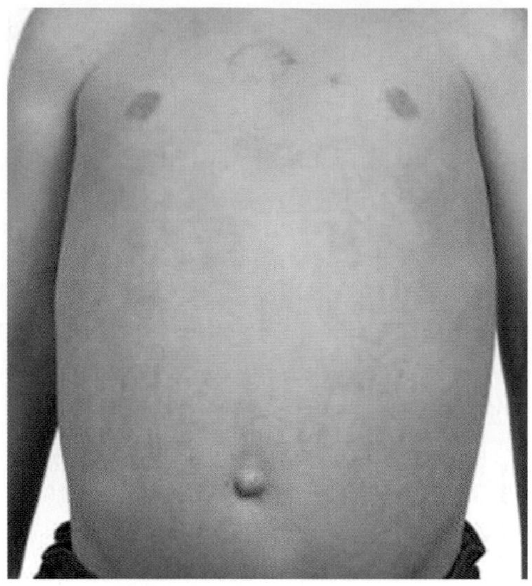

Figure 2.8 Abdominal distension with dilated superficial veins is suggestive of portal hypertension.

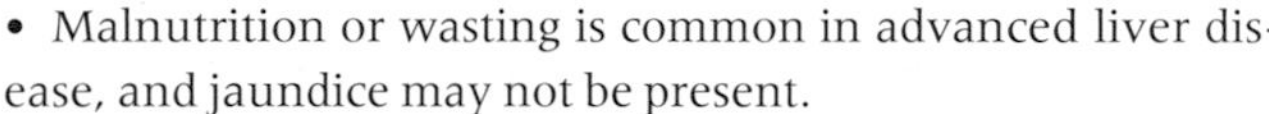

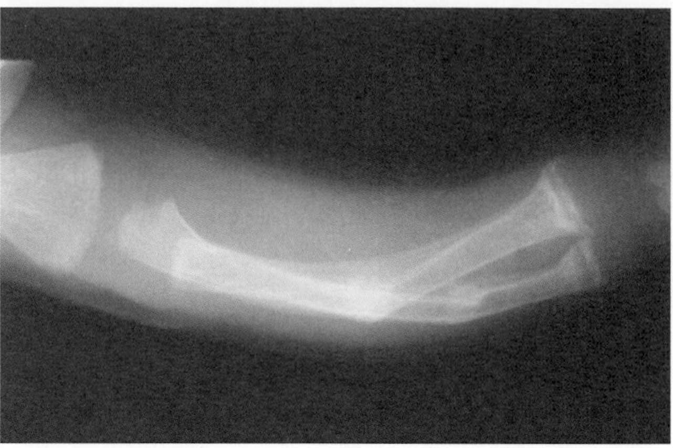

Figure 2.9 Fat malabsorption leads to fat-soluble vitamin deficiency and rickets. Note the splayed epiphyses and the pathological fracture.

- Malnutrition or wasting is common in advanced liver disease, and jaundice may not be present.

Investigating the liver

The principles of investigation should be to:
- Establish the diagnosis and exclude differential diagnoses.
- Stage disease and detect complications (Chapter 15).
- Detect associated conditions—e.g., celiac disease or inflammatory bowel disease (Chapter 16).

Biochemical liver function tests

Baseline investigations

Biochemical liver function tests (Table 2.2) reflect the severity of hepatic dysfunction, but rarely provide diagnostic

Table 2.2 Liver function tests.

Reference range of test	Abnormality
Conjugated bilirubin < 20 μmol/L	Elevated: hepatocyte dysfunction or biliary obstruction
Aminotransferases Aspartate (AST) < 50 U/L Alanine (ALT) < 40 U/L	Elevated: hepatocyte inflammation/damage
Alkaline phosphatase (ALP) < 600 U/L (age-dependent)	Elevated: biliary inflammation/obstruction
γ-Glutamyltransferase (GGT) < 30 U/L (age-dependent)	
Albumin 35–50 g/L	Reduced: chronic liver disease
Prothrombin time (PT) 12–15 s Partial thromboplastin time (PTT) 33–37 s	Prolonged: (i) Vitamin K deficiency (ii) Reduced hepatic synthesis
Ammonia < 50 μmol/L	Elevated: abnormal protein catabolism/urea cycle defect/other inherited metabolic disease
Glucose > 4 mmol/L	Reduced in: acute or chronic liver failure/metabolic disease/hypopituitarism

information on individual diseases. Conjugated bilirubin is nearly always elevated in liver disease and is a particularly important investigation in the differential diagnosis of neonatal jaundice (Chapter 4). The presence of bilirubin is always abnormal if it is detected in a fresh urine specimen.

Aminotransferases are intracellular enzymes that are present in the liver, heart, and skeletal muscle. Increases in aspartate aminotransferase (AST) and alanine aminotransferase (ALT) indicate hepatic necrosis, irrespective of etiology (Table 2.2). ALT is more liver-specific than AST, but has a longer plasma half-life. A rise in AST is an early indication of liver damage and is a useful marker of rejection after liver transplantation (Chapter 21). These enzymes may be normal in compensated cirrhosis. Elevated aminotransferases are often the first indication of the development of nonalcoholic fatty liver disease (NAFLD) in an obese child (Chapter 11).

Elevated aspartate aminotransferases and/or alanine are also found in muscular dystrophy, and this diagnosis should be considered if there are no other signs of liver disease.

Alkaline phosphatase is found in the liver, kidney, bone, placenta, and intestine. In pediatric liver disease, increases in this enzyme indicate biliary epithelial damage, malignant infiltration, cirrhosis, rejection, or osteopenia secondary to vitamin D deficiency. γ-Glutamyltransferase (GGT) is present in biliary epithelia and hepatocytes. The reference range is age-related, with higher levels in neonates. It is elevated in many forms of liver damage, but may be normal in certain forms of intrahepatic cholestasis (e.g., familial intrahepatic cholestasis types 1 and 2, Chapter 4).

The most useful tests of liver function are the plasma albumin concentration and coagulation time. Low serum albumin indicates chronicity of liver disease, while abnormal coagulation indicates significant hepatic dysfunction, either acute or chronic. Fasting hypoglycemia in the absence of other causes (e.g., hypopituitarism or hyperinsulinism) indicates poor hepatic function and is a guide to the prognosis in acute liver failure. If these baseline investigations suggest hepatic dysfunction, then it is appropriate to consider more specific investigations for metabolic disease (Table 2.3).[1–3]

Second-line investigations (Table 2.3)

Hepatic dysfunction may be secondary to sepsis, particularly urinary sepsis, inborn errors of metabolism, or endocrine disorders. It is usual to exclude sepsis by performing bacterial culture of the urine and/or blood cultures if appropriate, and to exclude known causes of viral hepatitis.

If the infant is unwell, or has evidence of acute liver failure, then galactosemia and tyrosinemia should be excluded (Chapter 5).

In neonates, hypopituitarism may be difficult to exclude, as thyroid function tests may be equivocal or in the low normal range. It is useful to perform a cortisol level test at 9 AM at the same time as measuring free thyroxine and thyroid-stimulating hormone (TSH).[4]

α_1-Antitrypsin deficiency is the commonest inherited metabolic liver disease and should always be excluded at any age. As α_1-antitrypsin is an acute-phase protein, it is necessary to measure both the concentration and phenotype in order to differentiate between homozygotes, heterozygotes, and an acute-phase response. Although cystic fibrosis is a rare cause of liver disease in the neonatal period, it should be considered in the differential diagnosis of neonatal liver disease, and excluded by performing an immunoreactive trypsin test, a sweat test, and mutation analysis if either is positive (Chapter 12).

Wilson's disease rarely presents before the age of 3 years, but may mimic any form of liver disease and should always be excluded in older children (Chapter 14). An autoimmune screen and immunoglobulin levels should detect 75% of children with autoimmune hepatitis (Chapter 8).

The development of new technology, such as fast atom bombardment mass spectrometry and tandem mass spectrometry, has made it possible to identify specific metabolites in the urine and blood in a number of rare diseases—e.g., primary bile salt deficiencies (Chapter 4). Other specific tests include measurement of carnitine and acylcarnitine in fatty acid oxidation disorders (Chapters 5 and 13). These investigations are essential steps in the differential diagnosis of unresolved neonatal hepatitis.

Serum cholesterol is usually elevated in children with severe cholestasis—for example, in Alagille's syndrome or biliary atresia—and provides supporting evidence of these diagnoses. In contrast, low or normal cholesterol is characteristic of bile acid transport disorders or of terminal liver disease (Chapters 4 and 21).

Plasma ammonia and amino acids (particularly phenylalanine, tyrosine, and methionine) may be raised in either acute or chronic liver failure and are nonspecific indications of hepatic dysfunction. An elevated plasma or urine tyrosine may indicate tyrosinemia type I, which should be confirmed by measurement of urinary succinylacetone. Definitive diagnosis requires assay of fumarylacetoacetase in skin fibroblasts or mutation analysis (Chapter 5). Primitive hepatic cells synthesize α-fetoprotein. The levels are highest in the newborn (> 1000 mg/L) and fall in the first few months of life. It may be a useful screening test in the diagnosis of tyrosinemia type I and hepatoblastoma, or for detection of hepatocellular carcinoma in chronic carriers of hepatitis B and C.

Imaging

Several imaging techniques provide valuable information in the investigation and diagnosis of pediatric liver disease, while the rapid development of interventional radiology has altered the management of many hepatic complications.[5]

Table 2.3 Investigation of liver disease.

Baseline investigations	*Neonate*
Bilirubin	Galactose 1-phosphate uridyltransferase
Conjugated	Free T_4, TSH
Unconjugated	9 AM cortisol
Aspartate aminotransferase	Chromosomes/DNA
Alanine aminotransferase	Sweat test (> 4 weeks)
Alkaline phosphatase	*Older child (> 2 years)*
γ-Glutamyl transpeptidase	Cu, ceruloplasmin, urinary Cu
Albumin	C3, C4, ANA, SMA, LKM
Glucose	Immunoglobulins
Full blood count and platelets	EBV
Prothrombin time	*If indicated*
Partial thromboplastin time	Radioisotope scan
Second-line investigations	Liver biopsy for:
Bacterial culture of blood and urine	Histology
TORCH screen	Electron microscopy
Hepatitis A, B, C	Enzyme analysis
α_1-Antitrypsin level and phenotype	Immunohistochemistry
Abdominal ultrasound	Culture
Metabolic investigations	Copper concentration
Immunoreactive trypsin	Skin biopsy
Plasma lactate, BOH, FFA	Ophthalmology
Ammonia	Cardiology
Acylcarnitine	Bone-marrow aspirate
Serum iron and ferritin	Endoscopy
Plasma amino acids	ERCP
Cholesterol, triglyceride	PTC
α-Fetoprotein	MRI
Parathyroid hormone	
Wrist for bone age/rickets	
Urine	
Reducing sugars	
Organic acids	
Amino acids	
Succinylacetone	
Bile salts	

ANA, antinuclear antibodies; BOH, β-hydroxybutyrate; C3, C4, complement components 3 and 4; EBV, Epstein–Barr virus; ERCP, endoscopic retrograde cholangiopancreatography; FFA, free fatty acids; LKM, liver/kidney microsomal antibodies; MRI, magnetic resonance imaging; PTC, percutaneous transhepatic cholangiography; SMA, smooth-muscle antibodies; T_4, thyroxine; TORCH, toxoplasmosis, other, rubella, cytomegalovirus, and herpes simplex; TSH, thyroid-stimulating hormone.

Radiography

Plain radiography of the abdomen will give an indication of liver and spleen size, but is rarely of diagnostic value and is not a routine investigation. Chest radiography may show skeletal abnormalities—for example, butterfly vertebrae in Alagille's syndrome, a dilated heart secondary to fluid overload in end-stage liver disease, or evidence of congenital heart disease. Wrist and knee radiography will demonstrate bone age and/or the development of osteopenia or rickets.

Ultrasound

The development of Doppler ultrasound has been an important advance in the investigation of liver disease. Ultrasonic investigation of the abdomen provides information on the size and consistency of the liver, spleen, pancreas, and kidneys, on the size of the gallbladder, and on the presence of gallstones. It may identify tumors, hemangiomas, abscesses, or cysts within the liver, and it allows targeting of lesions for liver biopsy. The gallbladder is best visualized after a 4–6-h fast. A small or absent gallbladder after fasting suggests either severe intrahepatic cholestasis or biliary atresia in the neonate (see Chapter 4, Figure 4.4), whereas an enlarged gallbladder may represent supportive evidence for primary sclerosing cholangitis. Extrahepatic bile ducts are usually identified, but intrahepatic bile ducts are rarely seen unless dilated as a result of biliary obstruction. Dilated intrahepatic bile ducts are not a feature of extrahepatic biliary atresia in the neonate.

Color-flow Doppler techniques allow rapid evaluation of vascular patency without the use of intravenous contrast material. They are particularly useful in pre- and post-transplant examinations to identify whether the portal vein, hepatic veins and artery, and splenic vessels are patent. Portal hypertension is suggested by the presence of ascites, splenomegaly, and splenic or gastric varices.

Ultrasound may be less sensitive in identifying hepatic outflow obstruction after transplantation. This problem is related to "kinking" of the hepatic vein, which may not be apparent in a prone fasted child. A high index of suspicion and a low threshold for hepatic venography are required if clinical symptoms exist.[6]

Radioisotope scanning

Soluble radioisotopes such as technetium trimethyl 1-bromoiminodiacetic acid (TEBIDA), which are taken up well by hepatocytes despite elevated bilirubin levels, have been used to demonstrate either hepatic uptake or biliary excretion. Pretreatment with phenobarbitone (5 mg/kg) for 3–5 days prior to the investigation improves hepatic uptake of the isotope. Hepatic uptake is an index of hepatic function and may be patchy in inflammatory conditions—e.g., neonatal hepatitis (see Chapter 4, Figure 4.5).

Radioisotope scanning is most useful in the assessment of biliary excretion in the differential diagnosis of neonatal cholestasis. Under normal conditions, biliary excretion is completed within 4 h. Delayed excretion or no excretion after 24 h suggests severe intrahepatic cholestasis or extrahepatic biliary atresia. Delayed biliary excretion or pooling in bile ducts is also a feature of cystic fibrosis liver disease (see Chapter 12, Figure 12.7).

In post-transplant patients, a TEBIDA scan may be of value in identifying the degree of biliary obstruction or a biliary leak.

Radioisotope scanning is of some value in the diagnosis of hepatic vein obstruction (Budd–Chiari syndrome), as poor uptake of the isotope is demonstrated in most of the liver except for the caudate lobe, which has a separate venous drainage. This method is rarely used now, as ultrasound or venography is preferred.

Interventional radiology

Interventional radiology has an important role in the modern management of hepatobiliary disorders and provides new treatment options. "Keyhole" or "pinhole" techniques using catheter-based technology are carried out under imaging guidance with radiography (including computed tomography), ultrasound, or magnetic resonance imaging. Useful diagnostic and therapeutic techniques are described below.

Computed tomography

Computed tomography (CT) of the liver is useful for identifying and taking biopsies from hepatic tumors or space-occupying lesions of the liver. Intravenous contrast medium causes enhancement of vascular lesions and of the walls of abscesses and may be helpful in differentiating tumors from other solid masses. An important recent advance is the introduction of helical or spiral CT scanning, in which both the table and the roentgen-ray tube move continuously to improve imaging. The use of CT angiography allows noninvasive evaluation of vascular structures. CT scans of the brain are helpful for the detection of cerebral edema in acute liver failure (Chapter 7) or for cerebral atrophy in certain metabolic conditions (Chapters 5 and 13).

Endoscopic retrograde cholangiopancreatography (ERCP)

In this endoscopic technique, a fiberoptic duodenoscope is passed into the first part of the duodenum, the ampulla of Vater is identified, the pancreatic and biliary ducts are cannulated, and radiographic contrast medium is injected. The technique has an 80% success rate in skilled hands and is invaluable for the assessment of extrahepatic biliary disease in older children (e.g., choledochal cysts, primary sclerosing cholangitis) and the assessment of chronic pancreatitis. Although this technique should be of value in the differential diagnosis of neonatal cholestasis, technical difficulties in cannulating the bile ducts in small infants may lead to equivocal information being obtained. The development of a prototype fiberoptic duodenoscope (7.5 mm in diameter) has improved the diagnostic yield in this group of patients. In general, the diagnostic value of this technique has been superseded by that of magnetic resonance imaging (MRI), which is noninvasive, but ERCP retains an important role in therapy[7] (see Chapter 8, Figure 8.4).

The removal of common bile duct stones, insertion of biliary and pancreatic stents, and sphincterotomy are useful therapeutic procedures that can be performed at the same time as the diagnostic procedure, but have limited application in children.

Endoscopic ultrasound

Endoscopic ultrasound (EUS) is a new imaging modality that visualizes the lower biliary tree. The technique uses mini-probes (external diameter 2.6 mm), which are small enough to be passed through the operating channel of conventional pediatric duodenoscopes. The technique is well established in adult practice, with a wide range of applications. It is a highly sensitive and specific method of visualizing the lower biliary

A

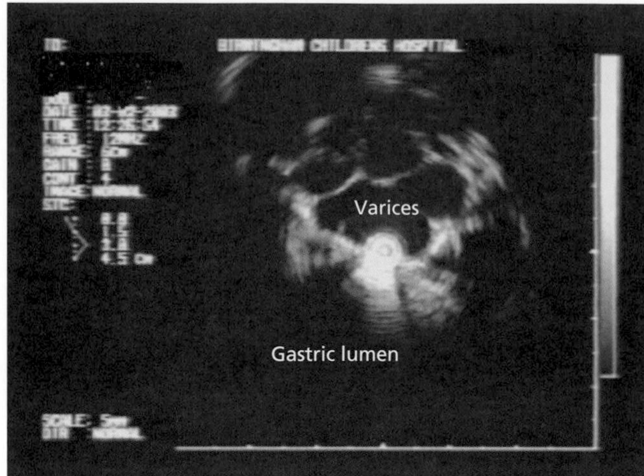

B

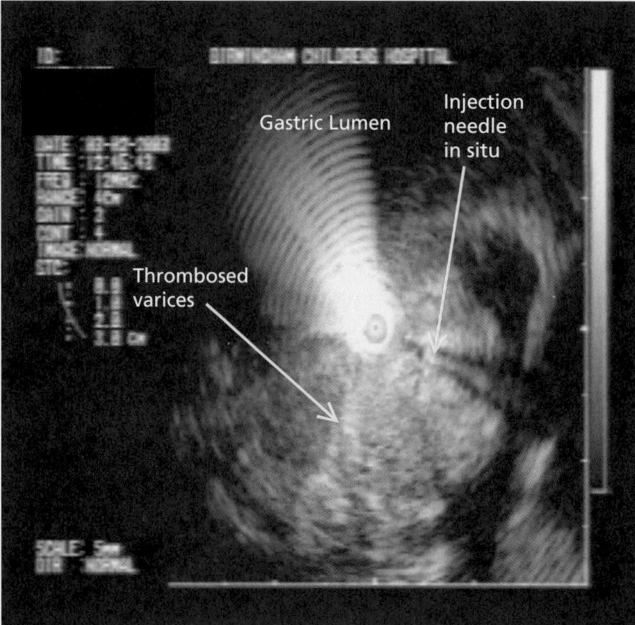

Figure 2.10 Endoscopic ultrasound is a useful way of detecting submucosal varices (**A**) before and (**B**) after injection with thrombin.

tree and demonstrating pathology in this area.[8,9] Although the technique has not yet been evaluated in pediatric practice, it may prove to be of value in the diagnosis of infants with neonatal cholestasis. Endoscopic ultrasound has also proved useful in the diagnosis of submucosal esophageal and gastric varices[10] (Figure 2.10).

Percutaneous transhepatic cholangiography (PTC)

This technique is useful for identifying biliary disease if the intrahepatic bile ducts are dilated secondary to obstruction and ERCP is impossible or unsuccessful. A thin needle (Chiba) is passed through the liver. The bile ducts or gallbladder are punctured and radiographic contrast medium is injected. External drainage of the biliary tree, dilation of biliary strictures, and the insertion of biliary stents are all possible using this technique and are useful both before and after transplantation.

Angiography

Catheter angiography is primarily undertaken in infants and children with the following disorders:

- Primary hepatic tumors for which complex surgical resection is being considered—e.g., in auto-transplantation.
- Cavernous transformation of the portal vein (also known as extrahepatic portal vein obstruction) prior to surgical shunting.
- Portal vein thrombosis in patients being considered for liver transplantation.
- If intervention is being considered for vascular stenoses or occlusion of the hepatic artery, vein, portal vein, or inferior vena cava following liver transplantation or in the Budd–Chiari syndrome.
- Hepatic vascular anomalies such as life-threatening hemangiomas, arterioportal fistulas, arteriovenous malformations, and congenital portosystemic shunts.
- Refractory or life-threatening bleeding from gastrointestinal disease or following blunt abdominal trauma or liver biopsy.
- Invasive diagnostic imaging when angiography is required as part of the procedure, such as transvenous (transjugular) liver biopsy, portal vein sampling, and arterially stimulated hepatic vein sampling.
- Thrombolysis to restore flow to occluded blood vessels by administration of recombinant tissue-plasminogen activator (tPA) (0.5 mg/kg/h for 6 h, or by direct clot infusion using a low-dose regimen).

Visualization of the celiac access and of the hepatic and splenic blood vessels is achieved by femoral artery catheterization and injection of radiographic contrast. This technique has two parts:

- The arterial phase, which provides information on the celiac axis, hepatic and splenic artery abnormalities, vascularization and anatomy of hepatic tumors, hepatic hemangiomas, or detection of hepatic artery thrombosis.
- The venous phase, which provides information about the patency of the portal, splenic, and superior mesenteric veins and the presence of portal hypertension by identification of mesenteric, esophageal, or gastric varices. In skilled hands, the investigation can be performed with little risk in infants.

Femoral artery spasm or thrombosis is an occasional side effect, but rarely requires operative treatment.

Hepatic artery embolization is indicated for the treatment of hepatic hemangiomas (see Chapter 10, Figure 10.7) or in the control of liver hemorrhage from trauma or needle biopsy. Angioplasty for portal or hepatic vein obstruction is also feasible using angiographic techniques.

Magnetic resonance imaging

Magnetic resonance imaging (MRI) has now replaced hepatic angiography as the best way to stage or diagnose hepatic tumors and identify their vascular supply. It may provide valuable information about liver or brain consistency and storage of heavy metals—for example, iron in hemochromatosis, copper in Wilson's disease, and cerebral edema in acute liver failure.[11,12] The recent development of MRI cholangiography, in which both intrahepatic and extrahepatic biliary duct abnormalities can be detected, has replaced ERCP as a diagnostic investigation[8] (see Chapter 8, Figure 8.5). ERCP or PTC will still be required for therapeutic procedures. Magnetic resonance spectroscopy is an emerging technique that may well be of value in the diagnosis of metabolic disorders, as intermediate metabolites such as lactate can be measured in the brain and other tissues.[13]

Splenoportography

This technique, in which the splenic and portal veins are visualized by the injection of radiological contrast into the spleen, has largely been replaced by hepatic angiography. It may be useful for measuring splenic pulse pressures in the evaluation of portal hypertension or if there is a post-transplant portal vein stenosis, but it carries a small risk of splenic rupture.

Transjugular intrahepatic portosystemic shunt

Life-threatening esophageal and gastric variceal bleeding occurs with portal hypertension secondary to liver disease. If the bleeding persists despite maximal medical and/or endoscopic therapy, a transjugular intrahepatic portosystemic shunt (TIPSS) can be carried out. TIPSS is an intrahepatic portosystemic shunt, created with radiographic assistance, between the high-pressure portal vein and the lower pressure hepatic vein. Since 1982, technological advances have made this technique possible in pediatric practice (see Chapter 15, Figure 15.8).

Central venous access and related venous occlusive disease

Intensive treatment regimens such as parenteral nutrition require long-term central venous access, particularly in patients undergoing small-bowel or combined liver and small-bowel transplantation. Interventional radiological techniques are useful in establishing percutaneous placement of tunneled central venous lines or Hickman lines, maintaining central venous access and managing the complications, such as thrombosis, in children of all ages.

Aspiration and drainage of fluid collections and abscesses

Imaging-guided (usually with ultrasound or occasionally CT) aspiration and drainage of fluid collections and abscesses in the peritoneal cavity, liver, spleen, pancreas, and retroperitoneum can be performed using percutaneous fine-needle aspiration in all age groups. Complicated fluid collections such as abscesses and pancreatic pseudocysts may require drainage over a period of time.

Histopathology

The diagnosis of most liver diseases requires histological confirmation, and liver biopsies are thus a routine procedure in specialist centers. An aspiration technique, using a Menghini needle (or disposable variant), has a complication risk of one in 1000 liver biopsies and may be performed under sedation with local anesthesia. In fibrotic or cirrhotic livers, a Tru-Cut needle, which removes a larger core, may be necessary. Transjugular liver biopsies, in which the liver is biopsied through a special catheter passed from the internal jugular vein into the hepatic veins, is now possible for children as small as 6 kg, and is the only safe way to perform a biopsy if coagulation times remain abnormal despite support (prothrombin time > 5 s prolonged over control value).[14] The complications of this potentially dangerous procedure (see below) are considerably reduced if it is performed by experts in specialized units under controlled conditions (Table 2.4).[15] It is essential to have information about liver size and consistency and the presence of cysts or dilated bile ducts from ultrasound, and if necessary to have a "spot" marked on the abdomen to ensure an accurate biopsy. Correct information about coagulation parameters is vital. Prothrombin time should be within 3 s of control values; the platelet count should be $> 80 \times 10^9$/L. The patient's blood group should be known, and it is prudent to cross-match a unit of blood prior to the procedure. Biopsy specimens should be obtained for routine histopathology, microbiology, electron microscopy, immunohistochemistry, and copper (if appropriate), and snap-frozen in liquid nitrogen for enzymatic or metabolic investigations. The interpretation of the histology may be difficult and requires considerable specialist expertise.

It is possible to carry out a liver biopsy as a day-case procedure in low-risk patients[16] if the following criteria apply:

- > 1 year old
- Bilirubin < 200 μmol/L*
- No other organ dysfunction
- No need for coagulation or platelet support
- Access to emergency facilities for 24 h after the procedure

Liver biopsy is contraindicated in the following circumstances:

- Abnormal coagulation parameters or thrombocytopenia (Table 2.4)
- Presence of grossly dilated bile ducts or large cysts
- Angiomatous malformation of the liver
- Extensive ascites

In these circumstances, image-guided or transjugular liver biopsies should be performed if the diagnosis will change the management.

* Bilirubin conversion factor: 1 mg/dL = 17 μmol/L

Table 2.4 Liver biopsy protocol.

• Establish blood group and save serum for cross-match
• Coagulation: prothrombin (PT, normal 12–15 s), partial thromboplastin (PTT, normal 33–37 s)
• Broad-spectrum antibiotics may be required if there are cardiac problems or concurrent dental extraction

Coagulation support	
PT: < 3 s prolonged	No action
> 3–6 s prolonged	15 mL/kg FFP over 2.5 h
> 6 s prolonged	Correct with FFP; recheck PT/PTT at 1 h Reassess risk–benefit if no correction
FBC and platelets	
Platelet count: > 80 x 10^9/L	No action
40–80 x 10^9/L	10 mL/kg platelet infusion over 1 h
< 40 μ/L	10 mL/kg platelet infusion, recheck Reassess risk–benefit if correction > 80 is impossible
Hemoglobin: < 8.0 g/L	Transfuse to Hb > 10 g/L prebiopsy
*Procedure and sedation**	
• Establish size of liver: +/– mark site after ultrasound	
• Apply local anesthetic cream to area of maximal dullness between 7th and 9th intercostal spaces (or ultrasound site)	
Oral midazolam	2.5 mg < 1 year old 5.0 mg > 1 year old
or	
Chloral hydrate 75 mg/kg	
Local anesthetic	Lignocaine 1–2%
Intravenous sedation	Pethidine 1–2 mg/kg Midazolam 0.1–0.75 mg/kg
Postbiopsy observations	
Blood pressure, pulse, respiration and temperature	
15 min for 2 h	
30 min for 2 h	
Hourly for 2 h	
4-hourly as required	
Chest radiograph/abdominal ultrasound may be required if bleeding is suspected. Laparotomy may be required	

*N.B., most units now carry out liver biopsies in children under a general anesthetic.

Complications of percutaneous liver biopsy

• The main complication is bleeding, and most deaths following a liver biopsy are due to intractable bleeding. However, subclinical bleeding (as evident on ultrasound imaging) is common, and intrahepatic and subcapsular hematomas with no hemodynamic compromise are seen in up to 23% of patients.[17,18] Significant nonfatal bleeding (as seen with evidence of active bleeding, shock, and a hemoglobin drop of 2.0 g/L) occurs more frequently in children than adults. In adults, significant hemorrhage occurs in 0.3–0.5% of cases, whilst bleeding requiring transfusion is seen in up to 2.8% of children.[15] Evidence of persistent bleeding following liver biopsy, despite medical support and blood transfusion, warrants urgent hepatic angiography and embolization or surgery.
• Pneumothorax or hemopneumothorax, which are treated in a standard way.
• Infection (particularly if the biopsy is combined with another procedure—e.g., dental extraction).
• Perforation of the gallbladder or bile ducts leading to biliary peritonitis and the need for emergency surgery.

Adequate monitoring of vital signs after biopsy is essential in order to detect complications such as hemorrhage or infection (Table 2.4).[19]

Metabolic investigations

Many inborn errors of metabolism present with hepatomegaly and/or liver disease. It is essential to screen for these diseases as part of the investigation of liver disease in neonates (Table 2.3) and in older children (Chapters 4, 5, and 13).

Bone-marrow aspiration

Bone-marrow aspiration should be performed in infants with undiagnosed neonatal hepatitis with both hepatomegaly and splenomegaly, in order to exclude Niemann–Pick type C or familial hemophagocytosis (Chapters 4 and 5), or at any age if a storage disorder is suspected.

Skin biopsy

This procedure should be performed if an inborn error of metabolism is being considered (e.g., Niemann–Pick type A, B, or C, or tyrosinemia type I) and the specimen should be stored frozen for future culture. It may also be necessary to obtain skin biopsies from parents or siblings.

Genetic tests (chromosome and DNA)

With the rapid development of molecular techniques for diagnosis and detection of genetic diseases, samples for DNA analysis and/or chromosomes from both child and parent are essential.

Endoscopy

Upper gastrointestinal endoscopy (gastroscopy) using a flexible fiberoptic endoscope is now the best way to diagnose peptic ulcer disease or esophageal and gastric varices secondary to portal hypertension. The technique is normally performed with the patient under sedation or general anesthetic. In children with hematemesis, gastroscopy not only provides rapid diagnosis, but also makes it possible to carry out therapy with variceal banding or endoscopic sclerotherapy for bleeding varices, or injection of bleeding ulcers with epinephrine or thrombin.

Capsule endoscopy

The clinical impact of wireless capsule endoscopy, which is a novel, noninvasive tool for the investigation of the small intestine, is being evaluated in children. In this technique, a wireless capsule is swallowed and images of the small intestine are obtained. It is of most value in the diagnosis of Crohn's disease, obscure or occult gastrointestinal bleeding, polyposis syndromes, and protein-losing enteropathy due to lymphangiectasia. In liver disease, it may be useful for diagnosing small-intestinal varices.[20]

Neurophysiology

Electroencephalography is mostly used in the assessment of hepatic encephalopathy. It will identify abnormal rhythms secondary to encephalopathy due to either acute or chronic liver failure or drug toxicity, such as post-transplant immunosuppression. It may also be of value for assessing brain death, as a flat electroencephalogram in the absence of sedation is an indication for withdrawal of therapy. CT or MRI scans of the brain (see above) may identify cerebral edema, infarction, or hemorrhage.

Ophthalmology

A number of inherited conditions have associated visual lesions—for example, Kayser–Fleischer rings in Wilson's disease, posterior embryotoxon or optic drusen in Alagille's syndrome, and cherry-red spot in Niemann–Pick type A. Ophthalmological examination may thus provide valuable diagnostic information and should be part of the assessment process. Children with Alagille's syndrome have a higher than normal incidence of benign intracranial hypertension, and annual fundoscopy for papilledema is therefore essential.[21]

Molecular biology

The development of molecular biology has revolutionized the methodology for many complex diagnostic procedures, transforming many techniques into routine laboratory procedures[22]—particularly in screening for rare neonatal diseases.[23]

Progress in identifying specific genes and DNA sequencing has made it possible to diagnose many inborn errors of metabolism and inherited disease (e.g., Alagille's syndrome, Wilson's disease, tyrosinemia type I) and has led to the identification of mitochondrial disorders.

Advances in methodology for gene cloning and molecular cloning have been helpful in identifying viruses such as hepatitis C and G, while the polymerase chain reaction has been used to diagnose active infection and monitor patients with many different viral diseases, such as hepatitis C, cytomegalovirus (CMV), and Epstein–Barr virus (EBV). Diagnosis for autoimmune disorders has improved, with specific assays that use recombinant protein antigens (e.g., antinuclear antigens and liver/kidney microsomal antibodies). The rapid development of molecular techniques is certain to lead to further improvements in diagnostic methods and to a better understanding of pediatric liver disease.

Emerging techniques

The FibroScan is a new noninvasive method for assessment of hepatic fibrosis. This device is based on one-dimensional transient elastography, a technique that uses both ultrasound (5 MHz) and low-frequency (50 Hz) elastic waves, whose propagation velocity is directly related to the elasticity. Liver elasticity measurements are reproducible and operator-independent and correlate well with the degree of fibrosis on histology. The method has been evaluated in adults with hepatitis C,[24] although not yet in children, but it has obvious advantages for the long-term follow-up of chronic disease.

References

1 Kelly DA, Green A. Investigation of paediatric liver disease. *J Inherit Metab Dis* 1991;**14**:531–7.
2 Kelly DA, Hull J. Investigation of prolonged neonatal jaundice. *Curr Paediatr* 1991;**1**:228–30.
3 McKiernan PJ. The infant with prolonged jaundice: investigation and management. *Curr Paediatr* 2001;**11**:83–9.
4 Spray CH, McKiernan P, Waldron KE, Shaw N, Kirk J, Kelly DA. Investigation and outcome of neonatal hepatitis in infants with hypopituitarism. *Acta Paediatr* 2000;**89**:951–4.
5 Saini S. Imaging of the hepatobiliary tract. *N Engl J Med* 1997;**336**:1889–94.
6 Lorenz JM, Van Ha T, Funaki B, *et al.* Percutaneous treatment of venous outflow obstruction in pediatric liver transplants. *J Vasc Interv Radiol* 2006;**17**:1753–61.
7 Halefoglu AM. Magnetic resonance cholangiopancreatography: a useful tool in the evaluation of pancreatic and biliary disorders. *World J Gastroenterol* 2007;**13**:2529–34.
8 Fernandez-Esparrach G, Gines A, Sanchez M, *et al.* Comparison of endoscopic ultrasonography and magnetic resonance cholangiopancreatography in diagnosis of pancreatobiliary diseases: a prospective study. *Am J Gastroenterol* 2007;**102**:1632–9.
9 Scheimann AO, Barrios JM, Al-Tawil YS, Gray KM, Gilger MA. Percutaneous liver biopsy in children: impact of ultrasonography and spring-loaded biopsy needles. *J Pediatr Gastroenterol Nutr* 2000;**31**:536–9.
10 Kuramochi A, Imazu H, Kakutani H, Uchiyama Y, Hino S, Urashima M. Color Doppler endoscopic ultrasonography in identifying groups at a high-risk of recurrence of esophageal varices after endoscopic treatment. *J Gastroenterol* 2007;**42**:219–24.
11 Wood JC. Magnetic resonance imaging measurement of iron overload. *Curr Opin Hematol* 2007;**14**:183–90.
12 Williams H, McKiernan P, Kelly D, Baumann U. Magnetic resonance imaging in neonatal hemochromatosis—are we there yet? *Liver Transpl* 2006;**12**:1725.
13 Cecil KM, Kos RS. Magnetic resonance spectroscopy and metabolic imaging in white matter diseases and pediatric disorders. *Top Magn Reson Imaging* 2006;**17**:275–93.
14 Furuya KN, Burrows PE, Phillips MJ, Roberts EA. Transjugular liver biopsy in children. *Hepatology* 1992;**15**:1036–42.

15 Cohen MB, A-Kader HH, Lambers D, Heubi JE. Complications of percutaneous liver biopsy in children. *Gastroenterology* 1992;**102**: 629–32.

16 Vivas S, Palacio MA, Rodriguez M, *et al.* Ambulatory liver biopsy: complications and evolution in 264 cases. *Rev Esp Enferm Dig* 1998;**90**:175–82.

17 McGill DB, Rakela J, Zinsmeister AR, Ott BJ. A 21-year experience with major hemorrhage after percutaneous liver biopsy. *Gastroenterology* 1990;**99**:1396–400.

18 Sugano S, Sumino Y, Hatori T, Mizugami H, Kawafune T, Abei T. Incidence of ultrasound-detected intrahepatic hematomas due to Tru-Cut needle liver biopsy. *Dig Dis Sci* 1991;**36**:1229–33.

19 Gonzalez-Vallina R, Alonso EM, Rand E, Black DD, Whitington PJ. Outpatient percutaneous liver biopsy in children. *J Pediatr Gastroenterol* 1993;**17**:370–5.

20 Anato B, Bishop J, Shawis R, Thomson M. Clinical application and diagnostic yield of wireless capsule endoscopy in children. *J Laparoendosc Adv Surg Tech A* 2007;**17**:364–70.

21 Narula P, Gifford J, Steggall MA, *et al.* Visual loss and idiopathic intracranial hypertension in children with Alagille's Syndrome. *J Pediatr Gastroenterol Nutr* 2006;**43**:348–52.

22 Worman HJ. Molecular biological methods in diagnosis and treatment of liver diseases. *Clin Chem* 1997;**43**:1476–86.

23 Dhondt JL. Neonatal screening: from the "Guthrie age" to the "genetic age." *J Inherit Metab Dis* 2007;**30**:418–22.

24 Sandrin L, Fourquet B, Hasquenoph JM, *et al.* Transient elastography: a new noninvasive method for assessment of hepatic fibrosis. *Ultrasound Med Biol* 2003;**29**:1705–13.

3 Liver Disease in Pregnancy

3 The Effects of Liver Disease on Mother and Child

Jane Hartley and Elwyn Elias

This chapter aims to cover:

- Hepatic conditions that are specifically related to pregnancy.
- Neonatal liver pathology secondary to maternal disease.
- Contraception and pregnancy in those with chronic liver disease and following liver transplantation.

There is an increasing trend for teenage pregnancy, one of the highest rates being in the United Kingdom, where in 2002 the incidence in 15–19-year-olds reached 30 per 1000 live births, in comparison with a rate of seven per 1000 live births in Sweden.[1] It is therefore important for pediatricians to consider the potential for conception in young women with chronic liver disease or those who have had a liver transplant, advise on contraception, and manage any ensuing pregnancy. Pediatricians should also be aware of hepatic complications specific to contraception and pregnancy, some of which require immediate action. Increased understanding of the pathophysiology of neonatal liver disease has led to a greater awareness of the influence of the mother on the neonatal liver, either via the fetal–placental unit or through inheritance.

Physiological changes to the liver and biliary system during normal pregnancy

Thirty-five percent of the cardiac output normally goes to the liver; however, due to the redirection of blood to the uterus during pregnancy, this drops to 28%, whilst the total blood volume increases, resulting in a relative decrease in the serum concentration of liver enzymes. Table 3.1 lists the liver-related changes seen in normal pregnancy.

Incidence of liver disease specific to pregnancy

Liver disease is a rare complication of pregnancy, but when it occurs, morbidity to both the mother and fetus can be severe and may prove fatal (Table 3.2).

Diseases of the Liver and Biliary System in Children, 3rd edition. Edited by Deirdre Kelly. © 2008 Blackwell Publishing, ISBN: 978-1-4051-6334-7.

Hepatic conditions specific to pregnancy

Hyperemesis gravidarum

In some pregnancies, the symptoms of nausea and vomiting in the first trimester are severe, leading to dehydration and malnutrition and requiring hospitalization. Raised transaminases (seldom exceeding 200 IU/dL)[2] occur in up to 50% of the hospitalized cohort. Both conjugated and unconjugated bilirubin may be mildly raised, as may alkaline phosphatase. Liver biopsy is not normally indicated and may be normal or have fatty changes.[3] Hypotheses to explain the transaminitis include a hepatic response to starvation,[4] which due to the associated increased fatty acid load may unmask a heterozygous defect of mitochondrial fatty acid oxidation in the mother.[5]

With hydration and nutritional therapy, the transaminases tend to settle without any further maternal pathology. The neonate may be small for gestational age, but no long-term detriment to the fetus has been reported.[6]

HELLP syndrome

This acronym was first coined in 1982 by Weinstein to describe patients with *h*emolysis, *e*levated *l*iver *e*nzymes and *l*ow *p*latelets.[7] It is associated with substantial maternal and perinatal morbidity and mortality. The diagnosis is made on clinical suspicion and supportive laboratory findings.

Pathogenesis

The exact cause of the condition is unknown. Hypotheses are:

- Placental ischemia, leading to the production of toxic factors damaging the endothelium.[8]
- A thrombotic tendency, with detection of anticardiolipin antibodies being the most common finding.[9]
- An immunological reaction that causes cytokine-mediated endothelial damage.[10]

Demographics

A pregnancy may be complicated by HELLP syndrome in a mother of any age or ethnicity. It affects primiparous or multiparous women, with an incidence of 0.11% of liveborn deliveries.[11] The majority (70%) are diagnosed in the third

Table 3.1 Physiological changes in liver investigations during normal pregnancy.

Clinical features	Liver and spleen are not palpable Palmar erythema and telangiectasia
Serum bilirubin	Normal or low
Serum albumin	Low
Prothrombin time	Normal
ALT, AST, and GGT	Normal
Alkaline phosphatase	Increases steadily throughout pregnancy, with a sharp rise in the last month. This reflects increased production by the placental syncytiotrophoblast and skeletal maturation of the fetus. It returns to normal within 2 weeks of delivery
Total bile acids	Normal or only mildly elevated
Urea	Low
Triglyceride and cholesterol	Increase throughout pregnancy
Gallbladder motility	Decreases Biliary lithogenicity increases
α-Fetoprotein	No changes
Liver biopsy	Normal histopathology Electron microscopy: proliferation of the smooth endoplasmic reticulum and giant mitochondria with increased paracrystalline inclusions, reflecting the increased protein and energy requirements

ALT, alanine aminotransferase; AST, aspartate aminotransferase; GGT, γ-glutamyltransferase.

Table 3.2 The incidence of liver disease specific to pregnancy and the trimesters in which each is most likely to occur.

Disease	Trimester	Incidence
Hyperemesis gravidarum	1 and 2	0.3–1.0%
Acute fatty liver of pregnancy	3	0.008%
HELLP syndrome	Late 2 and 3	0.1% (4–12% of those with preeclampsia)
Intrahepatic cholestasis of pregnancy	Mostly 3 and 2	0.1–20% (highest in Chile and Sweden and low in North America)

HELLP, hemolysis, elevated liver enzymes and low platelets.

trimester, while the remainder are identified during the first 72 h postpartum.

Maternal clinical features

- Malaise.
- Right upper quadrant pain or tenderness on palpation.
- Blood pressure is raised above the prepregnancy baseline (19% of mothers have preexisting chronic hypertension), but there may only be mildly raised nausea and vomiting.
- Features of hypertension, such as headache, edema, proteinuria, blurred vision, and hyperreflexia may be the presenting conditions in 10%.[12]
- Disseminated intravascular coagulation (DIC) and renal failure occur in severe disease (7%).
- Placental abruption (16%).
- Pulmonary edema (6%) is more common following abruption.
- Hepatic rupture presenting as profound shock occurs in 1% with HELLP syndrome.
- Postpartum bleeding may be severe in the setting of thrombocytopenia.

Laboratory findings

Hemolysis. The only constant diagnostic feature is decreased serum haptoglobins. Markers of microangiopathic hemolytic anemia (burr cells and schistocytes) and reticulocytosis with polychromasia, anisocytosis, and poikilocytosis are also frequently present.[13]

Liver transaminases. These are typically raised two to three standard deviations above the mean.[13–15]

Thrombocytopenia. A platelet count of < 100 000/μL is taken to define thrombocytopenia.[13,15,16] The platelet count continues to drop to a nadir at 24–48 h after delivery. Although the platelet count may respond to steroid therapy, other features (elevated liver enzymes, hemolysis, hypertension, and oliguria) are often not benefited.[17]

Histology of the liver

Liver biopsy is not necessary if there is no diagnostic uncertainty. Liver involvement is similar to the findings in preeclampsia. The main features are periportal neutrophilic infiltrates, hepatocyte necrosis, fibrin microthrombi in portal vessels, and fibrin deposition within the sinusoids (Figure 3.1). Fatty change in hepatocytes has also been described,[18] as in acute fatty liver of pregnancy, suggesting that the three entities may fall within the spectrum of the same disease.

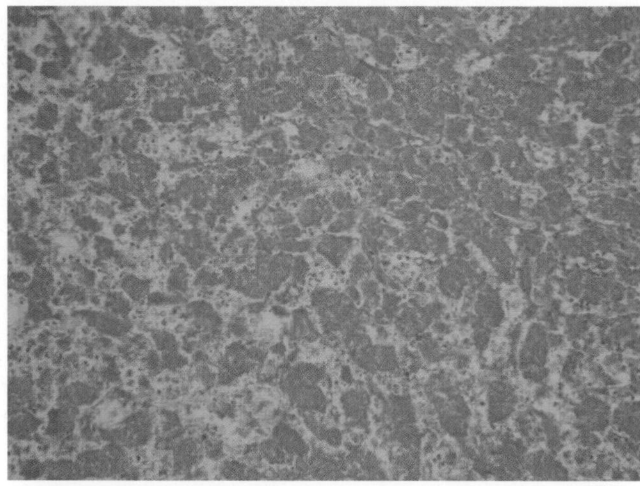

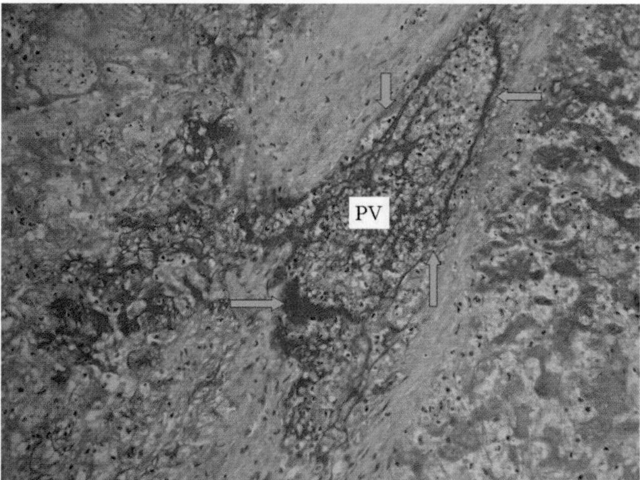

Figure 3.1 Liver histology from the resected infarcted liver in hemolysis, elevated liver enzymes and low platelets (HELLP) syndrome. **A** An area of coagulative ischemic-type necrosis and focal infiltration by neutrophils. (Hematoxylin–eosin, original magnification × 40). **B** Martius scarlet-blue stain, showing fibrin in the periportal sinusoids (stained red) and occluding a portal vein branch (PV).

Imaging

Ultrasonography and computed tomography (CT) are normal in HELLP syndrome unless it is complicated by hepatic rupture or infarction (Figure 3.2). Serial CT scans are the best method of monitoring the size and extent of the rupture. This will also aid planning of surgery if required.

Management of the mother

- The risk to the mother and the fetus increases with prolongation of the pregnancy, so that aggressive management and delivery are generally advisable. Vaginal delivery is possible, but a cesarean section is often necessary.[7,19] The majority of deliveries will be preterm via cesarean section (42–98%),[16,18] with an increased risk (7–14%) of wound hematoma and infection.[20,21] Complete normalization of laboratory indices has been reported in some women with continuation of pregnancy, but there is a higher risk of stillbirth.[20] In a study of 25 patients, it was found that steroids temporarily stabilized HELLP syndrome by increasing the platelet count, reducing liver enzymes, and increasing urine output.[22]
- Blood transfusions may be required. The indication for platelet support is controversial, as there is rapid platelet consumption, with no incremental rise. When Cesarean sections were studied, bleeding from the wound site was not seen to have diminished.[23]
- Hypertension should be controlled with standard medication.
- Renal support with continuous venovenous hemofiltration.
- In those who develop a liver hematoma, no intervention is required if the mother is hemodynamically stable. However, rupture is a major surgical emergency requiring evacuation and drainage of the blood, packing for tamponade, or suturing by experienced hepatobiliary surgeons.
- Hepatic infarction may lead to hepatic insufficiency, requiring management of acute liver failure.

Seventeen liver transplants for HELLP syndrome have been reported, the main indication being liver necrosis and liver failure following rupture. Two patients required total hepatectomy prior to transplantation, to control bleeding. Fourteen of the patients were alive at follow-up, suggesting that liver transplantation is appropriate in this setting.[24]

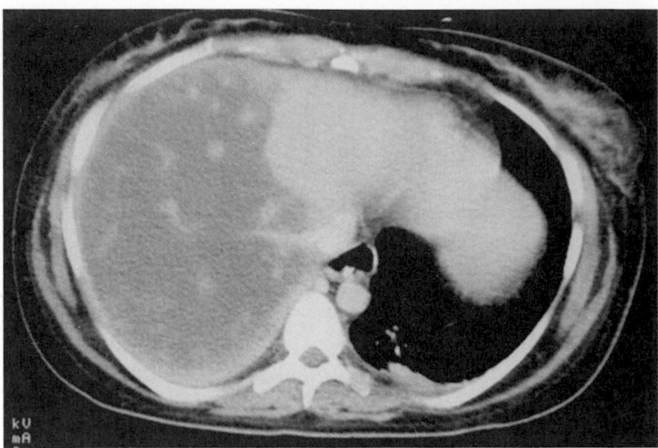

Figure 3.2 The liver in hemolysis, elevated liver enzymes and low platelets (HELLP) syndrome. Infarction of the liver is a rare complication of HELLP syndrome. This computed-tomographic image of the liver shows hemi-infarction of the right lobe. The main portal vein is patent, but the right portal vein branch has been occluded. Treatment is usually conservative.

Fetal presentation

- One-third will have intrauterine growth restriction.
- Placental abruption may lead to fetal death without expedient delivery.
- In those born alive, perinatal mortality has been reported as between 5–20%; it is related to the complications of preterm delivery,[25] and is comparable with those born preterm in the absence of maternal HELLP syndrome. The mean gestational age at delivery is 32 weeks, ranging from 24 to 39 weeks' gestation.[26]
- The neonate may have thrombocytopenia and leukopenia, but these findings are not specific to HELLP syndrome and may also be found in preeclampsia.[26]
- There is no increase in liver enzymes in neonates born to mothers with HELLP syndrome.[27]

Management of the neonate

As with preeclampsia, up to half of the babies born to mothers with HELLP syndrome will be small for gestational age. The long-term outcome for the infant depends on the extent of prematurity. The neonate should be managed initially on a neonatal intensive-care unit.

Risk in future pregnancies

There is a risk of recurrence in subsequent pregnancies of 3–19% for HELLP syndrome and a 23% risk for preeclampsia.[28,29]

Acute fatty liver of pregnancy

Acute fatty liver of pregnancy (AFLP) is a consequence of defective mitochondrial fatty acid β-oxidation in the infant, with a high potential for both maternal and fetal morbidity and mortality.

Mitochondrial β-oxidation

Mitochondrial long-chain fatty acid β-oxidation provides the major source of energy for cardiac and skeletal muscle and intermediary metabolism of ketone production by the liver in the fasting state. A trifunctional protein catalyses the final three steps in the formation of acetyl CoA from long-chain fats. Acetyl CoA then enters the tricarboxylic acid pathway, which results in energy generation by the liver. The three enzymatic steps for the trifunctional protein are:

1. 2,3-enoyl-CoA hydratase
2. Long-chain 3-hydroxyacyl-CoA dehydrogenase
3. Long-chain 3-keto-acyl-CoA thiolase

Two biochemical disease phenotypes have been described:

- Complete deficiency of all three enzymes of the trifunctional protein
- Isolated deficiency of long-chain 3-hydroxyacyl-CoA dehydrogenase (LCHAD deficiency)

Genetic analysis

A mutation resulting in a complete trifunctional protein of the fetus causes disease in the child only and has no effect on the mother.[30]

- Nineteen percent of infants born to women with AFLP have mutations leading to long-chain 3-hydroxyacyl-CoA dehydrogenase (LCHAD) deficiency in the fetus, which causes disease in the child and may result in AFLP in the mother.[31]
- A fetus carrying the G1528C mutation (amino acid residue E474Q; homozygous or compound heterozygote) results in disease in the child and AFLP in the mother in 79% of cases (whether the mutation was inherited from the mother or father).[30]
- A fetus with other hitherto detected mutations of long-chain 3-hydroxyacyl-CoA dehydrogenase does not cause AFLP in the mother.
- A heterozygous fetus (one wild type allele) does not cause AFLP in the mother.

Infants born to mothers with AFLP should always be screened for LCHAD deficiency.[32,33]

Not all cases of AFLP can be attributed to fetal LCHAD deficiency, and other causes of abnormal mitochondrial oxidation therefore need to be considered, including drugs (aspirin and tetracyclines have been reported as causing AFLP). A case report of carnitine palmitoyltransferase I (CPT I) deficiency identified two siblings with mild symptoms whose mother developed AFLP whilst carrying them.[34] AFLP has also been described as the presenting feature of maternal previously undiagnosed, medium-chain acyl-CoA dehydrogenase deficiency, with no effect on the fetus.[35]

Maternal presentation

AFLP usually affects women in the third trimester of pregnancy, although it has been reported exceptionally as early as 26 weeks' gestation.[36] It affects women of any ethnic group or age and can affect first or subsequent pregnancies.

The reported incidence has ranged from one in 13 000 pregnancies[37] to one in 6659,[38] and in a recent prospective study from Swansea, Wales, it reached one in 1000. In the latter study, six or more of the following features were accepted by Ch'ng *et al.* as being diagnostic of AFLP:[39]

- Vomiting
- Vague abdominal pain
- Polydipsia/polyuria
- Encephalopathy
- Elevated bilirubin (bilirubin rises in severe AFLP and in contrast to HELLP syndrome is not related to hemolysis)
- Hypoglycemia (profound)
- Elevated urate
- Leukocytosis (common)
- Ascites or bright liver on ultrasound scan
- Elevated transaminases—alanine aminotransferase (ALT) and aspartate aminotransferase (AST)—are moderately raised (rarely above 10 times normal)
- Elevated ammonia
- Renal impairment
- Coagulopathy (with DIC in 10%)
- Microvesicular steatosis on liver biopsy

Histology of the liver

Liver biopsy is not normally required in the acute situation, but if performed should be via the transjugular route. Biopsy within the week following parturition will allow confirmation of the diagnosis.

The liver is typically small, with microvesicular steatosis in a panacinar distribution or centrilobular with minimal inflammation (Figure 3.3). Other changes are intrahepatic cholestasis and extramedullary hemopoiesis, and when there is loss of hepatocytes, Kupffer cells aggregate.[40] Following delivery, the lipid rapidly mobilizes to become undetectable after a month, with normal hepatic architecture and no chronic changes.

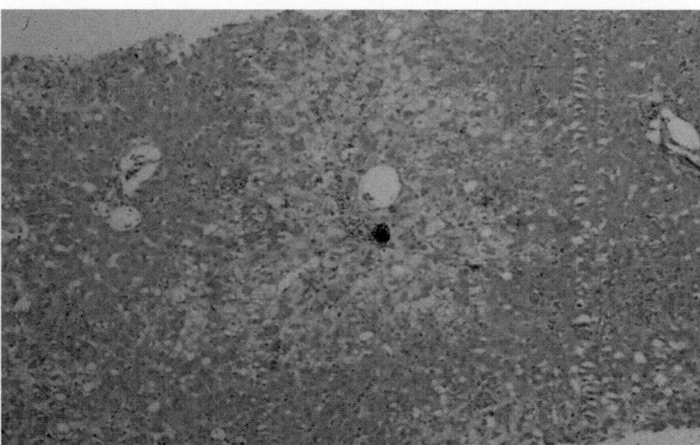

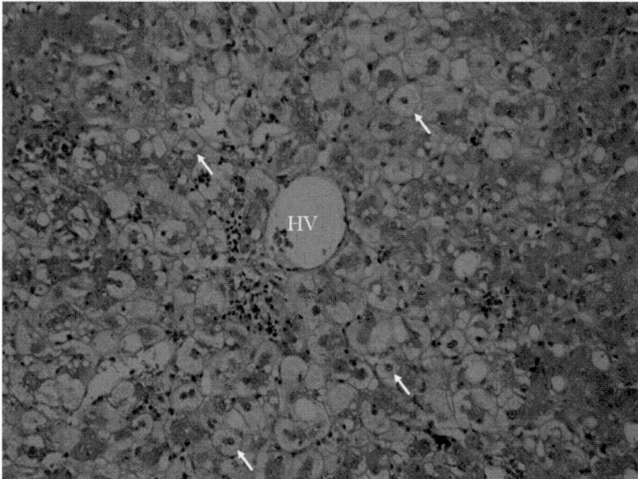

Figure 3.3 Acute fatty liver of pregnancy. **A** The typical distribution of fat accumulation in zones 2 and 3 surrounding the hepatic venule (HV), with relative sparing of zone 1 hepatocytes surrounding portal tracts (PT). **B** The microvesicular nature of the fatty droplets, which accumulate without displacing the nucleus from its central position (arrows). HV, hepatic venule.

Imaging

Ultrasonography. There is increased echogenicity, reflecting the increased fat in the liver.

CT scan. There is decreased attenuation of the liver in comparison with the spleen (usually the spleen is of lower attenuation than the liver).

Maternal management

Prompt diagnosis with expeditious delivery is recommended, as resolution of symptoms can only occur following delivery. Delivery may be vaginal, but in the face of acute liver failure requires emergency cesarean section. Meticulous management of liver failure and encephalopathy should lead to resolution of the symptoms with no long-term sequelae. Maternal death is related to the severity of liver disease, with raised intracranial pressure and gastrointestinal bleeding being reported as contributing to death in 12%.[41] In those who develop fulminant hepatic failure, successful liver transplantation has been performed.[42] Most mothers recover completely. Only rarely does recurrent AFLP affect subsequent pregnancies.[43]

Clinical features in the child

Fetal presentation. Late maternal diagnosis increases fetal mortality. There is an increased incidence of prematurity, asphyxia, intrauterine growth retardation, and intrauterine death, which may be related to uteroplacental insufficiency.[44]

Infancy. There is a genotype–phenotype correlation. Symptoms develop when there are periods of fasting or intercurrent illness.

Those with isolated LCHAD deficiency present with:

- Hepatic failure, which may lead to death
- Hepatomegaly

- Nonketotic hypoglycemia
- Encephalopathy
- Sudden death
- Hypocalcemia and cholestasis[45]

Those with complete trifunctional protein deficiency present with:

- Dilated cardiomyopathy
- Peripheral neuropathy and myopathy[46]
- Rhabdomyolysis
- Peripheral neuropathy and retinitis pigmentosa in long-term survivors

Laboratory investigations during the acute episode show:

- Hypoglycemia with low ketones
- Elevated transaminases
- Elevated prothrombin time
- Increased ammonia
- Increased urate and urea
- Elevated plasma acyl carnitines
- Urinary organic acids show an increase in 3-hydroxy dicarboxylic acids
- Secondary carnitine deficiency

Liver histology. There is usually microvesicular fat deposition in hepatocytes, although some macrovesicular deposition may be present.

Genetics. Mutation analysis of the trifunctional protein should be carried out.

Treatment of the child

All children born to mothers with AFLP should be treated as having LCHAD deficiency until the molecular investigations have been completed:

- Frequent feeding, which includes overnight nasogastric feeding to avoid prolonged fasting.
- Low-fat and high-carbohydrate diet to reduce the long chain fatty acid load.
- Medium-chain fats should replace most long-chain fats in the diet.
- Early intervention with intravenous fluids during intercurrent illness.
- Treatment of acute liver failure may be required.

Despite optimal treatment, sudden death can still occur and is most likely in the setting of an intercurrent illness, which may only be mild. Parents should be counseled as to the need for intravenous glucose even during mild infections.

Screening

All children born to mothers with AFLP should be screened for LCHAD deficiency by molecular analysis.

In mothers who's child is a compound heterozygote or homozygote for LCHAD deficiency, there is a 1 in 4 risk in future pregnancies. Chorionic villus sampling in subsequent at-risk pregnancies has been used to assess the risk of AFLP in pregnancy and LCHAD deficiency in the fetus[47] (see Chapters 5 and 13).

Intrahepatic cholestasis of pregnancy

Intrahepatic cholestasis of pregnancy (ICP) is characterized by pruritus, as the initial manifestation of cholestasis caused by pregnancy, and its complete resolution following delivery.

Diagnosis

- Pruritus is the main presenting symptom causing discomfort, insomnia and fatigue.
- Elevation of serum alanine aminotransferase (ALT/SGPT and serum bile acids > 10 μmol/L are the most sensitive laboratory indicators in confirming the diagnosis of cholestasis. Conventional liver function tests are initially normal, and it is in this circumstance that serum bile acid measurement may be needed to confirm the presence of cholestasis. Jaundice is uncommon, and γ-glutamyltransferase (GGT) remains normal in two-thirds of cases.[48]
- Spontaneous relief of signs and symptoms within 2–3 weeks after delivery.[49]

The resolution of symptoms and normalization of hepatic biochemistry after delivery help distinguish this from other liver conditions, such as primary biliary cirrhosis, that may first be unmasked in pregnancy. Interval liver function tests should be checked for confirmation that they have returned to normal.

Demographics

In Europe, ICP occurs in 0.1–1.5% of pregnancies.[50] The incidence is highest in Chile, the Baltic states, Scandinavia, and Bolivia, with up to 15% of pregnancies being associated with ICP.[51] Over the past decade, a trend toward lower incidence has been observed in Sweden and Chile, possibly due to increased micronutrients such as selenium in an improved diet.[52]

ICP is not influenced by parity, but is five times more common in multiple pregnancies. It may be sporadic or run in families.[53] There is seasonal variability, with more cases occurring in winter.

Pathogenesis

Estrogens and progestagens are naturally cholestatic. It is likely that in most instances, ICP occurs in individuals who have otherwise subclinical mutations within susceptibility genes for intrahepatic cholestasis, whose capacity for efficient biliary excretion is exceeded in the hormonal milieu of pregnancy.

Genetics

The increased incidence in certain populations, family clusterings, and recurrence in subsequent pregnancies supports a genetic etiology. This led to the investigation of genes involved in other cholestatic disorders, progressive familial intrahepatic cholestasis (PFIC) and benign recurrent intrahepatic cholestasis (BRIC).

• Familial intrahepatic cholestasis 1 (FIC-1) is caused by mutations in the *ATP8B1* gene. The gene encodes a P-type ATPase involved in bile salt transport across the canalicular membrane. In PFIC1 and BRIC1, γ-glutamyltransferase (GGT) is normal or low. Mullenbach *et al.* described two *ATP8B1* mutations (D70N and R867C) in four women with ICP and normal GGT. The development of ICP may be due to coinheritance of a second gene affecting cholestasis, or external influences such as changes in hormones.[54]

• Bile salt export pump (BSEP) deficiency is caused by mutations in the *ABCB11* gene leading to PFIC2 and BRIC2, also with low or normal GGT. Sequence variants (single-nucleotide polymorphisms) are more common in those with ICP than in the general population, suggesting increased susceptibility.[55]

• The multidrug resistance 3 *(MDR3)* or *ABCB4* gene encodes the hepatobiliary phospholipid transporter, mutations in which cause PFIC3, which differs from PFIC1 and 2 by having a raised GGT. In women with ICP and raised GGT, sequence variants have been identified in a small number of cases, including a frameshift deletion.[56] When women with ICP were screened for sequence-variant polymorphisms in the *ABCB4* gene in comparison with the normal population, there was a significant increase in specific variants in those with severe disease.[57] Mutations of the *ABCB4* gene leading to exon-splicing abnormalities may not be associated with raised GGT and should be considered in women with ICP and normal GGT.[58]

• The bile acid farnesoid X receptor (FXR) regulates bile acid homeostasis so as to reduce hepatocyte toxicity. It binds to DNA response elements in promoter regions of target genes, including *ABCB11* and *ABCB4*, to activate their transcription, thereby increasing bile acid secretion out of the hepatocyte. FXR also promotes genes for sulfonation and glucuronidation, reduces import and synthesis of bile salts in the hepatocyte, and also reduces ileal bile salt reabsorption. Functional variants in the gene are associated with a predisposition to ICP.[59]

Hormonal

A hormonal role in the etiology of ICP is suggested by the observation that symptoms are most prevalent in the third trimester, when estrogen levels are highest. When the hormone levels fall after delivery, symptoms tend to improve rapidly. Twin and triplet pregnancies, which have higher estrogen levels, have an increased incidence of ICP. Biliary excretion of estradiol-17β-D-glucuronide occurs via a canalicular multispecific conjugate export pump (multidrug resistance–related protein, MRP2) and exerts its cholestatic effect via a *trans*-inhibition of BSEP[60] from the canalicular side of the hepatocyte membrane. This causes a transient inhibition of BSEP.[61] Estradiol-17β-D-glucuronide also suppresses the expression of MRP2.[62]

There is a significant alteration in the ratio of different progesterone isomers in ICP in comparison with other causes of liver disease in pregnancy, the cause and effect of which are not known.[63]

Clinical presentation

ICP usally presents in the second or third trimester, but may occasonally occur as early as the first.

• Pruritus—often worst on the palms and soles—is characteristic and it may be intense, leading to discomfort and fatigue.

• Steatorrhea and fat-soluble vitamin malabsorption are observed.

• Excoriation is seen on clinical examination.

• There are no signs of chronic liver disease, and the liver is of normal size and not tender.

• Jaundice develops in 10%.

Histology

Liver biopsy is rarely undertaken unless there is diagnostic uncertainty.

Intracellular bile pigment and canalicular bile plugs are seen in the absence of any other histological abnormalities. Electron microscopy shows dilated canaliculi with loss of microvilli.

Maternal management

Management consists of:

• Relief of pruritus.

• A double-blind randomized controlled trial of ursodeoxycholic acid, dexamethasone, or placebo including 130 women with ICP showed a significant biochemical improvement in the ursodeoxycholic acid group and symptomatic improvement in those with initially high levels of bile salts (> 40 μmol/L). There were no changes in the fetal complication rate.[64] The meconium of neonates born to mothers with ICP has an increased concentration of bile acids in comparison with normal. In mothers with ICP who are treated with ursodeoxycholic acid, the neonatal meconium continued to have high levels of bile acids. This may explain the lack of a fetal response to ursodeoxycholic acid despite a good biochemical response in the mother. It may also suggest that subsequent changes in serum bile acid concentrations has little effect on those already accumulated in the meconium.[65] Cholestyramine is less effective in controlling the maternal symptoms, and no additional benefit to the fetus compared with ursodeoxycholic acid was observed.[66]

• Smaller controlled trials have suggested a benefit from treatment with *S*-adenosylmethionine and ursodeoxycholic acid, alone or in combination.[67,68]

• Dexamethasone and cholestyramine are not recommended. Rifampicin may be highly effective, but has not been subjected to a controlled trial.

- Fat-soluble vitamin supplementation should be given to those with cholestasis, alongside nutritional support. Postpartum bleeding has been reported in this group, which may be secondary to vitamin K deficiency.[69]
- Delivery of fetus. Due to the effect on the fetus, it is suggested that delivery should be induced at 38 weeks in those mildly affected and at 36 weeks in severe cases.[70] Prospective studies from Scandinavia have reported that the risk of fetal complications was largely confined to mothers with serum bile salt levels greater than 40 μmol/L.[71]

Effect on the child

Risks to the child include:

- Increased risk of preterm delivery (19–60%).[70]
- Fetal distress (22–41%), as indicated by meconium liquor and asphyxia.
- Fetal loss (0.4–1.6%).[70]
- A neonate with reduced BSEP expression, either due to the homozygous inheritance of SNP variants or known PFIC2 mutations, may present in the newborn period with liver disease (including liver failure). A history of maternal cholestasis should therefore lead to the consideration of BSEP deficiency in the differential diagnosis of liver disease of the neonate.

The pathogenesis of fetal complications is not fully understood. In stillborns, the postmortem findings are those of acute asphyxia.[71] The fetus is usually well grown, and surveillance of the fetoplacental unit is normal, suggesting that placental insufficiency is not the cause. Methods used to monitor the fetus, such as umbilical artery Doppler ultrasound, are poor predictors of fetal outcome.[72] Neonatal resuscitation facilities and intensive care should be available at delivery. In those neonates who are born healthy, there are no long-term complications.

Long-term maternal complications

ICP resolves within a few weeks of delivery, with no long-lasting effects. A retrospective study from Finland of 10 504 women with ICP found an increased rate of hepatitis C infection, gallstones, and nonalcoholic pancreatitis. On follow-up, 17 were found to have cirrhosis. It is unclear whether pregnancy enhances the symptoms of a previously undiagnosed chronic disorder leading to cirrhosis, or whether, in a very small minority, ICP may precipitate a chronic condition leading to fibrosis and cirrhosis.[73] Women who have experienced ICP have an increased risk of developing pruritus and jaundice whilst taking the combined oral contraceptive pill, due to the estrogen component. For contraception, women should be advised to use the progesterone-only pill.[74] Pregnancy has a natural tendency to increase the lithogenicity of bile, and the incidence of gallstones is increased. In a prospective study, biliary sludge was detected on ultrasound in 10.2% of women in the third trimester of pregnancy.[75]

Neonatal liver pathology secondary to maternal disease

Neonatal hemochromatosis

This severe disease causes liver failure with intrahepatic and extrahepatic siderosis in the newborn. The exact molecular pathogenesis is unknown. An alloimmune etiology has been suggested, due to the inheritance pattern and the high recurrence rate (up to 80%) in subsequent pregnancies.[76] The mother is well throughout the pregnancy. Normal neonates have been reported in between affected siblings[77] (see Chapter 5). Maternal factors that have also been associated are systemic lupus and anti-Ro anti-La antibodies.

The diagnosis is suspected in a neonate with liver failure that may have progressed to cirrhosis (confirming that the pathology was initiated *in utero*). The diagnosis is made by demonstrating siderosis in the liver and extrahepatic sites. Intracellular iron deposits are identified on biopsies of minor salivary glands. A liver biopsy demonstrates intracellular iron which spares the Kupffer cells.[78] Abdominal magnetic resonance imaging demonstrates loss of signal on T2-weighted images of the liver, indicating iron accumulation, whilst the spleen is normal (the reticuloendothelial system is spared). The signal intensity of the pancreas has been reported as variable.[78,79]

Untreated, the disease is fatal in up to 60% of neonates. If commenced early, an antioxidant cocktail (selenium, desferrioxamine, *N*-acetylcysteine, and prostaglandin E_1) improves outcome in those with mild features. Those with severe liver failure require liver transplantation for survival.[80]

Those who survive the neonatal period, either with antioxidants or liver transplantation, do not have long-term complications.

Postulation of an alloimmune etiology has led to the use of weekly intravenous infusions of immunoglobulin in the mother from the 18th week of subsequent pregnancies. This has been reported to modify the disease process, with either mild or no signs of neonatal hemochromatosis in the newborn.[81]

Viral hepatitis in pregnancy

Hepatitis A

Acute hepatitis A has no increased risk to the mother. Neonates born to mothers with acute hepatitis A in the month prior to delivery may acquire self-limiting infection.[82] Meconium peritonitis of the fetus has been reported following maternal infection, leading to ileal perforation and requiring resection in the newborn period.[83]

Hepatitis B

Hepatitis B vertical transmission occurs at the time of delivery on exposure to blood and rarely *in utero*.[84] The transmission rate is dependent on the mother's infectivity at the time of delivery. Mothers who are HbeAg-positive have a 70–90% risk of infecting their infants unless the infants are vaccinated. Mothers who develop acute hepatitis B in the last trimester have a 70% chance of infecting their infant and need similar prophylaxis (see Chapter 6). In mothers who are HBeAg-negative with low viral load, the transmission rate is lower, but vaccination is still recommended.[85] Without successful vaccination, the majority of infected infants become "healthy carriers," but a minority—born to mothers who despite being HBeAg-negative have high hepatitis B virus DNA titers due to the precore mutant form of the virus—have a high risk of fulminant hepatic failure from 6 weeks to 6 months of age.[86] Vaccination and hepatitis B immunoglobulins given to the neonate provide protection against perinatal transmission in over 95% of cases[87] (see Chapters 6 and 23).

Acute hepatitis in pregnancy may lead to preterm labor.[88] There is no increased maternal morbidity or mortality from hepatitis B with pregnancy.

Hepatitis C

There is a 5% transmission rate, with transmission occurring either *in utero* or during delivery.[89] Infectivity is related to the viral load.[90] Cesarean section does not reduce transmission rates.[91] Viral genotype does not alter infectivity,[92] but coinfection with human immunodeficiency virus may increase transmission.[93] Hepatitis C does not cause acute liver failure in infancy, but is likely to progress to a chronic hepatitis C virus infection, with the risk of fibrosis, cirrhosis, and hepatocellular carcinoma in adulthood.

Immunoprophylaxis for the newborn is not available. Pregnancy does not increase morbidity in the mother (see Chapter 6).

Hepatitis E

Hepatitis E is a self-limiting viral infection spread by the fecal–oral route, occurring sporadically or as epidemics in developing countries.[94] In pregnant women, hepatitis E has a high mortality rate, which increases throughout pregnancy up to 28% in the third trimester.[95] The fetal outcome is poor, with one series reporting a 70% mortality rate due to stillbirth and maternal death.[96]

Herpes simplex virus

Both herpes simplex virus-1 (HSV-1) and -2 can cause severe disease in the neonate, either through direct shedding at the time of delivery or in primary transplacental infection, leading to miscarriage, stillbirth, and congenital malformations.[97]

Primary herpes infection may be more severe in pregnant women, with dissemination leading to hepatitis, encephalitis, thrombocytopenia, coagulopathy, and a mortality rate of up to 50%.[98]

Genital herpes has the highest risk to the neonate at the time of delivery, due to direct viral shedding.

In the neonate, it may present as:

- Localized infection of the skin, eyes and mucous membranes
- Infection of the central nervous system, which has a 5% mortality rate, with 50% of survivors having neurological impairment
- Disseminated infection, presenting with acute liver failure, with a high mortality rate unresponsive to antiviral therapy in the setting of multiorgan failure

Neonatal herpes prevention

Active genital herpes should be treated with acyclovir or valacyclovir in the weeks prior to delivery.[99,100] Women with active genital infection at the time of delivery should be offered a cesarean section, as the likelihood of neonatal transmission is high.[101]

A high index of suspicion is needed in a septic neonate to commence acyclovir treatment early before the onset of multiorgan failure. Liver transplantation has been successful in herpes simplex infection isolated to the liver.[102]

Contraception and pregnancy

Contraception

Hepatic complications of combined oral contraceptives

The combined oral contraceptive pill (COCP) has an efficacy of 99.9%. It reduces menstrual irregularities and premenstrual tension, as well as reducing the risk of fibroids, benign breast disease, and ovarian and endometrial cancer.

No preexisting liver disease

Cholestasis. This occurs in 10 per 100 000 in the West, and as with ICP (see above), it has a higher incidence in Chile and Scandinavia (25 per 100 000). It is more common in those who have had ICP, or in whom there is a family history of jaundice in pregnancy or whilst taking the COCP. It tends to occur within 3 months of commencing an estrogen-containing COCP.

Hepatic adenomas. There is an increased risk of adenoma formation, which is associated with the length of use of the COCP and the strength of the estrogen component. With the introduction of COCPs containing lower estrogen levels, the incidence of adenoma has fallen. Adenomas may regress when the COCP is stopped but return again following reintroduction of the COCP or during pregnancy. Hepatic adenoma constitutes a contraindication to pregnancy, and in patients suitable for resection should be removed before conception occurs. Adenomas caused by estrogens are vascular and may rupture, with hemorrhage into the adenoma or peritoneal cavity.

Focal nodular hyperplasia (FNH). 50–75% of those with FNH use the COCP, suggesting that estrogen may be a contributing factor. FNH does not increase any risks during pregnancy.

Hepatocellular carcinoma (HCC). There is an increased risk of HCC with long-term use of COCPs containing high levels of estrogen.[103] Cofactors such as hepatitis B and alcohol may increase the risk. Tumors may regress following cessation of the COCP.

Budd–Chiari syndrome. The procoagulant effect of the COCP increases the risk of Budd–Chiari syndrome 2.5-fold.[104] Nine percent of cases of Budd–Chiari are attributed to COCP use.[105] In a case series of 13 women taking the COCP who developed hepatic vein thrombosis, 10 had an underlying prothrombotic condition, suggesting that the development of Budd–Chiari syndrome should prompt investigation for other thrombophilic disorders.[106]

Women with established liver disease

Fertility may be reduced in advanced chronic liver disease, but contraception is an important issue for the majority.

Gallstones. There is an alteration in the composition of bile in those taking the COCP, with an increase in cholic acid and a decrease in chenodeoxycholic acid, which may increase the risk of cholelithiasis.[107] There is no consensus from studies as to whether this is the case, but due to the potential risk it is advised that those with a history of biliary colic should avoid the COCP.[108]

Hepatocellular carcinoma. The cirrhotic liver is at risk of developing hepatocellular carcinoma. Some studies have reported an increased incidence of hepatocellular carcinoma in chronic liver disease in those using the COCP, but this has not been verified in subsequent studies.[109–111] Due to this uncertainty, it is recommended that COCPs should be avoided in chronic liver disease.

After transplantation. Following liver transplantation, COCPs have been used safely if there have been no thrombotic complications in the peritransplantation period. An increase in cyclosporine levels has been reported in concomitant use of the COCP, and levels should therefore be monitored closely.[112]

Other forms of contraception in liver disease

Progesterone-only oral and depot contraception is the preferred contraceptive in all forms of liver disease, as it avoids the estrogen component of the combined contraceptive. The pill has to be taken within the same 3 h every day to ensure efficacy. There are no hepatic complications. The progesterone-only pill is safe following liver transplantation and is recommended when there have been thrombotic complications after transplantation.

Intrauterine device. The intrauterine device (IUD) is 99% effective for 1–5 years. It can be used in all forms of liver disease except for Wilson's disease, in which the copper coil component of the IUD may potentially increase serum copper levels.[113] In the post-transplant patient, there have been reported cases of IUD failure due to immunosuppressants reducing the immunological mechanism of the IUD.[114] There is also a potentially increased risk of urinary tract infections.[115]

Barrier contraception. In the context of hepatitis B and C infection, this form of contraception should be advised in order to avoid sexual transmission of the infections. The efficacy is 80–95%. There are no contraindications to the use of this form of contraception.[116]

Pregnancy

Chronic liver disease

Evaluation before conception. Due to reduced fertility in advanced liver disease, pregnancy in the presence of cirrhosis and portal hypertension is rare. With advances in medical care, young people are surviving into adulthood with reproductive potential, with compensated cirrhosis. In general, the more advanced the liver disease, the higher the risk of complications to mother and child.[117]

Pregnancy is not contraindicated in liver disease, but should be planned for a time when the disease is in a steady state. If the disease is advanced, liver transplantation should be considered first.

Neonatal immunization and immunoglobulin to prevent transmission of hepatitis B should be discussed with mothers who are carriers. Although there is no vaccination to prevent the transmission of hepatitis C, mothers will want to know about transmission rates and management for their infants (see Chapter 6).

Drug therapy should be assessed for possible teratogens—e.g., in animal studies, spironolactone has caused genital abnormalities in males. It is essential that therapy with penicillamine for Wilson's disease and prednisolone and azathioprine for autoimmune hepatitis should be maintained.

Cirrhosis and portal hypertension. Although studies have not shown that pregnancy increases the risk of variceal bleeding, it is advisable that esophageal varices should be eradicated in advance of any pregnancy, as bleeding during pregnancy is associated with fetal loss.[118–120] The acute management is the same as in nonpregnant variceal bleeding, with hemodynamic stabilization, endoscopic banding, or sclerotherapy and octreotide. Vasopressin should be avoided if possible, as it causes decreased placental perfusion and potentiates placental abruption. It has also been associated with fetal digit necrosis and amputation.[121]

Pregnancy

In the presence of decompensated liver disease with ascites, encephalopathy, or liver failure, termination of pregnancy should be considered, because of the difficulties in bringing a normal infant to term.[122] Twenty-four percent of women with cirrhosis will decompensate during pregnancy,[123] requiring intensive care and possibly transplantation. Coagulopathy may lead to massive hemorrhage at delivery.[124] Splenic artery aneurysm rupture may occur in the third trimester,[125] with high maternal and fetal mortality rates (70% and 80%, respectively).

Labor and delivery

Delivery should be precipitated if there is life-threatening deterioration in the mother; otherwise, the pregnancy should go to term. Cesarean section should be avoided in women with cirrhosis unless absolutely necessary, due to the presence of intra-abdominal collaterals, leading to an increased risk of bleeding and infection.[126] Coagulation, fibrinogen, and platelet count should be assessed and blood product support should be available as required.

Epidural anesthesia may avoid the Valsalva maneuver, which may increase variceal pressure. However, if the platelet count is reduced, it may not be possible to provide this.

Postpartum

Thrombocytopenia and reduced synthetic clotting factors increase the risk of postpartum hemorrhage.[126]

Fetal complications

Prematurity is increased in the setting of cirrhosis and requires the delivery to be in a setting in which neonatal intensive-care facilities are available. Beta-blockers may cause growth restriction, and this should be monitored throughout the pregnancy. Fetal growth may also be reduced following a gastrointestinal bleed.

Pregnancy issues related to specific chronic liver diseases

Autoimmune hepatitis in pregnancy

Pregnancy tends to induce immune tolerance in autoimmune hepatitis (AIH), with improving liver function on baseline dosages of immunosuppression. Postpartum deterioration is common and should be anticipated.[127] With cirrhosis, decompensation requiring transplantation may complicate pregnancy.[128]

- *Steroids.* No teratogenic effects on the fetus have been reported in humans. In animal studies, high doses have led to cleft lip and palate, premature rupture of membranes, and adrenal insufficiency.[129]
- *Azathioprine.* In high doses, transient abnormalities in the neonate have been reported, including thymic atrophy, leukopenia, anemia, thrombocytopenia, reduced immunoglobulins, and transient chromosomal aberrations. No structural teratogenic effects have been reported. At dosages used for maintenance treatment in the mother, no adverse effects have been reported in the neonate
- *Tacrolimus.* Transient hyperkalemia has been reported in the neonate, but no specific teratogenicity.
- *Cyclosporine.* No specific teratogenicity.
- *Mycophenolate mofetil* (MMF). There are concerns regarding the safety of MMF in the developing fetus, with an increased risk of spontaneous abortion and serious malformations. MMF should be avoided in pregnancy.[130]

Wilson's disease

Pregnancy is not contraindicated in Wilson's disease. Fertility may be reduced in poorly controlled disease, with amenorrhea and frequent miscarriages.

Penicillamine as a chelating agent is well tolerated at conventional doses by both mother and child, with no increased incidence of fetal malformation.[131] Unnecessarily high doses may lead to cutis laxa.

Zinc has also been used safely during pregnancy, with no teratogenic effect on the developing fetus.[132]

Pregnancy following liver transplantation

Before conception

The menstrual irregularities that occur in chronic liver disease are reversed by liver transplantation, and fertility may return within 3 weeks of transplantation.[133] It is generally advisable that pregnancy should be avoided within the first year after transplantation, and contraception should therefore be carefully addressed in those of child-bearing age[134] (see above and Chapter 25).

Immunosuppressants in pregnancy

The largest experience of the use of immunosuppressive agents in pregnancy is with azathioprine and steroids. Information on the newer immunosuppressives in pregnancy is mainly from animal studies, as there are few data in humans (Table 3.3).

Pregnancy

Liver and renal function, cytomegalovirus (CMV) status and hemoglobin should be closely monitored.

Pregnancy should not alter graft function, so rejection and infection should be considered if liver function tests become abnormal (see Table 3.1 for the normal changes seen in liver function during pregnancy). Liver biopsy has no increased risk in comparison with the nonpregnant woman, and adjustments to immunosuppressives in the face of acute rejection should be the same as in the nonpregnant. There is an increased risk of hypertension, with the risk being greater in those receiving cyclosporine[135] and those with hypertension prior to conception.[136,137]

Preeclampsia, premature rupture of membranes, anemia, infection, and first-trimester abortion are all increased in pregnancies following transplantation.[138]

Table 3.3 Immunosuppressant use in pregnancy and breastfeeding.

Drug	Side effects in pregnancy	Effects on fetus	Breastfeeding recommendations
Steroids	Poor wound healing, hypertension, weight gain, gastric ulceration, osteoporosis and glucose intolerance	In animal studies, growth retardation and premature rupture of membranes. At high doses, may cause cleft palate in animal studies	Less than 10% enters breast milk, so considered safe at maintenance corticosteroid doses
Tacrolimus (FK506)	Nephrotoxicity, neurotoxicity, glucose intolerance, hyperkalemia, diarrhea	Transient hyperkalemia	50% enters breast milk. Manufacturers recommend avoiding breast feeding
Cyclosporine	Hypertension, nephrotoxicity, neurotoxicity, hyperkalemia, tremor, hirsutism, hypomagnesemia, glucose intolerance	Growth retardation Transient hyperkalemia	Secreted into breast milk, therefore not recommended
Mycophenolate mofetil	None known	Not recommended in pregnancy. Animal studies have shown malformations, intrauterine growth retardation and intrauterine death. Limited human experience also suggests teratogenicity[130]	No information available regarding secretion into breast milk, but the manufacturer recommends avoiding breast feeding
Azathioprine	Increased infections, alopecia, stomatitis, hepatotoxicity, fever, nausea and vomiting, pancreatitis, leukopenia, thrombocytopenia, and macrocytic anemia	At high doses, growth retardation, preterm delivery, bone-marrow suppression if this has occurred in the mother, and transient chromosomal abnormalities have been reported	Undetectable in breast milk, but potentially could be secreted, therefore avoid breast feeding
Sirolimus	None known	Delayed fetal ossification, but no teratogenic effects	No data available
Basiliximab	None known	In animal studies, there were no teratogenic effects. No human data are available	
Daclizumab, muromonab-CD3 (OKT3), and Thymoglobulin	No data available	No data available	No data available

Delivery

Normal vaginal delivery can occur. The risk of requiring a cesarean section is related to prolonged rupture of membranes or preeclampsia.

Effects on the fetus

Congenital malformations have not been reported. Fetal growth should be monitored by serial ultrasound scans, as there is an increased risk of intrauterine growth retardation from preeclampsia. Congenital CMV infection is the lead cause for neonatal death, and in one series all neonatal deaths in transplanted mothers were due to acute CMV infection.[139] The risk of maternal and therefore fetal CMV infection is greatest with high-dose immunosuppression—e.g., in the early post-transplantation period, when pregnancy should be avoided.[140]

Case study

A 28-year-old primigravida presented at 31 weeks of pregnancy when she developed raised blood pressure, edema, and proteinuria, which settled with bed rest. She and her husband were fit and healthy, with no significant medical history. She then remained well until 35 weeks, when she developed increased blood pressure (160/95). She had proteinuria and an increase in serum uric acid, but the full blood count and liver function tests remained normal. Two days, later she became tachycardic, edematous, and oliguric, and her blood results were as follows: hemoglobin 4.3 g/dL (reference range 11.5–16.6), platelets 18×10^9/L (reference range 150–450), AST 75 U/L (reference range 5–43). The fetus was also tachycardic, and she therefore underwent an emergency cesarean section under general anesthesia, delivering a well baby who did not require any resuscitation and remained well.

The mother was transferred to intensive care, complaining of right upper quadrant tenderness, and in the following 24 hours she developed acute liver failure (hypoglycemia, encephalopathy, acidosis, prothrombin time 27 seconds, albumin 29 g/L (reference range 34–51), bilirubin 371 μmol/L (reference range 1–22), alkaline phosphatase 1489 U/L (reference range 70–260), AST 4600 U/L and D dimers 2500 (reference range < 250). She required ventilatory support, inotropic support, (norepinephrine) and renal support (continuous venovenous filtration). The liver failure was treated with blood products, broad-spectrum antibiotics, antifungals, and *N*-acetylcysteine.

On day 6 postpartum, she developed low-grade pyrexia and an increasing white cell count. An ultrasound of the liver revealed changes in the right lobe, which on CT were identified as liver ischemia or infarction, with a possible thrombosis of the right portal vein (Figure 3.2). This was treated conservatively. During the next 48 h, she developed symptoms of systemic sepsis with pyrexia, rigors, tachycardia, an increased neutrophil count at 16.2×10^9/L (reference range 2.0–7.5) and increased inotropic requirements. No organisms were identified.

To control the systemic inflammatory response, she underwent a right hemihepatectomy. On microscopic examination, the resected right lobe showed vascular occlusion and infarction, which was in keeping with HELLP syndrome but more extensive than usually occurs in this condition (Figure 3.1).

A search for additional causes of portal vein thrombosis revealed a slightly low protein S level at 61 μ/dL (reference range 68–146) and heterozygosity for factor V Leiden.

During the initial postoperative period, her blood pressure was labile. Ventilatory and inotropic support was weaned over the following 48 h. She started to pass urine, and renal dialysis was reduced and then stopped 13 days post hemihepatectomy.

She had striking cholestasis from the onset of the HELLP syndrome, which peaked on day 12 postpartum, with serum bilirubin at 970 μmol/L. This slowly resolved to 505 μmol/L at discharge, and at 5 months postpartum was in the normal range. She has subsequently remained well, with no long-term liver complications.

Although she was concerned regarding bonding with her baby after such a long period on intensive care of time, this was not a problem when she was discharged home.

Comment. This case typifies a severe case of HELLP syndrome. It presented in the third trimester with right upper quadrant pain and features of preeclampsia. The patient developed renal failure, pulmonary edema, and disseminated intravascular coagulation. Liver failure developed following hepatic infarction, which was initially managed conservatively until it was clear that the ongoing systemic inflammatory response was not improving, requiring her to undergo a right hemihepatectomy. In other cases, complete hepatectomy has been required either in order to control bleeding or to remove an infarcted liver, as a temporary measure whilst awaiting organ donation and transplantation.

The liver histological features were in keeping with HELLP syndrome, but infarction was more extensive than is usually seen. This may have been the result of a heterozygous state for factor V Leiden deficiency, which may have precipitated portal vein thrombosis, increasing the hepatic infarction.

References

1 Kmietowicz Z. US and UK are top in teenage pregnancy rates. *BMJ* 2002;**324**:1354.

2 Wallstedt A, Riely CA, Shaver D, Leventhal S, Adamec TA, Nunnally J. Prevalence and characteristics of liver dysfunction in hyperemesis gravidarum. *Clin Res* 1990;**38**:970A.

3 Larry D, Rueff B, Feldman G, Degott C, Danan G, Benhamon J. Recurrent jaundice caused by recurrent hyperemesis gravidarum. *Gut* 1984;**25**:1414–5.

4 Morali G, Braveman D. Abnormal liver function enzymes and ketonuria in hyperemesis gravidarum. A retrospective review of 80 patients. *J Clin Gastroenterol* 1990;**12**:303–5.

5 Outlaw W, Ibdah J. Impaired fatty oxidation as a cause of liver disease associated with hyperemesis gravidarum. *Med Hypotheses* 2005;**65**:1150–3.

6 Conchillo J, Pijnenborg J, Peeters P, Stockbrugger R, Fevery J, Koeg G. Liver enzyme elevation induced by hyperemesis gravidarum: aetiology, diagnosis and treatment. *Neth J Med* 2002;**60**:374–8.

7 Weinstein L. Syndrome of hemolysis, elevated liver enzymes, and low platelet count: a severe consequence of hypertension in pregnancy. *Am J Obstet Gynecol* 1982;**142**:159–67.

8 Van Beek E, Peters L. Pathogenesis of preeclampsia: a comprehensive model. *Obstet Gynecol Surv* 1998;**53**:233–9.

9 Dekker G, de Vries J, Doelitzsch P, *et al.* Underlying disorders associated with severe early-onset preeclampsia. *Am J Obstet Gynecol* 1995;**173**:1042–8.

10 Haeger M, Undander M, Andersson B, Tarkowski A, Arnestad J, Bengtsson A. Increased release of tumor necrosis factor-alpha and interleukin-6 in women with the syndrome of hemolysis, elevated liver enzymes and low platelet count. *Acta Obstet Gynecol Scand* 1996;**75**:695–701.

11 Magann E, Perry K, Chauhan S, Graves G, Blake P, Martin J. Neonatal salvage by week's gestation in pregnancies complicated by HELLP syndrome. *J Soc Gynecol Investig* 1994;**1**:206–9.

12 Sibai B, Ramadan M, Usta I, Salama M, Mercer B, Friedman S. Maternal morbidity and mortality in 442 pregnancies with hemolysis, elevated liver enzymes, and low platelets. *Am J Obstet and Gynecol* 1993;**169**:1000–6.

13 Wilke G, Schutz E, Armstrong V, Kuhn W. Haptoglobin as a sensitive marker of hemolysis in HELLP-syndrome. *Int J Gynecol Obstet* 1992;**39**:29–34.

14 Sibai B. The HELLP syndrome (hemolysis, elevated liver enzymes and low platelets): much ado about nothing? *Am J Obstet Gynecol* 1990;**162**:311–6.

15 Paternoster DM, Stella A, Simioni P, Mussap M, Plebani M. Coagulation and plasma fibronectin parameters in HELLP syndrome. *Int J Gynecol Obstet* 1995;**50**:263–8.

16 Harms K, Rath W, Herting E, Kuhn W. Maternal hemolysis, elevated liver enzymes, low platelet count, and neonatal outcome. *Am J Perinatol* 1995;**12**:1–6.

17 Vigil-De Gracia P, Garcia-Cáceres E. Dexamethasone in the post-partum treatment of HELLP syndrome. *Int J Gynaecol Obstet* 1997;**59**:217–21.

18 Barton J, Riely C, Adamec T, Shanklin D, Khoury A, Sibai B. Hepatic histopathologic condition does not correlate with laboratory abnormalities in HELLP syndrome (hemolysis, elevated liver enzymes, and low platelet count). *Am J Obstet Gynecol* 1992;**167**:1538–43.

19 Van Pampus M, Westenberg S, van der Post J, Bonsel G, Treffers P. Maternal and perinatal outcome after expectant management of the HELLP syndrome compared with preeclampsia without HELLP syndrome. *Eur J Obstet Gynecol Reprod Biol* 1998;**76**:31–6.

20 Visser W, Wallenburg H. Temporising management of severe pre-eclampsia with and without the HELLP syndrome. *Br J Obstet Gynaecol* 1995;**102**:111–7.

21 Audibert F, Friedman S, Frangieh A, Sibai B. Clinical utility of strict diagnostic criteria for the HELLP syndrome (hemolysis, elevated liver enzymes, and low platelets). *Am J Obstet Gynecol* 1996;**175**:460–4.

22 Magann E, Bass D, Chauhan S, Sullivan D, Martin R, Martin J. Antepartum corticosteroids: disease stabilization in patients with the syndrome of hemolysis, elevated liver enzymes, and low platelets (HELLP). *Am J Obstet Gynecol* 1994;**171**:1148–53.

23 Roberts W, Perry K, Woods J, Files J, Blake P, Martin J. The intrapartum platelet count in patients with HELLP (hemolysis, elevated liver enzymes, and low platelets) syndrome: is it predictive of later hemorrhagic complications? *Am J Obstet Gynecol* 1994;**171**:799–804.

24 Shames B, Fernandez L, Sollinger H, *et al.* Liver transplantation for HELLP syndrome. *Liver Transpl* 2005;**11**:224–8.

25 Ganzevoort W, Rep A, de Vries JI, Bonsel GJ, Wolf H. Prediction of maternal complications and adverse infant outcome at admission for temporizing management of early-onset severe hypertensive disorders of pregnancy. *Am J Obstet Gynecol* 2006; **195**:495–503.

26 Raval D, Co S, Reid M, Pildes R. Maternal and neonatal outcome of pregnancies complicated with maternal HELLP syndrome. *J Perinatol* 1997;**17**:266–9.

27 Knapen M, van Schaiijk F, Mulder T, Peters W, Steegers E. Marker for liver damage in neonates born to mothers with HELLP syndrome. *Lancet* 1997;**349**:1519–20.

28 Sibai B, Ramadan M, Chari R, Friedman S. Pregnancies complicated by HELLP syndrome (hemolysis, elevated liver enzymes and low platelets): subsequent pregnancy outcome and long-term prognosis. *Am J Obstet Gynecol* 1995;**172**:125–9.

29 Sullivan C, Magann E, Perry K, Roberts W, Blake P, Martin J. The recurrence risk of the syndrome of hemolysis, elevated liver enzymes, and low platelets (HELLP) in subsequent gestations. *Am J Obstet Gynecol* 1994;**171**:940–3.

30 Ibdah J, Bennett M, Rinaldo P, *et al.* A fetal fatty acid oxidation disorder as a cause of liver disease in pregnant women. *N Engl J Med* 1999;**340**:1723–31.

31 Yang Z, Yamanda J, Zhao Y, Strauss A, Ibdah J. Prospective screening for pediatric mitochondrial trifunctional protein defects in pregnancy complicated by liver disease. *JAMA* 2002;**288**: 2163–6.

32 Treem W, Rinaldo P, Hale D, *et al.* Acute fatty liver of pregnancy and long-chain 3-hydroxyacyl-coenzyme A dehydrogenase deficiency. *Hepatology* 1994;**19**:339–45.

33 Ibdah JA. Acute fatty liver of pregnancy: an update on pathogenesis and clinical implications. *World J Gastroenterol* 2006; **12**:7397–404.

34 Innes A, Seargeant L, Balachandra K, *et al.* Hepatic carnitine palmitoyltransferase I deficiency presenting as maternal illness in pregnancy. *Pediatr Res* 2000;**47**:43–5.

35 Santos L, Patterson A, Moreea SM, Lippiatt CM, Walter J, Henderson M. Acute liver failure in pregnancy associated with maternal MCAD deficiency. *J Inherit Metab Dis* 2007;**30**:103.

36 Buytaert I, Elewaut A, van Kets H. Early occurrence of acute fatty liver in pregnancy. *Am J Gastroenterol* 1996;**91**:603–4.

37 Pockros P, Reynolds T. Acute fatty liver of pregnancy. *Dig Dis Sci* 1985;**30**:601–2.

38 Castro M, Fassett M, Reynolds T, Shaw K, Goodwin T. Reversible peripartum liver failure: a new perspective on the diagnosis, treatment, and cause of acute fatty liver of pregnancy, based on 28 consecutive cases. *Am J Obstet Gynecol* 1999;**181**:389–95.

39 Ch'ng C, Morgan M, Hainsworth I, Kingham J. Prospective study of liver dysfunction in pregnancy in Southwest Wales. *Gut* 2002;**51**:876–80.

40 Rolfes D, Ishak K. Liver disease in pregnancy. *Histopathology* 1986;**10**:555–570.

41 Rolfes D, Ishak K. Acute fatty liver of pregnancy: a clinicopathological study of 35 cases. *Hepatology* 1985;**5**:1149–58.

42 Ockner S, Brunt E, Cohn S, Krul E, Hanto D, Peters M. Fulminant hepatic failure caused by acute fatty liver of pregnancy treated by orthotopic liver transplantation. *Hepatology* 1990;**11**:59–64.

43 Sims H, Brackett J, Powell C, *et al.* The molecular basis of pediatric long chain 3-hydroxyacyl-CoA dehydrogenase deficiency associated with maternal acute fatty liver of pregnancy. *Proc Natl Acad Sci* 1995;**92**:841–5.

44 Moise K, Shah D. Acute fatty liver of pregnancy: etiology of fetal distress and fetal wastage. *Obstet Gynecol* 1987;**69**:482–5.

45 Ibdah J, Dasouki M, Strauss A. Long-chain 3-hydroxyacyl-CoA dehydrogenase deficiency: variable expressivity of maternal illness during pregnancy and unusual presentation with infantile cholestasis and hypocalcaemia. *J Inher Metab Dis* 1999;**22**: 811–4.

46 Ibdah J, Tein I, Dionisi-Vici C, *et al.* Mild trifunctional protein deficiency is associated with progressive neuropathy and myopathy and suggests a novel genotype-phenotype correlation. *J Clin Invest* 1998;**102**:1193–9.

47 Ibdah J, Yang Z, Bennett M. Liver disease in pregnancy and fetal fatty acid oxidation defects. *Mol Genet Metab* 2000;**71**: 182–9.

48 Milkiewicz P, Gallagher R, Chambers J, Eggington E, Weaver J, Elias E. Obstetric cholestasis with elevated gamma glutamyl

transpeptidase: incidence, presentation and treatment. *J Gastroenterol Hepatol* 2003;18:1283–6.

49 Beuers U, Pusl T. Intrahepatic cholestasis of pregnancy—a heterogeneous group of pregnancy-related disorders? *Hepatology* 2006;**43**:647–9.

50 Glanz A, Marschall H, Mattsson L. Intrahepatic cholestasis of pregnancy: relationship between bile acid levels and fetal complication rates. *Hepatology* 2004;**40**:467–74.

51 Lammert F, Marschall H, Glantz A, Matern S. Intrahepatic cholestasis of pregnancy: molecular pathogenesis, diagnosis and management. *J Hepatol* 2000;**33**:1012–21.

52 Reyes H, Baez M, Ganzalez M, Hernandez I, Palma J, Ribalta J. Selenium, zinc and copper plasma levels in intrahepatic cholestasis of pregnancy, in normal pregnancies and in healthy individuals. *J Hepatol* 2000;**32**:542–9.

53 Reyes H, Simon F. Intrahepatic cholestasis of pregnancy: an estrogen related disease. *Semin Liver Dis* 1993;**13**:289–301.

54 Mullenbach R, Bennett A, Tetlow N, *et al.* *ATP8B1* mutations in British cases with intrahepatic cholestasis of pregnancy. *Gut* 2005;**54**:829–34.

55 Eloranta M, Hakli T, Hiltunen M, Helisalmi S, Punnonen K, Heinonen S. Association of single nucleotide polymorphisms of the bile salt export protein gene with intrahepatic cholestasis of pregnancy. *Scand J Gastroenterol* 2003;**38**:648–52.

56 Jaquemin E, Cresteil D, Manouvrien S, Boute O, Hadchouel M. Heterozygous non-sense mutation of the *MDR3* gene in familial intrahepatic cholestasis of pregnancy. *Lancet* 1999;**353**:210–1.

57 Wasmuth H, Glantz A, Keppeler H, *et al.* Intrahepatic cholestasis of pregnancy: the severe form is associated with common variants of the hepatobiliary phospholipids transporter *ABCB4* gene. *Gut* 2007;**56**:265–70.

58 Schneider G, Paus T, Kullak-Ublick G, *et al.* Linkage between a new slicing site mutation in the *MDR3* alias *ABCB4* gene and intrahepatic cholestasis of pregnancy. *Hepatology* 2007;**45**: 150–8.

59 van Mil S, Milona A, Dixon P, *et al.* Functional variants of the central bile acid sensor *FXR* identified in intrahepatic cholestasis of pregnancy. *Gastroenterology* 2007;**133**:507–16.

60 Steiger B, Fattinger K, Madon J, Kullak-Ublick G, Meier P. Drug- and estrogen-induced cholestasis through inhibition of the hepatocellular bile salt export pump (Bsep) of a rat liver. *Gastroenterology* 2000;**118**:422–30.

61 Trauner M, Arrese M, Soroka C, Ananthanarayanan M, Koeppel T, Schlosser S. The rat canalicular conjugate export pump Mrp2 is down regulated in intrahepatic and obstructive cholestasis. *Gastroenterology* 1997;**113**:255–64.

62 Bacq Y. Intrahepatic cholestasis of pregnancy. *Clin Liver Dis* 1999;**3**:1–13.

63 Milkiewicz P, Elias E, Williamson C, Weaver J. Obstetric cholestasis. *BMJ* 2002;**324**:123–4.

64 Glanz A, Marschall H, Lammert F, Mattsson L. Intrahepatic cholestasis of pregnancy: a randomized controlled trial comparing dexamethasone and ursodeoxycholic acid. *Hepatology* 2005;**42**:1399–405.

65 Rodrigues C, Martin J, Brites D. Bile acid patterns in meconium are influenced by cholestasis of pregnancy and not altered by ursodeoxycholic acid treatment. *Gut* 1999;**45**:446–52.

66 Kondrackiene J, Beuers U, Kupcinskas L. Efficacy and safety of ursodeoxycholic acid versus cholestyramine in intrahepatic cholestasis of pregnancy. *Gastroenterology* 2005;**129**:894–901.

67 Nicastri P, Diaferia A, Tartagni M, Loizzi P, Fanelli M. A randomised placebo-controlled trial of ursodeoxycholic acid and *S*-adenosylmethionine in the treatment of intrahepatic cholestasis of pregnancy. *Br J Obstet Gynaecol* 1998;**105**:1205–7.

68 Roncaglia N, Locatelli A, Arreghini A, *et al.* A randomised controlled trial of ursodeoxycholic acid and *S*-adenosyl-l-methionine in the treatment of gestational diabetes. *BJOG* 2004;**111**:17–21.

69 Shaw D, Frohlich J, Wittman B, Wilms M. A prospective study of 18 patients with cholestasis of pregnancy. *Am J Obstet Gynecol* 1982;**142**:621–4.

70 Rioseco A, Ivankovic M, Manzur A, Hamed F, Kato S, Parer J. Intrahepatic cholestasis of pregnancy: a retrospective case-control study of perinatal outcome. *Am J Obstet Gynecol* 1994;**170**:890–5.

71 Fisk, N, Storey G. Fetal outcome in obstetric cholestasis. *Br J Obstet Gynaecol* 1988;**95**:1137–43.

72 Zimmermann P, Koskien J, Vaalamo P, Ranta T. Doppler umbilical artery velocimetry in pregnancies complicated by intrahepatic cholestasis. *J Perinat Med* 1991;**19**:351–5.

73 Ropponen A, Sund R, Riikonen S, Ylikorkala O, Aittomaki K. Intrahepatic cholestasis of pregnancy as an indicator of liver and biliary disease: a population-based study. *Hepatology* 2006;**43**: 723–8.

74 Connolly T, Zuckerman A. Contraception in the patient with liver disease. *Seminars in Perinatology* 1998;**22**:178–82.

75 Ko C, Beresford S, Schulte S, Matsumoto A, Lee S. Incidence, natural history, and risk factors for biliary sludge and stones during pregnancy. *Hepatology* 2005;**41**:359–65.

76 Whitington P, Malladi P. Neonatal hemochromatosis: is it an alloimmune disease? *J Pediatr Gastroenterol Nut* 2005;**40**:544–9.

77 Knisely A, Mieli-Vargani G, Whitington P. Neonatal hemochromatosis. *Gastroenterol Clin North Am* 2003;**32**:877–89.

78 Udell I, Barshes N, Voloyiannis T, *et al.* Neonatal hemochromatosis: radiological and histological signs. *Liver Transpl* 2005; **11**:998–1000.

79 Williams H, McKiernan P, Kelly D, Baumann U. Magnetic resonance imaging in neonatal hemochromatosis—are we there yet? *Liver Transpl* 2006;**12**:1725.

80 Flynn D, Mohan N, McKiernan P, *et al.* Progress in treatment and outcome for children with neonatal haemochromatosis. *Arch Dis Child Fetal Neonatal Ed* 2003;**88**:F124–7.

81 Whitington P, Hibbard J. High-dose immunoglobulins during pregnancy for recurrent neonatal haemochromatosis. *Lancet* 2004;**364**:1690–8.

82 Renge R, Dani V, Chitamber S, Arankalle V. Vertical transmission of hepatitis A. *Indian J Pediatr* 2002;**69**:535–6.

83 McDuffie R, Bader T. Fetal meconium peritonitis after maternal hepatitis A. *Am J Obstet Gynecol* 1999;**180**:1031–2.

84 Yao J. Perinatal transmission of hepatitis B virus infection and vaccination in China. *Gut* 1996;**38**:S37–8.

85 Aggarwal R, Ranjin P. Preventing and treating hepatitis B infection. *BMJ* 2004;**329**:1080–6.

86 Lee G, Gong Y, Brok J, Boxall E, Gluud C. Effects of hepatitis B immunisation in newborn infants of mothers positive for hepatitis B surface antigen: systematic review and meta-analysis. *BMJ* 2006;**332**:328–36.

87 Heiber J, Dalton D, Shorey J, Combes B. Hepatitis and pregnancy. *J Pediatr* 1977;**91**:545–9.

88 Chang M, Lee C, Chen D, Hsu H, Lai M. Fulminant hepatitis in children in Taiwan: the important role of hepatitis B virus. *J Pediatr* 1987;**111**:34–9.

89 Scwimmer J, Balistreri W. Transmission, natural history, and treatment of hepatitis C virus infection in the pediatric population. *Semin Liver Dis* 2000;**20**:37–46.

90 Ceci O, Margiotta M, Marello F, *et al.* Vertical transmission of hepatitis C virus in a cohort of 2447 HIV-seronegative pregnant women: a 24-month prospective study. *J Pediatr Gastroenterol Nutr* 2001;**33**:570–5.

91 McIntyre PG, Tosh K, McGuire W. Caesarean section versus vaginal delivery for preventing mother to infant hepatitis C virus transmission. *Cochrane Database Syst Rev* 2006;(**4**):CD005546.

92 Resti M, Jara P, Hierro L, Azzari C, Giachino R, Zuin G. Clinical features and progression of perinatally acquired hepatitis C virus infection. *J Med Virol* 2003;**70**:373–7.

93 Tovo P, Palomba E, Ferraris G, Principi N, Ruga E, Dallacasa P. Increased risk of maternal–infant hepatitis C virus transmission for women coinfected with human immunodeficiency virus type 1. Italian study group for HCV infection in children. *Clin Infect Dis* 1997;**25**:1121–4.

94 Reyes GR. Overview of the epidemiology and biology of the hepatitis E virus. In: Willson RA, ed. *Viral Hepatitis: Diagnosis, Treatment, Prevention.* New York: Decker, 1997: 239–58.

95 Kumar A, Beniwal M, Kar P, Sharma J, Murthy N. Hepatitis E in pregnancy. *Int Gynecol Obstet* 2004;**85**:240–4.

96 Banait V, Sandur V, Parikh F, *et al.* Outcome of acute liver failure due to acute hepatitis E in pregnant women. *Indian J Gastroenterol* 2007;**26**:6–10.

97 Duin L, Willekes C, Baldewijns M, Robben S, Offermans J, Vles J. Major brain lesions by intrauterine herpes simplex virus infection: MRI contribution. *Prenatal Diagnosis* 2007;**27**: 81–4.

98 Young E, Chafizadeh E, Oliveira V, Genta R. Disseminated herpes virus infection during pregnancy. *Clin Infect Dis* 1996; **22**:51–8.

99 Sheffield J, Hollier L, Hill J, Stuart G, Wendel G. Acyclovir prophylaxis to prevent herpes simplex virus recurrence at delivery: a systematic review. *Obstet Gynecol* 2007;**196**:89–94.

100 Sauerbrei A, Wutzler P. Herpes simplex and varicella-zoster infection during pregnancy: current concepts of prevention, diagnosis and therapy. Part 1: herpes simplex infection. *Med Microbiol Immunol* 2007;**196**:89–94.

101 Brown Z, Selke S, Zeh J, *et al.* The acquisition of herpes simplex during pregnancy. *N Engl J Med* 1997;**337**:509–15.

102 Verma A, Dhawan A, Zuzkerman M, Hadzic N, Baker A, Mieli-Vergani G. Neonatal herpes simplex virus infection presenting as acute liver failure: prevalent role of herpes simplex virus type 1. *J Pediatr Gastroenterol Nutr* 2006;**42**:282–6.

103 Giannitrapani L, Soresi M, La Spada E, Cervello M, D'Alessandro N, Mantalto G. Sex hormones and risk of liver tumor. *Ann N Y Acad Sci* 2006;**1089**:228–36.

104 O'Grady JG, Lake JR, Howdle PD. *Comprehensive Clinical Hepatology*. London: Mosby, 2000.

105 Mitchell MC, Boitnott JK, Kaufman S, Cameron JL, Maddrey WC. Budd–Chiari syndrome: etiology, diagnosis and management. *Medicine (Baltimore)* 1982;**61**:199–218.

106 Denninger M, Chait Y, Casadevall N, *et al.* Cause of portal or hepatic venous thrombosis in adults: the role of multiple concurrent factors. *Hepatology* 2000;**31**:587–91.

107 Bennion L, Ginsburg R, Gernick M, Bennett P. Effects of oral contraceptives on the gallbladder or normal women. *N Engl J Med* 1976;**294**:189–92.

108 Lindberg M. Hepatobiliary complications of oral contraceptives. *J Gen Intern Med* 1992;**7**:199–209.

109 Forman D, Doll R, Peto R. Trends in mortality from carcinoma of the liver and the use of oral contraceptives. *Br J Cancer* 1983;**48**:349–54.

110 Henderson B, Preston-Martin, Edmonson H, Peters R, Pike M. Hepatocellular carcinoma and oral contraceptives. *Br J Cancer* 1983;**48**:437–440.

111 [No authors listed.] Combined oral contraceptives and liver cancer. The WHO Collaborative Study of Neoplasia and Steroid Contraceptives. *Int J Cancer* 1989;**43**:254–9.

112 Deray G, Le Hoang P, Cacoub P, Assogba U, Grippon P, Baumelou A. Oral contraceptive interaction with cyclosporin [letter]. *Lancet* 1987:**i**:158–9.

113 Speroff L, Darney PD. *A Clinical Guide for Contraception.* Baltimore: Williams and Wilkins, 1992:171.

114 Zerner J, Doil KL, Drewry J, Leeber DA. Intrauterine contraceptive device failures in renal transplant patients. *J Reprod Med* 1981;**26**:99–102.

115 Laifer S, Guido R. Reproductive function and outcome of pregnancy after liver transplantation in women. *Mayo Clin Proc* 1995;**70**:388–94.

116 Alter M, Mast E. The epidemiology of viral hepatitis in the United States. *Gastroenterol Clin North Am* 1994;**23**:437–52.

117 Lee W. Pregnancy in patients with chronic liver disease. *Gastroenterol Clin North Am* 1992;**21**:889–903.

118 Pajor A, Lehoczky D. Pregnancy in liver cirrhosis. *Gynecol Obstet Invest* 1994;**38**:45–50.

119 Britton R. Pregnancy and esophageal varices. *Am J Surg* 1982;**143**:421–5.

120 Yip DM, Baker AL. Liver diseases in pregnancy. *Clin Perinatol* 1985;**12**:683–94.

121 Davies J, Robson JM. The effects of vasopressin, adrenaline and noradrenaline on the mouse foetus. *Br J Pharmacol* 1970;**38**:446P.

122 Fine R, Webber S, Harmon W, Kelly D, Olthoff K. *Pediatric Solid Organ Transplantation,* 2nd ed. Oxford: Blackwell, 2007.

123 Varma RR, Michelsohn NH, Borkowf HI, Lewis JD. Pregnancy in cirrhotic and noncirrhotic portal hypertension. *Obstet Gynecol* 1977;**50**:217–22.

124 Laifer SA, Darby MJ, Scantlebury VP, Harger JH, Caritis SN. Pregnancy and liver transplantation. *Obstet Gynecol* 1990;**76**:1083–8.

125 O'Grady JP, Day EJ, Toole AL, Paust JC. Splenic artery aneurysm rupture in pregnancy. A review and case report. *Obstet Gynecol* 1977;**50**:627–30.

126 Heriot JA, Steven CM, Sattin RS. Elective forceps delivery and extradural anaesthesia in a primigravida with portal hypertension and oesophageal varices. *Br J Anaesth* 1996;**76**:325–7.

127 Buchel E, Van Steenbergen W, Nevens F, Fevery J. Improvement of autoimmune hepatitis during pregnancy followed by a flare-up after delivery. *Am J Gastroenterol* 2002;**97**:3160–5.

128 Laifer S, Abu-Elmagd K, Fung J. Hepatic transplantation during pregnancy and the puerperium. *J Matern Fetal Med* 1997;**6**:40–4.

129 Fraser FC, Fainstat TD. Production of congenital defects in the off-spring of pregnant mice treated with cortisone; progress report. *Pediatrics* 1951;**8**:527–33.

130 Sifontis N, Coscia L, Constantinescu S, Lavelanet A, Moritz M, Armenti V. Pregnancy outcomes in solid organ transplant recipients with exposure to mycophenolate mofetil and sirolimus. *Transplantation* 2006;**82**:1698–702.

131 Sternlieb I. Wilson's disease and pregnancy. *Hepatology* 2000; **31**:531–2.

132 Brewer G, Johnson V, Dick R, Fink J, Kluin K. Treatment of Wilson's disease with zinc. XVII: treatment during pregnancy. *Hepatology* 2000;**31**:364–70.

133 Laifer S, Guido R. Reproductive function and outcome of pregnancy after liver transplantation in women. *Mayo Clin Proc* 1995;**70**:388–94.

134 Laifer S, Darby M, Scantlebury V, Harger J, Caritis S. Pregnancy and liver transplantation. *Obstet Gynecol* 1990;**76**:1083–8.

135 Pruvot F, Declerk N, Valat-Rigot A. Pregnancy after liver transplantation: focusing on risks to the mother. *Transpl Proc* 1997;**29**:2470–1.

136 Scantlebury V, Gordon R, Tzakis A. Childbearing after liver transplantation. *Transplantation* 1990;**49**:317–21.

137 Paternoster D, Floreani A, Burra P. Liver transplantation and pregnancy. *Int J Gynecol Obstet* 1995;**50**:199–200.

138 Ville Y, Fernandez, Samuel D, Bismuth H, Frydman R. Pregnancy in liver transplant recipients: course and outcome in 19 cases. *Am J Obstet Gynecol* 1993;**168**:896–902.

139 Cundy T, O'Grady J, Williams R. Recovery of menstruation and pregnancy after liver transplantation. *Gut* 1990;**31**:337–8.

140 Laifer S, Ehrlich G, Huff D, Balsan M, Scantlebury V. Congenital cytomegalovirus infection in offspring of liver transplant recipients. *Clin Infect Dis* 1995;**20**:52–5.

4 Neonatal liver disease

4 The Jaundiced Baby

Eve A. Roberts

Neonatal jaundice is a common finding. Many babies—as many as 30–50% of normal-term newborns—have transient jaundice 3–5 days after birth. This unconjugated hyperbilirubinemia is due to immaturity of the hepatic enzyme glucuronosyltransferase, which is responsible for glucuronidation of bilirubin. Unconjugated hyperbilirubinemia occurring later in the perinatal period may be associated with breastfeeding—so-called "breast-milk jaundice." Elevated blood levels of unconjugated bilirubin can be due to hemolysis, sepsis, hypothyroidism, or pyloric stenosis. In contrast, conjugated hyperbilirubinemia nearly always reflects hepatic dysfunction, which may be due to many different disorders, such as the neonatal hepatitis syndrome, biliary atresia, or duct paucity syndromes, all of which have different long-term outcomes. The nature of the liver disease must be determined as early as possible in order to start appropriate treatment or provide supportive therapies. The best current practice is to investigate jaundice in any term infant who is 14 days old, to determine whether unconjugated or conjugated hyperbilirubinemia is present.

Unconjugated hyperbilirubinemia

Bilirubin, a breakdown product of heme, is extremely toxic. When it binds to cellular macromolecules, as in neural tissue, it causes damage, disrupts metabolic processes, and leads to cell death. As bilirubin is normally tightly bound to albumin in the vascular compartment, concentrations of free bilirubin—which is capable of diffusing into brain tissue—are extremely low. Several parameters influence the level of free bilirubin: production of unconjugated bilirubin, the serum albumin concentration, and the concentration of bilirubin competitors that also bind to albumin. These include: commonly used drugs such as sulfonamides, furosemide, and benzoate; free fatty acids, including lipid infusions for total parenteral nutrition; and other breakdown products from red cell hemolysis. Premature infants are more vulnerable to bilirubin neurotoxicity than term infants, a tendency that may be potentiated by dehydration, which causes hyperosmolality, acidosis, and hypoxia. Kernicterus is the most serious consequence of severe unconjugated hyperbilirubinemia, and develops from binding of bilirubin in specific areas of the brain such as the basal ganglia. It may be fatal or may cause severe movement disorders (choreoathetosis), mental retardation, and deafness.

Physiological jaundice

Since hepatic bilirubin glucuronosyltransferase activity is low at the time of birth, nearly all newborn babies have hyperbilirubinemia in the first week of life. Unconjugated bilirubin predominates, whereas serum conjugated bilirubin is low or undetectable.[1] Approximately half of term babies are jaundiced; more severe jaundice (serum bilirubin ≥ 200 μmol/L) occurs in 8–20% in the first week of life.[2] Factors associated with severe jaundice include breastfeeding, exaggerated perinatal weight loss (> 7% of birth weight), maternal diabetes mellitus, bruising, and induction of labor with oxytocin. The severity and duration of jaundice may be increased in infants born prematurely. Infants of East Asian, Inuit, or North American Indian extraction tend to have more severe jaundice, with as many as 24–54% developing serum bilirubin > 200 μmol/L. In general, physiological jaundice peaks on day 3 of life, although hyperbilirubinemia may persist as long as 2 weeks.

The mechanism(s) of such severe physiological jaundice remain uncertain, and while environmental factors cannot be entirely excluded, genetic control of bilirubin production and clearance appears to be most important.[3] There may be an increased bilirubin load due to a shortened red blood cell lifespan,[4] increased activity of the enterohepatic circulation, and inefficient uptake of bilirubin by hepatocytes due to relatively immature expression of ligandin, which mediates the uptake of organic anions, in addition to immaturity of hepatic bilirubin glucuronosyltransferase. Infants who have abnormalities in bilirubin glucuronosyltransferase, which cause Gilbert syndrome[5,6]—alone or in addition to glucose-6-phosphatase dehydrogenase deficiency[7]—are at greater risk for severe physiological jaundice and breast-milk jaundice.

Diseases of the Liver and Biliary System in Children, 3rd edition. Edited by Deirdre Kelly. © 2008 Blackwell Publishing, ISBN: 978-1-4051-6334-7.

Treatment

Treatment may not be necessary in most cases. Phototherapy should be initiated for normal-term infants only when serum total bilirubin is > 300 μmol/L. The decision is complex and depends not only on the bilirubin concentration and its rate of increase, but also on the weight and gestational age of the infant, postnatal age, the rate at which bilirubin is generated, and the adequacy of bilirubin–albumin binding. Numerous clinical trials have demonstrated the effectiveness of phototherapy for decreasing unconjugated hyperbilirubinemia (bilirubin > 300 μmol/L) in term infants[8,9] and in premature babies with serum bilirubin > 200 μmol/L. Body temperature and fluid status must be monitored closely; fluid loss may be excessive, mainly because of increased insensible loss and additionally due to frequent watery stools. Eye patches are required. The baby may be more irritable, especially as normal parental interaction is often interrupted. For babies of ethnic extraction in whom severe unconjugated hyperbilirubinemia may commonly occur even in the absence of hemolysis, exchange transfusion remains a viable therapy to prevent kernicterus,[10] although tin-protoporphyrin treatment was used in the past.[11,12] Exchange transfusion may be required to prevent possible kernicterus in any baby with severe unconjugated hyperbilirubinemia. Outcomes are poorer for premature infants and those with an additional hemolytic anemia.[13]

Breast-milk jaundice

Moderately severe unconjugated hyperbilirubinemia associated with breastfeeding is common, occurring in 0.5–2.0% of healthy newborn babies. Jaundice may develop after the fourth day of life (early pattern) or towards the end of the first week of life (late pattern) and usually peaks around the end of the second week of life. Jaundice may overlap with physiological jaundice or be protracted and last 1–2 months.

The etiology remains uncertain. Contamination of breast milk with steroids such as pregnanediols appears unlikely. Breast milk may contain endogenous substances, such as free fatty acids, that displace bilirubin in the intestinal contents and enhance the enterohepatic circulation of bilirubin, although increased free fatty acids were not found in freshly expressed breast milk from mothers of infants with breast-milk jaundice.[14] An alternative hypothesis is that breast milk contains β-glucuronidase, leading to deconjugation of glucuronide moieties from conjugated bilirubin and subsequent reabsorption of bilirubin.[15] Breastfed babies have less frequent stools and eliminate less bile in feces than bottle-fed babies,[16] which may increase bilirubin reabsorption and contribute to hyperbilirubinemia. More frequent breastfeeding may enhance gut motility and stool output. Infants who actually have Gilbert syndrome may be at greater risk for breast-milk jaundice.[17]

The diagnosis is clinical: an exclusively breastfed infant with unconjugated hyperbilirubinemia, normal conjugated bilirubin, hemoglobin and reticulocyte counts, no maternal blood group incompatibility, and a normal physical examination except for jaundice. The condition is commoner in boys. The diagnosis is supported by a drop in serum bilirubin (≥ 50% in 1–3 days) if breastfeeding is interrupted for 48 h.[18] Breast-milk jaundice lasting 1–2 months requires surveillance by the physician to exclude liver disease. Pale stools, if noted, are highly suggestive of important liver disease, but monitoring serum conjugated bilirubin is a more reliable strategy.

Systemic disease

Unconjugated hyperbilirubinemia is frequently associated with systemic disease. Hemolysis of any etiology increases the bilirubin load and includes: rhesus and ABO incompatibility with Coombs positivity; glucose-6-phosphate dehydrogenase deficiency; erythrocyte membrane defects; and spherocytosis. Severe hemolytic disease of any etiology can result in severe jaundice associated with kernicterus and requires aggressive treatment with phototherapy and/or exchange transfusion. Bruising, hemorrhage into brain or lung tissue, and neonatal polycythemia also increase the bilirubin load.

The association of unconjugated hyperbilirubinemia with congenital hypothyroidism is based on early observations.[19] The mechanism of jaundice is not known, but thyroid function should be evaluated in any neonate with jaundice.

Unconjugated hyperbilirubinemia is also found with pyloric stenosis and other forms of upper intestinal obstruction, which resolves rapidly after pyloric myotomy.[20] The mechanism remains uncertain. A likely explanation is that these infants have Gilbert syndrome and develop unconjugated hyperbilirubinemia due to reduced oral intake.[21,22]

Other pathological conditions associated with unconjugated hyperbilirubinemia include sepsis, hypoxia, hypoglycemia, and galactosemia and fructose intolerance. With sepsis, inhibition of the constitutive androstane receptor (CAR) by inflammatory cytokines may lead to down-regulation of bilirubin conjugation.[23]

Inherited disorders

Crigler–Najjar syndromes

Crigler–Najjar syndromes type 1 and 2 are autosomal-recessive conditions that lead to unconjugated hyperbilirubinemia due to a deficiency of the enzyme bilirubin uridine diphosphate glucuronosyltransferase (UDPGT). In Crigler–Najjar type 1, there is effectively no UDPGT present; in type 2, the defect is partial.

The genetic basis for these diseases involves mutations in the *UGT1A1* gene, a member of the glucuronosyltransferase superfamily. The clinical phenotype of Crigler–Najjar type 1 can result from mutations in exons 2–5, resulting in a truncated nonfunctional enzyme, or in exon 1, resulting in complete loss of substrate recognition for bilirubin. Genetic heterogeneity in Crigler–Najjar type 1 is striking.[24–27] The genetic defect in Crigler–Najjar type 2 is somewhat subtler. Mutations leading to Crigler–Najjar type 2 appear to change the affinity of the enzyme for its substrate.[28–30]

Clinical features and diagnosis. Both conditions present early in the perinatal period with a rapid rise in bilirubin despite phototherapy. Kernicterus may develop in the perinatal period, particularly if treatment is delayed or if associated with dehydration or sepsis. Type 1 is much more severe than type 2, with peak serum bilirubin levels at 250–850 μmol/L. In Crigler–Najjar type 2, serum bilirubin is lower (200–300 μmol/L) and may reduce by 40–80% when phenobarbitone is administered.

Liver function tests, including conjugated bilirubin, are normal. Liver histology is normal, except for occasional bile plugs. Confirmation of the diagnosis may be obtained by detection of the enzyme deficiency in liver or estimation of bilirubin monoglucuronides and diglucuronides in bile aspirates. Bilirubin diglucuronides are not present in bile in type 1, but can be found in type 2;[31] however, these studies require cautious analysis in early infancy.[32]

Management. Treatment for Crigler–Najjar type 1 consists of aggressive use of measures to remove bilirubin with either phototherapy or exchange transfusion. Effective phototherapy depends on delivering radiant energy from light at a wavelength of 400–500 nm to the skin. Irradiance is not related to the brightness of the lights; the quantity of irradiation is inversely related to the distance between the lights and the infant. Skin pigmentation does not influence the effectiveness of treatment. The development of lighted mattresses[33] has facilitated treatment and permitted early discharge from hospital. The use of tin-protoporphyrin, which works by interfering with the generation of bilirubin from heme, was advocated as an alternative treatment, but is no longer used.[34,35]

The aim of therapy is to maintain bilirubin levels low enough (< 300 μmol/L) to prevent kernicterus, which may require up to 15 h of phototherapy a day.[36] Intercurrent infections with rapid increases in bilirubin should be managed with plasmapheresis or exchange transfusions. Drugs that displace bilirubin must be avoided.

Liver transplantation, including auxiliary transplantation, is a long-term option if damage to the nervous system has been avoided (Chapter 21) and may improve the quality of life. It is the only effective method for preventing kernicterus. Hepatocyte transplantation has limited success.[37,38]

In Crigler–Najjar type 2, prolonged treatment with phenobarbitone (5–10 mg/kg/day) may provide cosmetic improvement, but treatment is not usually required, since kernicterus is rare. In mice, the nuclear receptor CAR has been shown to up-regulate Ugt1a1.[39] Novel CAR agonists may provide a new treatment modality in the future.

Outcome. Sudden late neurological deterioration in Crigler–Najjar type 1 may occur even if management of hyperbilirubinemia has been meticulous. Late intrahepatic cholestasis has been reported. The outcome following liver transplantation is excellent. Heterozygote living donors have been used successfully.[40]

Gilbert syndrome

This condition manifests with mild variable unconjugated hyperbilirubinemia, with total serum bilirubin levels ranging from 30 to 90 μmol/L. It is a heterogeneous condition in which the responsible gene defect in has been identified: the presence of an extra TA tandem repeat in the promoter region of the bilirubin UDP glucuronosyltransferase gene (*UGT1A1*).[41,42] Instead of having the normal six repeats, seven or more are present; in other words, the normal $(TA)_6$TAA motif becomes $(TA)_7$TAA or $(TA)_8$TAA. Although this promoter region abnormality is the prevailing abnormality in individuals of European extraction, a different genetic picture exists in Asians, in whom mutations within the coding region of *UGT1A1* have been found associated with Gilbert syndrome.[5] Combinations of promoter and structural gene mutations may also be found in individuals with other ethnic origins.[43] A child with predominantly unconjugated hyperbilirubinemia has been described with mutations in both *UGT1A1* and *ABCC4*, the gene that is mutated in Dubin–Johnson syndrome.[44]

Clinical features. There is mild jaundice, which is exacerbated by dehydration, intercurrent illness, or fatigue. Patients often complain of vague abdominal pain, lethargy, and general malaise for which no good cause has been found. The condition is more common in males than females; most children present in adolescence. Serum aminotransferases are normal and biopsy is unnecessary. Infants homozygous for the genetic abnormality of Gilbert syndrome have a greater increase in jaundice in the first 2 days of life than heterozygotes or unaffected infants.[17,45,46] Asian infants with Gilbert syndrome associated with coding region mutations in the bilirubin glucuronosyltransferase gene are also more prone to physiological or breast-milk jaundice.[6,47–49] Compound heterozygotes may have more severe disease, as do children with Gilbert syndrome plus an identifiable form of hemolytic anemia. Gilbert syndrome may occur after liver transplantation, and it then has an atypical presentation.

Treatment. No treatment is required, but families often require reassurance. Irregular eating habits should be discouraged. A tendency to cholelithiasis in childhood has been identified in affected children.[50] *UGT1A1* (mainly with the promoter mutation) is a modifier gene for genetic hemolytic anemias, including sickle cell disease, and is associated with increased disease severity.

Conjugated hyperbilirubinemia

Conjugated hyperbilirubinemia indicates liver disease, which may be due to entities within the neonatal hepatitis syndrome, including biliary atresia and duct paucity syndromes. The predictive value of conjugated hyperbilirubinemia in the second week of life is robust enough to be the basis for infantile screening.[51] The importance of distinguishing jaundice due to liver disease from the more prevalent (and generally benign) types of neonatal jaundice with unconjugated hyperbilirubinemia cannot be overemphasized.

The nomenclature for neonatal liver disease is problematic. The term "neonatal jaundice" causes confusion with physiological jaundice, while "neonatal cholestasis" is imprecise. In the first 3–4 months of life, every infant has some degree of neonatal cholestasis on a physiological basis, which is multifactorial. Hepatocellular pathways of bile acid conjugation and biliary secretion are immature, and uptake of bile acids and other organic anions by hepatocytes is inefficient, leading to high concentrations of bile acids in blood; the circulating bile acid pool is contracted, and ileal uptake of bile acids is underdeveloped.[52,53] The term "neonatal hepatitis" is inadequate, as hepatic inflammation is not always prominent. The term "neonatal hepatitis syndrome" (NHS) conveys the similarity of the clinical illness in infants and suggests a broad spectrum of causative disease processes.

Neonatal hepatitis syndrome

"Neonatal hepatitis syndrome" is the term given to nonspecific hepatic inflammation, which develops due to many different causes, including intrauterine infection, endocrine disorders, and inborn errors of metabolism. Broadly, the term includes infantile biliary disorders, which have similar clinical features and may show some degree of inflammation on biopsy. Causes of the neonatal hepatitis syndrome and the diagnostic approach are summarized in Figure 4.1 and Table 4.1. Treatment is summarized in Table 4.5 (p. 90).

Clinical features

Conjugated hyperbilirubinemia may present at any time after birth. If it is detected in the first 24 h of life, infection is usually the cause. Most causes of the neonatal hepatitis syndrome have a similar presentation:

- Jaundice, which may not be obvious at first.
- Dark urine and pale yellow stools. Abnormal stool color, although suggestive of liver disease, is neither a specific nor a reliable feature.
- Infants may be small for gestational age, especially those with Alagille's syndrome, metabolic liver disease, and intrauterine infection (Figure 4.2).
- Failure to thrive or poor feeding.
- Dysmorphic features in trisomy 18, trisomy 21, Alagille's syndrome, Zellweger syndrome, and with certain congenital infections.
- Hypoglycemia in metabolic liver disease, hypopituitarism, or severe liver disease.
- Hypogonadism (in males) and optic dysplasia in hypopituitarism (Figure 4.3).
- Hepatomegaly.
- Splenomegaly (the spleen may also be palpated in healthy babies 1–2 cm below the left costal margin). An impalpable spleen in an infant with severe cholestatic jaundice may suggest extrahepatic biliary atresia with polysplenia.
- Ascites is rarely evident, except in metabolic liver disease (Chapter 5).
- Cardiac murmurs or neurological abnormalities are associated with specific congenital syndromes.
- Bleeding from vitamin K deficiency (particularly if the baby is breastfed) or thrombocytopenia.

Investigations

The following investigations and findings are used in determining a diagnosis of neonatal hepatitis syndrome:

- The cardinal feature is conjugated hyperbilirubinemia of any degree. Even a mildly elevated conjugated bilirubin ($\geq 10\ \mu mol/L$) in the absence of significant unconjugated hyperbilirubinemia may indicate significant hepatic disease.
- Serum aminotransferases are frequently elevated to two to four times the normal level, but they may be within normal limits for age. Higher elevations suggest an infectious process.
- Serum alkaline phosphatase may be normal or only mildly elevated. Higher levels may indicate biliary obstruction or rickets.
- Serum γ-glutamyltransferase (GGT) may be elevated, but reference values for GGT change dramatically during the first 3 months of life and may be difficult to gauge. GGT does not reliably distinguish bile duct obstruction from hepatocellular injury in the infant. Normal or low GGT suggests certain bile canalicular transporter defects (Byler disease or progressive familial intrahepatic cholestasis) (see below).
- Blood glucose may be normal or low. Hypoglycemia suggests metabolic liver disease, hypopituitarism, or poor hepatic reserve.
- Serum albumin is usually normal unless there is severe prenatal disease.
- Prothrombin and partial thromboplastin times are usually normal unless there is associated vitamin K deficiency (hemorrhagic disease of the newborn) or severe liver disease.
- Bilirubin is present in urine.
- Screening investigations for known causes of neonatal hepatitis syndrome may be diagnostic (Figure 4.1).
- Abdominal ultrasound scan (after a 4-h fast) to detect gallbladder size. Usually present unless there is severe intrahepatic cholestasis or biliary atresia (Figure 4.4). Improved technology now makes visualization of the common bile

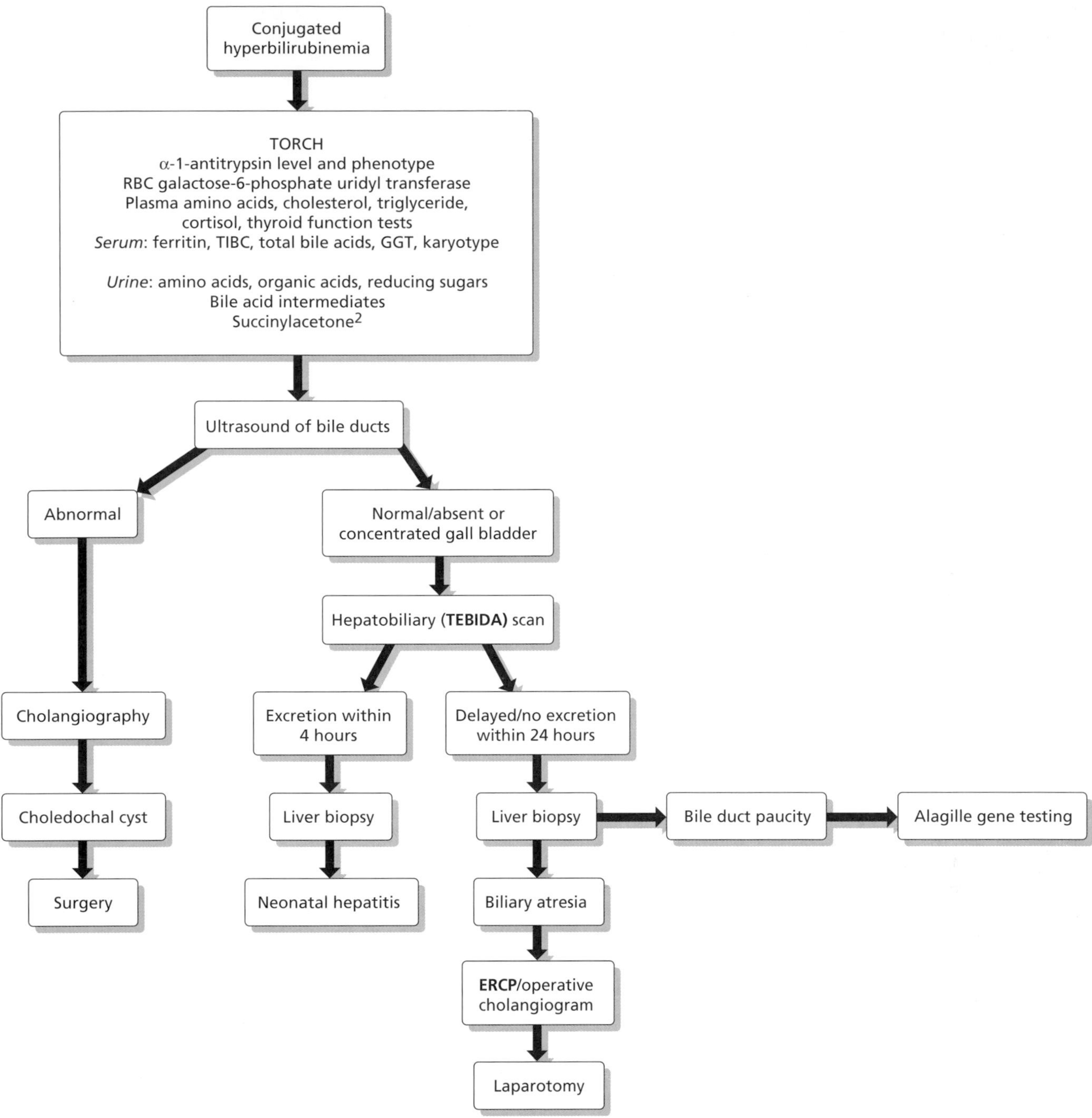

Figure 4.1 Investigation of conjugated hyperbilirubinemia in the neonate.
ERCP, endoscopic retrograde cholangiopancreatography; GGT, γ-glutamyltransferase; TEBIDA, technetium trimethyl-1-bromoiminodiacetic acid; TIBC, total iron-binding capacity; TORCH, toxoplasmosis, other, rubella, cytomegalovirus, and herpes simplex virus.

duct possible, but further verification of bile duct patency is almost always desirable.

- Radioisotope scan to demonstrate hepatic uptake (may be reduced in NHS) and biliary excretion (may be delayed more than 4–6 h in NHS if there is severe cholestasis, and more than 24 h, or indefinitely, in biliary atresia; Figure 4.5).
- Liver biopsy. This is frequently the most informative investigation in neonatal hepatitis syndrome.[54] If the liver is difficult to palpate, or if situs inversus abdominis is present, an ultrasound-guided biopsy should be performed. Information provided by liver biopsy includes: the severity of hepatocellular injury and extent of fibrosis; evidence for infiltrative

Table 4.1 Neonatal hepatitis syndrome: differential diagnosis and diagnostic approach.

Disease	Major diagnostic strategy
Congenital infection	
Toxoplasmosis	IgM-specific antibodies
Rubella	IgM-specific antibodies
Cytomegalovirus	Urine for viral culture, IgM antibodies
Herpes simplex	EM/viral culture of vesicle scraping
Syphilis	STS, VDRL, FTA-ABS, long-bone films
Human herpesvirus-6, herpes zoster	Serology, PCR
Hepatitis B	HB_sAg, anti-HB_c (IgM), HBV DNA
Hepatitis C	HCV RNA by RT-PCR
Human immunodeficiency virus	Anti-HIV, immunoglobulins, CD4 count
Parvovirus B19	IgM antibodies, PCR
Syncytial giant cell hepatitis	Giant cell hepatitis on liver biopsy
Enteric viral sepsis (echoviruses, Coxsackie A and B viruses, adenoviruses)	Appropriate serology or by PCR CSF for viral culture
Genetic	
Trisomy 18, (21), cat-eye syndrome	Karyotype
Endocrine	
Hypopituitarism (septo-optic dysplasia)	Low cortisol, TSH and T_4
Hypothyroidism	High TSH titer; low T_4, free T_4, T_3
Structural	
Biliary atresia	Delayed or absent excretion on hepatobiliary scan, biliary obstruction on histology
Caroli disease, choledochal cyst	Ultrasound, cholangiography
Neonatal sclerosing cholangitis	Cholangiogram
Hair-like bile duct syndrome	Cholangiogram
Spontaneous perforation of CBD	Ultrasound, paracentesis, biliary ascites
Inspissated bile syndrome	Coombs test, other evidence for hemolysis, dilated bile ducts
Duct paucity syndromes	
Alagille's syndrome	Echocardiogram, posterior embryotoxon, chest radiography for "butterfly vertebrae"
Nonsyndromic duct paucity	Bile duct paucity on histology
Metabolic	
α_1-Antitrypsin (AAT) deficiency	Serum AAT concentration, PI type
Cystic fibrosis	Sweat chloride, immunoreactive trypsin
Galactosemia	Galactose-1-phosphate uridylltransferase
Tyrosinemia	Serum tyrosine, methionine, α-fetoprotein, urine succinylacetone
Hereditary fructosemia	Liver biopsy: EM, enzyme activities
Citrin deficiency; citrullinemia, type II	Serum amino acids; genetic testing
Glycogen storage disease, type IV	Liver biopsy
Niemann–Pick, type A	Bone marrow aspirate, sphingomyelinase
Niemann–Pick, type C	Storage cells in BM aspirate, liver, rectal biopsy, fibroblast studies
Wolman disease	Abdominal radiography of adrenal glands
Primary defects in bile acid synthesis	Urinary bile acid intermediates by FAB-MS, total serum bile acids
Byler disease	GGT, total serum bile acids, genetic testing
Zellweger syndrome	Very-long-chain fatty acid studies
Immune	
Neonatal lupus erythematosus	Anti-Ro and anti-La antibodies (in infant and mother)
NH with autoimmune hemolytic anemia	Coombs test, giant cell hepatitis

AAT, α_1-antitrypsin; CBD, common bile duct; CSF, cerebrospinal fluid; EM, electron microscopy; FAB-MS, fast atom bombardment mass spectroscopy; FTA-ABS, fluorescent treponemal antibody, absorbed; GGT, γ-glutamyltransferase; Hb_sAg, hepatitis B surface antigen; HB_c, hepatitis B core antigen; HBV, hepatitis B virus; HCV, hepatitis C virus; HIV, human immunodeficiency virus; IgM, immunoglobulin M; NH, neonatal hepatitis; PCR, polymerase chain reaction; PI, protease inhibitor; RT-PCR, reverse transcriptase polymerase chain reaction; STS, standard test for syphilis; T_3, triiodothyronine; T_4, thyroxine; TSH, thyroid-stimulating hormone; VDRL, Venereal Disease Research Laboratory.

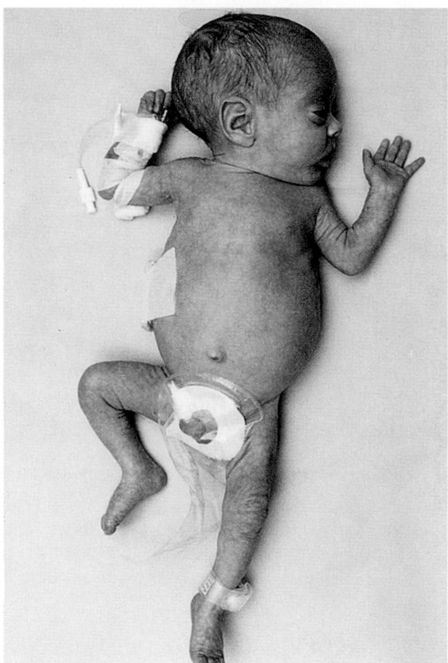

Figure 4.2 Infants with the neonatal hepatitis syndrome (NHS) present with prolonged jaundice. They may have intrauterine growth retardation or be small for gestational dates. Abdominal distension due to hepatosplenomegaly may be obvious.

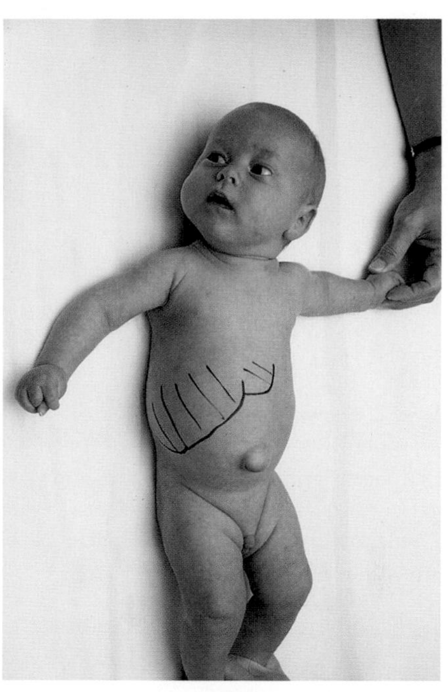

A

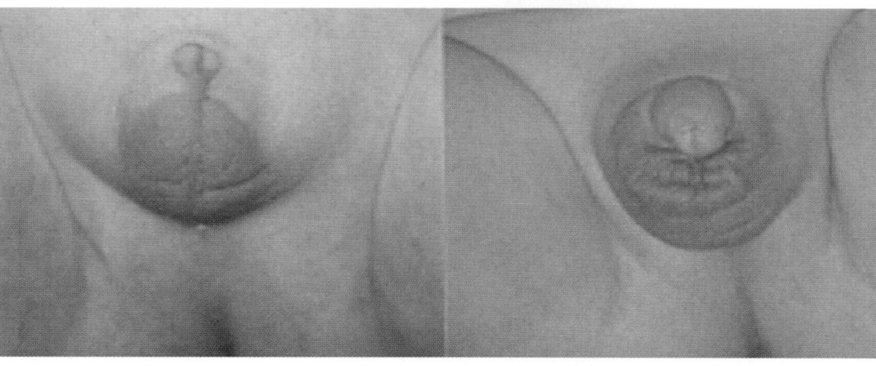

B

Figure 4.3 (**A**) Hypopituitarism may present with neonatal hepatitis and prolonged cholestasis. The diagnosis may be suspected by midline facial abnormalities, nystagmus, or (**B**) microgenitalia in males. Septo-optic dysplasia may be associated with the condition, and progresses despite endocrine replacement.

or storage disease; and type of biliary damage (bile duct reaction versus small duct paucity). Care should be taken to obtain a large enough specimen with adequate numbers of portal tracts to assess changes in the small bile ducts. Histological findings vary depending on the etiology. Most diseases will have conspicuous cholestasis with bile staining within the hepatocytes, and bile plugs within bile canaliculi and bile ductules. Hepatocytes may demonstrate a variable degree of multinucleated giant cell transformation and rosette formation on the hepatocytes. There may be a degree of extramedullary hemopoiesis. Although bile duct reaction is prominent in bile duct obstruction, it also occurs in children with other entities within the neonatal hepatitis syndrome, particularly those with α_1-antitrypsin deficiency, cystic fibrosis, and endocrine deficiency. Paucity of bile ducts is a feature in Alagille's syndrome, but occasionally duct reaction may occur early (Figures 4.6, 4.10).

Infection

TORCH infections

Congenital infections grouped under the acronym "TORCH" —toxoplasmosis, other (congenital syphilis and viruses), rubella, cytomegalovirus, and herpes simplex—often have very similar clinical features: hepatosplenomegaly, jaundice, pneumonitis, petechial or purpuric rash, and a tendency to prematurity or poor intrauterine growth. A presentation with acute-pattern liver failure in the newborn period is common with herpes simplex infection. Whenever possible,

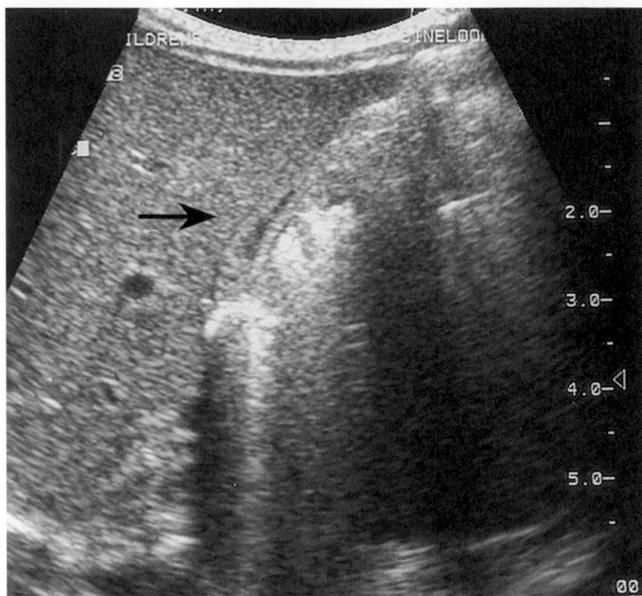

Figure 4.4 It is normal for a large gallbladder (arrow) to be visible on abdominal ultrasonography after a 4-h fast. In babies with intrahepatic cholestasis or extrahepatic biliary atresia, the gallbladder may be small or difficult to visualize.

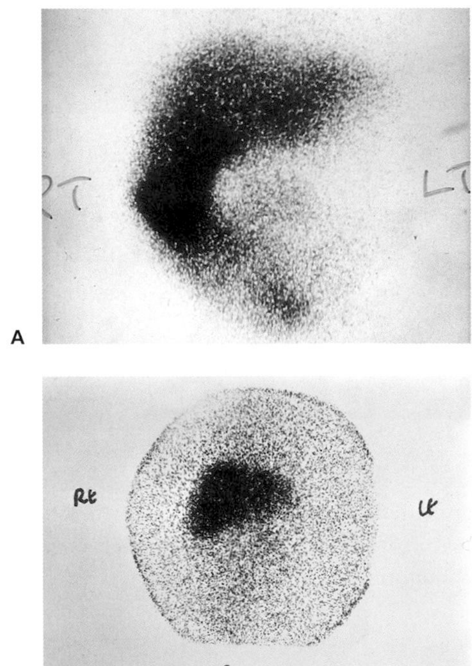

Figure 4.5 Hepatobiliary scanning with ^{99m}technetium trimethyl-1-bromoiminodiacetic acid (TEBIDA) provides good visualization of liver cells, especially after pretreatment with phenobarbitone (5 mg/kg/day for 3–5 days). This investigation may differentiate between neonatal hepatitis (**A**), in which there is patchy uptake of isotope but good excretion, in comparison with (**B**), in which there is no excretion of isotope from the liver, suggesting either extrahepatic biliary atresia or severe intrahepatic cholestasis.

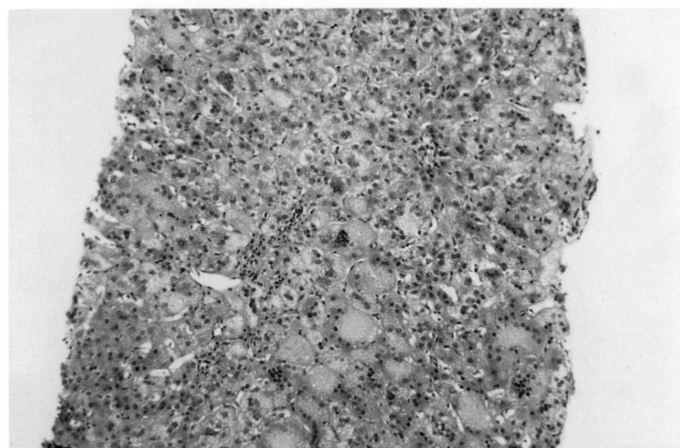

Figure 4.6 The characteristic histological features of neonatal or giant cell hepatitis are: conspicuous cholestasis with bile staining of hepatocytes, multinucleated giant cell transformation with rosette formation, and extramedullary hemopoiesis.

direct identification of viral infection by molecular methods or measurement of specific IgM antibodies should be sought for rapid diagnosis; relying on conventional TORCH titers is less preferable.

Toxoplasmosis. Congenital toxoplasmosis is comparatively rare. Maternal infection in the third trimester is more likely to cause fetal infection than infection earlier in pregnancy. Neonatal hepatitis is an important feature, but may be less obvious than central nervous system involvement with chorioretinitis (with large pigmented scars), hydrocephaly, or microcephaly. Intracranial calcification is usually prominent, leading to convulsions, nystagmus, and evidence of increased intracranial pressure. Pneumonitis may be severe.[55] Liver biopsy may demonstrate a nonspecific hepatitis or portal fibrosis with bile duct reaction. Spiramycin therapy may prevent progression of central nervous system and liver disease. Prognosis depends on the extent of neurological or optic disease.

Rubella. Congenital infection with rubella virus is now rare because of immunization. It may cause intrauterine growth retardation, anemia/thrombocytopenia, congenital heart disease (patent ductus arteriosus or pulmonary artery stenosis), cataracts, chorioretinitis ("salt-and-pepper" appearance), mental retardation, and sensorineural deafness. Hepatosplenomegaly is usual. Liver histology shows typical giant cell hepatitis. The disease may be self-limited or progress to cirrhosis.

Cytomegalovirus. Cytomegalovirus is the most common cause of congenital infection, affecting 1–2% of newborns, most of whom are asymptomatic. Those with evident disease may have intrauterine growth retardation or be premature.[56] Fetal ascites may occur.[57,58] Cytomegalovirus rarely causes acute-pattern liver failure in the newborn. Cytomegalovirus infection can be acquired postnatally via breast milk.[59] Although transient hepatitis with jaundice has been reported in a few premature infants, the overall outcomes appear to be benign.[60]

Clinical findings with congenital infection include: petechial rash, hepatosplenomegaly, and jaundice in 60–80%. Cytomegalovirus infection often affects the central nervous system, producing microcephaly, intracranial calcification, and chorioretinitis; progressive sensorineural deafness or cerebral palsy may develop later in childhood. Primary infection in the second and third trimesters appears to cause more severe fetal disease than recurrent infection.

Liver biopsy demonstrates giant cell hepatitis; the classical inclusion bodies are rarely seen in neonatal infection (see Figure 6.7, p. 154). In a study of liver tissue in infants with neonatal hepatitis or extrahepatic biliary atresia, Chang *et al.* found cytomegalovirus DNA in 23 of 50 infants with neonatal hepatitis by polymerase chain reaction, but in only two of 26 with extrahepatic biliary atresia, and in none of the control specimens.[61] Although differentiation from biliary atresia is usually easy, cytomegalovirus may be associated with extrahepatic biliary atresia. In one report of fraternal twins, both had congenital cytomegalovirus infection: one had hepatitis only, and the other presented with late-pattern extrahepatic biliary atresia.[56] In addition, 25% of infants with extrahepatic biliary atresia were found to have cytomegalovirus infection and were referred later than those without cytomegalovirus infection.[62] Cytomegalovirus is a candidate virus for causing late-presentation extrahepatic biliary atresia, as it can infect bile duct epithelial cells directly and increase expression of major histocompatibility complex (MHC) class II antigens.[63,64] Infants with congenital cytomegalovirus infection and persisting conjugated hyperbilirubinemia should have extrahepatic biliary atresia excluded. Congenital cytomegalovirus infection occasionally causes intrahepatic bile duct paucity.

Conclusive diagnosis requires identification of cytomegalovirus DNA in serum, or cytomegalovirus has to be cultured from the infant (usually from urine) within the first 4 weeks of life. Serological studies and clinical features provide support for the presence of cytomegalovirus infection, but do not distinguish congenital from early postnatal infection (Table 4.1). Guthrie card blood spots can be analyzed for presence of cytomegalovirus DNA and can thus diagnose congenital infection.[65]

In most children, cytomegalovirus hepatitis is mild and resolves completely. A few children develop hepatic fibrosis[66,67] or noncirrhotic portal hypertension.[68] Intrahepatic calcification has been reported.[69] Cirrhosis with chronic cholestasis necessitated liver transplantation in one child. Persisting neurodevelopmental abnormalities become the main problem in the majority of patients.[70] Treatment with ganciclovir is currently still controversial.[71]

Herpes simplex. In the newborn, this virus causes a severe multisystem disorder with encephalitis and severe hepatitis, or acute-pattern liver failure[72–74] (see Chapters 6 and 7). Either type 1 or type 2 virus is causative, although type 2 virus shed from the infected cervix at birth is more common. Liver biopsy shows areas of necrosis with viral inclusions in intact hepatocytes; however, profound coagulopathy may preclude biopsy. Scrapings from vesicular skin lesions reveal herpes simplex virus, but these typical herpetic skin, mouth, or eye lesions may not be present in neonates. Antiviral treatment with acyclovir should be administered to avert the otherwise high mortality.[75]

Syphilis

Congenital syphilis, once rare in the developed world, is once again increasing in frequency.[76] It causes a multisystem illness, which may include intrauterine growth retardation and subsequent failure to thrive, severe anemia and thrombocytopenia, nephrotic syndrome, periostitis, nasal discharge ("snuffles"), skin rash, diffuse lymphadenopathy, and hepatomegaly. Jaundice may be present within 24 h of birth or develop after treatment.[76] Jaundice may be severe.[13,77] Some babies with congenital syphilis never develop jaundice but present with a typical rash on the palms and soles or only with fever, as well as prominent hepatomegaly.[78] Central nervous system involvement occurs in up to 30% of infants.

Liver histology in untreated congenital syphilis may reveal numerous treponemes in hepatic tissue, but after treatment with penicillin, giant cell hepatitis without detectable treponemes is the usual finding. Bile duct paucity may develop. Diagnosis involves serological testing, including the Venereal Disease Research Laboratory (VDRL) test and confirmatory testing for specific antitreponemal antibodies. Radiographs of long bones may show typical bony abnormalities in the first 24 h of life and aid rapid diagnosis (Table 4.1). Penicillin is an effective treatment.

The recurrence of syphilis epidemics worldwide has lead to a World Health Organization global initiative to eradicate congenital syphilis.[79]

Varicella

Varicella may occur in newborn infants if maternal infection occurs within 14 days of delivery. It tends to be more severe in premature infants and is mild in term infants after 10 days of age. Early presentation or protracted disease in an infant of any gestational age may lead to a fatal outcome. This severe disease is characterized by jaundice and extensive skin and multisystem involvement, especially pneumonia. In severe or fatal cases, hepatic parenchymal involvement can be demonstrated.[80,81] Treatment with acyclovir may attenuate the infection or be curative.

Hepatotropic viruses: hepatitis A, B, and C

In general, infection with hepatotropic viruses in neonates

does not cause jaundice unless there is acute liver failure or severe hepatitis. Neither hepatitis A nor B has been associated with NHS or biliary atresia.[82]

Hepatitis A. Hepatitis A is rare in the neonate, but congenital infection may occur if the mother is infected 1–2 weeks before delivery.[83] The typical picture in the early neonatal period is a nonspecific diarrheal illness, as shown by rare outbreaks of transfusion-related hepatitis in premature infants.[84,85] Neonatal hepatitis syndrome is extremely rare.

Hepatitis B. Vertical hepatitis B infection is subclinical in the neonatal period; prompt administration of both hepatitis B immune globulin and hepatitis B immunization provides protection against chronic infection in 93% of infants at risk. Infants in whom this regimen fails may have been infected transplacentally. Without immunoprophylaxis, infants may become chronic carriers or develop acute hepatitis B or fulminant hepatic failure after a 3–4-month incubation period[86–89] (Chapters 6, 7, and 23).

Hepatitis C. Hepatitis C is not a cause of neonatal hepatitis syndrome. A study of 33 infants with either idiopathic neonatal hepatitis or extrahepatic biliary atresia revealed only one (with extrahepatic biliary atresia) positive for anti-hepatitis C virus (anti-HCV) antibodies and for virus by reverse transcriptase polymerase chain reaction (RT-PCR).[90] Similar studies in Taiwan, where hepatitis C is endemic, found no anti-HCV-positive infants among 42 with neonatal hepatitis and 11 with extrahepatic biliary atresia, using second-generation enzyme-linked immunoassay.[91] Vertical transmission of hepatitis is less common than in hepatitis B viral infection. Jaundice does not occur.

Human immunodeficiency virus (HIV) infection

Although infants with congenital HIV infection may present with hepatosplenomegaly,[92] conjugated hyperbilirubinemia in the neonatal period is rare. A case of neonatal hepatitis was attributed to HIV infection despite concomitant congenital cytomegalovirus infection;[93] an increased incidence of congenital cytomegalovirus infection has subsequently been found in HIV-infected infants. Congenital HIV infection may present clinically as hepatitis with jaundice although later than in the neonatal period, typically at around 6 months of age[94] (see Chapter 16).

Erythrovirus (parvovirus) B19 infection

Congenital parvovirus B19 infection may cause profound anemia, leading to hydrops[95] and fetal death. The spectrum includes conjugated hyperbilirubinemia, hepatomegaly, severe coagulopathy, dermal erythropoiesis ("blueberry muffin" rash), anemia, and perinatal distress.[96] Liver biopsy showed diffuse sinusoidal fibrosis, siderosis, and little giant cell transformation of hepatocytes but excessive extramedullary hemopoiesis.[97–99] Despite features of early hepatic insufficiency, serum aminotransferases may be low or near normal. The diagnosis is made by PCR for presence of parvovirus B19, although placental histology may suggest prenatal parvovirus infection. The outcome depends on the severity of the infection.

Human herpesvirus 6 (HHV-6) infection

Human herpesvirus 6 causes exanthema subitum, a common but usually benign febrile illness in infants; other HHV-6 infections are common and self-limited without a rash. Acute liver failure has been reported.[100,101]

Syncytial giant cell hepatitis

"Syncytial giant cell hepatitis" denotes severe liver disease attributed to paramyxovirus infection. The clinical liver disease varies with the age of the patient: in children, fulminant hepatic failure is common, while rapidly progressive chronic hepatitis occurs in adults. Older infants may have features of a chronic active hepatitis or autoimmune hemolytic anemia.

In neonates, syncytial giant cell hepatitis is associated with a severe hepatitis, which does not meet the criteria for fulminant liver failure (Chapters 5 and 7). Hepatitis with moderately elevated serum aminotransferases frequently progresses to chronic cholestasis and decompensated cirrhosis over 6–12 months.

Liver histology and electron microscopy show both the characteristic syncytial-type giant cells and viral inclusions consistent with the morphology of paramyxoviruses.[102–104] Formation of giant multinucleated hepatocytes is a characteristic response of infantile hepatocytes to injury, which is not often seen in hepatitis in adults. Syncytial giant cells differ from the giant cells of neonatal hepatitis because the outline of the liver cell plates remains evident, with indistinct, "smudged" borders between the cells. They may form because of cell fusion secondary to paramyxovirus, in the same way as with other viruses such as respiratory syncytial virus and measles virus.

Spontaneous recovery is uncommon. Treatment with the antiviral agent ribavirin appeared efficacious in one infantile case[105] and in a few adults. Most babies require liver transplantation before the end of the first year of life.

Enteric viral sepsis (echovirus, coxsackieviruses, adenoviruses)

The enteroviruses cause systemic viral infection in the newborn period, and severe hepatitis with acute liver failure may be a prominent feature. Incidence is greatest at the seasonal peak of echovirus infections (late summer to early autumn). The infant's mother may report that abdominal pain developed just prior to onset of labor. Vertical infection near the time of birth is associated with more severe disease in the infant. Most infants with enteric viral sepsis present between 1 and 5 weeks old. The infant is lethargic and jaundiced, with very high serum aminotransferases and severe coagulopathy; meningitis is usually present. Echovirus serotypes 3, 6, 7, 9, 11, 14, 19, and 21 have all been reported in severe infections with hepatitis.[106–109] Echovirus serotype 11 appears to be most virulent for newborns.

Coxsackie A and B viruses are capable of causing an identical clinical picture,[110,111] although myocarditis or heart failure suggests coxsackievirus infection. Adenoviruses[112] and herpes simplex infection (either type 1 or 2) also cause the same severe hepatitis.[73] The mortality with acute-pattern liver failure is of the order of 85–90%. Meticulous supportive care is essential (Chapters 7 and 15). Infants who recover may develop severe cholestatic jaundice. Subsequent hepatic function in survivors appears entirely normal.

Rapid identification of adenovirus may improve the outlook for infants with severe liver disease.[113]

Antiviral treatment may improve the dismal prognosis of neonatal enteroviral hepatitis. Pleconaril has been used successfully in some enteroviral infections.[114,115] Therapeutic drug monitoring is essential for safe use in this age group.

Bacterial infection outside the liver

Conjugated hyperbilirubinemia may occur with sepsis or localized extrahepatic infection, such as a urinary infection, that is inapparent.[116–118] This appears to occur because pro-inflammatory cytokines interfere with the function of bile canalicular transporters. Serum aminotransferases may be slightly elevated, but hepatosplenomegaly is uncommon. Jaundice may also occur with streptococcal and staphylococcal infections and Gram-negative bacterial septicemia (see also Chapter 16).

Infants with galactosemia may present initially with jaundice and Gram-negative septicemia, often due to *Escherichia coli* or *Klebsiella* species. Other typical features of galactosemia may not be obvious. Galactosemia should be investigated in any infant with conjugated hyperbilirubinemia associated with sepsis by measuring erythrocyte galactose-1-phosphate uridyltransferase.

Listeriosis

Congenital infection with *Listeria monocytogenes* typically involves the liver. Although meningitis is the predominant clinical feature of the systemic disease, infants have hepatosplenomegaly and are sometimes jaundiced. Pneumonia is usually present. A history of maternal illness is common. Liver biopsy may reveal simply a diffuse hepatitis or, more commonly, diffuse areas of focal necrosis. The diagnosis is made by isolating the organism from blood, cerebrospinal fluid (CSF), or liver. Treatment is with penicillin.

Tuberculosis

Congenital tuberculosis is rare, but since the prevalence of tuberculosis in women of child-bearing age has risen in the past few years, tuberculosis in infants may become more common. Newborn infants may be infected by aspirating infected amniotic fluid or cervical secretions at the time of delivery.

Practical criteria for diagnosis are a proven tuberculous infection in a newborn baby with at least one of the following: lesions in the first week of life; primary hepatic complex or caseating granulomas in the liver; tuberculous infection of the placenta or maternal genital organs; and exclusion of postnatal infection by investigation of contacts.[119,120]

Hepatomegaly is common in infants with tuberculosis, but jaundice is rare and indicates severe disease.[121] Respiratory distress, poor feeding, and fever are frequent. The mortality approaches 30%; a quadruple antitubercular antibiotic regimen *excluding* ethambutol is recommended. A high index of suspicion appears to be required for diagnosis, as tuberculosis in this age group often has atypical clinical features.[122]

Endocrine disorders

Hypothyroidism

Hypothyroidism is usually associated with an unconjugated hyperbilirubinemia, but may be associated with the neonatal hepatitis syndrome and should be excluded in every patient.

Hypopituitarism

Pituitary–adrenal dysfunction is associated with neonatal hepatitis syndrome in 30–70% of patients.[123–128] The cause of the hypopituitarism is variable. It is due to hypothalamic dysfunction in some; deficiency of anterior and/or posterior pituitary function may be present; a child with adrenal insensitivity to adrenocorticotropin has also been described.[129] Clinical features include: conjugated hyperbilirubinemia; hypoglycemia in the perinatal period, which is usually symptomatic and persistent; and septo-optic dysplasia,[130] which is a neuro-optical malformation that includes ventral midline developmental defect (absence of the septum pellucidum or corpus callosum) and hypoplasia of one or both optic nerves, associated with hypopituitarism. There may also be midline facial abnormalities, nystagmus and microgenitalia in boys (Figure 4.3).

The diagnosis is confirmed by detecting an extremely low random or 9 AM cortisol in association with low thyroid-stimulating hormone (TSH) and thyroxine (T_4) levels, although thyroid function tests may be in the low normal range initially.[131] Liver biopsy usually reveals typical giant cell hepatitis, but severe cholestasis may be present, with dilated bile canaliculi and hepatocellular necrosis. There may be delayed excretion on radioisotope scanning. Hormone replacement is essential and includes thyroxine, corticosteroids, and occasionally growth hormone. Progression of the disease to cirrhosis and portal hypertension has been reported in children in whom hormone replacement was delayed or not administered.

Adrenal injury

Damage to the adrenal glands may occur as a result of difficult delivery. This results in neonatal hepatitis syndrome with hypoglycemia. It may be more common with diabetic mothers.

Chromosomal disorders

Trisomy 18

Trisomy 18 is associated with growth retardation, skeletal abnormalities, and complex congenital heart disease. Both giant cell hepatitis and extrahepatic biliary atresia have been reported.[132,133] In one infant with trisomy 18, serial liver biopsies suggested late evolution from neonatal hepatitis to extrahepatic biliary atresia.

Other cytogenetic abnormalities, including trisomy 13, deletion of the short arm of chromosome 18 and 49 XXXXY,[134] have been reported in association with extrahepatic biliary atresia.

Trisomy 21

The association between trisomy 21 and neonatal cholestasis or extrahepatic biliary atresia[135] is not well substantiated. Recently, severe hepatic fibrosis associated with transient myeloproliferative disorder has been reported with Down syndrome,[136,137] raising the possibility that hepatic fibrogenesis might be due to high concentrations of growth factors derived from megakaryocytes. Infants with this transient leukemia have a poorer prognosis overall when there is jaundice and hepatic dysfunction.[138]

Cat-eye syndrome

Cat-eye syndrome is a highly variable malformation syndrome associated with a small supernumerary bisatellited marker chromosome derived from duplicated regions of chromosome 22. Major features may include coloboma of the iris and other facial malformations involving the eyes, anal atresia with fistula, complex congenital heart disease, and renal malformation. There is considerable phenotypic variability. Extrahepatic biliary atresia has been reported in association with this disorder. A candidate responsible gene in this condition has recently been identified as the human homologue of *CECR1*, which is an insect gene encoding growth factors. The expression pattern of *hCECR1* in the heart, cranial nerves, and notochord and later in fetal liver, lung, and kidney implicates it as leading to cat-eye syndrome when it is overexpressed.[139]

Idiopathic neonatal hepatitis

In a certain percentage of infants presenting with conjugated hyperbilirubinemia before 3 months of age, no etiology is found, and these infants are considered to have idiopathic neonatal hepatitis. Progress in identifying genetic defects causing hepatocellular metabolic defects and bile canalicular dysfunction has decreased the proportion of idiopathic neonatal hepatitis overall. Nevertheless, new observations continue to extend the range of idiopathic neonatal hepatitis —for example, with hydranencephaly[140] or in Seckel syndrome.[141] An important subset of idiopathic neonatal hepatitis includes instances in which more than one child in a single family is affected, accounting for 5–15% of cases in most series. In addition, heterozygosity for a bile canalicular transport disorder may predispose to idiopathic neonatal hepatitis.[142]

If cholestasis is severe, differentiation from extrahepatic biliary atresia and other cholestatic conditions is important. Infants with idiopathic neonatal hepatitis are more likely to be premature or small for gestational age than those with extrahepatic biliary atresia,[143] perhaps reflecting a genetic disorder or an intrauterine infection. Liver biopsy shows extensive giant cell transformation of hepatocytes with inflammation, but the bile ducts appear generally normal. A few infants with histologically severe inflammation also have small bile duct paucity. It is not always easy to differentiate between severe idiopathic neonatal hepatitis and extrahepatic biliary atresia. A cholangiogram may be required, and there is no evidence that diagnostic laparotomy for assessment of the extrahepatic biliary tree is adverse for infants with idiopathic neonatal hepatitis.

The prognosis is generally good. The estimate of mortality, at 13–25%, is based on older studies which may no longer be relevant.[144–146] Predictors of poor prognosis include: prolonged severe jaundice (beyond 6 months of age); acholic stools; familial occurrence; persistent hepatomegaly; and severe inflammation on biopsy. Peak bilirubin level is not necessarily predictive of outcome, and the prognostic importance of ductopenia has not been rigorously investigated. Septic complications may lead to decompensation. The long-term outlook for infants who survive the first year of life with little evidence of chronic liver disease is very good.

Neonatal hepatitis in preterm infants

Idiopathic neonatal hepatitis is a common referral in preterm babies, particularly as many more premature infants are resuscitated and survive. They may be prone to hypoglycemia and have a functionally immature gastrointestinal tract, resulting in difficulties with feeding. Most will have been maintained on parenteral nutrition (PN) initially and will be at increased risk of cholestasis due to immaturity of the biliary tree. It is important to differentiate this condition from other known causes of NHS, PN-associated liver disease, and in particular extrahepatic biliary atresia, which may have an atypical presentation in this age group, presenting at the corrected age for term. Examination of stools for pigment and a fasting ultrasound examination for gallbladder size are useful investigations to exclude biliary atresia in this age group. Liver biopsy is only indicated if there is persistent elevation of conjugated bilirubin and/or abnormal liver biochemistry. The prognosis is generally good.

Structural abnormalities

Biliary atresia

Extrahepatic biliary atresia (BA) is the cause of liver disease in approximately 25% of infants presenting with neonatal hepatitis syndrome and is the most important differential diagnosis. Early diagnosis is vital, as the Kasai portoenterostomy is less likely to be successful the later it is performed.[147,148] BA is found worldwide in all racial groups, with an incidence of one in 8000–18 000 live births.

BA involves a progressive destruction of the extrahepatic bile ducts, with scarring, obliteration, and concomitant ongoing damage to small and medium-sized intrahepatic bile ducts. For this reason, "extrahepatic" has been dropped from the terminology. The disease is classified according to the extent of damage at diagnosis. In type 1, damage is limited to the distal common bile duct (also known as "correctable"); in type 2, damage is limited to the common hepatic duct; in type 3, which is the most common, the entire extrahepatic biliary tree is involved. Type 1 accounts for approximately 10% of cases of BA, and type 2 is extremely rare (Chapter 19). Moreover, it has become evident that apart from this structural classification of BA, broad etiological groups can be defined that are relevant to the diagnosis. Most infants with BA appear to acquire the disease toward the end of gestation or shortly after birth (perinatal); a second BA group consists of babies with congenital malformations usually involving the spleen and often involving disorders of laterality, which may accompany either type 1 or type 3 BA (syndromic); a third group includes those with self-evident chromosomal abnormalities, such as trisomy 18; and the fourth group includes miscellaneous genetic disorders such as mutations in the villin gene and Martínez-Frías syndrome. Advances in molecular genetics with microarray technology have demonstrated differential gene expression in biliary atresia, suggesting up-regulation of inflammatory and immune regulatory genes.[149] For a discussion of the etiology and pathogenesis, see Chapter 19.

Clinical features

The clinical presentation of BA is unremitting and progressive jaundice in an infant who usually looks otherwise well. The main features are:

- Normal birth weight and gestational age in the majority. Preterm infants can have BA.
- Jaundice, which is present from shortly after birth, continuous with physiological jaundice. There may be some variability in intensity; however, jaundice can be readily identified in affected infants by 4 weeks of age.
- Yellow or dark urine with increasingly pale stools, which eventually become acholic. Initially, there may be variation in the stool color, which may be confusing.
- Hepatomegaly is always present; the liver is usually firm.
- Splenomegaly is a late sign and implies some degree of hepatic fibrosis; it is absent with polysplenia.
- Failure to thrive despite adequate feeding.
- Cardiovascular anomalies (ventricular or atrial septal defects) in 30%.
- Polysplenia syndrome; this includes preduodenal portal vein, situs inversus, absence of the inferior vena cava, and malrotation (Chapter 19).
- Bleeding from vitamin K–responsive coagulopathy, which is more common in breastfed infants who did not receive intramuscular vitamin K at birth.
- Ascites and pruritus are late complications.

Diagnosis

A diagnosis of BA involves the following investigations and findings:

- Serum conjugated bilirubin at presentation ranges from 40 to 200 μmol/L.
- Serum aminotransferases are always abnormal: concentrations of aspartate aminotransferase (AST) and alanine aminotransferase (ALT) are typically in the range of 80–200 U/L.
- Serum alkaline phosphatase is usually, but not invariably, elevated (range 500–800 U/L), due to biliary damage or rickets.
- γ-Glutamyltransferase (GGT) is usually elevated (10 times normal).
- Serum albumin is usually normal.
- Cholesterol may be elevated, but triglycerides are normal.
- Prothrombin time is normal, although 5–10% of cases present with vitamin K-responsive coagulopathy.
- Blood glucose is usually normal.
- Hepatic ultrasound, after a 4-h fast, may not demonstrate a gallbladder or only a misshapen gallbladder (Figure 4.4); it occasionally shows a dilated extrahepatic biliary tree, consistent with distal, "correctable" atresia; dilated intrahepatic bile ducts are uncommonly found. Abnormal vascular anatomy consistent with the polysplenia syndrome may be seen.
- Hepatobiliary scanning, using a technetium-labeled iminodiacetic acid derivative, following phenobarbitone pretreatment (5 mg/kg/day for 3–5 days) fails to demonstrate passage of the radiolabeled substance into the intestinal tract over a 24-h period (Figure 4.5b). Although hepatobiliary scanning has high sensitivity, scanning may appear normal if performed very early in the disease process in late-pattern extrahepatic biliary atresia.[149,150] It may also fail to show bile drainage in severe idiopathic neonatal hepatitis or bile duct paucity syndromes.
- Percutaneous liver biopsy is essential and has high diagnostic specificity. Features of bile duct obstruction (duct reaction, previously known as ductular proliferation; bile plugs in small bile ducts; portal tract edema) are usually obvious, along with variable fibrosis and some giant cell transformation

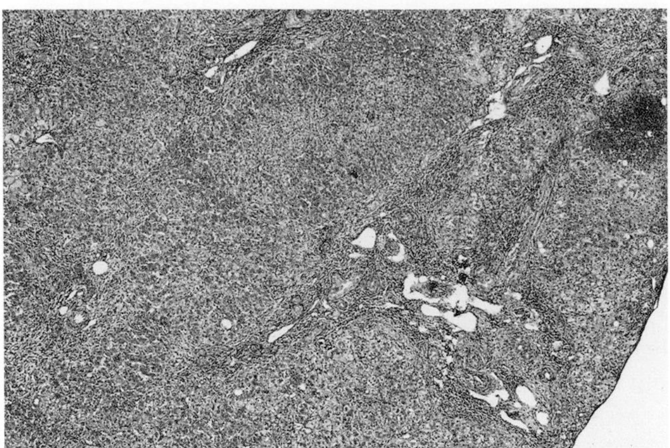

Figure 4.7 Features suggestive of biliary atresia are: cholestasis with bile duct reaction, bile plugs within bile canaliculi and bile ductules; and portal tract edema with variable fibrosis. There may be some giant cell transformation, but extramedullary hemopoiesis is unusual.

(Figure 4.7). The earlier the liver biopsy is performed, the more difficult it may be to interpret. When the hepatobiliary scan shows no drainage and the liver histology is ambiguous, close clinical surveillance and repeat liver biopsy are required to determine the evolution of disease.

• Cholangiography is required: with technical advances, endoscopic retrograde cholangiopancreatography (ERCP), percutaneous transhepatic cholangiography (PTC), and magnetic resonance cholangiography are becoming a reasonable alternative to intraoperative cholangiography[151,152] (Chapter 19).

Management

Therapy consists of nutritional and family support. Palliative surgery—the Kasai portoenterostomy—should be performed to establish biliary drainage unless liver disease is advanced. Chapter 19 describes the surgical details and postoperative management.

Optimally, the diagnosis of biliary atresia must be established before the infant is 5–7 weeks old, so that the Kasai portoenterostomy can be performed by 6–8 weeks of age. The operation should not be withheld from infants of 10–12 weeks of age, because successful palliation can be achieved in one-third of these patients. It is probably not indicated after 14 weeks of age, but every child should have a laparotomy to confirm the diagnosis and exclude unusual anatomy that might be amenable to surgical reconstruction. In one series, there was no improvement in outcome associated with carrying out the operation very early (before the infant is 40 days old),[153] but other series have shown benefit with early Kasai operations. Contrary to initial impressions, the presence of the polysplenia syndrome does not in itself predict that the Kasai operation is likely to fail.[154]

Complications and outcome

The complications include recurrent cholangitis, malnutrition due to malabsorption, and progression to cirrhosis and portal hypertension. Patients with a well-functioning portoenterostomy appear to have some risk of recurrent cholangitis at any age despite prophylaxis. In one series, children with correctable atresia appeared unusually susceptible to septicemia, presumably due to bacterial cholangitis.

Since damage to intrahepatic bile ducts is progressive, irrespective of whether or not bile drainage is reestablished, even children with a successful Kasai operation may be expected to develop biliary cirrhosis. Portal hypertension with variceal hemorrhage occurs in many long-term survivors, and endoscopic injection sclerotherapy or band ligation may be required. It is now clear that with expert surgical and medical management, 80% of children with successful Kasai portoenterostomy will survive 8–10 years without liver transplantation.[155,156]

In approximately 40% of children, a Kasai portoenterostomy fails to establish biliary drainage. These children remain cholestatic and develop the complications of fat malabsorption, with subsequent protein-energy malnutrition. They should be referred immediately for liver transplantation (Chapter 21). Treatment with ursodeoxycholic acid (20 mg/kg/day) may enhance the function of the portoenterostomy.

The 5-year survival after Kasai portoenterostomy is 40–60%.[57] Prolonged survival beyond childhood without liver transplantation occurs in 10–25%. Patients in Japan[157] and in France[158] have survived 20 years or more after a portoenterostomy without liver transplantation; most are well and asymptomatic, with normal growth and psychosocial development, but they have evidence of chronic liver disease and some are now being considered for liver transplantation. A few women have had babies after apparently uncomplicated pregnancies.

The majority of children will require liver transplantation at some stage, especially if the Kasai portoenterostomy has not been successful.

Biliary atresia with autosomal-recessive genetic diseases

Recent reports indicate that some rare autosomal-recessive genetic disorders may be associated with BA. Mutations in the villin gene were described in three children who clinically had BA.[159] Villin is an actin-binding protein essential for maintaining the integrity of the bile canalicular villus. Several infants have been described with a constellation of congenital abnormalities including BA; other features included low birth weight, tracheoesophageal fistula, intestinal atresias, hypoplastic pancreas, and hypospadias.[160–162] In some cases, the parents were consanguineous, and the genetic problem is thought to be an autosomal-recessive disorder affecting early development at the duodenal–biliary–pancreatic junction. The Kabuki make-up syndrome (Niikawa–Kuroki syndrome) features a distinctive facies and typically includes skeletal abnormalities, poor growth, and neurodevelopmental delay; BA has been found in some affected children.[163,164]

Choledochal cyst

Choledochal cyst refers to a group of congenital malformations of the biliary system. There are five major forms.[165,166] Choledochal cysts may be identified in the fetus by prenatal sonography[167–169] (see also Chapter 19).

Clinical features and diagnosis

The triad of symptoms associated with choledochal cyst consists of jaundice, abdominal mass, and pain, but this is an unusual presentation in the neonatal period. Some patients are referred with an antenatal diagnosis. There is female predominance (the female–male ratio is 5 : 1). Most affected infants have jaundice, abdominal mass or distension, and acholic stools,[168,170] and differentiation from biliary atresia or choledocholithiasis is important.

The diagnosis is made by identifying the choledochal cyst by ultrasound examination of the liver in a jaundiced infant (Figure 4.8). Cholangiography, either percutaneous or endoscopic, confirms the diagnosis (see Figure 19.5) or by hepatobiliary scanning (Figure 4.9). Liver function tests are consistent with biliary obstruction, and liver biopsy may demonstrate large bile duct obstruction and fibrosis, which is reversible after surgery.

Treatment and outcome

Treatment is aimed at removing the cyst as much as possible (Chapter 19). Excision of the cyst with hepaticoenterostomy offers the best outcome.[171–173] Complications are fewer with early surgical intervention. Surgery should be performed promptly in infants diagnosed prenatally who have conjugated hyperbilirubinemia. If the infant remains free of jaundice, elective surgical resection of the choledochal cyst may be postponed until the infant is around 1 month old, but it should not be greatly delayed. Although approximately 50% of infants with prenatally identified bile duct dilation have hepatic fibrosis, and a few have cirrhosis, most of these infants do well. A few of these infants have correctable biliary atresia, and close follow-up is warranted. Some infants with choledochal cyst not associated with biliary atresia later develop intrahepatic duct dilation, and they should therefore also be followed regularly.[174] Late development of cholangiocarcinoma is possible, but the risk is poorly quantified.[175]

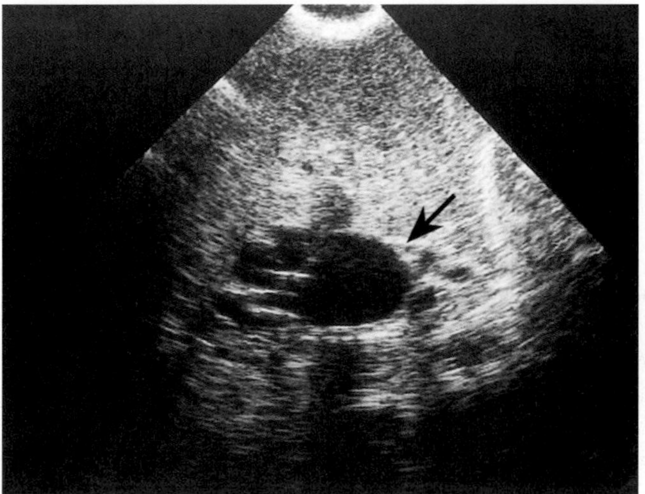

Figure 4.8 Choledochal cysts are usually diagnosed on abdominal ultrasound. A cystic structure (arrow) is visible here below the liver, close to the gallbladder.

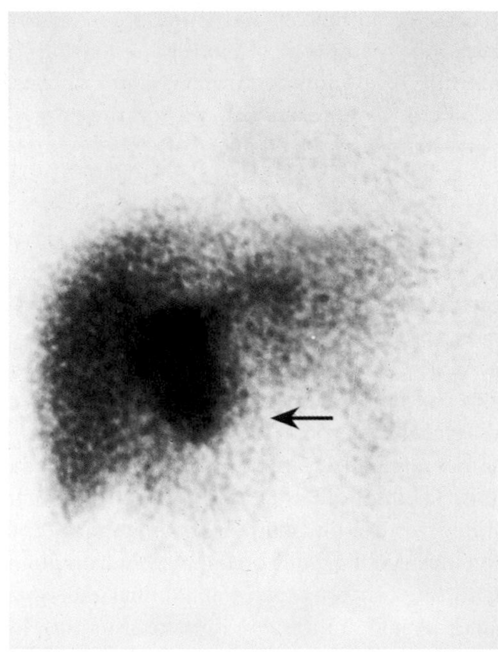

Figure 4.9 Hepatobiliary scanning with ^{99m}technetium trimethyl-1-bromoiminodiacetic acid (TEBIDA) provides good visualization of the radioisotope in a choledochal cyst (arrow), especially after pretreatment with phenobarbitone (5 mg/kg/day for 3–5 days).

Caroli disease

Caroli disease (also known as type 5 choledochal cyst) denotes congenital saccular dilations of the intrahepatic bile ducts, without hepatic fibrosis or portal hypertension. It may be limited to only one lobe of the liver, usually the left lobe. Caroli disease is rarely evident in infancy.[176] Associated jaundice may be due to acute cholangitis. Some newborn infants with severe autosomal-recessive polycystic kidney disease have extensive cystic bile duct changes, but renal insufficiency dominates the clinical picture. Ultrasound of the liver is often adequate for diagnosing Caroli disease; cholangiography is confirmatory. The outcome is related to the severity of renal disease, and/or the development of cholangitis and fibrosis with portal hypertension (Chapter 10).

Congenital hepatic fibrosis, often associated with the same bile duct abnormalities (Caroli syndrome), may present in infancy with hepatomegaly and either autosomal-recessive polycystic kidney disease or systemic hypertension. Jaundice and abnormal serum aminotransferases are uncommon.[177] The outcome is variable and depends on the progression of hepatic and renal disease (Chapter 10).

Cholelithiasis and choledocholithiasis

Choledocholithiasis was reported in four of 62 children with neonatal hepatitis syndrome.[178] Two of these infants had structural abnormalities of the extrahepatic bile ducts (correctable biliary atresia in one and choledochal cyst in the other). The stones were of the bilirubinate type. The stones were removed without difficulty with standard methods once the diagnosis was secured. Subsequent reports indicate that choledocholithiasis is not rare in infants.[179–181] Hemolysis, fasting, and total parenteral nutrition may be contributing factors, in addition to anatomical abnormalities. The obstructing gallstone may not contain enough calcium to be seen on a plain abdominal radiograph, but ultrasound usually (although not consistently) identifies the gallstone or shows dilation of the biliary tree due to obstruction.

Treatment may not be required if the stones are asymptomatic or pass into the duodenum without intervention.[182] Prolonged obstruction and cholangitis require surgery.[183,184] Alternatives to surgical treatment include ursodeoxycholic acid (20 mg/kg/day), percutaneous drainage after percutaneous transhepatic cholangiography with lavage of the bile ducts or combined with sphincterotomy in older infants.[185] Adequate antibiotic treatment is required to avoid bacterial cholangitis (Chapter 19).

Inspissated bile syndrome

"Inspissated bile syndrome" is the term traditionally given to conjugated hyperbilirubinemia complicating severe jaundice associated with hemolysis, usually due to rhesus factor or ABO incompatibility or erythrocyte membrane abnormalities.[186] A multifactorial cause cannot be entirely excluded, as these infants are often premature and present complex medical problems. Intrahepatic cholestasis is found on liver biopsy, and cholestasis may be due to direct hepatocellular toxicity of unconjugated bilirubin. The outlook is generally good, although early reports showed cirrhosis in some infants.

Obstruction of the extrahepatic biliary system with dried-out highly viscous bile has been reported in cystic fibrosis.[187,188] Diagnosis is usually made by demonstrating dilated bile ducts on ultrasound or cholangiography. Treatment includes ursodeoxycholic acid (20 mg/kg/day) or surgical or percutaneous lavage (Chapter 19).

Spontaneous perforation of the common bile duct

This condition usually presents as a severe acute illness resembling acute peritonitis with abdominal pain and distension, jaundice, and fever, but may present as neonatal hepatitis syndrome with abdominal distension in addition to jaundice and acholic stools.[189] Biliary ascites is pathognomonic. Bacterial superinfection greatly increases the morbidity of this condition. Hepatobiliary scanning may indicate the site of leakage and typically shows no drainage into the intestinal tract. In some cases, perforation is associated with distal choledocholithiasis. Surgical repair is usually curative[190] (Chapter 19).

Multiple intestinal atresias

Abnormalities of the digestive tract may be associated with neonatal hepatitis syndrome due to obstruction of extrahepatic bile ducts. These include intestinal atresias[191] and anterior abdominal wall defects.[192] Immunodeficiency syndromes may be associated.

Neonatal sclerosing cholangitis

Neonatal sclerosing cholangitis (NSC) was first described in 1987, and a few other reports followed subsequently.[193–197] Its etiology is unknown, but it may have a genetic basis.[197] Currently, the true nature of neonatal sclerosing cholangitis remains uncertain, although skepticism as to whether the entity exists is unwarranted. In one case, nonspecific autoantibodies were detected.[198] Identification of the genetic basis of a subset indicates that this is a heterogeneous clinical entity.

NSC is distinguished from childhood primary sclerosing cholangitis by the presentation in early infancy with conjugated hyperbilirubinemia, which then resolves. The clinical picture includes:

- Jaundice, which subsides within 3–6 months.[193] Although some children with childhood primary sclerosing cholangitis present as infants,[199] they have not had early cholestatic jaundice.
- Recurrent hyperbilirubinemia develops 1–2 years later or in mid-childhood (8–10 years old).
- Development of hepatosplenomegaly, biliary cirrhosis, and portal hypertension.

Laboratory investigations indicate obstructive biliary disease with elevated serum alkaline phosphatase and GGT. Endoscopic or percutaneous cholangiography demonstrates beaded irregularity of medium to large intrahepatic bile ducts in all patients, and in the extrahepatic ducts in 80%. Liver histology shows portal fibrosis with ductal proliferation, developing into biliary cirrhosis.

Surgical treatment with Kasai portoenterostomy is not indicated, but supportive management with attention to nutrition is required. The majority of children require liver transplantation at some stage.

The genetic basis of one form of NSC has been identified. Infants with neonatal ichthyosis–sclerosing cholangitis (NISCH) syndrome have mutations in the claudin-1 gene severe enough to interfere with production of claudin-1 protein and thus render tight junctions leaky. Cutaneous findings include decreased scalp hair, scarring alopecia, and ichthyosis.[200,201] Since only a few such patients have been identified, NSC must be a heterogeneous disease with more than one disease mechanism.

Hair-like bile duct syndrome

This very rare disorder is known as extrahepatic biliary hypoplasia or "hair-like bile duct syndrome."[202,203] Infants present with conjugated hyperbilirubinemia and features suggesting extrahepatic biliary atresia, but are found at laparotomy to have an intact but disproportionately small extrahepatic biliary tree. In some reports, the extrahepatic bile duct has been described as thickened. The clinical course is similar to that of neonatal sclerosing cholangitis: resolution of jaundice, development of biliary cirrhosis, progressive cholestasis with recurring jaundice, portal hypertension, and hepatic insufficiency. A Kasai portoenterostomy is not indicated for these children.

Bile duct paucity syndromes

Alagille's syndrome

Alagille's syndrome (syndromic duct paucity, Watson–Miller syndrome, arteriohepatic dysplasia) is a genetic disorder with autosomal-dominant transmission but highly variable expression. Alagille's syndrome was identified in the early 1970s[204,205] because of the unusual association of congenital heart disease—usually peripheral pulmonary artery stenosis —with neonatal cholestasis. Alagille's syndrome is thought to be rare, occurring in one in 100 000 live births. This is probably a gross underestimate, reflecting only those with disease severe enough to be recognized clinically.

Genetic basis. Contrary to the original expectation that Alagille's syndrome was due to a contiguous gene defect, it has proven to be due to mutations in genes whose gene products influence cell differentiation and tissue development. The vast majority (approximately 95%) of patients have mutations in *JAG1* (Jagged 1). Inheritance is autosomal-dominant, with essentially complete penetrance but highly variable expression, suggesting the role of genetic modifiers. There is no evidence for anticipation or imprinting in the pattern of expression. The proportion of new mutations is uncertain, estimated at 15% to 50% or more.[206,207] The gene defect has been localized to the human *JAG1* gene, which is on the short arm of chromosome 20 (specifically, 20p12).[208,209] Alagille's syndrome is genetically heterogeneous, however, and can arise with mutations in *NOTCH2*.[210]

JAG1 is the human homologue of the rat gene *Jagged 1*. It codes for a ligand of Notch 1, which is one of four members in a family of transmembrane proteins with epidermal growth factor–like motifs. Alagille's syndrome is the first childhood disorder identified with a mutation in a ligand for a Notch protein. The expression of Notch 1 and its ligand includes many of the organs potentially abnormal in Alagille's syndrome. *JAG1* is expressed in adult heart and kidney; it is not expressed in adult liver, but it is in fetal liver.[208,211] Haploinsufficiency of *JAG1* causes Alagille's syndrome. Mutations result in truncated and thus inactive proteins; residual gene expression cannot compensate, leading to the phenomenon of haploinsufficiency.[212] Various dominant negative effects may also operate in some patients.[213] Dosage of Notch ligands is critical in development, and this may contribute to the clinical diversity of Alagille's syndrome. Many mutations (approximately 70%) are sporadic. No clear relationship between genotype and phenotype has been found, although the Delta/Serrate/Lag-2 (DSL) domain in the Jag1 protein may influence the severity of liver disease.[214–217]

The disease mechanism of Alagille's syndrome is still being elucidated. The expression patterns of Jagged 1 and various Notch proteins in the portal tracts of the fetal liver suggest that they mediate the interaction of portal tract mesenchyme and hepatic arterial endothelium for ductal plate remodeling and development of intrahepatic bile ducts.[218] Zebrafish with various Jagged and Notch genes knocked down have numerous features of Alagille's syndrome, and studies suggest that Notch may promote biliary epithelial cell evolution from bipotential precursor cells.[219] Accumulating data suggest that in Alagille's syndrome, bipotential precursor cells do not progress to biliary epithelial cells[220,221] and that bile duct formation is inhibited.[222,223]

Clinical features. Alagille's syndrome is fairly benign in the majority of children. The majority of patients with clinically important Alagille's syndrome have conjugated hyperbilirubinemia in the neonatal period.[224,225] The main clinical features are as follows (Figure 4.10):

- Cholestasis, which may be sufficiently severe to produce acholic stools and dark urine.
- Characteristic facies, which consists of a broad forehead, deep-set eyes, mild hypertelorism, straight nose and small pointed chin. The facies may not be evident in the first months of life and the classic childhood appearance differs from the adult form.
- Skeletal abnormalities, which include "butterfly" vertebrae due to failure of fusion on the anterior arch of the vertebral body, are commonly found in the thoracic spine.[226] There may also be a decrease in the interpedicular distance in the lumbar spine, spina bifida occulta, short distal phalanges and fifth finger clinodactyly, and short ulna.
- Eye findings may be very diverse.[227] Posterior embryotoxon, an abnormal prominence of Schwalbe's line (junction of Descemet's membrane with the uvea at the angle of the anterior chamber), is most common and requires slit-light examination for detection. It is not pathognomonic, since it occurs in 8–15% of normal persons. Optic disk drusen, which are calcific deposits in the extracellular space of the

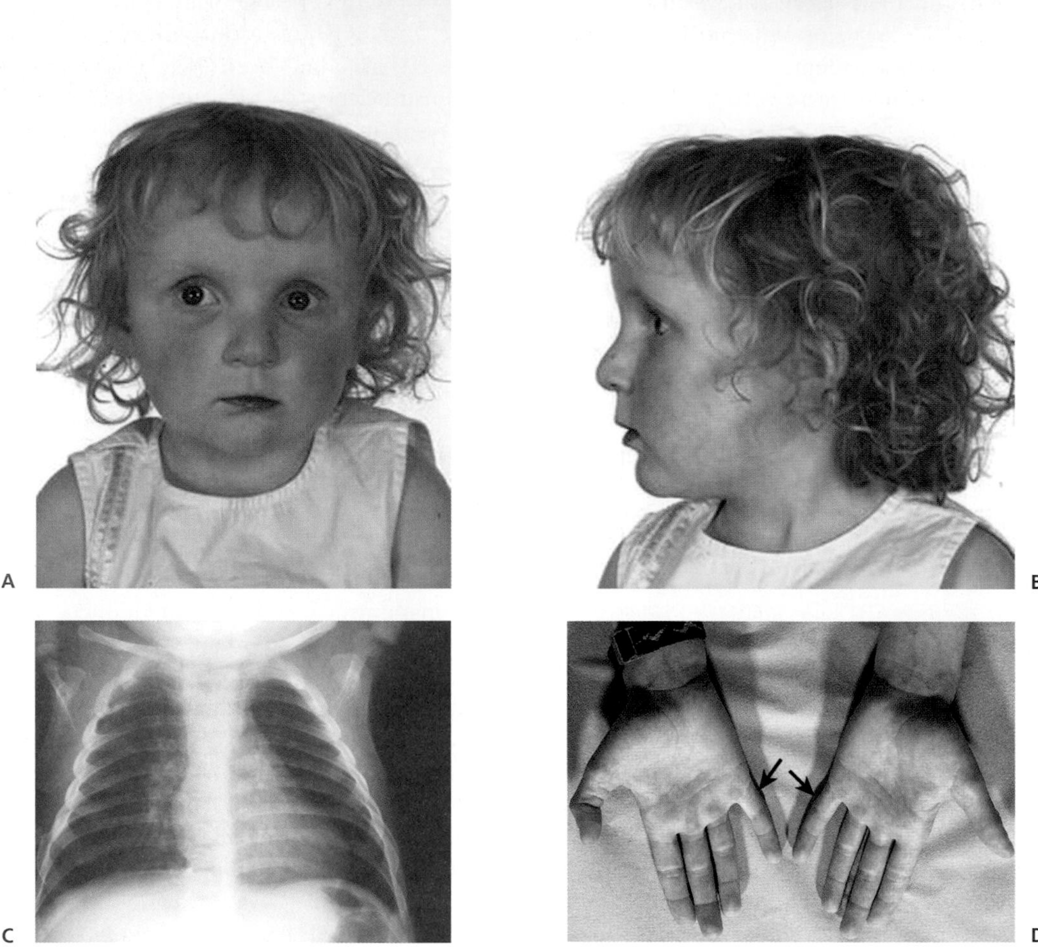

Figure 4.10 Alagille's syndrome is a genetic disorder with characteristic facies (**A**, **B**), consisting of a broad forehead, deep-set eyes, mild hypertelorism, straight nose, and a pointed chin. It is associated with skeletal abnormalities, such as butterfly vertebrae (**C**) and curved distal phalanges (**D**).

optic nerve head, are common in Alagille's syndrome and are not found in other cholestatic conditions. They are detected by ocular ultrasound examination.[228] Abnormal retinal pigmentation without evidence of functional retinal degeneration may occur. Strabismus, ectopic pupil, and hypotrophic optic disks with or without abnormal retinal vessels have also been reported.

• Cardiac disease includes peripheral pulmonary artery stenosis, severe hypoplasia of the pulmonary artery branches,[229,230] Fallot's tetralogy, pulmonary valve stenosis, aortic stenosis, ventricular septal defect, atrial septal defect and anomalous pulmonary venous return. The severity of cardiac disease varies between patients and careful assessment is required, particularly if liver transplantation is contemplated.

• Chronic cholestasis with pruritus and fat malabsorption, occasionally exacerbated by exocrine pancreatic insufficiency.

• Failure to thrive in association with intrauterine retardation.

• Severe malnutrition, present in approximately 50% of patients, may be part of the syndrome or secondary to fat malabsorption or gastroesophageal reflux.

Minor features. Apart from the main aspects of Alagille's syndrome outlined above, a number of other features may be present. These are:

• Renal disease, which includes defects in urinary concentrating function, nephrolithiasis, or structural abnormalities such as small kidneys or congenital single kidney, or renal cystic disease. Histological examination may reveal a membranous nephropathy or lipid accumulation in the kidney (mesangiolipidosis).

• Intracranial vasculopathy, which may present as catastrophic acute intracranial bleeding, with or without head trauma.[231] Some children have angiographic findings consistent with moyamoya disease.[232]

• Delayed puberty or hypogonadism.

• Abnormal cry or voice.

• Vascular anomalies, including decreased intrahepatic portal vein radicals, coarctation of the aorta and other arterial abnormalities.[233]

• Bleeding diathesis in addition to spontaneous intracerebral bleeds, despite normal coagulation profile, probably due to vascular abnormalities.[234]

• Neurological problems, such as peripheral neuropathy and disconjugate gaze, may be related to vitamin E deficiency from severe chronic cholestasis.
• Visual impairment associated with intracranial hypertension diagnosed by the development of papilledema.[235]
• Mental retardation, learning difficulties, or antisocial behavior.
• Hypothyroidism and pancreatic insufficiency.
• Recurrent otitis media.[236]
• Recurrent chest infections, perhaps secondary to gastrointestinal reflux and aspiration pneumonia.
• Xanthomas from hypercholesterolemia and other skin disorders.[237]

Diagnosis. The diagnosis of Alagille's syndrome is based on the characteristic clinical features, but laboratory investigations may indicate:
• Conjugated hyperbilirubinemia in neonates, which may improve with age.
• Serum aminotransferases and alkaline phosphatase concentrations are usually elevated (up to 10 times normal).
• γ-Glutamyltransferase (GGT) concentration elevated 3–20 times normal.
• Serum cholesterol and triglyceride may be raised to values three times the upper limit of normal.
• Serum albumin and prothrombin time are normal, except in decompensated disease.
• Abdominal ultrasound may be normal or show a small contracted gallbladder.
• Radioisotope scanning may show delayed or no excretion if intrahepatic cholestasis is severe.
• Liver biopsy classically shows reduced numbers of small (i.e., portal) bile ducts, and in neonates there may be giant cell transformation and cholestasis. It is essential to obtain a liver biopsy specimen with sufficient intact portal tracts (at least 10). In some infants (up to 20%), ongoing damage to small bile ducts may be found, or duct reaction suggestive of extrahepatic bile duct obstruction. The diagnostic histological findings may become obvious only with age.[238] Alternatively, the number of portal tracts may be reduced. Periportal or centrilobular fibrosis is usually absent in infancy, but progressive disease with biliary cirrhosis develops in 15–20% of patients. Differentiation from extrahepatic biliary atresia may be difficult on histological grounds alone, particularly if there is significant duct reaction (Figure 4.11).
• Genetic diagnosis may be required; consistent genotype–phenotype correlations have not yet been established.

Management. It is essential to exclude extrahepatic biliary atresia, which may be difficult in infants with severe cholestasis, acholic stools, and nonexcreting hepatobiliary scanning. Endoscopic or operative cholangiography may identify a patent extrahepatic biliary tree. Portoenterostomy is not indicated, as this rarely improves bile flow and may increase portal fibrosis because of recurrent cholangitis.

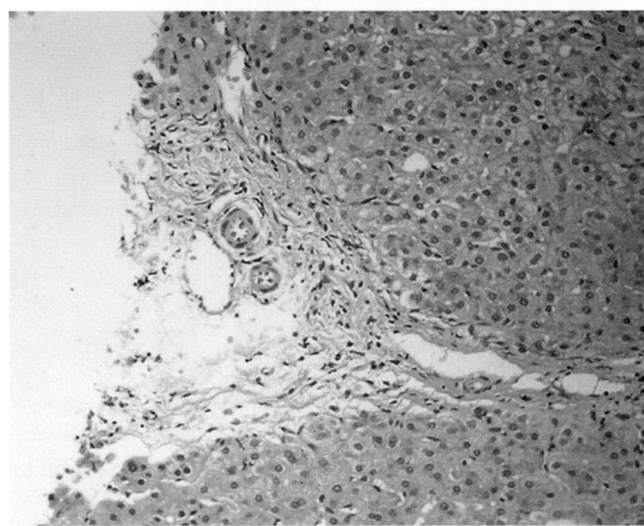

Figure 4.11 In Alagille's syndrome, liver histology demonstrates a paucity of intrahepatic bile ducts in the portal tract. In the neonate, there may be giant cell hepatitis and the bile duct paucity may not be obvious until later in life.

Specific management of Alagille's syndrome is dependent on the distribution and severity of associated disease. Severe cholestasis requires supportive management (see Chapters 15 and 25). Nutritional support with feeding via a gastric tube may be highly effective.[239] Hypercholesterolemia usually responds to a modified fat diet or cholestyramine (0.5–2.0 g/day); gastroesophageal reflux requires standard medical or surgical management. Cardiac anomalies may require corrective surgery, with balloon dilation or surgical correction of pulmonary valve or pulmonary artery stenosis. Children with Alagille's syndrome are prone to bleeding episodes, without necessarily having definite abnormalities of coagulation.[234,240] Renal disease requires specific management as indicated.

Caution must be exercised with respect to intracranial bleeding, which may occur spontaneously even when there is no coagulopathy. Head trauma and dehydration should be avoided. The risk seems to be greatest in pre-schoolers, but it can occur at any age. In view of the potential blindness with intracranial hypertension, fundoscopy should be part of routine monitoring.[235]

Outcome. The outcome of Alagille's syndrome depends on the hepatic and extrahepatic disease. The majority of children have a relatively benign course. Most estimates put the overall mortality at 20–30%, due to cardiac disease, intercurrent infection, or progressive liver disease.[225,241,242]

Hepatocellular carcinoma may complicate Alagille's syndrome, especially in older children surviving with their native liver, although hepatocellular carcinoma has been reported in infancy.[243–245] Hepatoblastoma, focal nodular hyperplasia and isolated fatty infiltration have been reported. Surveillance is appropriate, but hepatic masses require complete evaluation (see Chapter 20).

Early reports of outcome minimize the role for liver transplantation. Liver transplantation should be reserved for patients with hepatic failure, intolerable pruritus unresponsive to medical treatment, and severe growth failure. Liver transplantation can be complicated by associated heart disease, renal impairment, or vascular anomalies.[246] Catch-up growth after transplantation may occur[247–249] (Chapter 21).

Nonsyndromic duct paucity

In a full-term neonate with small bile duct paucity in whom Alagille's syndrome has been excluded, various disorders may cause portal ductopenia (small-duct paucity), known as "nonsyndromic duct paucity." These disorders (Table 4.2) fall into the broad categories of infection, genetic (with chromosomal abnormalities), and metabolic diseases.[250,251] When idiopathic neonatal hepatitis is clinically severe, bile duct paucity may also be present.

Among congenital infections, cytomegalovirus is the most important cause,[252,253] and cytomegaloviral inclusions may occasionally be found in bile duct epithelial cells. Chromosomal abnormalities associated with duct paucity include trisomy 18 and 21. Congenital syphilis can also cause duct paucity. Metabolic disorders associated with duct paucity in the infant are diverse and include α_1-antitrypsin deficiency (which usually indicates more severe liver disease and a poor prognosis), ATP8B1 (FIC-1) deficiency, and rarely cystic fibrosis or Zellweger syndrome. Duct paucity may also develop in late stages of extrahepatic biliary atresia following a Kasai portoenterostomy, or in primary sclerosing cholangitis.

Small bile duct paucity may develop in infants as a result of graft-versus-host disease[254] or other immunological injury complicating allogeneic bone-marrow transplant or a stem cell transplant in the perinatal period. Occasionally, this develops without features of graft-versus-host disease.[255]

When no specific associated condition can be found, isolated nonsyndromic bile duct paucity can be diagnosed. These children are supposed to have a less favorable outlook than children with Alagille's syndrome, with persistent severe cholestasis and progressive liver damage. The relationship of childhood nonsyndromic duct paucity to idiopathic adult ductopenia, which may be familial, remains uncertain.[256,257] Individuals with HNF-1β mutations may develop nonsyndromic duct paucity as infants, well before the constellation of features defining MODY-5 are apparent.[258] While this is probably not the genetic basis for idiopathic adult ductopenia, it establishes the possibility that a genetic mechanism or mechanisms can be defined.

Table 4.2 Causes of nonsyndromic paucity of bile ducts in infants.

Prematurity
Infection
Cytomegalovirus (CMV)
Rubella
Syphilis
Hepatitis B
Metabolic
α_1-antitrypsin deficiency
Cystic fibrosis
Zellweger syndrome
ATP8B1 deficiency (PFIC1, Byler disease)
Ivemark syndrome
Prune belly syndrome
Hypopituitarism
HNF-1β mutations
Genetic: chromosomal disorders
Trisomy 18, 21
Partial trisomy 11
Monosomy X
Immune-related: graft-versus-host disease
Severe idiopathic neonatal hepatitis
Isolated/idiopathic (? familial)

Metabolic disorders

α_1-Antitrypsin deficiency

This autosomal-recessive condition is the most common inherited cause of neonatal hepatitis syndrome. Deficiency occurs in one in 1600–2000 live births in North American and European populations, but it is less common in people of other ethnic backgrounds. The protease inhibitor, α_1-antitrypsin, is a glycoprotein that is produced mainly in the liver. Only a small proportion of individuals with α_1-antitrypsin deficiency ever develop liver disease, but it is the main cause of emphysema in early adulthood.

Etiology and genetics. A member of the serpin superfamily, α_1-antitrypsin binds and inactivates leukocyte elastase. More than 75 variants have been reported. The deficiency status is caused by a mutation in the α_1-antitrypsin gene on chromosome 14. There is impaired secretion of the mutant gene product, which can be demonstrated in the hepatocyte—with periodic acid–Schiff (PAS)-positive diastase-resistant granules. The most important deficiency variant is "Z," a slow-moving protein on electrophoresis, with a point mutation resulting in a single amino acid substitution (lysine replacing glutamic acid at position 342). Some variants such as M_{Malton} and M_{Duarte} show only subtle electrophoretic differences from the normal "M," and may be difficult to recognize.

Structural variants of α_1-antitrypsin are classified according to the protease inhibitor (PI phenotype) system. More than 75 variants have been reported, most of which are not associated with clinical disease. Inheritance is co-dominant, not autosomal-recessive. Liver disease is associated with protease inhibitor ZZ (PI ZZ) in the majority of cases. It may occur with PI SZ at a relatively young age and with PI FZ and PI MZ later in adulthood.[259]

The full pathogenesis of α_1-antitrypsin liver disease is unknown, although clearly liver injury is caused by accumulation of the abnormal α_1-antitrypsin gene product in hepatocytes. The Z and M_{Malton} mutations cause abnormal folding of the α_1-antitrypsin molecule, so that it becomes stuck in the endoplasmic reticulum.[260,261] Since not everyone with PI ZZ α_1-antitrypsin develops liver disease, additional factors such as increased production and decreased removal of abnormal α_1-antitrypsin within hepatocytes might accelerate liver damage. Because α_1-antitrypsin is an acute-phase reactant, any inflammatory process may increase its production. Defects in hepatocellular proteasome action or other mechanisms for removing abnormal proteins from the endoplasmic reticulum might account for excessive accumulation of abnormal α_1-antitrypsin in hepatocytes. New treatments are envisioned on the basis of these mechanisms, including administration of chemical chaperones.[262,263] Recent observations indicate that the protein gp78 is important for Z-variant α_1-antitrypsin degradation.[264]

Clinical features

Neonates with α_1-antitrypsin deficiency who develop liver disease present with:

- Conjugated hyperbilirubinemia (Figure 4.2).
- Intrauterine growth retardation.
- Severe cholestasis with totally acholic stools; differentiation from extrahepatic biliary atresia may be difficult. The rare infant has been reported with both α_1-antitrypsin deficiency and extrahepatic biliary atresia.[265]
- Hepatomegaly is usual at presentation, but splenomegaly is unusual unless significant hepatic fibrosis develops.

Approximately 2% of infants present with a vitamin K-responsive coagulopathy, which is more likely in those infants not given prophylactic vitamin K at birth or who are breastfed. The coagulopathy may be obvious, with bruising and bleeding from the umbilicus, or the initial presentation may be an intraventricular hemorrhage. There is a rapid response to intravenous vitamin K.

Diagnosis

Biochemical findings are typical of neonatal hepatitis syndrome. Radiological investigation may demonstrate a contracted gallbladder on abdominal ultrasound and delayed or absent excretion of radioisotope on hepatobiliary scanning.

In homozygotes, the diagnosis is confirmed by demonstrating low serum α_1-antitrypsin levels (normal > 1.0 g/L) and determining the phenotype (PI type) by isoelectric focusing. Confusion may arise if α_1-antitrypsin levels are

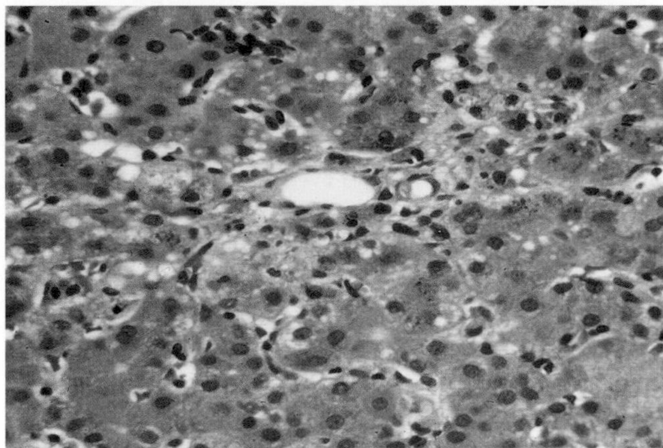

Figure 4.12 α_1-Antitrypsin deficiency can be differentiated from other causes of neonatal hepatitis by identifying periodic acid–Schiff (PAS)-positive granules of α_1-antitrypsin within hepatocytes.

increased secondary to hepatic inflammation because it is an acute-phase reactant, but in practice this is rarely a problem with homozygotes. Nevertheless, PI typing should be performed.[266] Genetic diagnosis is possible and can be facilitated.[267]

Liver biopsy typically demonstrates a giant cell hepatitis in which the characteristic PAS-positive diastase-resistant (PASD) granules are detected in the hepatocytes, often noted as early as 6–8 weeks (Figure 4.12). Occasionally, PASD-positive inclusions are found in individuals without the Z allele because of an M variant associated with hepatocellular α_1-antitrypsin retention.[268]

Management

Management consists of nutritional support, fat-soluble vitamin supplementation, treatment of pruritus, and cholestasis as required. Patients and parents should not be permitted to smoke, and PI ZZ individuals should be protected from passive smoking. It is usual to offer family screening for families wishing to have further children. Parents are obligate heterozygotes, so that there is a 25% chance of each subsequent fetus being affected. Antenatal diagnosis by chorionic villus sampling is now available using synthetic oligonucleotide probes specific for the M and Z gene, or by restriction fragment length polymorphism.[269]

Prognosis

The prognosis is variable. The long-term outlook for many infants with α_1-antitrypsin deficiency is good, although a certain proportion of infants with early jaundice develop chronic liver disease.[270] The outcome falls into four general categories.[271] Approximately half do well; of these infants, half become entirely normal and the other half have mildly abnormal serum aminotransferases but no progression of liver disease. The other half do poorly. Among the infants with a poor prognosis, half develop persisting cholestasis with progressive hepatic decompensation and may die or require live transplantation in the first year of life. In the other half, jaundice resolves, but serum aminotransferases are abnormal; the liver and spleen remain enlarged. These infants develop cirrhosis with eventual hepatic insufficiency. The few children with α_1-antitrypsin deficiency who present later in infancy or in childhood with hepatomegaly, but without any neonatal jaundice, are usually cirrhotic and have a poor prognosis.

Early prognostication of individual infants with α_1-antitrypsin deficiency is difficult. Standard indicators of hepatic decompensation—such as persistent or recurring jaundice, hepatosplenomegaly, prolonged prothrombin time (PT), and elevated serum aminotransferases—are only helpful later in the course of disease.[272] A retrospective analysis of 85 children with neonatal hepatitis and α_1-antitrypsin deficiency showed that very elevated serum alanine aminotransferase, prolonged PT, and very low serum α_1-antitrypsin concentration at presentation were associated with a poor outcome; girls generally had a worse outcome than boys.[273] In another study of children with neonatal hepatitis, persisting elevation of serum aminotransferases and serum GGT through 6–12 months of age, or presence of bile duct reaction, bridging fibrosis, or cirrhosis on the initial liver biopsy presaged rapidly progressive liver disease.[274] Infants in whom jaundice or hepatomegaly resolves before the age of 6 months are likely to have a good outcome, but those with prolonged jaundice, cirrhosis, or bile duct paucity pursue a downhill course. Infants whose liver disease appears to resolve should still be monitored for development of splenomegaly, as this may herald advancing hepatic fibrosis. Children with α_1-antitrypsin–associated cirrhosis remain stable for some time, but may decompensate precipitously. Hepatopulmonary syndrome is an indication for liver transplantation, and evaluation for transplantation should be considered early for these children. The outcome following liver transplantation is good, although attention to potential kidney disease associated with α_1-antitrypsin deficiency is required through the early postoperative period.[275]

Heterozygotes for one normal allele and a deficiency allele have no important neonatal or childhood liver disease. PI MS results in mildly decreased α_1-antitrypsin levels (approximately 80% of normal) and PI MZ levels are lower yet. With PI MZ, α_1-antitrypsin inclusions are found in the liver, and liver disease is occasionally reported.

Cystic fibrosis

Abnormalities of liver function tests or hepatic pathology are found in one-third of infants with cystic fibrosis (Chapter 12). The spectrum of hepatic disorder is highly variable, but the clinical presentation is with jaundice, hepatomegaly, and failure to thrive. Some infants have only giant cell hepatitis. Extrahepatic bile duct obstruction may be due to inspissated bile actually plugging the common bile duct;[187] the blockage can be removed by choledochotomy. Some infants have a lesion resembling that of biliary atresia, where the common hepatic and common bile ducts are apparently damaged by the abnormal bile so that portoenterostomy is required to restore bile flow.[276] Another rare lesion in cystic fibrosis in infancy is paucity of intrahepatic bile ducts ("nonsyndromic duct paucity"),[277] raising the possibility that there is an inherent abnormality in the small bile ducts in cystic fibrosis. Severe hepatic steatosis has been reported in infants with cystic fibrosis who are typically not jaundiced. In one case, carnitine deficiency was found, and the steatosis improved with carnitine supplementation.[278] One child has been reported with chronic-pattern liver failure and iron overload;[279] however, hepatic parenchymal iron tends to be increased anyway in cystic fibrosis.

Early studies suggested that infants with severe liver disease had meconium ileus, and this is supported by more recent data obtained at autopsy in patients similar with respect to pulmonary function, nutritional status, and Shwachman score.[280] Children with cirrhosis had a statistically significant relationship between the incidence of mucous plugs in liver tissue histologically and meconium ileus in infancy or distal intestinal obstruction syndrome later in life. Occurrence of neonatal hepatitis syndrome in itself does not necessarily predict early development of cirrhosis.

Bile canalicular transport disorders (Byler disease/syndrome; progressive familial intrahepatic cholestasis)

Byler disease was originally described as a disorder of intrahepatic cholestasis in an American Amish kindred named "Byler." Clinical features included pruritus, steatorrhea, poor growth, and inexorable progression to cirrhosis in early childhood.[281] Non-Amish children were later reported with similar clinical characteristics.[282–286] A prominent finding was a low or normal serum GGT, which was discordant with the severe cholestasis. Nomenclature is problematic: a more inclusive term, "progressive familial intrahepatic cholestasis" (PFIC), has been proposed for these pediatric disorders but is not entirely satisfactory. A preferable term is "bile canalicular transport disorders," especially as it has become apparent that these disorders have numerous clinical phenotypes across all age brackets. For example, intrahepatic cholestasis of pregnancy can occur in association with abnormalities in any of these genes. The two infantile disorders with low serum GGT are ATP8B1 (FIC-1) deficiency (PFIC-1) and bile salt export pump (BSEP) deficiency (PFIC-2). One disorder has high serum GGT: MDR3 deficiency (PFIC-3). Genetic diagnosis and differentiation are possible.[267,287,288] Other high-GGT disorders exist and require further definition genetically,[289] but not all of these will prove to be bile canalicular transport disorders as such.

ATP8B1 (FIC-1) deficiency (PFIC-1)

Genetics

Most patients with classic Byler disease have a mutation on chromosome 18q21-22 in ATP8B1 gene.[290,291] ATP8B1 encodes FIC-1, a P-type ATPase (ATP8B1, previously known as FIC-1) involved in aminophospholipid transport between membrane leaflets. It is phospholipid flippase. When it is deficient, changes in bile canalicular membrane occur—specifically, a loss of phospholipid asymmetry, so that bile acid transport is impaired.[292] The nuclear receptor FXR (farnesoid X-receptor) is also down-regulated, which may have adverse effects on the function of other bile canalicular transporters. Moreover, ATP8B1 is highly expressed in biliary epithelial cells, and when it is abnormal, production of bile is abnormal and CFTR is down-regulated.[293] ATP8B1 is also expressed in numerous tissues, including the gastrointestinal tract, pancreas, and lung. Inheritance is autosomal-recessive. Mutations in ATP8B1 are also responsible for Greenland Eskimo cholestasis.[294–296] Low or normal serum cholesterol is also characteristic and may identify patients reported prior to 1969.[297] Mutations in ATP8B1 are often the cause of benign recurrent intrahepatic cholestasis, a disease mainly of adults but sometimes symptomatic in childhood.[298–300] ATP8B1 mutations are associated with some cases of intrahepatic cholestasis of pregnancy.[301]

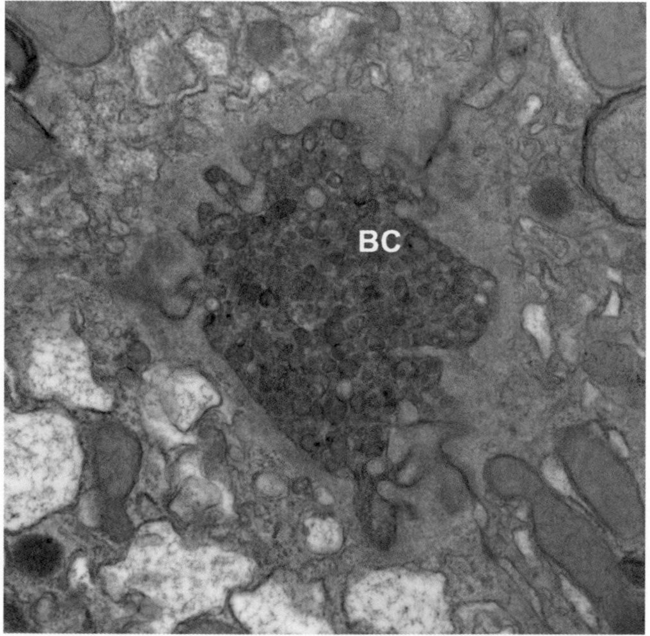

Figure 4.13 In FIC-1 deficiency (ATP8B1 deficiency; progressive familial intrahepatic cholestasis type 1, PFIC-1) abnormal particulate ("chunky') bile may be found within the lumen of the bile canaliculus by electron microscopy. Other features shown here include loss of microvilli and thickening of pericanalicular hyaloplasm. BC, bile canaliculus. (Kindly provided by Dr. Ernest Cutz, Hospital for Sick Children, Toronto)

Clinical features

ATP8B1 deficiency presents with conjugated hyperbilirubinemia in the first 3–6 months of life. The degree of jaundice may vary. Hepatomegaly persists, although the rate of progression to cirrhosis is variable. Fat-soluble vitamin deficiencies, including rickets, may be severe. Pruritus is problematic and refractory to most treatment. Growth retardation may not be evident initially. Children with ATP8B1 deficiency have extrahepatic disorders, including persistent diarrhea with fat malabsorption and protein loss, bouts of pancreatitis, and poor growth leading to short stature. Recurrent pneumonia may also compromise growth. Sensorineural hearing loss may occur. Cirrhosis usually develops in early childhood, and liver transplantation is required. After liver transplantation, pancreatitis may still occur, and the diarrhea may get worse.

Diagnosis

The serum GGT is repeatedly normal, as is serum cholesterol. The total serum bile acid concentration is elevated. However, the concentration of chenodeoxycholic acid in bile from these patients is extremely low.[282,302] Liver biopsy shows cholestasis with almost no inflammation. Canalicular bile plugs of distinctive color are found on routine hematoxylin and eosin staining, with a characteristic granular appearance on electron microscopy ("chunky bile") (Figure 4.13). Small-duct paucity may be present. The main differential diagnosis is from an inborn error of bile salt metabolism (see below).

Treatment and outcome

Many patients respond to treatment with cholestyramine and rifampicin for pruritus. Some may have excellent relief of pruritus following biliary diversion,[303] provided the procedure is performed before the development of significant hepatic fibrosis. Ursodeoxycholic acid (20 mg/kg/day) is the usual treatment, but some patients appear to have increased pruritus when treated with it. Most require liver transplantation during childhood.

BSEP deficiency (PFIC-2)

Genetics and clinical features

Some children with intrahepatic cholestasis and normal serum GGT have a mutation in a gene found on chromosome 2q24.[304] The gene encodes the human bile salt export pump (BSEP, *ABCB11*), an ATP-binding cassette transporter formerly known as sister of P-glycoprotein (SPGP).[305,306] Functional disturbances in bile salt excretion lead to clinical disease. Different mutations may cause different kinds of BSEP dysfunction, including protein lack, misfolded protein, or protein not delivered from the Golgi to the bile canalicular membrane.[307] Inheritance is autosomal-recessive. Affected children differ from those with ATP8B1 deficiency in some important respects; they do not have extrahepatic involvement such as pancreatitis or diarrhea. Cirrhosis usually develops in early childhood, and liver transplantation is required.

Diagnosis

The serum GGT is repeatedly normal. On liver biopsy, there is inflammation with giant cell hepatitis, fibrosis, and duct reaction. On electron microscopy, bile appears unremarkable. Lack of immunoperoxidase staining for BSEP protein may be found, and this supports the diagnosis (Figure 4.14).[307,308] Genetic diagnosis remains the definitive diagnostic technique.

Treatment and outcome

Routine interventions for chronic cholestatic liver disease are required. Treatment with ursodeoxycholic acid (20 mg/kg/day) appears to be beneficial. Partial biliary diversion surgery is sometimes used successfully. Although variability in the disease course is becoming evident, liver damage is often unremittingly progressive. Many patients require liver transplantation during childhood.[309] Early development of hepatocellular carcinoma in the first 5 years of life has been reported.[308] Cholangiocarcinoma was found in two children in the 5–10-year-old age bracket.[310]

MDR3 deficiency (PFIC-3)

Genetics and clinical features

A further group of children has been identified who have a bile canalicular transport disorder, with intrahepatic cholestasis but an elevated serum GGT.[311] Mutations in the P-glycoprotein MDR-3 gene (*ABCB4*) have been identified, and mutations resulting in a truncated protein appear to be associated with more severe disease than missense mutations.[312] The affected protein is the bile canalicular membrane translocator of phospholipids, known as the phospholipid export pump or translocase. Children with MDR3 deficiency have bile phospholipid concentrations which are < 15% of normal. Inheritance is autosomal-recessive. The onset may occur later in childhood, and older children may develop cholelithiasis; however, presentation in infancy is common. In children with MDR3 deficiency, jaundice may be less prominent than pruritus; despite the clinical features of biliary tract obstruction (jaundice, itching, high GGT), imaging reveals a normal biliary tree. Portal fibrosis with or without bile duct reaction is prominent on liver biopsy.

Treatment and outcome

Treatment is supportive. Treatment with ursodeoxycholic acid (20 mg/kg/day) is the usual strategy. Recent observations in a mouse model suggest that treatment with lecithin may be effective in retarding liver damage.[313] Most children with severe disease require liver transplantation during childhood. Disease expression is quite variable and includes low-phospholipid cholelithiasis in adults; heterozygote females may experience intrahepatic cholestasis of pregnancy.

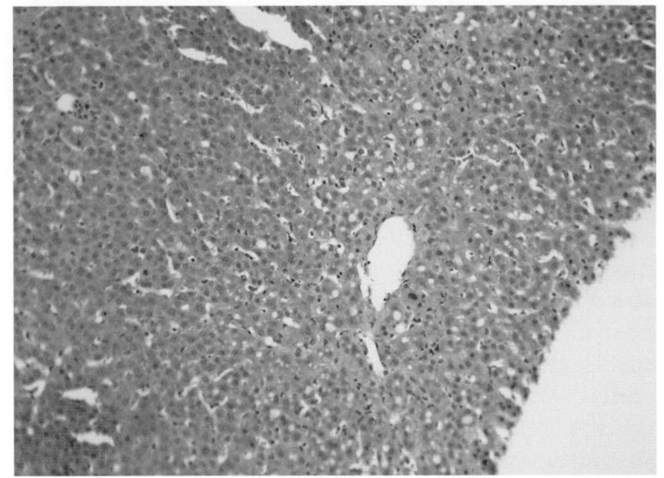
A

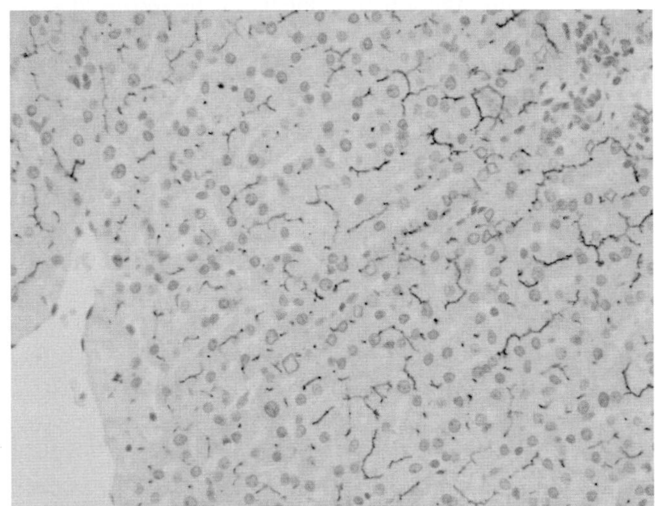
B

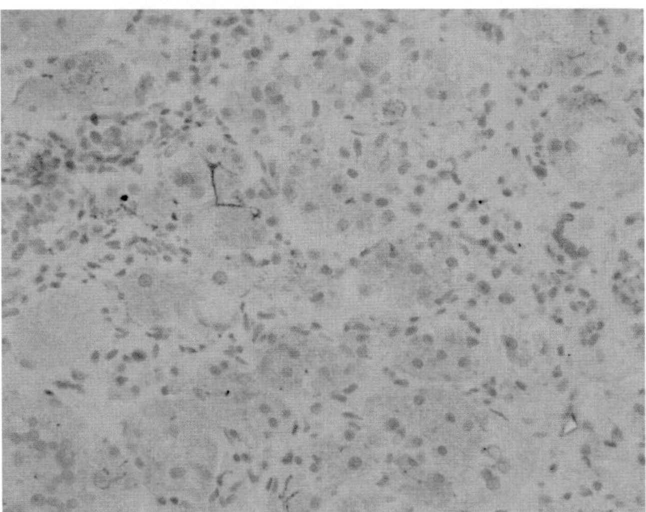
C

Figure 4.14 BSEP deficiency (Progressive familial intrahepatic cholestasis type 2, PFIC 2) presents with neonatal cholestasis and biliary hypoplasia (**A**). It is due to a defect in *ACB11*, the gene that encodes the bile salt export pump (BSEP) protein. This can now be demonstrated by immunostaining using specific antibodies to demonstrate BSEP in bile canaliculi (**B**), which are not expressed in affected patient (**C**). (Reproduced by kind permission of Dr. Alex Kniseley.[307])

Hypercholanemia

Jaundice is uncommon in infants with familial hypercholanemia: infants usually present with growth failure, fat and fat-soluble vitamin malabsorption, including rickets and bleeding diathesis. Pruritus may be prominent, with elevated serum bile acids and normal GGT. The condition is an example of oligogenic inheritance. It is due to mutations in *TJP2* (formerly known as *ZO-2*), which encodes a protein that ensures bile canalicular tight junction integrity to bile acids, but the effect of this genetic defect is enhanced when mutations in *BAAT*—which encodes bile acid coenzyme A: amino acid acyltransferase—are also present.[314] Mutations in the microsomal epoxide hydrolase gene (*EPHX1*) may also occur.[315]

North American Indian childhood cirrhosis (NAIC)

Severe chronic cholestatic liver disease was described in 14 North American Indians living in northwestern Quebec, Canada. Nine of the 14 presented with neonatal conjugated hyperbilirubinemia, and in these infants jaundice disappeared during the first year of life. Chronic cholestatic disease was similar in all 14: hepatosplenomegaly, pruritus, facial telangiectasia, and eventually portal hypertension. Serum aminotransferases, alkaline phosphatase, and bile acids were elevated, but serum cholesterol was normal in most patients. Serum GGT data were not reported. Electron microscopy revealed widening of the pericanalicular microfilament cuff, not unlike changes due to phalloidin intoxication.[316] A subsequent report indicated that most had moderate elevation of serum cholesterol and elevated GGT.[317] Liver disease typically progresses to biliary cirrhosis in this disorder, although liver transplantation is often not required in the first decade of life. The gene mutated in this disorder has recently been identified: it is *FLJ14728*, conventionally called *CIRH1A*, on chromosome 16q22.[318] Its gene product, cirhin, is a protein that was originally thought to localize to mitochondria; however, it proves to be nucleolar protein.[319]

A second, apparently different, cholestatic disease has been described in North American Indians from various regions of Ontario, Canada.[320] Most belong to a single extended kindred and presented as infants with conjugated hyperbilirubinemia and hepatomegaly; in some, jaundice was transient and chronic cholestatic disease developed later in childhood. Two unrelated North American Indian children appeared to have extrahepatic biliary atresia clinically and at laparotomy. Increased concentrations of zinc were found in hepatic parenchyma obtained at the time of liver transplantation in all patients. The pathogenesis of this zinc-overload cholestatic liver disease remains to be determined.

Citrin deficiency (citrullinemia type II)

Genetics

Citrin is a mitochondrial aspartate glutamate carrier associated with the urea cycle, encoded by the gene *SLC25A13*, found on chromosome 7q21. It is expressed mainly in the liver, also in the kidney and heart, and it is structurally similar to another protein, aralar (encoded by *SLC25A12* on chromosome 2), which is expressed in the brain and heart but not in the liver. Lack of citrin leads to liver-specific dysfunction of argininosuccinate synthetase. It plays an important role in reduced nicotinamide adenine dinucleotide (NADH) disposition, because it transports reducing equivalents into mitochondria as part of the malate aspartate shuttle, which is critical for aerobic glycolysis. In adults, this disorder—termed citrullinemia type II—presents with fatty liver, hepatitis, and iron accumulation; episodic neurological symptoms associated with hyperammonemia may also occur. Infants with type II citrullinemia typically present with NHS. This disorder has been termed "neonatal intrahepatic cholestasis with citrin deficiency" (NICCD). It occurs mainly in East Asians, but not exclusively.[321] Inheritance is autosomal-recessive. Numerous mutations have been found.[322–325]

Clinical features

The typical infant presents with jaundice and diverse metabolic abnormalities. These include defects in gluconeogenesis, aerobic glycolysis, urea synthesis and possibly in fatty acid synthesis; galactose metabolism is abnormal due to decreased UDP-galactose epimerase activity.[326] Clinically, the infant may seem to have galactosemia with increased plasma levels of galactose; plasma levels of citrulline and methionine are elevated.[327] Features of compromised liver synthetic function such as ascites and coagulopathy may be found; hypoglycemic seizures have been reported. Poor growth or outright failure to thrive is frequent. Occasionally, the infant has failure to thrive without jaundice; one such infant had a pronounced coagulation disorder.[328] Liver biopsy shows neonatal hepatitis with steatosis and iron deposition.

Diagnosis

The diagnosis should be suspected in an infant who has NHS with hypoglycemia or hypergalactosemia, and routine measurements of serum amino acids in NHS should facilitate the diagnosis. Steatosis on liver biopsy may be suggestive. Genetic screening is possible in high-risk populations.[329,330] The diagnosis can be confirmed genetically, or citrin protein can be measured in peripheral mononuclear cells.[331] Curiously, older children and adults are said to have peculiar food preferences: they avoid sweets and rice, and they prefer peanuts and beans.

Treatment and outcome

Best treatment strategies are still being established. A lactose-free formula appears to be preferable, since lactose may be cytotoxic while the infant still has NHS.[327] Cataracts have been found in some infants. A formula low in aromatic amino acids (as used for hereditary tyrosinemia type 1) may not be required. Medium chain triglycerides and fat-soluble vitamins should be supplied. A high-protein, low-carbohydrate formula has been used successfully.[328]

The NHS associated with citrin deficiency appears to resolve spontaneously in most affected infants, usually within the first year of life; however, clinical features of citrullinemia may then develop from adolescence onward.[332,333] Social drinking may provoke hepatic deterioration. Occasionally, the neonatal liver disease is very severe and progresses to liver failure, requiring liver transplantation.[327,334] Living donor transplants with a heterozygote donor appear to be successful.

Arthrogryposis, renal dysfunction, and cholestasis (ARC syndrome)

ARC syndrome includes skeletal abnormalities resembling contractures (arthrogryposis), a Fanconi-like renal tubular dysfunction, and cholestasis. Affected infants can also have ichthyosis, lissencephaly, and poor growth. It can be incomplete, in which case the arthrogryposis is not found and the infant appears to have NHS with renal tubulopathy.[335,336] This multisystemic disorder is due to germline mutations in the gene *VPS33B* on chromosome 15q26.[337] The gene product, VPS33B, helps regulate vesicular membrane fusion by interacting with soluble *N*-ethylmaleimide-sensitive fusion protein attachment receptor (SNARE) proteins; abnormal polarized membrane protein trafficking has been found in some patients with ARC.[338] This gene is similar to the zebrafish *vps18*, which influences bile canalicular membrane function.[339,340]

Affected infants may have striking ichthyosis. Hypotonia may be obvious. ARC appears to be a normal-GGT cholestatic disorder: most, though not all, infants have had a normal serum GGT.[341] The clinical phenotype of 62 ARC syndrome patients was recently analyzed.[340] In addition to the classical features described previously, all patients had severe failure to thrive, which was not adequately explained by the degree of liver disease, and 10% had structural cardiac defects. Almost half of the patients, who underwent diagnostic organ biopsy (seven of 16), developed life-threatening hemorrhage despite normal platelet count and morphology. Although liver biopsy may be informative, it can be hazardous in ARC because of intrinsic platelet dysfunction,[342] and so *VPS33B* mutation analysis should replace organ biopsy as a first-line diagnostic test for ARC syndrome. Liver histology demonstrates duct paucity with some degree of neonatal hepatitis.[341,343] The outlook for survival beyond the first year of life is poor. Liver disease may progress to cirrhosis.

Aagenaes syndrome

Aagenaes syndrome is a very rare disorder with cholestasis and lower limb edema. It was initially reported in a Norwegian kindred, but has also been reported in children of Norwegian descent and in other ethnic groups.[344–348] The principal features are neonatal hepatitis syndrome with elevated GGT, evolving to a chronic cholestatic condition and a lymphatic disorder. The lymphatic abnormalities may present clinically later than the jaundice and include localized lower-limb lymphedema—such as Milroy disease, a more subtle disorder with generalized edema despite normal serum albumin, or hemangioma(s) and/or lymphangioma(s).

The neonatal hepatitis evolves into a cholestatic problem, with pruritus and fat-soluble vitamin deficiencies that require treatment. Rapid evolution to chronic liver failure requiring liver transplantation is uncommon.[349] In most patients, the initial cholestasis resolves in early childhood, but recurrent bouts of cholestasis, similar to benign recurrent cholestasis, and lymphedema become a prominent problem in adulthood. Chronic liver disease with portal hypertension has not been reported, and life expectancy is often normal.[349] Abnormal development of hepatic lymphatics has been postulated as part of the pathogenesis of this condition. The genetic basis of this familial cholestatic disorder remains unknown, but the genetic locus has been mapped to chromosome 15q.[350]

Bile acid synthetic defects

Inherited defects in the enzymes involved in bile acid synthesis lead to neonatal hepatitis syndrome or to chronic cholestasis later in childhood. A number of new entities have been identified (Table 4.3), largely facilitated by fast atom bombardment mass spectroscopy (FAB-MS) of urine to identify unusual intermediates arising from deranged bile acid synthesis. These diseases are autosomal-recessive. Although rare (1–2% of childhood cholestatic disorders), they can be treated by supplementation of critical bile acids if the diagnosis is made early in the course of the disease.

Etiology

Bile acid synthesis involves the conversion of cholesterol to the primary bile acids, cholic and chenodeoxycholic acid. This takes place in hepatocytes, and enzymes in the process are variously located in the endoplasmic reticulum ("microsomal"), the cytoplasm ("cytosolic"), mitochondria, or peroxisomes. The initial, and rate-limiting, step is a change in the steroid nucleus: hydroxylation of cholesterol at the C_7 position by the microsomal enzyme 7α-hydroxylase. Further modifications can then be categorized as involving the steroid nucleus or the side chain. The major bile acid synthetic defect disorders involve 3β-Hydroxy-Δ^5-C_{27}-steroid dehydrogenase/isomerase (microsomal) and Δ^4-3-oxosteroid 5β-reductase (cytosolic). Side-chain abnormalities are found mainly with mitochondrial or peroxisomal disorders. Cerebrotendinous xanthomatosis is due to deficiency of the mitochondrial enzyme C_{27}-hydroxylase, leading to abnormal side-chain modifications. NHS has recently been identified in this disease.[351] NHS occurs infrequently with Smith–Lemli–Opitz disease (7-dehydrocholesterol reductase deficiency).

Autosomal-recessive mutations in two enzymes associated with steroid nucleus modifications at early stages of bile acid synthesis have been associated with severe neonatal liver

Table 4.3 Primary disorders of bile acid synthesis.

Enzyme	Cellular location	Features	Treatment
3α-Hydroxy-Δ^5-C_{27}-steroid dehydrogenase/isomerase	Endoplasmic reticulum ("microsomal")	Severe neonatal hepatitis; normal serum GGT; low serum total bile acid concentrations; no pruritus	Cholic acid ± UDCA initially
Δ^4-3-Oxosteroid 5β-reductase	Cytoplasm ("cytosolic")	Severe cholestasis, coagulopathy; elevated serum total bile acid concentrations	Cholic acid
24,25-Dihydroxycholanoic cleavage enzyme	Endoplasmic reticulum	Severe giant cell hepatitis; normal serum GGT; elevated serum cholesterol; low serum total bile acid concentrations	Cholic acid
C_{27}-Hydroxylase	Mitochondria	Cerebrotendinous xanthomatosis; rarely, liver disease	–

GGT, γ-glutamyltransferase; UDCA, ursodeoxycholic acid.

disease. Other inborn errors of bile acid metabolism have been described in single patients presenting with neonatal liver disease. An infant with NHS progressing rapidly to biliary cirrhosis with a low to normal serum GGT was found to have oxysterol 7α-hydroxylase deficiency: the liver disease did not improve with cholic acid treatment, and liver transplantation was required.[352] Rather mild NHS with profound fat-soluble vitamin deficiencies was found with deficiency of peroxisomal 2-methylacyl-CoA racemase.[353] The bile acid profile was similar to that found with Zellweger syndrome (alligator bile), and treatment with cholic acid was effective. NHS with a defect in bile acid conjugation (ligase deficiency) has also been observed.[354]

3β-Hydroxy-Δ^5-C_{27}-steroid dehydrogenase/isomerase (3βHSD) deficiency. This microsomal enzyme is the second in the bile acid synthetic pathway. Infants lacking it present with jaundice and acholic stools in the first few days of life;[355] neonatal hepatitis may be histologically severe,[356] or the cholestatic disease may be somewhat more indolent, resembling a bile canalicular transport disorder and presenting later in childhood.[357–359] One patient was described with rickets and fat-soluble vitamin deficiencies in the absence of jaundice.[360] Typically affecting infants and children, this deficiency produces excessive amounts of C_{24} bile acids with a 3α-hydroxy-β5 structure. Biochemically, they have normal serum GGT and low serum total bile acid concentrations, and clinically have no pruritus. Treatment with chenodeoxycholic acid[358,361] or ursodeoxycholic acid[359] has been reported, but the preferred treatment strategy is cholic acid with or without ursodeoxycholic acid. This may improve bile flow and prevent cirrhosis and hepatic decompensation. Chenodeoxycholic acid appears to be potentially toxic.

Δ^4-3-Oxosteroid 5β-reductase deficiency. Δ^4-3-Oxosteroid 5β-reductase is an important cytosolic enzyme in the bile acid synthetic pathway. The original description of this disorder included two infants with early severe cholestasis and coagulopathy;[362] subsequent reports have included infants with a clinical presentation of chronic-pattern neonatal liver failure resembling perinatal hemochromatosis.[363,364] In this disorder, Δ^4-3-oxo bile acids are overproduced and may be hepatotoxic. Serum GGT is usually, but not invariably, normal. Liver biopsy may reveal abnormal bile canaliculi in a focal, "mosaic" pattern. Treatment with cholic acid (with or without ursodeoxycholic acid) appears beneficial in patients without iron overload.[365,366]

There is a diagnostic subtlety in identifying patients with this genetic disorder, because hepatocellular levels of Δ^4-3-oxosteroid 5β-reductase drop with progressive severe liver disease.[367] Thus, for diagnostic reasons as well as therapeutic ones, diagnostic testing should be performed as early as possible.

24,25-Dihydroxycholanoic cleavage enzyme deficiency. Infants have been described with a defect in the 25-hydroxylase pathway[368] and excess production of a bile alcohol with an abnormal, eight-carbon side chain. Jaundice and hepatomegaly were noted in the first week of life; serum GGT was normal, but alkaline phosphatase and cholesterol were elevated; biliary and serum bile acid concentrations were low; hepatobiliary scanning showed no drainage; pruritus later developed. Liver biopsy revealed severe giant cell hepatitis with cholestasis. Treatment with chenodeoxycholic plus cholic acid appeared beneficial.

Treatment

Treatment for all bile acid synthetic defect disorders consists of nutritional support and therapy for cholestasis. The specific intervention is supplementation with specific bile acids, aimed at compensating for or unloading a defective synthetic pathway (see above). The objective is to avoid production of toxic bile acids and the need for liver transplantation.

McCune–Albright syndrome

McCune–Albright syndrome consists of café-au-lait spots, polyostotic fibrous dysplasia, and endocrine abnormalities (precocious puberty or hyperfunctioning endocrinopathy). It is due to an activating mutation in the α-subunit of the protein Gs, which increases cyclic adenosine monophosphate (cAMP) formation.[369] Several infants with neonatal hepatitis syndrome have been described,[370] and liver disease may occur in as many as 10% of those affected. Neonatal hepatitis may be severe, with a nondraining hepatobiliary scan. The serum GGT is elevated. Other features of the syndrome, notably café-au-lait spots, may not be evident in the early neonatal period. The mutation should be sought in total genomic DNA preparations or in the liver tissue. The long-term outcome of the liver disease has not been established.

Niemann–Pick disease, type A or type C

There are two types of Niemann–Pick disease (A and C) associated with neonatal liver disease. Type B is defined as a juvenile–adult form of sphingomyelinase deficiency without neurological features (see also Chapter 13).

Niemann–Pick type A

This is due to lysosomal sphingomyelinase deficiency. Clinical features include hepatosplenomegaly, failure to thrive, and progressive neurological deterioration. Jaundice is unusual. Fetal ascites has been reported.[371]

Niemann–Pick type C

Niemann–Pick type C is due to a disorder of cholesterol esterification.[372] There are two subtypes, characterized by different mutations.[373,374] Correlation of the genotype with the phenotype is complex.[375,376] The gene product of *NPC1* appears to mediate trafficking of sterols and various other substrates out of lysosomes to other subcellular compartments.[377] Numerous animal models exist for type C Niemann–Pick disease. Recent studies in a mutant mouse strain suggest that in addition to abnormal cholesterol homeostasis, peroxisomal function is impaired. This appears to develop at an early stage of the disease and may influence disease progression.[378] Some infants may have a similar pattern of disease.[379] As a cause of severe NHS, Niemann–Pick type C appears to be being diagnosed more often than previously.

Clinical features and diagnosis

Two-thirds of infants present with prolonged cholestasis, hepatomegaly, and a particularly prominent splenomegaly; some may have fetal ascites.[380,381] Chronic-pattern liver failure may occur with clinical similarities to perinatal hemochromatosis. The affected infants appear neurologically normal at birth, although subsequent motor and speech development may lag.[381–383] In one Indo-Pakistani kindred, type C Niemann–Pick disease was associated with extrahepatic biliary atresia and meconium ileus in two of three affected infants.[384] The remainder of the affected children present with isolated splenomegaly, with or without neurological symptoms.

Liver biopsy shows a histologically severe neonatal hepatitis, pericellular fibrosis, and pseudoacinar formation.[385] The diagnosis is confirmed by identifying the characteristic PASD-resistant material in Kupffer cells and hepatocytes, which may be difficult to identify in neonates (Figure 4.15A). It may be easier to detect the foamy storage cells in bone-marrow aspirate (Figure 4.15B). Neuronal storage is usually present at birth and may be demonstrated in the ganglion cells of a suction rectal biopsy, which demonstrate typically pleomorphic lamella cytoplasmic inclusions (Figure 4.16).[381]

In vitro studies of cholesterol esterification in the patient's cultured fibroblasts are definitive.

Management and prognosis

In most infants, liver disease resolves and jaundice disappears in the first year of life. Neurological symptoms become obvious by 5 years of age. Most children develop loss of upward gaze due to vertical supranuclear ophthalmoplegia, which is regarded as a pathognomonic sign. Other neurological complications include ataxia, convulsions, developmental delay, and dementia. Most children die in early adolescence from bronchial pneumonia rather than liver failure. There is no specific treatment. Low-cholesterol diets have not been effective, but OGT-918 (*n*-butyl-deoxynojirimycin, miglustat) —which inhibits glucosyltransferase, impairs the synthesis of glycosphingolipids, and crosses the blood–brain barrier—is under evaluation. Liver and bone-marrow transplantation are ineffective. Genetic counseling is essential, and antenatal diagnosis is available by chorionic villus biopsy[386] or by gene analysis.[387] A first diagnosis of Niemann–Pick type C in adults[388] raises the possibility of different outcomes for individuals who do not have early liver disease.

Williams syndrome

Neonatal hepatitis syndrome may rarely occur with Williams syndrome and may predate the development of hypercalcemia typically found. A case with bile duct paucity has been reported.[389]

Zellweger syndrome

Zellweger syndrome is the prototype of the peroxisomal biogenesis disorders, characterized by multiple abnormalities of peroxisome function. The molecular and cell biology of these disorders is complex, involving multiple *PEX* genes, which encode peroxins—proteins required for peroxisome assembly. Zellweger syndrome is most often associated with mutations in *PEX1* and *PEX6*.[390–392] Bile acid synthesis is abnormal because of selective or generalized deficiency of the peroxisomal enzymes involved in side-chain modification. In Zellweger syndrome, C_{27} bile acids accumulate; these are principally trihydroxycoprostanic acid (THCA) and dihydroxycoprostanic acid (DHCA). These would ordinarily undergo side-chain

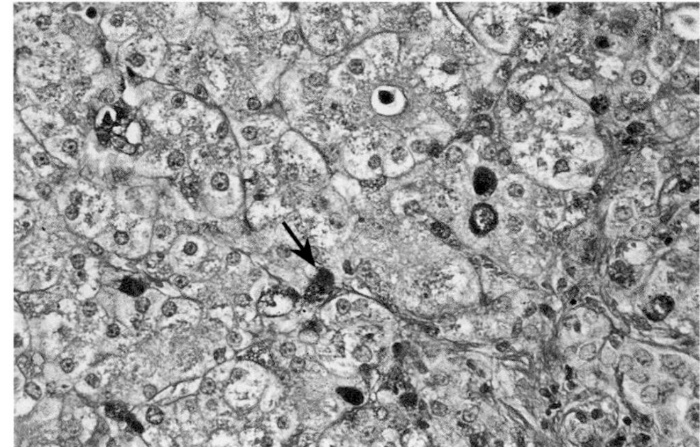
A

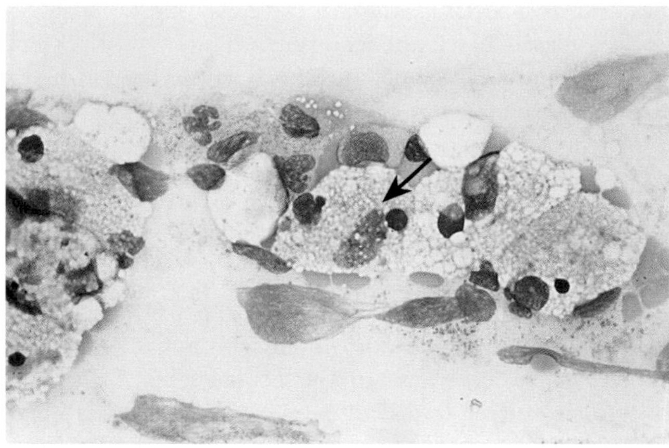
B

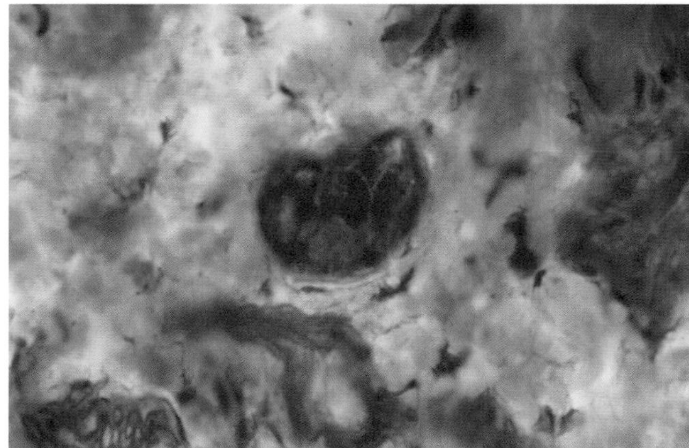
C

Figure 4.15 Niemann–Pick C typically presents with prolonged cholestasis and hepatomegaly in infancy. Foamy storage cells are difficult to see, but may be identified by experts in both Kupffer cells and hepatocytes (**A**, arrow) or in bone-marrow aspirate (**B**, arrow). **C** Neuronal storage in ganglion cells is present at birth.

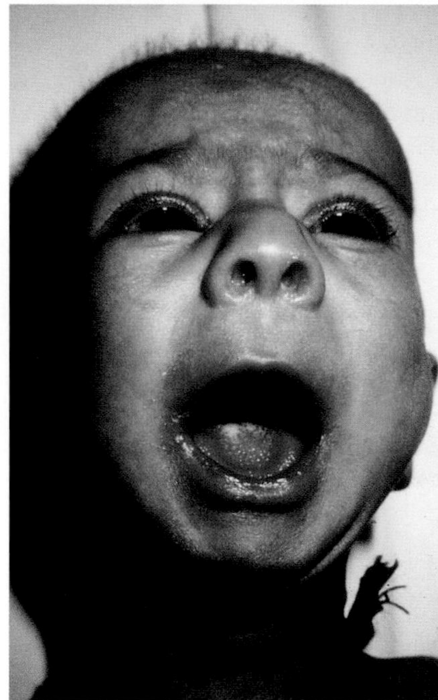

Figure 4.16 Zellweger syndrome includes profound hypotonia and facial dysmorphism, with a high forehead and large fontanelle. Note the hypotonia of the lower jaw. Most infants die within the first year of life.

modification in the peroxisome to chenodeoxycholic acid and cholic acid. It is a rare disorder, with an incidence of one in 100 000. The sexes are affected equally.

Clinical features and diagnosis

Multiple systems besides the liver are affected. Features include profound hypotonia, facial dysmorphism with a high forehead and large fontanelles, developmental delay, seizures, bony abnormalities such as epiphyseal calcifications, and cystic malformations in the brain and kidneys (Figure 4.16). Failure to thrive and feeding difficulties are common. In the first 3 months of life, hepatic involvement may not be prominent, although some babies have persistent conjugated hyperbilirubinemia.[393,394] Fifty percent of infants are not jaundiced but have hepatosplenomegaly with evidence of poor hepatic synthetic function.

The diagnosis is confirmed by demonstrating abnormal bile salt metabolites using FAB-MS, or by the detection of very long-chain fatty acids in serum. Hepatic histology may be normal, although there may be excess iron deposition. Hepatic fibrosis is typical. Paucity of the small (portal) bile ducts may be found. Electron-microscopic studies of the liver reveal an absence of peroxisomes in the hepatocytes. Mitochondria may appear abnormal. These infants may develop cirrhosis, although extrahepatic features of the syndrome typically overshadow the hepatic disease.

Treatment and outcome

Treatment is supportive, as death is inevitable. Liver transplantation is contraindicated because of the multisystem disease. Primary bolus therapy with cholic and chenodeoxycholic acid may produce some initial improvement, but does not prolong life.[395]

Wolman disease

Wolman disease and the associated milder condition, cholesterol ester storage disease, are both due to deficiency of lysosomal acid lipase (also known as acid esterase, cholesterol esterase, or sterol esterase). Inheritance is autosomal-recessive; some mutations in the lysosomal acid esterase gene capable of causing severe functional deficiency have been identified.[396] Babies with Wolman disease are not usually jaundiced but have deranged liver function, hepatosplenomegaly, persistent diarrhea, and poor growth; calcified adrenal glands are found radiologically. The majority die in early infancy. Bone-marrow transplantation was curative in one infant.[397]

Gaucher disease

Although this is rarely associated with neonatal hepatitis syndrome, an infant has been described with neonatal Gaucher disease and cholestasis, as well as prominent thrombocytopenia.[398]

Mucopolysaccharidoses

Neonatal hepatitis syndrome is unusual with most forms of mucopolysaccharidosis. It has also been reported with type VI mucopolysaccharidosis, Maroteaux–Lamy disease, in which the lysosomal enzyme arylsulfatase B is abnormal.[399] The infant also had typical facies and a cherry-red spot. Type VII mucopolysaccharidosis (β-glucuronidase deficiency) has also been reported with NHS.[400]

Toxic injury

Total parenteral nutrition-associated cholestasis

Progressive cholestasis in infants receiving total parenteral nutrition without any enteral nutrition occurs mainly in critically ill infants who are premature or have a low birth weight or are suffering from repeated sepsis.

Etiology

Total parenteral nutrition-associated cholestasis is more likely to develop in very premature infants who require a long duration of exclusive total parenteral nutrition (TPN) to meet nutritional needs. Severe gastrointestinal disease (such as recurrent necrotizing enterocolitis, gastroschisis, or intestinal atresias), with recurrent septicemia, surgical resection(s), or short gut syndrome is a difficult situation, since these infants cannot avoid protracted use of total parenteral nutrition. An important factor is the immaturity of the liver. The more premature the infant, the more underdeveloped are hepatocellular mechanisms of bile formation, predisposing to the development of total parenteral nutrition-associated cholestasis. Factors that amplify this physiological inefficiency by interfering with enterohepatic circulation of bile acids may contribute to the pathogenesis of the cholestasis. Depending on the gestational age, fetal patterns of bile acid biosynthesis may persist; synthesis of the toxic bile acid, lithocholic acid, may be higher than in older infants.

Fasting interrupts the enterohepatic circulation, diminishes the output of gut hormones needed for normal hepatobiliary function, and may promote small-bowel overgrowth by bacteria that are capable of producing endotoxin or modifying endogenous bile acids to more toxic chemicals. Bacterial translocation may occur, especially if there is a short gut. All these mechanisms are compounded by systemic factors such as hypoxia or hypoperfusion, localized infection, or septicemia, and medications used to treat these sick infants. Specific nutritional deficiencies may also play a role—lack of taurine, essential fatty acids, carnitine, and antioxidants such as vitamin E, selenium, and glutathione.[401] The possible benefits of providing supplemental taurine in the parenteral nutrition formulation remain unproven.

It is not clear whether specific components in the total parenteral nutrition solution are toxic. High concentrations of amino acids do not necessarily promote more rapid protein synthesis and may be toxic to hepatocytes. Data regarding the inherent toxicity of intravenous lipid preparations are conflicting;[402] however, accumulation of lipofuscin in Kupffer cells appears to be due mainly to the lipid component. Some sources of lipid may be tolerated better than others.[403] Vitamins in the parenteral formulation may oxidize and become toxic.[404] This has not been shown to initiate cholestatic liver damage,[405] but it may lead to hepatic steatosis.[406]

Recurrent septicemia accelerates the progression of total parenteral nutrition-associated cholestatic liver damage, possibly by further down-regulating bile canalicular transporters. Septicemia is frequently related to problems with central venous access.

Clinical features and diagnosis

Most infants present with conjugated hyperbilirubinemia and hepatomegaly in the context of prolonged parenteral nutrition. Cholestasis may be so severe that the stools are acholic, and the condition has to be differentiated from extrahepatic biliary tract obstruction. Serum aminotransferases, alkaline phosphatase, and GGT are usually elevated, whereas albumin and coagulation times are usually normal unless affected by extrahepatic disease.

The diagnosis is relatively straightforward. A careful history, mapping out feeding history, all other medications, and intercurrent illnesses is essential. Other causes of neonatal hepatitis syndrome should be considered and excluded. Abdominal ultrasound may be normal or demonstrate a contracted gallbladder. If cholestasis is severe, excretion on a hepatobiliary scan may be delayed or absent. Liver biopsy shows cholestasis with hepatocellular necrosis, abundant lipofuscin, some fatty infiltration, mild giant cell transformation, portal inflammatory infiltrate, and some bile duct reaction,

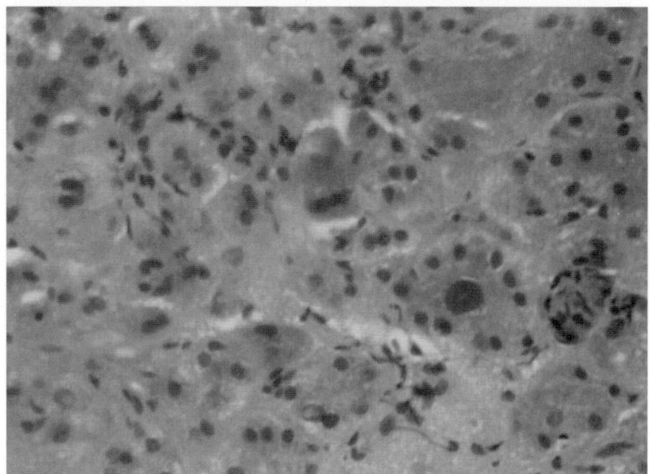

Figure 4.17 The early histological changes that take place in total parenteral nutrition cholestasis are centrilobular cholestasis without inflammation, necrosis, or fatty infiltration. Fibrosis is a late sign.

with or without portal fibrosis (Figure 4.17). Electron microscopy may reveal cholesterol crystals in hepatocytes.

Treatment

Treatment is empirical. If possible, some oral nutrition should be introduced: even dextrose in water given in very small boluses (2–5 mL) every few hours is beneficial. Oral or nasogastric feeding with a highly digested formula should be commenced concurrent with continued total parenteral nutrition. The components of the total parenteral nutrition solution should be reviewed carefully to ensure that amino acid requirements are being met but not exceeded and that essential fatty acids and trace metals are supplied. Taurine and carnitine can be supplemented. Protecting the total parenteral nutrition solution from light, and cycling total parenteral nutrition administration are other simple strategies. Extreme care to avoid central venous catheter sepsis is critically important. There may be benefit from treating small-bowel overgrowth with metronidazole, although no controlled trials are available; metronidazole is preferable to gentamicin. Erythromycin may be beneficial to improve intestinal motility and enteral tolerance.[407] Once some oral intake is established, ursodeoxycholic acid (20 mg/kg/day) may promote bile flow and improve cholestasis, but there are few reports in children.[408]

An emerging therapy is the provision of omega-3 fatty acids (fish oil) intravenously. Improvement in the degree of cholestasis has been reported,[409] but reports are still very preliminary. Whether hepatic fibrosis is decreased or not remains an unanswered question.

In general, recovery is slow, unless parenteral nutrition can be discontinued. Infants totally dependent on total parenteral nutrition because of massive bowel dysfunction due to severe inherited disorders of motility or short gut syndrome will develop progressive liver disease, cirrhosis, and portal hypertension, which may be exacerbated by intercurrent portal vein thrombosis. Cirrhosis may be averted by either innovative bowel surgery or successful intestinal transplantation, and this should be considered at an early stage before a combined liver–intestine transplant may be needed (Chapter 22).

Other complications of total parenteral nutrition

Other complications of total parenteral nutrition include: generation of "biliary sludge" (material appreciated by sonography as echogenic, resembling a stone but without typical acoustic shadowing);[410] cholelithiasis;[411,412] or acalculous cholecystitis[413] (Chapter 19). Extensive abdominal surgery leading to short gut syndrome or resection of the ileocecal valve, as well as longer duration of parenteral nutrition, may predispose to biliary tract disease. Regular ultrasound examination of the biliary tree at 4–6-week intervals during prolonged use of total parenteral nutrition may be of value in such patients. Spontaneous resolution of gallstones sometimes occurs in infancy, and thus surveillance of the asymptomatic infant is often appropriate, instead of immediate surgery.[179]

Drug-induced hepatotoxicity

Drug hepatotoxicity as a cause of neonatal hepatitis syndrome is poorly documented. Prolonged chloral hydrate administration is associated with conjugated hyperbilirubinemia in newborns, without other signs of liver toxicity.[414] Fluconazole may cause conjugated hyperbilirubinemia in preterm infants.[415] Octreotide has been associated with cholestasis.[416]

Cholelithiasis in infants has been attributed to certain drug therapies, including prolonged use of furosemide[411,417] or various antibiotics such as ceftriaxone.[418,419] Without choledocholithiasis, jaundice is unusual.

Prenatal exposure to drugs has been implicated in NHS in some infants. This has been reported with coumarin.[420] Drug exposure might occur via breast milk, which has been reported for carbamazepine.[421,422]

Immune causes

Neonatal lupus erythematosus

Neonatal lupus erythematosus is due to passage of maternal anti-Ro and anti-La antibodies across the placenta, leading to damage to fetal tissues, which express Ro and La antigenic determinants. Other susceptibility factors remain undefined. The heart, skin, and liver are most likely to be involved, rarely with thrombocytopenia and leukopenia.[423] Congenital heart block is the most dramatic cardiac manifestation. A rash resembling discoid lupus erythematosus may be present in the newborn period or may develop some weeks later. Hepatic involvement, evident in approximately 10% of cases, is often limited to elevated serum aminotransferases, but neonatal hepatitis syndrome is found.[424,425] Occasionally this is severe enough to mimic extrahepatic biliary tract obstruction, with acholic stools and nondraining hepatobiliary scan.[426] In severe cases, a clinical phenotype of neonatal hemochromatosis may be found.[427] Deposits of associated antibodies (anti-Ro and/or anti-La) may be found in affected liver tissue on immunofluorescence.[428] Transient unexplained isolated conjugated hyperbilirubinemia in the perinatal period, and later presentation at 2–3 months of age with transient elevations of serum aminotransferases, are other possible clinical presentations.[429] In most infants, the liver disease resolves completely between 6 and 12 months of age, as the maternal antibodies are degraded. Mild fibrosis was found in one child on repeat liver biopsy.

The diagnosis of neonatal lupus erythematosus is difficult in the child who does not have congenital heart block, a typical skin rash, or a history of maternal systemic lupus erythematosus or Sjögren syndrome. The risk of neonatal lupus erythematosus in subsequent pregnancies appears variable, estimated at 10–50%.

Autoimmune hemolytic anemia with giant cell hepatitis

This condition is rare and poorly defined, as only about 20 children with this disorder have been reported. Most are infants aged 6–24 months or more. Pallor, jaundice, and hepatosplenomegaly are the important clinical findings. The autoimmune hemolytic anemia is Coombs-positive, but autoantibodies typical of autoimmune hepatitis are not present.[430] Viral studies are generally negative, although it is possible that the disease is related to syncytial giant cell hepatitis, attributed to paramyxoviral infection.[102] Liver biopsy reveals extensive giant cell transformation with fibrosis. Some patients have responded to treatment with prednisolone and azathioprine,[431] but the disease has frequently been refractory to immunosuppressive treatment and may recur following liver transplantation.

Miscellaneous causes

Vascular disorders

Budd–Chiari syndrome

Budd–Chiari syndrome is rarely diagnosed in infants,[432–434] but may be due to endophlebitis from a venous catheter or associated with neoplasia, septicemia, or fungal infection;[435] membranous obstruction of the inferior vena cava probably represents previous thrombosis of the vessel. A prothrombotic disorder may be present.[436] Hepatic vein thrombosis may rarely occur due to other intra-abdominal congenital abnormalities.[437] Affected children usually have hepatomegaly, splenomegaly, or ascites; jaundice is more common in infants.

Budd–Chiari syndrome must be differentiated from veno-occlusive disease, in which the vascular blockage is at the level of the terminal hepatic venules, as opposed to larger hepatic veins. Veno-occlusive disease is rarely reported in infants, although an infant with congenital leukemia developed veno-occlusive disease after treatment with antineoplastic drugs.

Severe congestive heart failure

The role of chronic passive congestion, or functional hepatic venous obstruction, in neonatal hepatitis syndrome is difficult to assess. Babies with severe chronic congestive heart failure may develop moderate hepatomegaly or hepatosplenomegaly, as well as ascites. Jaundice is uncommon (Chapter 16). Infants with acute circulatory failure associated with severe congenital heart disease or shock may develop elevated serum aminotransferases, coagulopathy, and jaundice with mild to moderate conjugated hyperbilirubinemia,[438] which resolves rapidly once hepatic perfusion is restored.

Neonatal asphyxia

Neonatal conjugated hyperbilirubinemia with mild elevations of aminotransferases is associated with severe neonatal asphyxia.[439–441] In these series, conjugated hyperbilirubinemia developed within 6 days of birth, and was protracted. Hepatobiliary scanning showed bile drainage. In other infants, the serum aminotransferase profile was characteristic of ischemic hepatitis.[442] Spontaneous resolution typically occurs. Infants who develop hemodynamically significant tachyarrhythmias during gestation may have neonatal hepatitis syndrome, which generally resolves spontaneously. Those with fetal atrioventricular block appear to have a very poor prognosis, sometimes with neonatal liver failure.[443]

Neoplasia

Primary hepatic neoplasms rarely present with the neonatal hepatitis syndrome, although mesenchymal hamartoma may present with hyperbilirubinemia in the neonatal period (Chapter 20). Rhabdomyosarcoma of the biliary tree rarely presents in infancy, but jaundice and acholic stools are the major clinical features. Hepatoblastoma occasionally presents under 6 months of age and should be differentiated from a hemangioma, particularly as the α-fetoprotein is elevated in the neonate. However in normal neonates it will fall rapidly, but will continue to rise in infants with hepatoblastoma.

Any neoplasm that obstructs bile flow may cause jaundice.[444] Langerhans cell histiocytosis is associated with sclerosing cholangitis in children and may present in early infancy with jaundice.[445] Jaundice rarely occurs with neuroblastoma, erythrophagocytic lymphohistiocytosis, or neonatal leukemia. Systemic juvenile xanthogranuloma has been reported with neonatal hepatitis.[446]

Consequences of cholestasis

Many infants with neonatal liver disease will have a mild

Table 4.4 Consequences of chronic cholestasis and cirrhosis.

Etiology	Clinical manifestations
Reduced excretion of bilirubin, bile acids	Pruritus, jaundice
Fat malabsorption	Steatorrhea, loss of fat stores
Essential fatty acid deficiency	Peeling skin rash
Vitamin A deficiency	Conjunctival and corneal drying, abnormal retinal function, night blindness
Vitamin E deficiency	Peripheral neuropathy, ophthalmoplegia, ataxia, hemolysis
Vitamin D deficiency	Osteopenia, rickets, fractures
Vitamin K deficiency	Bruising, epistaxis, coagulopathy
Hypercholesterolemia	Xanthomas
Increased protein catabolism	Muscle wasting, motor development delay, growth failure

self-limiting disease, but those children with progressive disease, or following unsuccessful Kasai portoenterostomy, will develop significant fat malabsorption with consequent protein malnutrition. It is important to establish baseline anthropometric examinations in order to detect and prevent early malnutrition. This is best evaluated by using a combination of weight (which may be imprecise because of fluid retention), height (which may be useful for assessing chronic malnutrition), triceps skin fold (to evaluate fat stores), and mid-arm muscle area (to evaluate protein stores). Mid-arm circumference is a reliable marker of malnutrition in children under 5 years old.

The effects of chronic cholestasis are extensive: failure of biliary excretion of bilirubin, bile salts, and cholesterol leads to jaundice, pruritus, and xanthomas; a decrease in bile salts in the intestine leads to malabsorption of long-chain triglycerides and consequent fat malnutrition. Malabsorption of fat-soluble vitamins is inevitable (Table 4.4). If cirrhosis develops, then protein malnutrition and muscle wasting are likely.

Management of neonatal liver disease

Management should be supportive and, whenever possible, definitive. Disorders for which specific medical or surgical therapies are available are summarized in Table 4.5.

Nutritional support

The main aim of nutritional support is to provide sufficient caloric intake to reverse or prevent fat malabsorption and protein malnutrition. In biliary atresia, resting energy expenditure runs approximately 30% higher than in normal infants of the same age and sex.[447] An aggressive approach to feeding is therefore required, including nasogastric supplementation if oral feeding cannot meet caloric needs.[448] Increased energy expenditure is not the only cause of malnutrition; anorexia, behavioral feeding, and gastroesophageal reflux are additional reasons, particularly in Alagille's syndrome.

Infants with severe cholestatic jaundice require special formulas to ensure that calorie intake is 120–150% of the estimated average requirement (EAR), using either a standard infant formula with appropriate supplements or a modular feed in which individual constituents can be added according to requirement. A nearly elemental formula containing medium-chain triglyceride (MCT), which can be absorbed regardless of the luminal concentrations of bile acids, is preferable. Caloric density can be increased further by concentrating the formula or adding starch powder (glucose polymer). If the infant is breastfeeding satisfactorily, this should be encouraged with supplementation using a highly digestible high-caloric-density formula. Since their metabolism is somewhat deranged, providing increased amounts of branched-chain amino acids may improve nutritional status.[449,450] Deficiency of essential fatty acids may occur with prolonged cholestasis after maternal stores are depleted approximately 3 months after birth. It may also develop in infants who receive feeds that are high in MCT, so all feeds need to include some long-chain fat (Chapter 15).

Fat-soluble vitamin supplementation

All infants with chronic cholestasis, whether jaundiced or not, require supplementation with fat-soluble vitamins. Clinical deficiency of vitamin A may require special assessment with electroretinograms.[451] Deficiency in vitamin K is related to cholestasis with abnormal coagulation status.[452] These vitamins can be provided as water-soluble preparations of vitamins A, D, E, and K given orally,[448,452] or less commonly as parenteral supplementation (Table 4.6). Vitamin levels should be monitored to ensure adequate absorption and prevent toxicity.

Vitamin A. This is provided in a water-soluble preparation. Toxic levels may lead to hepatic fibrosis or pseudotumor cerebri.

Vitamin D. This is provided as 1,25-dihydroxyvitamin D or 25-hydroxyvitamin D.[453] Vitamin D production in the skin can be enhanced through sunlight or sunlamp exposure, even for babies who are jaundiced.[454] Absorption of water-soluble vitamin D may be enhanced by simultaneous administration of an α-tocopheryl polyethylene glycol succinate formulation of vitamin E.[455]

Vitamin E. Vitamin E transferred via the placenta to the fetus may keep the infant replete until the age of 3 months, but

Table 4.5 Neonatal hepatitis syndrome: specific treatments.

Disease	Major diagnostic strategy
Infection	
Toxoplasmosis	Spiramycin
Cytomegalovirus	Ganciclovir, if severe
Herpes simplex	Acyclovir
Enteric virus	Pleconaril
Syphilis	Penicillin
Bacterial infection elsewhere (sepsis)	Appropriate antibiotic(s)
Tuberculosis	Quadruple antitubercular therapy (no ethambutol)
Syncytial giant cell hepatitis	Ribavirin (unproven benefit)
Endocrine	
Panhypopituitarism (septo-optic dysplasia)	Corticosterone, thyroxine, growth hormone
Structural	
Extrahepatic biliary atresia	Kasai portoenterostomy by 100 days old (preferably)
Choledochal cyst	Surgical resection
Choledocholithiasis	Surgical removal
Spontaneous perforation of CBD	Surgical repair
Metabolic	
Bile canalicular transport disorders	Ursodeoxycholic acid; rifampicin
Galactosemia	Lactose-free formula uridyltransferase
Tyrosinemia	NTBC, low-tyrosine formula
Hereditary fructosemia	Fructose-free diet
Citrin deficiency; citrullinemia, type II	Lactose-free low-protein high-carbohydrate formula
Primary defects in bile acid synthesis	Bile acid supplementation
Toxic	
TPN-associated cholestasis	Enteral feeding; metronidazole; ursodeoxycholic acid
Drug-induced	Stop causative drug
Immune	
Neonatal hepatitis with autoimmune hemolytic anemia	Prednisolone + azathioprine

CBD, common bile duct; NTBC, 2-(2-nitro-4-trifluoromethylbenzoyl)-1,3-cyclohexanedione (nitisinone); TPN, total parenteral nutrition.

Table 4.6 Oral regimens for supplementation of fat-soluble vitamins in infants with chronic cholestasis.

Vitamin	Regimen	Features of toxicity
A	Water-soluble preparation 5000–25 000 units/day	Hepatotoxicity; pseudotumor cerebri; dermatitis
D	Vitamin D 800–5000 units/day or 25-hydroxyvitamin D_3 3–5 mg/kg/day	Hypercalcemia: lethargy, cardiac arrhythmia, nephrocalcinosis
E	TPGS 15–25 IU/kg/day or α-tocopheryl 25–200 IU/day	(None known) (Polyethylene glycol: hyperosmolarity if renal impairment)
K	2.5 mg twice per week 5 mg daily	(Clotting diathesis?)

TPGS, α-tocopheryl polyethylene glycol succinate.

the sufficiency of maternal stores varies from baby to baby. Most babies require supplementation after 2 months of age, or earlier if the baby was born preterm. Vitamin E linked to polyethylene glycol 1000 through succinate linkage (α-tocopheryl polyethylene glycol succinate, TPGS), has the best bioavailability in severe cholestasis,[456,457] as its absorption depends on simple passive absorption of polyethylene glycol independent of bile acids in the intestinal lumen. This formulation is not universally available, and the more traditional oral supplement vitamin E acetate may not be as effectively absorbed.

Vitamin K. Coagulation should be monitored closely in all infants with cholestasis, who should receive oral vitamin K prophylactically. Infants receiving rifampicin for pruritus should receive extra vitamin K.

Other dietary measures

It is reasonable to place an infant with conjugated hyperbilirubinemia on lactose-free formula until the results of testing for galactosemia are known; however, interrupting breastfeeding is problematic. Brief use of a more restrictive diet is sometimes justifiable: an infant with severe neonatal hepatitis syndrome might be placed on a lactose-free/low-protein formula (to minimize aromatic amino acid intake) until the results of tests for both galactosemia and hereditary tyrosinemia type I are available.

Special diets are used lifelong for children with inborn errors of carbohydrate and amino acid metabolism. Supplementation with specific bile acids may arrest liver damage in inborn errors of bile acid metabolism.[366]

Pruritus

Pruritus due to severe cholestasis interferes with the infant's sleep and compromises quality of life. It is often difficult to treat; local measures such as nonperfumed skin cream may help. For infants with some duct patency and bile flow, medical therapy includes:

- Cholestyramine (0.5–4 g/day) is effective but unpalatable. The mechanism of action is to bind bile salts in the intestinal lumen, thus interrupting the enterohepatic circulation and reducing bile salt concentration. Side effects include malabsorption of fat-soluble vitamins and drugs, folic acid deficiency, constipation and acidosis. Cholestyramine can cause intestinal obstruction or hypernatremia in small infants; adequate fluids must be given with it.
- Ursodeoxycholic acid (UDCA) may be effective when given at a dosage of 20–30 mg/kg/day. It is thought to have a choleretic action, but is not universally effective. UDCA may transiently increase pruritus.
- Phenobarbitone (5–10 mg/kg/day) may stimulate bile salt–independent bile flow and decrease jaundice and control pruritus. However, it is relatively ineffective, causes sedation, and may exacerbate rickets.
- Biliary diversion may be effective in some conditions, including PFIC and Alagille's syndrome.[458,459] Ileal exclusion is a newly described alternative,[460] which avoids an ostomy and can be reversed.
- Rifampicin (5–10 mg/kg/day) relieves pruritus in at least 50% of cases, producing a significant improvement in the remainder.[461] The results are variable and experience in young infants is limited.[462,463] Rifampicin induces certain cytochromes P450 in hepatocytes, and it is an agonist for pregnane X receptor (PXR).[464,465] It thus has multiple actions on bile acid disposition and metabolism. Side effects include hepatotoxicity in 5–10% of cases and thrombocytopenia. It appears to be well tolerated and effective in adults.[466,467] The urine may turn an orange-red color.
- Phototherapy with infrared or ultraviolet radiation may improve pruritus if given for 3–10 min daily.
- Antihistamines are largely ineffective, but as they cause drowsiness, they may be useful at night. Toxic side effects include cardiac dysrhythmias.

Family and psychological support

Specific attention to the infant's developmental needs is beneficial. Physiotherapy may improve gross motor development, while infant stimulation programs enhance mental development in infants who require frequent hospitalization. Family education and support are essential, particularly for children with progressive illness requiring liver transplantation.

Indications for liver transplantation

The indications for liver transplantation are severe cholestasis, failure to thrive not responsive to intensive nutrition, decompensated liver disease, and intractable pruritus (Chapter 21). With emerging data on the occurrence of hepatocellular carcinoma in some metabolic conditions causing NHS, liver tumors are also an indication. Orthotopic liver transplantation is often the only definitive treatment for severe infantile liver disease, and it can be performed safely in the first year of life,[468–470] especially if nutrition has been maintained well. In those who are malnourished, including patients with Alagille's syndrome, catch-up growth occurs after liver transplantation.[248,471] Heterozygous living donors can often be utilized safely for metabolic diseases.[40,472] The roles of hepatocyte transplantation and gene transfer therapies for genetic disorders causing the neonatal hepatitis syndrome require further clarification.

Inherited disorders of bilirubin conjugation

These rare disorders are characterized by benign conjugated hyperbilirubinemia and an unexplained abnormality of coproporphyrin metabolism. Clinical features include jaundice, which may be exacerbated by stress, intercurrent illness, pregnancy, and oral contraceptives. There are no other clinical or laboratory features of liver disease. The diagnosis is made as described below.

Dubin–Johnson syndrome

Dubin–Johnson syndrome is due to mutations in the human gene *MRP2* (equivalent to *ABCC2*), which encodes the bile canalicular membrane transporter for anion conjugates.[473,474] (Some initial reports used the term "canalicular multispecific organic anion transporter" or cMOAT for this transporter.) Numerous mutations have been described, most of which cause functional deficits though defects in protein maturation and localization.[475,476] Neonatal hepatitis syndrome has been reported rarely in Dubin–Johnson syndrome.[477,478] Treatment of severely affected neonates with ursodeoxycholic acid may be beneficial. Diagnosis is hampered by the difficulty of recognizing the typical melanin-containing pigment in the liver during infancy, as little accumulates until later in childhood. Sulfobromophthalein sodium retention in the serum at 45 min is generally between 10% and 20%. Coproporphyrin excretion in urine is normal, but the ratio of coproporphyrin III to coproporphyrin I is reversed, with coproporphyrin I accounting for > 75% of the total urinary coproporphyrins.[479] Abdominal computed tomography showing high attenuation in the liver may provide important supporting evidence for the diagnosis in an infant.[480] Liver histology in older children demonstrates a typical melanin-containing pigment, which is found predominantly in the centrolobular region.

Rotor syndrome

Rotor syndrome is also characterized by conjugated hyperbilirubinemia without cholestasis, but does not have pigment accumulation in the liver. The pathogenesis of Rotor syndrome remains unclear, but it is related to a defect in bilirubin secretion. It does not appear to be a variant genetic defect affecting *ABCC2*.[481] Neonatal hepatitis syndrome has not been reported in infants with Rotor syndrome. The diagnosis is made by estimating the sulfobromophthalein sodium retention in serum, which is 30–50% at 45 min after injection, or by measuring urinary coproporphyrin excretion, which is generally increased, with a particular increase in coproporphyrin I. No treatment is required for either disorder, apart from reassurance.

Case history

An infant girl presented at the age of 2 months with jaundice. She had been born at term after a pregnancy that was apparently normal, except that the mother had contracted malaria during the pregnancy and had been treated with chloroquine. Uncomplicated premature rupture of membranes occurred. The infant weighed 2400 g and appeared normal. Oral vitamin K was given at birth. Jaundice was first noted when she was 3–4 weeks old, but the physical examination was normal and breastfeeding was continued. She developed bruising and poor feeding.

The physical examination at presentation showed jaundice, hepatomegaly, and bruising over her back and chest. Laboratory tests:

- Hemoglobin 8.3 g/L (baby A+ and mother B+, Coombs test negative)
- Total bilirubin 172 μmol/L, conjugated bilirubin 85 μmol/L
- AST 522 U/L (upper limit of normal: 115 U/L)
- ALT 132 U/L (upper limit of normal: 60 U/L)
- Alkaline phosphatase (ALP) 500 U/L (upper limit of normal: 550 U/L)
- GGT 600 U/L (upper limit of normal: 250 U/L)
- Albumin 37 g/L
- Glucose 4.0 mmol/L (normal)
- International normalized ratio (INR) 4.0 (normal 1.0), which corrected on intravenous vitamin K 2 mg

TORCH screen and serological tests for hepatitis B and C were all negative.

Urine culture was negative; urinary succinylacetone was negative.

Liver ultrasonography showed an enlarged liver and spleen, but the gallbladder was not seen well. Hepatobiliary scanning showed suboptimal uptake, but no excretion of tracer into the gastrointestinal tract after 24 h.

A liver biopsy was performed, which showed a moderate degree of giant cell transformation of hepatocytes; periodic acid–Schiff (PAS)–positive granules were seen in the hepatocytes, consistent with α_1-antitrypsin deficiency (see Figure 4.12).

The α_1-antitrypsin level was 0.3 g/L (normal 1.0–2.0) and the phenotype was PI ZZ.

She was treated with nutritional support and fat-soluble vitamins. She became less jaundiced in time, but developed hepatosplenomegaly. She developed decompensated liver disease at the age of 4 and underwent successful transplantation.

Comment. This infant had α_1-antitrypsin deficiency, which presented with severe cholestasis and vitamin K–responsive coagulopathy. Breastfed infants with cholestasis of any cause are prone to develop vitamin K deficiency, because breast milk contains very little vitamin K. This is exacerbated by prophylaxis with oral vitamin K, which is malabsorbed. It is effectively prevented by administering intramuscular vitamin K (1 mg) at birth.

α_1-Antitrypsin deficiency may develop with severe cholestasis similar to biliary atresia, and it is important to differentiate the conditions. Rarely, they may coexist. The diagnosis is confirmed by histology and measurement of the level and phenotype. Children with severe cholestasis at birth often have a poorer prognosis and require liver transplantation in childhood.

References

1 Keffler S, Kelly DA, Powell JE, Green A. Population screening for neonatal liver disease: a feasibility study. *J Pediatr Gastroenterol Nutr* 1998;**27**:306–11.

2 Maisels MJ, Gifford K, Antle CE, Leib GR. Jaundice in the healthy newborn infant: a new approach to an old problem. *Pediatrics* 1988;**81**:505–11.

3 Kaplan M, Muraca M, Hammerman C, *et al.* Imbalance between production and conjugation of bilirubin: a fundamental concept in the mechanism of neonatal jaundice. *Pediatrics* 2002;**110**:e47.

4 Kaplan M, Hammerman C, Rubaltelli FF, *et al.* Hemolysis and bilirubin conjugation in association with UDP-glucuronosyltransferase 1A1 promoter polymorphism. *Hepatology* 2002;**35**: 905–11.

5 Burchell B, Hume R. Molecular genetic basis of Gilbert's syndrome. *J Gastroenterol Hepatol* 1999;**14**:960–6.

6 Akaba K, Kimura T, Sasaki A, *et al.* Neonatal hyperbilirubinemia and a common mutation of the bilirubin uridine diphosphate-glucuronosyltransferase gene in Japanese. *J Hum Genet* 1999; **44**:22–5.

7 Kaplan M, Beutler E, Vreman HJ, *et al.* Neonatal hyperbilirubinemia in glucose-6-phosphate dehydrogenase-deficient heterozygotes. *Pediatrics* 1999;104(1 Pt 1):68–74.

8 Tan KL. Comparison of the effectiveness of phototherapy and exchange transfusion in the management of non-hemolytic neonatal hyperbilirubinemia. *J Pediatr* 1975;**87**:609–12.

9 Brown AK, Kim MH, Wu PY, Bryla DA. Efficacy of phototherapy in prevention and management of neonatal hyperbilirubinemia. *Pediatrics* 1985;**75** (Suppl):393–400.

10 Yeung CY. Kernicterus in term infants. *Austral Paediatr J* 1985; **21**:273–4.

11 Rubaltelli FF, Guerrini PG, Reddi E, Jori G. Tin-protoporphyrin in the management of children with Crigler–Najjar disease. *Pediatrics* 1989;**84**:728–31.

12 Galbraith RA, Drummond GS, Kappas A. Suppression of bilirubin production in the Crigler–Najjar type 1 syndrome: studies with the heme oxygenase inhibitor tin-mesoporphyrin. *Pediatrics* 1992;**89**:175–82.

13 Wolf MJ, Beunen G, Casaer P, Wolf B. Extreme hyperbilirubinaemia in Zimbabwean neonates: neurodevelopmental outcome at 4 months. *Eur J Pediatr* 1997;**156**:803–7.

14 Jalili F, Garza C, Huang CTL, Nichols BL. Free fatty acids in the development of breast milk jaundice. *J Pediatr Gastroenterol Nutr* 1985;**4**:435–40.

15 Gourley GR, Arend RA. β-Glucuronidase and hyperbilirubinaemia in breast-fed and formula-fed babies. *Lancet* 1986;**i**:644–6.

16 De Carvalho M, Robertson S, Klaus M. Fecal bilirubin excretion and serum bilirubin concentrations in breast-fed and bottle-fed infants. *J Pediatr* 1985;**107**:786–90.

17 Monaghan G, McLellan A, McGeehan A, *et al.* Gilbert's syndrome is a contributory factor in prolonged unconjugated hyperbilirubinemia of the newborn. *J Pediatr* 1999;**134**:441–6.

18 Lascari AD. "Early" breast-feeding jaundice: clinical significance. *J Pediatr* 1986;**108**:156–8.

19 Weldon AP, Danks DM. Congenital hypothyroidism and neonatal jaundice. *Arch Dis Child* 1972;**47**:469–71.

20 Bleicher MA, Reiner MA, Rapaport SA, Track NS. Extraordinary hyperbilirubinemia in a neonate with idiopathic hypertrophic pyloric stenosis. *J Pediatr Surg* 1979;**14**:527–9.

21 Labrune P, Myara A, Huguet P, Trivin F, Odievre M. Jaundice with hypertrophic pyloric stenosis: a possible early manifestation of Gilbert syndrome. *J Pediatr* 1989;**115**:93–5.

22 Trioche P, Chalas J, Francoual J, *et al.* Jaundice with hypertrophic pyloric stenosis as an early manifestation of Gilbert syndrome. *Arch Dis Child* 1999;**81**:301–3.

23 Assenat E, Gerbal-Chaloin S, Larrey D, *et al.* Interleukin 1beta inhibits CAR-induced expression of hepatic genes involved in drug and bilirubin clearance. *Hepatology* 2004;**40**:951–60.

24 Aono S, Yamada Y, Keino H, *et al.* Identification of defect in the genes for bilirubin UDP-glucuronosyl-transferase in a patient with Crigler–Najjar syndrome type II. *Biochem Biophys Res Comm* 1993;**197**:1239–44.

25 Labrune P, Myara A, Hadchouel M, *et al.* Genetic heterogeneity of Crigler–Najjar syndrome type I: a study of 14 cases. *Hum Genet* 1994;**94**:693–7.

26 Koshy A, Bosma PJ, Oude-Elferink RP. Crigler–Najjar syndrome type 1 associated with combined 1070A—>G, Q357R and (TA)7 mutation in Kuwaiti Bedouin families indicate a founder effect in Arabs. *J Clin Gastroenterol* 2004;**38**:465–7.

27 Petit FM, Gajdos V, Parisot F, *et al.* Paternal isodisomy for chromosome 2 as the cause of Crigler–Najjar type I syndrome. *Eur J Hum Genet* 2005;**13**:278–82.

28 Seppen J, Bosma PJ, Goldhoorn BG, *et al.* Discrimination between Crigler–Najjar type I and II by expression of mutant bilirubin uridine diphosphate-glucuronosyltransferase. *J Clin Invest* 1994;**94**:2385–91.

29 Guldutuna S, Langenbeck U, Bock KW, Sieg A, Leuschner U. Crigler–Najjar syndrome type II. New observation of possible autosomal recessive inheritance. *Dig Dis Sci* 1995;**40**: 28–32.

30 Huang CS, Tan N, Yang SS, Sung YC, Huang MJ. Crigler–Najjar syndrome type 2. *J Formos Med Assoc* 2006;**105**:950–3.

31 Sinaasappel M, Jansen PLM. The differential diagnosis of Crigler–Najjar disease, types I and II, by bile pigment analysis. *Gastroenterology* 1991;**100**:783–9.

32 Lee WS, McKiernan PJ, Beath SV, *et al.* Bile bilirubin pigment analysis in disorders of bilirubin metabolism in early infancy. *Arch Dis Child* 2001;**85**:38–42.

33 Hughes-Benzie R, Uttley DA, Heick HM. Crigler–Najjar syndrome type I: management with phototherapy crib mattress. *Arch Dis Child* 1993;**69**:470.

34 Kappas A, Drummond GS, Manola T, Petmezaki S, Valaes T. Sn-Protoporphyrin use in the management of hyperbilirubinemia in term newborns with direct Coombs-positive ABO incompatibility. *Pediatrics* 1988;**81**:485–97.

35 McDonagh AF. Purple versus yellow: preventing neonatal jaundice with tin-porphyrins. *J Pediatr* 1988;**113**:777–81.

36 Strauss KA, Robinson DL, Vreman HJ, Puffenberger EG, Hart G, Morton DH. Management of hyperbilirubinemia and prevention of kernicterus in 20 patients with Crigler–Najjar disease. *Eur J Pediatr* 2006;**165**:306–19.

37 Fox IJ, Chowdhury JR, Kaufman SS. Treatment of the Crigler–Najjar syndrome type I with hepatocyte transplantation. *N Engl J Med* 1998;**338**:1422–6.

38 Dhawan A, Mitry RR, Hughes RD. Hepatocyte transplantation for liver-based metabolic disorders. *J Inherit Metab Dis* 2006;**29**:431–5.

39 Wagner M, Halilbasic E, Marschall HU, *et al.* CAR and PXR agonists stimulate hepatic bile acid and bilirubin detoxification and elimination pathways in mice. *Hepatology* 2005;**42**:420–30.

40 Morioka D, Takada Y, Kasahara M, *et al.* Living donor liver transplantation for noncirrhotic inheritable metabolic liver diseases: impact of the use of heterozygous donors. *Transplantation* 2005;**80**:623–8.

41 Bosma PJ, Chowdhury JR, Bakker C, *et al.* The genetic basis of the reduced expression of bilirubin UDP-glucuronosyltransferase 1 in Gilbert's syndrome. *N Engl J Med* 1995;**333**:1171–5.

42 Monaghan G, Ryan M, Seddon R, Hume R, Burchell B. Genetic variation in bilirubin UPD-glucuronosyltransferase gene promoter and Gilbert's syndrome. *Lancet* 1996;**347**:578–81.

43 Costa E, Vieira E, Martins M, *et al.* Analysis of the UDP-glucuronosyltransferase gene in Portuguese patients with a clinical diagnosis of Gilbert and Crigler–Najjar syndromes. *Blood Cells Mol Dis* 2006;**36**:91–7.

44 Cebecauerova D, Jirasek T, Budisova L, *et al.* Dual hereditary jaundice: simultaneous occurrence of mutations causing Gilbert's and Dubin–Johnson syndrome. *Gastroenterology* 2005;**129**:315–20.

45 Bancroft JD, Kreamer B, Gourley GR. Gilbert syndrome accelerates development of neonatal jaundice. *J Pediatr* 1998;**132**: 656–60.

46 Roy-Chowdhury N, Deocharan B, Bejjanki HR, *et al.* Presence of the genetic marker for Gilbert syndrome is associated with increased level and duration of neonatal jaundice. *Acta Paediatr* 2002;**91**:100–1.

47 Maruo Y, Nishizawa K, Sato H, Doida Y, Shimada M. Association of neonatal hyperbilirubinemia with bilirubin UDP-glucuronosyltransferase polymorphism. *Pediatrics* 1999;**103**: 1224–7.

48 Maruo Y, Nishizawa K, Sato H, Sawa H, Shimada M. Prolonged unconjugated hyperbilirubinemia associated with breast milk and mutations of the bilirubin uridine diphosphate-glucuronosyltransferase gene. *Pediatrics* 2000;**106**:E59.

49 Sutomo R, Laosombat V, Sadewa AH, *et al.* Novel missense mutation of the *UGT1A1* gene in Thai siblings with Gilbert's syndrome. *Pediatr Int* 2002;**44**:427–32.

50 Kitsiou-Tzeli S, Kanavakis E, Tzetis M, Kavazarakis E, Galla A, Tsezou A. Gilbert's syndrome as a predisposing factor for idiopathic cholelithiasis in children. *Haematologica* 2003;**88**:1193–4.

51 Powell JE, Keffler S, Kelly DA, Green A. Population screening for neonatal liver disease: potential for a community-based programme. *J Med Screen* 2003;**10**:112–6.

52 Suchy FJ, Balistreri WF, Heubi JE, Searcy JE, Levin RS. Physiologic cholestasis: elevation of the primary serum bile acid concentrations in normal infants. *Gastroenterology* 1981;**80**: 1037–41.

53 Balistreri WF, Heubi JE, Suchy FJ. Immaturity of the enterohepatic circulation in early life: factors predisposing to "physiologic" maldigestion and cholestasis. *J Pediatr Gastroenterol Nutr* 1983;**2**:346–54.

54 Lichtman S, Guzman C, Moore DL, Weber JL, Roberts EA. Morbidity after percutaneous liver biopsy. *Arch Dis Child* 1987; **62**:901–4.

55 Armstrong L, Isaacs D, Evans N. Severe neonatal toxoplasmosis after third trimester maternal infection. *Pediatr Infect Dis J* 2004;**23**:968–9.

56 Hart MH, Kaufman SS, Vanderhoof JA, *et al.* Neonatal hepatitis and extrahepatic biliary atresia associated with cytomegalovirus infection in twins. *Am J Dis Child* 1991;**145**:302–5.

57 Binder ND, Buckmaster JW, Benda GI. Outcome for fetus with ascites and cytomegalovirus infection. *Pediatrics* 1988;**82**: 100–3.

58 Sun CCJ, Keene CL, Nagey DA, Hepatic fibrosis in congenital cytomegalovirus infection: with fetal ascites and pulmonary hypoplasia. *Pediatr Pathol* 1990;**10**:641–6.

59 Schleiss MR. Role of breast milk in acquisition of cytomegalovirus infection: recent advances. *Curr Opin Pediatr* 2006;**18**: 48–52.

60 Neuberger P, Hamprecht K, Vochem M, *et al.* Case–control study of symptoms and neonatal outcome of human milk-transmitted cytomegalovirus infection in premature infants. *J Pediatr* 2006;**148**:326–31.

61 Chang MH, Huang HH, Huang ES, Kao CL, Hsu HY, Lee CY. Polymerase chain reaction to detect human cytomegalovirus in livers of infants with neonatal hepatitis. *Gastroenterology* 1992;**103**:1022–5.

62 Tarr PI, Haas JE, Christie DL. Biliary atresia, cytomegalovirus, and age at referral. *Pediatrics* 1996;**97**:828–31.

63 Fischler B, Ehrnst A, Forsgren M, Orvell C, Nemeth A. The viral association of neonatal cholestasis in Sweden: a possible link between cytomegalovirus infection and extrahepatic biliary atresia. *J Pediatr Gastroenterol Nutr* 1998;**27**:57–64.

64 Domiati-Saad R, Dawson DB, Margraf LR, Finegold MJ, Weinberg AG, Rogers BB. Cytomegalovirus and human herpesvirus 6, but not human papillomavirus, are present in neonatal giant cell hepatitis and extrahepatic biliary atresia. *Pediatr Dev Pathol* 2000;**3**:367–73.

65 Barbi M, Binda S, Caroppo S. Diagnosis of congenital CMV infection via dried blood spots. *Rev Med Virol* 2006;**16**:385–92.

66 Zuppen CW, Bui HD, Grill BG. Diffuse hepatic fibrosis in congenital cytomegalovirus infection. *J Pediatr Gastroenterol Nutr* 1986;**5**:489–91.

67 Le Luyer B, Menager V, Le Roux P, *et al.* [Neonatal cytomegalovirus infection with development of liver fibrosis; in French.] *Arch Fr Pediatr* 1990;**47**:361–4.

68 Ghishan FK, Greene HL, Halter S, Barnard JA, Moran JR. Noncirrhotic portal hypertension in congenital cytomegalovirus infection. *Hepatology* 1984;**4**:684–6.

69 Alix D, Castel PY, Gouedard H. Hepatic calcification in congenital cytomegalic inclusion disease. *J Pediatr* 1978;**92**:856.

70 Conboy TJ, Pass RF, Stagno S, *et al.* Early clinical manifestations and intellectual outcome in children with symptomatic congenital cytomegalovirus infection. *J Pediatr* 1987;**111**:343–8.

71 Vancíková Z, Kucerová T, Pelikán L, Zikmundová L, Priglová M. Perinatal cytomegalovirus hepatitis: to treat or not to treat with ganciclovir. *J Paediatr Child Health* 2004;**40**:444–8.

72 Miller DR, Hanshaw JB, O'Leary DS, Hnilicka JV. Fatal disseminated herpes simplex virus infection and hemorrhage in the neonate. *J Pediatr* 1970;**76**:409–15.

73 Benador N, Mannhardt W, Schranz D, *et al.* Three cases of neonatal herpes simplex infection presenting as fulminant hepatitis. *Eur J Pediatr* 1990;**149**:555–9.

74 Meerbach A, Sauerbrei A, Meerbach W, Bittrich HJ, Wutzler P. Fatal outcome of herpes simplex virus type 1-induced necrotic hepatitis in a neonate. *Med Microbiol Immunol* 2006;**195**:101–5.

75 Fidler KJ, Pierce CM, Cubitt WD, Novelli V, Peters MJ. Could neonatal disseminated herpes simplex virus infections be treated earlier? *J Infect* 2004;**49**:141–6.

76 Yarlagadda S, Acharya S, Goold P, Ward DJ, Ross JD. A syphilis outbreak: recent trends in infectious syphilis in Birmingham, UK, in 2005 and control strategies. *Int J STD AIDS* 2007;**18**: 410–2.

77 Filippi L, Serafini L, Dani C, *et al.* Congenital syphilis: unique clinical presentation in three preterm newborns. *J Perinat Med* 2004;**32**:90–4.

78 Hossain M, Broutet N, Hawkes S. The elimination of congenital syphilis: a comparison of the proposed World Health Organization action plan for the elimination of congenital syphilis with existing national maternal and congenital syphilis policies. *Sex Transm Dis* 2007;**34**(7 Suppl):S22–30.

79 Dorfman DH, Glaser JH. Congenital syphilis presenting in infants after the newborn period. *N Engl J Med* 1990;**323**:1299–302.

80 Feldman S. Varicella zoster infections of the fetus, neonate and immunocompromised child. *Adv Pediatr Infec Dis* 1986;**1**:99–115.

81 Yu HR, Huang YC, Yang KD. Neonatal varicella frequently associated with visceral complications: a retrospective analysis. *Acta Paediatr Taiwan* 2003;**44**:25–8.

82 Balistreri WF, Tabor E, Gerety RJ. Negative serology for hepatitis A and B viruses in 18 cases of neonatal cholestasis. *Pediatrics* 1980;**66**:269–71.

83 Watson JC, Fleming DW, Borella AJ, Olcott ES, Conrad RE, Baron RC. Vertical transmission of hepatitis A resulting in an outbreak in a neonatal intensive care unit. *J Infect Dis* 1993;**167**:567–71.

84 Klein BS, Michaels JA, Rytel MW, Berg KG, Davis JP. Nosocomial hepatitis A. A multinursery outbreak in Wisconsin. *JAMA* 1984;**252**:2716–21.

85 Noble RC, Kane MA, Reeves SA, Roeckel I. Posttransfusion hepatitis A in a neonatal intensive care unit. *JAMA* 1984;**252**: 2711–5.

86 Dupuy JM, Frommel D, Alagille's D. Severe viral hepatitis type B in infancy. *Lancet* 1975;**i**:191–4.

87 Mollica F, Musumeci S, Fischer A. Neonatal hepatitis in five children of a hepatitis B surface antigen carrier woman. *J Pediatr* 1977;**90**:949–51.

88 Shiraki K, Yoshihara BN, Sakurai M, Acute hepatitis B in infants born to carrier mothers with the antibody to the hepatitis B e antigen. *J Pediatr* 1980;**97**:768–70.

89 Delaplane D, Yogev R, Crussi F, Shulman ST. Fatal hepatitis B in early infancy: the importance of identifying HBsAg positive pregnant women and providing immunoprophylaxis to their newborns. *Pediatrics* 1983;**72**:176–80.

90 A-Kader HH, Nociki MJ, Kuramoto KI, Baroudy B, Zeldis JB, Balistreri WB. Evaluation of the role of hepatitis C virus in biliary atresia. *Pediatr Infect Dis J* 1994;**13**:657–9.

91 Chang MH, Lee CY, Chen DS. Minimal role of hepatitis C virus infection in childhood liver diseases in an area hyperendemic for hepatitis B infection. *J Med Virol* 1993;**40**:322–5.

92 Godfried MH, Boer K, Beuger S, Scherpbier HJ, Kuijpers TW. A neonate with macrosomia, cardiomyopathy and hepatomegaly born to an HIV-infected mother. *Eur J Pediatr* 2005;**164**:190–2.

93 Witzleben CL, Marshall GS, Wenner W, Piccoli DA, Barbour SD. HIV as a cause of giant cell hepatitis. *Hum Pathol* 1988;**19**: 603–5.

94 Persaud D, Bangaru B, Greco MA, *et al.* Cholestatic hepatitis in children infected with the human immunodeficiency virus. *Pediatr Infect Dis J* 1993;**12**:492–8.

95 Essary LR, Vnencak-Jones CL, Manning SS, Olson SJ, Johnson JE. Frequency of parvovirus B19 infection in nonimmune hydrops fetalis and utility of three diagnostic methods. *Hum Pathol* 1998;**29**:696–701.

96 Silver MM, Hellmann J, Zielenska M, Petric M, Read S. Anemia, blueberry-muffin rash, and hepatomegaly in a newborn infant. *J Pediatr* 1996;**128**:579–86.

97 Metzman R, Anard A, DeGiulo P, Knisely AS. Hepatic disease associated with intrauterine parvovirus B19 infection in a newborn premature infant. *J Pediatr Gastroenterol Nutr* 1989;**9**: 112–4.

98 Langnas AN, Markin RS, Cattral MS, Naides SJ. Parvovirus B19 as a possible causative agent of fulminant liver failure and associated aplastic anemia. *Hepatology* 1995;**22**:1661–5.

99 White FV, Jordan J, Dickman PS, Knisely AS. Fetal parvovirus B19 infection and liver disease of antenatal onset in an infant with Ebstein's anomaly. *Pediatr Pathol* 1995;**15**:121–9.

100 Asano Y, Yoshikawa T, Suga S, Yazaki T, Kondo K, Yamanishi K. Fatal fulminant hepatitis in an infant with human herpesvirus-6 infection. *Lancet* 1990;**335**:862–3.

101 Aita K, Jin Y, Irie H, *et al.* Are there histopathologic characteristics particular to fulminant hepatic failure caused by human herpesvirus-6 infection? A case report and discussion. *Hum Pathol* 2001;**32**:887–9.

102 Phillips MJ, Blendis LM, Poucell S, *et al.* Syncytial giant cell hepatitis: sporadic hepatitis with distinctive pathology, severe clinical course and paramyxoviral features. *N Engl J Med* 1991;**324**:455–60.

103 Sussman NL, Finegold MJ, Barish JP, Kelly JH. A case of syncytial giant-cell hepatitis treated with an extracorporeal liver assist device. *Am J Gastroenterol* 1994;**89**:1077–82.

104 Hicks J, Barrish J, Zhu SH. Neonatal syncytial giant cell hepatitis with paramyxoviral-like inclusions. *Ultrastruct Pathol* 2001;**25**: 65–71.

105 Roberts E, Ford-Jones EL, Phillips MJ. Ribavirin for syncytial giant cell hepatitis. *Lancet* 1993;**341**:640–1.

106 Modlin JF. Fatal echovirus 11 disease in premature neonates. *Pediatrics* 1980;**66**:775–9.

107 Gillam GL, Stokes KB, McLellan J, Smith AL. Fulminant hepatic failure with intractable ascites due to an echovirus 11 infection successfully managed with a peritoneo-venous (LeVeen) shunt. *J Pediatr Gastroenterol Nutr* 1986;**5**:476–80.

108 Modlin JF, Kinney JS. Perinatal echovirus infection: insights from a literature review of 61 cases and 16 outbreaks in nurseries. *Rev Infect Dis* 1986;**8**:918–26.

109 Huang QS, Carr JM, Nix WA, *et al.* An echovirus type 33 winter outbreak in New Zealand. *Clin Infect Dis* 2003;**37**:650–7.

110 Kao YH, Hung HY, Chi H. Congenital coxsackievirus B5 infection: report of one case. *Acta Paediatr Taiwan* 2005;**46**:321–3.

111 Cheng LL, Ng PC, Chan PK, Wong HL, Cheng FW, Tang JW. Probable intrafamilial transmission of coxsackievirus b3 with vertical transmission, severe early-onset neonatal hepatitis, and prolonged viral RNA shedding. *Pediatrics* 2006;**118**:e929–33.

112 Matsuoka T, Naito T, Kubota Y, *et al.* Disseminated adenovirus (type 19) infection in a neonate. *Acta Paediatr Scand* 1990;**79**: 568–71.

113 Rocholl C, Gerber K, Daly J, Pavia AT, Byington CL. Adenoviral infections in children: the impact of rapid diagnosis. *Pediatrics* 2004;**113**:e51–6.

114 Abzug MJ. Presentation, diagnosis, and management of enterovirus infections in neonates. *Paediatr Drugs* 2004;**6**:1–10.

115 Bryant PA, Tingay D, Dargaville PA, Starr M, Curtis N. Neonatal coxsackie B virus infection—a treatable disease? *Eur J Pediatr* 2004;**163**:223–8.

116 Hamilton JR, Sass-Kortsak A. Jaundice associated with severe bacterial infection in young infants. *J Pediatr* 1963;**63**:121–32.

117 Franson TR, Hierholzer WJ, LaBrecque DR. Frequency and characteristics of hyperbilirubinemia associated with bacteremia. *Rev Infect Dis* 1985;**7**:1–9.

118 Garcia FJ, Nager AL. Jaundice as an early diagnostic sign of urinary tract infection in infancy. *Pediatrics* 2002;**109**:846–51.

119 Cantwell MF, Shehab ZM, Costello AM, *et al.* Brief report: congenital tuberculosis. *N Engl J Med* 1994;**330**:1051–4.

120 Chou YH. Congenital tuberculosis proven by percutaneous liver biopsy: report of a case. *J Perinat Med* 2002;**30**:423–5.

121 Berk DR, Sylvester KG. Congenital tuberculosis presenting as progressive liver dysfunction. *Pediatr Infect Dis J* 2004;**23**:78–80.

122 Gögüş S, Umer H, Akçören Z, Sanal O, Osmanlioglu G, Cimbiş M. Neonatal tuberculosis. *Pediatr Pathol* 1993;**13**:299–304.

123 Herman SP, Baggenstoss AH, Cloutier MD. Liver dysfunction and histologic abnormalities in neonatal hypopituitarism. *J Pediatr* 1975;**87**:892–5.

124 Leblanc A, Odievre M, Hadchouel M, Gendrel D, Chaussain JL, Rappaport R. Neonatal cholestasis and hypoglycemia: possible role of cortisol deficiency. *J Pediatr* 1981;**99**:577–80.

125 Kraehe J, Hauffa BP, Wollmann HA, Kaeser H. Transient elevation of urinary catecholamine excretion and cholestatic liver disease in a neonate with hypopituitarism. *J Pediatr Gastroenterol Nutr* 1992;**14**:153–9.

126 Sheehan AG, Martin SR, Stephure D, Scott RB. Neonatal cholestasis, hypoglycemia and congenital hypopituitarism. *J Pediatr Gastroenterol Nutr* 1992;**14**:426–30.

127 Ellaway CJ, Silinik M, Cowell CT, *et al.* Cholestatic jaundice and congenital hypopituitarism. *J Paediatr Child Health* 1995;**31**: 51–3.

128 Karnsakul W, Sawathiparnich P, Nimkarn S, Likitmaskul S, Santiprabhob J, Aanpreung P. Anterior pituitary hormone effects on hepatic functions in infants with congenital hypopituitarism. *Ann Hepatol* 2007;**6**:97–103.

129 Lacy DE, Nathavitharana KA, Tarlow MJ. Neonatal hepatitis and congenital insensitivity to adrenocorticotropin (ACTH). *J Pediatr Gastroenterol Nutr* 1993;**17**:438–40.

130 Fahnehjelm KT, Fischler B, Jacobson L, Nemeth A. Optic nerve hypoplasia in cholestatic infants: a multiple case study. *Acta Ophthalmol Scand* 2003;**81**:130–7.

131 Spray CH, McKiernan P, Waldron KE, Shaw NJ, Kirk J, Kelly DA. Investigation and outcome of neonatal hepatitis in infants with hypopituitarism. *Acta Paediatr* 2000;**89**:951–4.

132 Alpert LI, Strauss L, Hirschhorn K. Neonatal hepatitis and biliary atresia associated with trisomy 17–18 syndrome. *N Engl J Med* 1969;**280**:16–20.

133 Ikeda S, Sera Y, Yoshida M, *et al.* Extrahepatic biliary atresia associated with trisomy 18. *Pediatr Surg Int* 1999;**15**:137–8.

134 Silveira TR, Salzano FM, Howard ER, Mowat AP. Congenital structural abnormalities in biliary atresia: evidence for etiopathogenic heterogeneity and therapeutic implications. *Acta Paediatr Scand* 1991;**80**:1192–9.

135 Henriksen NT, Drablos PA, Aagenaes O. Cholestatic jaundice in infancy. The importance of familial and genetic factors in aetiology and prognosis. *Arch Dis Child* 1981;**56**:622–7.

136 Ruchelli ED, Uri A, Dimmick JE, *et al.* Severe perinatal liver disease and Down syndrome: an apparent relationship. *Hum Pathol* 1991;**22**:1274–80.

137 Becroft DM. Fetal megakaryocytic dyshemopoiesis in Down syndrome: association with hepatic and pancreatic fibrosis. *Pediatr Pathol* 1993;**13**:811–20.

138 Massey GV, Zipursky A, Chang MN, *et al.* A prospective study of the natural history of transient leukemia (TL) in neonates with Down syndrome (DS): Children's Oncology Group (COG) study POG-9481. *Blood* 2006;**107**:4606–13.

139 Riazi MA, Brinkman-Mills P, Nguyen T, *et al.* The human homolog of insect-derived growth factor, CECR1, is a candidate gene for features of cat eye syndrome. *Genomics* 2000;**64**:277–85.

140 Kawashima H, Watanabe C, Nishimata S, *et al.* Hydranencephaly with cholestasis and giant hepatitis. *J Clin Gastroenterol* 2006;**40**:956–8.

141 Deniz K, Kontaş O, Akçakuş M. Neonatal hepatitis in 2 siblings with Seckel syndrome. *Pediatr Dev Pathol* 2006;**9**:81–5.

142 Hermeziu B, Sanlaville D, Girard M, Léonard C, Lyonnet S, Jacquemin E. Heterozygous bile salt export pump deficiency: a possible genetic predisposition to transient neonatal cholestasis. *J Pediatr Gastroenterol Nutr* 2006;**42**:114–6.

143 Mowat AP, Psacharopoulos HT, Williams R. Extrahepatic biliary atresia versus neonatal hepatitis. Review of 137 prospectively investigated infants. *Arch Dis Child* 1976;**51**:763–70.

144 Deutsch J, Smith AL, Danks DM, Campbell PE. Long term prognosis for babies with neonatal liver disease. *Arch Dis Child* 1985;**60**:447–51.

145 Chang MH, Hsu HC, Lee CY, Wang TR, Kao CL. Neonatal hepatitis: a follow-up study. *J Pediatr Gastroenterol Nutr* 1987;**6**:203–7.

146 Suita S, Arima T, Ishii K, Yakabe S, Matsuo S. Fate of infants with neonatal hepatitis: pediatric surgeons' dilemma. *J Pediatr Surg* 1992;**27**:696–9.

147 Mieli-Vergani G, Howard ER, Portmann B, Mowat AP. Late referral for biliary atresia—missed opportunities for effective surgery. *Lancet* 1989;**i**:421–3.

148 Chardot C, Carton M, Spire-Bendelac N, Le Pommelet C, Golmard JL, Auvert B. Prognosis of biliary atresia in the era of liver transplantation: French national study from 1986 to 1996. *Hepatology* 1999;**30**:606–11.

149 Bezerra JA. The next challenge in pediatric cholestasis: deciphering the pathogenesis of biliary atresia. *J Pediatr Gastroenterol Nutr.* 2006;**43**(Suppl 1):S23–9.

150 Gilmour SM, Hershkop M, Reifen R, Gilday D, Roberts EA. Outcome of hepatobiliary scanning in neonatal hepatitis syndrome. *J Nucl Med* 1997;**38**:1279–82.

151 Norton KI, Glass RB, Kogan D, Lee JS, Emre S, Shneider BL. MR cholangiography in the evaluation of neonatal cholestasis: initial results. *Radiology* 2002;**222**:687–91.

152 Nwomeh BC, Caniano DA, Hogan M. Definitive exclusion of biliary atresia in infants with cholestatic jaundice: the role of percutaneous cholecysto-cholangiography. *Pediatr Surg Int* 2007;**23**:845–9.

153 Davenport M, Kerkar N, Mieli-Vergani G, Mowat AP, Howard ER. Biliary atresia: the King's College Hospital experience (1974–1995). *J Pediatr Surg* 1997;**32**:479–85.

154 Vasquez J, Lopez Gutierrez JC, Gamez M, *et al.* Biliary atresia and the polysplenia syndrome: its impact on final outcome. *J Pediatr Surg* 1995;**30**:485–7.

155 McKiernan PJ, Baker AJ, Lloyd C, Mieli-Vergani G, Kelly DA. The BPSU study of biliary atresia: outcome at 13 years. *Arch Dis Child* 2007;**92**(Suppl 1):A4–A5.

156 Shneider BL, Brown MB, Haber B, *et al.* Biliary Atresia Research Consortium. A multicenter study of the outcome of biliary atresia in the United States 1997 to 2000. *J Pediatr* 2006;**148**: 467–74.

157 Nio M, Ohi R, Hayashi Y, Endo N, Ibrahim M, Iwani D. Current status of 21 patients who have survived more than 20 years since undergoing surgery for biliary atresia. *J Pediatr Surg* 1996;**31**:381–4.

158 Lykavieris P, Chardot C, Sokhn M, Gauthier F, Valayer J, Bernard O. Outcome in adulthood of biliary atresia: a study of 63 patients who survived for over 20 years with their native liver. *Hepatology* 2005;**41**:366–71.

159 Hadzić N, Davenport M, Tizzard S, Singer J, Howard ER, Mieli-Vergani G. Long-term survival following Kasai portoenterostomy: is chronic liver disease inevitable? *J Pediatr Gastroenterol Nutr* 2003;**37**:430–3.

160 Phillips MJ, Azuma T, Meredith SL, *et al.* Abnormalities in villin gene expression and canalicular microvillus structure in progressive cholestatic liver disease of childhood. *Lancet* 2003;**362**:1112–9.

161 Annerén G, Meurling S, Lilja H, Wallander J, von Döbeln U. Lethal autosomal recessive syndrome with intrauterine growth retardation, intra- and extrahepatic biliary atresia, and esophageal and duodenal atresia. *Am J Med Genet* 1998;**78**:306–7.

162 Galán-Gómez E, Sánchez EB, Arias-Castro S, Cardesa-García JJ. Intrauterine growth retardation, duodenal and extrahepatic biliary atresia, hypoplastic pancreas and other intestinal anomalies: further evidence of the Martínez-Frías syndrome. *Eur J Med Genet* 2007;**50**:144–8.

163 Matsumoto N, Niikawa N. Kabuki make-up syndrome: a review. *Am J Med Genet C Semin Med Genet* 2003 2003;**117**:57–65.

164 Galán-Gómez E, Cardesa-García JJ, Campo-Sampedro FM, Salamanca-Maesso C, Martínez-Frías ML, Frías JL. Kabuki make-up (Niikawa–Kuroki) syndrome in five Spanish children. *Am J Med Genet* 1995;**59**:276–82.

165 Todani T, Watanabe Y, Narusue M, Tabuchi K, Okajima K. Congenital bile duct cysts. Classification, operative procedures, and review of thirty-seven cases including cancer arising from choledochal cyst. *Am J Surg* 1977;**134**:263–9.

166 Todani T, Watanabe Y, Toki A, Morotomi Y. Classification of congenital biliary cystic disease: special reference to type Ic and IVA cysts with primary ductal stricture. *J Hepatobiliary Pancreat Surg* 2003;**10**:340–4.

167 Bancroft JD, Bucuvalas JC, Ryckman FC, Dudgeon DL, Saunders RC, Schwarz KB. Antenatal diagnosis of choledochal cyst. *J Pediatr Gastroenterol Nutr* 1994;**18**:142–5.

168 Stringer MD, Dhawan A, Davenport M, Mieli-Vergani G, Mowat AP, Howard ER. Choledochal cysts: lessons from a 20 year experience. *Arch Dis Child* 1995;**73**:528–31.

169 Burnweit CA, Birken GA, Heiss K, The management of choledochal cysts in the newborn. *Pediatr Surg Int* 1996;**11**:130–3.

170 Todani T, Urushihara N, Morotomi Y, *et al.* Characteristics of choledochal cysts in neonates and early infants. *Eur J Pediatr Surg* 1995;**5**:143–5.

171 Lipsett PA, Pitt HA, Colombani PM, Boitnott JK, Cameron JL. Choledochal cyst disease. A changing pattern of presentation. *Ann Surg* 1994;**220**:644–52.

172 Miyano T, Yamataka A. Choledochal cysts. *Curr Opin Pediatr* 1997;**9**:283–8.

173 Yamataka A, Ohshiro K, Okada Y, *et al.* Complications after cyst excision with hepaticoenterostomy for choledochal cysts and their surgical management in children versus adults. *J Pediatr Surg* 1997;**32**:1097–1102.

174 Lee HC, Yeung CY, Fang SB, Jiang CB, Sheu JC, Wang NL. Biliary cysts in children—long-term follow-up in Taiwan. *J Formos Med Assoc* 2006;**105**:118–24.

175 de Vries JS, de Vries S, Aronson DC, *et al.* Choledochal cysts: age of presentation, symptoms, and late complications related to Todani's classification. *J Pediatr Surg* 2002;**37**:1568–73.

176 Keane F, Hadzic N, Wilkinson ML, *et al.* Neonatal presentation of Caroli's disease. *Arch Dis Child Fetal Neonatal Ed* 1997;**77**: F145–6.

177 Alvarez F, Bernard O, Brunelle F, *et al.* Congenital hepatic fibrosis in children. *J Pediatr* 1981;**99**:370–5.

178 Lilly JR. Common bile duct calculi in infants and children. *J Pediatr Surg* 1980;**15**:577–80.

179 Debray D, Pariente D, Gauthier F, Myara A, Bernard O. Cholelithiasis in infancy: a study of 40 cases. *J Pediatr* 1993; **122**:385–91.

180 Bohle AS. Cholelithiasis with common bile duct obstruction in a 20-week-old infant. *Eur J Pediatr Surg* 1995;**5**:57–8.

181 Rescorla FJ. Cholelithiasis, cholecystitis, and common bile duct stones. *Curr Opin Pediatr* 1997;**9**:276–82.

182 Monnerie JL, Soulard D. [Cholelithiasis in infants with spontaneously favourable course; in French.] *Arch Pediatr* 1995;**2**:654–6.

183 Ishitani MB, Shaul DB, Padua EA, McAlpin CA. Choledocholithiasis in a premature neonate. *J Pediatr* 1996;**128**:853–5.

184 Wilcox DT, Casson D, Bowen J, Thomas A, Bruce J. Cholelithiasis in early infancy. *Pediatr Surg Int* 1997;**12**:198–9.

185 Wilkinson ML. Sphincterotomy for jaundice in a neonate. *J Pediatr Gastroenterol Nutr* 1996;**23**:507–9.

186 Allgood C, Bolisetty S. Severe conjugated hyperbilirubinaemia and neonatal haemolysis. *Int J Clin Pract* 2006;**60**:1513–4.

187 Davies C, Daneman A, Stringer DA. Inspissated bile in a neonate with cystic fibrosis. *J Ultrasound Med* 1986;**5**:335–7.

188 Evans JS, George DE, Mollit D. Biliary infusion therapy in the inspissated bile syndrome of cystic fibrosis. *J Pediatr Gastroenterol Nutr* 1991;**12**:131–5.

189 Stringel G, Mercer S. Idiopathic perforation of the biliary tract in infancy. *J Pediatr Surg* 1983;**18**:546–50.

190 Lloyd DA, Mickel RE. Spontaneous perforation of the extrahepatic bile ducts in neonates and infants. *Br J Surg* 1980;**67**:621–3.

191 Darwish AA, Debauche C, Clapuyt P, Feruzi Z, de Ville de Goyet J, Reding R. Pyloric obstruction, duodenal dilatation, and extrahepatic cholestasis: a neonatal triad suggesting multiple intestinal atresias. *J Pediatr Surg* 2006;**41**:1771–3.

192 Teoh L, Wong CK, Martin H, O'Loughlin EV. Anterior abdominal wall defects and biliary obstruction. *J Paediatr Child Health* 2005;**41**:143–6.

193 Amedee-Manesme O, Bernard O, Brunelle F, *et al.* Sclerosing cholangitis with neonatal onset. *J Pediatr* 1987;**111**:225–9.

194 Sisto A, Feldman P, Garel L, *et al.* Primary sclerosing cholangitis in children: study of five cases and review of the literature. *Pediatrics* 1987;**80**:918–23.

195 Maggiore G, De Giacomo C, Ugazio AG. Sclerosing cholangitis in childhood [letter]. *Gastroenterology* 1988;**94**:551–2.

196 Mulberg AE, Arora S, Grand RJ, Vinton N. Expanding the spectrum of neonatal cholestatic liver disease. *Hepatology* 1992; **16**:192A.

197 Baker AJ, Portmann B, Westaby D, Wilkinson M, Karani J, Mowat AP. Neonatal sclerosing cholangitis in two siblings: a category of progressive intrahepatic cholestasis. *J Pediatr Gastroenterol Nutr* 1993;**17**:317–22.

198 Bar Meir M, Hadas-Halperin I, Fisher D, *et al.* Neonatal sclerosing cholangitis associated with autoimmune phenomena. *J Pediatr Gastroenterol Nutr* 2000;**30**:332–4.

199 Wilschanski M, Chait P, Wade JA, *et al.* Primary sclerosing cholangitis in 32 children: clinical, laboratory, and radiographic features, with survival analysis. *Hepatology* 1995;**22**:1415–22.

200 Hadj-Rabia S, Baala L, Vabres P, *et al.* Claudin–1 gene mutations in neonatal sclerosing cholangitis associated with ichthyosis: a tight junction disease. *Gastroenterology* 2004;**127**:1386–90.

201 Feldmeyer L, Huber M, Fellmann F, Beckmann JS, Frenk E, Hohl D. Confirmation of the origin of NISCH syndrome. *Hum Mutat* 2006;**27**:408–10.

202 Krant SM, Swenson O. Biliary duct hypoplasia. *J Pediatr Surg* 1973;**8**:301–7.

203 Lilly JR. The surgery of biliary hypoplasia. *J Pediatr Surg* 1976;**11**:815–9.

204 Watson GH, Miller V. Arteriohepatic dysplasia. Familial pulmonary arterial stenosis with neonatal liver disease. *Arch Dis Child* 1973;**48**:459–66.

205 Alagille's D, Odievre M, Gautier M, Dommergues JP. Hepatic ductular hypoplasia associated with characteristic facies, vertebral malformations, retarded physical, mental, and sexual development, and cardiac murmur. *J Pediatr* 1975;**86**:63–71.

206 Dhorne-Pollet S, Deleuze JF, Hadchouel M, Bonaiti-Pellie C. Segregation analysis of Alagille's syndrome. *J Med Genet* 1994;**31**: 453–7.

207 Elmslie FV, Vivian AJ, Gardiner H, Hall C, Mowat AP, Winter RM. Alagille's syndrome: family studies. *J Med Genet* 1995;**32**: 264–8.

208 Li L, Krantz ID, Deng Y, *et al.* Alagille's syndrome is caused by mutations in human Jagged1, which encodes a ligand for Notch1. *Nat Genet* 1997;**16**:243–51.

209 Oda T, Elkahloun A, Pike B, *et al.* Mutations in the human Jagged1 gene are responsible for the Alagille's syndrome. *Nat Genet* 1997;**16**:235–42.

210 McDaniell R, Warthen DM, Sanchez-Lara PA, *et al.* NOTCH2 mutations cause Alagille's syndrome, a heterogeneous disorder of the notch signaling pathway. *Am J Hum Genet* 2006;**79**: 169–73.

211 Pollet N, Boccaccio C, Dhorne-Pollet S, *et al.* Construction of an integrated physical and gene map of human chromosome 20p12 providing candidate genes for Alagille's syndrome. *Genomics* 1997;**42**:489–92.

212 Spinner NB, Colliton RP, Crosnier C, Krantz ID, Hadchouel M, Meunier-Rotival M. Jagged1 mutations in Alagille's syndrome. *Hum Mutat* 2001;**17**:18–33.

213 Boyer J, Crosnier C, Driancourt C, *et al.* Expression of mutant *JAGGED1* alleles in patients with Alagille's syndrome. *Hum Genet* 2005;**116**:445–53.

214 Crosnier C, Driancourt C, Raynaud N, *et al.* Mutations in *JAGGED1* gene are predominantly sporadic in Alagille's syndrome. *Gastroenterology* 1999;**116**:1141–8.

215 Crosnier C, Driancourt C, Raynaud N, Hadchouel M, Meunier-Rotival M. Fifteen novel mutations in the *JAGGED1* gene of patients with Alagille's syndrome. *Hum Mutat* 2001;**17**:72–3.

216 Colliton RP, Bason L, Lu FM, Piccoli DA, Krantz ID, Spinner NB. Mutation analysis of Jagged1 (JAG1) in Alagille's syndrome patients. *Hum Mutat* 2001;**17**:151–2.

217 Yuan ZR, Okaniwa M, Nagata I, *et al.* The DSL domain in mutant JAG1 ligand is essential for the severity of the liver defect in Alagille's syndrome. *Clin Genet* 2001;**59**:330–7.

218 Flynn DM, Nijjar S, Hubscher SG, *et al.* The role of Notch receptor expression in bile duct development and disease. *J Pathol* 2004;**204**:55–64.

219 Lorent K, Yeo SY, Oda T, *et al.* Inhibition of Jagged-mediated Notch signaling disrupts zebrafish biliary development and generates multi-organ defects compatible with an Alagille's syndrome phenocopy. *Development* 2004;**131**:5753–66.

220 Yuan ZR, Kobayashi N, Kohsaka T. Human Jagged 1 mutants cause liver defect in Alagille's syndrome by overexpression of hepatocyte growth factor. *J Mol Biol* 2006;**356**:559–68.

221 Fabris L, Cadamuro M, Guido M, *et al.* Analysis of liver repair mechanisms in Alagille's syndrome and biliary atresia reveals a role for notch signaling. *Am J Pathol* 2007;**171**:641–53.

222 Libbrecht L, Spinner NB, Moore EC, Cassiman D, Van Damme-Lombaerts R, Roskams T. Peripheral bile duct paucity and cholestasis in the liver of a patient with Alagille's syndrome: further evidence supporting a lack of postnatal bile duct branching and elongation. *Am J Surg Pathol* 2005;**29**:820–6.

223 Loomes KM, Russo P, Ryan M, *et al.* Bile duct proliferation in liver-specific Jag1 conditional knockout mice: effects of gene dosage. *Hepatology* 2007;**45**:323–30.

224 Deleuze JF, Dhorne-Pollet S, Pollet N, Meunier-Rotival M, Hadchouel M. [Alagille's syndrome in 1995. Clinical and genetic data; in French.] *Gastroenterol Clin Biol* 1995;**19**:587–96.

225 Emerick KM, Rand EB, Goldmuntz E, Krantz ID, Spinner NB, Piccoli DA. Features of Alagille's syndrome in 92 patients: frequency and relation to prognosis. *Hepatology* 1999;**29**:822–9.

226 Sanderson E, Newman V, Haigh SF, Baker A, Sidhu PS. Vertebral anomalies in children with Alagille's syndrome: an analysis of 50 consecutive patients. *Pediatr Radiol* 2002;**32**:114–9.

227 Hingorani M, Nischal KK, Davies A, *et al.* Ocular abnormalities in Alagille's syndrome. *Ophthalmology* 1999;**106**:330–7.

228 Nischal KK, Hingorani M, Bentley CR, *et al.* Ocular ultrasound in Alagille's syndrome. A new sign. *Ophthalmology* 1997;**104**:79–85.

229 Silberbach M, Lashley D, Relier MD, Kinn WFJ, Terry A, Sunderland CO. Arteriohepatic dysplasia and cardiovascular malformations. *Am Heart J* 1991;**127**:695–9.
230 McElhinney DB, Krantz ID, Bason L, *et al.* Analysis of cardiovascular phenotype and genotype-phenotype correlation in individuals with a JAG1 mutation and/or Alagille's syndrome. *Circulation* 2002;**106**:2567–74.
231 Emerick KM, Krantz ID, Kamath BM, *et al.* Intracranial vascular abnormalities in patients with Alagille's syndrome. *J Pediatr Gastroenterol Nutr* 2005;**41**:99–107.
232 Connor SE, Hewes D, Ball C, Jarosz JM. Alagille's syndrome associated with angiographic moyamoya. *Childs Nerv Syst* 2002; **18**:186–90.
233 Kamath BM, Spinner NB, Emerick KM, *et al.* Vascular anomalies in Alagille's syndrome: a significant cause of morbidity and mortality. *Circulation* 2004;**109**:1354–8.
234 Lykavieris P, Crosnier C, Trichet C, Meunier-Rotival M, Hadchouel M. Bleeding tendency in children with Alagille's syndrome. *Pediatrics* 2003;**111**:167–70.
235 Narula P, Gifford J, Steggall MA, *et al.* Visual loss and idiopathic intracranial hypertension in children with Alagille's syndrome. *J Pediatr Gastroenterol Nutr* 2006;**43**:348–52.
236 Quiros-Tejeira RE, Ament ME, Heyman MB, *et al.* Variable morbidity in Alagille's syndrome: a review of 43 cases. *J Pediatr Gastroenterol Nutr* 1999;**29**:431–7.
237 Garcia MA, Ramonet M, Ciocca M, *et al.* Alagille's syndrome: cutaneous manifestations in 38 children. *Pediatr Dermatol* 2005; **22**:11–4.
238 Deutsch GH, Sokol RJ, Stathos TH, Knisely AS. Proliferation to paucity: evolution of bile duct abnormalities in a case of Alagille's syndrome. *Pediatr Dev Pathol* 2001;**4**:559–63.
239 Duche M, Habes D, Lababidi A, Chardot C, Wenz J, Bernard O. Percutaneous endoscopic gastrostomy for continuous feeding in children with chronic cholestasis. *J Pediatr Gastroenterol Nutr* 1999;**29**:42–5.
240 Berard E, Triolo V. Intracranial hemorrhages in Alagille's syndrome. *J Pediatr* 2000;**136**:708–10.
241 Hoffenberg EJ, Narkewicz MR, Sondheimer JM, Smith DJ, Silverman A, Sokol RJ. Outcome of syndromic paucity of interlobular bile ducts (Alagille's syndrome) with onset of cholestasis in infancy. *J Pediatr* 1995;**127**:220–4.
242 Lykavieris P, Hadchouel M, Chardot C, Bernard O. Outcome of liver disease in children with Alagille's syndrome: a study of 163 patients. *Gut* 2001;**49**:431–5.
243 Bhadri VA, Stormon MO, Arbuckle S, Lam AH, Gaskin KJ, Shun A. Hepatocellular carcinoma in children with Alagille's syndrome. *J Pediatr Gastroenterol Nutr* 2005;**41**:676–8.
244 Kim B, Park SH, Yang HR, Seo JK, Kim WS, Chi JG. Hepatocellular carcinoma occurring in Alagille's syndrome. *Pathol Res Pract* 2005;**201**:55–60.
245 Schwarzenberg SJ, Grothe RM, Sharp HL, Snover DC, Freese D. Long-term complications of arteriohepatic dysplasia. *Am J Med* 1992;**93**:171–6.
246 Englert C, Grabhorn E, Burdelski M, Ganschow R. Liver transplantation in children with Alagille's syndrome: indications and outcome. *Pediatr Transplant* 2006;**10**:154–8.
247 Cardona J, Houssin D, Gauthier F, *et al.* Liver transplantation in children with Alagille's syndrome—a study of twelve cases. *Transplantation* 1995;**60**:339–42.
248 Holt RIG, Broide E, Buchman CR, *et al.* Orthotopic liver transplantation reverse the adverse nutritional changes of end-stage liver disease in children. *Am J Clin Nutr* 1997;**65**:534–42.
249 Quiros-Tejeira RE, Ament ME, Heyman MB, *et al.* Does liver transplantation affect growth pattern in Alagille's syndrome? *Liver Transpl* 2000;**6**:582–7.
250 Kahn E, Daum F, Markowitz J, *et al.* Nonsyndromic paucity of interlobular bile ducts: light and electron microscopic evaluation of sequential liver biopsies in early childhood. *Hepatology* 1986;**6**:890–901.
251 De Tommaso AM, Kawasaki AS, Hessel G. Paucity of intrahepatic bile ducts in infancy—experience of a tertiary center. *Arq Gastroenterol* 2004;**41**:190–2.
252 Finegold MJ, Carpenter RJ. Obliterative cholangitis due to cytomegalovirus: a possible precursor of paucity of intrahepatic bile ducts. *Hum Pathol* 1982;**13**:662–5.
253 Dimmick JE. Intrahepatic bile duct paucity and cytomegalovirus infection. *Pediatr Pathol* 1993;**13**:847–52.
254 Shulman HM, Sharma P, Amos D, Fenster LF, McDonald GB. A coded histologic study of hepatic graft-versus-host disease after human bone marrow transplantation. *Hepatology* 1988;**8**:463–70.
255 Wulffraat NM, Haddad E, Benkerrou M, *et al.* Hepatic GVHD after HLA-haploidentical bone marrow transplantation in children with severe combined immunodeficiency: the effect of ursodeoxycholic acid. *Br J Haematol* 1997;**96**:776–80.
256 Ludwig J, Wiesner RH, LaRusso NF. Idiopathic adulthood ductopenia: a cause of chronic cholestatic liver disease and biliary cirrhosis. *J Hepatol* 1988;**7**:193–9.
257 Bruguera M, Llach J, Rodes J. Nonsyndromic paucity of intrahepatic bile ducts in infancy and idiopathic ductopenia in adulthood: the same syndrome? *Hepatology* 1992;**15**:830–4.
258 Beckers D, Bellanne-Chantelot C, Maes M. Neonatal cholestatic jaundice as the first symptom of a mutation in the hepatocyte nuclear factor-1beta gene (HNF-1beta). *J Pediatr* 2007;**150**: 313–4.
259 Primhak RA, Tanner MS. Alpha-1 antitrypsin deficiency. *Arch Dis Child* 2001;**85**:2–5.
260 Lomas DA, Evans DL, Finch JT, Carrell RW. The mechanism of Z α1-antitrypsin accumulation in the liver. *Nature* 1992;**357**: 605–7.
261 Perlmutter DH. Alpha-1-antitrypsin deficiency: biochemistry and clinical manifestations. *Ann Med* 1996;**28**:385–94.
262 Burrows JA, Willis LK, Perlmutter DH. Chemical chaperones mediate increased secretion of mutant alpha 1-antitrypsin (alpha 1-AT) Z: a potential pharmacological strategy for prevention of liver injury and emphysema in alpha 1-AT deficiency. *Proc Natl Acad Sci U S A* 2000;**97**:1796–801.
263 Perlmutter DH. Chemical chaperones: a pharmacological strategy for disorders of protein folding and trafficking. *Pediatr Res* 2002;**52**:832–6.
264 Shen Y, Ballar P, Fang S. Ubiquitin ligase gp78 increases solubility and facilitates degradation of the Z variant of alpha-1-antitrypsin. *Biochem Biophys Res Commun* 2006;**349**:1285–93.
265 Nord KS, Saad S, Joshi VV, McLoughlin LC. Concurrence of a1-antitrypsin deficiency and biliary atresia. *J Pediatr* 1987;**111**: 416–8.
266 Lang T, Mühlbauer M, Strobelt M, Weidinger S, Hadorn HB. Alpha-1-antitrypsin deficiency in children: liver disease is not

reflected by low serum levels of alpha-1-antitrypsin—a study on 48 pediatric patients. *Eur J Med Res* 2005;**10**:509–14.

267 Liu C, Aronow BJ, Jegga AG, *et al.* Novel resequencing chip customized to diagnose mutations in patients with inherited syndromes of intrahepatic cholestasis. *Gastroenterology* 2007; **132**:119–26.

268 Roberts EA, Cox DW, Medline A, Wanless IR. Occurrence of alpha-1-antitrypsin deficiency in 155 patients with alcoholic liver disease. *Am J Clin Pathol* 1984;**82**:424–7.

269 Povey S. Genetics of alpha 1-antitrypsin deficiency in relation to neonatal liver disease. *Mol Biol Med* 1990;**7**:161–72.

270 Volpert D, Molleston JP, Perlmutter DH. Alpha$_1$-antitrypsin deficiency-associated liver disease progresses slowly in some children. *J Pediatr Gastroenterol Nutr* 2000;**31**:258–63.

271 Psacharopoulos HT, Mowat AP, Cook PJ, Carlile PA, Portmann B, Rodeck CH. Outcome of liver disease associated with alpha 1 antitrypsin deficiency (PiZ). Implications for genetic counselling and antenatal diagnosis. *Arch Dis Child* 1983;**58**:882–7.

272 Nebbia G, Hadchouel M, Odievre M, Alagille's D. Early assessment of evolution of liver disease associated with alpha 1-antitrypsin deficiency in childhood. *J Pediatr* 1983;**102**:661–5.

273 Ibarguen E, Gross CR, Savik SK, Sharp HL. Liver disease in alpha-1-antitrypsin deficiency: prognostic indicators. *J Pediatr* 1990;**117**:864–70.

274 Francavilla R, Castellaneta SP, Hadzic N, *et al.* Prognosis of alpha-1-antitrypsin deficiency-related liver disease in the era of paediatric liver transplantation. *J Hepatol* 2000;**32**:986–92.

275 Prachalias AA, Kalife M, Francavilla R, *et al.* Liver transplantation for alpha-1-antitrypsin deficiency in children. *Transpl Int* 2000;**13**:207–10.

276 Greenholz SK, Krishnadasan B, Marr C, Cannon R. Biliary obstruction in infants with cystic fibrosis requiring Kasai portoenterostomy. *J Pediatr Surg* 1997;**32**:175–180.

277 Furuya KN, Roberts EA, Canny GJ, Phillips MJ. Neonatal hepatitis syndrome with paucity of interlobular bile ducts in cystic fibrosis. *J Pediatr Gastroenterol Nutr* 1991;**12**:127–30.

278 Treem WR, Stanley CA. Massive hepatomegaly, steatosis, and secondary plasma carnitine deficiency in an infant with cystic fibrosis. *Pediatrics* 1989;**83**:993–7.

279 Sergi C, Himbert U, Weinhardt F, *et al.* Hepatic failure with neonatal tissue siderosis of hemochromatotic type in an infant presenting with meconium ileus. Case report and differential diagnosis of the perinatal iron storage disorders. *Pathol Res Pract* 2001;**197**:699–709.

280 Maurage C, Lenaerts C, Weber A, Brochu P, Yousef I, Roy CC. Meconium ileus and its equivalent as a risk factor for the development of cirrhosis: an autopsy study in cystic fibrosis. *J Pediatr Gastroenterol Nutr* 1989;**9**:17–20.

281 Clayton RJ, Iber FL, Ruebner BH, McCusick VA. Byler disease: fatal familial cholestasis in an Amish kindred. *Am J Dis Child* 1969;**117**:112–24.

282 Tazawa Y, Yamada M, Nakagawa M, Konno T, Tada K. Bile acid profiles in progressive intrahepatic cholestasis: absence of biliary chenodeoxycholate. *J Pediatr Gastroenterol Nutr* 1985;**4**:32–7.

283 Maggiore G, Bernard O, Riely CA, Hadchouel M, Lemonnier A, Alagille's D. Normal serum gamma-glutamyl-transpeptidase activity identifies groups of infants with idiopathic cholestasis with poor prognosis. *J Pediatr* 1987;**111**:251–2.

284 Winklhofer-Roob BM, Shmerling DH, Soler R, Briner J. Progressive idiopathic cholestasis presenting with profuse watery diarrhea and recurrent infections (Byler's disease). *Acta Paediatr* 1992;**81**:637–40.

285 Whitington PF, Freese DK, Alonso EM, Schwarzenberg SJ, Sharp HL. Clinical and biochemical findings in progressive familial intrahepatic cholestasis. *J Pediatr Gastroenterol Nutr* 1994;**18**:134–41.

286 Bourke B, Goggin N, Walsh D, Kennedy S, Setchell KDR, Drumm B. Byler-like familial cholestasis in an extended kindred. *Arch Dis Child* 1996;**75**:223–7.

287 Nobili V, Di Giandomenico S, Francalanci P, Callea F, Marcellini M, Santorelli FM. A new *ABCB11* mutation in two Italian children with familial intrahepatic cholestasis. *J Gastroenterol* 2006;**41**:598–603.

288 Jung C, Driancourt C, Baussan C, *et al.* Prenatal molecular diagnosis of inherited cholestatic diseases. *J Pediatr Gastroenterol Nutr* 2007;**44**:453–8.

289 Chen HL, Chang PS, Hsu HC, *et al.* Progressive familial intrahepatic cholestasis with high gamma-glutamyltranspeptidase levels in Taiwanese infants: role of *MDR3* gene defect? *Pediatr Res* 2001;**50**:50–5.

290 Bull LN, van Eijk MJ, Pawlikowska L, *et al.* A gene encoding a P-type ATPase mutated in two forms of hereditary cholestasis. *Nat Genet* 1998;**18**:219–24.

291 Klomp LW, Vargas JC, van Mil SW, *et al.* Characterization of mutations in *ATP8B1* associated with hereditary cholestasis. *Hepatology* 2004;**40**(1):27–38.

292 Paulusma CC, Groen A, Kunne C, *et al.* Atp8b1 deficiency in mice reduces resistance of the canalicular membrane to hydrophobic bile salts and impairs bile salt transport. *Hepatology* 2006;**44**:195–204.

293 Demeilliers C, Jacquemin E, Barbu V, *et al.* Altered hepatobiliary gene expressions in PFIC1: *ATP8B1* gene defect is associated with CFTR downregulation. *Hepatology* 2006;**43**:1125–34.

294 Klomp LW, Bull LN, Knisely AS, *et al.* A missense mutation in FIC1 is associated with Greenland familial cholestasis. *Hepatology* 2000;**32**:1337–41.

295 Nielsen IM, Eiberg H. Cholestasis familiaris groenlandica: an epidemiological, clinical and genetic study. *Int J Circumpolar Health* 2004;**63**(Suppl 2):192–4.

296 Eiberg H, Norgaard-Pedersen B, Nielsen IM. Cholestasis familiaris groenlandica/Byler-like disease in Greenland—a population study. *Int J Circumpolar Health* 2004;**63**(Suppl 2):189–91.

297 Gray OP, Saunders RA. Familial intrahepatic cholestatic jaundice in infancy. *Arch Dis Child* 1966;**41**:320–8.

298 Carleton VE, Knisely AS, Freimer NB. Mapping of a locus for progressive familial intrahepatic cholestasis (Byler disease) to 18q21-q22, the benign recurrent intrahepatic cholestasis region. *Hum Mol Genet* 1995;**4**:1049–53.

299 Bull LN, Stricker NL, Baharloo S, *et al.* Genetic and morphological findings in progressive familial intrahepatic cholestasis (Byler disease [PFIC-1] and Byler syndrome): evidence for heterogeneity. *Hepatology* 1997;**26**:155–64.

300 van Ooteghem NA, Klomp LW, van Berge-Henegouwen GP, Houwen RH. Benign recurrent intrahepatic cholestasis progressing to progressive familial intrahepatic cholestasis: low GGT cholestasis is a clinical continuum. *J Hepatol* 2002;**36**:439–43.

301 Müllenbach R, Bennett A, Tetlow N, *et al.* *ATP8B1* mutations in British cases with intrahepatic cholestasis of pregnancy. *Gut* 2005;**54**:829–34.

302 Jacquemin E, Dumont M, Bernard O, Erlinger S, Hadchouel M. Evidence for defective primary bile acid secretion in children with progressive familial intrahepatic cholestasis (Byler disease). *Eur J Pediatr* 1994;**153**:424–8.

303 Melter M, Rodeck B, Kardorff R, *et al.* Progressive familial intrahepatic cholestasis: partial biliary diversion normalizes serum lipids and improves growth in noncirrhotic patients. *Am J Gastroenterol* 2000;**95**:3522–8.

304 Strautnieks SS, Kagalwalla AF, Tanner MS, *et al.* Identification of a locus for progressive familial intrahepatic cholestasis PFIC2 on chromosome 2q24. *Am J Hum Genet* 1997;**61**:630–3.

305 Strautnieks SS, Bull LN, Knisely AS, *et al.* A gene encoding a liver-specific ABC transporter is mutated in progressive familial intrahepatic cholestasis. *Nat Genet* 1998;**20**:233–8.

306 Jansen PL, Strautnieks SS, Jacquemin E, *et al.* Hepatocanalicular bile salt export pump deficiency in patients with progressive familial intrahepatic cholestasis. *Gastroenterology* 1999;**117**:1370–9.

307 Wang L, Soroka CJ, Boyer JL. The role of bile salt export pump mutations in progressive familial intrahepatic cholestasis type II. *J Clin Invest* 2002;**110**:965–72.

308 Knisely AS, Strautnieks SS, Meier Y, *et al.* Hepatocellular carcinoma in ten children under five years of age with bile salt export pump deficiency. *Hepatology* 2006;**44**:478–86.

309 Jansen PL, Sturm E. Genetic cholestasis, causes and consequences for hepatobiliary transport. *Liver Int* 2003;**23**:315–22.

310 Scheimann AO, Strautnieks SS, Knisely AS, Byrne JA, Thompson RJ, Finegold MJ. Mutations in bile salt export pump (*ABCB11*) in two children with progressive familial intrahepatic cholestasis and cholangiocarcinoma. *J Pediatr* 2007;**150**:556–9.

311 Jacquemin E, de Vree JML, Sturm E, *et al.* Mutations in the *MDR3* gene are responsible for a subtype of progressive familial intrahepatic cholestasis (PFIC) [abstract]. *Hepatology* 1997;**26**:248A.

312 Jacquemin E. Role of multidrug resistance 3 deficiency in pediatric and adult liver disease: one gene for three diseases. *Semin Liver Dis* 2001;**21**:551–62.

313 Lamireau T, Bouchard G, Yousef IM, *et al.* Dietary lecithin protects against cholestatic liver disease in cholic acid-fed Abcb4-deficient mice. *Pediatr Res* 2007;**61**:185–90.

314 Carlton VE, Harris BZ, Puffenberger EG, *et al.* Complex inheritance of familial hypercholanemia with associated mutations in *TJP2* and *BAAT*. *Nat Genet* 2003;**34**:91–6.

315 Zhu QS, Xing W, Qian B, *et al.* Inhibition of human m-epoxide hydrolase gene expression in a case of hypercholanemia. *Biochim Biophys Acta* 2003;**1638**:208–16.

316 Weber AM, Tuchweber B, Yousef I, *et al.* Severe familial cholestasis in North American Indian children: a clinical model of microfilament dysfunction? *Gastroenterology* 1981;**81**:653–62.

317 Drouin E, Russo P, Tuchweber B, Mitchell G, Rasquin-Weber A. North American Indian cirrhosis in children: a review of 30 cases. *J Pediatr Gastroenterol Nutr* 2000;**31**:395–404.

318 Chagnon P, Michaud J, Mitchell G, *et al.* A missense mutation (R565W) in cirhin (FLJ14728) in North American Indian childhood cirrhosis. *Am J Hum Genet* 2002;**71**:1443–9.

319 Yu B, Mitchell GA, Richter A. Nucleolar localization of cirhin, the protein mutated in North American Indian childhood cirrhosis. *Exp Cell Res* 2005;**311**:218–28.

320 Phillips MJ, Ackerley CA, Superina RA, Roberts EA, Filler RM, Levy GA. Excess zinc associated with severe progressive cholestasis in Cree and Ojibwa-Cree children. *Lancet* 1996;**347**:866–8.

321 Ben-Shalom E, Kobayashi K, Shaag A, *et al.* Infantile citrullinemia caused by citrin deficiency with increased dibasic amino acids. *Mol Genet Metab* 2002;**77**:202–8.

322 Tazawa Y, Kobayashi K, Ohura T, *et al.* Infantile cholestatic jaundice associated with adult-onset type II citrullinemia. *J Pediatr* 2001;**138**:735–40.

323 Saheki T, Kobayashi K. Mitochondrial aspartate glutamate carrier (citrin) deficiency as the cause of adult-onset type II citrullinemia (CTLN2) and idiopathic neonatal hepatitis (NICCD). *J Hum Genet* 2002;**47**:333–41.

324 Lu YB, Kobayashi K, Ushikai M, *et al.* Frequency and distribution in East Asia of 12 mutations identified in the *SLC25A13* gene of Japanese patients with citrin deficiency. *J Hum Genet* 2005;**50**:338–46.

325 Yeh JN, Jeng YM, Chen HL, Ni YH, Hwu WL, Chang MH. Hepatic steatosis and neonatal intrahepatic cholestasis caused by citrin deficiency (NICCD) in Taiwanese infants. *J Pediatr* 2006;**148**:642–6.

326 Lee NC, Chien YH, Kobayashi K, *et al.* Time course of acylcarnitine elevation in neonatal intrahepatic cholestasis caused by citrin deficiency. *J Inherit Metab Dis* 2006;**29**:551–5.

327 Ohura T, Kobayashi K, Tazawa Y, *et al.* Clinical pictures of 75 patients with neonatal intrahepatic cholestasis caused by citrin deficiency (NICCD). *J Inherit Metab Dis* 2007;**30**:139–44.

328 Dimmock D, Kobayashi K, Iijima M, *et al.* Citrin deficiency: a novel cause of failure to thrive that responds to a high-protein, low-carbohydrate diet. *Pediatrics* 2007;**119**:e773–7.

329 Tamamori A, Fujimoto A, Okano Y, *et al.* Effects of citrin deficiency in the perinatal period: feasibility of newborn mass screening for citrin deficiency. *Pediatr Res* 2004;**56**:608–14.

330 Ohura T, Kobayashi K, Abukawa D, *et al.* A novel inborn error of metabolism detected by elevated methionine and/or galactose in newborn screening: neonatal intrahepatic cholestasis caused by citrin deficiency. *Eur J Pediatr* 2003;**162**:317–22.

331 Tokuhara D, Iijima M, Tamamori A, *et al.* Novel diagnostic approach to citrin deficiency: analysis of citrin protein in lymphocytes. *Mol Genet Metab* 2007;**90**:30–6.

332 Saheki T, Kobayashi K, Iijima M, *et al.* Pathogenesis and pathophysiology of citrin (a mitochondrial aspartate glutamate carrier) deficiency. *Metab Brain Dis* 2002;**17**:335–46.

333 Takaya J, Kobayashi K, Ohashi A, *et al.* Variant clinical courses of 2 patients with neonatal intrahepatic cholestasis who have a novel mutation of *SLC25A13*. *Metabolism* 2005;**54**:1615–9.

334 Tamamori A, Okano Y, Ozaki H, *et al.* Neonatal intrahepatic cholestasis caused by citrin deficiency: severe hepatic dysfunction in an infant requiring liver transplantation. *Eur J Pediatr* 2002;**161**:609–13.

335 Coleman RA, Van Hove JL, Morris CR, Rhoads JM, Summar ML. Cerebral defects and nephrogenic diabetes insipidus with the ARC syndrome: additional findings or a new syndrome (ARCC-NDI)? *Am J Med Genet* 1997;**72**:335–8.

336 Bull LN, Mahmoodi V, Baker AJ, *et al.* *VPS33B* mutation with ichthyosis, cholestasis, and renal dysfunction but without arthrogryposis: incomplete ARC syndrome phenotype. *J Pediatr* 2006;**14**:269–71.

337 Gissen P, Johnson CA, Morgan NV, *et al.* Mutations in *VPS33B*, encoding a regulator of SNARE-dependent membrane fusion, cause arthrogryposis-renal dysfunction-cholestasis (ARC) syndrome. *Nat Genet* 2004;**36**:400–4.

338 Gissen P, Tee L, Johnson CA, *et al.* Clinical and molecular genetic features of ARC syndrome. *Hum Genet* 2006;**120**:396–409.

339 Sadler KC, Amsterdam A, Soroka C, Boyer J, Hopkins N. A genetic screen in zebrafish identifies the mutants vps18, nf2 and foie gras as models of liver disease. *Development* 2005;**132**: 3561–72.

340 Matthews RP, Plumb-Rudewiez N, Lorent K, *et al.* Zebrafish vps33b, an ortholog of the gene responsible for human arthrogryposis-renal dysfunction-cholestasis syndrome, regulates biliary development downstream of the onecut transcription factor hnf6. *Development* 2005;**132**:5295–306.

341 Abu-Sa'da O, Barbar M, Al-Harbi N, Taha D. Arthrogryposis, renal tubular acidosis and cholestasis (ARC) syndrome: two new cases and review. *Clin Dysmorphol* 2005;**14**:191–6.

342 Hayes JA, Kahr WH, Lo B, Macpherson BA. Liver biopsy complicated by hemorrhage in a patient with ARC syndrome. *Paediatr Anaesth* 2004;**14**:960–3.

343 Yehezkely-Schildkraut V, Munichor M, Mandel H, *et al.* Nonsyndromic paucity of interlobular bile ducts: report of 10 patients. *J Pediatr Gastroenterol Nutr* 2003;**37**:546–9.

344 Aagenaes O, van der Hagen CB, Refsum S. Hereditary recurrent intrahepatic cholestasis from birth. *Arch Dis Child* 1968;**43**:646–57.

345 Sharp HL, Krivit W. Hereditary lymphedema and obstructive jaundice. *J Pediatr* 1971;**78**:491–6.

346 Vajro P, Romano A, Fontanella A, Oggero V, Vecchione R, Shmerling DH. Aagenaes's syndrome in an Italian child. *Acta Paediatr Scand* 1984;**73**:695–6.

347 Morris AA, Sequeira JS, Malone M, Slaney SF, Clayton PT. Parent–child transmission of infantile cholestasis with lymphoedema (Aagenaes syndrome). *J Med Genet* 1997;**34**:852–3.

348 Aagenaes O. Hereditary cholestasis with lymphoedema (Aagenaes syndrome, cholestasis-lymphoedema syndrome). New cases and follow-up from infancy to adult age. *Scand J Gastroenterol* 1998;**33**:335–45.

349 Drivdal M, Trydal T, Hagve TA, Bergstad I, Aagenaes O. Prognosis, with evaluation of general biochemistry, of liver disease in lymphoedema cholestasis syndrome 1 (LCS1/Aagenaes syndrome). *Scand J Gastroenterol* 2006;**41**:465–71.

350 Bull LN, Roche E, Song EJ, *et al.* Mapping of the locus for cholestasis-lymphedema syndrome (Aagenaes syndrome) to a 6.6-cM interval on chromosome 15q. *Am J Hum Genet* 2000;**67**: 994–9.

351 von Bahr S, Björkhem I, Van't Hooft F, *et al.* Mutation in the sterol 27-hydroxylase gene associated with fatal cholestasis in infancy. *J Pediatr Gastroenterol Nutr* 2005;**40**:481–6.

352 Setchell KD, Schwarz M, O'Connell NC, *et al.* Identification of a new inborn error in bile acid synthesis: mutation of the oxysterol 7alpha-hydroxylase gene causes severe neonatal liver disease. *J Clin Invest* 1998;**102**:1690–703.

353 Setchell KD, Heubi JE, Bove KE, *et al.* Liver disease caused by failure to racemize trihydroxycholestanoic acid: gene mutation and effect of bile acid therapy. *Gastroenterology* 2003;**124**:217–32.

354 Bove KE. Liver disease caused by disorders of bile acid synthesis. *Clin Liver Dis* 2000;**4**:831–48.

355 Buchmann MS, Kvittingen EA, Nazer H, *et al.* Lack of 3β-hydroxy-C_{27}-steroid dehydrogenase/isomerase in fibroblasts from a child with urinary excretion of 3b-hydroxy bile acids. *J Clin Invest* 1990;**12**:2034–7.

356 Clayton PT, Leonard JV, Lawson AM, *et al.* Familial giant cell hepatitis associated with synthesis of 3β,7α-dihydroxy- and 3β,7α,12α-trihydroxy-5-cholenoic acids. *J Clin Invest* 1987;**79**: 1031–8.

357 Witzleben CL, Piccoli DA, Setchell K. A new category of causes of intrahepatic cholestasis. *Pediatr Pathol* 1992;**12**:269–74.

358 Horslen SP, Lawson AM, Malone M, Clayton PT. 3beta-hydroxy-delta5-C_{27}-steroid dehydrogenase deficiency; effect of chenodeoxycholic acid therapy on liver histology. *J Inherit Metab Dis* 1992;**15**:38–46.

359 Jacquemin E, Setchell KD, O'Connell NC, *et al.* A new cause of progressive intrahepatic cholestasis: 3-beta-hydroxy-C_{27}-steroid dehydrogenase/isomerase deficiency. *J Pediatr* 1994; **125**:379–84.

360 Akobeng AK, Clayton PT, Miller V, Super M, Thomas AG. An inborn error of bile acid synthesis (3beta-hydroxy-delta5-C_{27}-steroid dehydrogenase deficiency) presenting as malabsorption leading to rickets. *Arch Dis Child* 1999;**80**:463–5.

361 Ichimiya H, Nazer H, Gunasekaran T, Clayton P, Sjovall J. Treatment of chronic liver disease caused by 3β-hydroxy-Δ5-C_{27}-steroid dehydrogenase deficiency with chenodeoxycholic acid. *Arch Dis Child* 1990;**65**:1121–4.

362 Setchell KD, Suchy FJ, Welsh MB, Zimmer-Nechemias L, Heubi J, Balistreri WF. Delta 4-3-oxosteroid 5 beta-reductase deficiency described in identical twins with neonatal hepatitis. A new inborn error in bile acid synthesis. *J Clin Invest* 1988;**82**:2148–57.

363 Shneider BL, Setchell KD, Whitington PF, Neilson KA, Suchy FJ. Delta 4-3-oxosteroid 5 beta-reductase deficiency causing neonatal liver failure and hemochromatosis. *J Pediatr* 1994;**124**: 234–8.

364 Siafakas CG, Jonas MM, Perez-Atayde AR. Abnormal bile acid metabolism and neonatal hemochromatosis: a subset with poor prognosis. *J Pediatr Gastroenterol Nutr* 1997;**25**:321–6.

365 Daugherty CC, Setchell KD, Heubi JE, Balistreri WF. Resolution of liver biopsy alterations in three siblings with bile acid treatment of an inborn error of bile acid metabolism (delta 4-3oxosteroid 5 beta reductase deficiency). *Hepatology* 1993;**18**: 1096–101.

366 Bove KE, Heubi JE, Balistreri WF, Setchell KD. Bile acid synthetic defects and liver disease: a comprehensive review. *Pediatr Dev Pathol* 2004;**7**:315–34.

367 Clayton PT. Delta 4-3-oxosteroid 5 beta-reductase deficiency and neonatal hemochromatosis. *J Pediatr* 1994;**125**:845–6.

368 Clayton PT, Casteels M, Mieli-Vergani G, Lawson AM. Familial giant cell hepatitis with low bile acid concentration and increased urinary excretion of specific bile alcohols: a new inborn error of bile acid synthesis? *Pediatr Res* 1995;**37**:424–31.

369 Lumbroso S, Paris F, Sultan C. Activating Gsalpha mutations: analysis of 113 patients with signs of McCune–Albright

syndrome—a European Collaborative Study. *J Clin Endocrinol Metab* 2004;**89**:2107–13.

370 Silva ES, Lumbroso S, Medina M, Gillerot Y, Sultan C, Sokal EM. Demonstration of McCune–Albright mutations in the liver of children with high gammaGT progressive cholestasis. *J Hepatol* 2000;**32**:154–8.

371 Meizner I, Levy A, Carmi R, Robinsin C. Niemann–Pick disease associated with nonimmune hydrops fetalis. *Am J Obstet Gynecol* 1990;**163**:128–9.

372 Pentchev PG, Comly ME, Kruth HS, *et al.* A defect in cholesterol esterification in Niemann–Pick disease (type C) patients. *Proc Nat Acad Sci U S A* 1985;**82**:8247–51.

373 Millat G, Marcais C, Rafi MA, *et al.* Niemann–Pick C1 disease: the I1061T substitution is a frequent mutant allele in patients of Western European descent and correlates with a classic juvenile phenotype. *Am J Hum Genet* 1999;**65**:1321–9.

374 Naureckiene S, Sleat DE, Lackland H, *et al.* Identification of HE1 as the second gene of Niemann–Pick C disease. *Science* 2000;**290**:2298–301.

375 Millat G, Marcais C, Tomasetto C, *et al.* Niemann–Pick C1 disease: correlations between NPC1 mutations, levels of NPC1 protein, and phenotypes emphasize the functional significance of the putative sterol-sensing domain and of the cysteine-rich luminal loop. *Am J Hum Genet* 2001;**68**:1373–85.

376 Millat G, Chikh K, Naureckiene S, *et al.* Niemann–Pick disease type C: spectrum of HE1 mutations and genotype/phenotype correlations in the NPC2 group. *Am J Hum Genet* 2001;**69**:1013–21.

377 Neufeld EB, Wastney M, Patel S, *et al.* The Niemann–Pick C1 protein resides in a vesicular compartment linked to retrograde transport of multiple lysosomal cargo. *J Biol Chem* 1999;**274**:9627–35.

378 Schedin S, Sindelar PJ, Pentchev P, Brunk U, Dallner G. Peroxisomal impairment in Niemann–Pick type C disease. *J Biol Chem* 1997;**272**:6245–51.

379 Sequeira JS, Vellodi A, Vanier MT, Clayton PT. Niemann–Pick disease type C and defective peroxisomal beta-oxidation of branched-chain substrates. *J Inherit Metab Dis* 1998;**21**:149–54.

380 Maconochie IK, Chong S, Mieli-Vergani G, Lake BD, Mowat AP. Fetal ascites: an unusual presentation of Niemann–Pick disease type C. *Arch Dis Child* 1989;**64**:1391–3.

381 Kelly DA, Portmann B, Mowat AP, Sherlock S, Lake BD. Niemann–Pick disease type C: diagnosis and outcome in children, with particular reference to liver disease. *J Pediatr* 1993;**123**:242–7.

382 Semeraro LA, Riely CA, Kolodny EH, Dickerson GR, Gryboski JD. Niemann–Pick variant lipidosis presenting as "neonatal hepatitis". *J Pediatr Gastroenterol Nutr* 1986;**5**:492–500.

383 Yerushalmi B, Sokol RJ, Narkewicz MR, Smith D, Ashmead JW, Wenger DA. Niemann–Pick disease type C in neonatal cholestasis at a North American center. *J Pediatr Gastroenterol Nutr* 2002;**35**:44–50.

384 Adam G, Brereton RJ, Agrawal M, Lake BD. Biliary atresia and meconium ileus associated with Niemann–Pick disease. *J Pediatr Gastroenterol Nutr* 1988;**7**:128–31.

385 Rutledge JC. Progressive neonatal liver failure due to type C Niemann–Pick disease. *Pediatr Pathol* 1989;**9**:779–84.

386 Vanier MT, Rousson RM, Mandon G, Choiset A, Lake BD, Pentchev PG. Diagnosis of Niemann–Pick disease type C on chorionic villus cells. *Lancet* 1989;**i**:1014–5.

387 Vanier MT. Prenatal diagnosis of Niemann–Pick diseases types A, B and C. *Prenat Diagn* 2002;**22**:630–2.

388 Imrie J, Vijayaraghaven S, Whitehouse C, *et al.* Niemann–Pick disease type C in adults. *J Inherit Metab Dis* 2002;**25**:491–500.

389 O'Reilly K, Ahmed SF, Murday V, McGrogan P. Biliary hypoplasia in Williams syndrome. *Arch Dis Child* 2006;**91**:420–1.

390 Moser HW. Genotype–phenotype correlations in disorders of peroxisome biogenesis. *Mol Genet Metab* 1999;**68**:316–27.

391 Gould SJ, Valle D. Peroxisome biogenesis disorders: genetics and cell biology. *Trends Genet* 2000;**16**:340–5.

392 Preuss N, Brosius U, Biermanns M, Muntau AC, Conzelmann E, Gartner J. *PEX1* mutations in complementation group 1 of Zellweger spectrum patients correlate with severity of disease. *Pediatr Res* 2002;**51**:706–14.

393 Naidu S, Moser AE, Moser HW. Phenotypic and genotypic variability of generalized peroxisomal disorders. *Pediatr Neurol* 1988;**4**:5–12.

394 Zeharia A, Ebberink MS, Wanders RJ, *et al.* A novel *PEX12* mutation identified as the cause of a peroxisomal biogenesis disorder with mild clinical phenotype, mild biochemical abnormalities in fibroblasts and a mosaic catalase immunofluorescence pattern, even at 40 degrees C. *J Hum Genet* 2007;**52**:599–606.

395 Setchell KD, Bragetti P, Zimmer-Nechemias L, *et al.* Oral bile acid treatment and the patient with Zellweger syndrome. *Hepatology* 1992;**15**:198–207.

396 Anderson RA, Byrum RS, Coates PM, Sando GN, *et al.* Mutations at the lysosomal acid cholesteryl ester hydrolase gene locus in Wolman disease. *Proc Nat Acad Sci USA* 1994;**91**:2718–22.

397 Krivit W, Peters C, Dusenbery K, *et al.* Wolman disease successfully treated by bone marrow transplantation. *Bone Marrow Transplant* 2000;**26**:567–70.

398 Roth P, Sklower Brooks S, Potaznik D, Cooma R, Sahdev S. Neonatal Gaucher disease presenting as persistent thrombocytopenia. *J Perinatol* 2005;**25**:356–8.

399 Arslan N, Mavi A, Kalkan S, *et al.* Findings of hepatobiliary scintigraphy and liver biopsy in Maroteaux–Lamy syndrome presenting as neonatal cholestasis. *Pediatr Int* 2006;**48**:498–500.

400 Gillett PM, Schreiber RA, Jevon GP, *et al.* Mucopolysaccharidosis type VII (Sly syndrome) presenting as neonatal cholestasis with hepatosplenomegaly. *J Pediatr Gastroenterol Nutr* 2001;**33**:216–20.

401 Sokol RJ, Taylor SF, Devereaux MW, *et al.* Hepatic oxidant injury and glutathione depletion during total parenteral nutrition in weanling rats. *Am J Physiol* 1996;**270**:G691–700.

402 Shin JI, Namgung R, Park MS, Lee C. Could lipid infusion be a risk for parenteral nutrition-associated cholestasis in low birth weight neonates? *Eur J Pediatr* 2008;**167**:197–202.

403 Socha P, Koletzko B, Demmelmair H, *et al.* Short-term effects of parenteral nutrition of cholestatic infants with lipid emulsions based on medium-chain and long-chain triacylglycerols. *Nutrition* 2007;**23**:121–6.

404 Chessex P, Laborie S, Lavoie JC, Rouleau T. Photoprotection of solutions of parenteral nutrition decreases the infused load as well as the urinary excretion of peroxides in premature infants. *Semin Perinatol* 2001;**25**:55–9.

405 Lavoie JC, Chessex P, Gauthier C, *et al.* Reduced bile flow associated with parenteral nutrition is independent of oxidant load and parenteral multivitamins. *J Pediatr Gastroenterol Nutr* 2005;**41**:108–14.

406 Chessex P, Lavoie JC, Rouleau T, *et al.* Photooxidation of parenteral multivitamins induces hepatic steatosis in a neonatal guinea pig model of intravenous nutrition. *Pediatr Res* 2002;**52**: 958–63.
407 Ng PC, Lee CH, Wong SP, *et al.* High-dose oral erythromycin decreased the incidence of parenteral nutrition-associated cholestasis in preterm infants. *Gastroenterology* 2007;**132**:1726–39.
408 Cocjin J, Vanderhal A, Sehgal S, Rosenthal P. Ursodeoxycholic acid therapy for total parenteral nutrition-associated cholestasis in the neonate [abstract]. *Gastroenterology* 1993:A615.
409 Gura KM, Duggan CP, Collier SB, *et al.* Reversal of parenteral nutrition-associated liver disease in two infants with short bowel syndrome using parenteral fish oil: implications for future management. *Pediatrics* 2006;**118**:e197–201.
410 Matos C, Avni EF, Van Gansbeke D, Pardou A, Struyven J. Total parenteral nutrition (TPN) and gallbladder diseases in neonates. *J Ultrasound Med* 1987;**6**:243–8.
411 Whitington PF, Black DD. Cholelithiasis in premature infants treated with parenteral nutrition and furosemide. *J Pediatr* 1980;**97**:647–9.
412 Roslyn JJ, Berquist WE, Pitt HA, *et al.* Increased risk of gallstones in children receiving total parenteral nutrition. *Pediatrics* 1983;**71**:784–9.
413 Thurston WA. Acute acalculous cholecystitis in a premature infant treated with parenteral nutrition. *Can Med Assoc J* 1986;**135**:332–4.
414 Lambert GH, Muraskas J, Anderson CL, Myers TF. Direct hyperbilirubinemia associated with chloral hydrate administration in the newborn. *Pediatrics* 1990;**86**:277–81.
415 Aghai ZH, Mudduluru M, Nakhla TA, *et al.* Fluconazole prophylaxis in extremely low birth weight infants: association with cholestasis. *J Perinatol* 2006;**26**:550–5.
416 Andreou A, Papouli M, Papavasiliou V, Badouraki M. Postoperative chylous ascites in a neonate treated successfully with octreotide: bile sludge and cholestasis. *Am J Perinatol* 2005;**22**:401–4.
417 Callahan J, Haller JO, Cacciarelli AA, Slovis TL, Friedman AP. Cholelithiasis in infants: association with total parenteral nutrition and furosemide. *Pediatr Radiol* 1982;**143**:437–9.
418 Schaad UB, Wedgwood-Krucko J, Tschaeppeler H. Reversible ceftriaxone-associated biliary pseudolithiasis in children. *Lancet* 1988;**ii**:1411–3.
419 Araz N, Okan V, Demirci M, Araz M. Pseudolithiasis due to ceftriaxone treatment for meningitis in children: report of 8 cases. *Tohoku J Exp Med* 2007;**211**:285–90.
420 Hetzel PG, Glanzmann R, Hasler PW, Ladewick A, Bührer C. Coumarin embryopathy in an extremely low birth weight infant associated with neonatal hepatitis and ocular malformations. *Eur J Pediatr* 2006;**165**:358–60.
421 Merlob P, Mor N, Litwin A. Transient hepatic dysfunction in an infant of an epileptic mother treated with carbamazepine during pregnancy and breastfeeding. *Ann Pharmacother* 1992; **26**:1563–5.
422 Frey B, Braegger CP, Ghelfi D. Neonatal cholestatic hepatitis from carbamazepine exposure during pregnancy and breast feeding. *Ann Pharmacother* 2002;**36**:644–7.
423 Silverman ED, Laxer RM. Neonatal lupus erythematosus. *Rheum Dis Clin North Am* 1997;**23**:599–618.
424 Laxer RM, Roberts EA, Gross KR, *et al.* Liver disease in neonatal lupus erythematosus. *J Pediatr* 1990;**116**:238–42.
425 Evans N, Gaskin K. Liver disease in association with neonatal lupus erythematosus. *J Paediatr Child Health* 1993;**29**:478–80.
426 Rosh JR, Silverman ED, Groisman G, Dolgin S, LeLeiho NS. Intrahepatic cholestasis in neonatal lupus erythematosus. *J Pediatr Gastroenterol Nutr* 1993;**17**:310–2.
427 Schoenlebe J, Buyon JP, Zitelli BJ, Friedman D, Greco MA, Knisely AS. Neonatal hemochromatosis associated with maternal antibodies against Ro/SS-A and La/SS-B ribonucleoproteins. *Am J Dis Child* 1993;**147**:1072–5.
428 Selander B, Cedergren S, Domanski H. A case of severe neonatal lupus erythematosus without cardiac or cutaneous involvement. *Acta Paediatr* 1998;**87**:105–7.
429 Lee LA, Sokol RJ, Buyon JP. Hepatobiliary disease in neonatal lupus: prevalence and clinical characteristics in cases enrolled in a national registry. *Pediatrics* 2002;**109**:E11.
430 Bernard O, Hadchouel M, Scotto J, Odievre M, Alagille's D. Severe giant cell hepatitis with autoimmune hemolytic anemia in early childhood. *J Pediatr* 1981;**99**:704–11.
431 Brichard B, Sokal E, Gosseye S, Buts JP, Gadisseux JF, Cornu G. Coombs-positive giant cell hepatitis of infancy: effect of steroids and azathioprine therapy. *Eur J Pediatr* 1991;**150**:314–7.
432 Jaffe R, Yunis EJ. Congenital Budd–Chiari syndrome. *Pediatr Pathol* 1983;**1**:187–92.
433 McClead RE, Birken G, Wheller JJ, Hansen NB, Bickers RG, Menke JA. Budd–Chiari syndrome in a premature infant receiving total parenteral nutrition. *J Pediatr Gastroenterol Nutr* 1986;**5**:655–8.
434 Gentil-Kocher S, Bernard O, Brunelle F, *et al.* Budd–Chiari syndrome in children: report of 22 cases. *J Pediatr* 1988;**113**:30–8.
435 Brocart M, Tchernia G, Martin E, Thibert M, Lemerle M, Schweisguth O. Syndrome de Budd–Chiari relevant un lymphosarcome de l'enfant. *Arch Fr Pediatr* 1974;**31**:887–900.
436 Dahms BB, Boyd T, Redline RW. Severe perinatal liver disease associated with fetal thrombotic vasculopathy. *Pediatr Dev Pathol* 2002;**5**:80–5.
437 Yonekura T, Kubota A, Hoki M, *et al.* Intermittent obstruction of the inferior vena cava by congenital anteromedial diaphragmatic hernia: an extremely rare case of Budd–Chiari syndrome in an infant. *Surgery* 1998;**124**:109–11.
438 Jacquemin E, Saliba E, Blond MH, Chantepie A, Laugier J. Liver dysfunction and acute cardiocirculatory failure in children. *Eur J Pediatr* 1992;**151**:731–4.
439 Vajro P, Amelio A, Stagni A, *et al.* Cholestasis in newborn infants with perinatal asphyxia. *Acta Paediatr* 1997;**86**:895–8.
440 Jacquemin E, Lykavieris P, Chaoui N, Hadchouel M, Bernard O. Transient neonatal cholestasis: origin and outcome. *J Pediatr* 1998;**133**:563–7.
441 Herzog D, Chessex P, Martin S, Alvarez F. Transient cholestasis in newborn infants with perinatal asphyxia. *Can J Gastroenterol* 2003;**17**:179–82.
442 Karlsson M, Blennow M, Nemeth A, Winbladh B. Dynamics of hepatic enzyme activity following birth asphyxia. *Acta Paediatr* 2006;**95**:1405–11.
443 Sant'Anna AM, Fouron JC, Alvarez F. Neonatal cholestasis associated with fetal arrhythmia. *J Pediatr* 2005;**146**:277–80.
444 Finegold MJ. Tumors of the liver. *Semin Liver Dis* 1994;**14**:270–81.

445 Leblanc A, Hadchouel M, Jehan P, Odievre M, Alagille's D. Obstructive jaundice in children with histiocytosis X. *Gastroenterology* 1981;**80**:134–9.
446 Hu WK, Gilliam AC, Wiersma SR, Dahms BB. Fatal congenital systemic juvenile xanthogranuloma with liver failure. *Pediatr Dev Pathol* 2004;**7**:71–6.
447 Pierro A, Koletzko B, Carnielli V, *et al.* Resting energy expenditure in infants and children with extrahepatic biliary atresia. *J Pediatr Surg* 1989;**24**:534–8.
448 Kaufman SS, Murray ND, Wood RP, Shaw, BW Jr, Vanderhoof JA. Nutritional support for the infant with extrahepatic biliary atresia. *J Pediatr* 1987;**110**:679–86.
449 Mager DR, Wykes LJ, Roberts EA, Ball RO, Pencharz PB. Mild-to-moderate chronic cholestatic liver disease increases leucine oxidation in children. *J Nutr* 2006;**136**:965–70.
450 Mager DR, Wykes LJ, Roberts EA, Ball RO, Pencharz PB. Branched-chain amino acid needs in children with mild-to-moderate chronic cholestatic liver disease. *J Nutr* 2006;**136**:133–9.
451 Feranchak AP, Gralla J, King R, *et al.* Comparison of indices of vitamin A status in children with chronic liver disease. *Hepatology* 2005;**42**:782–92.
452 Mager DR, McGee PL, Furuya KN, Roberts EA. Prevalence of vitamin K deficiency in children with mild to moderate chronic liver disease. *J Pediatr Gastroenterol Nutr* 2006;**42**:71–6.
453 Heubi JE, Hollis BW, Specker B, Tsang RC. Bone disease in chronic childhood cholestasis. I. Vitamin D absorption and metabolism. *Hepatology* 1989;**9**:258–64.
454 Kooh SW, Roberts EA, Fraser D, *et al.* Ultraviolet irradiation for hepatic rickets. *Arch Dis Child* 1989;**64**:617–9.
455 Argao EA, Heubi JE, Hollis BW, Tsang RC. d-Alpha-tocopheryl polyethylene glycol-1000 succinate enhances the absorption of vitamin D in chronic cholestatic liver disease of infancy and childhood. *Pediatr Res* 1992;**31**:146–50.
456 Sokol RJ, Heubi JE, Butler-Simon N, McClung HJ, Lilly JR, Silverman A. Treatment of vitamin E deficiency during chronic childhood cholestasis with oral d-alpha-tocopheryl polyethylene glycol-1000 succinate. *Gastroenterology* 1987;**93**:975–85.
457 Sokol RJ, Butler-Simon NA, Bettis D, Smith, DJ, Silverman A. Tocopheryl polyethylene glycol 1000 succinate therapy for vitamin E deficiency during chronic childhood cholestasis: neurologic outcome. *J Pediatr* 1987;**111**:830–6.
458 Emerick KM, Whitington PF. Partial external biliary diversion for intractable pruritus and xanthomas in Alagille's syndrome. *Hepatology* 2002;**35**:1501–6.
459 Mattei P, von Allmen D, Piccoli D, Rand E. Relief of intractable pruritus in Alagille's syndrome by partial external biliary diversion. *J Pediatr Surg* 2006;**41**:104–7.
460 Modi BP, Suh MY, Jonas MM, Lillehei C, Kim HB. Ileal exclusion for refractory symptomatic cholestasis in Alagille's syndrome. *J Pediatr Surg* 2007;**42**:800–5.
461 Yerushalmi B, Sokol RJ, Narkewicz MR, Smith D, Karrer FM. Use of rifampin for severe pruritus in children with chronic cholestasis. *J Pediatr Gastroenterol Nutr* 1999;**29**:442–7.
462 Banks L, Pares A, Elena M, Piera C, Rodes J. Comparison of rifampicin with phenobarbitone for treatment of pruritus in biliary cirrhosis. *Lancet* 1989;**i**:574–6.
463 Gregorio GV, Ball CS, Mowat AP, Mieli-Vergani G. Effect of rifampin in the treatment of pruritus in hepatic cholestasis. *Arch Dis Child* 1993;**69**:141–3.
464 Kliewer SA, Willson TM. Regulation of xenobiotic and bile acid metabolism by the nuclear pregnane X receptor. *J Lipid Res* 2002;**43**:359–64.
465 Marschall HU, Wagner M, Zollner G, *et al.* Complementary stimulation of hepatobiliary transport and detoxification systems by rifampicin and ursodeoxycholic acid in humans. *Gastroenterology* 2005;**129**:476–85.
466 Khurana S, Singh P. Rifampin is safe for treatment of pruritus due to chronic cholestasis: a meta-analysis of prospective randomized-controlled trials. *Liver Int* 2006;**26**:943–8.
467 Tandon P, Rowe BH, Vandermeer B, Bain VG. The efficacy and safety of bile acid binding agents, opioid antagonists, or rifampin in the treatment of cholestasis-associated pruritus. *Am J Gastroenterol* 2007;**102**:1528–36.
468 Colombani PM, Cigarroa FG, Schwarz K, Wise B, Maley WE, Klein AS. Liver transplantation in infants younger than 1 year of age. *Ann Surg* 1996;**223**:658–62.
469 Bonatti H, Muiesan P, Connelly S, *et al.* Hepatic transplantation in children under 3 months of age: a single centre's experience. *J Pediatr Surg* 1997;**32**:486–8.
470 Grabhorn E, Schulz A, Helmke K, *et al.* Short- and long-term results of liver transplantation in infants aged less than 6 months. *Transplantation* 2004;**78**:235–41.
471 D'Antiga L, Moniz C, Buxton-Thomas M, *et al.* Bone mineral density and height gain in children with chronic cholestatic liver disease undergoing transplantation. *Transplantation* 2002;**73**:1788–93.
472 Cutillo L, Najimi M, Smets F, *et al.* Safety of living-related liver transplantation for progressive familial intrahepatic cholestasis. *Pediatr Transplant* 2006;**10**:570–4.
473 Kartenbeck J, Leuschner U, Mayer R, Keppler D. Absence of the canalicular isoform of the MRP gene-encoded conjugate export pump from the hepatocytes in Dubin–Johnson syndrome. *Hepatology* 1996;**23**:1061–6.
474 Paulusma CC, Kool M, Bosma PJ, *et al.* A mutation in the human canalicular multispecific organic anion transporter gene causes the Dubin–Johnson syndrome. *Hepatology* 1997;**25**:1539–42.
475 Hashimoto K, Uchiumi T, Konno T, *et al.* Trafficking and functional defects by mutations of the ATP-binding domains in *MRP2* in patients with Dubin–Johnson syndrome. *Hepatology* 2002;**36**:1236–45.
476 Keitel V, Nies AT, Brom M, Hummel-Eisenbeiss J, Spring H, Keppler D. A common Dubin–Johnson syndrome mutation impairs protein maturation and transport activity of *MRP2* (*ABCC2*). *Am J Physiol Gastrointest Liver Physiol* 2003;**284**:G165–74.
477 Shieh CC, Chang MH, Chen CL. Dubin–Johnson syndrome presenting with neonatal cholestasis. *Arch Dis Child* 1990;**65**:898–9.
478 Regev RH, Stolar O, Raz A, Dolfin T. Treatment of severe cholestasis in neonatal Dubin–Johnson syndrome with ursodeoxycholic acid. *J Perinat Med* 2002;**30**:185–7.
479 Haimi-Cohen Y, Merlob P, Marcus-Eidlits T, Amir J Dubin–Johnson syndrome as a cause of neonatal jaundice: the importance of coproporphyrins investigation. *Clin Pediatr (Phila)* 1998; **37**:511–3.
480 Shimizu T, Tawa T, Maruyama T, Oguchi S, Yamashiro Y, Yabuta K. A case of infantile Dubin–Johnson syndrome with high CT attenuation in the liver. *Pediatr Radiol* 1997;**27**:345–7.
481 Hrebícek M, Jirásek T, Hartmannová H, *et al.* Rotor-type hyperbilirubinaemia has no defect in the canalicular bilirubin export pump. *Liver Int* 2007;**27**:485–91.

5 The Acutely Ill Baby

Patrick J. McKiernan

The majority of patients presenting with liver disease in infancy will have either cholestatic liver disease (Chapter 4) or acute liver failure with multisystem disease. Recent advances in biochemical techniques and molecular genetics have dramatically improved the diagnosis of many of these conditions, whilst significant developments in therapy have altered management and outcome. This chapter outlines the clinical presentation and approach to diagnosis and management for infants presenting with an acute illness.

Approach to diagnosis and management

Infants and neonates have limited responses to severe illness, irrespective of etiology, but important diagnostic information may be obtained from simple clinical and laboratory observations obtained at the time of presentation.

Age at presentation is important, with three risk periods recognizable: at birth, in the neonatal period, and later in infancy. Conditions presenting at birth imply an intrauterine process, while early neonatal presentation may imply a toxic process, often infective or metabolic in origin (Table 5.1).

In establishing etiology, the clinical history should inquire about preceding symptoms and precipitants. In infants presenting soon after birth, information about pregnancy and delivery is of obvious relevance. In all age groups, a dietary history is crucial, with particular attention being paid to symptoms on weaning or on fasting, and recent changes in diet. In neonates, the first sign of altered consciousness may be difficulty in feeding, whereas in older infants vomiting is a frequent accompaniment of encephalopathy. A history of consanguinity or of any previously affected siblings should be sought.

Clinical assessment should first concentrate on the airway–breathing–circulation (ABC) of resuscitation, followed by a complete physical examination. Particular attention should be paid to the presence of hepatomegaly, neurological abnormalities, tachypnea, and unusual odors. It is important to recognize intercurrent illnesses such as pneumonia, septicemia, or congenital heart disease, which may have precipitated the acute episode and will require specific treatment.

Table 5.1 Differential diagnosis of acutely ill infants.

Conditions presenting at birth
Hydrops fetalis
Lysosomal storage disease
Conditions presenting in the neonatal period
Infection:
Coxsackie A or B
Herpes simplex
Adenovirus
Cytomegalovirus
Parvovirus
Echovirus
Neonatal hemochromatosis
Mitochondrial cytopathy
Galactosemia
Organic acidemia
Urea cycle defects
Disorder of fatty acid oxidation
Conditions presenting later in infancy
Tyrosinemia type 1
Glycogen storage disease
Hereditary fructose intolerance

Table 5.2 lists the investigations that are required immediately. Additional samples of each biological fluid should be separated and frozen, with subsequent analysis depending on the results of the initial screen. An algorithm for the diagnosis of the acutely ill infant is given in Figure 5.1, with appropriate second-line investigations outlined in Table 5.3.

Until the diagnosis is established, management is supportive, with correction of hypoglycemia, acid–base imbalance, electrolyte imbalance, and coagulopathy as required (Chapter 7). It is prudent to exclude lactose, fat, and protein from the diet during the first 24 h of acute illness while awaiting specific diagnostic information, but restriction should be

Diseases of the Liver and Biliary System in Children, 3rd edition. Edited by Deirdre Kelly. © 2008 Blackwell Publishing, ISBN: 978-1-4051-6334-7.

Table 5.2 Initial investigations in the acutely ill infant.

*Blood**	*Urine**
Bacterial culture	pH
Prothrombin time, partial thromboplastin time,	Microscopy and culture
fibrinogen, D-dimers	Reducing substances
Bilirubin, alkaline phosphatase, transaminases,	Ketones
albumin, GGT	Organic acids
Acid–base balance	Amino acids
Glucose	
Lactate	*CSF* (if coagulation and neurological
Ammonia, amino acids	state allow)
Full blood count and film	Gram stain and culture
Urea, sodium, potassium, calcium	Protein, glucose
Acylcarnitine profile	Lactate
	Imaging
	Chest and wrist radiography
	Echocardiography

* Store plasma, serum and urine samples for further investigations (see Table 5.3).
CSF, cerebrospinal fluid; GGT, γ-glutamyltransferase.

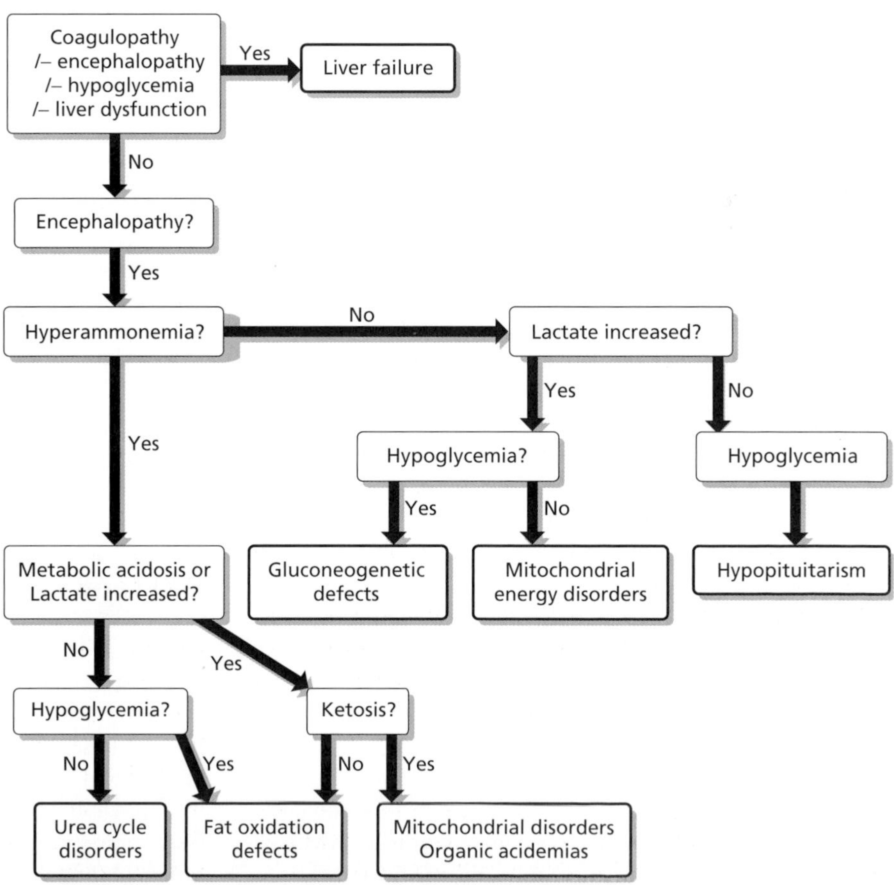

Figure 5.1 Algorithm for the initial investigation/diagnosis of the acutely ill infant. The bold boxes represent phenotypic groups. For each phenotypic group, second-line investigations are summarized in Table 5.3.

Table 5.3 Second-line investigations following initial assessment.

Phenotypic group	Second-line investigations
Liver failure	Fe, transferrin, ferritin Cholesterol and triglycerides Galactose-1-phosphate uridyltransferase Plasma amino acids Urinary organic acids and succinylacetone Specific urine and stool viral culture Respiratory chain enzymes
Mitochondrial energy disorders*	Pre-/post-prandial plasma lactate, glucose, FFA, and 3-OH Plasma carnitine, acylcarnitine Plasma amino acids, creatine kinase Urinary organic acids CSF lactate Muscle biopsy for RCE Brain MRI EEG and visual evoked potentials
Urea cycle disorders	Plasma amino acids Carnitine and acylcarnitines Lactate, glucose, FFA, and 3-OH Creatine kinase Urinary amino, organic and orotic acids
Fat oxidation defects*	Carnitine and acylcarnitines; lactate, glucose, FFA, 3-OH Creatine kinase Urinary organic acids
Gluconeogenetic defects	Lactate, glucose, FFA, 3-OH Creatine kinase, urate, cholesterol, triglycerides Urinary organic acids and oligosaccharides Specific enzyme assays (see text)
Organic acidemias*	Plasma amino acids Carnitine and acylcarnitines Urinary organic acids
Hypopituitarism	9 AM cortisol, thyroid function tests, growth hormone, IGF-1

CSF, cerebrospinal fluid; EEG, electroencephalography; Fe, iron; FFA, free fatty acids; IGF-1, insulin-like growth factor-1; MRI, magnetic resonance imaging; 3-OH, 3-hydroxybutyrate; RCE, respiratory chain enzyme.

* Fibroblast culture for specific enzymatic diagnosis.

for as short a time as possible. Parenteral empirical broad-spectrum antibiotic treatment should be commenced once initial samples have been obtained, and it should be continued until sepsis has been excluded.

Infection

Intrauterine or postnatal infection is an important and common cause of acute illness in the neonate; it is fully discussed in Chapters 4, 6 and 7 (see also Tables 5.1 and 5.2).

Fetal and neonatal ascites

Fetal or neonatal ascites is a rare presentation that occurs in about one in 3000 pregnancies and is associated with intrauterine infection, inborn errors of metabolism, or rhesus hemolytic disease. As the rate of fetal loss is high, few infants present with this complication. The widespread use of anti-D immunoglobulin has reduced the incidence of hemolytic disease, and the majority of cases are now secondary to disorders of cardiac structure or rhythm, hematological, gastro-

Table 5.4 Causes of neonatal ascites.

Congenital infection
Cytomegalovirus
Toxoplasmosis
Syphilis
Metabolic
Lysosomal storage disorders:
Salla disease
Sialidosis type II
Niemann–Pick type A and C
Infantile GM_1 gangliosidosis
Mucopolysaccharidosis VII
Wolman disease
Gaucher disease
Tyrosinemia type 1
Neonatal hemochromatosis
Carbohydrate deficient glycoprotein syndrome
Mitochondrial DNA mutation
Other
Cardiac disease
Hepatoblastoma
Hemangioendothelioma
Mesenchymal hamartoma

intestinal, or genitourinary disease. Hepatic and metabolic causes account for about 4% of cases, with lysosomal storage disorders being the commonest of this group, which may even include mitochondrial disorders (Table 5.4). It is particularly important to recognize these, as they may recur and early prenatal diagnosis may be possible.[1,2]

A number of pathogenic mechanisms may contribute to the development of ascites: cardiac failure; anemia due to infiltration of the reticuloendothelial system; hepatic infiltration or insufficiency producing hypoalbuminemia; or mass effects resulting in vascular and lymphatic obstruction.

The diagnosis may be suspected on antenatal ultrasound, or at birth because of abdominal distension. Hepatosplenomegaly is usually present.

Investigation

If this is fatal, the placenta and fetus should have a comprehensive radiological and pathological examination. It is necessary to exclude the commoner infective, cardiovascular, and hematological causes, and search for storage disorders as follows:

- Blood film for vacuolated lymphocytes
- Bone-marrow aspirate for storage cells
- Plasma transferrin electrophoresis for carbohydrate-deficient glycoprotein syndrome
- Urinary oligosaccharidases and glycosaminoglycans
- White cell or fibroblast culture or placental cell line for lysosomal enzyme studies

Treatment

This should be started prenatally, if possible, with close obstetric liaison with regard to the mode and place of delivery. Resuscitation may require immediate paracentesis and transfusion in the labor suite. Subsequent management and prognosis depend on the etiology. The prognosis is poor for storage diseases presenting in this manner. Symptomatic relief may be gained by the use of spironolactone (3 mg/kg/day), fluid restriction (50–75% maintenance) and 4.5% albumin transfusion (5–10 mL/kg).

Galactosemia

This autosomal-recessive disorder is caused by a deficiency of galactose-1-phosphate uridyl/transferase and has an incidence of one in 45 000. Several different allelic variants with varying degrees of residual activity have been recognized, and a database for these has been established.[3] The commonest mutation (Q188R) accounts for > 70% of abnormal alleles, while N314D is associated with a milder form, the Duarte variant.[4] Much more rarely, a defect of the epimerase enzyme can occur with a similar clinical presentation.[5] Galactose, galactitol, and galactose-1-phosphate (Gal-1-P) accumulate following feeding. While accumulation of galactitol causes cataract, it is unclear which metabolites cause liver dysfunction.

Clinical presentation and diagnosis

Infants may present with collapse with hypoglycemia and encephalopathy in the first few days of life, or with progressive jaundice and liver failure. Vomiting, diarrhea, jaundice, and poor weight gain are common in early infancy. Cataracts (characteristically "oil-drop") are present shortly after birth and may be associated with intraocular hemorrhage and retinal detachment. There is a high incidence of Gram-negative sepsis, which is usually associated with a severe coagulopathy. Renal tubular dysfunction is common.

The diagnosis is classically suggested by the detection of urinary reducing substances without glycosuria, but urinary tests are neither sensitive nor specific. An associated proximal renal tubular defect may result in aminoaciduria and glycosuria, while reducing substances in the urine are a frequent nonspecific finding in other forms of neonatal liver disease.[6] Alternatively, galactosuria may not be detected in an infant with galactosemia who is severely ill and no longer taking a lactose-containing formula.

The diagnosis should be confirmed by demonstration of reduced enzyme activity in blood. Misleading results may be obtained if the baby has been transfused (false-negative) or in glucose-6-phosphate dehydrogenase deficiency (false-positive). Where there is confusion, other diagnostic options include measuring erythrocyte Gal-1-P, testing for the Q188R mutation, or measuring parental-erythrocyte galactose-1-phosphate uridyltransferase.

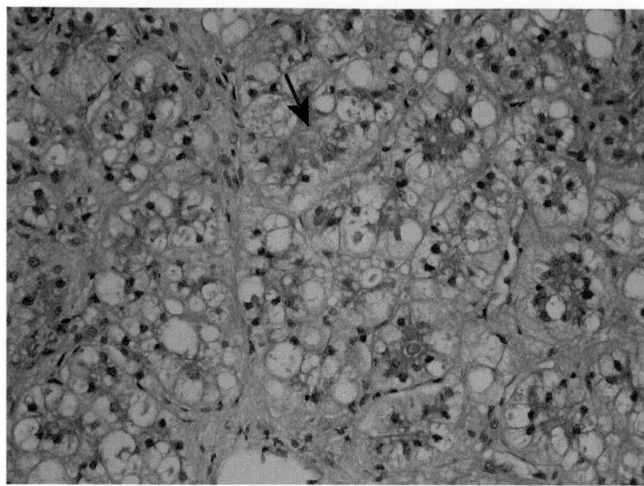

Figure 5.2 Galactosemia may present with acute liver failure or cholestasis with a giant cell hepatitis. This 6-week-old baby presented with both, as she developed cholestasis from biliary obstruction due to biliary sludge. Note the bile plugs (arrow).

Hepatic pathology initially demonstrates fatty change, periportal bile duct proliferation, and iron deposition, with extramedullary hemopoiesis (Figure 5.2). If galactose ingestion persists, hepatic fibrosis and cirrhosis may develop, although cirrhosis may be present at birth.[7]

Management and prognosis

Liver function improves within days following exclusion of galactose from the diet, unless liver failure or cirrhosis is already established. Progressive liver disease is very rare. Cataracts may improve if treatment is started early enough. Galactose elimination should be lifelong, but long-term complications such as cognitive impairment, speech defects, hypergonadotropic hypogonadism, and motor abnormalities are common despite dietary treatment. This probably results from ongoing endogenous synthesis of galactose-1-phosphate and generalized glycoprotein hypoglycosylation, rather than dietary indiscretion.[8]

Neonatal screening

Neonatal screening for galactosemia is not universally available, but leads to early detection except in those babies who present with fulminant hepatitis. Antenatal diagnosis is possible by chorionic villus sampling.

Infantile liver failure

Acute liver failure in infancy usually presents with multisystem involvement (Figure 5.3). The diagnosis may initially be difficult, as jaundice may be a late feature. Infants may be small for gestational dates or have intrauterine growth retardation. The clinical presentation includes hypotonia, hypoglycemia, and hypotension. Coagulopathy is invariable in association with liver dysfunction and moderate hyperammonemia. Encephalopathy is frequent, but not inevitable, in infants and may be difficult to recognize (Chapter 7). Neurological problems such as nystagmus and convulsions may be secondary to cerebral disease or encephalopathy. Renal tubular acidosis and lactic acidosis are common.

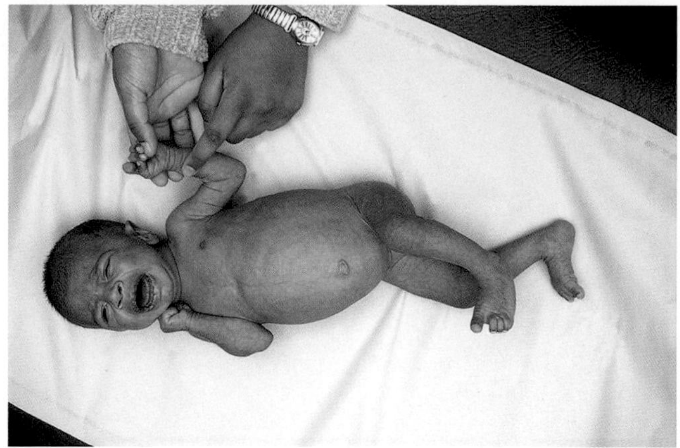

Figure 5.3 Infants with acute liver failure present with multiorgan failure, coagulopathy, encephalopathy, and jaundice.

Physical examination and investigations should be directed at identifying and excluding multiorgan disease and pathology.

General measures include intravenous dextrose to maintain blood glucose at 4–8 mmol/L, prophylactic antibiotics and intravenous acyclovir, antifungal therapy, intravenous ranitidine to prevent gastric bleeding, correction of coagulopathy with fresh frozen plasma and/or exchange transfusions (Chapter 7). Once baseline and essential investigations have been conducted (Table 5.2), galactose and protein should be excluded from the diet until the underlying diagnosis is confirmed or galactosemia is specifically excluded. As spontaneous recovery is unlikely, all children should be assessed for liver transplantation unless there is irreversible multiorgan disease.

Neonatal hemochromatosis (NNH)

This disorder—also known as perinatal hemochromatosis or neonatal iron storage disease—is the commonest cause of acute liver failure in the neonate.

The disease is characterized by prenatal liver disease combined with extrahepatic siderosis, with sparing of the reticuloendothelial system.[9] Fetal liver disease appears to be the primary event, with siderosis being a secondary phenomenon.[10,11] It is unclear whether the hemochromatosis phenotype is due to redistribution of fetal liver iron as a consequence of liver damage, or whether there is increased body iron due to increased placental iron transfer.[9] In the majority of cases, the liver disease appears to be alloimmune. Maternal antibodies to an uncharacterized fetal antibody have been detected, the recurrence pattern is characteristic of other gestational alloimmune diseases, and early prenatal immunoglobulin treatment modifies the disease.[9]

Recurrence

There is no association with mutations in the genes for hereditary hemochromatosis or juvenile hemochromatosis.[12] NNH is extremely rare in first pregnancies, and once one affected child has been born, the risk of recurrence in subsequent pregnancies is 80%. Of seven reported cases in which half-siblings were born to the same mother, NNH occurred in both sibships in six, but recurrence has never been reported in children born to the same father with different mothers.[13,14] This pattern is strongly suggestive of a maternal alloimmune disorder.

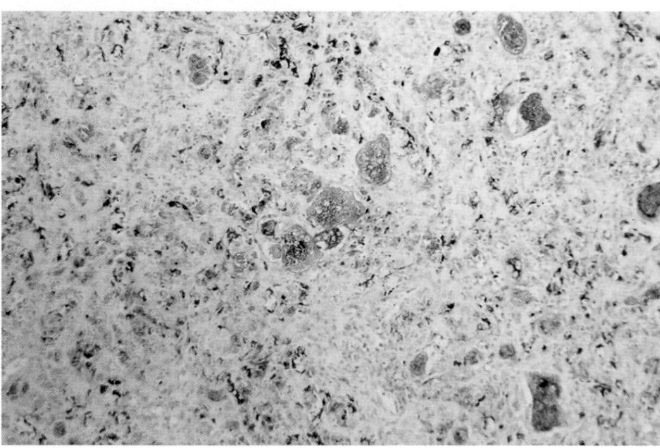

Figure 5.4 Neonatal hemochromatosis. This rare disorder is characterized by elevated serum iron and ferritin and hypersaturation of iron-binding capacity. Histology shows hepatic necrosis, with iron deposition in hepatocytes and Kupffer cells.

Presentation and diagnosis

Intrauterine growth retardation is common, and the majority of affected infants are delivered prematurely. Children present with hypoglycemia, jaundice, and coagulopathy, often on the first day of life, although the presentation may be delayed until up to 3 months of age.[9,15] Ascites may be present. Encephalopathy is variable and may present with irritability and drowsiness. The clinical course is usually rapidly progressive, with most infants dying in the first month of life.

Laboratory features include:

- Mild elevation of transaminases
- Low albumin
- Elevated conjugated bilirubin
- Prothrombin time grossly elevated (> 50 s)
- Low transferrin, with hypersaturation of iron-binding capacity (95–105%)
- Grossly elevated ferritin levels (2000–3000 μg/L).

These laboratory features, including iron status markers, are sensitive but nonspecific, being found in neonatal liver failure of any cause.[16] For definitive diagnosis, liver biopsy is rarely feasible in life, but extrahepatic siderosis can be safely demonstrated in minor salivary glands obtained by lip biopsy.[15] Magnetic resonance imaging may also provide evidence of hepatic and extrahepatic siderosis, although interpretation may be difficult.[17] Where feasible, liver histology demonstrates cirrhosis, pericellular fibrosis, giant cell transformation, ductular proliferation, and regenerative nodules (Figure 5.4).[15]

Management and outcome

Infants should be managed in a neonatal intensive-care setting in a transplant center. In addition to the usual supportive regimen for acute liver failure (Chapter 7), an antioxidant cocktail should be commenced once the diagnosis is suspected. This includes three antioxidants:

- *N*-acetylcysteine (140 mg/kg by mouth or nasogastric tube as a loading dose; then 70 mg/kg every 4 h to a total of 17–21 doses)
- Selenium (3 μg/kg/day intravenously over 24 h)
- α-Tocopheryl polyethylene glycol succinate (20–30 IU/kg/day orally in two divided doses)
- Prostaglandin E_1, given as a continuous intravenous infusion (0.4–0.6 μg/kg/h daily for 2–4 weeks)
- Desferrioxamine (30 mg/kg/day as an intravenous infusion over 8 h until serum ferritin is < 500 μg/L).

The response to the antioxidant cocktail is variable and difficult to predict. The antioxidant cocktail is more effective if begun within 24–48 h of birth and in infants with a less severe phenotype.[18,19] Even in children who do not completely respond to treatment, the use of this cocktail may produce sufficient stabilization of their condition to allow liver transplantation. Children who survive without liver transplantation develop an inactive fibrosis or cirrhosis.

Double-volume exchange transfusion in combination with immunoglobulin treatment has been reported to be successful, and it is a logical treatment, given the alloimmune etiology.

Liver transplantation remains the definitive treatment. Children should be listed for transplantation at diagnosis, while the antioxidant cocktail is continuing, as suitable donor organs are scarce in this age group and the major cause of mortality is progressive liver failure while awaiting transplantation. Recent reports have demonstrated that liver transplantation is successful in this group of infants, despite technical difficulties.[18–20] In only one case has there been clinically significant recurrence.[21]

Prevention of recurrent disease in siblings

The recurrence risk in subsequent pregnancies is 80%. On the basis of the likely alloimmune background, Whitington and Hibbard proposed prenatal maternal treatment with immunoglobulin.[22] The regimen tested was a weekly infusion of 1 g/kg from the 18th week of pregnancy until delivery. This appears to be extremely effective in preventing severe recurrent disease, and no child born after treatment with the complete protocol has developed liver failure or required liver transplantation.[13,22,23] This should now be considered the standard of care. Irrespective of antenatal treatment, all subsequent siblings should be carefully assessed for evidence of NNH and as a minimum should have iron status (iron, transferrin, and ferritin) and coagulation checked and medical management instituted if necessary.

Disorders of mitochondrial energy metabolism

This rare group of disorders may present with acute liver failure, multiorgan disease, and Alpers syndrome. There is a wide range of clinical phenotypes with any mode of inheritance—autosomal-recessive, autosomal-dominant, or transmission through maternal DNA. The pathological effects are secondary to dysfunction of the electron transport chain, resulting in cellular adenosine triphosphate (ATP) deficiency, impaired fat oxidation, and the generation of toxic free radicals. Clinical symptoms are variable, depending on the nature of the primary defect, its tissue distribution and abundance, and the importance of aerobic metabolism in the affected tissue. The constituent proteins of the electron transport chain are encoded by autosomally inherited nuclear DNA (nDNA) and by mitochondrial DNA (mtDNA), which is maternally inherited.[24] In the acutely ill infant, three entities are most relevant: isolated deficiencies of the electron transport chain enzymes, mtDNA depletion syndromes, and Alpers syndrome.

Deficiencies of the electron transport chain enzymes

The most common isolated defects involve complexes IV and I. It appears that multiple respiratory chain defects are usually part of a deletion syndrome.[25] There is often a family history of consanguinity, and presumably many of these disorders result from nuclear gene mutations, but the primary genetic defect is rarely found when the presentation is with liver failure.[26]

Mitochondrial DNA depletion syndrome

Mitochondria normally contain 2–10 copies of mtDNA. Replication of mtDNA is regulated by a number of factors encoded by nuclear genes. Mutations in these nuclear genes lead to reduction in copy numbers of mtDNA, resulting in mitochondrial DNA depletion with autosomal-recessive inheritance. Mutations have been found in genes encoding the mitochondrial enzymes DNA polymerase gamma,[27] thymidine kinase,[28] deoxyguanosine kinase,[28] and succinyl CoA-ligase,[29] and in the *MPV17* gene.[30]

Alpers syndrome

Alpers syndrome is an autosomal-recessive, developmental mtDNA depletion disorder characterized by degenerative brain and liver disease, which may be precipitated by valproate treatment.[27] The liver disease may rarely present with infantile liver failure, but may evolve from asymptomatic biochemical liver dysfunction. Seizures, which are focal and refractory, usually precede liver disease but may follow it, especially in infancy. Also in infancy, the developmental regression may not be appreciated.

Clinical presentation

The clinical presentation is varied, and the onset may be prenatal, with structural brain abnormalities. Nonspecific dysmorphic features are not uncommon. Neurological features are prominent, and lethargy and hypotonia are almost invariable. Cardiac involvement includes hypertrophic cardiomyopathy, and there may be proximal renal tubulopathy. Hepatic involvement is unpredictable and includes isolated hepatomegaly, neonatal cholestasis, and acute liver failure with coagulopathy.

Diagnosis

The diagnostic hallmark of these disorders is elevated blood lactate, but even this may be intermittent and is nonspecific. Useful secondary investigations to identify the cause of lactic acidosis include:

- Increased plasma 3-OH-butyrate/acetoacetate ratio (> 2)
- Increased plasma lactate and/or ketone bodies, either postprandially or following a glucose load (2 g/kg)
- Detection of specific organic acids such as urinary 3-methylglutaconic acid or other Krebs cycle intermediates.[31]

A comprehensive evaluation is required, including renal tubular function, electrocardiography and echocardiography, electroretinography and visual evoked potentials, and brain magnetic resonance imaging (MRI). An elevated cerebrospinal fluid (CSF)/plasma lactate ratio or elevated CSF protein suggests central nervous system involvement.

Hepatic pathology is characterized by both microvesicular and macrovesicular steatosis, with hepatocyte degeneration and micronodular cirrhosis (Figure 5.5a). Electron microscopy may reveal an abnormal structure or number of mitochondria, although this is not invariable. Muscle histology usually shows increased lipid droplets with variation in fiber size; the presence of ragged red fibers on the Gomori stain is strongly suggestive of mtDNA abnormalities (Figure 5.5b).

The definitive diagnosis is based on demonstrating dysfunction of electron transport chain function in affected tissue by histochemistry and direct measurement of enzyme activity, combined with demonstration of reduced mtDNA copy number (< 35% of control).[25] Deficiencies of some respiratory chain subunits can be detected by immunocytochemistry. It is helpful to identify whether or not these defects are encoded in mtDNA or nDNA, as this facilitates genetic counseling. The most useful tissue to sample is usually muscle, as it is easily accessible with well-established normal ranges. In the presence of liver failure, demonstration of extrahepatic involvement will preclude liver

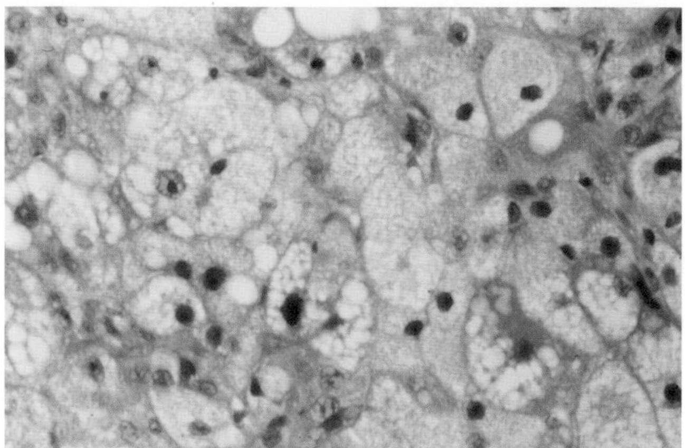
A

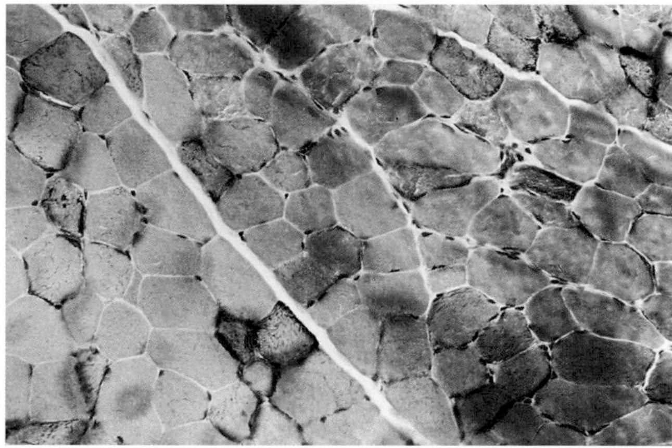
B

Figure 5.5 Mitochondrial deletions or depletions. These rare inherited defects present with acute liver failure with multisystem involvement. Hepatic histology may demonstrate microvesicular steatosis (**A**), while muscle biopsy demonstrates ragged red fibers due to a deficiency of the respiratory chain enzymes (**B**). (Gomori one-step trichrome stain, original magnification × 25.)

transplantation, and abnormalities in muscle correlate highly with neurological involvement. The exception is Alpers syndrome, in which muscle biopsy is usually normal at presentation and lactic acidosis is infrequent. In this disorder, visual evoked responses and brain MRI are often abnormal and the electroencephalogram may be characteristic. This disorder is commonly caused by mutations in *POLG*, and demonstrating these may well prove to be an important diagnostic method.

Management and prognosis

Supportive management for acute liver failure may be the only therapeutic option. If valproate has been used, it should be immediately discontinued. Dichloroacetate may lower lactate concentrations, but clinical benefit has not been established and there are concerns about side effects. Liver transplantation may be successful if the defect is confined to the liver,[32,33] which is highly unusual if the presentation is with infantile liver failure. Transplantation is contraindicated if multisystem involvement is demonstrated, or in Alpers syndrome, as neurological deterioration continues after transplantation, with eventual death.[27,34]

Antenatal diagnosis

Inheritance is most commonly autosomal-recessive, but in individual families it is impossible to exclude spontaneous mutations. Antenatal diagnosis is occasionally possible if the underlying mutation is known.

Tyrosinemia type I

Tyrosinemia type I is an autosomal-recessive disorder due to a defect of fumarylacetoacetase (FAA), which is the terminal enzyme in tyrosine degradation. Intermediate metabolites such as maleylacetoacetate and fumarylacetoacetate are highly reactive compounds that are locally toxic and mutagenic within the liver. The secondary metabolite succinylacetone has local and systemic effects (Figure 5.6), including inhibition of porphobilinogen synthase, accounting for the porphyria-like neurological crises seen.

The gene for FAA is on the short arm of chromosome 15. More than 40 mutations have been described to date,[35,36] although in some populations a single mutation may be prevalent. A hallmark of the condition is the extremely high lifetime risk of developing hepatocellular carcinoma (HCC), which historically is at least 40%.[37,38]

Clinical presentation

The disease is found worldwide, but is particularly common in the Saguenay–Lac St. Jean region of Canada (incidence one in 500) and in parts of Pakistan and northern Europe. In Birmingham (England), the incidence is one in 20 000, reflecting the mixed ethnic population.[39]

The clinical presentation is heterogeneous, even within the same family.[35] Acute liver failure is a common presentation in infants between 1 and 6 months of age; these patients present with mild jaundice, coagulopathy, encephalopathy, and ascites, with inguinal hernias. Hypoglycemia is common and may be secondary to liver dysfunction or hyperinsulinism due to pancreatic islet cell hyperplasia.[40]

In older infants, failure to thrive, coagulopathy, hepatosplenomegaly, hypotonia, and rickets are common. Older children may present with chronic liver disease, cardiomyopathy, renal failure or a porphyria-like syndrome with self-mutilation (Figure 5.7). Neurological symptoms include muscle weakness, particularly respiratory muscle weakness. Renal tubular dysfunction is almost invariable, and hypophosphatemic rickets may occur at any age.

Diagnosis

Investigations and diagnostic findings include:

- Mildly elevated bilirubin.
- Mildly abnormal transaminases (100–200 IU/L).

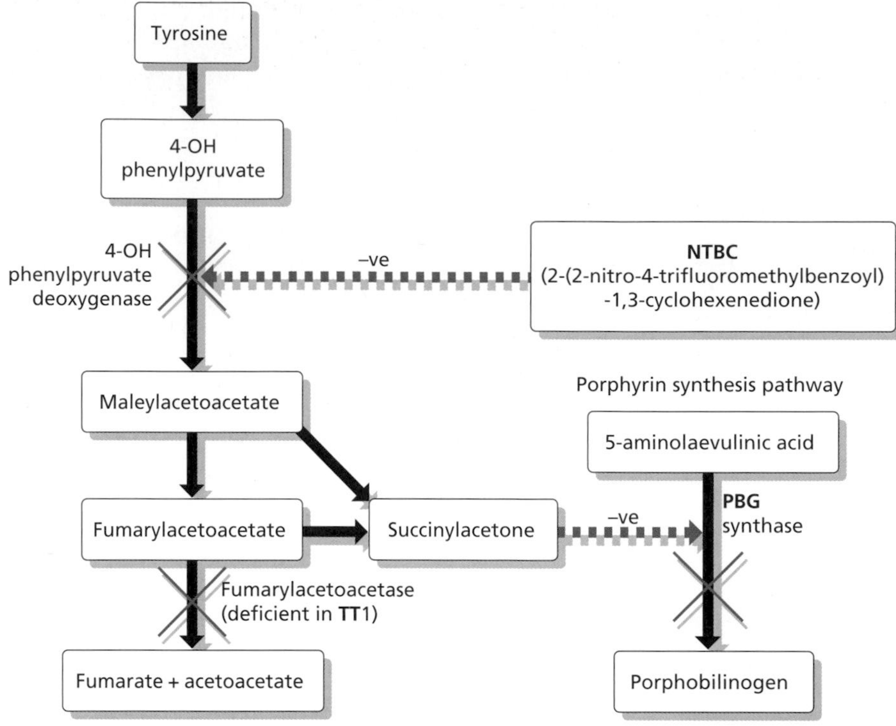

Figure 5.6 The metabolic pathway for tyrosine metabolism. 4-OH, 4-hydroxybutyrate; PBG, porphobilinogen; TT1, tyrosinemia type 1.

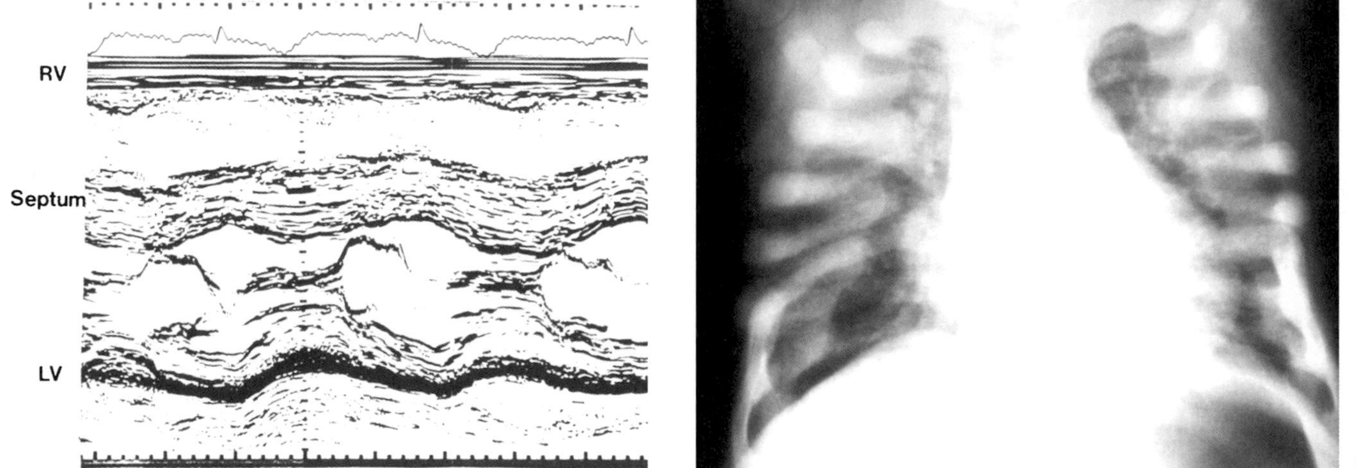

Figure 5.7 Tyrosinemia type1 may present with acute or chronic liver failure. Hypertrophic cardiomyopathy (**A**) and rickets (**B**) are common.

- Elevated alkaline phosphatase (> 600 IU/L).
- Low albumin (< 30 g/L).
- Prolonged prothrombin time (> 20 s).
- Grossly elevated α-fetoprotein levels (> 40 000–2 000 000 μg/L).
- Increased plasma tyrosine, phenylalanine, and methionine (three times normal, depending on age).
- Significant urinary succinylacetone is a pathognomonic but not invariable finding, although this compound should be estimated in order to exclude a nonspecific elevation of amino acids secondary to liver dysfunction.
- Increased urinary delta-aminolevulinic acid.
- Proximal tubular dysfunction with phosphaturia and aminoaciduria is invariable.
- Echocardiography may reveal a hypertrophic cardiomyopathy.
- Radiographic evidence of rickets.

Hepatic histology is nonspecific, with steatosis and siderosis. Cirrhosis is almost always established at the time of clinical presentation (Figure 5.8).

The diagnosis is usually confirmed by mutation analysis, but FAA activity can be measured in fibroblasts or lymphocytes.

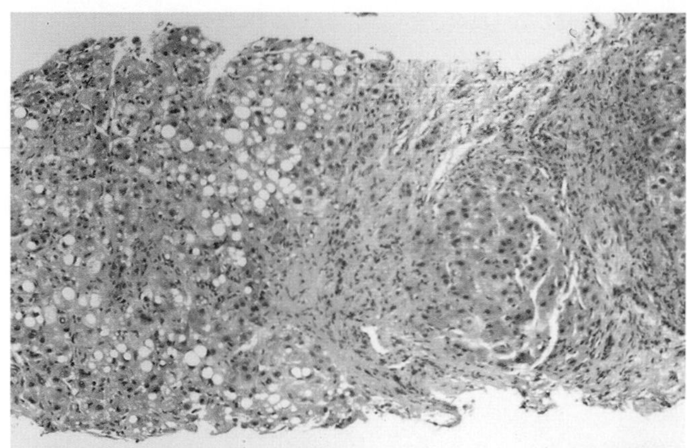

Figure 5.8 Liver histology in tyrosinemia type 1 is nonspecific, with steatosis, fibrosis, or cirrhosis.

Management

The recent introduction of nitisinone, which prevents the formation of toxic metabolites (Figure 5.2), has transformed the natural history of this disease.[41]

Treatment with nitisinone (1 mg/kg/day) in addition to a phenylalanine-restricted and tyrosine-restricted diet leads to rapid reduction of toxic metabolites within days, with disappearance within 1 month. Over 400 patients worldwide have been treated with nitisinone, with normalization of renal tubular function, complete control of porphyria-like crises, and improvement in both nutritional status and liver function.[42] In Birmingham, we have treated 26 children with nitisinone. Twelve of these children presented with acute liver failure, of whom 11 responded to nitisinone with correction of coagulopathy and encephalopathy. All responders showed an improvement in prothrombin time within 1 week of treatment, and the single nonresponder underwent successful liver transplantation.

Nitisinone therapy requires close monitoring of plasma amino acids. Tyrosine levels should be kept < 500 μmol/L, with the phenylalanine level within the normal range. Nitisinone clearly protects against the development of HCC, but this is related to the age at which treatment is started. If started at < 6 months, the risk of late HCC is negligible, while if treatment is commenced at > 2 years a significant risk of HCC remains.[42,43]

Due to the risk of hepatocellular carcinoma, we suggest that α-fetoprotein levels should be monitored every 3 months, abdominal ultrasound every 6 months, and hepatic MRI annually (unless ultrasound is abnormal) (Figure 5.9). A sustained rise in α-fetoprotein, or a failure to fall with treatment, is an indication for consideration of liver transplantation. Liver transplantation remains a highly effective treatment for tyrosinemia, but has become second-line since the introduction of nitisinone. In addition, it has become clear that the residual metabolic defect due to renal fumarylacetoacetate hydrolase is more extensive than originally believed.[42]

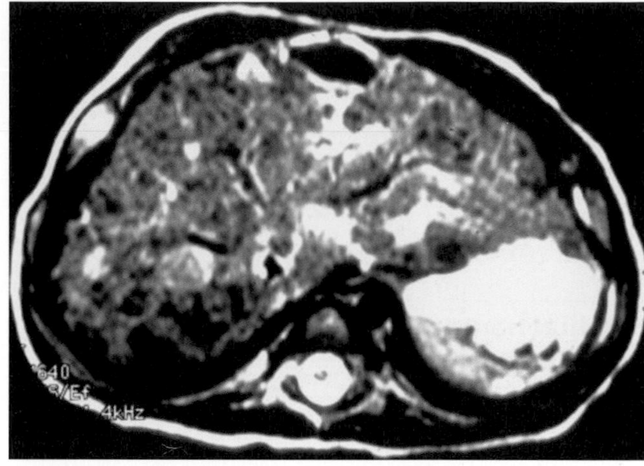

Figure 5.9 Despite treatment with nitisinone, there is a risk of hepatocellular carcinoma, which is best documented by computed tomography or magnetic resonance imaging to detect nodularity and early tumors.

Current indications for liver transplantation include:

- Unresponsive liver failure
- Established HCC
- Chronic liver disease with future risk of HCC
  —At development of first nodule
  —If abnormal α-fetoprotein evolution

Prognosis

More than 90% of children presenting with acute liver failure respond to nitisinone. Most of these children will have chronic liver disease and hence some risk of developing HCC. However, if treatment is started before 6 months, > 80% will be well on treatment at 10 years. The likelihood of remaining well on treatment diminishes with increasing age at commencement.

In Birmingham, seven children have been treated preemptively following neonatal screening. They remain clinically normal, with no biochemical or radiographic evidence of liver dysfunction (unpublished data). Similar findings have been reported with a much larger experience in Quebec, where neonatal screening is routine, with a significant decrease in the need for liver transplantation.[44]

For those who require rescue, liver transplantation is associated with 5-year survival rate of more than 80%, with a good quality of life.[45–47] It results in a functional "cure," although renal production of succinylacetone continues.

Screening

Neonatal screening programs have been established in populations with relatively high incidences of tyrosinemia. The improved outcome following preemptive nitisinone treatment makes the case for universal screening compelling. Experience has shown that blood tyrosine is a poor screening target and that succinylacetone or porphobilinogen synthase detection, combined with mutation detection in homogeneous populations, is the most effective strategy.[48]

Antenatal diagnosis

Antenatal diagnosis is possible either by chorionic villus sampling to measure FAA directly, or from mutation analysis if the genotype is known. Alternatively, succinylacetone can be measured in amniotic fluid.

Familial hemophagocytic lymphohistiocytosis

This rare disorder is a clinical syndrome due to a variety of underlying inherited disorders. It is characterized by uncontrolled proliferation of activated lymphocytes and histiocytes secreting large amounts of inflammatory cytokines.[49] The disease is classified in accordance with the location of the primary genetic defect:

- Familial hemophagocytic lymphohistiocytosis 1 (FHL1), unknown
- FHL2, perforin gene (*PRF1*)
- FHL3, *UNC13D* gene
- FHL4 syntaxin 11 gene (*STX11*)

These are all autosomal-recessive. In addition, the defect may be caused by inherited immune deficiencies, which are usually autosomal-recessive, although some show X-linked inheritance. If the disease presents in later infancy or in older childhood, the distinction between familial and infection-associated hemophagocytic syndrome may be extremely difficult to make.

Clinical presentation and diagnosis

Infants present with malaise, jaundice, hepatosplenomegaly, relapsing fever, and skin rash.

Laboratory investigations show:

- Consumptive coagulopathy with hypofibrinogenemia
- Cytopenia (two or more cell lines)
- Elevated plasma triglycerides
- Increased serum ferritin and lactate dehydrogenase
- Low albumin and sodium
- Impaired natural killer and cytotoxic T cell function
- Erythrophagocytosis in bone marrow or liver (Figure 5.10)
- CSF lymphocytic infiltration and/or increased protein

Treatment and prognosis

The condition is fatal without treatment, but 50% may recover with current management.[50] Etoposide, cyclosporine, and steroids are used to induce remission with maintenance cyclosporine to maintain remission. Relapse is frequent and stem cell transplant is necessary for long-term survival. Matched unrelated donor transplants are as effective as matched sibling transplants and offer a 70% 3-year survival.[50] Liver transplantation is contraindicated and inappropriate.[51]

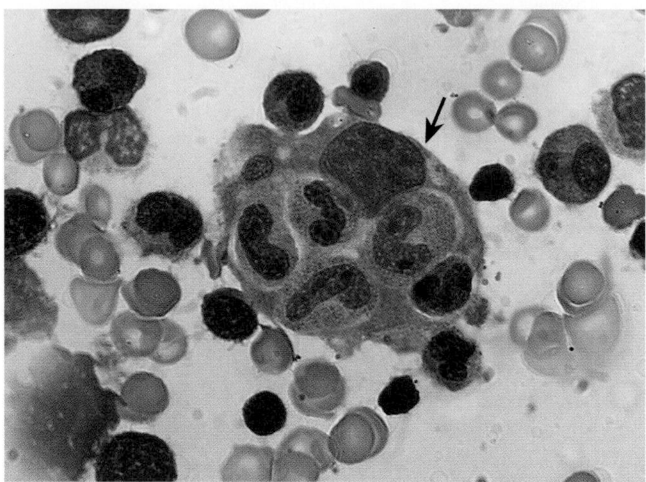

Figure 5.10 Familial erythrophagocytic syndrome presents with jaundice, liver failure, and pancytopenia. The diagnosis is made by demonstrating erythrophagocytosis (arrow) in liver or bone-marrow aspirate.

Inborn errors of metabolism associated with hepatic enzyme deficiency

There are a number of inborn errors of metabolism associated with defective hepatic enzymes, which are characterized by profound acidosis, hyperammonemia, or disorders of fatty acid oxidation. The relevance of these disorders is that presentation is usually in the neonatal period with an acute illness, which may be associated with abnormal liver function tests, hepatomegaly, and very rarely liver failure.[52] A brief overview of these disorders is provided here.

Urea cycle disorders

There are four main disorders in which defects in enzymes of the urea cycle lead to neurotoxicity due to an accumulation of ammonia and glutamine. These defective enzymes are:

- Carbamoyl phosphate synthetase (CPS)
- Ornithine transcarbamylase (OTC)
- Arginosuccinic acid synthetase (citrullinemia)
- Arginosuccinate lyase (ASA).

These disorders are autosomal-recessive, apart from OTC, which is X-linked. Females with OTC may be heterozygotes and have varying degrees of deficiency and clinical involvement.[53]

Clinical features and diagnosis

There is a wide range of clinical features, which are associated with increased plasma ammonia. Hepatomegaly and abnormal transaminases are usual. Neonates present shortly after birth and are extremely ill, with vomiting, lethargy, seizures, and coma. The diagnosis may be suspected if there is a low urea and alkalosis.

Females with OTC may present later in infancy or even in adult life. Clinical features include episodic vomiting with neurological dysfunction, which may be precipitated by intercurrent infection or ingestion of protein. A history of natural avoidance of high-protein foods is common.

Investigations include:

- Hyperammonemia.
- Plasma amino acids, which demonstrate abnormal citrulline levels—elevated in citrullinemia, low in ASA, and undetectable in OTC and CPS.
- Argininosuccinic acid is also high in ASA.
- Orotic aciduria is present in OTC, ASA and citrullinemia.
- Glutamine and alanine concentrations may also be elevated.
- Prothrombin time may be increased.

The biochemical features are diagnostic in citrullinemia and ASA. The diagnosis is confirmed by finding pathogenic mutations or by measuring specific enzyme activity in liver tissue for CPS and OTC.

The main differential diagnoses for an elevated ammonia in the newborn periods include poor sampling, organic acidemia, liver dysfunction, including acute liver failure (Chapter 7), or transient hyperammonemia of the newborn.[53]

Treatment

Emergency management of hyperammonemia. The initial aim of treatment is to reduce ammonia as quickly as possible, to prevent further neurotoxicity. Dietary protein should be withdrawn. Initial management is pharmacological (Table 5.5), with dialysis if hyperammonemia is severe. Intravenous dextrose, in combination with insulin, is provided to minimize catabolism. Phenylbutyrate and sodium benzoate form conjugates with glutamine and glycine, respectively, which are excreted in the urine and provide an alternative route for elimination of nitrogenous compounds. Arginine, which corrects the arginine deficiency resulting from the block in the urea cycle, also acts as a source of ornithine for reconstitution of the cycle if there is residual activity.

Table 5.5 Emergency management of hyperammonemia.

Stop all dietary protein
If ammonia > 200 μmol/L, then:
1 Intravenous dextrose 10%
2 Sodium benzoate:
Loading dose 250 mg/kg
Continuous infusion 250 mg/kg/day
3 Arginine in 10%:
Loading dose 350 mg/kg over 2 h
Continuous infusion 350 mg/kg/day
If ammonia > 400 μmol/L or rising despite treatment, then:
1 Dialysis
2 Continuous infusion of sodium phenylbutyrate (250 mg/kg/day)
3 Repeat loading dose of sodium benzoate and arginine

Continuous venovenous hemodialysis is more rapidly effective than hemofiltration or peritoneal dialysis, especially in the newborn period.[54] Dialysis should be continued until ammonia is < 150 μmol/L. The intravenous dextrose and insulin are continued until the ammonia is < 100 μmol/L and the child is neurologically normal. Protein can slowly be reintroduced at this stage.

Maintenance treatment. This consists of dietary restriction of protein (0.7 g/kg), supplemented with essential amino acids and a high-calorie diet sufficient to allow normal growth. Oral sodium benzoate (0.1–0.25 g/kg/day) and/or phenylbutyrate (0.25–0.6 g/kg/day) are given. Frequent nutritional assessment and monitoring of plasma ammonia and amino acids are required. Plasma glutamine should be maintained at < 800 μmol/L to minimize the risk of acute decompensation. The need for protein restriction may be less severe in children with ASA and citrullinemia, and arginine rather than benzoate is used for maintenance treatment.

Due to the poor prognosis and severity of the nutritional regimen, liver transplantation is often indicated and has been successful in selected patients with OTC, CPS, and citrullinemia.[55] The indications for liver transplantation in urea cycle disorders are:

- Very severe disease with a poor prognosis
- Progressive liver disease that will ultimately result in liver failure
- Major complications that are life-threatening and cannot be controlled satisfactorily by other means[55]

Liver transplantation should not be performed as emergency rescue from neonatal coma. Liver transplantation results in complete functional correction of the defect, although some residual biochemical abnormalities may persist.[55] These residual abnormalities do not appear to have any functional consequences. Hepatocyte transplantation has been proposed for high-risk infants presenting in the neonatal period. To date, this has had an inconsistent effect, but it may prove to be a useful bridge to liver transplantation.[56,57] The potential applications of hepatocyte transplantation are discussed below.

Prognosis and outcome

Without treatment, the disease is usually fatal, and most children still die during the acute neonatal illness. The most important determinant of outcome is the degree of hyperammonemia and duration of neonatal coma; coma lasting longer than 5 days is associated with severe neurological abnormality. Children remain at lifelong risk of hyperammonemic coma, either during intercurrent illness or following dietary indiscretion. Families and patients should be taught an emergency regimen and have open access to hospital treatment.

Table 5.6 Recognized defects of fatty acid oxidation.

Fatty acid transporter
Carnitine transporter
Carnitine palmitoyltransferase 1
Acylcarnitine translocase
Carnitine palmitoyltransferase 2 (neonatal and late onset)
Very-long-chain acyl-CoA dehydrogenase
Long-chain 3-hydroxyacyl-CoA dehydrogenase
Trifunctional protein
Medium-chain acyl-CoA dehydrogenase
Short-chain acyl-CoA dehydrogenase
Short-chain 3-hydroxyacyl-CoA dehydrogenase (3 different types)
Multiple acyl-CoA dehydrogenases—electron transport flavoprotein (α and β) and electron transport flavoprotein dehydrogenase)
Riboflavin-responsive multiple acyl-CoA dehydrogenase
2,4-Dienoyl-CoA reductase deficiency
HMG-CoA synthase
HMG-CoA lyase

Defects in fatty acid oxidation

Fatty acid oxidation provides an important source of energy during fasting, especially in childhood, when glycogen stores are limited. Hepatic fatty acid oxidation produces ketone bodies, which are an important secondary energy source for many tissues, including the brain. Defects in any of the proteins in this pathway may lead to disease, and more than 20 individual defects have been recognized to date (Table 5.6).[58] All have autosomal-recessive inheritance. The principles of pathophysiology, diagnosis, and treatment will be discussed here.

Pathophysiology

The first step in fatty acid metabolism is lipolysis in response to fasting, resulting in circulating free fatty acids (FFAs). Fatty acids are then transported across the plasma membrane and are transformed to coenzyme A (CoA) esters in the cytosol before entry to the mitochondria for further metabolism. Long-chain acyl-CoA esters are transported into the mitochondrion by a three-step carnitine-dependent pathway. Defects in each of these steps and in carnitine uptake have been recognized. Within the mitochondria, acyl-CoA esters undergo β-oxidation. This is a four-step cyclical process in which fatty acids are sequentially degraded to acetyl-CoA, with a molecule of acetyl-CoA being released at each step. β-Oxidation results in a continuous flow of electrons to the electron transport chain by electron transfer flavoprotein (ETF) and its dehydrogenase (ETF-DH). The first two cycles of β-oxidation of long-chain fatty acids take place at the inner mitochondrial membrane using very-long-chain acyl-CoA dehydrogenase (VLCAD) and the associated trifunctional protein (which contains the other three enzymes needed to complete a cycle, including long-chain 3-hydroxyacyl-CoA dehydrogenase, LCHAD). Shorter-chain fatty acids are oxidized within the mitochondrial matrix by length-specific enzymes. Within the liver, acetyl-CoA is used for ketone body synthesis.

Defects at any stage in the pathway will result in failure of energy production and inadequate ketone body production. Moreover, when β-oxidation is defective, FFAs undergo omega-oxidation in microsomes, producing dicarboxylic acids.

Clinical features and diagnosis

These disorders are characterized by hypoketotic hypoglycemia, which may become evident on weaning or in association with the increased metabolic needs of intercurrent infection. Other clinical features include:

- Hypotonia
- Cardiomyopathy
- Rhabdomyolysis
- Metabolic acidosis
- Maternal fatty liver of pregnancy or HELLP (hemolysis, elevated liver enzymes, and low platelet count) syndrome

The most dramatic presentation may be with a Reye-like syndrome or an apparent sudden infant death syndrome, but patients may be clinically and biochemically normal between episodes. These disorders have not been thought of as common causes of liver failure. However, a recent study has recognized a subgroup of children with acute liver failure with a poor outlook who had abnormal bile acylcarnitine species.[59] Whether this represents a newly recognized presentation of fatty acid oxidation defects or is an effect of liver failure in those with genetic susceptibility to such defects is currently unclear.

The best diagnostic yield will be from the blood acylcarnitine profile and urinary organic analysis at the time of decompensation.

Biochemical investigations reveal:

- Elevated aminotransferases
- Low plasma carnitine
- Abnormal acylcarnitine profile, especially during decompensation or following a controlled fast
- Elevated ratio of free fatty acids : 3-hydroxybutyrate
- Increased urinary ratio of dicarboxylic acids : 3-hydroxybutyrate
- Mild to moderate hyperammonemia
- Metabolic acidosis
- Elevated plasma creatinine kinase.

Confirmation of specific defects may be difficult, due to the variety of potential enzyme defects. In selected patients, loading tests with medium-chain or long-chain triglyceride may be helpful. In medium-chain acyl-CoA dehydrogenase deficiency and LCHAD, common single mutations make the diagnosis simpler.[58] All recognized defects are expressed in skin fibroblasts. In vitro analysis with labeled myristate, palmitate, and oleate are useful for diagnostic screening, and in vitro acylcarnitine profiling can provide very specific diagnostic information.[60]

A fascinating aspect of this group of disorders is the association with maternal illness during pregnancy (see also Chapter 1). This association was first noted when a mother with acute fatty liver of pregnancy delivered an infant with LCHAD deficiency.[61] Recently it has become clear that this association is not limited to fetal LCHAD deficiency, but may occur in any fatty acid oxidation defect, including medium- and short-chain defects.[62] The maternal illness may be part of a spectrum ranging from acute fatty liver to the HELLP syndrome. The mechanism of the maternal illness is unclear, but presumably results from a limited ability to detoxify metabolites produced by the fetus in an obligate heterozygote. The incidence of fatty acid oxidation defects in unselected pregnancies complicated by HELLP is low,[63] but recognition of susceptible infants is important, as prospective treatment can be offered to the affected infant and the maternal illness may recur in future pregnancies.[61]

Treatment and prognosis

The primary aim of treatment is to avoid excess fasting and suppress lipolysis. This may require the use of overnight nasogastric tube feeds or nocturnal uncooked cornstarch. In some disorders of long-chain fat oxidation, dietary long-chain fat should be restricted with medium-chain triglyceride supplementation. Routine carnitine supplementation is controversial (100 mg/kg/day), but should be used during acute episodes.

The prognosis for infants with a neonatal presentation is poor, with overall mortality in the first episode as high as 60%. In patients who survive to diagnosis, the prognosis is good. Physical and intellectual development is usually normal, as long as acute crises can be avoided.

Carnitine palmitoyltransferase 1 deficiency

This disorder is due to a defect in the carnitine palmitoyltransferase enzyme at the outer mitochondrial membrane. This defect prevents mitochondrial uptake of long-chain fatty acyl-CoA, the rate-limiting step in fat oxidation. Presentation is usually in the first year of life, with acute hypoketotic hypoglycemia following an episode of fasting or intercurrent illness. Hepatomegaly, renal tubular acidosis, convulsions, and coma are reported.

Investigations demonstrate the typical features of fat oxidation defects (see above), except:

- Plasma carnitine may be normal or increased.
- The acylcarnitine profile is normal.
- Liver histology demonstrates microvesicular and macrovesicular steatosis.
- Muscle biopsy may show an accumulation of glycogen and lipid.

The diagnosis is confirmed by demonstrating impaired oxidation of palmitate in fibroblast culture.

Treatment consists of the avoidance of fasting and provision of a low-fat diet with medium-chain triglyceride supplements. The prognosis is good, and normal growth and development can be achieved.

Multiple acyl-coenzyme A dehydrogenase defect (glutaric acidemia type 2)

This rare disease is due to a deficiency of electron transfer flavoprotein (ETF; two types are recognized) or its dehydrogenase (ETF-DH), which interferes with the function of all acyl-CoA dehydrogenases. There is no strict genotype–phenotype correlation.[58]

Distinguishing features include:

- Severe neonatal illness with profound metabolic acidosis
- Congenital malformations, including polycystic kidneys, defects in the anterior abdominal wall, and genital abnormalities
- Dysmorphic features, including low-set ears, high forehead, rocker-bottom feet, single palmar creases, and defects in the anterior abdominal wall

Biochemical investigations and diagnostic findings include:

- Increased urinary organic acids, including ethylmalonic and adipic acids
- Hypoglycemia without ketonuria
- Mild to moderate elevation of ammonia
- Metabolic acidosis
- Hepatic dysfunction with elevated bilirubin and transaminases
- Plasma lactate (usually elevated)

The diagnosis is confirmed by demonstrating the enzyme deficiency in fibroblast cultures.

Treatment consists of providing a diet low in protein and fat.

Patients who present later should be assessed for riboflavin responsiveness, and treated with 100–300 mg/day riboflavin. Carnitine (100–200 mg/kg/day) may be helpful and should be used in acute episodes.

Most infants with structural abnormalities die within the first week of life. Some respond to initial treatment, but often succumb to cardiomyopathy in infancy.

Long-chain 3-hydroxyacyl-CoA dehydrogenase (LCHAD) deficiency

The enzyme long-chain 3-hydroxyacyl-CoA dehydrogenase (LCHAD) is a component of the trifunctional protein of the inner mitochondrial membrane and has optimal activity for C_{12} to C_{16} chain length fatty acids. A common mutation (G1528C) has been recognized, accounting for 70% of abnormal alleles.[58]

The clinical presentation is similar to that of other disorders of fatty acid oxidation, with infantile hypoketotic hypoglycemia, sudden infant death syndrome, or a Reye-like illness.

Distinguishing features include:

- Severe cardiomyopathy.
- Marked hypotonia.
- Diarrhea and failure to thrive.
- Peripheral neuropathy and retinitis pigmentosa.
- Neonatal cholestasis or acute liver failure.
- Hepatic histology demonstrates microvesicular steatosis, but progression to cirrhosis is frequent.[64]

The diagnosis is confirmed either by mutation detection or by specific enzymatic diagnosis from cultured fibroblasts.

As in other fatty acid oxidation defects, fasting should be avoided. Long-chain fat should be restricted, with the addition of medium-chain triglycerides. Riboflavin (100 mg/day) and carnitine (100 mg/kg/day) have also been used. Previously, many children have died in crises, but with early recognition and treatment, medium-term survival can be expected.[65] The neuropathy and retinopathy do not appear to respond to dietary treatment.

Maternal acute fatty liver of pregnancy may develop when a heterozygote mother carries a fetus with LCHAD deficiency, particularly if the fetus carries the G1528C mutation[61,62] (see also Chapter 1).

Organic acidemias

Inborn errors of organic acid metabolism produce life-threatening illness early in life. They should be suspected in any patient with metabolic acidosis. Propionic acidemia and methylmalonic acidemia (MMA) are the commonest of the organic acidemias.

Propionic acidemia

Propionic acidemia is due to an autosomal-recessive defect in the enzyme propionyl-CoA carboxylase. The gene has been cloned and mapped to chromosome 13q32 (α-subunit) and 3913.3-22 (β-subunit). A number of mutations have been defined, with some genotype–phenotype correlation.[66,67] Most propionate is derived from catabolism of the essential amino acids valine and isoleucine, and to a lesser extent from threonine and methionine. Odd-chain fatty acids are synthesized from the 3-carbon propionyl-CoA and subsequently act as a propionate source when they are oxidized during catabolism or fasting. Anaerobic bacterial metabolism contributes approximately 20% of propionate turnover. Biotin is a coenzyme for this pathway.

Methylmalonic acidemia

Methylmalonic acidemia is part of a group of disorders with abnormal metabolism of branch-chain amino acids due to defective activity of methylmalonyl-CoA mutase. The gene has been localized to chromosome 6q12-21.2, and more than 20 mutations have been identified.[68] The methylmalonyl-CoA mutase enzyme has a vitamin B_{12}–derived cofactor, 5′-deoxyadenosylcobalamin.

There is considerable genetic heterogeneity, as some patients are B_{12}-responsive due to defects in the synthesis of the cofactor, while unresponsive patients have defects in the mutase enzyme itself.

Clinical presentation and diagnosis

Both disorders have a wide clinical spectrum of severity. The most severely affected patients present in the newborn period with encephalopathy, hypotonia, hepatomegaly, and subsequent coma. Some children present later with recurrent illness characterized by bouts of lethargy, abnormal behavior, and altered consciousness, or occasionally with a slowly progressive form with failure to thrive and developmental delay. In general, patients are more susceptible to infection.

First-line investigations demonstrate:

- Metabolic acidosis and ketosis (arterial pH < 6.9; serum bicarbonate < 10 mEq/L).
- Neutropenia and thrombocytopenia.
- Hyperammonemia, which may be profound
- Plasma amino acids show hyperglycinemia (> 600 μmol/L).
- Urinary organic acids reveal either the characteristic propionyl-CoA derivatives, including glycine and carnitine conjugates, methylcitrate and 3-hydroxypropionate, or urinary methylmalonate.

The definitive diagnosis is achieved by demonstrating the relevant enzyme defect in cultured fibroblasts. Liver histology may show fatty change or mild biliary changes.

Management and prognosis

Initial management of the acute crisis involves intravenous 10% dextrose and sodium bicarbonate and dietary protein restriction. Carnitine (200 mg/kg/day) and metronidazole (20 mg/kg/day) help to detoxify and decrease the production of propionate, respectively. Insulin may be useful, especially if hyperglycemia occurs. Hyperammonemia requires specific treatment with sodium benzoate or dialysis (see "Urea cycle disorders" above).

In MMA, higher fluid intakes are necessary and all patients should have a trial of pharmacological doses of vitamin B_{12} (1 mg/day).

Maintenance treatment consists of an individually titrated low-protein, high-calorie diet with overnight nasogastric tube feeding. Amino acid supplementation may be necessary. Carnitine supplementation is continued. Metronidazole may be used continuously or intermittently as required. Sodium benzoate is useful in those with a recurrent hyperammonemia.[69]

In B_{12}-responsive MMA, treatment should be lifelong, with little need for dietary restriction. With the exception of those patients with MMA who respond to B_{12}, patients remain at risk of recurrent metabolic decompensation, often in association with intercurrent illness. The outlook for patients with neonatal presentation is poor. Neurological abnormalities are common, with severe hypotonia, progressive neurodevelopmental delay, and learning difficulties. Basal ganglia damage and stroke-like symptoms are common in patients who presented early, but all affected patients are vulnerable to neurological damage.[70] Nutritional progress is difficult, and systemic complications such as pancreatitis, cardiomyopathy, and osteoporosis occur. Tubulointerstitial nephritis with progressive renal impairment occurs in MMA and may lead to renal failure in adolescence.

Appreciation of this poor outlook has led to consideration of early liver transplantation to correct the defect before the onset of systemic complications. Initial experience demonstrates that liver transplantation results in useful partial correction of propionic acidemia. Diet is normalized, with decreased metabolite excretion and nutritional and developmental catch-up. There is complete protection against recurrent crises.[71,72] Experience in Birmingham has confirmed that successful liver transplantation improves the quality of life for affected children and their families.[73] However, the risks of early liver transplantation in those with neonatal presentation are very high. In this group, transplantation is best deferred until the patient is at least 3 years old, when the risks of perioperative instability are less.[72] Indications for liver transplantation would be recurrent metabolic instability despite maximal medical treatment.

The situation is not as clear in severe MMA. Liver transplantation in infancy has a poor outcome but also results in a useful functional correction of the metabolic defect, albeit less than in propionic acidemia. However, transplantation does not appear to prevent vulnerability to neurological damage or renal damage, particularly the development of metabolic stroke.[74–76] In addition, children with MMA are at high risk for developing renal failure. Considering combined liver–kidney transplantation at this juncture is reasonable and can be effective.[77] However, the risk is higher than in other candidates for combined transplantation, and isolated renal transplantation may be a reasonable option for some children with MMA in renal failure.[72,78,79]

Antenatal diagnosis

Prenatal diagnosis is possible for both conditions by enzymatic measurement in cultured amniocytes or amniotic fluid measurement of methylcitrate or methylmalonate. DNA analysis from chorionic villi is feasible in families with known mutations. In adenosylcobalamin synthetic defects, prenatal B_{12} treatment may be given.

Other organic acidemias

Isovaleric acidemia and multiple carboxylase deficiency are rarer organic acidemias due to deficiencies in isovaleryl-CoA dehydrogenase and holocarboxylase synthetase, respectively.

Clinical presentation and diagnosis

Both conditions present with severe neonatal illness, with similar presentation to other organic acidemias. Distinguishing features include a "sweaty feet" odor in isovaleric acidemia. Diagnostic biochemical features include elevated plasma isovaleric acid and urinary isovaleryl glycine in isovaleric acidemia, and urinary 3-methylcrotonylglycine and 3-hydroxyvaleric acid in multiple carboxylase deficiency. Enzymatic diagnosis is confirmed in cultured fibroblasts in both disorders.

Management and prognosis

Emergency management is similar to the other organic acidemias. Most patients with multiple carboxylase deficiency are responsive to pharmacological doses of biotin (10 mg/day), and in the majority no other treatment is required other than an "emergency regimen" for use during intercurrent illness. In isovaleric acidemia, a low-protein, high-calorie diet should be used in combination with glycine supplementation.

Hepatocyte transplantation

With improvements in cell handling techniques, it is now possible to isolate functionally relevant masses of hepatocytes, and even to cryopreserve these for urgent use.[80] A small number of humans with acute or chronic liver disease or metabolic disease have been treated. In OTC, 2 male infants with a very poor outlook have been treated using reconstituted cryopreserved cells transfused via the umbilical vein in the early neonatal period.[56,57] Both infants tolerated the procedure, but the metabolic effect was inconstant, requiring repeat transfusions and high-dose immunosuppression.[56,57] However, both infants survived to receive liver transplantation at 6 and 7 months. A similar experience was found with factor VII deficiency[81]—i.e., a partial correction that was in itself insufficient to justify the long-term risks of immunosuppression. At present, therefore, this technique has a role as a bridge to transplantation in high-risk newborns with metabolic disease that can be corrected by liver transplantation. More widespread application of the technique will depend on developing techniques to allow the transplanted hepatocytes to have a survival advantage over native hepatocytes, to promote immune tolerance, and to identify alternative hepatocyte sources.[56,80]

Screening for inborn errors of metabolism

The advent of tandem mass spectrometry has changed the paradigm for neonatal screening. This technique has the potential to detect more than 30 inborn metabolic disorders simultaneously from a single blood spot, with a high degree of sensitivity. The method has been used for disorders of amino acids, organic acids, and fatty acids to date, and it has the potential to be applied to disorders such as lysosomal disorders.[82] However, the potential technical, logistic, and ethical difficulties posed by application of this technique to mass screening programs should not be underestimated. The technique has to date been validated in only a small number of individual disorders, and the challenge in the coming years will be to learn how to harness the potential of this technique for mass neonatal screening. The applications chosen will likely differ from country to country and may change depending on clinical developments. For example, the excellent outcome for presymptomatic use of nitisinone makes the case for screening for tyrosinemia much stronger.[42,44] The role for screening in the diagnosis of liver disease has yet to be established.

Case report

Patient J, weighing 3.74 kg, was born after a normal pregnancy. He was the first child of nonconsanguineous parents and has three older half siblings who were well.

He was fed on bottle milk and became jaundiced from day 2. Serum bilirubin was 140 μmol/L (normal 0–24), mostly unconjugated. He was allowed home, as he was feeding well.

At the age of 7 days, he was admitted to his local hospital with marked jaundice and dehydration and was transferred to a specialist unit. On examination, he was drowsy and had a high-pitched cry and no dysmorphic features. Ophthalmic examination showed a normal red reflex. He was jaundiced and had a firm hepatomegaly and no splenomegaly. He had no ascites.

Initial investigations showed:

- Prothrombin time 23 s (normal 11–15 s)
- Electrolytes normal
- Urea 1.5 mmol/L (normal 1.7–6.7)
- Creatinine 81 μmol/L (normal 26–63)
- Total bilirubin 303 μmol/L (normal 0–24)
- Unconjugated 163 μmol/L (normal 3–17)
- Alanine aminotransferase (ALT) 113 U/L (normal 5–54)
- Aspartate aminotransferase (AST) 1108 U/L (normal 0–80)
- γ-Glutamyl transferase (GT) U/L = 61 (normal 0–80)
- Albumin 33 g/L (normal 34–42)
- Hemoglobin 16.6 g/L
- Platelets 125 × 10^9 g/L
- White cells 6.4 × 10^9 g/L
- Burr cells noted on the blood film
- Blood glucose 3.2 mmol/L (fasting range 3.5–6.0)
- Ammonia 37 μmols/L (normal < 100)

Abdominal ultrasound confirmed hepatomegaly, no splenomegaly, no ascites, and no structural abnormalities.

Initial management consisted of administering intravenous fluid, a lactose-free diet, intravenous antibiotics, intravenous acyclovir, and the antioxidant cocktail for suspected neonatal hemochromatosis.

On the following day, further investigations showed ferritin > 1000 mg/L (normal 4–405). Arrangements were made for a lip mucosal biopsy.

Forty-eight hours after admission, there was a significant improvement, with:

- Bilirubin 72 μmol/L (normal 0–24)
- Unconjugated bilirubin 37 μmol/L (normal 3–17)
- ALT 58 U/L (normal 5–45)
- AST 94 U/L (normal 0–80)
- Albumin 29 g/L (normal 34–42)
- Ammonia 35 μmol/L (normal < 100)
- Electrolytes normal
- Prothrombin time 15 s (normal 11–15)

The lip biopsy result became available and showed no salivary siderosis; in view of the significant improvement, the hemochromatosis antioxidant regimen was discontinued. The lactose-free diet and antibiotics were continued.

Metabolic investigations showed a normal lactate value of 1.0. Organic acids showed tyrosine metabolites only.

An ophthalmology assessment was obtained, which showed bilateral small subcapsular cataracts.

Management was continued to day 5, when the results of galactose-1-phosphatase uridyltransferase became available and confirmed the diagnosis of galactosemia. Subsequent DNA analysis showed that the patient was a compound heterozygote.

The lactose-free diet was continued. Antiviral treatment was stopped and antibiotics were stopped after 5 days. He maintained a continuing clinical improvement; by 1 week, his hepatomegaly was just visible and liver function tests showed:

- Normal coagulation
- Bilirubin 38 μmol/L (normal 0–24)
- Alkaline phosphatase 452 U/L (normal 250–1000)
- AST 94 U/L (normal 0–80)
- Albumin 35 g/L (normal 43–42)

Fat-soluble vitamin treatment was continued for a further month. A review at 6 weeks showed that he was clinically normal. Hepatomegaly had resolved, and he was making developmental progress.

Subsequent follow-up was by the metabolic pediatrician and he remains on a galactose-free diet. He is clinically normal. A repeat ultrasound at age 2 years showed no hepatic abnormality.

The final diagnosis is classical galactosemia. The important management point is to stop galactose-containing feeds immediately in neonatal liver failure. The additional point is that the early improvement suggests that something in the initial generic regimen was working. If there are diagnostic doubts, it is easy to continue the galactose-free diet until these are resolved. Never consider a galactose challenge as a diagnostic test.

A galactose-free diet results in improvement in liver function within days, with eventual normal hepatic function being the rule. Ironically, dietary treatment is less successful in preventing other systemic manifestations of the disease, due to the existence of significant endogenous galactose-1-phosphate production independent of dietary treatment.

References

1 Meulemans A, Seneca S, Smet J, *et al.* A new family with the mitochondrial tRNAGLU gene mutation m.14709T>C presenting with hydrops fetalis. *Eur J Paediatr Neurol* 2007;**11**:17–20.

2 Wraith JE. Lysosomal disorders. *Semin Neonatol* 2002;**7**:75–83.

3 Calderon FR, Phansalkar AR, Crockett DK, Miller M, Mao R. Mutation database for the galactose-1-phosphate uridyltransferase (*GALT*) gene. *Hum Mutat* 2007;**28**:939–43.

4 Elsas LJ, Lai K. The molecular biology of galactosemia. *Genet Med* 1998;**1**:40–8.

5 Walter JH, Roberts RE, Besley GT, *et al.* Generalised uridine diphosphate galactose-4-epimerase deficiency. *Arch Dis Child* 1999;**80**:374–6.

6 Vajro P, Fontanella A, Tedesco M, Vecchione R, D'Armiento M. Fulminant hepatitis B and neonatal hepatitis with galactosemia-like presentation. *Clin Pediatr (Phila)* 1991;**30**:191–3.

7 Holton JB. Galactosaemia: pathogenesis and treatment. *J Inherit Metab Dis* 1996;**19**:3–7.

8 Bosch AM. Classical galactosaemia revisited. *J Inherit Metab Dis* 2006;**29**:516–25.

9 Whitington PF. Fetal and infantile hemochromatosis. *Hepatology* 2006;**43**:654–60.

10 Hoogstraten J, de Sa DJ, Knisely AS. Fetal liver disease may precede extrahepatic siderosis in neonatal hemochromatosis. *Gastroenterology* 1990;**98**:1699–701.

11 Witzleben CL, Uri A. Perinatal hemochromatosis: entity or end result? *Hum Pathol* 1989;**20**:335–40.

12 Kelly AL, Lunt PW, Rodrigues F, *et al.* Classification and genetic features of neonatal haemochromatosis: a study of 27 affected pedigrees and molecular analysis of genes implicated in iron metabolism. *J Med Genet* 2001;**38**:599–610.

13 Whitington PF, Malladi P. Neonatal hemochromatosis: is it an alloimmune disease? *J Pediatr Gastroenterol Nutr* 2005;**40**:544–9.

14 Verloes A, Temple IK, Hubert AF, *et al.* Recurrence of neonatal haemochromatosis in half sibs born of unaffected mothers. *J Med Genet* 1996;**33**:444–9.

15 Knisely AS, Mieli-Vergani G, Whitington PF. Neonatal hemochromatosis. *Gastroenterol Clin North Am* 2003;**32**:877–vii.

16 Lee WS, McKiernan PJ, Kelly DA. Serum ferritin level in neonatal fulminant liver failure. *Arch Dis Child Fetal Neonatal Ed* 2001;**85**:F226.

17 Williams H, McKiernan P, Kelly D, Baumann U. Magnetic resonance imaging in neonatal hemochromatosis—are we there yet? *Liver Transpl* 2006;**12**:1725.

18 Flynn DM, Mohan N, McKiernan P, *et al.* Progress in treatment and outcome for children with neonatal haemochromatosis. *Arch Dis Child Fetal Neonatal Ed* 2003;**88**:F124–7.

19 Heffron T, Pillen T, Welch D, *et al.* Medical and surgical treatment of neonatal hemochromatosis: single center experience. *Pediatr Transplant* 2007;11:374–8.

20 Noujaim HM, Mayer DA, Buckles JA, *et al.* Techniques for and outcome of liver transplantation in neonates and infants weighing up to 5 kilograms. *J Pediatr Surg* 2002;**37**:159–64.

21 Egawa H, Berquist W, Garcia-Kennedy R, Cox K, Knisely AS, Esquivel CO. Rapid development of hepatocellular siderosis after liver transplantation for neonatal hemochromatosis. *Transplantation* 1996;**62**:1511–3.

22 Whitington PF, Hibbard JU. High-dose immunoglobulin during pregnancy for recurrent neonatal haemochromatosis. *Lancet* 2004;**364**:1690–8.

23 Carrabin N, Cordier MP, Gaucherand P. [High-dose immunoglobulin during pregnancy for two patients with risk of recurrent neonatal haemochromatosis; in French.] *J Gynecol Obstet Biol Reprod (Paris)* 2007;**36**:409–12.

24 Leonard JV, Schapira AH. Mitochondrial respiratory chain disorders, II: neurodegenerative disorders and nuclear gene defects. *Lancet* 2000;**355**:389–94.

25 Sarzi E, Bourdon A, Chretien D, *et al.* Mitochondrial DNA depletion is a prevalent cause of multiple respiratory chain deficiency in childhood. *J Pediatr* 2007;**150**:531–4.

26 Valnot I, Osmond S, Gigarel N, *et al.* Mutations of the *SCO1* gene in mitochondrial cytochrome c oxidase deficiency with neonatal-onset hepatic failure and encephalopathy. *Am J Hum Genet* 2000;**67**:1104–9.

27 Nguyen KV, Ostergaard E, Ravn SH, *et al.* *POLG* mutations in Alpers syndrome. *Neurology* 2005;**65**:1493–5.

28 Saada A, Shaag A, Mandel H, Nevo Y, Eriksson S, Elpeleg O. Mutant mitochondrial thymidine kinase in mitochondrial DNA depletion myopathy. *Nat Genet* 2001;**29**:342–4.

29 Elpeleg O, Miller C, Hershkovitz E, *et al.* Deficiency of the ADP-forming succinyl-CoA synthase activity is associated with encephalomyopathy and mitochondrial DNA depletion. *Am J Hum Genet* 2005;**76**:1081–6.

30 Spinazzola A, Viscomi C, Fernandez-Vizarra E, *et al.* MPV17 encodes an inner mitochondrial membrane protein and is mutated in infantile hepatic mitochondrial DNA depletion. *Nat Genet* 2006;**38**:570–5.

31 Poggi-Travert F, Martin D, Billette de Villemeur T, *et al.* Metabolic intermediates in lactic acidosis: compounds, samples and interpretation. *J Inherit Metab Dis* 1996;**19**:478–88.

32 Dubern B, Broue P, Dubuisson C, *et al.* Orthotopic liver transplantation for mitochondrial respiratory chain disorders: a study of 5 children. *Transplantation* 2001;**71**:633–7.

33 Sokal EM, Sokol R, Cormier V, *et al.* Liver transplantation in mitochondrial respiratory chain disorders. *Eur J Pediatr* 1999;**158** (Suppl 2):S81–S84.

34 Thomson M, McKiernan P, Buckels J, Mayer D, Kelly D. Generalised mitochondrial cytopathy is an absolute contraindication to orthotopic liver transplant in childhood. *J Pediatr Gastroenterol Nutr* 1998;**26**:478–81.

35 Mitchell GA, Grompe M, Lambert M, Tanguay RM. Hypertyrosinemia. In: Scriver CR, Beaudet AR, Sly W, Valle D, eds. *The Metabolic and Molecular Bases of Inherited Disease*, 8th ed. New York: McGraw-Hill, 2001: 1777–805.

36 Heath SK, Gray RG, McKiernan P, Au KM, Walker E, Green A. Mutation screening for tyrosinaemia type I. *J Inherit Metab Dis* 2002;**25**:523–4.

37 Weinberg AG, Mize CE, Worthen HG. The occurrence of hepatoma in the chronic form of hereditary tyrosinemia. *J Pediatr* 1976;**88**:434–8.

38 van Spronsen FJ, Thomasse Y, Smit GP, *et al.* Hereditary tyrosinemia type I: a new clinical classification with difference in prognosis on dietary treatment. *Hepatology* 1994;**20**:1187–91.

39 Hutchesson AC, Hall SK, Preece MA, Green A. Screening for tyrosinaemia type I. *Arch Dis Child Fetal Neonatal Ed* 1996;**74**: F191–4.

40 Baumann U, Preece MA, Green A, Kelly DA, McKiernan PJ. Hyperinsulinism in tyrosinaemia type I. *J Inherit Metab Dis* 2005;**28**:131–5.
41 Lindstedt S, Holme E, Lock EA, Hjalmarson O, Strandvik B. Treatment of hereditary tyrosinaemia type I by inhibition of 4-hydroxyphenylpyruvate dioxygenase. *Lancet* 1992;**340**:813–7.
42 McKiernan PJ. Nitisinone in the treatment of hereditary tyrosinaemia type 1. *Drugs* 2006;**66**:743–50.
43 Holme E, Lindstedt S. Nontransplant treatment of tyrosinemia. *Clin Liver Dis* 2000;**4**:805–14.
44 Alvares F, Bussières JF, Dallaire L, *et al.* Nitisinone (NTBC) treatment of hepatorenal tyrosinaemia in Quebec. *J Inherit Metab Dis* 2005;**28**(Suppl 1):49.
45 Herzog D, Martin S, Turpin S, Alvarez F. Normal glomerular filtration rate in long-term follow-up of children after orthotopic liver transplantation. *Transplantation* 2006;**81**:672–7.
46 Pierik LJ, van Spronsen FJ, Bijleveld CM, van Dael CM. Renal function in tyrosinaemia type I after liver transplantation: a long-term follow-up. *J Inherit Metab Dis* 2005;**28**:871–6.
47 Mohan N, McKiernan P, Preece MA, *et al.* Indications and outcome of liver transplantation in tyrosinaemia type 1. *Eur J Pediatr* 1999;**158**(Suppl 2):S49–S54.
48 Sander J, Janzen N, Peter M, *et al.* Newborn screening for hepatorenal tyrosinemia: tandem mass spectrometric quantification of succinylacetone. *Clin Chem* 2006;**52**:482–7.
49 Janka GE. Familial and acquired hemophagocytic lymphohistiocytosis. *Eur J Pediatr* 2007;**166**:95–109.
50 Durken M, Finckenstein FG, Janka GE. Bone marrow transplantation in hemophagocytic lymphohistiocytosis. *Leuk Lymphoma* 2001;**41**:89–95.
51 Parizhskaya M, Reyes J, Jaffe R. Hemophagocytic syndrome presenting as acute hepatic failure in two infants: clinical overlap with neonatal hemochromatosis. *Pediatr Dev Pathol* 1999;**2**:360–6.
52 Mustafa A, Clarke JT. Ornithine transcarbamoylase deficiency presenting with acute liver failure. *J Inherit Metab Dis* 2006;**29**:586.
53 Brusilow S, Horwich AL. Urea cycle enzymes. In: Scriver CR, Beaudet AL, Sly WS, Valle D, eds. *The Metabolic and Molecular Bases of Inherited Disease,* 8th ed. New York: McGraw-Hill, 2001: 1909–64.
54 Schaefer F, Straube E, Oh J, Mehls O, Mayatepek E. Dialysis in neonates with inborn errors of metabolism. *Nephrol Dial Transplant* 1999;**14**:910–8.
55 Leonard JV, McKiernan PJ. The role of liver transplantation in urea cycle disorders. *Mol Genet Metab* 2004;**81**(Suppl 1):S74–S78.
56 Mitry RR, Dhawan A, Hughes RD, *et al.* One liver, three recipients: segment IV from split-liver procedures as a source of hepatocytes for cell transplantation. *Transplantation* 2004;**77**:1614–6.
57 Horslen SP, McCowan TC, Goertzen TC, *et al.* Isolated hepatocyte transplantation in an infant with a severe urea cycle disorder. *Pediatrics* 2003;**111**:1262–7.
58 Rinaldo P, Matern D, Bennett MJ. Fatty acid oxidation disorders. *Annu Rev Physiol* 2002;**64**:477–502.
59 Shneider BL, Rinaldo P, Emre S, *et al.* Abnormal concentrations of esterified carnitine in bile: a feature of pediatric acute liver failure with poor prognosis. *Hepatology* 2005;**41**:717–21.
60 Roe DS, Vianey-Saban C, Sharma S, Zabot MT, Roe CR. Oxidation of unsaturated fatty acids by human fibroblasts with very-long-chain acyl-CoA dehydrogenase deficiency: aspects of substrate specificity and correlation with clinical phenotype. *Clin Chim Acta* 2001;**312**:55–67.
61 Ibdah JA. Acute fatty liver of pregnancy: an update on pathogenesis and clinical implications. *World J Gastroenterol* 2006;**12**:7397–404.
62 Browning MF, Levy HL, Wilkins-Haug LE, Larson C, Shih VE. Fetal fatty acid oxidation defects and maternal liver disease in pregnancy. *Obstet Gynecol* 2006;**107**:115–20.
63 den Boer ME, Ijlst L, Wijburg FA, *et al.* Heterozygosity for the common LCHAD mutation (1528g>C) is not a major cause of HELLP syndrome and the prevalence of the mutation in the Dutch population is low. *Pediatr Res* 2000;**48**:151–4.
64 Tyni T, Rapola J, Paetau A, Palotie A, Pihko H. Pathology of long-chain 3-hydroxyacyl-CoA dehydrogenase deficiency caused by the G1528C mutation. *Pediatr Pathol Lab Med* 1997;**17**:427–47.
65 den Boer ME, Wanders RJ, Morris AA, Ijlst L, Heymans HS, Wijburg FA. Long-chain 3-hydroxyacyl-CoA dehydrogenase deficiency: clinical presentation and follow-up of 50 patients. *Pediatrics* 2002;**109**:99–104.
66 Kennerknecht I, Suormala T, Barbi G, Baumgartner ER. The gene coding for the alpha-chain of human propionyl-CoA carboxylase maps to chromosome band 13q32. *Hum Genet* 1990;**86**:238–40.
67 Desviat LR, Perez B, Perez-Cerda C, Rodriguez-Pombo P, Clavero S, Ugarte M. Propionic acidemia: mutation update and functional and structural effects of the variant alleles. *Mol Genet Metab* 2004;**83**:28–37.
68 Adjalla CE, Hosack AR, Gilfix BM, *et al.* Seven novel mutations in mut methylmalonic aciduria. *Hum Mutat* 1998;**11**:270–4.
69 Walter JH, Wraith JE, Cleary MA. Absence of acidosis in the initial presentation of propionic acidaemia. *Arch Dis Child Fetal Neonatal Ed* 1995;**72**:F197–9.
70 Nicolaides P, Leonard J, Surtees R. Neurological outcome of methylmalonic acidaemia. *Arch Dis Child* 1998;**78**:508–12.
71 Schlenzig JS, Poggi-Travert F, Laurent J, *et al.* Liver transplantation in two cases of propionic acidaemia. *J Inherit Metab Dis* 1995;**18**:448–61.
72 Leonard JV, Walter JH, McKiernan PJ. The management of organic acidaemias: the role of transplantation. *J Inherit Metab Dis* 2001;**24**:309–11.
73 Gissen P, Chakrapani A, Wraith JE, *et al.* Long term survival post early liver transplantation in organic acidaemias. *Gut* 2001;**48**:71A.
74 Nyhan WL, Gargus JJ, Boyle K, Selby R, Koch R. Progressive neurologic disability in methylmalonic acidemia despite transplantation of the liver. *Eur J Pediatr* 2002;**161**:377–9.
75 Chakrapani A, Sivakumar P, McKiernan PJ, Leonard JV. Metabolic stroke in methylmalonic acidemia five years after liver transplantation. *J Pediatr* 2002;**140**:261–3.
76 Kasahara M, Horikawa R, Tagawa M, *et al.* Current role of liver transplantation for methylmalonic acidemia: a review of the literature. *Pediatr Transplant* 2006;**10**:943–7.
77 van't Hoff W, McKiernan PJ, Surtees RA, Leonard JV. Liver transplantation for methylmalonic acidaemia. *Eur J Pediatr* 1999;**158**(Suppl 2):S70–4.

78 Van Calcar SC, Harding CO, Lyne P, *et al.* Renal transplantation in a patient with methylmalonic acidaemia. *J Inherit Metab Dis* 1998;**21**:729–37.

79 Coman D, Huang J, McTaggart S, *et al.* Renal transplantation in a 14-year-old girl with vitamin B_{12}-responsive cblA-type methylmalonic acidaemia. *Pediatr Nephrol* 2006;**21**:270–3.

80 Fisher RA, Strom SC. Human hepatocyte transplantation: worldwide results. *Transplantation* 2006;**82**:441–9.

81 Dhawan A, Mitry RR, Hughes RD, *et al.* Hepatocyte transplantation for inherited factor VII deficiency. *Transplantation* 2004;**78**: 1812–4.

82 Wilcken B. Recent advances in newborn screening. *J Inherit Metab Dis* 2007;**30**:129–33.

5 Acute Liver Disease

6 Infective Disorders of the Liver

Suzanne Davison and Elizabeth H. Boxall

Infective disorders of the liver may be generalized, causing hepatitis; localized, with abscess formation; or confined to the biliary tree (cholangitis). Inflammatory processes may be acute or chronic. There is considerable overlap in the clinical presentation, particularly since exacerbations of chronic disease may mimic acute infection. However, some infections have characteristic features that aid diagnosis.

Infective disorders, particularly hepatitis, may also mimic noninfective disorders, including autoimmune hepatitis, and thus the differential diagnosis in children is wide. In assessing a child with a possible infective liver disorder, the following may be of value in determining the diagnosis and likely pathogens:

- Age of the child: neonates, younger children and teenagers have different susceptibilities—e.g., herpes simplex liver failure in neonates and Epstein–Barr virus (EBV) hepatitis in teenagers.
- Ethnicity, history of foreign travel, contact with travelers, residency abroad.
- Vaccination status.
- Local epidemics, household contacts.
- Presence of immunosuppression: opportunistic pathogens and coinfection must be considered.
- Extrahepatic intestinal diseases—e.g., Crohn's disease and appendicitis may lead to portal pyemia and hepatic abscess formation.
- Preexisting biliary disease—e.g., biliary atresia, choledochal cyst, primary sclerosing cholangitis, Caroli's disease: infective cholangitis is rare in immunocompetent individuals unless there is an underlying biliary abnormality.
- Risk of parenteral infection: hospitalization, recreational activity, body piercing.
- Risk of vertical transmission: maternal history and risk factors.
- Exposure to animals/household pets.
- Exposure to contaminated water.
- Comorbidity—e.g., thalassemia.

In this chapter, the clinical features, differential diagnosis, and investigation of acute and chronic hepatic infections in general will be considered, followed by a more detailed description of specific infections, including their molecular characteristics, epidemiology, pathogenesis, diagnosis, and management.

Diseases of the Liver and Biliary System in Children, 3rd edition. Edited by Deirdre Kelly. © 2008 Blackwell Publishing, ISBN: 978-1-4051-6334-7.

Acute infective hepatitis

Acute infection of the liver may be due to a wide range of pathogens. The outcome of the infection is dependent not only on the cause but on the host immune response; complete recovery depends on elimination of the infecting agent, resolution of the inflammatory changes and prevention of reinfection by effective antibody production.

Viruses are the major cause of acute infective hepatitis. Viral hepatitis may be due to infection with hepatotropic viruses (Table 6.1), a heterogeneous group with differing modes of transmission that cause disease primarily affecting the liver, or with viruses predominantly associated with disease manifestations outside the liver (Table 6.2). Nonviral causes of hepatitis (Table 6.3) are less common, but must be considered in the differential diagnosis.

Infection may occur more frequently, severely, or atypically in the presence of immunosuppression, or according to the age of the host.

Clinical features

The clinical presentation varies according to the infecting organism, the presence of extrahepatic disease, and host immunocompetence.

Table 6.1 Hepatotropic viruses.

Virus	Family	Type	Route of spread	Disease
HAV	Picornaviridae	RNA	Orofecal	Acute
HBV	Hepadnaviridae	DNA	Parenteral	Acute/chronic
HCV	Flaviviridae	RNA	Parenteral	Acute/chronic
HDV	Incomplete virus	RNA	Parenteral	Acute/chronic
HEV	Hepevirus	RNA	Orofecal	Acute

Table 6.2 Nonhepatotropic viruses associated with hepatocellular damage.

RNA viruses	DNA viruses
Paramyxovirus (measles)	Parvovirus B19
Togavirus (rubella)	Adenovirus
Enteroviruses	Herpesviruses
Echovirus	Herpes simplex type 1
Coxsackievirus	Herpes simplex type 2
Flaviviruses	Varicella-zoster virus
Yellow fever flavivirus	Cytomegalovirus
Dengue fever flavivirus	Epstein–Barr virus
Filoviruses	Human herpesvirus 6
Marburg virus	
Ebola virus	
Arenavirus (Lassa fever)	
Retrovirus (HIV)	

Table 6.3 Nonviral causes of hepatic infection.

Bacteria
Bartonella henselae, B. quintana
Brucella melitensis
Coxiella burnetii (Q fever)
Legionella pneumophila
Leptospira interrogans serovar *icterohaemorrhagiae*
Listeria monocytogenes
Mycobacterium tuberculosis
Salmonella typhi
Treponema pallidum (syphilis)
Protozoa
Toxoplasma gondii
Helminths (worms)
Cestodes (tapeworms)
Echinococcus multilocularis
Echinococcus granulosus
Nematodes (roundworms)
Ascaris lumbricoides
Toxocara canis, T. cati
Trematodes (flukes)
Schistosoma mansoni
Schistosoma japonicum
Fasciola hepatica

Typical symptoms may include:

- A prodrome of malaise
- Anorexia
- Nausea
- Vomiting
- Fever
- Tender hepatomegaly
- Splenomegaly
- Lymphadenopathy
- Rash
- Jaundice

Differential diagnosis

A clinical picture resembling acute infective hepatitis may be the presenting illness in both noninfective acute liver disease and underlying chronic disease, including:

- Metabolic liver disease
- Drug-induced hepatitis
- Autoimmune hepatitis
- Chronic infective hepatitis

Laboratory investigations

Specific features are discussed with each infection, but some investigations are of general application.

Biochemical features. The main biochemical finding in hepatitis is typically raised aminotransferases. Serum bilirubin may be normal despite significant inflammation. Hepatic synthetic function, measured by serum albumin and coagulation, is normal unless there is extensive hepatocellular necrosis, underlying chronic disease or disseminated intravascular coagulation.

Hematological features. The blood count may be normal or reveal pancytopenia (viral infection), eosinophilia (helminth infection), or polymorphonuclear leukocytosis (bacterial infection, hepatic abscess).

Histology. Histology is rarely required unless the diagnosis is in doubt, but in acute viral hepatitis it may demonstrate inflammation, ballooning of hepatocytes, lobular disarray, and reticulin collapse (Figure 6.1).

Management of acute hepatitis

The principles of management of acute hepatitis are to treat the causative agent if possible, ameliorate the inflammatory process, limit histological progression, and minimize the complications of both the disease and the treatment. Identification of the precise etiology and prognostic factors and knowledge of the natural history of the disease process are crucial for implementing the appropriate therapy. Specific treatment strategies are described in the following sections, according to the etiology.

Chronic infective hepatitis

A diagnosis of chronic hepatitis encompasses a wide range of diseases, with distinct etiologies, which typically lead to

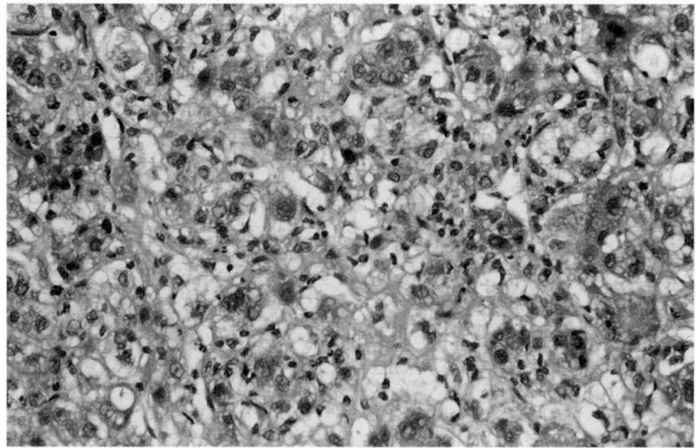

Figure 6.1 Acute viral hepatitis. Histology is rarely required for diagnosis, but demonstrates inflammation, ballooning of hepatocytes, lobular disarray, and reticulin collapse (hematoxylin–eosin, original magnification × 25).

slowly progressive inflammatory damage and fibrosis. The process of chronic hepatitis is one of continuing inflammation centered on the hepatocyte, which leads to hepatocellular damage. It requires a trigger, a target, and a mechanism of persistence. The trigger may be a microbial antigen, the target a component of the cell structure, and persistence may be due for example to viral mechanisms for immune escape or an ineffective host immune response.

Despite the chronicity of the underlying disease process, the duration of signs and symptoms at diagnosis may be short, and the clinical presentation may resemble that of an acute hepatitic illness. In addition, hepatitis due to viral infection may evolve from an acute inflammatory process to chronicity.

Viral infections account for at least 90% of chronic hepatitis, with hepatitis B virus (HBV) and hepatitis C virus (HCV) as the leading causative agents. Chronic viral hepatitis is the principal cause of chronic liver disease in the world. Individual viruses may lead to similar clinical symptoms, signs, biochemical abnormalities, and histological characteristics. However, even for a single agent, the natural history following infection and the rate of progression may be variable. This is exemplified by HCV infection, which may lead to rapid progression to cirrhosis within 2 years, but more typically slowly progresses over decades.

There are also considerable differences in the response to therapy, influenced not only by the infecting virus, but also by host factors, including the route of acquisition, ethnic origin, and coexisting disease.

A diagnosis of chronic viral hepatitis must be supplemented by characterization not only of the viral agent, but also of specific viral and host factors that may influence the natural history and prognosis.

Clinical features

The clinical presentation of chronic hepatitis may be varied, even for a specific etiology.

Asymptomatic presentation. The diagnosis may be made following incidental detection of abnormal liver enzymes, or during screening of those at risk.

Insidious onset/complications of cirrhosis. This is characterized by a gradual onset of fatigue, anorexia and weight loss, and abdominal discomfort, which may be intermittent. Jaundice, if present, may be variable or fluctuating. Symptoms may have been present for many years, and histological progression to cirrhosis may already be apparent at diagnosis. Complications of cirrhosis, such as ascites or bleeding varices, may be the presenting symptom.

Acute onset. An acute illness mimicking acute viral hepatitis may occur. Although hepatitis B or C virus infection may occasionally present during the acute infection, presentation in this way may also be precipitated by superimposed infection by a different infective agent—for example, delta virus in hepatitis B infection.

Diagnosis

Depending on the mode of clinical presentation, the differential diagnosis of chronic infective hepatitis may include:
- Acute infective hepatitis
- Autoimmune hepatitis
- Sclerosing cholangitis
- Drug-induced liver disease
- Metabolic liver disease
- Cystic fibrosis

Laboratory investigations

Biochemical abnormalities are nonspecific:
- Serum aminotransferases—alanine aminotransferase (ALT) and aspartate aminotransferase (AST)—are usually raised, may fluctuate spontaneously to normal levels, and do not always correlate with histological severity.
- Serum alkaline phosphatase and γ-glutamyltransferase (GGT) are usually normal or mildly elevated, except in the presence of cirrhosis.
- Serum bilirubin is variable, and may be normal.

Management of chronic hepatitis

The principles of management of chronic hepatitis are, as with acute hepatitis, to remove the causative agent, ameliorate the inflammatory process, limit histological progression, and minimize the complications of both the disease and the treatment. Identification of the precise etiology and prognostic factors and a knowledge of the natural history of the disease process are crucial for implementing the appropriate therapy. Specific treatment strategies are described in the following sections, according to the etiology.

Laboratory diagnosis of viral infections

Traditionally, the diagnosis of acute or persistent viral infection depended on either the identification of infecting organisms by viral growth in tissue culture or the demonstration of viral antigens or antibodies by immunological techniques. In the last 10–20 years, laboratory techniques have moved to molecular methods, first for the identification of hepatitis C and more recently to the quantitation of viral DNA and RNA as diagnostic methods for assessing infectivity and to assess the response to antiviral chemotherapy.

Molecular methods are now essential to the management of chronic hepatitis B and C, and genome sequencing plays an important role in identifying drug-resistant variants and investigating the relatedness of isolates.

Serology

Serological assays are still the first-line approach to the diagnosis of virus infections. The assays are sensitive and specific and can give rapid results on the same day as the sample is taken. There are different approaches for each virus, but the principle behind each assay is the demonstration of an antigen or antibody in the patient's serum by laboratory reaction with a defined antibody or antigen, using a detection system to demonstrate the reaction—enzyme immunoassays (EIAs). Automated methods using detection systems involving fluorescent or luminescent substrates have been developed improving the availability of rapid results. As serological methods are sensitive, weak reactions may be misleading and should be discussed with the virologist, as some antigens are transient, some antibodies take longer to develop, and follow-up samples may be required for clarification. With the diagnosis of blood-borne viruses, it is recommended that such diagnoses are confirmed by reference tests and confirmed by a second sample to ensure the patient's identity.

Molecular methods (Table 6.4)

The viruses normally associated with infectious hepatitis do not grow well in tissue culture, and few in vitro culture systems are available. Infectivity is therefore determined by virus replicative ability, genome organization, and virus gene products. Recombinant DNA technology played a role in the production of hepatitis B vaccine and in the discovery of hepatitis C virus and the viruses grouped as hepatitis G or GB virus type C.

Hybridization

The first methods to be introduced were those based on hybridization, where single-stranded viral DNA or RNA was targeted with a complementary cloned or synthetic probe of complementary DNA, which was labeled either with a radioactive on chemical molecule. This allows the demonstration of virus nucleic acid using radioactive or enzyme detection systems. Such assay systems include dot blot hybridization and in situ hybridization, which allows localization of virus in fixed tissue sections. Quantitative methods are based on a range of standards with the patient's samples using the separation of single-stranded and double-stranded DNA, such as the Abbott Genostics method,[1] which has a lower limit of detection of 2 pg/mL (equivalent to about 1 000 000 genome copies per milliliter).

Signal amplification

A modification of the hybridization method to provide greater sensitivity and dynamic range in quantitative assays is to introduce an amplification of the detection system or the signal. Examples of assays using signal amplification are the branched-chain DNA or bDNA assay (Chiron)[2] and the Hybrid Capture System (Digene).[3,4]

bDNA assays. The first step in these assays is to bind sample single-stranded DNA to virus-specific oligonucleotide probes bound to plastic microwells. Bound hybrids are detected by specially designed probes with multiple copies of a DNA sequence, which is then detected by another probe, attached to an enzyme. As multiple copies of the enzyme are present, the signal produced is enhanced, allowing a greater level of sensitivity.

Hybrid capture assays. The first step in these assays is to hybridize the patient's DNA to a complementary RNA probe. These hybrids are then bound to a solid phase by antibodies to

Table 6.4 Genome assays.

Assay	Principle	Lower limit of detection (hepatitis B DNA)
Genostics	Hybridization	1 000 000 (1 x 10^6) genome copies/mL)
bDNA	Signal Amplification	700 000 (7 x 10^5) genome copies/mL)
Hybrid capture	Signal Amplification	5000 (5 x 10^3) genome copies/mL)
PCR	Target Amplification	200 (2 x 10^2) genome copies/mL)

bDNA, branched-chain DNA; PCR, polymerase chain reaction.

DNA–RNA hybrids. Detection antibodies bound to multiple enzyme molecules produce a chemiluminescent signal, which is detected photometrically with a high level of sensitivity. However, the demand for the increased sensitivity of direct genome amplification methods has resulted in a range of commercial assays based on the polymerase chain reaction (PCR).

Qualitative and quantitative PCR

The development of PCR assays revolutionized the laboratory diagnosis and monitoring of viral infections. The principle is to produce single-stranded DNA (a reverse transcriptase step is required first if looking for an RNA virus), which reacts with single-stranded DNA primers designed to hybridize with a conserved region of the target genome, producing double-stranded regions, and then extend from the double-stranded regions by adding nucleotides, thereby making copies of the original DNA, which can then be detected.

A variety of polymerase enzyme systems have been used by commercial diagnostics manufacturers in order to avoid patent issues. Most PCR methods use repeated rounds of thermal cycling and use a heat-stable DNA polymerase enzyme, but some use novel systems and enzymes that go through the amplification process without thermal cycling.

The technology has also advanced in the meantime, and methods using small volumes of sample with short cycling times have been developed.

Real-time PCR

Real-time PCR is a development of the technique that introduces a quantitation step at each cycle through the detection of fluorescent products. These developments have improved the dynamic range of assays at the same time as improving the speed with which samples are tested and reported.

Detection of variant viruses

Variant or "mutant" viruses are increasingly important as new antiviral agents are introduced and become widely used. Specific variants and their clinical importance will be discussed in the appropriate section of this chapter, but the following section describes how some variants might be detected.

Point mutation assays. When the exact location of the mutation is known, it is possible to devise point mutation assays in which a single-stranded DNA (similar to the first part of a PCR reaction, above) is annealed with a specific probe that stops short of the exact nucleotide location of the mutation. The reaction is then provided with all four nucleotides, one of which is labeled with a detection system such as an enzyme or a fluorescent or radioactive marker, which will be specific for the mutation and allow detection of either the mutant or wild type.

Sequencing. Detection of point mutations is useful, but direct sequencing of PCR products gives more information about the nature of the virus and can detect a wider range of variations. Sequencing is now the method of choice for the identification of antiviral drug-resistant variants and is also one of the methods used for identifying genotypes.

Genotyping. As well as genotyping by direct sequencing, a range of "line probe" assays are available for easy laboratory use. These are based on the absorption of specific oligonucleotide probes onto a solid-phase strip and allowing PCR products from patient material to hybridize to the strips. The patterns of bands produced are compared with a chart produced from standard independently validated samples.

Histology of acute and chronic infective hepatitis

Liver biopsy is not essential in every child with infective hepatitis, particularly if the underlying cause is known. Furthermore, it may be contraindicated—for example, in those with significant liver impairment, biliary obstruction, ascites, or uncontrolled sepsis. However, liver histology may be helpful in revealing diagnostic features, including granulomas and viral inclusion bodies, or detection of viral products by immunohistochemistry—e.g., cytomegalovirus (CMV), EBV, and hepatitis B surface antigen (HBsAg; see below).

- Chronic HBV infection—detectable in hepatocytes by immunostaining and hepatitis B core antigen (HBcAg) by orcein staining.
- Hepatitis D virus (HDV) infection—HDV antigen in hepatocytes is detectable by immunofluorescence or immunoperoxidase stains.

Hepatitis, both acute and chronic, is characterized histologically by:

- Inflammatory cell infiltrates of predominantly lymphocytes and plasma cells
- Hepatocellular damage, manifest by swelling (balloon degeneration) or shrinkage
- Hepatocellular necrosis, which may be:
  - —Spotty (focal)
  - —Bridging (confluent): either portal–portal or portal–central
  - —Piecemeal (at the interface of parenchyma and connective tissue): periportal or periseptal

In chronic hepatitis, staging depends on the degree of fibrosis, which may be:

- Mild: expansion of portal tracts;
- Moderate: portoportal or periportal septa
- Severe: portocentral septa, with architectural distortion
- Cirrhosis: fibrous septa surrounding parenchymal nodules

In chronic viral hepatitis, histological assessment is also of value in assessing the degree of inflammation and fibrosis, which will guide the timing of antiviral therapy.

Hepatitis A virus

Hepatitis A virus (HAV) is the most common form of acute

viral hepatitis in much of the world. HAV usually gives rise to an asymptomatic infection, with less than 5% of infected people having an identifiable illness. Due to its high prevalence worldwide, however, HAV alone accounts for 20–25% of clinically apparent hepatitis, with 1.5 million clinical cases reported worldwide annually.[5] The likelihood of symptomatic infection increases with the age of acquisition, with most children under 6 years of age being asymptomatic.[6] The HAV-associated mortality of 0.2–0.4% of symptomatic cases is increased in individuals older than 50 years or less than 5 years of age at acquisition. The significant morbidity and mortality of HAV infection in childhood are due to its high worldwide prevalence, the development of fulminant hepatic failure, and hepatic and extrahepatic complications.

A significant change in the epidemiology of HAV infection has occurred over recent decades. This is due to both improved public health hygiene measures and also the introduction of vaccination programs. These are discussed in detail in the prevention section below and in Chapter 23.

Molecular virology

Hepatitis A is a member of the picornavirus family and is a small, spherical virus approximately 27 nm in diameter. The virus particle contains single-stranded positive-sense RNA of 7487 nucleotides (with a molecular weight of 2.25×10^6) that codes for four structural proteins. Although initially classed with the enteroviruses, its genome is sufficiently different from the other members of the group and has been assigned its own genus, *Hepatovirus*. Although up to seven genotypes have been recognized, the surface protein classes all of the isolates as a single serotype, making the universal application of diagnostic tests and the production of effective vaccines possible. The virus grows slowly in tissue culture, but in sufficient quantity for the production of an inactivated vaccine.[7]

Replication and pathogenesis

The virus attaches to hepatocytes via a glycoprotein receptor.[8] The uncoated RNA acts as a messenger and codes for a polyprotein through cleavages, and further processing, to produce four structural proteins (VP1-4) and several non-structural proteins required for RNA replication. Further understanding of the complex replication process[9] may lead to the identification of targets for intervention with antiviral agents, which are rarely needed as the infection is usually self-limiting.

Pathophysiology

Studies of the virus in tissue culture show that the virus is not directly cytopathogenic. During the incubation period of acute hepatitis A, there is very little evidence of histopathological change. It is generally accepted that liver damage and subsequent recovery from infection are mediated by the host's immune response. Animal models appear to indicate that the liver is the only organ in which the virus replicates; an intermediate replication site in the gut has been suggested, but not proven. The virus is shed into the blood and into the gut through the bile, and peak excretion occurs before the onset of disease. Viremia lasts for several weeks following the onset of symptoms, and virus may be excreted in the feces for a similar time period but at a much lower level than during the incubation phase.[10] A cellular immune response is responsible for recovery through a subset of virus-specific $CD8^+$ T cells, which also produce interferon gamma.[11] $CD4^+$ T cells also have a role, as do natural killer cells. Overwhelming elimination of infected hepatocytes by T cell–mediated lysis, where nearly all hepatocytes are infected, results in fulminant hepatitis. Complete recovery is the norm, but there are reports of recurrent hepatitis or relapsing hepatitis, with elevated hepatic transaminase enzymes,[12] giving the appearance of a biphasic illness.[13]

Risk factors

The majority of cases in the United Kingdom and the developed world are sporadic and not associated with any known risk factor. However, the risk of sporadic HAV acquisition is increased by:

- *Travel.* Hepatitis A is the most frequently diagnosed form of hepatitis imported from the developing world,[14] with 36% of imported cases occurring in children.[6]
- *Household contact* with HAV infection. Household spread is the predominant route of transmission; symptomatic secondary cases occur in up to 50% of household members. Young children are important sources of infection in both household-acquired and community-acquired infection.

Crowding, poor social hygiene, and mixing of children in institutions such as day-care centers and schools increase the risk of community outbreaks. However, no significant increased risk was identified in nursery nurses, childminders, health-care workers, or teachers.[15] Outbreaks may also occur following exposure of large groups to a common source such as contaminated drinking water or food, particularly bivalve molluscs.

Parenteral acquisition is uncommon. Acquisition by individuals with high-risk behavior, such as intravenous drug abuse, may relate to poor hygiene and crowding in addition to exposure to infected blood. Transfusion-associated HAV is uncommon, but has been reported in patients exposed to factor concentrates[16] and following neonatal transfusion.[17,18] Vertical transmission is reported but rare.[19]

Clinical features

HAV infection has an incubation period of 2–6 weeks, following which symptoms become evident. A prodromal illness is characterized by nonspecific symptoms, including anorexia, nausea, malaise, and fever. In children, gastrointestinal symptoms such as diarrhea and vomiting may predominate. Within a few days to a week, jaundice, pale stools, and dark urine become apparent, and the prodromal symptoms usually subside. There may be tender hepatic enlargement, splenomegaly, and posterior cervical lymphadenopathy. Rarely, extrahepatic manifestations such as arthritis and vasculitis may accompany the acute illness.

The infectivity of HAV due to fecal shedding typically begins during the prodromal phase, peaks at the onset of symptoms, and then rapidly declines. However, fecal shedding of HAV RNA may persist for up to 3 months, with a prolonged risk of transmission.[20] Furthermore, HAV RNA may be detected in blood during the incubation period and up to 30 days after the onset of the illness.[21] Precautions to minimize transmission are therefore advisable during this period.

Extrahepatic manifestations

Extrahepatic manifestations rarely occur, but include:

- Neurological involvement: Guillain–Barré syndrome, transverse myelitis, postviral encephalitis and mononeuritis multiplex
- Renal disease: acute interstitial nephritis, mesangioproliferative glomerulonephritis, nephrotic syndrome, and acute renal failure
- Acute pancreatitis: described in children in both the acute and convalescent phase
- Hematological disorders: autoimmune hemolytic anemia, red cell aplasia, and thrombocytopenic purpura

Diagnosis

Laboratory diagnosis of HAV infection is by the demonstration of hepatitis A–specific immunoglobulin M (IgM) class antibodies, usually by an EIA technique or by a laboratory platform providing random access capability. Peak levels occur during the acute illness or early convalescent phase. HAV IgM persists for 4–6 months after infection. HAV RNA is not routinely offered as a laboratory test, but may be available in some reference laboratories, particularly for the investigation of foodstuffs implicated in transmission events.

Biochemical indices of HAV infection are nonspecific and include elevated conjugated bilirubin and aminotransferase enzymes (ALT and AST). The degree of elevation does not correlate with the severity of the illness or likelihood of complications. The prothrombin time is usually normal and is a good guide to severity. Persistently abnormal coagulation is an indication for referral to a specialist center.

Ultrasound examination is not essential in uncomplicated HAV infection if the diagnosis is not in doubt. Ultrasound features include hepatomegaly with periportal echogenicity, periportal lymphadenopathy, and splenomegaly. The gallbladder may be distended, with a thickened wall.

Liver biopsy is not indicated if the diagnosis is known or the disease has an uncomplicated course.

Management and outcome

The majority of symptomatic children will have an uncomplicated course, with complete resolution of the infection. Supportive treatment with rest, analgesia, and ensuring adequate hydration is needed during the acute phase. Complete recovery is usual within 3–6 months. However, the course may be complicated by:

- Fulminant hepatic failure
- Prolonged cholestasis
- Recurrent hepatitis and extrahepatic manifestations
- Preexisting chronic liver disease

Fulminant hepatic failure. This affects approximately 0.1% of symptomatic infected children. Deterioration in liver function may not be apparent clinically, and may occur either rapidly following the onset of symptoms or after an interval of several weeks. Frequent vomiting or deterioration in the conscious level, even if only intermittent, should prompt careful clinical assessment and evaluation of hepatic function, particularly coagulation. Those with a rapid onset of liver failure from the onset of jaundice are most likely to undergo spontaneous recovery. In children with encephalopathy, the predictors of a poor outcome are bilirubin > 400 mmol/L or a significantly elevated prothrombin time, irrespective of the grade of encephalopathy.[22] Children with fulminant HAV infection should be transferred to a center where liver transplantation is available (see also Chapter 7).

Prolonged cholestasis. In a series of nine adults with prolonged cholestasis due to HAV infection, the mean duration of cholestasis was 77 days (range 30–120 days) and the mean bilirubin level was 265 mmol/L (range 51–560 mmol/L).[23] Histological features were intralobular cholestasis and portal tract infiltrates, associated with dystrophy and paucity of bile ducts. A course of corticosteroids may shorten the duration of cholestasis, but spontaneous recovery is usual. Fat-soluble vitamin supplementation should be provided, together with antipruritic treatment.

Recurrent hepatitis. A biphasic or relapsing course may occur in up to 25% of symptomatic cases and may be associated with extrahepatic manifestations. Complete recovery is usual; HAV infection does not give rise to chronic liver disease.

Hepatitis A infection in chronic liver disease. Acute HAV infection in children with preexisting chronic liver disease may lead to more severe acute hepatitis, with an increased risk of fulminant hepatic failure and increased mortality. This has been reported in both chronic hepatitis B infection[24] and hepatitis C infection.[25] Immunization is recommended in all patients with chronic liver disease (see below).

Prevention

Global strategies to minimize epidemics of HAV infection include improving sanitation and providing education to improve standards of basic hygiene. These have led to a decrease in the incidence of hepatitis A in childhood, with a shift to the acquisition of infection at an older age (see Chapter 23).

Prevention of HAV may be by active or passive immunization. Routine vaccination of children has been introduced in some areas of the world, including the United States. When immunization has been targeted to high-risk populations, a decreased incidence has occurred in the nonimmunized population, due to herd immunity.

Active immunization

There are four monovalent vaccines available; all are inactivated and can be used interchangeably. The recommended regimen is a single dose of 1440 enzyme-linked immunosorbent assay (ELISA) units in adults and 720 ELISA units in children. In 90% of those vaccinated, protective levels of antibodies are achieved and persist for at least 1 year. A second dose given after an interval of 6–12 months may increase the duration of protection to up to 10 years. Postvaccination testing is not indicated; antibody assays are not sufficiently sensitive to detect the low but protective level of antibody.[6] HAV vaccine is both safe and immunogenic for protection of patients with underlying chronic liver disease.[24]

The vaccine is not licensed for children under 1 year of age; passively transferred maternal antibody may lead to a suboptimal response to the vaccine. HAV vaccine can be given concurrently with passive immunization.

A combination vaccine for protection against both hepatitis A virus and hepatitis B virus (with a three-dose schedule) is available, and also a combined hepatitis A and typhoid vaccine (single dose).

The Department of Health for England recommends preexposure vaccination in the following groups, of relevance to children:[26]

- Travelers to areas of high-prevalence or intermediate-prevalence endemicity
- Patients with chronic liver disease
- Patients with hemophilia

Passive immunization

Human normal immunoglobulin, given by intramuscular injection, offers up to 3–6 months of protection against HAV. It may be used alone or with active immunization in management of contacts and offers more rapid protection than can be achieved with active immunization.

Hepatitis B virus

Introduction

Hepatitis B virus (HBV) infection may lead to an acute, symptomatic hepatitic illness, or a chronic disease without any initial symptoms. Acute HBV infection presents with viral symptoms and jaundice and may be indistinguishable from other causes of acute hepatitis. It may occasionally precipitate fulminant liver failure or be associated with extrahepatic manifestations. After recovery, however, viral eradication and protective immunity are usually achieved. Although persistent or chronic HBV infection is usually clinically silent during childhood, it may eventually lead to chronic liver disease with cirrhosis and hepatocellular carcinoma.

Chronic HBV infection and its prevention pose a major health challenge worldwide: chronic HBV carriers comprise 5% of the world population.[27] The likelihood of remaining a chronic carrier after HBV infection is highest in infancy.[28] The risk of developing cirrhosis and primary hepatocellular carcinoma is related to the duration of chronic infection, and acquisition in infancy is associated with an estimated 25% lifetime risk of cirrhosis or primary hepatocellular carcinoma. The particular challenges that HBV poses in childhood, therefore, are the prevention of HBV acquisition and the prevention of progressive liver disease in those who become infected.

Molecular virology

Hepatitis B has a unique partly single-stranded and partly double-stranded circular DNA genome of 3200 nucleotides (with a molecular weight of 2.3×10^6) The Hepatovirus group includes the human hepatitis B virus and similar viruses infecting a wide variety of species such as ducks, woodchucks, and ground squirrels. In humans, eight different genotypes (A to H) have been described and characterized by genome sequencing. These genotypes have a distinct geographical distribution (Table 6.5).[29] The genotypes do not correlate with previously described serotypes.

The virus particles are 42 nm in diameter and consist of an outer coat protein, the hepatitis B surface antigen (HBsAg), and an inner hepatitis B core antigen (HBcAg). In the replication cycle, excess HBsAg accumulates and aggregates into virus-like small particles and filaments with a 22-nm diameter (Figure 6.2). The small 22-nm particles are highly immunogenic and were the source of HBsAg for the first hepatitis B vaccines.

Replication and pathogenesis

The receptor for hepatitis B binding to the hepatocyte has not yet been clearly identified, but once bound, the virus fuses with the plasma membrane and is internalized and uncoated. The virus carries its own DNA polymerase, which completes the shorter DNA strand to complete the circular structure. Within 24 h, viral DNA can be found in the nucleus as covalently closed circular molecules (cccDNA). This acts as a template for mRNAs and pregenomic RNA, which is transcribed with a reverse transcriptase enzyme into DNA (virus-coded HBV DNA polymerase) for assembly into new virions. This step in the replication cycle provides a target for the inhibition of replication of the virus using antiretroviral drugs, which inhibit reverse transcriptase enzymes. A large open reading frame coding for the polymerase overlaps three others,

Table 6.5 Geographical distribution of HBV genotypes.

Genotype	Geographical distribution
A	Europe, North America, Australia, Africa
B	Far East
C	Far East, Pacific
D	West Asia, Mediterranean, worldwide
E	Africa
F	South America
G	Europe, North America
H	Central America

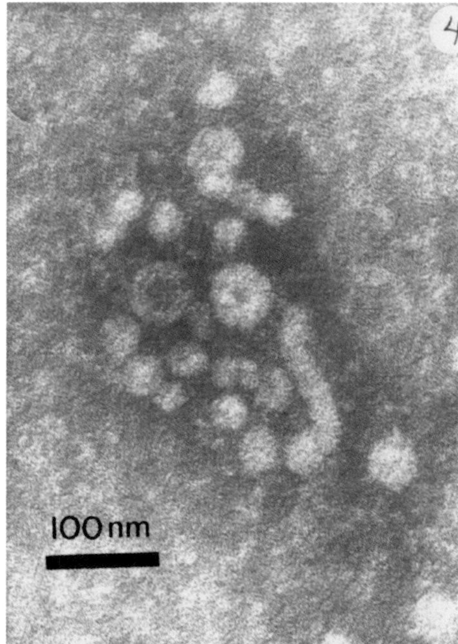

Figure 6.2 Electron micrograph of hepatitis B, showing the morphological forms—small spherical and tubular particles, 20–22 nm in diameter, and double-shelled virus particles, 42 nm in diameter.

which code for the three forms of the surface antigen (S, preS1 and preS2), the core antigen, and the X protein (which transactivates transcription). The pregenomic RNA is packed into particles with polymerase enzyme and surrounded by core protein; through a process of genome maturation, RNA is reverse-transcribed into DNA, and some of these progeny genomes cycle back into the nucleus to maintain the pool of infected hepatocytes. The majority of the core particles are then coated with surface antigen in three forms: small S (HBsAg), medium M (HBsAg + PreS1) and large L (HBsAg + preS1 + preS2). Excess small protein aggregates into 22-nm spheres and variable-length filaments, which can also contain small amounts of M and L protein. The stem loop structure of the pregenomic RNA is important in the packing of the genome into core particles and therefore in the replication of the viral DNA. Mutations that destroy the integrity of the stem loop structure are not viable. Within the key hairpin bend of the pregenomic RNA is the region of the precore gene that codes for hepatitis B e antigen (HBeAg). However, as long as the mutations that prevent the synthesis of HBeAg do not compromise the hairpin structure, the virus remains viable. HBeAg-negative variants either arise from mutations in the precore region of the genome or from mutations in the core promoter region, the location of the specific mutations is genome-dependent. Genomes B, C, and D are likely to have HBeAg-negative variants due to mutations in the precore region, whereas genotype A is more likely to have a mutation in the core promoter region. Mature virus particles, HBsAg particles, and soluble HBeAg are secreted from the infected cells, but the cccDNA remains within the cell to continue the replication cycle. The soluble HBeAg is produced in excess during periods of active viral replication and can be easily detected in serum. The presence of HBeAg coincides with high levels of replication and therefore high levels of HBV DNA, which led to its use as a surrogate marker for virus infectivity until the advent of direct measurement of HBV DNA.

Pathophysiology

Most HBV infections in older children and adults with hepatitis B are self-limiting, and the virus is cleared with resultant long-term immunity. The human immune system, both innate and adaptive, is important in eliminating the infection and for the acute symptoms. The appearance of antibody to the core component of the virus coincides with liver cell damage as measured by increases in serum transaminase enzymes. The cellular immune response plays an important role in the initial pathogenesis of the virus and in eliminating virus-infected cells. The elimination of infected cells containing cccDNA is important in clearing the infection from the liver. If these cells are not cleared, they remain a source of virus and are important in the development of persistent infection. The balance between the roles of cytokines, cytotoxic T lymphocytes, natural killer (NK) cells, and the host's genetic susceptibility is complex, and the factors that lead to a resolving infection or a persistent infection are still not understood.[30]

HBV transmission

Perinatal transmission. Exposure to maternal blood efficiently transmits HBV to offspring. Transmission may occur through placental tears, trauma during delivery, and contact of the infant mucous membranes with infected maternal fluids. Intrauterine transmission may occur, but this does not appear to be a major route. Mothers who are HBeAg-positive have the highest infectivity and a 70–90% risk of transmitting infection to their offspring. Those who are e antibody (anti-HBe)-positive have a lower risk of transmitting infection.

However, if the offspring are infected, they are at risk of developing fulminant liver failure.[31]

Horizontal transmission. HBV is present in infected individuals in high concentrations in blood, serum and serous exudates, semen, vaginal fluid, and saliva. Parenteral and sexual exposure routes are effective for transmission. Although HBV is also found in low concentrations in feces and breast milk, these are not associated with a significant risk of transmission. Children at high risk include those requiring frequent transfusions (e.g., with hemolytic anemia, thalassemia, hemophilia), those with high-risk sexual behavior, and intravenous drug users.

Environmental transmission in childhood may occur by exposure to infected body fluids through a broken skin surface, either directly by biting or by accidental contamination. Household transmission of HBV from infected family members may occur; up to 40% of children who are born to carrier mothers but not infected at birth acquire infection in the first 5 years of life.[32] An increased risk of environmental transmission also occurs in residential institutions and hemodialysis centers.

Clinical presentation and diagnosis

HBV infection may be acquired in unimmunized children who are exposed to HBV through perinatal transmission, household contact, infected needles or blood products, or through sexual contact. A small proportion of those receiving an appropriate vaccination course (approximately 5%) will fail to achieve adequate protection and thus remain at risk. Children who have received hospital care in countries with inadequate HBV prevention strategies are at risk of acquiring HBV. As infection is often clinically silent, identifying these risk factors is crucial for appropriate screening and diagnosis. In the UK, perinatal infection is still the most common route of infection in children, either because of failed vaccination or in immigrants from endemic countries.

Acute infection. Symptomatic acute HBV infection is unusual in childhood. It may present with malaise, anorexia, and abdominal discomfort, which usually precedes the onset of jaundice and occurs weeks to months after exposure. Raised aminotransferase enzymes are detected in serum, and the typical serological markers of acute infection are present (Table 6.6). Acute infection is rarely a severe illness, although fulminant hepatic failure may occur in up to 1% of infected patients. Patients with severe symptoms during acute infection are least likely to develop persistent infection, and those requiring liver transplantation for fulminant infection are less likely to have recurrence in the transplanted liver. Mild or asymptomatic acute infection is more likely to progress to chronicity.

Chronic infection. Chronic carriers of HBV are often asymptomatic, but fatigue and anorexia may occur. The only biochemical abnormality may be mild transaminitis. Presentation may be delayed until the onset of complications of cirrhosis and portal hypertension or with hepatocellular carcinoma. Because of the typical lack of symptoms, the diagnosis is usually made by screening those known to be at risk. An acute exacerbation of hepatitis or more rapid progression of chronic disease may occur with hepatitis delta infection, coinfection with hepatitis C, or emergence of the precore mutation.

Extrahepatic manifestations. Manifestations of HBV infection outside the liver, often due to deposition of circulating immune complex, may occur in both acute and chronic hepatitis and include:

- Polyarteritis nodosa (rare)
- Essential mixed cryoglobulinemia (uncommon, more frequently associated with HCV)
- Glomerulonephritis
- Arthralgia/arthritis
- Rashes

Table 6.6 Serological and biochemical markers of hepatitis B virus infection.

Host HBV status	ALT	HBV DNA	Anti-HBc	HBsAg	Anti-HBs	HBeAg	Anti-HBe
Acute infection	Raised	Detectable	IgM then IgG	+	–	+	–
Chronic infection							
Immune tolerance	Normal	High	IgG	+	–	+	–
Immune clearance	Raised	Variable	IgG	+	–	+	–
Nonreplicative	Normal	Undetectable	IgG	+	–	–	+
Reactivation	Raised	Detectable	IgG	+	–	–	+
Resolved infection	Normal	Undetectable	IgG	–	+	–	–

ALT, alanine aminotransferase; anti-HBc, core antibody; anti-HBe, antibody to e antigen; anti-HBs, surface antibody; HBeAg, nonstructural e antigen; HBsAg, surface antigen; HBV, hepatitis B virus; IgG, immunoglobulin G; IgM, immunoglobulin M.

Polyarteritis nodosa, a vasculitis of medium-sized arteries, is the only type of vasculitis reported to be associated with HBV infection. It most frequently involves the kidneys, peripheral nervous system, and gastrointestinal tract, leading to hypertension, mononeuropathy multiplex, and abdominal pain. Cutaneous involvement may occur. It is rare in childhood; a case has been reported of a 2-year-old who presented with hypertensive encephalopathy.[33] Glomerulonephritis complicates HBV infection most frequently in children, and predominantly in areas of the world in which HBV is endemic. Membranous and membranoproliferative glomerulonephritis are the most common pathological types seen in association with HBV, with nephrotic syndrome the usual clinical presentation. The natural history is generally benign, with up to 85% of affected children in spontaneous remission within 2 years and only a small risk of chronic renal insufficiency.[34] Symptoms may resolve with reduction in viral load and be an indication for therapy.

Laboratory diagnosis (Table 6.6)

Acute infection

Laboratory diagnosis of HBV relies on sensitive EIAs for the detection of HBsAg, which is the major marker of HBV infection. HBsAg and HBeAg are present during the late incubation phase before the onset of symptoms. At the time of onset, anti-HBc can be detected, mostly as IgM antibody (IgM anticore).

IgM class anti-HBc can also be detected by sensitive methods in persistent infection and is therefore not always a reliable marker of an acute infection. With the diagnosis of all blood-borne infections, it is customary laboratory practice to test a second sample for confirmation and for follow-up as the infection progresses. During an acute infection, HBeAg will disappear and be replaced by anti-HBe; HBsAg will clear and be replaced by anti-HBs, with long-term immunity.

Chronic infection

In chronic infection, the initial serological response is as for an acute infection. In the absence of symptoms, however, this phase may not be detected. Chronic infection is defined as persistent HBsAg for at least 6 months, and anti-HBs is not produced. Ongoing viral replication is accompanied by persistence of eAg, although loss of HBeAg and anti-HBe seroconversion may occur despite ongoing chronic infection.

Measurement of HBV DNA is a useful indicator of viral load, which can be quantified. HBV DNA levels can be used to assess the course of viremia in response to treatment. This is of particular value in monitoring infection in e antigen–negative chronic hepatitis or occult infection (see below), when other markers may be absent.

Occult HBV infection

Occult HBV infection is described when HBsAg is not detectable using standard techniques. Such infections occur in immunosuppressed patients and those who have undergone chemotherapy. The diagnosis is made by recognizing HBsAg-negative, anti-HBc-positive serology, and it is confirmed by detecting HBV DNA. Such infections may be described as non-A–E infections, but more importantly the blood and transplant services may fail to detect potentially infectious donations. For this reason, all potential liver transplant donations are also screened for anti-HBc, to avoid the risk of transplanting a liver with intracellular cccDNA within the hepatocytes, which would reactivate to cause an active infection after transplantation in the presence of immunosuppression. The clinical outcomes of such infections in children have not been described, although a study from a high-prevalence country (Taiwan) showed evidence of transmission of occult hepatitis B to children, which led to self-limiting subclinical infections.[35]

Histology

Chronic HBV infection may lead to a wide spectrum of histological severity, ranging from minimal inflammatory infiltrate to piecemeal necrosis, and from mild fibrosis to established cirrhosis (Figure 6.3). Pathognomonic features of HBV are the detection by immunohistochemistry of HBV core antigen (HBcAg), demonstrable in hepatocyte nuclei and cytoplasm, and HBsAg, most abundant in "ground-glass" hepatocytes. The characteristic ground-glass appearance is due to the granular appearance of hepatocytes in which the cytoplasm is rich in endoplasmic reticulum and HBV surface material (Figure 6.4).

Natural history

Asymptomatic chronic infection is the most likely outcome following acquisition in infancy and early childhood, occurring in more than 95% of infants infected and 85–95% of those aged 1–5 years. It is defined by the persistence of HBsAg in peripheral blood for at least 6 months, irrespective of

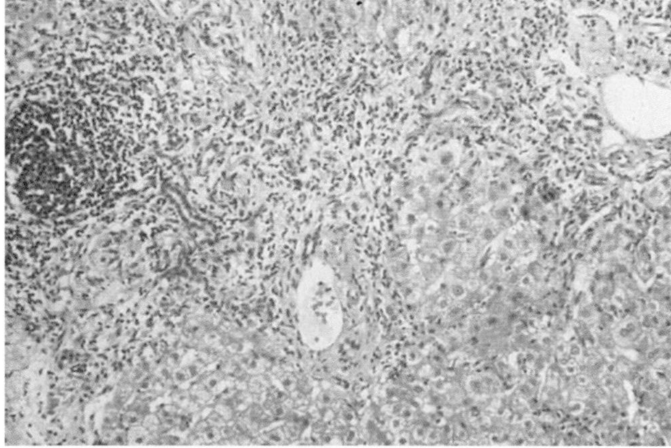

Figure 6.3 Chronic hepatitis B is characterized histologically by portal inflammation, consisting predominantly of lymphocytes and plasma cells. It may be limited to the portal tract or may spill out into the lobule.

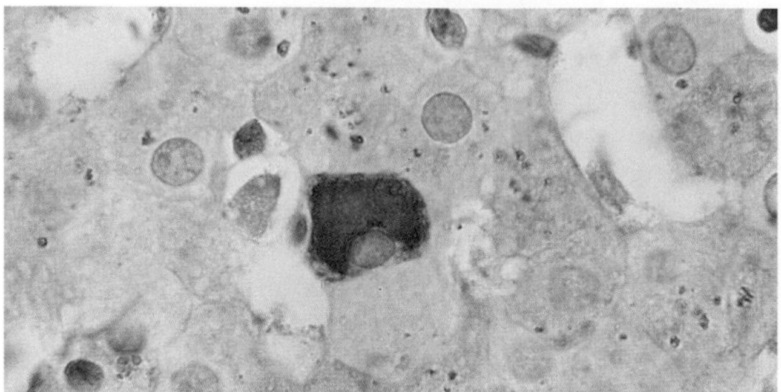

Figure 6.4 Hepatitis B infection may be suggested by the detection of hepatitis B surface antigen (orcein, original magnification × 1000).

HBeAg/anti-HBe status. The natural seroconversion rate is low in children, although girls may seroconvert earlier than boys.

Chronic HBV infection is characterized by three stages:[36,37] immune tolerance, immune clearance, and residual non-replicative infection (Table 6.6).

Immune tolerance. In the initial stage of chronic infection, infected hepatocytes express viral proteins (HBcAg, HBeAg, HBsAg) and there is a high level of replicating virus, with high levels of HBV DNA detectable in the circulating blood. The host T-cell response is actively suppressed. As there is no immune-mediated destruction of infected hepatocytes, there is no elevation of hepatic aminotransferase enzymes and no significant hepatic inflammation. The affected individual is usually asymptomatic. This state may persist for several decades, particularly after perinatal acquisition, before the immune response becomes active and immune clearance is attempted.

Immune clearance (HBeAg-positive chronic hepatitis). During this stage, a T-cell–mediated inflammatory response is directed against infected hepatocytes, leading to cell necrosis and hepatic fibrosis. This is characterized by elevation in aminotransferase enzymes. Continued viral replication and immune destruction during this stage lead to progressive liver damage and ultimately cirrhosis. Progression to cirrhosis is accompanied by a risk of liver failure and hepatocellular carcinoma. Although the evolution of liver damage is typically slow, both these sequelae have been reported in childhood.

Levels of circulating DNA fall with immune clearance of infected cells, eventually becoming undetectable ($< 10^3$ IU/mL). When viral replication ceases, there is clearance of HBeAg and emergence of anti-HBe. Seroconversion may be accompanied by an increase in liver inflammation, manifest by a transient rise in hepatic transaminases.

Residual nonreplicative infection (inactive carrier state). If successful seroconversion is achieved, either spontaneously or by successful treatment, aminotransferase enzymes return to normal and disease progression is halted. The risk of end-stage liver disease is reduced, and even if cirrhosis is already present, there may be clinical improvement. Following resolution of both viral replication and immune-mediated damage, HBV DNA remains integrated in the hepatocyte genome and surface antigen expression may continue. Another gene product, termed the X protein, is also produced and may have a role in malignant transformation. There is a continued risk of hepatocellular carcinoma, even after replicative infection has been eliminated. This risk is reduced further if HBsAg is cleared and seroconversion to surface antibody (anti-HBs) occurs, although this is rare.

Reactivation

Reactivation of HBV replication may occur, either spontaneously or as a result of immunosuppression. In this phase of HBeAg-negative chronic hepatitis, most patients have mutations in HBV that prevent HBeAg production despite active replication. This phase is accompanied by ongoing necroinflammation and raised ALT. Reactivation of eAg-negative chronic hepatitis is uncommon in children, but is an increasing problem in adults with chronic infection.

Management

Despite their apparent well-being, chronic HBV carriers should remain under medical supervision in order to:

- *Assess virological factors.* Monitoring HBeAg persistence or anti-HBe in order to consider antiviral therapy or assess infectivity. HBV DNA levels provide additional evidence, and are essential to detect relapse in anti-HBe-positive children.
- *Assess disease progression.* Monitoring hepatic transaminases provides indirect evidence of inflammatory damage. ALT may be normal despite histological evidence of inflammation and fibrosis. Annual liver ultrasound assessment and serum α-fetoprotein assessments facilitate early detection of hepatocellular carcinoma. Liver biopsy provides a more accurate assessment of inflammation and fibrosis, particularly when treatment is being considered.
- *Provide emotional and psychological support and education.* Support and education are needed for the whole family regarding minimizing transmission while avoiding social isolation or stigmatization. All family members should be counseled regarding the need for screening and immunization. All HBV-infected children should be immunized against hepatitis A virus.

Treatment

The ultimate goal of treatment is to reduce the risk of morbidity and mortality from cirrhosis and hepatocellular carcinoma. The first step is the eradication of replicative infection; clearance of HBeAg is associated with improved survival[38,39] and a reduction in the transmission risk. Natural seroconversion occurs at a variable rate, depending on age at acquisition and ethnic origin, and is in the order of 10–20%. The impact of any treatment strategy must be compared with this background rate. Successful eradication of HBV infection requires effective immune-mediated clearance of infected hepatocytes and cessation of viral replication before end-stage disease, i.e. cirrhosis, has occurred. To date, treatment is rarely completely successful because of side effects, poor efficacy, and viral resistance. There are two main strategies for treating chronic HBV infection:

- Immune-modulatory therapy—e.g., interferon
- Antiviral agents—e.g., lamivudine

The decision to treat and the type of treatment require consideration of:

- Host/disease factors:
  —ALT level
  —Histological activity and severity
  —Comorbidity/coinfection
  —Route of acquisition
  —Ethnic origin
  —Gender
- Viral factors:
  —Serological markers: presence/absence of HBeAg
  —HBV DNA level
  —Genotype
- Treatment factors:
  —Likelihood of response
  —Durability of response
  —Treatment-associated side effects
  —Previous treatment

Immune-modulatory therapy

Interferon alpha (IFN-α) is the treatment of which there has been the most experience. The mode of action is to augment the preexisting host immune response by:

- Stimulating lymphocyte proliferation
- Increasing major histocompatibility complex (MHC) antigen expression and thus T-cell recognition
- Increasing natural killer cell activity

IFN has an antiviral effect by degrading viral mRNA and inhibiting viral protein synthesis, and also protects non-infected cells from viral invasion.

A meta-analysis of studies of IFN-α in adults reported 33% eAg clearance in comparison with 12% in controls.[40] Improved tolerability of interferon may be achieved by pegylated interferon: the conjugation of the polyethylene glycol molecule (PEG) with interferon alpha leads to reduced clearance, thereby reducing the injection frequency from thrice to once weekly. Pegylated interferon has similar efficacy to conventional interferon and has superseded its role.

In children, the response rates to IFN-α therapy are very variable, but not dissimilar to those reported in adult studies. Differences in the response rates depend on the route of acquisition, ethnic origin, disease activity, and the treatment regimen. Sustained clearance varies between 0% and 50% of those treated, and is usually around twice that of untreated controls.[41]

Predictors of IFN responsiveness include:

- Active histology
- Low HBV DNA levels
- Elevated serum aminotransferase enzymes (more than twice the upper limit of normal)
- Short duration of the disease
- Non-Oriental ethnic origin
- Horizontal transmission

Interferon therapy is therefore unlikely to be of benefit in children with perinatally acquired infection who have normal or minimally elevated aminotransferase enzymes.

Limitations of interferon therapy. In addition to its limited efficacy, interferon is limited by its adverse profile of side effects, although children tolerate the treatment better than adults. Fever and flu-like symptoms are invariable during initiation of treatment, and bone-marrow suppression is common. Autoimmune thyroid disease and alopecia are frequent, and mental disturbance, including severe depression, may occur. Furthermore, interferon treatment is potentially hazardous in patients with cirrhosis, as a flare of immune activity with increased immune damage occurs prior to seroconversion, which may lead to decompensation of liver function.

Steroid priming prior to interferon treatment. The transient rise in transaminases that occurs during treatment is associated with increased likelihood of HBeAg clearance. Pretreatment with corticosteroids ("priming") and their withdrawal prior to commencing IFN-α may exacerbate the host immune response, facilitating seroconversion. In a study of the long-term effects of IFN treatment with a 5-year follow-up, those who had received steroid priming had a significantly higher chance of seroconversion, with almost 50% becoming eAg-negative and HBV DNA–negative.[42] However, the benefit remains unproven[43,44] and is associated with a risk of precipitating fulminant liver failure.

Antiviral agents

Antiviral agents directed predominantly against viral replication include nucleoside or nucleotide analogs. These are usually phosphorylated within infected cells to their active form, and are effective by incorporation into viral DNA, leading to inhibition of viral replication. The drug must be selective for viral DNA to minimize toxicity; the safety of early agents being evaluated was limited by their effects on mitochondrial DNA. Approved therapies for adults are lamivudine, adefovir dipivoxil, entecavir, and telbivudine.[45] Of these, only lamiviudine and adefovir have been evaluated in clinical studies in children.

Lamivudine

Lamivudine is a pyrimidine nucleoside analog. It prevents replication of HBV in infected hepatocytes; it is incorporated into viral DNA, leading to chain termination, and competitively inhibits viral reverse transcriptase. In adult studies, significant histological improvement following lamivudine therapy, with resolution or reduced progression of fibrosis, has been demonstrated.[46] In three large placebo-controlled trials in adults,[47–49] histological improvement occurred in 52–56% of treated patients in comparison with 23–25% in controls. Loss of HBeAg after 1 year of treatment occurred in 17–33% of those receiving lamivudine in comparison with 11–13% of those receiving the placebo, with loss of detectable DNA in 40–44%. As with IFN, response rates are related to low pretreatment serum HBV DNA levels and raised aminotransferase enzymes. Chien *et al.* report 65% seroconversion after 52 weeks' treatment in those with ALT over five times the upper limit of normal, in comparison with 38% of those with ALT only over twice the upper limit of normal.[50] However, there does not appear to be any variation in the response relative to ethnic origin or the duration of infection, and it is safe to use lamivudine in patients with cirrhosis, as an immune-mediated flare does not occur. Prolongation of treatment for up to 3 years may improve the seroconversion rate, but it increases resistance.

Limitations of lamivudine. Relapse. Unfortunately, rebound to pretreatment levels is almost invariable after cessation of therapy. The ccc intermediate of HBV DNA is stable and persists during treatment; the formation of cccDNA may be dependent on cellular rather than viral polymerase, and thus is not inhibited by lamivudine.[51,52] Furthermore, elimination of the infected cells remains dependent on T-cell–mediated lysis: in the absence of effective clearance, infection may persist for many years due to the long half-life of infected cells.[53]

Resistance. HBV may acquire resistance to lamivudine due to a specific HBV mutation (tyrosine–methionine–aspartate–aspartate or YMDD mutation) in the polymerase gene.[54] The mutant virus has an altered tertiary structure that reduces the ability of lamivudine, rather than viral nucleoside, to be incorporated. The YMDD variant emerges in 15–20% after 1 year of treatment and increases with time. Due to the survival advantage of the wild type due to more effective replication, the mutant virus may revert to the wild type after lamivudine therapy is withdrawn.

Experience with lamivudine in children. A preliminary dose-ranging study of lamivudine in children demonstrated that it is well tolerated, with a dose of 3 mg/kg/day (maximum 100 mg) providing levels of exposure and trough concentrations similar to those in adults receiving 100 mg.[55] A subsequent international randomized, double-blind, placebo-controlled trial in 286 children with chronic HBV showed a complete response (HBeAg clearance and undetectable HBV DNA after 52 weeks' treatment) in 23% in comparison with 13% with the placebo.[56] In those with ALT over twice the upper limit of normal, the response rates were 34% and 16%, respectively. The YMDD variant emerged in 18%. This study confirmed the safety of lamivudine and its superiority in comparison with placebo, but also highlighted its limited efficacy and the problem of resistance. Although prolonging the treatment from 1 year to 3 years led to an improved viral response, the prevalence of YMDD mutations also increased to 64%, limiting the efficacy.[57]

Adefovir dipivoxil

Adefovir is a purine analog. In addition to inhibition of viral replication, it may also augment natural killer cell activity and endogenous interferon activity.[58] Furthermore, HBV strains resistant to lamivudine may be susceptible to adefovir.[59] In adult studies, loss of HBeAg occurs in 24% (11% placebo) after 48 weeks' treatment, with seroconversion rates increasing with increased duration of treatment. Although resistance is uncommon after 1 year, a 30% resistance rate at 5 years has been described.[45] In a trial of adefovir in children, it proved to be well tolerated, with 20% of 12–18-year-olds after 1 year achieving HBV DNA < 1000 copies and normal ALT in comparison with 0% with the placebo.[60] In younger children, however, there was no statistically significant benefit over placebo, although there was a significant fall in HBV DNA.

Other antivirals

Entecavir is a nucleoside analog of 2′-deoxyguanosine. It has been shown to be superior in efficacy to lamivudine,[61] with similar tolerability. Resistance after 3 years is very low in adults. A multicenter clinical trial is planned in children.[62] Although telbivudine has similar efficacy to adefovir, its use may be limited by resistance. There are currently no studies in children. Antivirals under evaluation include tenofovir (structurally similar to adefovir) and emtricitabine (structurally similar to lamivudine). Both are currently approved for use in human immunodeficiency virus (HIV) infection.

Combination strategies

To date, there has been no consistent evidence of an additive or synergistic antiviral activity when antiviral drugs with a common target (HBV polymerase), such as lamivudine and adefovir, are used in combination.[45] There is some evidence to support the use of lamivudine/interferon combination therapy, with improved HBeAg clearance in comparison with monotherapy.[63,64] In a pilot study of lamivudine and interferon alpha in children, many of whom were immunotolerant with normal ALT, 78% became HBV DNA–negative at the end of treatment and 17% achieved complete viral control (HBsAg-negative).[65]

Recommendations for children

In all children with HBV infection, the role of treatment should be considered.

Treatment should be considered for those with persistent infection without HBeAg seroconversion. Treatment is more likely to be successful during the immune clearance phase, or if there is significant hepatic inflammation with elevated ALT and HBV DNA positivity. IFN is the only currently licensed treatment, although lamivudine is licensed for children over the age of 12 years. The consensus recommendations for interferon, based on short-term efficacy, are as follows:[66]

- The rationale for treatment is to accelerate HBeAg clearance in a subgroup of patients.
- Candidates for treatment are children with HBeAg and HBV DNA positivity, with low to intermediate HBV DNA levels and abnormal aminotransferase enzymes, aged 2 years or more.
- IFN is contraindicated in children with decompensated liver disease, cytopenia, severe renal or cardiac disorders, and autoimmune disease.
- The standard treatment regimen is 5 mU/m^2 thrice weekly for 6 months. Repeat treatment in nonresponders is not indicated.

It should be noted, however, that pegylated interferon is likely to replace standard interferon in future recommendations for children.

Lamivudine also merits consideration. With similar efficacy, oral administration, and better tolerability than interferon, it has significant advantages, which are counterbalanced by the problem of resistance. It also has a role in treating those with contraindications to interferon, such as cirrhosis or severe renal impairment.

Other treatment strategies

Hepatitis B in the immunosuppressed patient. Patients coinfected with HBV and HIV, organ transplant recipients, and chronic carriers requiring chemotherapy—for example, for hematological malignancies—present a problem. Immunodeficiency potentiates HBV replication, with increased serum levels of HBV DNA and HBeAg. Although there may be no clinical manifestations other than a rise in ALT, it may lead to acute hepatitis and fulminant hepatic failure. Furthermore, if immunosuppressive therapy is withdrawn, the return in immune function may lead to rapid destruction of infected hepatocytes, acute hepatitis, and liver failure. Lamivudine has been shown to be effective in ameliorating these effects,[41] both with preemptive treatment[67,68] and in the treatment of acute or fulminant hepatitis in this setting.[69,70] Lamivudine may also have a role in the treatment of hepatitis B–associated nephrotic syndrome.

Liver transplantation. Indications for liver transplantation are considered in Chapter 21. Chronic HBV-related disease is an infrequent indication for transplantation in children. Although transplantation transiently reduces the viral titer in the circulation, persistence of HBV in extrahepatic sites leads to reinfection of the graft,[71] and treatment with anti-HBV human immunoglobulin (HBIG) and lamivudine after transplantation is required.[72] In fulminant HBV infection, HBV replication appears to be interrupted, and recurrence after transplantation is infrequent.[73]

Further developments. These will include evaluation of combination strategies and long-term data regarding the outcome of current therapies. Strategies involving gene therapy are being developed in animal models. These include interferon gene transfer to control HBV replication in mice, RNA interference strategies to degrade viral replication intermediates, and the vector transfer of viral genes combined with immunostimulatory genes, promoting an antiviral immune response.[74]

Prevention of HBV infection

Strategies to prevent HBV transmission include:

- Strategies aimed at minimizing spread from carriers:
  —Health education of high-risk populations
  —Specific advice to identified carriers
  —Screening of blood/organ donors
  —Screening personnel in occupations at high risk of transmission
- Strategies aimed at conferring immunity in those at risk, including vaccination of:
  —Health-care workers
  —Family members and sexual partners of identified carriers
  —Infants born to carrier mothers
  —All infants
  —Adolescents
  —Intravenous drug users
  —Active homosexuals

Hepatitis B vaccines are inactivated, and contain HBsAg prepared by recombinant DNA techniques. The recombinant protein is absorbed onto an adjuvant (aluminum hydroxide). The schedule of vaccination consists of three doses. Effective immunization is defined as the development of a protective antibody level above 100 IU/L. Poor responders (10–100 IU/L) should receive a booster dose, and nonresponders (< 10 IU/L) should be revaccinated. The duration of protective levels is dependent on the anti-HBs titer achieved by immunization. The rate of disappearance of protective antibody has been studied in a large cohort of children vaccinated in infancy following the implementation of universal HBV vaccination in Taiwan.[75] Protective levels waned at a rate of approximately 10% per year, with a rise in anti-HBs titer occurring following a booster dose. Similar findings were reported in the UK.[76]

Prevention of perinatal transmission

HBV transmission to the newborn may be successfully prevented by immunization, with an effective response to vaccine in up to 97% of newborn infants. Strategies for preventing perinatal transmission include *immunization of at-risk infants,* identified either by selective screening of

Table 6.7 Current United Kingdom recommendations for immunization against hepatitis B virus in neonates.[26]

Maternal status			HBIG	HBV vaccine
HBsAg	HBeAg	anti-HBe		
+	+	–	Yes	Yes
+	–	–	Yes	Yes
+	Not determined		Yes	Yes
+	–	+	No	Yes
Acute HBV during pregnancy			Yes	Yes

Anti-HBe, antibody to e antigen; HBeAg, nonstructural e antigen; HBsAg, surface antigen; HBIG, hepatitis B immunoglobulin HBV, hepatitis B virus.

at-risk women or by universal screening of all women during pregnancy; or *universal immunization of all infants*.

Immunization of at-risk infants. Comparison of selective versus universal screening of women in Britain revealed that selective screening failed to identify about half of the women with babies at risk,[77] and in 1995 less than one-third of pregnancies occurred in districts with a universal screening policy.[78] Since April 2000, all women in England and Wales have been screened during pregnancy. Current immunization recommendations, according to maternal serological status, are shown in Table 6.7. In a systematic review of hepatitis B prevention strategies, 29 randomized clinical trials were identified, five of which were considered to be of high quality. This review reported evidence that hepatitis B vaccine, hepatitis B immunoglobulin, and vaccine plus immunoglobulin prevented hepatitis B occurrence in newborn infants of mothers positive for HBsAg and HBeAg. The combination of HBIG and vaccine provided more protection in comparison with vaccine alone. There is insufficient evidence to support or refute the use of hepatitis B vaccine with HBIG in babies of mothers who are HBsAg-positive but HBeAg-negative. In countries in which HBIG can be easily and safely resourced, a combination of HBIG and vaccine at birth with a further two or three doses of vaccine later provides optimal protection, irrespective of maternal status. However, a vaccine-alone protocol starting at birth was almost as effective as the combination and may be more appropriate for countries with high endemicity.[79]

As vaccination strategies have become more effective, the rate of perinatally acquired infection has fallen. Sadly, children still become infected perinatally from failed vaccination, either because of a poor response (5%) or because of failure to administer the program correctly.

Universal immunization. In 1992, an assembly of the World Health Organization recommended that all countries should integrate hepatitis B vaccination into their national immunization programs by 1997. Economic and epidemiological evaluation suggested that this was cost-effective even in countries with low HBV endemicity (i.e., with less than 2% of the population being carriers). Furthermore, in 1994 a target of reducing the incidence of new carrier children by 80% by the year 2001 was set. There is already evidence of the success of universal HBV vaccination. Since its introduction in Taiwan in 1984, the incidence of hepatocellular carcinoma in children has declined from an average annual rate of 0.7 to 0.36 per 100 000,[80] with a decreased carrier rate in15-year-olds[80] (see Chapter 23).

Prevention of horizontal transmission

Children with chronic HBV infection are at risk of social isolation and stigmatization if inappropriate guidance is given to their families, carers, health workers, and other professionals. There is no obligation for parents to inform schools and nurseries of their child's HBV status; the same precautions should apply in dealing with blood/body fluid spillage of all children. Staff at schools and other institutions, as well as health-care workers, should adhere to the Universal Infection Control Precautions,[81] which recommend:

- Treating all blood and body fluids as potential sources of infection
- Wearing protective clothing when dealing with body fluids
- Using good hand hygiene
- Covering any broken skin
- Using and disposing of sharps appropriately
- Disinfecting body fluid spillages correctly
- Disposing of waste and excreta carefully

During hospital admission, children with HBV infection do not need to be nursed in isolation. At home and in school, children's social and sporting activities should not be restricted on account of their HBV status. Immunization should be offered to all nonimmune family members.

Immunization of adolescents. In low-endemicity populations, acute HBV is related to high-risk sexual behavior or intravenous drug use. Pilot studies indicate that vaccination of adolescents at school may be an effective strategy.[82] It has also been shown that teenagers may maintain protective antibody levels longer than those vaccinated during infancy.[83–86]

Hepatitis C virus

Hepatitis C virus (HCV) infection emerged as the major cause of transfusion-acquired non-A, non-B hepatitis when it was first characterized in the 1980s. It is now known to be a major cause of chronic liver disease and a risk factor for hepatocellular carcinoma.

In children, HCV infection is prevalent in recipients of infected blood products—particularly in those with hemophilia, leukemia, and thalassemia. Since 1990, strategies for virtually eliminating HCV-infected blood have been successful. Parenteral acquisition remains a risk worldwide, especially in countries that do not have effective screening policies. Currently, most new cases of HCV infection in childhood are due to vertical transmission from infected mothers, as demonstrated in the UK and Italy.[87,88]

Recognition of HCV as a major health burden and improved antiviral therapy have changed the emphasis from treating those with advanced disease to the promotion of HCV awareness, encouraging testing of at-risk populations in order to facilitate earlier management and treatment.

Epidemiology and transmission

The worldwide prevalence of chronic HCV infection is estimated at 3%, with 150 million people being chronic HCV carriers. The prevalence varies considerably between different populations, and is higher in eastern and southern Europe than in the north and west. The estimated prevalence in England and Wales is 0.4%, with rates varying from 0.04% in blood donors to 50% in intravenous drug users.[89]

Prior to the introduction of HCV antibody (anti-HCV) screening of blood products and organ donors in 1990, HCV accounted for up to 90% of transfusion-associated hepatitis. Parenteral transmission is so effective that almost every individual receiving a blood transfusion or solid organ from an anti-HCV–positive donor was likely to become infected.[90,91] The risk of parenteral acquisition of HCV infection was increased in children exposed to multiple donors, either by receiving multiple blood transfusions or by repeated infusion of pooled products. In children with hemophilia, anti-HCV seroprevalence ranged from 50% to 82%.[92] This route of acquisition should now have been eliminated by appropriate screening of blood products and health-care procedures.

Other routes of transmission include parenteral transmission in intravenous drug users, sexual transmission, nosocomial spread, and vertical transmission. At least 50% of the infected population has no identifiable risk factor.

Vertical transmission

In contrast to hepatitis B, vertical transmission of HCV from an infected mother is infrequent, occurring in only 5–10% of deliveries. The seroprevalence of HCV infection in pregnant women in the UK is estimated to be 0.2%, with an estimated 1150 pregnancies occurring each year in women infected with HCV and 70 infants acquiring infection.[93] The risk of transmission is increased by coexistent maternal HIV infection and high maternal HCV RNA titers. In a systematic review of 77 studies published between 1992 and 2000, the rate of vertical transmission was 22.1% in women with HIV coinfection and 4.3% in those without.[94] In a European study of 1474 HCV-infected women, the rates of transmission with and without HIV were 13.9% and 6.6%, respectively.[95]

In a study of infants born in the UK and Ireland, the vertical transmission rate was 6.7% overall, and 3.8 times higher in HIV-coinfected than in HIV-negative women.[96]

Infection may occur in utero[97] or at the time of delivery.[96] Other factors, such as placental breakdown and birth order, may also be important, as discordant outcomes in twin pregnancies have been observed.[98] There is conflicting evidence regarding the benefit of delivery by cesarean section in reducing transmission risk in both HIV-infected and noninfected mothers.[96,97,99–101]

There is also currently insufficient evidence to discourage breastfeeding, as there is little evidence of an increased risk of transmission, despite HCV RNA being frequently detectable in colostrum.[102]

Molecular virology

HCV is a positive-sense single-stranded RNA virus with a genome structure similar to that of the Flaviviridae and is now classed as a genus within the Flavivirus family. The genome is about 9500 nucleotides in length and codes for 10 proteins—two core (C and p7) and two envelope proteins (E1 and E2) and six nonstructural proteins (NS2, NS3, NS4A, NS4 B, NS5A, NS5B), with a wide variety of enzymic functions. The virus particle is enveloped and is about 45–65 nm in diameter, although there are very few published electron micrographs of the virus. The free genomic RNA is infectious in cultured chimpanzee hepatocytes. The virus can be grouped into a range of genotypes, based on sequencing, with distinct geographical distributions (Table 6.8) and prognoses.

Replication and pathogenesis

The E2 glycoprotein binds to the CD81 receptor molecule, which is found on a variety of cell types, including hepatocytes and B cells, which explains some of the extrahepatic pathologies of hepatitis C. The virus has a single open reading frame coding for a polyprotein, which is subsequently cleaved into at least 10 polypeptides. The structural glycoproteins E1 and E2 are processed in the endoplasmic reticulum, and E2 is cleaved to produce p7, a fusion protein. The nonstructural proteins have a variety of molecular functions

Table 6.8 Geographical distribution of hepatitis C virus genotypes.

Genotype	Geographical distribution
1 (a, b, c, d, e, f)	America, Europe, Africa
2 (a, b, c, d, e, f, g, h)	Europe, south-east Asia
3 (a, b, c, d, e, f, g)	Worldwide, south Asia, south-east Asia
4 (a, b, c, d, e, f, g, h)	Egypt, Central Africa, Middle East
5	South Africa
6 (a, b)	Far East
7 (a, b, c, d)	South-east Asia
8, 9, 10, 11	South-east Asia

involved in the replication of the genome, including RNA-dependent RNA polymerase (NS5B), helicase (NS3 NTPase/helicase), protease (NS3/NS4A), and cleavage (NS2). The protease NS3 may be a promising target for new antiviral agents in the treatment of hepatitis C.[103]

Pathophysiology

There is no evidence that the virus has a direct cytopathic effect on the liver cell, and there is no direct correlation between the level of viremia and the level of liver damage. Immune-mediated damage, as with hepatitis B, is thought to be important. Cytotoxic T cells (CD8) levels rise with elevations in liver damage (observed through raised liver enzymes). Despite active T-cell responses, the virus is not easily cleared from the liver and the resulting chronicity is higher than with hepatitis B. The production of neutralizing antibody to the hepatitis C structural proteins (E1 and E2) is a late event in the natural history of acute hepatitis C. During the evolution of infection, many quasi-species are produced, and these may contribute to making the clearance of infection difficult.

Laboratory diagnosis

Serological assays

Serological assays are available for antibody to hepatitis C (anti-HCV) and hepatitis C core antigen. Although IgM antibody assays were developed, they failed to find a useful diagnostic role. Anti-HCV is produced a few months after the patient develops viremia, and so is invariably negative in the acute phase of infection. Furthermore, the value of antibody testing alone is limited by the following:

- Anti-HCV may persist for many years after clearance of viremia and resolution of infection.
- Anti-HCV may be absent in patients with HCV infection who are immunocompromised.
- Maternal anti-HCV may persist in the newborn for up to 18 months (see below).

A variety of serological assays for HCV core antigen have been produced; some measure "free" antigen and include an antigen/antibody dissociation step, while others measure both antigen and antibody in the same assay (combination assays). The former can be quantitative and correlate well with assays for RNA, but with a lower sensitivity; the latter can be used as a screening assay to increase the sensitivity for incident infections.

Molecular testing for HCV RNA

Molecular testing for HCV RNA by PCR has several uses. It is valuable in making the diagnosis before anti-HCV has become detectable (the window period), either during the first few months of infection or in screening blood donations, and also in testing those who are exposed to infection with hepatitis C–positive material (e.g., inoculation accidents or infants of HCV positive mothers). Following perinatal transmission, HCV RNA may not reach detectable levels for up to 3 months, so testing should be deferred. It is also useful for monitoring the response to antiviral therapy.

An algorithm to guide diagnosis in infants and older children is outlined in Figure 6.5.[104]

Clinical presentation and monitoring

The incubation period ranges from 6 to 12 weeks. Signs and symptoms are usually absent, but when they occur they include fever, malaise, nausea, abdominal discomfort, and jaundice.

Chronic infection is usually asymptomatic for decades, or may be accompanied by fatigue. Of 606 children with chronic HCV infection, only 8% had symptoms or signs, which included anorexia, weight loss, abdominal pain, hepatomegaly and splenomegaly.[87]

Aggressive disease with progression to cirrhosis and end-stage liver disease has been described in childhood[105] but is uncommon, as the complications of cirrhosis rarely develop within 10–15 years.

A diagnosis of HCV infection should be suspected in the following clinical settings:

- Unexplained elevation of aminotransferase enzymes
- Acute hepatitic illness
- Unexplained chronic liver disease
- Children born to infected mothers
- Children exposed to potentially infected blood products or contaminated equipment
- Children offered for adoption, particularly from endemic areas

The diagnosis should be accompanied by careful consideration of the factors that may influence the natural history, prognosis, decision to treat, and likely therapeutic response:

- Mode of acquisition
- Duration of infection
- Coinfection with HIV/HBV
- Underlying disease (thalassemia, leukemia, etc.)
- Associated extrahepatic manifestations
- Complications of chronic liver disease

Histology

Histological features of chronic HCV infection are not pathognomonic, and may resemble autoimmune hepatitis (Figure 6.6). The most characteristic features are mild portal tract inflammation with lymphoid aggregates, inflammatory bile duct damage, and mild steatosis. Episodes of increased inflammatory activity are associated with piecemeal necrosis and fibrosis is variable. Viral proteins may be detected by immunohistochemical stains.[106] A giant-cell hepatitis in association with HCV infection has been described.[107] The histological severity is considered under natural history (below).

Natural history

The majority of adults and children with HCV infection do not

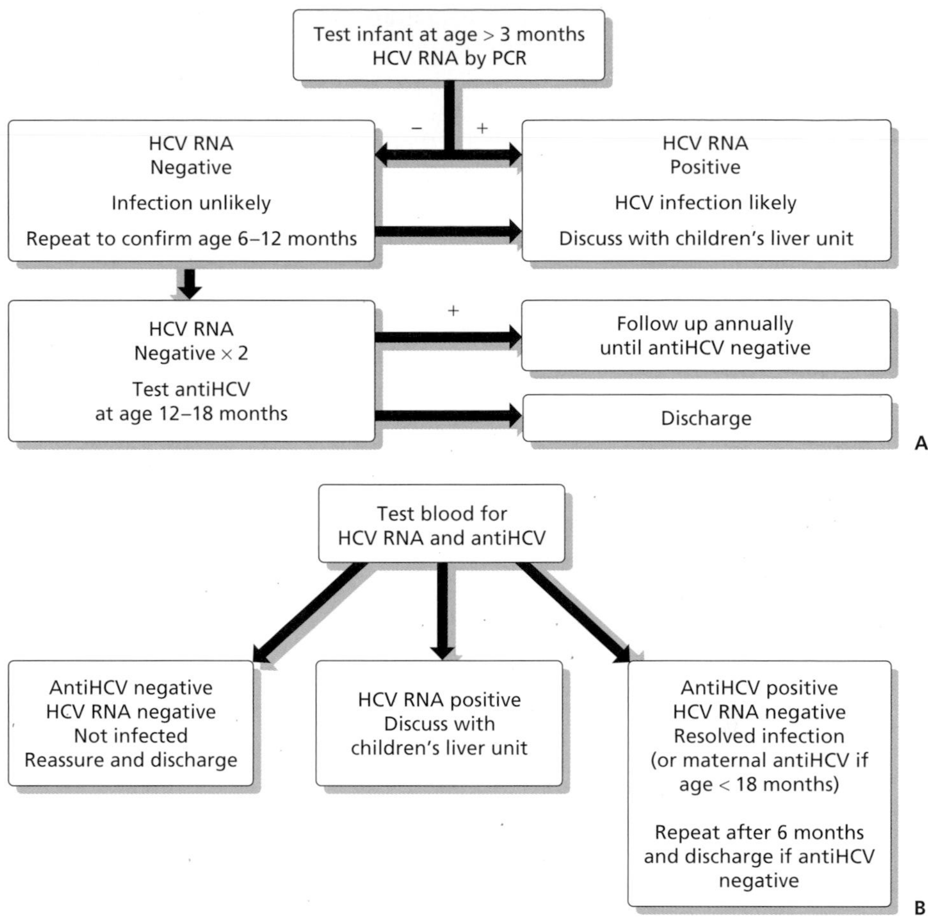

Figure 6.5 Algorithm for the diagnosis of hepatitis C virus (HCV) infection in **A** infants at risk of perinatal infection. **B** child age 12 months or older.

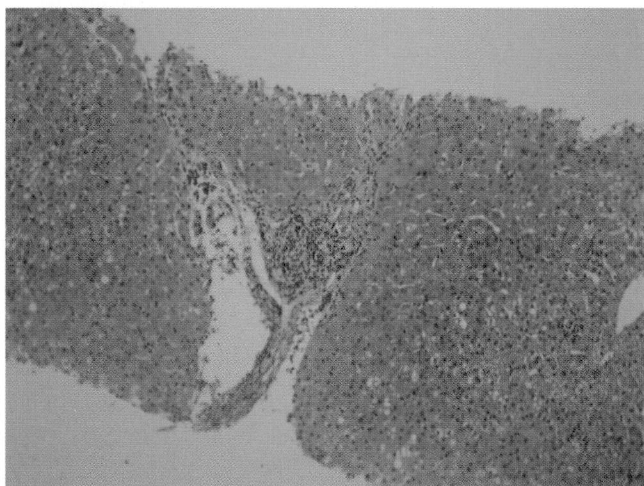

Figure 6.6 Chronic hepatitis C has a mild inflammatory infiltrate in the portal tract. Fatty change with glycogenated nuclei and cytoplasmic eosinophilia is characteristic.

have effective immune clearance and become chronically infected. The severity of disease and/or rate of progression are adversely affected by:

- Age > 40 years at acquisition
- Duration of infection
- Comorbidity (alcohol, coinfection with HBV/HIV, immunodeficiency, iron overload

The natural history can be studied by monitoring several different parameters:

- Persistence/clearance of HCV RNA
- Clinical/laboratory abnormalities
- Histological progression
- Morbidity/mortality

These parameters do not always correlate. For example, in the absence of cirrhosis, chronic HCV infection in adults may cause a significant reduction in the quality of life.[108] However, the presence of severe histological disease may not be accompanied by clinical symptoms or biochemical evidence of inflammation.

The natural history may also be influenced according to the route of acquisition and comorbidity. For transfusion-acquired HCV, a UK National Register has provided a resource for further study of the natural history.[109] After a mean duration of infection of 11 years (range 8–20 years) in 924 people, including children, 37% had abnormal liver enzymes, but only 14% had signs or symptoms. Of the 363 who underwent biopsy, 10% had cirrhosis.[110] Other populations may have a more favorable outcome: of 1980 women acquiring HCV from anti-D immunoglobulin, only

46% remained HCV RNA positive after 25 years and only 0.5% developed cirrhosis.[111]

Natural history in childhood

Studies of the outcome following HCV infection acquired in childhood are currently limited by the heterogeneity of the populations included, the route of acquisition, the presence of coexisting disease, and also by the limited number of children with histological assessment. There are conflicting opinions as to whether this is a benign and more slowly progressive disease than in adults, or one in which significant progression frequently occurs early but insidiously.

HCV RNA persistence. Spontaneous resolution is defined by sustained disappearance of HCV RNA from the serum. In children, this appears to be infrequent, occurring overall in 5–10% of those infected.[112–114] The rates of clearance in individual small studies confined to specific populations are more optimistic, with long-term clearance rates of up to 50% reported both after vertical infection and after neonatal blood transfusion. In a large study of 266 infants with vertical infection, 20% became HCV RNA–negative.[115]

Histology. The minority of children with HCV infection have been evaluated by liver biopsy, and it is likely that they represent those with clinical evidence of active inflammation or more severe disease. The reported high prevalence of histological disease may therefore overemphasize the actual spectrum of severity. Most studies suggest that children with chronic HCV infection have histological features of mild to moderate inflammation. In a study of histology 20 years after transfusion-acquired HCV infection, most had only minimal inflammation, and those with significant fibrosis or cirrhosis had a coexisting disease.[116] Similarly, after transfusion-related HCV infection in neonates, most had mild histological disease after long follow-up periods of 35 years, with none having cirrhosis.[117]

In a study examining histological progression in nine children who underwent two sequential biopsies, progression of fibrosis occurred in five over a median period of 2.8 years. The predicted median time to cirrhosis was estimated as 17.14 years.[118] However, progression of fibrosis is not linear and it is thus not a reliable prognostic indicator.[119] Factors influencing the prevalence of significant fibrosis include age and the duration of infection and comorbidity.[96,120,121] Severe fibrosis is unusual in infection of less than 10 years' duration.[119]

Clinical progression. Chronic HCV infection in infancy and childhood is usually asymptomatic, although nonspecific symptoms or mild hepatomegaly may be apparent. Most vertically infected infants will have raised aminotransferase enzymes, particularly in the first few years of life, which do not correlate with clinical severity. Although rare, rapid progression to cirrhosis may occur, and decompensated cirrhosis has been reported in three children with vertically acquired infection,[105] all of whom required liver transplantation.

Extrahepatic disorders

HCV infection appears to be strongly associated with autoimmune disorders, including essential mixed cryoglobulinemia, membranoproliferative glomerulonephritis (with HCV probably having a direct pathogenic role), and also porphyria cutanea tarda. There is also a suggested association with autoimmune thyroiditis. Signs and symptoms of these disorders should be sought in patients with chronic HCV infection.[122] Although HCV infection may precipitate anti-liver-kidney microsomal antibody-1 (LKM-1)–positive chronic hepatitis (type 2b), this appears to be uncommon in children.

Management

Children with HCV infection should be seen at intervals of 6–12 months. Outpatient review should include an assessment of:
- Clinical signs and symptoms
- Disease progression/resolution (liver function tests, HCV RNA, α-fetoprotein, ultrasound)
- Comorbidity
- Timing of treatment

A liver biopsy is helpful in assessing the severity of histological disease, which may influence the decision to treat or continue "watchful waiting."

Regular follow-up should also provide an opportunity to counsel families regarding the risk of transmission and treatment options.

All children with HCV should undergo vaccination against HAV and HBV, to reduce the risk of coinfection.

Treatment

The aims and benefits of treatment are:
- Eradication of HCV infection (loss of HCV RNA in peripheral blood)
- Reduction of hepatic inflammatory damage and progression of fibrosis
- Reduction of the risk of complications of cirrhosis, including hepatocellular carcinoma
- Normalization of liver function
- Improved quality of life
- Reduced transmission risk

However, the decision to treat will depend on the genotype, the balance between efficacy and treatment side effects, and the family's individual circumstances.

Current treatment options are with pegylated interferon in combination with ribavirin.

Interferon

See above (under HBV treatment) for the mode of action of interferon.

Interferon monotherapy was the first established treatment for hepatitis C. Studies in children have shown similar efficacy to that seen in adults. A meta-analysis of 19 trials of IFN-α for children with HCV infection examined the effect of treatment in 366 children in comparison with 105 untreated controls.[123] A response to treatment occurred in a mean of 54% (range 0–91%), with a sustained response in 36% (0–73%). Genotype 1 adversely affected the likelihood of response, with a sustained response in 27% of children, in comparison with 70% in those with other genotypes. The spontaneous clearance rate in untreated children was 5%. Treatment regimens varied, with the duration of therapy ranging from 6 to 18 months. Most studies used 3 MU/m^2 by subcutaneous injection three times weekly, although higher and lower doses were also used.

PEG interferon. The covalent attachment of a polyethylene glycol (PEG) moiety to IFN-α enhances its half-life and removes its immunogenicity.[124] This has similar side effects, but the efficacy is enhanced and the treatment has the benefit of once-weekly rather than thrice-weekly injections. It has superseded interferon in combination therapy regimens. It is undergoing trials as monotherapy in children and has a potential role in those in whom ribavirin is contraindicated. Pilot studies are encouraging.[125]

Combination therapy

The addition of ribavirin has improved the response rates in comparison with interferon monotherapy. Ribavirin is a guanosine nucleoside analog, which although ineffective as monotherapy[126] appears to have synergy with IFN-α. Its mode of action is uncertain, but may include enhancement of T-cell–mediated immunity and direct inhibition of viral polymerase. As in adults, studies of combination therapy in children support its efficacy in achieving sustained HCV RNA clearance (sustained viral response, SVR) and improved likelihood of a response in comparison with IFN-α alone.[127–132]

Combination therapy with ribavirin and pegylated interferon is now the recommended treatment for adults.[133] The duration is 6 months' initial treatment, with a further 24 weeks in patients with genotype 1 if an initial response (clearance of HCV RNA) occurs. The likelihood of SVR is highest in genotypes 2 and 3 (76%) and lower in genotype 1 (46%).[134] In a pilot study in children, the response rates were 100% with genotype 2 and 3 and 53% with genotype 1.[135] A multicenter pediatric study of pegylated interferon and ribavirin is in progress.

Treatment side effects

Contraindications must be carefully considered prior to starting treatment.

Side effects of interferon or pegylated interferon are common—particularly flu-like symptoms, fatigue, and neutropenia. Alopecia, pruritus, rash, and gastrointestinal disturbances (diarrhea, anorexia, nausea, and abdominal pain) leading to weight loss may also occur. Mood disturbances, including irritability, insomnia, and somnolence can occur. More severe side effects, including depression and suicidal ideation, are more common in those with preexisting mood disturbances or those receiving treatment during adolescence. Abnormalities of thyroid function and reversible hypothyroidism also occur.

Ribavirin is teratogenic. A reversible hemolytic anemia is the most common side effect of treatment, due to the accumulation of phosphorylated ribavirin in erythrocytes, which shortens their lifespan.

Up to 74% of adults experience a drop in hemoglobin of 2 g/dL, but falling to less than 10 g/dL in only 10%. In children with normal bone-marrow function, there is a rapid reticulocyte response within 12 weeks, and hemoglobin returns to normal. Ribavirin and pegylated interferon should be used cautiously in children with previous aplastic anemia or thalassemia.[136]

All of these side effects are less prominent in younger children, who tolerate the combination therapy well.

Who to treat

The recommendations have been modified over the years, reflecting improved tolerability and efficacy of treatment and the recognition that earlier, less severe, disease may respond better. Treatment is no longer restricted to adults with biopsy-proven moderate or severe disease; those with mild hepatitis should also be considered for treatment. Factors in adult studies that increase the likelihood of a response include:

- Genotype other than 1
- Baseline viral load < 3.5 million copies/mL
- Minimal histological disease
- Female gender
- Age < 40 years

All children over the age of three should be considered for treatment, as they tolerate treatment better than adults and may have better response rates in view of milder disease. Furthermore, treatment with interferon-based strategies may be cost-effective in comparison with no treatment.[137] As side effects may be troublesome, especially during adolescence, the timing of treatment should take into account both age and the stage of schooling, avoiding stressful times. If treatment is deferred, monitoring of the disease should continue in order to identify those with histological progression that would further influence the decision to treat.

HCV and thalassemia

Children with HCV and thalassemia are more likely to develop progressive liver disease, due to the coexistence of hepatic iron overload. Significant fibrosis and cirrhosis are more common at an earlier age.

Treatment with pegylated interferon and ribavirin appears to have similar efficacy to that in children without thalassemia. However, hemolytic anemia due to ribavirin may increase transfusion requirements. Although this may be tolerated without extra chelation therapy,[138,139] monotherapy with pegylated interferon is an alternative strategy.

Future treatment strategies

Ribavirin analogs such as viramidine are undergoing clinical studies. Viramidine is a prodrug of ribavirin. It is more liver-specific and may reduce the risk of hemolytic anemia.[140] A recombinant protein of interferon alfa 2b genetically fused with albumin is undergoing clinical trials. This may have the advantage of further reducing the frequency of injection.[141]

New drugs in development continue to target both viral replication, through specific inhibition of viral replication enzymes, and modulation of the host immune response by toll-like receptor agonists. Toll-like receptors (TLRs) are expressed by a range of immune cells. After stimulation by a microorganism, they initiate an acute inflammatory response through antimicrobial gene and cytokine induction. Agonists of TLRs are currently undergoing clinical evaluation.[142]

Vaccine prospects

There is currently increasing optimism regarding vaccination for hepatitis C. Recent developments that have facilitated progress include an HCV culture model, which is infectious for chimpanzees. Vaccine efficacy data in chimpanzees indicate that it appears feasible to impede progression to chronic infection.[143–145] Furthermore, characterization of the natural immune response resulting in viral clearance has informed vaccine development. Candidate vaccines are currently undergoing phase 1 and 2 treatment trials.[146]

Future studies

Global priorities for hepatitis C[147] include:

- More detailed natural history studies
- Promotion of public awareness regarding transmission
- Multicenter clinical studies of antiviral therapies
- Guidelines for implementing safe medical practices for health-care workers

Hepatitis D virus

Hepatitis D or delta virus infection (HDV) only occurs in chronic HBV carriers. HDV is a defective RNA virus that can only replicate in the presence of HBsAg. The route of transmission is mainly parenteral, with infection occurring either at the same time or subsequent to HBV acquisition. There is considerable regional variation in HDV infection; environmental and genetic factors, as well as viral genotypes, may have a role. HDV increases the risk of hepatocellular carcinoma and increases the mortality rate in HBV carriers with cirrhosis.[148] In children with hepatitis B, it has been associated with an increased risk of histological deterioration.[149]

Molecular virology

Delta virus is a small RNA virus with a circular single-stranded RNA genome of about 1700 nucleotides which is bound within a delta-specific antigen and coated with HBsAg. The virus is dependent on HBV for its existence. There are three genotypes: type I is found in many parts of the world; type II is restricted to the Far East; and type III was found in South America associated with a severe form of the infection.

Replication and pathogenesis

The viral RNA is replicated by a host RNA polymerase. Delta antigen exists in two forms in the cell—a smaller form, which binds to the genome and is essential for replication; and a larger form, which plays an important part in the self-regulation of its own mRNA synthesis by a feedback mechanism. The virions are coated with both SHBsAg and MHBsAg, including preS1, which is required for the attachment of the virus to hepatocytes.

Pathophysiology

There are two circumstances in which a delta infection can occur:

- *Superinfection*: when an individual with an existing HBV infection is infected with a source that contains both HBV and delta. These circumstances can lead to increased liver damage and fulminant hepatitis.
- *Dual infection*: such infections may present as for acute hepatitis B and may never be recognized as delta infections. There may be a tendency toward more severe illness.

The delta antigen may be cytopathic, but this has been difficult to prove. It may be that the pathology is due to HBV, since dual-infected patients with transplanted livers do not produce symptoms until the HBV reactivates.[150]

Clinical presentation

HDV infection in HBV carriers may:

- Be asymptomatic, with complete resolution of infection
- Lead to acute hepatitis or fulminant hepatic failure
- Develop rapid progression of chronic hepatitis
- Be responsible for persistent low-grade transaminitis

The presence of HDV should be assessed in HBV carriers, particularly during acute exacerbation or clinical progression.

Laboratory diagnosis

A diagnosis of HDV infection is made by detecting HDV antibodies and HBsAg in serum. Serological enzyme immunoassays are available for delta antigen and for immunoglobulin G (IgG) and IgM antibodies. The presence of delta antigen and IgM antibody may indicate an acute or active infection, but a delta-specific RNA assay is the most useful laboratory test for monitoring the treatment response. This is not widely available, and the response to treatment is therefore monitored with biochemical parameters.

Prevention/treatment

The prevention of HBV infection and eradication of chronic HBV carriage will prevent the disease associated with HDV infection. Identification of HBV-infected mothers and immunization of their babies should therefore prevent HDV infection in children. The incidence of acute hepatitis delta virus infection in Italy has markedly decreased, with universal anti-hepatitis B vaccination being an important contributing factor.[151]

Successful treatment of HDV hepatitis with interferon requires high doses (5 million units daily or 9–10 million units three times weekly), with lower doses having no lasting benefit.[152]

Hepatitis E virus

Hepatitis E virus (HEV) infection is a major public health problem in many developing countries. It is the cause of 50% of cases of acute viral hepatitis in young to middle-aged adults in the developing world (see Chapter 23). Although it is less common in children, outbreaks have been described.[153]

The global impact of HEV is now beginning to emerge, as sporadic cases not associated with travel are increasingly reported. HEV infection may be unrecognized if lack of a travel history precludes appropriate diagnostic testing; among 333 patients in south-west England with unexplained hepatitis, 21 were found to have autochthonous HEV.[154]

Molecular virology

HEV is an unenveloped virus about 32–34 nm in diameter with a positive-sense, single-stranded RNA virus genome of about 7200 nucleotides. It was originally classed with the Caliciviruses, but has now been given a separate genus, the Hepeviridae. There are three open reading frames: one codes for the enzymes required to replicate the virus genome open reading frame (ORF1); the second codes for the major capsid protein (ORF2); and the function of the last one (ORF3) has not yet been elucidated. The virus exists in several genotypes, which like the other hepatitis viruses have a distinct geographical distribution (Table 6.9). The recent recognition of indigenous HEV infection in developed countries of genotype 3, closely related to swine strains, has led to increased interest in possible routes of transmission associated with potential zoonoses or through food.

Table 6.9 Geographical distribution of hepatitis E virus genotypes.

Genotype	Geographical distribution
1	Far East, South Asia, Africa
2	Mexico, Africa
3	North America, Europe, and swine strains
4	Swine strains in Far East

Replication and pathogenesis

It is thought that the virus enters through the gut mucosa and migrates to the liver, where the cell receptor has not yet been identified. The virion RNA acts as messenger RNA to produce a polyprotein from the ORF1, which is cleaved to produce the replicative enzymes. This process produces a negative strand, from which more genomic RNA and the mRNA for the structural proteins (ORF2) is produced. The product of ORF3 is thought to serve a regulatory role. Structural proteins and new positive-strand RNA are assembled into new virions, which are released into the bile canaliculi and thereafter into the bile for excretion in the feces.

Prevalence/transmission

HEV is transmitted orofecally, usually by contaminated water. Epidemics most frequently occur in developing countries, particularly after the rainy season, with people aged between 15 and 40 most commonly affected. A striking and unexplained feature is the severity of HEV infection in pregnant women, with a mortality rate as high as 20%. Vertical transmission has been described, with significant perinatal morbidity and mortality[155] (see Chapter 23).

Although sporadic cases were initially linked to travel from endemic areas, increasing reports are now emerging from developed countries of infection occurring without travel as a risk factor. Of 186 cases serologically diagnosed in England and Wales between 1996 and 2003, 31% were not associated with travel. In comparison with travel-acquired infection, these cases were more likely in older patients (> 55 years) infected by genotype 3. The genomic sequences were unique and closely related to those seen in British pigs, supporting the role of pigs as a viral reservoir.[156] More than 80% of pigs in the UK are seropositive for anti-HEV antibody.[157] Other routes of transmission suggested in industrialized countries include exposure to sewage-contaminated water.

Clinical features

HEV infection resembles HAV infection, often with very high hepatic transaminase enzyme levels, and should be considered in the differential diagnosis of acute hepatitis. The incubation period is 2–9 weeks, with symptomatic illness lasting up to 4 weeks. Although it is usually mild and self-limiting, especially in children, fulminant hepatitis, anicteric hepatitis, and prolonged cholestasis have also been observed. Acute hepatitis E complicated by acute pancreatitis[158] in a young adult and precipitating hemolysis in undiagnosed glucose-6-phosphate dehydrogenase deficiency in a child[159] has been described.

Superinfection with HEV in patients with chronic liver disease may cause severe decompensation,[160] but chronic liver disease and persistent viremia due to HEV have not been observed. The frequency of secondary cases in household members is low. Chronic or persistent infection does not occur.

Histological features in sporadic acute hepatitis E include severe intralobular necrosis, polymorphonuclear leukocyte inflammation, and acute cholangitis with numerous neutrophils.[161]

Laboratory diagnosis

Serological assays for IgG and IgM antibodies to hepatitis E are commercially available and suitable for the diagnosis of acute infections. IgM appears during the early phase of symptoms and disappears after 4–5 months.[162] IgG appears soon after IgM, and the titer continues to increase into the convalescent phase and may remain high for several years. The interpretation of weak IgM results can be difficult in the absence of IgG antibody; in such cases, a follow-up sample can often clarify the results.

The use of HEV RNA assays can be a useful adjunct when the results of IgM assays have been equivocal in the absence of IgG antibody. HEV RNA is present in the incubation and early acute phase and can also be detected during the period of cholestasis that can follow the acute infection. Genotyping of such samples allowed the identification of indigenous virus in patients who had not traveled abroad.

Management

As for HAV, management is supportive. Fulminant liver failure is rare, but may be an indication for liver transplantation.

Vaccination

An HEV recombinant protein vaccine (rHEV) has been evaluated in a phase 2 clinical trial in a high-risk population.[163] The efficacy of a three-dose vaccination course was 95.5%. The profile of adverse events was similar to that in the placebo group, except for injection-site pain.

Other candidate viral hepatitis viruses

Hepatitis F virus

Viral particles have been observed in the explanted livers of children and adults undergoing liver transplantation for fulminant non-A, non-B hepatitis. In some of these cases, small viruses 60–70 nm in diameter, possibly related to the togaviruses or bunyaviruses, have been observed and termed "hepatitis F."[164,165] However, these particles are only rarely seen, and their clinical and diagnostic significance has not been established.

Hepatitis G virus

Hepatitis G virus (HGV) or GB virus type C is a transfusion-transmissible agent.[166] HGV has been described in a wide range of symptomless patients, particularly those exposed to blood or blood products. It has a high prevalence in those at risk from parenteral acquisition and may coexist with HCV. Vertical transmission has also been described.[167] Although HGV infection is described in association with acute, fulminant, and chronic hepatitis, its precise role in causing liver disease is not established. In a series of pediatric liver transplant recipients, the HGV prevalence was 30% and infection was persistent, although not associated with graft dysfunction.[168] In the majority of infected people, there is no biochemical evidence of liver disease, and the role of this group of viruses in hepatitis, particularly in children, has yet to be established. The only laboratory diagnostic tools for the investigation of HGV are molecular methods for detecting HGV RNA. There are no commercial reagents for the detection of either the antigen or antibody, and investigations for these agents are only at the research level.

Other transfusion-transmissible viruses

Other potential transfusion-transmissible agents, such as SEN virus[169] and torquetenovirus (TTV),[170] have yet to become established as significant human pathogens. Mother-to-baby transmission of SEN virus, with and without coinfecting HCV, has been described, but without any clinical evidence of liver disease on follow-up.[171] TTV is common in many parts of the world at very high prevalence, but has still not been associated with significant human pathology.[172]

Non-A–E hepatitis

It is apparent that there are other, currently unidentified viruses that may cause acute hepatitis. This diagnosis of exclusion, previously termed non-A, non-B hepatitis, has now been renamed non-A–E hepatitis or non-A–G hepatitis.

Although there may be more than one infectious agent to account for non-A–E hepatitis, a characteristic clinical picture has emerged. Children and young adults are predominantly affected, the hepatitic illness is usually severe, and there is a low rate of spontaneous recovery. Non-A–E hepatitis is the commonest cause of acute hepatic failure in children, accounting for 37–48%, and the commonest viral cause of liver failure requiring liver transplantation.[173,174]

Management is supportive, with early consideration of liver transplantation in view of the poor chance of spontaneous recovery.

Non-A–E hepatitis may be complicated by transient bone-marrow suppression or aplastic anemia. Although other viruses (e.g., parvovirus B19, EBV, echovirus, HBV, and HAV) may also be implicated in hepatitis with bone marrow suppression, non-A–E is most frequent. In a population with non-A–E liver failure requiring liver transplantation, aplastic anemia occurred in 23.2%, with a mean age of 10 years and male preponderance.[175] Early evidence of bone-marrow dysfunction may be apparent prior to liver transplantation. Treatment options for aplastic anemia, if there is no spontaneous recovery, include antithymocyte globulin, cyclophosphamide, cyclosporine, and bone-marrow transplantation.

Measles

Hepatic involvement with measles is more common in adolescents and adults than in children. Measles-associated hepatobiliary disease has been described in 27 patients, ranging in age from 9 to 59 years,[176] with two distinct patterns emerging:

- *Asymptomatic hepatocellular dysfunction,* with aminotransferase elevation occurring early in measles infection and resolving within days
- *Cholestasis and jaundice,* becoming apparent as measles resolves and persisting for 2 weeks or longer

In children hospitalized with measles, hepatic dysfunction with elevated aminotransferase enzymes is described in 5–11% of cases[177,178] and is usually subclinical, with spontaneous and rapid resolution. Type 1 autoimmune hepatitis occurring within 3 months of measles infection has been reported, with measles virus being proposed as the viral trigger.[179]

Rubella

Rubella is associated with liver disease in children following intrauterine infection, as part of the congenital rubella syndrome (Chapter 4). Hepatic involvement in congenital rubella may range from a mild hepatitis with focal necrosis to severe disease with massive necrosis, and progression to cirrhosis may occur. In acquired rubella infection, acute hepatitis has been described.

Parvovirus B19

Human parvovirus (HPV) B19 infection in childhood typically presents with erythema infectiosum, or in the presence of an underlying hemolytic anemia leads to an aplastic crisis. Infection during pregnancy may lead to hydrops fetalis. HPV B19 infection is, however, becoming increasingly associated with a wide range of systemic manifestations, including hepatic dysfunction:

- *Raised hepatic aminotransferase enzymes*—median aspartate aminotransferase (AST) 865 IU/L, alanine aminotransferase (ALT) 993 IU/L—associated with HPV B19 infection were described in seven children, three of whom had erythema infectiosum, with complete biochemical recovery occurring within 3 weeks.[180]
- *Fulminant liver failure* (with and without aplastic anemia) in association with HPV B19 has been described, with evidence of productive HPV B19 infection in the liver.

The hematological and fetal effects of HPV B19 infection are due to the erythrocyte P antigen, present on erythroid and fetal liver cells, acting as a receptor for the virus. The pathogenesis of hepatocellular damage is not known. It is proposed that a nonstructural protein of HPV B19 may be hepatotoxic, or that a specific defect in the immune response may contribute. Immune-mediated destruction of the hepatocytes is thought unlikely, due to the lack of cellular infiltration seen in affected liver tissue.[181]

Laboratory diagnosis

Serological assays for both IgG and IgM antibodies to HPV B19 are available commercially, with good specificity and sensitivity. As with all IgM assays, weakly reactive samples without IgG require a follow-up sample for confirmation. The detection of HPV DNA in blood can be useful in immunecompromised patients, in whom the infection can become persistent. Such investigations are usually only available in reference or specialist research laboratories.

Herpesviruses

The herpesviruses are a family of icosahedral double-stranded DNA viruses, all of which may cause acute hepatitis. They have a propensity to latency, persisting in the host after primary infection despite high levels of neutralizing antibody. Reactivation may occur particularly in the presence of immunosuppression. Replication by herpesvirus DNA polymerase may be inhibited by antiviral agents, providing effective therapy for severe disease (see below).

Herpes simplex viruses 1 and 2

Herpes simplex virus (HSV) hepatitis is very rare outside the neonatal period in an immunocompetent host. In perinatally acquired infection, a severe, disseminated disease typically manifests at day 4 or 5 of life and may be associated with severe hepatic dysfunction and fulminant hepatitis. In 90% of cases, this is due to HSV type 2, with a clear history of maternal herpetic vulvovaginitis, although occasionally type 1 HSV is implicated. HSV may be detected in affected tissue by electron microscopy or specific anti-HSV antibody by immunoassay.

Laboratory diagnosis

The diagnosis of a perinatal HSV infection is by direct identification of virus either by virus isolation in tissue culture, direct immunofluorescence of swabs or tissue or by molecular techniques. Serology is of no value in diagnosis of perinatal infections because of the presence of maternal IgG to HSV.

Varicella-zoster virus

Varicella-zoster virus (VZV) infection typically causes chickenpox, with a characteristic rash. Dissemination may occur in the first week of infection, particularly in the immunocompromised host, to involve the lungs, brain, and liver. The prognosis is determined by the lung involvement; varicella hepatitis in the absence of pneumonitis usually resolves.

Laboratory diagnosis

Diagnosis may be made by detecting specific IgM antibody by EIA methods or by detecting VZV in vesicle fluid by electron microscopy, direct immunofluorescence, or by molecular techniques. In the early stages of infection, the IgM may be negative and would require repeat testing for confirmation. However, for the diagnosis of chickenpox in a child, a lesion swab from the base of the lesion or vesicle fluid are the optimal specimens.

Cytomegalovirus

Cytomegalovirus (CMV) infection is usually a mild illness in childhood, but is of great significance following congenital infection, and in the immunocompromised host (Chapters 4, 21, and 22).

In the immunocompetent, acquired infection is usually asymptomatic or associated with mild nonspecific symptoms. In less than 1%, a clinically apparent syndrome that resembles infectious mononucleosis may occur. Hepatic involvement is frequent and usually mild, with raised transaminases, alkaline phosphatase, and bilirubin. The condition has a good prognosis, and a chronic course is unusual. Treatment is usually not required.

In the presence of immunosuppression, there may be more diffuse and severe disease involving in particular the respiratory system, gastrointestinal tract, and central nervous system. In liver transplant recipients, the transplanted liver is the most frequent site of CMV disease, with the donor organ the likely mode of transmission (see Chapter 21).

Histology

Histological features of CMV infection may be diagnostic (Figure 6.7). Cytomegalovirus is so named because it leads to a characteristic cytopathic effect after infection, with the appearance of:

- Cellular enlargement
- Enlarged rounded nuclei with a prominent rim
- Intranuclear "owl's-eye" inclusion bodies
- Cytoplasmic granules

Immunostaining of biopsy material using monoclonal antibody and in situ DNA hybridization may permit a rapid and specific diagnosis, even in the absence of suggestive histological changes. Inflammatory changes, especially in the immunocompetent, may be mild.

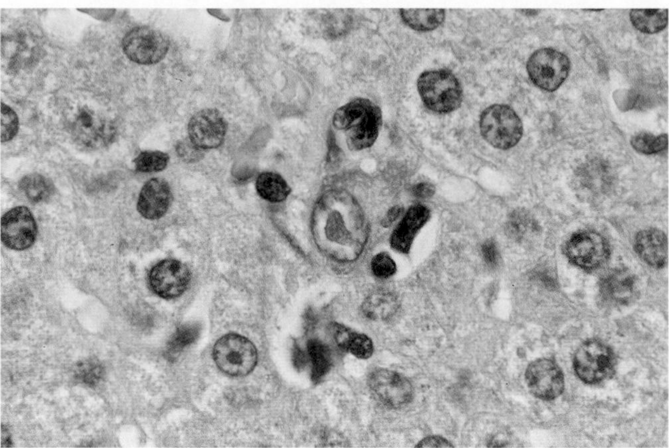

Figure 6.7 The histological features of cytomegalovirus infection may be diagnostic, demonstrating hepatocellular enlargement, an enlarged nucleus and an "owl's-eye" appearance due to intranuclear inclusion bodies.

Laboratory diagnosis

Acute CMV infection is characterized by specific IgM production and reactivation by a fourfold increase in IgG titer or by IgM production. As with all serological diagnosis, care needs to be taken over the interpretation of weak IgM reactions, and IgG avidity may help distinguish recent (low avidity) from past (high avidity) infections. CMV early antigen may be detected in infected urine, peripheral blood leukocytes, serum, sputum, or other tissue by immunofluorescence or latex agglutination. Viral genome detection by PCR is now widely available, leading to more rapid diagnosis, and quantitative PCR allows the course of the infection or disease and its resolution or the treatment response to be monitored. Congenital CMV is best diagnosed by PCR on a urine sample taken from the infant while under 3 weeks old.

Epstein–Barr virus

Epstein Barr virus is a significant pathogen, causing liver disease in both the immunocompetent and immunosuppressed host. The severity of Epstein–Barr virus (EBV) infection depends on the age of acquisition and the immune status of the host. In early childhood, EBV infection is frequent and usually asymptomatic or associated with mild, nonspecific symptoms. Primary infection occurring in adolescence or early adulthood, however, is typically associated with acute infectious mononucleosis (IM) or "glandular fever."

Clinical presentations of EBV include the following:

- Infectious mononucleosis
- Acute hepatitis and fulminant liver failure
- Chronic active EBV infection

Infectious mononucleosis (IM) is characterized by pharyngitis and malaise. Splenomegaly and lymphadenopathy are present in almost 50%, liver enlargement in up to 20%, and jaundice in 5%. Although elevated aminotransferase enzymes (up to five times normal) are detected in up to 80%, hepatitis is usually mild, with a complete recovery likely. Pancytopenia is frequent. Although predominantly infecting B-lymphocytes, the manifestations of EBV seen in IM are due to T-cell proliferation and infiltration of lymphoid tissue. Treatment is supportive.

Acute hepatitis may be severe and accompanied by cholestasis and ascites. Fulminant liver failure may occur, even in the immunocompetent. It may be the initial clinical presentation of EBV, or develop after a clinical presentation resembling IM, known as sporadic fatal infectious mononucleosis (SFIM). SFIM occurs in approximately one in 3000 cases of IM,[182] with a median age at presentation of 13 years. Treatment for acute liver failure is required (see Chapter 7).

Chronic active EBV infection (CAEBV) is characterized by chronic or recurrent IM-like symptoms. Skin rashes, uveitis, and diarrhea may also occur. Other terms used have included "chronic symptomatic EBV infection" and "chronic mononucleosis syndrome." In a nationwide study in Japan of 82 cases, the mean age at onset was 11.3 years, with males and females equally affected.[183] CAEBV has high morbidity and mortality rates and may lead to a wide range of systemic complications, including hemophagocytosis and hepatic failure. It is accompanied by extremely high EBV levels in peripheral blood, and either a predominance of infected T cells or NK cells in peripheral blood. Unusual antibody profiles, including extremely high viral capsid antigen IgG or absence of anti-Epstein–Barr virus-associated nuclear antigen, have been described but are not invariable.[184]

In the presence of immunodeficiency or immunosuppression, proliferation of EBV-infected B-cells is not controlled by the specific T-lymphocyte response. Clinical syndromes associated with unchecked B-cell proliferation range in severity from benign lymphoid hyperplasia to malignant monoclonal lymphoma (see Chapters 21 and 22).

Histology

The features of acute infectious mononucleosis are:[182]

- Mild predominantly lymphocytic portal inflammation
- Mild hepatocellular ballooning
- Prominent hepatocellular mitoses
- Panlobular canalicular cholestasis

Laboratory diagnosis

The diagnosis of EBV rests on serological assays, as virus culture is difficult. The pattern of antibody detection in acute and previous infection is as follows:

- Antibody to viral capsid antigen: IgM is positive in early acute infection; IgG is usually present at clinical presentation and then declines but persists for life.
- Antibody to Epstein–Barr nuclear antigen increases during convalescence, persists for life, and may increase during reactivation.
- Antibody to early antigen transiently increases during infection and reactivation.

The Paul–Bunnell test demonstrates acute nonspecific antibody production in response to EBV infection. In contrast to adults, in whom the Paul–Bunnell test is usually diagnostic of IM, the heterophile antibodies are not detectable in up to 50% of children or in the presence of immunosuppression.

Detection of EBV-encoded products—including latent membrane protein (LMP), Epstein–Barr nuclear antigen (EBNA), and EBV-encoded RNA (EBER)—by immunohistochemistry, and detection of EBV genome by in situ hybridization, allow specific detection of EBV in infected tissues, and these techniques are currently used as research tools. PCR detection and quantitation of EBV DNA in blood samples allows the monitoring of viral load, which is of particular value in organ-transplant recipients so that immunosuppressive therapy can be tailored appropriately.

Human herpesvirus 6

Most children are infected with human herpesvirus 6 (HHV6) in the first year of life.[185] The only disease for which a causal link is definitely established is roseola infantum (exanthem subitum), characterized by a fever for 3–5 days, which subsides as a rose-pink macular rash becomes apparent.

Liver dysfunction in association with HHV6 infection has been described, and includes an infectious mononucleosis-like syndrome, isolated hepatitis, and fulminant hepatic failure.

Laboratory diagnosis

Diagnostic tests for HHV6 are not available in all laboratories, as there is not a great diagnostic imperative to provide diagnosis for a very common, self-limiting childhood infection. The most specific test is for HHV6 DNA in blood, but the interpretation of the results can be difficult, as the infection —like all herpesvirus infections—is persistent and can be reactivated by a variety of other infections.

Treatment of herpesvirus infections

Antiviral therapy is effective against the herpes viruses by inhibition of viral DNA synthesis. As the majority of infections in the immunocompetent host are mild and self-limiting, specific treatment is only warranted in certain circumstances in which the disease is likely to be severe or disseminated, or in the presence of immunosuppression.

Antiviral agents effective against herpes viruses include:

- Acyclovir and valacyclovir
- Ganciclovir and valganciclovir
- Foscarnet
- Cidofovir

Acyclovir

Acyclovir, a nucleoside analog, is safe and relatively nontoxic, and has the best therapeutic index of all currently available antiviral agents. Its activation by phosphorylation to acyclovir triphosphate is catalyzed by a virus-encoded thymidine kinase, and thus only occurs in infected cells. Acyclovir triphosphate has a higher affinity for viral DNA polymerase than the natural substrate, and when incorporated into DNA terminates replication.

The susceptibility of herpesviruses to acyclovir is as follows:

- HSV 1 and 2: very susceptible.
- VZV: less effective phosphorylation of acyclovir occurs by VZV thymidine kinase, but with intravenous administration, adequate antiviral activity is achieved and may prevent dissemination.
- CMV: limited susceptibility, as CMV has no thymidine kinase: ganciclovir is a more effective alternative (see below).
- EBV: acyclovir is effective against EBV replication, but has no effect on latent virus. It may therefore reduce viral shedding in infectious mononucleosis, but has no effect on the symptoms or course.
- HHV6: resembles CMV in its susceptibility, being relatively resistant to acyclovir.

Valacyclovir

Valacyclovir is an ester of acyclovir with valine, with good absorption and bioavailability. Following oral administration, valacyclovir may achieve levels equivalent to intravenous acyclovir. Its safety profile appears to be similar to that of acyclovir. Pharmacokinetic studies in children support the use of oral valacyclovir instead of intravenous acyclovir for mucositis in immunosuppressed children, but clinical application is limited by palatability and the lack of an oral suspension.[186]

Ganciclovir

Ganciclovir is 100 times more active than acyclovir in its action against CMV replication. It is activated by phosphorylation in CMV-infected cells, despite the lack of viral thymidine kinase. It is more toxic than acyclovir, with 25% of patients experiencing reversible bone-marrow suppression, and intravenous therapy (5 mg/kg/dose i.v. twice daily for 2–3 weeks) should therefore be reserved for specific indications, which include prophylaxis against CMV in organ-transplant recipients and CMV disease in immunocompromised hosts.

Ganciclovir resistance due to lack of phosphorylation is rare, but emergence of resistant strains may be facilitated by prolonged ganciclovir use. The role of ganciclovir in congenital CMV infection or acquired neonatal hepatitis is not established.

Oral ganciclovir is poorly absorbed and has poor bioavailability, but at appropriate dosages may be as effective as intravenous treatment. In a study in children with HIV infection, 30 mg/kg body weight three times a day was well tolerated and achieved drug levels similar to the effective adult dose of 1 g three times a day.[187] High-dose oral ganciclovir has been successful in the management of symptomatic CMV infection in a child with acute lymphoblastic leukemia.[188]

Valganciclovir

As for acyclovir, ganciclovir linked to the amino acid valine increases its bioavailability tenfold. It has been shown in adults to be as effective as intravenous ganciclovir in the treatment of CMV disease, and as effective as oral ganciclovir for prophylaxis in immunosuppressed patients, with limited data available in children. It has the advantages of a once-daily regimen and provides greater systemic exposure to ganciclovir than oral ganciclovir. It is being evaluated for a potential role in perinatal CMV infection.

Foscarnet

Foscarnet acts by directly binding to pyrophosphate binding sites of DNA polymerases, leading to noncompetitive inhibition. As it does not require activation by cellular or viral kinases, it is of value in ganciclovir-resistant CMV disease. Its usefulness, however, is limited by its toxicity, with major adverse effects being renal impairment, electrolyte disturbance, and seizures.

Cidofovir

Cidofovir is an acyclic nucleoside phosphonate (as are adefovir and tenofovir). It has activity against all the herpesviruses and also against adenovirus. It has been successfully used for CMV disease with resistance to ganciclovir or foscarnet,[189] and in invasive adenovirus disease. It has significant nephrotoxicity and is therefore not recommended as first-line treatment. It has a potential role in treating herpesvirus and adenovirus infections in immunosuppressed patients when there is resistance to first-line agents.

Adenovirus

Adenovirus is a double-stranded DNA virus that typically causes pharyngitis and conjunctivitis. In the presence of immunosuppression, it has been implicated in both sporadic hepatitis and fulminant hepatic failure and may be rapidly fatal. Three immunosuppressed children have been reported with biopsy features of cholangiohepatitis caused by adenovirus.[190] In one, there was marked necrotizing cholangitis, with adenoviral inclusions in the biliary epithelium. All three had adenovirus gastrointestinal infection.

Diagnosis is by immunoassay or PCR to detect virus in stool, blood, or liver tissue. Although asymptomatic viremia is common, increasing viremia measured by quantitative PCR may preempt clinical disease.[191]

The antiviral agent cidofovir (see above) may be of value. Otherwise, treatment is supportive, with reduction of immunosuppression.

Enteroviruses

Echoviruses and coxsackieviruses (A and B) are the most frequent causes of viral meningitis, and Coxsackie B virus may cause myocarditis. Hepatitis due to these enteroviruses has also been described, however.

Coxsackie B viruses, particularly B1, may be acquired in the newborn period and cause acute hepatitis[192] associated with thrombocytopenia. The spectrum of disease may range from a mild nonspecific illness to overwhelming multiorgan involvement, with fulminant hepatic failure.

Laboratory diagnosis

Diagnosis may be made by virus isolation or virus antigen detection in throat swabs, stool, or cerebrospinal fluid using immunofluorescence with monoclonal antibody. Coxsackie B–specific IgM assay is a rapid but less sensitive method of diagnosis.[193] PCR for the Enterovirus group of viruses will now be available in many diagnostic virology laboratories for samples including cerebrospinal fluid, throat swabs, and nasopharyngeal aspirates.

Treatment is supportive.

Human immunodeficiency virus (HIV) and the liver

Liver dysfunction in children with HIV infection is common. It may be a presenting feature or due to coinfection, particularly with HBV or HCV, or subsequent opportunistic infection. Drug-induced liver disease due to antiretroviral therapy must also be considered.

Nonimmune hydrops with hepatitis in a neonate[194] and cholestatic hepatitis during infancy[195] have been reported as the initial clinical manifestations. Of 31 children with perinatally acquired HIV infection, 58% had liver disease with either acute or chronic hepatitis, for which CMV and hepatitis B and C were predisposing factors.[196] Those with liver disease had a poor prognosis.

Chronic liver disease due to HBV or HCV infection in adults with HIV coinfection progresses more rapidly than in those without,[197] and antiviral treatment should be considered. For HBV/HIV coinfection, there are limited data on interferon therapy; lamivudine is well tolerated, although its efficacy is limited by resistance. Newer drugs such as tenofovir and emtricitabine have efficacy against both HBV and HIV and would be the initial treatment of choice.

For HCV/HIV coinfection, combination therapy with pegylated interferon is recommended. Adverse effects are similar to those occurring in non–HIV-infected patients, except for hyperlactatemia/lactic acidosis and hepatic decompensation.[198] Little is known of the way in which HIV affects the course of HCV in children.

Viral hemorrhagic fever

Imported viral hemorrhagic fevers are characterized by fever, circulatory collapse, and hemorrhage. There may be diffuse organ involvement with severe hepatocellular necrosis.

Yellow fever

This is due to a flavivirus, which is transmitted to man, the main animal reservoir, by mosquitoes. It is endemic in West and Central Africa and may also occur in South America. The incubation period is between 3 and 6 days. In endemic areas, symptoms may be mild, with fever, proteinuria, leukopenia, and occasionally jaundice. In the severe form, after 3–4 days of fever, rigors, and headache, there is a transient improvement for less than 24 h before the onset of cutaneous and gastrointestinal hemorrhage and renal failure. Jaundice may become apparent during recovery.

Treatment is supportive. The mortality rate is in the order of 5%, with death usually occurring 7–10 days after the onset of symptoms. Immunization with a live attenuated vaccine is effective.

Dengue hemorrhagic fever

There have been recent epidemics of dengue fever, both in endemic areas and in travelers.

The distribution area of dengue fever and dengue hemorrhagic fever (DHF) is south-east Asia, the Pacific islands, India, Africa, and the Caribbean. Children are most frequently infected. After 4–8 days' incubation, there is either a mild febrile illness or a more severe infection with generalized aches, especially arthralgia, nausea, vomiting, painful eye movements, and depression, accompanied by petechiae and often tender hepatomegaly. Fever subsides after 3 days, to recur 1–2 days later accompanied by circulatory collapse. Treatment is supportive, with improvement usual after 48 h.

Hepatitis with mild to moderate elevation in aminotransferase enzymes are common: in an epidemic in Brazil in 2002, of 1585 patients with confirmed dengue, 65% had hepatitis. Acute liver failure is uncommon, but in Thailand dengue infection is the leading cause of acute liver failure in children, accounting for 12 of 35 cases[199] (see Chapter 23).

Lassa fever

This Arenavirus infection is endemic in rats and is transmitted by water contaminated with their urine or saliva. In endemic areas, infection may be limited to a mild febrile illness. In others, after 7–17 days' incubation there is persistent fever, pharyngitis with tonsillar exudate, lethargy, gastrointestinal symptoms, and maculopapular rash. In the second week, encephalopathy, circulatory collapse, and diffuse hemorrhage into skin and organs may develop. Diagnosis is by isolation of virus from the throat, urine or blood, or by detection of specific Lassa antibodies—present in the second week of illness—by immunofluorescence. Infected patients must be treated in strict isolation. Intravenous ribavirin may be effective in reducing the mortality.[200]

Marburg and Ebola viruses

These are endemic in Africa. After an initial flu-like illness, massive hepatocellular necrosis and disseminated intravascular coagulation occur, with a high mortality rate of up to 90%.

Nonviral causes of hepatic infection

Nonviral hepatic infections (Table 6.3) may be manifest by:
- Hepatitis with inflammatory destruction of hepatocytes, resembling acute viral hepatitis
- Invasion and infiltration leading to hepatomegaly (e.g., hydatid disease)
- Abscess formation, either single or multiple, which may be secondary to extrahepatic sepsis (Table 6.10)
- Cholangitis: infection limited to the biliary tree

Tuberculosis and malaria

See Chapter 23.

Leptospirosis

Leptospira interrogans serovar *icterohaemorrhagiae* is a spirochete that is carried in the kidneys of both wild and domestic animals, particularly the rat, with contamination of streams and rivers occurring through infected urine. Human exposure occurs in veterinarians and farm workers, and by swimming in contaminated water. Transmission occurs via skin abrasions or mucous membranes, with person-to-person spread being rare.

Table 6.10 Bacterial causes of hepatic abscess.

Common	Uncommon
Coliform organisms, particularly:	*Mycobacterium tuberculosis*
Escherichia coli	*Actinomycosis*
Klebsiella pneumoniae	*Brucella melitensis*
Streptococcus milleri	*Salmonella typhi*
Anaerobic streptococci	*Yersinia enterocolitica*
	Bacteroides species
	Listeria monocytogenes
	Staphylococcus aureus

Clinical features

Following an incubation period of 1–2 weeks, bacteremia is established and leads in the majority of cases to a subclinical infection or a mild flu-like illness with fever and myalgia. Symptoms usually persist for 1 week, with their severity relating to the number of infecting organisms and the immune status of the host. In less than 10% of symptomatic cases, a severe systemic disease known as Weil disease occurs. Symptoms are due to damage to the endothelium of small vessels and to seeding of the leptospires in meninges, liver, or kidneys. They include:
- Fever, headache, myalgia.
- Extensive vasculitic rash and circulatory collapse.
- Renal failure.
- Myocarditis.
- Pneumonitis.
- Hepatitis: jaundice and hepatomegaly are characteristic, and transaminases are usually only mildly elevated. Fulminant liver failure may occur.

In Egypt, 16% of 392 patients with undiagnosed acute hepatitis had serological evidence of leptospira IgM.[201]

Diagnosis

Diagnosis is made by:
- Demonstrating leptospires by dark-ground microscopy in:
  —Blood during the bacteremic phase
  —Urine during the phase of organ involvement
- Detection in serum of specific IgM antibody or a rising titer of IgG antibody

Treatment

Treatment with penicillin G (200 000–250 000 U/kg/day i.v. in six divided doses for 1 week) may have a beneficial effect on the illness if given in the first 4–7 days. Tetracycline or erythromycin is also effective. Most patients recover without long-term sequelae. In those with liver failure, support with the molecular adsorbent recirculating system (MARS; see Chapter 7) has led to a successful outcome.[202]

Bartonella infection

Bartonella henselae or *B. quintana* infection leading to hepatic disease has been described in both immunosuppressed and immunocompetent children. Almost all reported cases in children are linked to likely transmission from cats by bites or scratches.

Two histopathological types are described: vascular proliferative disease with cystic blood-filled spaces and foci of necrosis within the liver and spleen; and a necrotizing granulomatous type. In both, ultrasonography reveals low-attenuation lesions within the liver and spleen. A giant, solitary hepatic granuloma, mimicking a hepatic tumor, has also been described.[203]

The diagnosis may be confirmed by serological (EIA) testing for antibodies to *B. henselae* or *B. quintana*, or by specific stains applied to biopsy material or culture. The outcome is good, with a dramatic response to erythromycin or doxycycline.

Listeria monocytogenes

Almost all cases of hepatic involvement with *Listeria* infection occur in the presence of immunosuppression. A hepatitic illness with fever, raised transaminases, and jaundice may occur, and the diagnosis is confirmed by isolating listeria organisms from blood cultures. Treatment with antibiotics (ampicillin 200–400 mg/kg/day i.v. for 14 days) is usually effective. Hepatic abscess formation due to *L. monocytogenes* infection has also been described (see below).

Other bacterial infections

Legionella pneumophila has also been associated with a hepatitic illness in the immunosuppressed host, and *Salmonella typhi* infection may give rise to a hepatitis that clinically resembles viral hepatitis. Brucellosis and tuberculosis may give rise to a granulomatous hepatitis with fever and hepatosplenomegaly in which jaundice is uncommon and transaminases are only mildly elevated, but alkaline phosphatase is typically raised.

Other organisms

Toxoplasmosis

Toxoplasma gondii is a protozoan parasite whose animal reservoir is the cat. Excretion of cysts by cats contaminates the soil and leads to infection in other animals, particularly sheep. Infection in humans occurs following ingestion of meat contaminated by *Toxoplasma* cysts, or due to prenatal acquisition (Chapter 4).

The majority of acquired infections are asymptomatic and unrecognized. Symptomatic acute infection is manifest by fever, fatigue, and lymphadenopathy, resembling infectious mononucleosis, and may be accompanied by hepatitis. Lymph-node biopsy may be characteristic and may permit isolation of the parasite.

Recovery can be prolonged over several weeks, but is usually complete.

Treatment is only indicated in the immunocompetent with acquired infection if there is clinically overt visceral involvement or severe or persistent symptoms.[204] A good response may be seen with pyrimethamine and sulfadiazine. The optimal duration of therapy is not determined, but should be from 1 to 4 months, until symptoms resolve. Folinic acid (5–10 mg every 1–2 days) should be given to prevent significant bone-marrow suppression occurring due to pyrimethamine.

Helminthic infections

Helminths, or parasitic worms, lead to a wide range of liver diseases, the type and severity of which depends not only on the type of worm but also on the intensity of the infection and the host response. Simultaneous infection with more than one type of worm may occur. Children are particularly at risk, as infection may occur following close contact with infected animals, ingestion of infected soil, or contaminated food.

Echinococcus multilocularis (alveolar echinococcosis) and *E. granulosus* (hydatid disease)

The primary host for the adult *Echinococcus* tapeworm is the dog. Ova are excreted in feces, and although sheep are the usual intermediate host, humans may become infected following close contact with infected dogs. In the UK, hydatid disease is most prevalent in Wales. Following ingestion of ova, the embryo develops and penetrates the stomach wall, reaching the liver via the portal venous circulation.

Hydatid disease. In hydatid disease, cysts develop most frequently within the lungs and liver. Hepatic cysts are usually slow-growing and lead to asymptomatic hepatomegaly, but may become manifest due to secondary infection or because of their size. Aspiration of the cysts is hazardous, due to the risk of dissemination and hypersensitivity to the daughter cysts contained within the fluid-filled parent cysts.

Serological diagnosis is highly sensitive. Treatment is by careful surgical excision if the cysts lead to symptoms, or with daily mebendazole for at least 3 months.

Alveolar echinococcosis. In alveolar echinococcosis, the cysts resemble a slow-growing tumor, with symptoms due to local pressure and parenchymal infiltration. As growth is slow, the clinical symptoms may be delayed for decades, but presentation in childhood has been reported and may be associated with immunodeficiency.[205] Metastatic spread to the lung and brain may occur.

Ultrasound reveals a typical solid, heterogeneous mass, which may resemble a malignant lesion, with a necrotic center. If complete surgical excision is not possible, mebendazole 40 mg/kg/day may arrest the growth of the lesion.

Ascaris lumbricoides

Ascaris has a worldwide distribution and often may cause no symptoms. Heavy infestation may lead to intestinal obstruction. Migration into the biliary tree, gallbladder, and liver may lead to obstructive jaundice and secondary pyogenic infection with cholangitis and abscess formation.[206] Diagnosis is made following recognition of *Ascaris* eggs or mature worms in infected feces. Treatment is with levamisole (single dose), mebendazole (twice daily for 3 days), or piperazine (single dose) and is effective in 90% of cases.

Toxocara canis and *T. cati*

Adult worms of *Toxocara* are found in the intestine of dogs (*T. canis*) or cats (*T. cati*). Infection in humans follows ingestion of ova due to food contaminated by infected feces. Larvae develop in the small intestine, invade the portal circulation, and lead to tissue damage, with granulomas in the liver and other organs. Infection is characterized by fever, hepatosplenomegaly, and eosinophilia—"visceral larva migrans." The diagnosis is presumptive or by serology. Treatment is with thiabendazole 25 mg/kg/day for 5 days or diethylcarbamazine 6 mg/kg/day for 21 days.[207]

Schistosoma mansoni (Middle East and Africa) and *S. japonicum* (Far East)

The ova of these flukes infect snails and emerge in water as cercariae, which then gain access to humans as the intermediate host by penetrating the skin. Following invasion into the circulation, ova may embolize to the liver, become impacted in presinusoidal portal veins, and give rise to a granulomatous hepatitis with progressive fibrosis and portal hypertension. The diagnosis is made by detecting the ova in stools or in rectal biopsy material. Treatment is a one-day course of praziquantel, with two doses given for *S. mansoni* and three for *S. japonicum*.[208]

Fasciola hepatica

This sheep liver fluke inhabits large bile ducts. The eggs, after excretion in feces, hatch in water and infect snails. Cercariae emerge from the snail and thus contaminate water and vegetation such as watercress. Human infection is common where watercress is eaten.

Following ingestion, *F. hepatica* may invade the biliary tree by migration through the gastrointestinal mucosa, peritoneal cavity, and hepatic parenchyma. This may be accompanied by fever, tender hepatic enlargement, anorexia, nausea, and vomiting, and with allergic symptoms, urticaria and eosinophilia. Severe infection may lead to biliary tract involvement, including hyperplasia, necrosis, dilation, and inflammation.

The diagnosis is by recognition of the ova in infected feces. Serological tests are also of value. Treatment is with bithionol 30–50 mg/kg, given on alternate days for a total of 10–15 doses.[208] Recovery is usually complete.

Liver abscesses

Abscess formation within the hepatic parenchyma may be due to pyogenic, fungal, or amebic infection (Table 6.10). As the symptoms may be nonspecific, a high index of suspicion, particularly in those with underlying risk factors (see below), is needed.

Clinical features

Symptoms and signs present in a series of 48 adults with pyogenic hepatic abscesses included the following:[209]

- Fever (77%)
- Abdominal pain (66%)
- Nausea (62%)
- Chest pain/cough (51%)
- Vomiting (43%)
- Right upper quadrant tenderness (42%)
- Right upper quadrant pain (27%)
- Hepatomegaly (25%)
- Jaundice (22%).

The duration of symptoms was less than 2 weeks in 63% of cases. Patients with amebic abscesses were more likely to have abdominal pain (90%), nausea (85%), right upper quadrant tenderness (67%), and a short duration of symptoms (86%), and were less likely to have respiratory symptoms (24%).

Predisposing factors for pyogenic abscess

Various conditions increase the likelihood of a pyogenic abscess developing in the liver. These include:

- Complications of prematurity
- Intra-abdominal sepsis

A history of gastrointestinal symptoms should be sought in order to identify a predisposing disorder—e.g., appendicitis, pancreatitis, Crohn's disease, trauma.

- Diabetes (especially with *Klebsiella pneumoniae*)
- Primary hemochromatosis (*Yersinia enterocolitisca* is an iron-dependent bacterium species, requiring high iron for growth)
- Hemoglobinopathy
- Immunodeficiency, including chronic granulomatous disease (fungi, staphylococci): in chronic granulomatous disease (CGD), abscesses may be multiple and recurrent.

Laboratory features

Although there may be no detectable abnormality, the majority of patients with either pyogenic or amebic abscesses have:

- Raised serum alkaline phosphatase
- Reduced serum albumin
- Mildly elevated aminotransferase enzymes (40–100 U/L)
- Leukocytosis

Imaging

Ultrasonography may permit detection of abscesses with a diameter of at least 1 cm within the hepatic parenchyma. The typical appearance is of a hypoechoic area with ring enhancement (Figure 6.8). Computed tomography, where necessary, permits confirmation and more precise localization of the lesion (Figure 6.9). Lesions that may mimic an abscess include malignant metastatic disease and the necrotizing hepatic lesions of fulminant herpes hepatitis.[210] There are no reliable ultrasonographic features to distinguish amebic from pyogenic abscesses.[209] In patients with CGD, the radiographic appearance may differ from that of sporadic abscesses. The abscesses typically show homogeneous and multiseptal enhancement on computed tomography and magnetic resonance imaging.[211] Imaging should also evaluate a predisposing disease, particularly in the gastrointestinal tract.

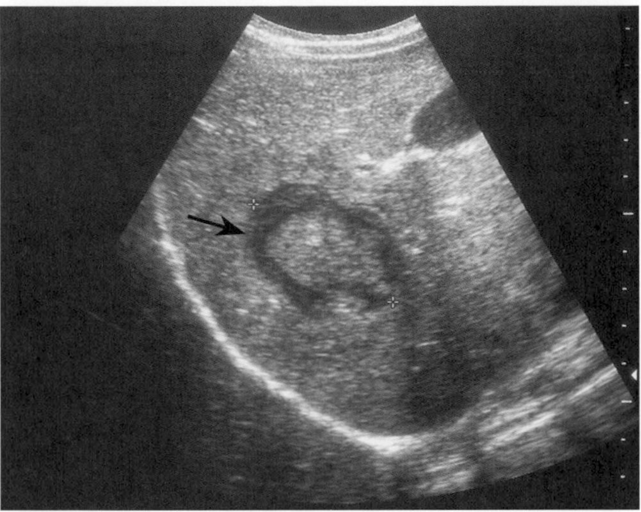

Figure 6.8 This hepatic ultrasound image demonstrates an abscess (arrow) in a patient with abdominal pain and hepatic tenderness.

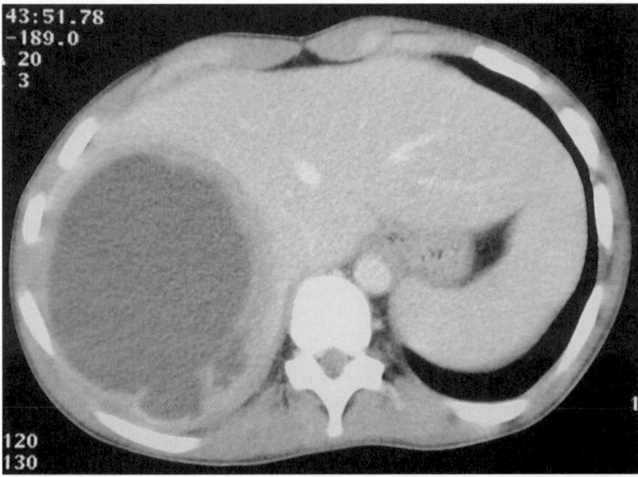

A

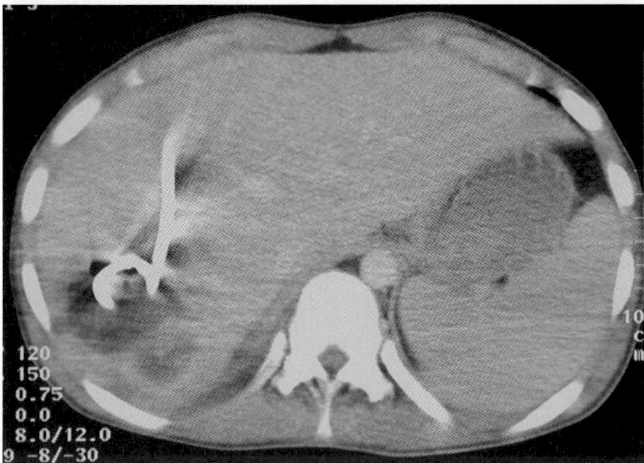

B

Figure 6.9 The diagnosis of a hepatic abscess is best confirmed by computed tomography—here showing a thick-walled right hepatic abscess (**A**). Abscesses are best treated by percutaneous aspiration and drainage through the liver parenchyma, to avoid local spillage from the cavity (**B**).

Microbiology

Aspiration of the abscess will yield the causative organism in almost all cases of pyogenic infection, with almost 50% of infected patients having the same organism isolated from peripheral blood culture.[209,212] *Streptococcus milleri* and *Klebsiella pneumoniae* are the most common infecting microorganisms. Recently, abscesses secondary to *Ascaris* have been described.[206] Staphylococci are the most common organisms isolated in CGD.

Amebic abscess may be diagnosed by negative bacterial culture and positive serology, with antibody to *Entamoeba histolyticum* detectable by indirect hemagglutination assay, complement fixation, or indirect fluorescence.

Neonatal pyogenic abscess

Hepatic abscesses occurring in the neonatal period are usually solitary and associated with an underlying predisposition due to:

- Prematurity
- Umbilical vessel catheterization
- Necrotizing enterocolitis

Signs and symptoms may be absent or nonspecific, with irritability and a mildly distended, tender abdomen. Fever may be absent. Liver function may remain normal, leukocytosis is not invariable and abdominal radiography may be unhelpful. The diagnosis rests on a high index of suspicion and ultrasonography (see above).

In a review of 18 cases,[212] the following bacteria were identified, isolated from the abscess in the majority:

- Gram-negative coliforms
- Staphylococcal species
- Streptococcal species

Multiple pathogens were isolated in 24% of cases.

Treatment

Percutaneous aspiration and drainage of the abscess cavity should be performed, and intravenous antibiotic therapy should be administered for 2–6 weeks. Antimicrobial treatment should be directed against the most likely organisms, and thus include a penicillin, aminoglycoside, and metronidazole. Amebic abscesses usually respond to metronidazole. Serial ultrasonography should be performed to document a reduction in the size of the abscess cavity prior to stopping antibiotic therapy. Complete resolution over a few months, with eventual calcification of the lesion, can be expected, with no long-term sequelae.

In patients with CGD, more aggressive treatment—including early surgical excision—may be required.[213]

Infective cholangitis

Infection of the biliary tree in the immunocompetent usually signifies an underlying structural abnormality. Predisposing disorders (see Chapters 4, 10, and 20) include:

- Primary sclerosing cholangitis
- Choledochal cyst
- Biliary atresia (after portoenterostomy)
- Cholelithiasis
- Caroli's disease
- Portal vein cavernoma with biliary obstruction
- Biliary strictures

The presentation may be with fever, jaundice, and biliary obstructive symptoms such as pale stools and dark urine, accompanied by tenderness in the right hypochondrium. Occasionally, the only symptom may be fever. Blood cultures may yield bacterial pathogens, but are frequently negative, and treatment with broad-spectrum antibiotics is indicated, such as:

- Ceftazidime: 30 mg/kg three times a day for 10 days
- Amoxicillin: 20 mg/kg three times a day for 10 days
- Ciprofloxacin 4–7 mg/kg/12 h i.v. for 10 days

If there is persistent biliary obstruction and sepsis, external biliary drainage or biliary dilation may be required.

Unusual organisms that may cause cholangitis include *Ascaris* infection and *Aspergillus*.[214] *Cryptosporidium* and microsporidia may cause cholangitis in those with immunodeficiency. Recent treatment options include azithromycin, nitazoxanide, and paromomycin.

Case study 1

A 13-year-old presented with jaundice, abdominal pain, and fever. Five weeks previously, he had had severe abdominal pain localized to the right iliac fossa, which then became more generalized, associated with fever. It was initially thought to be a viral illness, but the fever continued, although the pain became intermittent. The onset of jaundice prompted reassessment and transfer to a pediatric liver unit. There was no significant history or family history and no recent travel.

The examination revealed fever, weight loss, palpable hepatosplenomegaly, and ascites. Laboratory investigations showed:

- Anemia, neutrophil leukocytosis, raised C-reactive protein (CRP)
- Abnormal liver function—ALT 146 IU/L (normal < 40), bilirubin 41 mmol/L (normal < 20), albumin 20 g/L (normal 35–45 g/L), international normalized ratio (INR) 1.3 (normal)

Ultrasound revealed a liver with a heterogeneous echotexture, containing hypoechoic areas (Figure 6.8). The portal vein and superior mesenteric vein were distended by thrombus. Ascites was present.

Computed tomography confirmed the ultrasound appearances (Figure 6.9).

A Barium small-bowel follow-through suggested edema of the ileocecum. A large liver abscess (15 × 11 cm) was drained percutaneously, and three separate lesions were aspirated. No microorganisms were detected in the blood or abscess contents. Treatment was with intravenous antibiotics and anticoagulation.

Nutritional support with nasogastric feeding was required. Symptoms and ultrasound appearances gradually improved. After 4 weeks of intravenous antibiotics, the patient was discharged on oral antibiotics for a further 2 weeks and anticoagulation with warfarin. Chronic granulomatous disease was excluded by neutrophil function testing.

Subsequently, an appendicectomy was performed electively and revealed fibrous obliteration of the lumen, in keeping with previous acute appendicitis. At follow-up, the main portal vein appeared to be recanalized, with collaterals present, the spleen remained enlarged, and at endoscopy esophageal varices were present, in keeping with portal hypertension.

The final diagnosis was acute appendicitis leading to portal and mesenteric pyemia and thrombosis with multiple hepatic abscesses. Long-term sequelae include portal hypertension, leading to esophageal varices.

Comment. Hepatic abscesses in children are unusual, but may be secondary to intra-abdominal sepsis. This young boy developed extensive sepsis from an undiagnosed appendicitis or appendix abscess. A common organism for this would be *Streptococcus milleri,* which might have been cultured from the liver abscess. Although the organism is sensitive to antibiotics, he would not recover without drainage of the abscesses. He also developed portal pyemia, which caused extensive intravascular thrombosis and portal hypertension, an unusual occurrence. It needs vigorous therapy with antibiotics, anticoagulants, and—if the diagnosis is made soon enough—infusion of tissue plasminogen activator to dissolve the clots.

Case study 2

A 7-year-old child of Pakistani origin with β thalassemia was screened for hepatitis C infection in view of multiple blood transfusions. She required blood transfusion every 4 weeks and received antichelation therapy with desferrioxamine.

She was HCV RNA–positive with genotype 3a. She was immune to hepatitis B following immunization. ALT was mildly elevated (86–261 IU/L; normal < 40). Liver biopsy showed bridging fibrosis, marked Kupffer cell hemosiderosis, and mild hepatitis.

Treatment for HCV infection was considered, in view of her advanced fibrosis and favorable genotype. However, ribavirin might be contraindicated in view of her hemolytic anemia. Hemolytic anemia due to ribavirin may increase transfusion requirements and aggravate existing iron overload. Although there are reports of combination therapy being used in children with thalassemia, there is also evidence supporting pegylated interferon monotherapy.

A decision was made to treat initially with pegylated interferon monotherapy, with a view to adding ribavirin after 12 weeks if there was no reduction in viral load. The viral load did reduce and became undetectable at 24 weeks. She tolerated the treatment well and remains in remission.

Comment. HCV genotype 3a is very sensitive to combination therapy with pegylated interferon and ribavirin, with a 90% chance of clearing the virus. Treatment with ribavirin in children with hemolysis is difficult and can only be managed by increasing the rate of transfusions or by accepting a lower hemoglobin level. This young girl responded to monotherapy with pegylated interferon. Pegylated interferon is more effective than ribavirin in reducing the viral load, but ribavirin is thought to be necessary for prolonged viral remission. She may have a higher risk of relapse in the future.

References

1 Kuhns M, Thiers V, Courouce A, Scotto J, Tiollais P. Quantitative detection of HBV DNA in human sera. In: Vyas GN, Dienstag SL, Hoofnagle JH, eds. *Viral Hepatitis and Liver Disease*. Orlando, FL: Grune and Stratton, 1984: 665–6.

2 Urdea MS, Horn T, Fultz TJ, *et al.* Branched DNA amplification multimers for the sensitive, direct detection of human hepatitis viruses. *Nucleic Acids Symp Ser* 1991;**24**:197–200.

3 Barlet V, Cohard M, Thelu MA, *et al.* Quantitative detection of hepatitis B DNA in serum using chemiluminescence: comparison with radioactive solution hybridization assay. *J Virol Methods* 1994;**49**:141–51.

4 Pawlotsky JM. Molecular diagnosis of viral hepatitis. *Gastroenterology* 2002;**122**:1554–68.

5 Martin A, Lemon SM. Hepatitis A virus: from discovery to vaccines. *Hepatology* 2006;**43**:S164–72.

6 Bell BP. Hepatitis A vaccine. *Pediatr Infect Dis J* 2000;**19**:1187–8.

7 Provost PJ, Hilleman MR. Propagation of human hepatitis A virus in cell culture in vitro. *Proc Soc Exp Biol Med* 1979;**160**: 213–21.

8 Kaplan G, Totsuka A, Thompson P, Akatsuka T, Moritsugu Y, Feinstone SM. Identification of a surface glycoprotein on African green monkey kidney cells as a receptor for hepatitis A virus. *EMBO J* 1996;**15**:4282–96.

9 Lemon SM, Martin A. Structure and molecular virology of hepatitis A. In: Thomas HC, Lemon SM, Zuckerman AJ, eds. *Viral Hepatitis*. 3rd ed. Oxford: Blackwell, 2005: 79–91.

10 Bower WA, Nainan OV, Han X, Margolis HS. Duration of viraemia in hepatitis A virus infection. *J Infect Dis* 2000;**182**:12–7.

11 Maier K, Gabriel P, Koscielniak, *et al.* Human gamma interferon production by cytotoxic T lymphocytes sensitized during hepatitis A virus infection. *J Virol* 1988;**62**:3756–63.

12 Gruer LD, McKendrick MW, Beeching NJ, Gedded AM. Relapsing hepatitis associated with hepatitis A. *Lancet* 1982;**2**:163.

13 Cobden I, James OFW. A biphasic illness associated with acute hepatitis A virus infection. *J Hepatol* 1986;**2**:19–23.

14 Steffen R, Kane MA, Shapiro CN, Billo N, Shoellhorn KJ, van Damme P. Epidemiology and prevention of hepatitis A in travelers. *JAMA* 1994;**272**:885–9.

15 Maguire HC, Handford S, Perry KR, *et al.* A collaborative case control study of sporadic hepatitis A in England. *Commun Dis Rep CDR Rev* 1995;**5**:R33–40.

16 Mannucci PM, Gdovin S, Gringeri A, *et al.* Transmission of hepatitis A to patients with hemophilia by factor VIII concentrates treated with organic solvent and detergent to activate viruses. *Ann Intern Med* 1993;**120**:1–7.

17 Noble RC, Kane MA. Posttransfusion hepatitis A in neonatal intensive care unit. *JAMA* 1984;**252**:2711–5.

18 Lee KK, Vargo LR, Lê CT, Fernando L. Transfusion-acquired hepatitis A outbreak from fresh plasma in a neonatal intensive care unit. *Pediatr Infect Dis J* 1992;**11**:122–3.

19 Urganci N, Arapoglu M, Akyildiz B, Nuhoglu A. Neonatal cholestasis resulting from vertical transmission of hepatitis A infection. *Pediatr Infect Dis J* 2003;**22**:381–2.

20 Yotsuyanagi H, Koike K, Yasuda K, *et al.* Prolonged fecal excretion of hepatitis A virus in adult patients with hepatitis A as determined by polymerase chain reaction. *Hepatology* 1996;**24**:10–3.

21 Fujiwara K, Yokosuka O, Ehata T, *et al.* Frequent detection of hepatitis A viral RNA in serum during the early convalescent phase of acute hepatitis A. *Hepatology* 1997;**26**:1634–9.

22 Debray D, Cullufi P, Devictor D, Fabre M, Bernard O. Liver failure in children with hepatitis A. *Hepatology* 1997;**26**:1018–22.

23 Corpechot C, Cadranel JF, Hoang C, *et al.* [Cholestatic viral hepatitis A in adults. Clinical, biological and histopathological study of 9 cases; in French.] *Gastroenterol Clin Biol* 1994;**18**:743–50.

24 Keeffe E. Hepatitis A in patients with chronic liver disease—severity of illness and prevention with vaccination. *J Viral Hepat* 2000;**7**(Suppl 1):15–7.

25 Vento S, Garofano T, Renzini C, *et al.* Fulminant hepatitis associated with hepatitis A virus superinfection in patients with chronic hepatitis C. *N Engl J Med* 1998;**338**:286–90.

26 Salisbury D, Ramsay M, Noakes K, eds. *Immunisation against Infectious Disease*. 3rd ed. London: TSO, 2006.

27 Kane MA, Clements J, Hu D. Hepatitis B. In: Jamison DT, Mosley WH, Measham AR, Bobadilla J. *Disease Control Priorities in Developing Countries.* New York: Oxford University Press, 1993: 321–30.

28 McMahon BJ, Alward WLM, Hall DB, *et al.* Acute hepatitis B infection: relation of age to the clinical expression of disease and subsequent development of the carrier state. *J Infect Dis* 1985;**151**:599–603.

29 Echevarria JM, Avellon A. Hepatitis B virus genetic diversity. *J Med Virol* 2006;**78**:S36–S42.

30 Thursz MR, Howard HC. Pathogenesis of chronic hepatitis B virus infection. In: Thomas HC, Lemon SM, Zuckerman AJ, eds. *Viral Hepatitis*. 3rd ed. Oxford: Blackwell, 2005: 308–22.

31 Beath SV, Boxall EH, Watson RM, Tarlow MJ, Kelly DA. Fulminant hepatitis B in infants born to anti-HBe hepatitis B carrier mothers. *BMJ* 1992;**304**:1169–70.

32 Beasley RP, Hwang LY. Postnatal infectivity of hepatitis B surface antigen-carrier mothers. *J Infect Dis* 1987;**147**:185–90.

33 Balkaran BN, Teelucksingh S, Singh VR. Hepatitis B-associated polyarteritis nodosa and hypertensive encephalopathy. *West Indian Med J* 2000;**49**:170–1.

34 Wilson's RA. Extrahepatic manifestations of chronic viral hepatitis. *Am J Gastroenterol* 1997;**92**:3–17.

35 Liu CJ, Lo SC, Kao JH, *et al.* Transmission of occult hepatitis B virus by transfusion to adult and pediatric recipients in Taiwan. *J Hepatol* 2006;**44**:39–46.

36 Chu CM, Karayiannis P, Fowler MJ, *et al.* Natural history of chronic hepatitis B virus infection in Taiwan: studies of hepatitis B virus DNA in serum. *Hepatology* 1985;**5**:431–4.

37 Chu CM, Liaw YF. Natural history of chronic hepatitis B virus infection: an immunopathological study. *J Gastroenterol Hepatol* 1997;**12**: S218–222.

38 Niederau C, Heintges T, Lange S, *et al.* Long-term follow-up of HBeAg-positive patients treated with interferon alfa for chronic hepatitis B. *N Engl J Med* 1996;**334**:1422–7.

39 Lau DTY, Everhart J, Kleiner DE, *et al.* Long-term follow-up of patients with chronic hepatitis B treated with interferon alfa. *Gastroenterology* 1997;**113**:1660–7.

40 Wong DKH, Cheung AM, O'Rourke K, Naylor CD, Detsky AS, Heathcote J. Effect of alpha-interferon treatment in patients with hepatitis B e antigen-positive chronic hepatitis B: a meta-analysis. *Ann Intern Med* 1993;**119**:312–23.

41 Merican I. Management of chronic hepatitis B. Treatment of chronic hepatitis B virus infection in special groups of patients: decompensated cirrhosis, immunosuppressed and paediatric patients. *J Gastroenterol Hepatol* 2000;**15**(Suppl):E71–8.

42 Sira JK, Boxall E, Sleight E, Ballard A, Yoong AK, Kelly DA. Long-term treatment of chronic hepatitis B carrier children in the UK [abstract]. *Hepatology* 1997;**26**:427A.

43 Gregorio GV, Jara P, Hierro L, *et al.* Lymphoblastoid interferon alfa with or without steroid pre-treatment in children with chronic hepatitis B: a multicenter controlled trial. *Hepatology* 1996;**23**:700–7.

44 Yokosuka O. Role of steroid priming in the treatment of chronic hepatitis B. *J Gastroenterol Hepatol* 2000;**15**(Suppl):E41–5.

45 Lok A. Navigating the maze of hepatitis B treatments. *Gastroenterology* 2007;**132**:1586–94.

46 Leung, N. Liver disease—significant improvement with lamivudine. *J Med Virol* 2000;**61**:380–5.

47 Lai CL, Chien RN, Leung NW, *et al.* A one year trial of lamivudine for chronic hepatitis B. *N Engl J Med* 1998;**339**:61–8.

48 Schiff E, Karayalcin S, Grimm I, *et al.* A placebo controlled study of lamivudine and interferon alpha-2b in patients with chronic hepatitis B who previously failed interferon therapy. *Hepatology* 1998;**28**:388A.

49 Deinstag JL, Schiff ER, Wright TL, *et al.* Lamivudine as initial treatment for chronic hepatitis B in the United States. *N Engl J Med* 1999;**341**:1256–63.

50 Chien RN, Liaw YF, Atkins M. Pretherapy alanine transaminase level as a determinant for hepatitis B e antigen seroconversion during lamivudine therapy in patients with chronic hepatitis B. *Hepatology* 1999;**30**:770–4.

51 Moraleda G, Saputelli J, Aldrich CE, Averett, D, Condreay L, Mason WS. Lack of effect of antiviral therapy in non-dividing hepatocyte cultures on the closed circular DNA of woodchuck hepatitis virus. *J Virol* 1997;**71**:9392–9.

52 Kock J, Schlicht HJ. Analysis of the earliest steps of hepadnavirus replication: genome repair after infectious entry into hepatocytes does not depend on viral polymerase activity. *J Virol* 1993;**67**:4867–74.

53 De Jong MD, Boucher CAB, Danner SA, *et al.* Summary of the international consensus symposium on management of HIV, CMV and hepatitis virus infections. *Antiviral Res* 1998;**37**: 1–16.

54 Ling R, Mutimer D, Ahmed M, *et al.* Selection of mutations in the hepatitis B virus polymerase during therapy of transplant recipients with lamivudine. *Hepatology* 1996;**24**:711–3.

55 Sokal EM, Roberts EA, Mieli-Vergani G, *et al.* A dose ranging study of the pharmacokinetics, safety, and preliminary efficacy of lamivudine in children and adults with chronic hepatitis B. *Antimicrob Agents Chemother* 2000;**44**:590–7.

56 Jonas MM, Kelly DA, Mizerski J, *et al.* Clinical trial of lamivudine in children with chronic hepatitis B. *N Engl J Med* 2002;**346**:1706–13.

57 Sokal EM, Kelly DA, Mizerski J, *et al.* Long-term lamivudine therapy for children with HBeAg-positive chronic hepatitis B. *Hepatology* 2006;**43**:225–32.

58 Calio R, Villani E, Balestra E, *et al.* Enhancement of natural killer activity and interferon induction by different acyclic nucleoside phosphonates. *Antiviral Res* 1994;**23**:77–89.

59 Perillo R, Schiff E, Magill A, Murray A. In vivo demonstration of sensitivity of YMDD variants to adefovir. *Gastroenterology* 1999;**116**:A1261.

60 Sokal E, Jonas M, Kelly D, *et al.* Safety, efficacy and pharmacokinetics of adefovir dipivoxil in children and adolescents (age 2 to < 18) with chronic hepatitis B [abstract]. *J Pediatr Gastroenterol Nutr* 2007;**44**:e28.

61 Robinson DM, Scott LJ, Plosker GL. Entecavir: a review of its use in chronic hepatitis B. *Drugs* 2006;**66**:1605–22.

62 Colonno R, Rose R, Pokornowski K, *et al.* Assessment at three years shows high barrier to resistance is maintained in entecavir-treated nucleoside naïve patients while resistance emergence increases over time in lamivudine refractory patients [abstract]. *Hepatology* 2006;**44**:229A–230A.

63 Mutimer D, Dowling D, Cane O, *et al.* Additive antiviral effects of lamivudine and alpha-interferon in chronic hepatitis B infection. *Antiviral Ther* 2000;**5**:273–7.

64 Schalm SW, Heathcote J, Cianciara J, *et al.* Lamivudine and alpha interferon combination treatment of patients with chronic hepatitis B infection: a randomised trial. *Gut* 2000;**46**: 562–8.

65 D'Antiga L, Aw M, Atkins M, Moorat A, Vergani D, Mieli-Vergani G. Combined lamivudine/interferon-alpha treatment in "immunotolerant" children perinatally infected with hepatitis B: a pilot study. *J Pediatr* 2006;**148**:228–33.

66 Jara P, Bortolotti F. Interferon-(alpha) treatment of chronic hepatitis B in childhood: a consensus advice based on experience in European children. *J Pediatr Gastroenterol Nutr* 1999;**29**: 163–70.

67 Al-Taie OH, Mörk H, Gassel AM, Wilhelm M, Weissbrich B, Scheurlen M. Prevention of hepatitis B flare-up during chemotherapy using lamivudine: case report and review of the literature. *Ann Hematol* 1999;**78**:247–9.

68 Xunrong L, Yan AW, Liang R, Lau GK. Hepatitis B virus reactivation after cytotoxic or immunosuppressive therapy—pathogenesis and management. *Rev Med Virol* 2001;**11**:287–99.

69 Kawai Y, Ikegaya S, Hata M, *et al.* Successful lamivudine therapy for post-chemotherapeutic fulminant hepatitis B in a hepatitis B virus carrier with non-Hodgkin's lymphoma: case report and review of the literature. *Ann Hematol* 2001;**80**:482–4.

70 Saif MW, Little RF, Hamilton JM, Allegra CJ, Wilson's WH. Reactivation of chronic hepatitis B infection following intensive

chemotherapy and successful treatment with lamivudine: a case report and review of the literature. *Ann Oncol* 2001;**12**: 123–9.

71 Demetris AJ, Jaffe R, Sheahan DG, *et al.* Recurrent hepatitis B in liver allograft recipients: differentiation between viral hepatitis B and rejection. *Am J Pathol* 1986;**125**:161–72.

72 Mutimer D. Review article: hepatitis B and liver transplantation. *Aliment Pharmacol Ther* 2006;**23**:1031–41.

73 Brechot C, Bernuau J, Thiers V, *et al.* Multiplication of hepatitis B virus in fulminant hepatitis B. *BMJ* 1984;**288**:270–1.

74 Schmitz V, Qian C, Ruiz J, *et al.* Gene therapy for liver disease: recent strategies for treatment of viral hepatitis and liver malignancies. *Gut* 2002;**50**:130–5.

75 Lin YC, Chang MW, Ni YH, Hsu HY, Cheng DS. Long-term immunogenicity and efficacy of universal hepatitis B virus vaccination in Taiwan. *J Infect Dis* 2003;**187**:134–8.

76 Boxall EH, Sira J, El-Shukri N, Kelly DA. Long-term persistence of immunity to hepatitis B after vaccination during infancy in a country where endemicity is low. *J Infect Dis* 2004;**190**:1264–9.

77 Banatvala JE, Chrystie IL, Palmer SJ, Kenney A. Retrospective study of HIV, hepatitis B and HTLV–1 at a London antenatal clinic. *Lancet* 1990;**335**:859–60.

78 Boxall EH. Antenatal screening for carriers of hepatitis B virus. *BMJ* 1995;**311**:1178–9.

79 Lee C, Gong Y, Brok J, Boxall EH, Gluud C. Effect of hepatitis B immunisation in newborn infants of mothers positive for hepatitis B surface antigen: systematic review and meta-analysis. *BMJ* 2006;**332**:328–36.

80 Chang MH, Chen CJ, Lai MS, *et al.* Universal hepatitis B vaccination in Taiwan and the incidence of hepatocellular carcinoma in children. *N Engl J Med* 1997;**336**:1855–9.

81 Great Britain. Expert Advisory Group on AIDS. *Guidance for Clinical Health Care Workers: Protection against Infection with Blood-Borne Viruses: Recommendations of the Expert Advisory Group on AIDS and the Advisory Group on Hepatitis.* London: Department of Health, 1998.

82 Van Damme P, Vorsters A. Hepatitis B control in Europe by universal vaccination programmes: the situation in 2001. *J Med Virol* 2002;**67**:433–9.

83 Zanetti AR, Mariano A, Romano L, *et al.* Long-term immunogenicity of hepatitis B vaccination and policy for booster: an Italian multicentre study. *Lancet* 2005;**366**:1379–84.

84 Wallace LA, Young D, Brown A, *et al.* Costs of running a universal adolescent hepatitis B vaccination programme. *Vaccine* 2005;**23**: 5624–31.

85 Zuckerman J, van Hattum J, Cafferkey M, *et al.* Should hepatitis B vaccination be introduced into childhood immunisation programmes in northern Europe? *Lancet Infect Dis* 2007;**7**:410–9.

86 Rubin L, Hefer E, Dubnov Y, Warman S, Rishpon S. An evaluation of the efficacy of the national immunization programme for hepatitis B. *Public Health* 2007;**121**:529–33.

87 Bortolotti F, Iorio R, Resti M, *et al.* An epidemiological survey of hepatitis C virus infection in Italian children in the decade 1990–1999. *J Pediatr Gastroenterol Nutr* 2001;**32**:562–6.

88 Bunn SK, Sira J, Kelly DA. Paediatric hepatitis C—a single centre experience. *J Pediatr Gastroenterol Nutr* 2002;**32**:432.

89 National Institute for Clinical Excellence. *Guidance on the Use of Ribavirin and Interferon Alpha for Hepatitis C.* London: National Institute for Clinical Excellence, 2000. (Technology appraisal guidance, no. 14.)

90 Wreghitt TG, Gray JJ, Allain JP, *et al.* Transmission of hepatitis C virus by organ transplantation in the United Kingdom. *J Hepatol* 1994;**20**:768–72.

91 Tillmann HL, Manns MP. Mode of hepatitis C virus infection, epidemiology, and chronicity rate in the general population and risk groups. *Dig Dis Sci* 1996;**41**:27S–40S.

92 Tedder RS, Briggs M, Ring C, *et al.* Hepatitis C antibody profile and viraemia prevalence in adults with severe haemophilia. *Br J Haematol* 1991;**79**:512–5.

93 Ades AE, Parker S, Walker J, Cubitt WD, Jones R. HCV prevalence in pregnant women in the UK. *Epidemiol Infect* 2000; **125**:399–405.

94 Yeung LTF, King SM, Roberts EA. Mother-to-infant transmission of hepatitis C virus. *Hepatology* 2001;**34**:223–9.

95 European Paediatric Hepatitis C Virus Network. Effects of mode and delivery and infant feeding on the risk of mother-to-child transmission of hepatitis C virus. *BJOG* 2001;**108**:371–7.

96 Gibb DM, Goodall RL, Dunn DT, *et al.* Mother-to-child transmission of hepatitis C virus: evidence for preventable peripartum transmission. *Lancet* 2000;**356**:904–7.

97 Resti M, Azzari C, Mannelli F, *et al.* Mother to child transmission of hepatitis C virus: prospective study of risk factors and timing of infection in children born to women seronegative for HIV-1. *BMJ* 1998;**317**:437–41.

98 Boxall EH, Baumann K, Price N Sira J, Brown M, Kelly D. Discordant outcome of perinatal transmission of hepatitis C in twin pregnancies. *J Clin Virol* 2007;**38**:91–5.

99 Maccabruni A, Bossi G, Caselli D, *et al.* High efficiency of vertical transmission of hepatitis C virus among babies born to human immunodeficiency virus-negative women. *Pediatr Infect Dis J* 1995;**14**:921–2.

100 Paccagnini S, Principi N, Massironi E, *et al.* Perinatal transmission and manifestation of hepatitis C virus infection in a high risk population. *Pediatr Infect Dis J* 1995;**14**:195–9.

101 Tovo PA, Palombo E, Ferraris G, *et al.* Increased risk of maternal–infant hepatitis C virus transmission for women co-infected with human immunodeficiency virus type 1. *Clin Infect Dis*1997; **25**:1121–4.

102 Ruiz-Extremera A, Salmeron J, Torres C, *et al.* Follow-up of transmission of hepatitis C to babies of human immunodeficiency virus-negative women: the role of breast-feeding in transmission. *Pediatr Infect Dis J* 2000;**19**:511–6.

103 Macias J, Mira JA, López-Cortés LF, *et al.* Antiretroviral therapy based on protease inhibitors as a protective factor against liver fibrosis progression in patients with chronic hepatitis. *Antivir Ther* 2006;**11**:839–46.

104 Davison SM, Mieli-Vergani G, Sira J, Kelly DA. Perinatal hepatitis C virus infection: diagnosis and management. *Arch Dis Child* 2006;**91**:781–5.

105 Birnbaum AH, Shneider BL, Moy L. Hepatitis C in children. *N Engl J Med* 2000;**342**:290–1.

106 Fischer HP, Willsch E, Bierhoff E, Pfeifer U. Histopathologic findings in chronic hepatitis C. *J Hepatol* 1996;**24**(2 Suppl):35–42.

107 Thaler MM, Hu F, Heyman, M.B. Giant cell hepatitis due to hepatitis C infection. *Hepatology* 1992;**16**:74A.

108 Foster GR, Goldin RD, Thomas HC. Chronic hepatitis C virus infection causes a significant reduction in quality of life in the absence of cirrhosis. *Hepatology* 1998;**27**:209–12.
109 Harris HE, Ramsay ME, Heptonstall J, Soldan K, Eldridge KP. The HCV National Register: towards informing the natural history of hepatitis C infection in the UK. *J Viral Hepat* 2000;**7**: 420–7.
110 Harris HE, Ramsay ME, Andrews N, Eldridge KP. Clinical course of hepatitis C virus during the first decade of infection: cohort study. *BMJ* 2002;**324**:450–3.
111 Wiese M, Grungieff K, Guthoff W, *et al.* Outcome in a hepatitis C (genotype 1b) single source outbreak in Germany—a 25-year multicentre study. *J Hepatol* 2005;**43**:590–6.
112 Tovo PA, Pembrey LJ, Mewell ML. Persistence rate and progression of vertically acquired hepatitis C infection. *J Infect Dis* 2000;**181**:419–24.
113 Jara P, Resti M, Hierro L, *et al.* Chronic hepatitis C virus infection in childhood: clinical patterns and evolution in 224 white children. *Clin Infect Dis* 2003;**36**:275–80.
114 Bortolotti F, Resti M, Marcellini M, *et al.* Hepatitis C virus (HCV) genotypes in 373 Italian children with HCV infection; changing distribution and correlation with clinical features and outcome. *Gut* 2005;**54**:825–7.
115 European Paediatric Hepatitis C Virus Network. Three broad modalities in the natural history of vertically acquired hepatitis C virus infection. *Clin Infect Dis* 2005;**41**:45–51.
116 Vogt M, Lang T, Frosner G, *et al.* Prevalence and clinical outcome of hepatitis C infection in children who underwent cardiac surgery before the implementation of blood donor screening. *N Engl J Med* 1999;**341**:866–70.
117 Casiraghi MA, De Paschale M, Romano L, *et al.* Long-term outcome (35 years) of hepatitis C after acquisition of infection through mini transfusions of blood given at birth. *Hepatology* 2004;**39**:90–6.
118 Bunn S, Hubscher S, Kelly, D. The progression of hepatic inflammation and fibrosis in children with hepatitis C. *J Pediatr Gastroenterol Nutr* 2000;**31**:203.
119 Guido M, Bortolotti F, Leandro G, *et al.* Fibrosis in hepatitis C acquired in infancy: is it only a matter of time? *Am J Gastroenterol* 2003;**98**:660–3.
120 Badizadegan K, Jonas MM, Ott JJ, *et al.* Histopathology of the liver in children with chronic hepatitis C viral infection. *Hepatology* 1998;**28**:1416–23.
121 Harris HE, Mieli-Vergani G, Kelly D, Davison S, Gibb DM, Ramsay ME. A national sample of individuals who acquired hepatitis C virus infections in childhood or adolescence: risk factors for advanced disease. *J Pediatr Gastroenterol Nutr* 2007; **45**:335–41.
122 Gumber SC, Chopra S. Hepatitis C: a multifaceted disease. Review of extrahepatic manifestations. *Ann Intern Med* 1995; **123**:615–20.
123 Jacobson KR, Murray K, Zellos A, Schwarz KB. An analysis of published trials of interferon monotherapy in children with chronic hepatitis C. *J Pediatr Gastroenterol Nutr* 2002;**34**:52–8.
124 Nieforth KA, Nadeau R, Patal IH, Mould D. Use of an indirect pharmacodynamic simulation model of MX protein induction to compare in vivo activity of interferon alfa-2a and a polyethylene glycol-modified derivative in healthy subjects. *Clin Pharmacol Ther* 1996;**59**:636–46.
125 Schwarz KB, Mohan P, Narkewicz MR, *et al.* Safety, efficacy and pharmacokinetics of peginterferon alpha2a (40 kd) in children with chronic hepatitis C. *J Pediatr Gastroenterol Nutr* 2006;**43**: 499–505.
126 Kjaergard LL, Krogsgaard K, Gluud C. Ribavirin with or without alpha interferon for chronic hepatitis C. *Cochrane Database Syst Rev* 2002;(**2**):CD002234.
127 Lackner H, Moser A, Deutsch J, *et al.* Interferon-alpha and ribavirin in treating children and young adults with chronic hepatitis C after malignancy. *Pediatrics* 2000;**106**:E53.
128 Christensson B, Wiebe T, Akesson A, Widell A. Interferon-alpha and ribavirin treatment of hepatitis C in children with malignancy in remission. *Clin Infect Dis* 2000;**30**:585–6.
129 Woynarowski M, Socha J, Kuydowicz J, *et al.* Interferon and ribavirin versus interferon alone in treatment of chronic HCV infection in children. *J Pediatr Gastroenterol Nutr* 2001;**32**:48.
130 Gonzalez-Peralta RP, Kelly DA, Haber B, *et al.* Interferon alfa-2b in combination with ribavirin for children with chronic hepatitis C in children: efficacy, safety and pharmacokinetics. *Hepatology* 2005;**42**:1010–8.
131 Suoglu D, Elkabes B, Sokucu S, Saner G. Does interferon and ribavirin combination therapy increase the rate of treatment response in children with hepatitis C? *J Pediatr Gastroenterol Nutr* 2002;**34**:199–206.
132 Wirth S, Gehring S, Lang T, Gerner P. Treatment with alfa-interferon and ribavirin improves the response rate in children with chronic hepatitis C. *J Pediatr Gastroenterol Nutr* 2002;**34**: 439.
133 National Institute for Health and Clinical Excellence (Great Britain). *Peginterferon Alfa and Ribavirin for the Treatment of Mild Chronic Hepatitis C.* London: National Institute for Health and Clinical Excellence, 2006. (NICE Technology Appraisal Guidance, Quick Reference Guide 106.)
134 Fried MW, Shiffman ML, Reddy KR, *et al.* Peginterferon alfa-2a plus ribavirin for chronic hepatitis C infection. *N Engl J Med* 2002;**347**:975–83.
135 Wirth S, Pieper-Boustani H, Lang T, *et al.* Peginterferon alfa-2b plus ribavirin treatment in children and adolescents with chronic hepatitis C. *Hepatology* 2005;**41**:1013–8.
136 McHutchison JG, Manns MP, Brown RS, *et al.* Strategies for managing anemia in hepatitis C patients undergoing antiviral therapy. *Am J Gastroenterol* 2007;**102**:880–9.
137 Sinha M, Das A. Cost effectiveness analysis of different strategies of management of chronic hepatitis C infection in children. *Pediatr Infect Dis J* 2000;**19**:22–30.
138 Inati A, Taher A, Ghorra S, *et al.* Efficacy and tolerability of peginterferon alpha-2a with or without ribavirin in thalassaemia major patients with chronic hepatitis C virus infection. *Br J Haematol* 2005;**130**:644–6.
139 Butensky E, Pakbaz Z, Foote D, Walters MC, Vichinsky EP, Harmatz P. Treatment of hepatitis C virus infection in thalassemia. *Ann N Y Acad Sci* 2005;**1054**:290–9.
140 Gish RG. Treating HCV with ribavirin analogues and ribavirin-like molecules. *J Antimicrob Chemother* 2006;**57**:8–13. Erratum in *J Antimicrob Chemother* 2006;**58**:488.
141 Bain VG, Kaita KD, Yoshida EM, *et al.* A phase 2 study to evaluate the antiviral activity, safety and pharmacokinetics of recombinant human albumin-interferon alfa fusion protein in genotype 1 chronic hepatitis C patients. *J Hepatol* 2006;**44**:671–8.

142 De Francesco R, Migliaccio G. Challenges and successes in developing new therapies for hepatitis C. *Nature* 2005;**436**: 953–60.

143 Wakita T, Pietschmann T, Kato T, *et al.* Production of infectious hepatitis C virus in tissue culture from a cloned viral genome. *Nat Med* 2005;**11**:791–6.

144 Zhong J, Gastaminza P, Cheng G, *et al.* Robust hepatitis C virus infection in vitro. *Proc Natl Acad Sci USA* 2005;**102**:9294–9.

145 Lindenbach BD, Evans MJ, Syder AJ, *et al.* Complete replication of hepatitis C virus in cell culture. *Science* 2005;**309**:623–626.

146 Houghton M, Abrignani S. Prospects for a vaccine against the hepatitis C virus. *Nature* 2005;**436**:961–6.

147 Chang MH, Hadzic D, Rouassant SH, *et al.* Acute and chronic hepatitis: Working Group report of the second World Congress of Pediatric Gastroenterology, Hepatology, and Nutrition. *J Pediatr Gastroenterol Nutr* 2004;**39**(Suppl 2):S584–8.

148 Fattovich G, Giustina G, Christensen E, *et al.* Influence of hepatitis delta virus infection on morbidity and mortality in compensated cirrhosis type B. The European Concerted Action on Viral hepatitis (Eurohep) *Gut* 2000;**46**:420–6.

149 Farci P, Barbera C, Navone C, *et al.* Infection with delta agent in children. *Gut* 1985;**26**:4–7.

150 Ottobrelli A, Marzano A, Smedile A, *et al.* Patterns of hepatitis delta virus reinfection and disease in liver transplantation. *Gastroenterology* 1991;**101**:1649–55.

151 Mele A, Mariano A, Tosti ME, *et al.* Acute hepatitis delta virus infection in Italy: incidence and risk factors after the introduction of the universal anti-hepatitis B vaccination campaign. *Clin Infect Dis* 2007;**44**:e17–24.

152 Hoofnagle JH, Di Bisceglie AM. The treatment of chronic viral hepatitis. *N Engl J Med* 1997;**336**:347–56.

153 Arora NK, Panda SK, Nanda SK, *et al.* Hepatitis E infection in children: study of an outbreak. *J Gastroenterol Hepatol* 1999;**14**: 572–7.

154 Dalton HR, Thurairajah PH, Fellows HJ, *et al.* Autochthonous hepatitis E in southwest England. *J Viral Hepat* 2007;**14**:304–9.

155 Khuroo MS, Kamili S, Jameel S. Vertical transmission of hepatitis E virus. *Lancet* 1995;**345**:1025–6.

156 Ijaz S, Arnold E, Banks M, *et al.* Non-travel-associated hepatitis E in England and Wales: demographic, clinical and molecular epidemiological characteristics. *J Infect Dis* 2005;**192**:1166–72.

157 Banks M, Heath GS, Grierson SS, *et al.* Evidence for the presence of hepatitis E virus in pigs in the United Kingdom. *Vet Rec* 2004;**154**:223–7.

158 Jaroszewicz J, Flisiak R, Kalinowska A, Wierzbicka I, Prokopowicz D. Acute hepatitis E complicated by pancreatitis: a case report and literature review. *Pancreas* 2005;**30**:382–4.

159 Zamvar V, McClean P, Odeka E, Richards M, Davison S. Hepatitis E virus infection with non-immune haemolytic anemia. *J Pediatr Gastroenterol Nutr* 2005;**40**:1–3.

160 Hamid SS, Atiq M, Shehzad F, *et al.* Hepatitis E virus superinfection in patients with chronic liver disease. *Hepatology* 2002;**36**:474–8.

161 Peron JM, Danjoux M, Kamar N, *et al.* Liver histology in patients with sporadic acute hepatitis E: a study of 11 patients from South-West France. *Virchows Archiv* 2007;**450**:405–10.

162 Favorov MO, Fields HA, Purdy MA, *et al.* Serologic identification of hepatitis E virus infections in epidemic and endemic settings. *J Med Virol* 1992;**36**:246–50.

163 Shrestha MP, Scott RM, Joshi DM, *et al.* Safety and efficacy of a recombinant hepatitis E vaccine. *N Engl J Med* 2007;**356**;895–903.

164 Fagan EA, Ellis DS, Tovey GM, *et al.* Toga-like virus as a cause of fulminant hepatitis attributed to sporadic non-A, non-B. *J Med Virol* 1989;**28**:150–5.

165 Fagan EA, Ellis DS, Tovey GM, *et al.* Toga virus-like particles in acute liver failure attributed to sporadic non-A, non-B hepatitis and recurrence after liver transplantation. *J Med Virol* 1992;**38**: 71–7.

166 Linnen J, Wages J Jr, Zhang-Keck ZY, *et al.* Molecular cloning and disease association of hepatitis G virus: a transfusion-transmissible agent. *Science* 1996;**271**:505–8.

167 Lin HH, Kao JH, Chen PJ, Chen DS. Mechanism of vertical transmission of hepatitis G [letter]. *Lancet* 1996;**347**:1116.

168 Davison SM, Skidmore SJ, Collingham KE, Irving WL, Hubscher SG, Kelly DA. Chronic hepatitis in children after liver transplantation: role of hepatitis C virus and hepatitis G virus infections. *J Hepatol* 1998;**28**:764–70.

169 Sottini A, Mattioli S, Fiordalisis G, Imberti L, Moratto D, Primi D. Molecular and biological characterisation of SEN viruses: a family of viruses remotely related to the original TTV isolates. In: Margolis HS, Alter MJ, Liang TJ, Deinstag JL, eds. *Proceedings of the 10th International Symposium on Viral Hepatitis and Liver Disease.* Atlanta: International Medical Press, 2002:449–452.

170 Nishizawa T, Okamoto M, Konishi K, Yoshizawa H, Miyakawa Y, Mayumi M. A novel DNA virus (TTV) associated with elevated transaminase levels in posttransfusion hepatitis of unknown origin. *Biochem Biophys Res Commun* 1997:**241**:92–7.

171 Moriondo M, Resti M, Betti L, *et al.* SEN virus co-infection among HCV-RNA-positive mothers, risk of transmission to the offspring and outcome of child infection during a 1-year follow-up. *J Viral Hepat* 2007;**14**:355–9.

172 Hino S, Miyata H. Torque teno virus (TTV): current status. *Rev Med Virol* 2007;**17**:45–57.

173 Lee WS, McKiernan P, Kelly DA. Etiology, outcome and prognostic indicators of childhood fulminant hepatic failure in the United Kingdom. *J Pediatr Gastroenterol Nutr* 2005;**40**:575–81.

174 Squires RH, Shneider B, Bucuvalas J, *et al.* Acute liver failure in children: the first 348 patients in the pediatric acute liver failure study group. *J Pediatr* 2006;**148**:652–8.

175 Iterbeek P, Vandenberghe P, Nevens F, *et al.* Aplastic anaemia after transplantation for non-A, non-B, non-C fulminant hepatic failure: case report and review of the literature. *Transpl Int* 2002;**15**:117–23.

176 Khatib R, Siddique M, Abbass M. Measles-associated hepatobiliary disease: an overview. *Infection* 1993;**21**:112–4.

177 Makhene MK, Diaz PS. Clinical presentation and complications of suspected measles in hospitalized children. *Pediatr Infect Dis J* 1993;**12**:836–40.

178 Papadopoulou AL, Theodoridou M, Syriopoulou V, Mostron G, Kattamis CH. Hepatitis in children hospitalized with measles: the experience acquired after a Greek epidemic. *J Paediatr Child Health* 2001;**37**:55–7.

179 Vento S, Cainelli F, Ferraro T, Concia E. Autoimmune hepatitis type 1 after measles. *Am J Gastroenterol* 1996;**91**:2618–20.

180 Yoto Y, Kudoh T, Haseyama K, Suzuki N, Chiba S. Human parvovirus B 19 infection associated with acute hepatitis. *Lancet* 1996;**347**:868–9.

181 Naides SJ, Karetnyi YV, Cooling LL, Mark RS, Langnas AN. Human parvovirus B19 infection and hepatitis. *Lancet* 1996; **347**:1563–4.

182 Markin RS. Manifestations of Epstein–Barr virus-associated disorders in liver. *Liver* 1994;**14**:1–13.

183 Kimura H, Morishima T, Kanegane H, *et al.* Prognostic factors for chronic active Epstein–Barr virus infection. *J Infect Dis* 2003;**187**:527–33.

184 Kimura H. Pathogenesis of chronic active Epstein–Barr virus infection: is this an infectious disease, lymphoproliferative disorder, or immunodeficiency? *Rev Med Virol* 2006;**16**:251–61.

185 Kimberlin DW. Human herpesviruses 6 and 7: identification of newly recognized viral pathogens and their association with human disease. *Pediatr Infect Dis J* 1998;**17**:59–68.

186 Eksborg S, Pal N, Kalin M, Palm C, Söderhäll S. Pharmacokinetics of acyclovir in immunocompromised children with leukopenia and mucositis after chemotherapy: can intravenous acyclovir be substituted by oral valacyclovir? *Med Pediatr Oncol* 2002;**38**:240–6.

187 Frenkel LM, Capparelli EV, Dankner WM, *et al.* Oral ganciclovir in children: pharmacokinetics, safety, tolerance, and antiviral effects. The Pediatric AIDS Clinical Trials Group. *J Infect Dis* 2000;**182**:1616–24.

188 Castagnola E, Cristina E, Dufour C. High-dose oral ganciclovir for management of CMV-symptomatic infection in a child with acute lymphoblastic leukemia. *Med Pediatr Oncol* 2002;**38**:295–6.

189 Ljungman P, Deliliers GL, Platzbecker U, *et al.* Cidofovir for cytomegalovirus infection and disease in allogeneic stem cell transplant recipients. The Infectious Diseases Working Party of the European Group for Blood and Marrow Transplantation. *Blood* 2001;**97**:388–92.

190 Brundler MA, Rodriguez BN, Jaffe R, Weinberg AG, Rogers BB. Adenovirus ascending cholangiohepatitis. *Pediatr Dev Pathol* 2003;**6**:156–9.

191 Seidemann K, Heim A, Pfister ED, *et al.* Monitoring of adenovirus infection in pediatric transplant recipients by quantitative PCR: report of six cases and review of the literature. *Am J Transplant* 2004;**4**:2102–8.

192 Chou LL, Chang CP, Wu LC. Neonatal coxsackievirus B1 infection associated with severe hepatitis: report of three cases. *Zhonghua Min Guo Xiao Er Ke Yi Xue Hui Za Zhi* 1995;**36**:296–9.

193 Haddad J, Gut JP, Wendling MJ, *et al.* Enterovirus infection in neonates. A retrospective study of 21 cases. *Eur J Med* 1993;**2**:209–14.

194 Kadrofske M, Parimi P, Myers M, Kumar ML, Abughali N. Nonimmune hydrops fetalis and hepatitis in a neonate with congenital human immunodeficiency virus infection. *Pediatr Infect Dis J* 2006;**25**:952–4.

195 Persaud D, Bangaru B, Greco MA, *et al.* Cholestatic hepatitis in children infected with the human immunodeficiency virus. *Pediatr Infect Dis J* 1993;**12**:492–8.

196 Nigro G, Taliani G, Krzysztofiak A, *et al.* Multiple viral infections in HIV infected children with chronically evolving hepatitis. *Arch Virol* 1993;**8**:237–48.

197 Haydon GH, Mutimer DJ. Hepatitis B and C virus infections in the immune compromised. *Curr Opin Infect Dis* 2003;**16**:473–9.

198 Mauss S. Treatment of viral hepatitis in HIV-coinfected patients—adverse events and their management. *J Hepatol* 2006;**44**(1 Suppl):S114–8.

199 Poovorawan Y, Hutagalung Y, Chongsrisawat V, Boudville I, Bock HL. Dengue virus infection: a major cause of acute hepatic failure in Thai children. *Ann Trop Paediatr* 2006;**26**:17–23.

200 McCormick JB, King IJ, Webb PA, *et al.* Lassa fever: effective therapy with ribavirin. *N Engl J Med* 1986;**314**:20–6.

201 Ismail TF, Wasfy MO, Abdul RB, *et al.* Retrospective serosurvey of leptospirosis among patients with acute febrile illness and hepatitis in Egypt. *Am J Trop Med Hyg* 2006;**75**:1085–9.

202 Covic A, Maftei ID, Gusbeth TP. Acute liver failure due to leptospirosis successfully treated with MARS dialysis. *Int Urol Nephrol* 2007;**39**:313–6.

203 Murano I, Yoshii H, Kurashige K, Sugio Y, Tsukahara M. Giant hepatic granuloma caused by *Bartonella henselae. Pediatr Infect Dis J* 2001;**20**:319–20.

204 Craft JC, Ruff AJ. Protozoan infections. In: Nelson BC, ed. *Current Therapy in Paediatric Infectious Disease,* vol. 2. Toronto: Decker, 1988: ??–??.

205 Sailer M, Soelder B, Allerberger F, Zaknun D, Feichtinger H, Gottstein B. Alveolar echinococcosis of the liver in a six-year-old girl with acquired immunodeficiency syndrome. *J Pediatr* 1997;**130**:320–3.

206 Bari S, Sheikh KA, Ashraf M, Hussain Z, Hamid A, Mufti GN. *Ascaris* liver abscess in children. *J Gastroenterol* 2007;**42**:236–40.

207 Pawlowski ZS. Roundworm infections. In: Nelson BC, ed. *Current Therapy in Paediatric Infectious Disease,* vol. 2. Toronto: Decker, 1988: ??–??.

208 Markell EK. Trematode infections. In: Nelson BC, ed. *Current Therapy in Paediatric Infectious Disease,* vol. 2. Toronto: Decker, 1988: ??–??.

209 Barnes PF, De Cock KM, Reynolds TN, Ralls PW. A comparison of amebic and pyogenic abscess of the liver. *Medicine* 1987;**66**: 472–83.

210 Wolfsen HC, Bolen JW, Bowen JL, Fenster LF. Fulminant herpes hepatitis mimicking hepatic abscesses. *J Clin Gastroenterology* 1993;**16**:61–4.

211 Garcia-Eulate R, Hussain N, Heller T, *et al.* CT and MRI of hepatic abscess in patients with chronic granulomatous disease. *AJR Am J Roentgenol* 2006;**187**:482–90.

212 Doerr CA, Demmler GJ, Garcia-Prats JA, Brandt ML. Solitary pyogenic liver abscess in neonates: report of three cases and review of the literature. *Pediatr Infect Dis J* 1994;**13**:64–9.

213 Lublin M, Bartlett DL, Danforth DN, *et al.* Hepatic abscess in patients with chronic granulomatous disease. *Ann Surg* 2002;**235**:383–91.

214 Erdman SH, Barber BJ, Barton LL. *Aspergillus* cholangitis: a late complication after Kasai portoenterostomy. *J Pediatr Surg* 2002;**37**:923–5.

7 Acute Liver Failure

Peter F. Whitington, Estella M. Alonso, and Robert H. Squires

Definition

The broadest definition of acute liver failure (ALF) is hepatic necrosis resulting in loss of liver function within weeks or a few months of the onset of clinical liver disease.[1–3] ALF is the current preferred name for such disease, although other terms—such as "fulminant hepatic failure" and "fulminant hepatitis"—have been used in the medical literature to describe this condition. The narrow definition of ALF that is currently accepted includes the onset of hepatic encephalopathy and coagulopathy (which defines failure of liver function) within 8 weeks of the onset of liver disease and the absence of preexisting liver disease in any form.[4] It is important to realize that there are several problems with this definition in children. First, some patients with acute hepatocellular disease develop encephalopathy later than 8 weeks into the course of the illness and are defined as having subacute hepatic failure, subacute hepatic necrosis, or late-onset hepatic failure. Second, acute liver failure may be the first presentation of a previously unrecognized autoimmune or metabolic liver disease—e.g., Wilson's disease or tyrosinemia type I. Third, many cases of hepatic failure in neonates are secondary to an inborn metabolic error or an intrauterine insult, which would represent a preexisting disease. In addition, encephalopathy may be difficult to detect in infants and small children and may be less severe than coagulopathy. Finally, some important pediatric disorders—such as Reye syndrome and inborn errors of metabolism mimicking Reye syndrome—produce a syndrome similar to acute liver failure in which the encephalopathy is metabolic and secondary to liver failure. A consensus of the members of the Pediatric Acute Liver Failure (PALF) Study Group, a multicenter and multinational consortium, resulted in a working definition for ALF that is the summation of clinical and biochemical parameters, as follows:

- The acute onset of liver disease with no known evidence of chronic liver disease
- Biochemical and/or clinical evidence of severe liver dysfunction:

Diseases of the Liver and Biliary System in Children, 3rd edition. Edited by Deirdre Kelly. © 2008 Blackwell Publishing, ISBN: 978-1-4051-6334-7.

—Hepatic-based coagulopathy, with a prothrombin time (PT) $\geq$ 20 s or international normalized ratio (INR) $\geq$ 2.0, that is not corrected by parenteral vitamin K
—And/or hepatic encephalopathy (must be present if the PT is 15.0–19.9 s or INR 1.5–1.9, but not if PT $\geq$ 20 s or INR $\geq$ 2.0)

In the United Kingdom, the unique difficulty in detecting encephalopathy in infants means that this is no longer a criterion for super-urgent listing for transplantation.

Etiology

The etiology of acute liver failure is age-dependent (Table 7.1).[5] While acute viral hepatitis is the most common identifiable cause in all series, there is a distinct geographical impact on the frequency of diagnosis, particularly with regard to the frequency with which hepatitis A and B infections are implicated. Table 7.2 details the causes of ALF in children enrolled in the PALF study, representing the incidence of causation in 19 pediatric sites in the United States, Canada, and the United Kingdom (see also Chapter 24).

Infectious disease

Hepatitis virus infection

Early reports of ALF in children suggest that viral hepatitis accounts for the largest proportion of ALF in children of all age groups. In a series of 31 children with ALF in London,[6] 26 (84%) had presumed viral hepatitis, and all 33 children reported from Cape Town[7] had viral hepatitis. In a recent series of 97 children with ALF in the United Kingdom, 47 (48%) had infectious causes, including indeterminate hepatitis.[8] However, in the 348 children enrolled in the PALF study, identified viral infection accounted for less than 6% of cases, with the most common viral causes being herpes simplex virus in children < 3 years of age and Epstein–Barr infection in children $\geq$ 3 years of age. There were three cases of hepatitis A and one case of hepatitis C.[9] Acute hepatitis A virus (HAV) infection is a relatively frequently diagnosed cause of ALF, particularly where HAV is endemic or in the setting of a regional outbreak of HAV. The prevalence of HAV among patients of all ages with acute liver failure in

Table 7.1 Causes of acute hepatic failure in children.

Etiology	Disease	Incidence
Neonates		
Infectious	Herpesviruses, echovirus, adenovirus, HBV	Frequent
Metabolic*	Galactosemia,* tyrosinemia,* neonatal Hemochromatosis,* mitochondrial disease	Moderately frequent
Ischemia	Congenital heart disease, cardiac surgery, myocarditis, severe asphyxia	Rare
Older children		
Infectious	HAV, HBV, NA–G, herpesviruses, sepsis,* other	Frequent
Drugs	Valproate, isoniazid, acetaminophen, carbamazepine, halothane	Moderately frequent
Toxins	*Amanita phalloides,* carbon tetrachloride, phosphorus	Rare
Metabolic*	Hereditary fructose intolerance,* Wilson's disease†	Rare
Autoimmune	Hepatitis	Rare
Ischemia	Congenital heart disease, cardiac surgery, myocarditis, severe asphyxia, Budd–Chiari syndrome	Rare
Other	Malignancy	Rare

HAV, hepatitis A virus; HBV, hepatitis B virus; NA–G, non-A–G virus.
* These diseases do not fulfill the definition of ALF.
† Rare under 3 years.

published series has varied from as low as 1.5% to as high as 31%. Not surprisingly, HAV is a frequent cause of acute liver failure in reports from developing countries, but also in pediatric series from developed countries.[8,10] In the United States, HAV generally causes < 5% of cases of acute liver failure. New indications for using the hepatitis A vaccine may reduce the incidence of ALF in certain regions.[11]

The prevalence of acute hepatitis B virus (HBV) infection in large series of acute liver failure ranges from 25% to 75%, making it the commonest cause worldwide.[12–14] The overall rate of acute liver failure in acute HBV infection is estimated to be about 1%. It is uncommon to document HBV infection in children with acute liver failure from western Europe and the United States, as demonstrated in the PALF study, except in infants born to mothers who are positive for HBV and negative for hepatitis B e antigen (HB_eAg), while in endemic areas it plays a much greater role.[15] The prognosis in HBV-related acute liver failure is generally worse than with other etiologies, with spontaneous recovery occurring in fewer than 20% of cases.[16] Fortunately, universal hepatitis B vaccination in endemic areas of the world, such as Taiwan, has resulted in a significant decline in the mortality associated with ALF secondary to HBV.[17]

Hepatitis C virus (HCV) is a very unusual cause for acute liver failure.[18] Hepatitis D virus and hepatitis E virus have rarely been associated with acute liver failure in children, although hepatitis E infection is common in endemic areas and in returning travelers. Hepatitis G virus and transfusion-transmitted virus do not cause acute liver failure (see also Chapter 24).

Infection with viruses other than hepatitis viruses

The viruses in the herpes family are highly cytopathic and can cause severe hepatic necrosis, often in the absence of significant inflammation. Herpes simplex virus (HSV), varicella-zoster virus, cytomegalovirus, and Epstein–Barr virus (EBV) have been reported to cause acute liver failure, almost always in immunocompromised hosts, with EBV most frequently implicated.[19] Paramyxovirus, parvovirus B19, and togavirus have been identified in some cases.

Acute liver failure in the neonate may result from infection with many different viruses that do not characteristically cause severe hepatitis in older individuals. HSV, cytomegalovirus, EBV, echovirus (principally type 11), adenovirus, and coxsackievirus have been observed to cause acute liver failure in infants. The reasons for this susceptibility are poorly understood.

Nonviral infectious hepatitis

Infectious agents other than viruses rarely lead to acute liver

Table 7.2 Final diagnosis in children with acute liver failure in the Pediatric Acute Liver Failure (PALF) Study registry.

Diagnosis	Age group		
	< 3 years (%)	> 3 years (%)	Total (%)
	162 (39)	256 (6)	418
Acetaminophen (n = 48)	2 (2)	46 (21)	48 (14)
Indeterminate (n = 169)	68 (54)	101 (46)	169 (49)
Autoimmune (n = 22)	6 (5)	16 (7)	22 (6)
Infectious (n = 20)	9 (7)	11 (5)	20 (6)
Adenovirus (n = 2)	1 (1)	1 (0)	2 (1)
Cytomegalovirus (n = 1)	1 (1)	0 (0)	1 (0)
Epstein–Barr virus (n = 6)	1 (1)	5 (2)	6 (2)
Enterovirus (n = 1)	1 (1)	0 (0)	1 (0)
Hepatitis A (n = 3)	0 (0)	3 (1)	3 (1)
Hepatitis C (n = 1)	0 (0)	1 (0)	1 (0)
Herpes simples virus (n = 6)	5 (4)	1 (0)	6 (2)
Non-acetaminophen drug–induced liver disease (n = 17)	1 (1)	16 (7)	17 (5)
Mushroom (n = 2)	0 (0)	2 (1)	2 (1)
Anesthetic (n = 1)	0 (0)	1 (0)	1 (0)
Co-trimoxazole (Bactrim) (n = 1)	0 (0)	1 (0)	1 (0)
Pemoline (Cylert) (n = 1)	0 (0)	1 (0)	1 (0)
Cyclophosphamide (Cytoxan)/phenytoin (Dilantin) (n = 1)	0 (0)	1 (0)	1 (0)
Phenytoin (Dilantin) (n = 1)	0 (0)	1 (0)	1 (0)
Isoniazid (n = 2)	0 (0)	2 (1)	2 (1)
Iron (n = 1)	0 (0)	1 (0)	1 (0)
Methotrexate (n = 1)	0 (0)	1 (0)	1 (0)
Minocycline (n = 1)	0 (0)	1 (0)	1 (0)
Pravastatin (n = 1)	0 (0)	1 (0)	1 (0)
Valproate (n = 3)	1 (1)	2 (1)	3 (1)
Metabolic (n = 36)	23 (18)	13 (6)	36 (10)
α_1-Antitrypsin (n = 1)	1 (1)	0 (0)	1 (0)
Fatty acid oxidation defect (n = 4)	4 (3)	0 (0)	4 (1)
Galactosemia (n = 2)	2 (2)	0 (0)	2 (1)
Fructose intolerance (n = 1)	1 (1)	0 (0)	1 (0)
Mitochondrial disorder (n = 4)	2 (2)	2 (1)	4 (1)
Niemann–Pick type C (n = 1)	1 (1)	0 (0)	1 (0)
Respiratory chain defect (n = 7)	7 (6)	0 (0)	7 (2)
Reye syndrome (n = 1)	0 (0)	1 (0)	1 (0)
Tyrosinemia (n = 4)	4 (3)	0 (0)	4 (1)
Urea cycle defect (n = 2)	1 (1)	1 (0)	2 (1)
Wilson's disease (n = 9)	0 (0)	9 (4)	9 (3)
Other (n = 20)	11 (9)	9 (4)	20 (6)
Budd–Chiari (n = 2)	0 (0)	2 (1)	2 (1)
Hemophagocytic syndrome (n = 4)	2 (2)	2 (1)	4 (1)
Leukemia (n = 2)	1 (1)	1 (0)	2 (1)
Neonatal hemochromatosis (n = 6)	6 (5)	0 (0)	6 (2)

failure. These include: congenital syphilis, leptospirosis, and —in endemic areas—*Coxiella burnetii* (Q fever), *Plasmodium falciparum*, and *Entamoeba histolytica*. Systemic sepsis may occasionally present as acute liver failure[20] (see also Chapter 17).

Indeterminate hepatitis

Hepatitis of indeterminate cause, formerly referred to as sporadic non-A–E hepatitis, is diagnosed when there is evidence of acute hepatitis in the absence of markers for hepatitis virus infection, the absence of clinical and/or serological evidence of systemic infection with other infectious agents, no exposure to drugs or toxins, and negative markers of autoimmune disease.[2] It is clearly the most important cause of acute liver failure in children in Western developed countries, comprising the vast majority of pediatric acute liver failure cases in series from western Europe and the United States.[8,21] In the PALF series, 169 of 300 non-acetaminophen cases were attributed to acute hepatitis of indeterminate cause. The prognosis in indeterminate acute liver failure is poor, with a rate of spontaneous recovery ranging from 5% to 43%,[8,9,21,22] indicating the need for early referral to a liver transplant center.

Drug and toxin-related hepatic injury

(see also Chapter 10)

After viral hepatitis, liver injury due to drugs and toxins is the most common etiology of acute liver failure in children and adults.[22] Table 7.3 lists the drugs and toxins that have been associated with acute liver failure in children, grouped according to their mechanism of action.[23] The three most common drugs implicated in children are acetaminophen,[24] isoniazid, and propylthiouracil. Halothane hepatitis is more frequent in adults, but has also been observed in children. Fourteen percent of cases in the PALF study were the result of acetaminophen overdose. Acetaminophen may also be responsible for some cases of ALF in which a cause is not readily identified. The role of fasting and alcohol consumption in potentiating acetaminophen toxicity in patients exposed to high doses (60–100 mg/kg) remains controversial,[24,25] but they appear to increase liver damage in children. New techniques for identifying serum markers of acetaminophen hepatotoxicity in patients with ALF may help unravel this question.[26] Patients with hepatic injury secondary to acetaminophen ingestion have a higher rate of recovery than do patients with viral hepatitis and should be observed as long as possible before liver transplantation is considered.[27,28] Drugs that cause steatosis (sodium valproate, amiodarone) may cause liver failure. The complex chemotherapy that is used to treat childhood cancer may occasionally result in hepatic failure.

Table 7.3 Drugs and toxins associated with acute liver failure.

*Hepatotoxic agents**
Acetaminophen overdose
Chlorinated hydrocarbons
Amanita species
Salicylate (overdose)
$FeSO_4$ (overdose)
2-Nitropropane
Yellow phosphorus
Solvents
Drugs associated with idiosyncratic reactions
Isoniazid
Propylthiouracil
Sodium valproate
Halothane
Amiodarone
Nonsteroidal anti-inflammatory agents
Tetracycline
Carbamazepine
Lamotrigene
Recreational drugs associated with hepatic injury
Cocaine
Ecstasy

* Listed in approximate order of frequency as causes of acute liver failure in children. Mechanism of action according to Arundel and Lewis.[23]

Autoimmune hepatitis

Autoimmune hepatitis has been reported as a common cause of liver failure in patients referred for liver transplantation.[29] Children with both type I and type II autoimmune hepatitis have been reported with acute liver failure, although it is more common in type II.[20,30,31] In the PALF study, autoimmune hepatitis accounted for 6% of pediatric patients registered. Many of these patients will respond to medical therapy (corticosteroid and azathioprine), avoiding the need for transplantation. Liver biopsy shows signs of chronic hepatitis (portal fibrosis and piecemeal necrosis), in addition to severe lobular hepatitis. The majority of patients have titers of antinuclear, anti-smooth muscle, or anti-liver–kidney microsomal antibodies in serum and elevated immunoglobulin G (IgG).

Inherited and metabolic diseases

In the PALF study, metabolic disease—including α_1-antitrypsin deficiency and Wilson's disease—accounted for 10% of pediatric patients registered. The metabolic disorders that present in the neonatal period or infancy with hepatic failure are galactosemia, hereditary fructose intolerance, tyrosinemia type I, and neonatal hemochromatosis.[32] Inborn errors of bile acid synthesis can rarely present as acute liver failure in infancy. Zellweger disease and Alpers disease cause cerebral degeneration and disordered hepatic function, and may present with acute liver failure and be confused with primary hepatic failure if the neurological symptoms characteristic of these disorders are not obvious.[33,34] Disorders of fatty acid oxidation and of oxidative phosphorylation produce episodes of recurrent hepatic dysfunction and coma that can be confused with Reye syndrome or severe hepatitis at any age. Wilson's disease is most likely to produce acute liver failure in the older child.

Other causes of acute hepatic failure in children are listed in Table 7.1.

Pathology

The pathological features of acute liver failure differ depending on the etiology. There are three basic lesions.

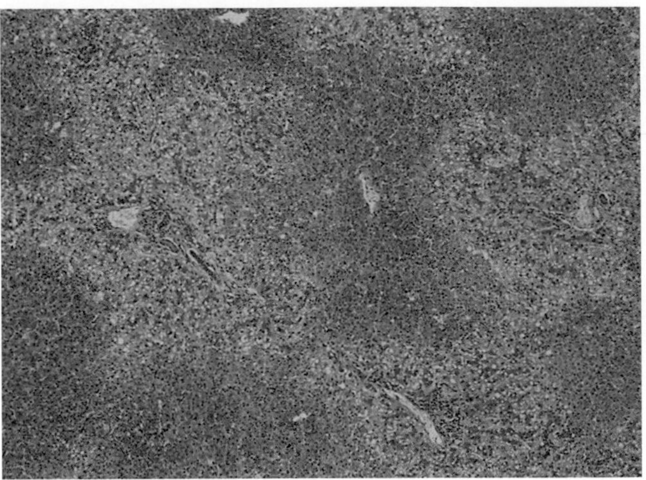

Figure 7.1 Liver histology is usually obtained postmortem or at transplantation. There is usually severe hepatic necrosis with reticulin collapse and biliary proliferation, irrespective of etiology.

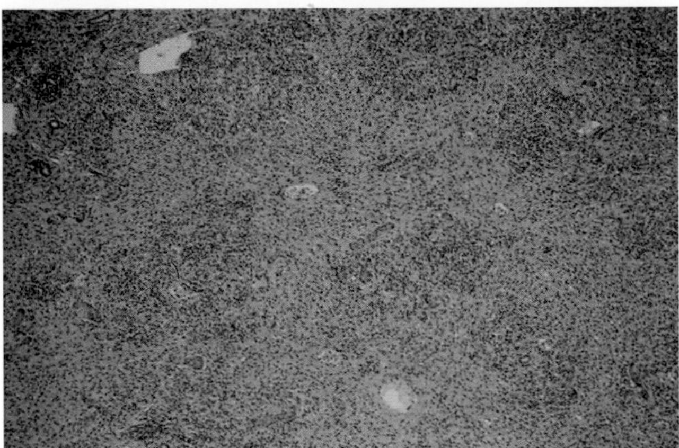

Figure 7.2 Acute liver failure secondary to viral hepatitis may show significant lobular inflammation, which may differentiate it from drug toxicity.

Hepatic necrosis

Severe hepatitis with loss of lobular architecture, secondary to extensive hepatocyte necrosis with collapse of the reticulin framework, characterizes the pathological lesion seen in either viral infection[35] or an idiosyncratic drug reaction (Figure 7.1). In viral hepatitis, necrosis tends to be panacinar in distribution, while in toxic injury it is zonal (Figure 7.2). There may be diffuse necrosis of individual hepatocytes, or pericentral sublobular necrosis. Most acute liver failure is associated with massive confluent necrosis.[36–39] In many cases, it is difficult to identify any remaining viable hepatocytes. The reticulin framework of the lobule is collapsed, and the mass of the liver is small. A moderate acute inflammatory infiltrate may be evident, and this may be helpful in establishing the etiology. In indeterminate hepatitis, for instance, there may be lymphoid aggregates around the bile ducts, with congestion of centrilobular sinusoids. In HBV hepatitis, there is a minimal inflammatory infiltrate, while in EBV fulminant hepatitis, centrilobular necrosis with bridging and collapse may be obvious, with cholestasis and lymphoid "blast cells." In some cases, no evidence of regeneration can be found,[40] while in others there is a proliferation of duct-like structures that probably results from attempts at regeneration. The degree and pattern of necrosis do not correlate with the development of encephalopathy or cerebral edema.[36,38]

Hepatocellular degeneration

In ALF due to metabolic or toxic injuries in children, the prominent lesion is hepatocellular degeneration with diffuse fatty infiltration of hepatocytes.[23,41] There is minimal hepatocyte necrosis or inflammatory infiltrate. In Reye syndrome and similar disorders, the intracellular fat is microvesicular and does not displace the nuclei. This lesion is seen in association with toxic injury (valproic acid, aspirin) and inborn errors of metabolism (disorders of fatty acid oxidation). Rarely, macrovesicular steatosis is seen with drug and toxic injury (hydrocarbon ingestion, amiodarone therapy). The absence of cell necrosis in association with failure of liver function implies organelle failure as the etiology. The hepatic mass is usually increased, and hepatomegaly is evident. Serum aminotransferase levels are usually elevated, but only to a mild to moderate degree (usually < 400 IU/L), indicating that hepatocytes generally remain intact. Jaundice is minimal (serum bilirubin usually < 200 μmol/L), which suggests that some organelle function remains intact and also that bilirubin production is probably not increased. Full histological recovery is the rule if the patient survives.[32]

Patients with acute liver failure due to hereditary fructose intolerance, acute-onset tyrosinemia type I, and—to a lesser degree—galactosemia have a lesion characterized by diffuse swelling of hepatocytes with condensation of organelles and cytoplasmic elements. Hepatocyte necrosis is spotty and usually not prominent. Macrovesicular fat with displacement of nuclei is seen in a variable proportion of hepatocytes, sometimes a majority. This lesion suggests organelle injury, probably resulting from chemical alteration of macromolecules that is severe enough to cause the death of some hepatocytes. Aminotransferase levels and serum bilirubin levels are moderately elevated. Full histological recovery is the rule if the metabolic injury can be controlled.

Underlying cirrhosis

In acute liver failure due to either tyrosinemia type I or Wilson's disease, the pathological features will include preexisting cirrhosis (see Chapters 5 and 14).

Recovery

Spontaneous recovery from acute liver failure is usually associated with complete histological recovery, even when extensive necrosis is present. Recovery from massive confluent necrosis is distinctly unusual, but when it occurs, postnecrotic cirrhosis often remains.[37,38]

Biochemistry

The serum aminotransferase levels (alanine aminotransferase, aspartate aminotransferase) are usually markedly elevated in children with acute liver failure. Levels are almost always above 1000 IU/L and may reach values above 10 000. Peak values tend to be higher in nonsurvivors, but aminotransferase values are not predictive of outcome.[42] Rapidly falling aminotransferase values signify "exhaustion" of the hepatocyte mass and terminal hepatic failure, unless associated with evidence of functional recovery such as improved coagulation and reduced encephalopathy.[43]

Marked jaundice is typically seen with severe hepatic necrosis.[44] Serum bilirubin concentrations typically range from 200 to 1200 μmol/L. The rate of increase in serum bilirubin often exceeds that expected with a normal rate of production and zero clearance. Increased production may result from catabolism of hepatic heme proteins or from hemolysis. Early in the course, most of the serum bilirubin is in the conjugated form, indicating excretory dysfunction of viable hepatocytes. Later, most of the bilirubin may be unconjugated, indicating loss of conjugating ability. Children with acetaminophen poisoning, fulminant hepatitis secondary to hepatitis B, and metabolic disease may be anicteric or only mildly jaundiced.

Pathogenesis

Fulminant hepatitis leads to multisystem organ failure, particularly affecting the brain and kidney. The process leading to hepatic injury is not known, but it is multifactorial and dependent on the balance between the following factors:

- Susceptibility of the host—e.g., neonate who develops fulminant HBV
- Severity and nature of hepatic injury—e.g., dose of acetaminophen
- The ability of the liver to regenerate

Liver regeneration

The ability of the liver to regenerate is a crucial factor for survival. Many patients who die with fulminant hepatic failure show some evidence of hepatic regeneration, while in others there is no sign of regeneration. It is possible that failure of regeneration is due to prolonged viral injury and persistent viral replication, with failure of eradication of the virus, as patients with ALF due to acetaminophen or other drug poisoning or hepatitis A have a better prognosis than those with indeterminate hepatitis.

Encephalopathy

Encephalopathy is a unique feature of ALF that occurs in the majority of children with acute liver failure. It results from an indirect effect of hepatocyte failure on the function of the brain,[45–47] although the neuropharmacological events that lead to clinical hepatic encephalopathy are complex and not yet completely understood. In acute liver failure, the presumption is that hepatocyte dysfunction has progressed to a point following which the liver fails to produce appropriate amounts of neuroregulatory substances, and/or fails to eliminate neurotoxins, resulting in brain dysfunction. Over the years, there have been many candidates for potential neurotransmitters or neurotoxins; these have included ammonia, glutamine, short-chain fatty acids, amino acids, mercaptans and octopamine, and more recently γ-aminobutyric acid (GABA). No neuropathological abnormalities associated with acute hepatic encephalopathy are considered irreversible. Cerebral edema is a separate entity that complicates acute liver failure and may be reversible in the early stages only.[46]

Clinical manifestations

Clinical presentation

The clinical presentation varies depending on the etiology, but essentially there is hepatic dysfunction with hypoglycemia, coagulopathy, and encephalopathy. Jaundice may be a late feature, particularly in metabolic disease. The clinical onset may be within hours or weeks. Most pediatric patients who develop acute liver failure are previously healthy, with no history of major medical problems and no clear exposure to hepatitis or toxins.

All forms of viral hepatitis have similar clinical features. There may be a prodromal illness, with a "flu-like" syndrome of malaise, myalgia, nausea, vomiting, and diarrhea, and subsequent jaundice. While these findings may be typical of acute viral hepatitis, they are not specific for a viral etiology. The disease may progress rapidly at this stage, or deterioration may occur after a period of improvement.

Warning signs of progressive disease are:

- Prolonged prothrombin time that is unresponsive to vitamin K (particularly at presentation)
- Persistent jaundice, with a rapid increase in bilirubin in association with a progressive decline in serum aminotransferase levels
- Decreasing liver size
- Increasing lethargy or occasionally hallucinations
- Rarely, hemorrhagic diathesis and systemic collapse

By the time the disease is established, the patient is deeply jaundiced and fetor hepaticus is often evident. Features of encephalopathy such as drowsiness, confusion, aggression, incontinence, and lack of response to painful stimuli are common. The liver size may be large, normal or small, depending on the stage of the disease. The patient may bleed from needle puncture sites, the nose, or the gastrointestinal tract.

Laboratory evaluation will demonstrate:

• Marked conjugated hyperbilirubinemia. Occasional exceptions are observed—as in some cases of drug-induced hepatitis, fulminant hepatitis B, and in idiopathic anicteric fulminant failure.[48]
• Aminotransferases—alanine aminotransferase (ALT), aspartate aminotransferase (AST)—may be very high (> 1000 IU/L), or may have fallen precipitously since their last measurement (in concert with a decreasing liver size, reflecting severe necrosis and collapse of hepatic mass).
• Plasma ammonia is usually elevated by two to eight times (> 100 μmol/L).
• Serum creatinine may be elevated secondary to renal complications, while the urea may be high (renal dysfunction, increased production from blood in the gastrointestinal tract, dehydration) or low (failure of hepatic synthesis).
• Hypoglycemia may be present and difficult to correct.
• Arterial blood gas analysis may show a wide spectrum of abnormalities, ranging from respiratory alkalosis to mixed respiratory and metabolic acidosis, usually in association with hypoxemia.
• Electrolyte abnormalities are associated with vomiting and dehydration.
• Coagulation profiles demonstrate deficiencies of clotting factors and often evidence of consumptive coagulopathy.
• The platelet count is often reduced, due to consumption or reduced production (aplastic anemia occurs in 10–20% of cases of indeterminate hepatitis).
• The white blood cell count varies from high (stress response, secondary bacterial infection) to low (aplastic anemia).

Diagnosis

The diagnosis is established by the combination of clinical and biochemical features and specific diagnostic tests (Table 7.4). A histological diagnosis by liver biopsy is not critical for patient management and may be dangerous because of the abnormal coagulation. The risk of biopsy can only be justified when atypical clinical features exist or a potentially treatable condition, such as autoimmune hepatitis, is likely. Transjugular biopsy to reduce the risk of bleeding is technically possible in children other than infants.

Table 7.4 Investigations in acute severe hepatitis.

Baseline essential investigations
Biochemistry
Bilirubin, transaminases
Alkaline phosphatase
Albumin
Urea and electrolytes
Creatinine
Calcium, phosphate
Ammonia
Acid–base, lactate
Glucose
Hematology
Full blood count, platelets
PT, PTT
Factors V or VII
Blood group cross-match
Septic screen
Omitting lumbar puncture
Imaging
Chest radiograph
Abdominal ultrasound
Head CT scan or MRI
Neurophysiology
EEG
Diagnostic investigations
Serum
Acetaminophen levels
Cu, ceruloplasmin (> 3 years)
Autoantibodies
Immunoglobulins
Amino acids
Hepatitis A, B, C, E
EBV, CMV, HSV
Leptospira (if clinically relevant)
Other viruses
Urine
Toxic metabolites
Amino acids, succinylacetone
Organic acids
Reducing sugars

CMV, cytomegalovirus; CT, computed tomography; EBV, Epstein–Barr virus; EEG, electroencephalography; HSV, herpes simplex virus; MRI, magnetic resonance imaging; PT, prothrombin time; PTT, partial thromboplastin time.

Management

There is no specific therapy for ALF except hepatic replacement. Management is therefore directed towards early consideration for liver transplantation, hepatic support, and the prevention and treatment of complications, while awaiting recovery or a suitable donor for liver transplantation.[49–51] The key elements are medical support in the setting of an intensive-care unit and rapid referral to a transplant center.

It is essential to take a full history from the parents, which would include establishing appropriate risk factors such as information on intravenous injections, infusions of blood products, drugs, foreign travel, or contact with jaundice. It is important to establish which medications family members are taking, and in adolescents to enquire about drug addiction and sexual contact. Over-the-counter medications, particularly those containing acetaminophen, should be queried specifically, as the family may not consider these to be significant enough to volunteer the information that they are being used. The use of herbal teas and availability of potentially toxic mushrooms should be included in the history.

The initial physical examination should establish hepatic, cerebral, cardiovascular, respiratory, renal, and acid–base status. The patient's conscious state and degree of coma should be established and a complete central nervous system examination performed.

Evidence of chronic liver disease or other signs that may indicate etiology, such as Kayser–Fleischer rings, cataracts, and needle marks, should be established. Liver size should be measured and marked on the abdomen.

The presence of impaired central nervous system function with acute liver disease is an indication for immediate hospitalization, independent of any other clinical or biochemical findings.

General measures

Management should be in an intensive-care unit setting with routine intensive-care monitoring. Until a diagnosis is made, it is assumed that all children are infectious and that all blood, excretions, and secretions are potentially capable of transmitting viral hepatitis. Enteric isolation procedures must be enforced (Table 7.5).

A central venous catheter is useful for assessment of central venous pressure and volume status, but may require surgical placement with coagulation support. An indwelling arterial line for continuous measurement of blood pressure and for biochemical and acid–base monitoring is essential. A nasogastric tube is passed and placed to gravity, with regular gentle saline lavage to detect upper gastrointestinal hemorrhage. The urinary bladder is catheterized and strict output records are maintained to help in the evaluation of fluid status and renal function.

Baseline biochemical and other investigations should be performed (Table 7.4) and management instigated as in Table 7.5 and Figure 7.2. Frequency of monitoring will depend on the severity of illness, ranging from daily in mild cases to 4-hourly to 6-hourly in patients in stage III and IV coma, and should include:

- Complete blood count
- Blood gases and electrolytes
- Aminotransferases
- Prothrombin time
- Daily monitoring of plasma creatinine, bilirubin, and ammonia

It is useful to take a chest radiograph to diagnose left ventricular failure or aspiration. An abdominal ultrasound may indicate liver size and patency of the hepatic and portal veins, particularly if liver transplantation is being considered.

Table 7.5 Management of acute liver failure.

No sedation except for procedures
Minimal handling
Monitor:
Heart and respiratory rate
Arterial BP, CVP
Core/toe temperature
Neurological observations
Gastric pH (> 5.0)
Blood glucose (> 4 mmol/L)
Acid–base
Electrolytes
PT, PTT
Fluid balance
75% maintenance
Dextrose 10–50%
Sodium (0.5–1.0 mmol/L)
Potassium (2–4 mmol/L)
Maintain circulating volume with colloid/FFP
Coagulation support only if required
Drugs
Vitamin K
H_2-antagonist
Antacids
Lactulose
N-acetylcysteine
Broad-spectrum antibiotics
Antifungals
Nutrition
Enteral feeding (1–2 g protein/day)
Parenteral nutrition if ventilated

BP, blood pressure; CVP, central venous pressure; FFP, fresh frozen plasma; PN, parenteral nutrition; PT, prothrombin time; PTT, partial thromboplastin time.

Fluid balance

The aim of fluid balance is to maintain hydration and renal function while not provoking cerebral edema. Maintenance fluids consist of 10% dextrose in 0.25 N saline, and intake should be 75% of normal maintenance requirements unless cerebral edema develops. A total sodium intake of 0.5–1 mmol/kg/day is usually adequate. Potassium requirements may be large, 3–6 mmol/kg/day, as guided by the serum concentration. As patients may become hypophosphatemic, intravenous phosphate may be given as potassium phosphate.

Attempts should be made to maintain urinary output using loop diuretics in large doses (furosemide at 1–3 mg/kg every 6 h) and colloid/fresh frozen plasma (FFP) to maintain renal perfusion. Should profound oliguria occur, consideration should be given to hemofiltration or dialysis.

Anemia should be corrected, maintaining the hemoglobin concentration above 10 g/dL to provide maximum oxygen delivery to tissues. Coagulopathy should be managed conservatively; the massive requirements for FFP may result in fluid overload.

Other therapy

It is usual to prescribe vitamin K (2–10 mg i.v.), although it is not usually effective. H_2-antagonists and antacids (see below) should be administered prophylactically to prevent gastrointestinal hemorrhage from stress erosions. The role of *N*-acetylcysteine (70 mg/kg 4-hourly) in the management of ALF other than acetaminophen poisoning is unproven, but anecdotal results suggest that it may have a role. A multicenter study, supported by the National Institutes of Health, of its role in the management of acute liver failure is in progress.

Antibiotic therapy

The results of surveillance cultures can be used to guide antibiotic therapy in the event of suspected infection, but broad-spectrum antibiotics (amoxicillin, cefuroxime, metronidazole, and prophylactic fluconazole) are only prescribed if sepsis is suspected or liver transplantation is anticipated.[52]

Nutritional support

The role of parenteral nutrition in the management of patients with acute liver failure is controversial. The main aims of therapy are:

• To maintain blood glucose (> 4 mmol/L) and ensure sufficient carbohydrates for energy metabolism. The glucose infusion rate required to maintain an acceptable serum glucose may vary between patients, but rates as high as 12–15 mg/kg/min can be required. A catheter placed in a central vein will be necessary to deliver such a concentrated glucose solution.

• To reduce protein intake to 1–2 g/kg/day, either enterally or parenterally.

• To provide sufficient energy intake to reverse catabolism, either enterally or parenterally.

Children who are mechanically ventilated should have parenteral nutrition, as it may be 7–10 days before a full normal diet is resumed following transplantation.

Central nervous system monitoring

A baseline electroencephalogram (EEG) is helpful for staging coma and providing information on the prognosis (Figure 7.3). Computed tomography (CT) scans are probably not useful early in encephalopathy, but may provide information on cerebral edema, hemorrhage, or irreversible brain damage later in the disease (Figure 7.4). Frequent evaluation of neurological function and blood ammonia is essential to follow the progress of hepatic encephalopathy. The role of intracranial pressure monitoring remains controversial. There are many systems in use: extradural monitors (e.g., Ladd transducers), which are easy to insert but inaccurate; subdural systems (e.g., Gaeltec transducers), which may also be inaccurate; and Camino catheters, which are inserted into the brain or dura. All forms of intracranial monitoring are potentially hazardous in patients with severe coagulopathy, but they may provide helpful information on changes in intracranial pressure and improve selection for liver transplantation.

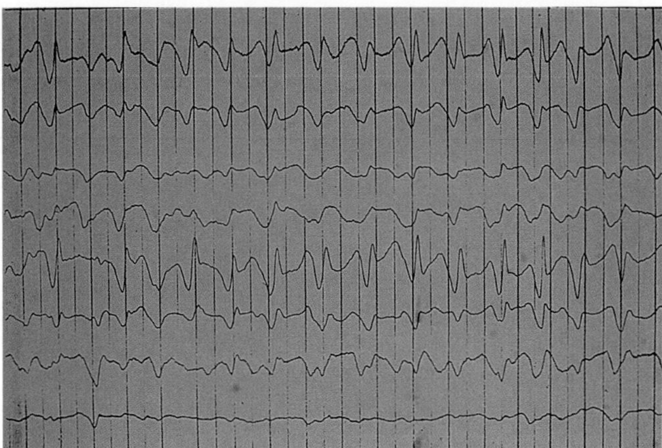

Figure 7.3 Acute hepatic encephalopathy may be difficult to detect in infants or older children. Electroencephalography demonstrates a slow rhythm and reduced amplitude, with characteristic triphasic waves.

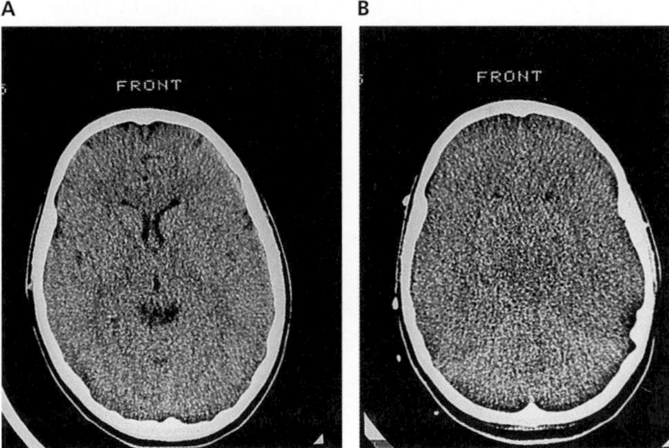

Figure 7.4 The rapid development of cerebral edema in acute liver failure is a poor prognostic sign. This is best demonstrated by computed tomography, which shows a reduction in the size of the ventricles (**A**) and reversal of gray/white matter (**B**); however, it is a very late sign.

Prevention and management of complications

The clinical course is dominated by the complications of hepatic failure, and therapy should be focused on their prevention and management.

Hypoglycemia

Hypoglycemia (blood glucose < 400 mg/L) develops in the majority of children. It may contribute to central nervous system impairment and other organ dysfunction. Factors contributing to hypoglycemia include:

- Failure of hepatic glucose synthesis and release
- Hyperinsulinemia (due to failure of hepatic degradation)
- Increased glucose utilization (due to anaerobic metabolism)
- Secondary bacterial infection[53–56]

Frequent bedside monitoring of blood glucose concentrations (every 2–4 h) and intravenous administration of glucose (10–50% dextrose) are required to prevent this complication. Increased insulin production, secondary to excess glucose infusion, leads to increased glucose need, and can be avoided by permitting blood glucose to remain between 400 and 600 mg/L. Profound refractory hypoglycemia carries a grave prognostic implication and often heralds the imminent death of the patient.

Coagulopathy and hemorrhage

The management of coagulopathy and hemorrhage is a major part of the overall care of the child with ALF. Profound disturbances in hemostasis develop secondary to failure of hepatic synthesis of clotting factors and fibrinolytic factors, reduction in platelet numbers and function, or intravascular coagulation. The coagulation factors synthesized by hepatocytes include factors I (fibrinogen), II (prothrombin), V, VII, IX, and X, and a reduction in synthesis leads to the prolongation of prothrombin and partial thromboplastin time.

The prothrombin time is the most clinically useful measure of hepatic synthesis of clotting factors. Prolongation of the prothrombin time often precedes other clinical evidence of hepatic failure, such as encephalopathy, and may alert the clinician to the severity of acute hepatitis; it is a guide to the urgency of liver transplantation. Administering vitamin K parenterally ensures a sufficiency of this essential cofactor, but rarely improves coagulation in ALF.

The prothrombin time depends on the availability of factor VII, which has a shorter half-life than other factors and decreases more rapidly than other liver-derived clotting factors. As a result, measurement of factor VII may be a more sensitive indicator than the prothrombin time. Fibrinogen concentrations are usually normal unless there is also disseminated intravascular coagulation (DIC). The level of factor VIII may help differentiate between DIC and ALF, as it is synthesized by vascular endothelium and therefore in ALF is normal or increased, possibly as an acute-phase response or due to decreased utilization. Decreased levels of factor XIII may contribute to poor clot stabilization.

A reduction in platelet numbers (80×10^9/L) occurs in up to half of adult patients, although thrombocytopenia is less of a problem in pediatric experience. Severe thrombocytopenia, requiring platelet transfusion, suggests hypersplenism, intravascular coagulation, or aplastic anemia. The use of extracorporeal support devices may also contribute.

Intravascular coagulation, as detected by abnormal concentrations of fibrin degradation products, is present in almost all patients, indicating ongoing clot deposition and dissolution, most probably as a consequence of tissue necrosis in the liver. DIC is rarely significant, but can contribute to organ damage. The administration of commercial concentrates containing activated clotting factors may precipitate DIC.

Bleeding from needle puncture sites and line insertion is common, while pulmonary or intracranial hemorrhage may be terminal events. Petechiae reflect decreased platelet function, disturbed vascular integrity, or DIC.

Although in the early stages of assessment prolongation of prothrombin time is a sensitive guide to prognosis and the need for liver transplantation, life-threatening coagulopathy should be corrected with FFP, cryoprecipitate, and platelets as needed. It is not necessary to maintain coagulation parameters (prothrombin time) in the normal range. In general, mild to moderate coagulopathy (prothrombin time < 25 s) requires no therapy except support for procedures. Marked coagulopathy (prothrombin time > 40 s) should be corrected (10 mL/kg of FFP every 6 h) to prevent the risk of bleeding, particularly intracranial hemorrhage. If major bleeding occurs, additional attempts should be made to correct coagulation using 15–20 mL/kg FFP every 6 h, or continuous infusions at a rate of 3–5 mL/kg/h. Administration of recombinant factor VII (80 µg/kg) reliably corrects the coagulation defect in patients with ALF for a period of 6–12 h and may be useful in preparation for invasive procedures. Double-volume exchange transfusion may temporarily improve coagulation and DIC and control hemorrhage. Hemofiltration may be necessary to control fluid balance if much coagulation support is required. Platelet counts should be maintained above 50×10^9/L by infusion of platelets. DIC is rarely severe enough to require heparin infusion.

Prevention of gastrointestinal hemorrhage. Gastrointestinal tract hemorrhage may be life-threatening due to gastritis or stress ulceration. High-dose H_2-antagonists (ranitidine 1–3 mg/kg 8-hourly) or proton-pump inhibitors (omeprazole 10–20 mg/kg/day, pantoprazole 25 mg/m^2/day) should be administered intravenously, and sucralfate (1–2 g 4-hourly) may be given by nasogastric tube to reduce upper gastrointestinal tract bleeding.

Encephalopathy

Clinically, acute hepatic encephalopathy is defined as any brain dysfunction that occurs as a result of acute hepatic dysfunction[47] and may be exacerbated by sepsis, gastrointestinal bleeding, electrolyte disturbances, or sedation, particularly benzodiazepine administration. Clinical manifestations and progression are highly variable, but acute hepatic encephalopathy usually evolves over days through definable stages. It may progress rapidly, with coma developing within hours of the earliest detectable signs.

A scale for grading clinical encephalopathy is presented in Table 7.6.[4,57] This scale is useful for assessing encephalopathy

Table 7.6 Clinical stages of hepatic encephalopathy.

Stage	Asterixis	EEG changes	Clinical manifestations
I (prodrome)	Slight	Minimal	Mild intellectual impairment, disturbed sleep–wake cycle
II (impending)	Easily elicited	Usually generalized slowing of rhythm	Drowsiness, confusion, coma, inappropriate behavior, disorientation, mood swings
III (stupor)	Present if patient cooperative	Grossly abnormal slowing	Drowsy, unresponsive to verbal commands, markedly confused, delirious, hyperreflexia, (+) Babinski sign
IV (coma)	Usually absent	Appearance of delta waves, decreased amplitudes	Unconscious, decerebrate or decorticate response to pain present (IVA) or absent (IVB)

Adapted from refs. 4, 35.

in older patients, but has less value in assessing neonates and infants, particularly in the early stages of encephalopathy. Although alterations in the EEG are not specific, the EEG is useful for monitoring progression in hepatic encephalopathy (Table 7.6).

The earliest abnormalities may not be detectable by clinical assessment, but are apparent to family members. These include:

• Personality changes—reflecting forebrain dysfunction—include regression, irritability, apathy, and occasionally euphoria. Younger children are more likely to be irritable and apathetic.

• Sleep disturbances, such as insomnia or sleep inversion, are often observed. Intellectual deterioration, observed in stage I of chronic hepatic encephalopathy, is usually not evident in acute encephalopathy.

• Constructional apraxia related to disturbed spatial recognition may be present. Simple age-related tasks may be clinically useful tools for the day-to-day assessment of inattentiveness and apraxia. Subtraction of serial 7s, recall of events (such as recently viewed videos), handwriting, and figure drawing are appropriate tasks that older children can be asked to repeat daily in order to assess early encephalopathy.

• Drowsiness and lethargy are readily apparent as the patient progresses into stage II hepatic encephalopathy.

• Asterixis develops and is a useful sign, but it cannot be elicited with regularity in children less than 8–10 years of age.

• Progressive motor impairment becomes evident, including ataxia, dysarthria, and apraxia. Other neuromotor disturbances that can be detected as patients progress to stage III encephalopathy include hyperreflexia and sustained clonus. EEG abnormalities are detectable at this stage. Infants exhibit increasing irritability and often produce high-pitched, ear-piercing screams. They may refuse to suckle or eat.

• Stage III hepatic encephalopathy is characterized by deepening somnolence and stupor. The patient is arousable by vigorous physical stimuli, but does not respond to commands. Patients are disoriented and often do not recognize family members. School-aged children and teenagers in deepening stage II and stage III coma often exhibit extreme agitation and rage. Seizures may develop. Neurological findings are more profound (Table 7.6).

• Progression into stage IV hepatic encephalopathy is heralded by the onset of coma. The patient responds only to painful stimuli. At first, the patient is flaccid, but in deeper stage IV the patient will assume decerebrate posturing, and brainstem reflexes are lost.

Acute hepatic encephalopathy is completely reversible after resolution of the hepatic dysfunction. Although the role played by ammonia in the development of encephalopathy is controversial, therapy to reduce ammonia production or accumulation is indicated. The components of therapy are:

• Restriction of dietary protein
• Enteral antibiotics
• Enteral lactulose
• Controlling the complications of acute liver failure that contribute to ammonia accumulation.

In the early stages of hepatic encephalopathy, conventional measures are taken to minimize the formation of nitrogenous substances by the intestine. A cathartic, such as sodium-free magnesium sulphate and/or a nonabsorbable disaccharide (lactulose 1–2 mL/kg every 4–6 h) may be administered orally or via the nasogastric tube. Neomycin (50–100 mg/kg/day) may also be used to prevent ammonia production if diarrhea secondary to lactulose is a problem. Protein intake should be limited to 0.5–1 g/kg/day and may be administered enterally or parenterally to limit the production of ammonia. Caloric intake is maintained in the early stages with glucose polymers and supplemented by infusion of 10% dextrose solution, with frequent monitoring of blood glucose.

The older patient with aggressive delirium is at risk for self-injury, as well as being a risk to care providers. Sedation is not usually needed, except in violent patients. Elective ventilation should be considered if the encephalopathy progresses. If sedation is required, either for restraint or during procedures, short-acting barbiturates or opiates can be safely utilized, but benzodiazepines should be avoided. There are potential therapeutic implications related to the GABA receptor, which has been implicated in encephalopathy. Flumazenil, a benzodiazepine antagonist, may produce temporary reversal of hepatic encephalopathy.[58] Administration is followed in minutes by a clinical response, which may last for several hours, and it has been suggested that a lack of response to flumazenil may indicate a poor prognosis.

Many of the complications of ALF, such as gastrointestinal hemorrhage, increase the potential for ammonia accumulation and its consequent neurotoxicity. Measures should be taken to prevent and control hemorrhage. Dehydration, electrolyte, and acid–base disturbances should be corrected, and blood glucose concentration should be maintained by administering a 10–25% glucose solution.

Cerebral edema

Brain death associated with cerebral edema is the most frequent cause of death in acute liver failure and contributes to reduced survival after liver transplantation.[46,59] Every effort should be made to prevent this complication, since the prognosis is poor once it is evident.

Cerebral edema may develop between stage III and stage IV encephalopathy and present within hours of the onset of coma. It is heralded by changes in the neurological examination—abnormally reacting or unequal pupils, muscular rigidity and decerebrate posturing, mild clonus and/or focal seizures, and loss of brainstem reflexes. There may be alteration of respiratory pattern, bradycardia, and an increase in blood pressure. It is associated with a rise in intracranial pressure (ICP) > 30 mmHg.[60] CT or magnetic resonance imaging (MRI) scans of the brain will show flattening of the gyri and reduction of the size of the ventricles, but they are not helpful for early diagnosis (Figure 7.4). Loss of the definition of gray/white matter is an ominous sign. Fixed, dilated pupils indicate brainstem coning and irreversible brain damage, but care in interpretation is required if sedative drugs have been used.

The etiology of cerebral edema is not known, but iatrogenic factors may contribute. These include: fluid overload from therapeutic efforts to improve coagulopathy and hypotension; failure to maintain blood glucose concentrations, leading to anaerobic brain metabolism, which can result in cerebral fluid shifts; and failure to maintain systemic blood pressure, which can lead to cerebral ischemia and secondary edema.[61]

Management. Current treatment for cerebral edema in ALF is inadequate, so every effort must be made to prevent it. The key strategy is fluid restriction (< 75% of maintenance), maintaining circulating volume with colloid. The intravenous infusion of mannitol (0.5 g/kg every 4–6 h) helps control acute increases in intracranial pressure and may reverse acute neurological changes. Serum osmolarity should be monitored during mannitol therapy and should not exceed 320 mosmol/L. Hemofiltration to prevent or remove fluid overload is an important strategy, particularly while awaiting a suitable donor, if diuretic therapy is ineffective or hepatorenal failure develops.

Elective ventilation should be performed if cerebral edema is suspected. Intubation may be carried out using a short-acting agent (atracurium 300–600 µg/kg i.v. and then 100–200 µg/kg as required), to prevent the rise in ICP associated with the gag reflex. Further sedation may be required with physiotherapy and suction. Hyperventilation ($P\text{CO}_2$ < 3.5 kPa) may have a temporary effect in reducing ICP, but metabolic compensation limits this to 24 h. Diligent efforts should be made to maintain cerebral perfusion pressure (mean arterial pressure minus intracranial pressure) by administering blood products, albumin, and inotropic agents (epinephrine or norepinephrine). Controlled hypothermia also shows promise in preventing and perhaps treating cerebral edema in ALF.[62,63]

Corticosteroids are of no value in preventing or reducing cerebral edema. Barbiturate coma (thiopentone 0.5–1.0 mg/kg i.v. followed by an infusion of 0.5–3.0 mg/kg/h) may maintain cerebral perfusion while a donor liver is awaited, but has no proven value in ALF. Convulsions should be treated promptly. Monitoring intracranial pressure is controversial,[64] as it has no therapeutic role and does not improve overall outcome; however, it may improve selection for liver transplantation.

Electrolyte and acid–base disturbances

Disturbances in sodium homeostasis—either hyponatremia and/or hypernatremia—are observed in virtually all children.[65] Hyponatremia is more common, despite sodium retention by the kidney. It may result from decreased water excretion, increased antidiuretic hormone, disturbances in the sodium/potassium pump, or the excess administration of hypotonic saline. Hypernatremia is less common, but is related to the administration of sodium-rich intravenous fluids and the vigorous use of lactulose or mannitol.

Hypokalemia occurs secondary to increased retention of sodium by the kidney from secondary hyperaldosteronism, the vigorous use of diuretics, excessive vomiting, or nasogastric suction. Occasionally, hyperkalemia is observed in patients with massive hepatic necrosis and/or hemolysis. Hypocalcemia and hypomagnesemia frequently occur and should be corrected.

Acid–base disturbances are common and may be secondary to liver failure, sepsis, or the underlying disease. Respiratory alkalosis is observed in the early stages of encephalopathy, due to central hyperventilation. Metabolic alkalosis is seen with hypokalemia and vigorous use of diuretics, particularly furosemide. Metabolic acidosis may be multifactorial and develop secondary to metabolic liver disease, with accumulation of organic acids, including lactate and free fatty acids, although ketosis is usually minimal. Other factors include: administration of blood preserved with citrate, tissue hypoxia and anaerobic metabolism, renal failure, or acetaminophen poisoning.[66] Severe metabolic acidosis requires intravenous sodium bicarbonate (8.4%), elective ventilation, or bicarbonate dialysis. Respiratory failure and respiratory acidosis develop as coma deepens, requiring mechanical ventilation.

Renal dysfunction

Renal insufficiency complicates the course in 75% of children,[67,68] and may be due to prerenal uremia, acute tubular necrosis, and functional renal failure.

Prerenal uremia may be due to dehydration or gastrointestinal bleeding because of absorption of nitrogenous substances from the gut. A marked increase in the blood creatinine concentration may develop from decreased glomerular filtration and/or increased muscle breakdown.

Acute tubular necrosis is seen in a minority of patients and may occur due to hypovolemia or dehydration related to mannitol infusion or diuretic therapy. Features include: abnormal urinary sediment; urinary sodium concentration > 20 mmol/L, reduction in creatinine clearance (urine/plasma creatinine ratio < 10); and oliguria (urine output < 0.5 mL/kg/h).

Functional renal failure (hepatorenal syndrome) is the commonest cause of renal insufficiency. Features include sodium retention (urinary sodium concentration < 20 mmol/L), normal urinary sediment, and reduced urinary output (< 1 mL/kg/h). The etiology is multifactorial, and electrolyte imbalance, sepsis, and hypovolemia all play a part. Endotoxemia may contribute to renal injury.

The aim of management is to maintain circulating volume to prevent prerenal hypovolemia and ensure that urine output is > 0.5 mL/kg/h. A fluid challenge (10 mL/kg) may be successful unless central venous pressure indicates fluid overload (> 8–10 cmH_2O), when the use of furosemide (1–2 mg/kg i.v. or 0.25 mg/kg/h by infusion) may be effective. Established renal failure requires hemodialysis or filtration for fluid overload.

While functional renal failure recovers quickly after liver transplantation, acute tubular necrosis may severely complicate the postoperative management.[69] Although 50% of patients require hemodialysis or hemofiltration support, renal function returns to normal after successful liver transplantation.

Ascites

The use of ultrasound in the pretransplant assessment has demonstrated excessive peritoneal fluid in most patients, probably due to acute portal hypertension, from lobular collapse, vasodilation, poor vascular integrity, and reduced oncotic pressure. Clinically evident ascites occurs in less than half the patients, but may be a site for secondary bacterial or fungal infection, indicating the necessity for paracentesis in septic patients without an obvious focus of infection. Therapy is not indicated, other than for correction of oncotic pressure with albumin infusion and general fluid management.

Cardiovascular and pulmonary complications

Cardiac output is increased secondary to reduced vascular resistance and arteriovenous shunting.[68] Reduced vascular resistance may be due to gut-derived endotoxin or to substances released from the necrotic liver, as removal of the liver improved hemodynamic stability in a few cases. Patients frequently exhibit clinical evidence of warm extremities, facial flush, and erythema of palms and soles despite profound hypotension ("warm shock").

Hypotension due to hemorrhage, bacteremia, or increased capillary permeability is a frequent event and may be refractory to volume replacement and to administration of pressor agents.

Sinus tachycardia is present in 75% of patients,[6] while inappropriate bradycardia is a late sign that may be associated with a rise in intracranial pressure, suggesting a failure of central regulatory mechanisms, which may occur in the absence of clinically evident cerebral edema.

The combination of hypotension, evidence of peripheral vasodilation, and metabolic acidosis (or elevated blood lactate) is an indication of imminent death.

Respiratory problems

Defective ventilation and ventilatory response to chemical stimuli are commonly observed. Hyperventilation often accompanies stage II–III encephalopathy and results in respiratory alkalosis. Patients in stage IV coma develop hypoventilation, hypoxia, and hypercapnia. Arterial blood gas analysis usually reveals a mixed respiratory–metabolic acidosis. Although these patients may increase ventilation in response to transient hypoxia, ventilation is not maintained if hypoxia is prolonged. Elective mechanical ventilation guided by arterial blood gas analysis should be initiated at the first sign of respiratory failure. Unfortunately, positive-pressure ventilation, with positive end-expiratory pressure, may reduce hepatic perfusion and exacerbate metabolic acidosis.

Poor oxygenation despite adequate (mechanical) ventilation can be the result of intrapulmonary shunting of blood—a secondary ventilation–perfusion mismatch due to microvascular dilation. Necropsy findings include diffuse dilation of the pulmonary vascular bed and occasional spider nevi. Intrapulmonary shunting resolves promptly after liver transplantation or spontaneous recovery.

About one-third of adult patients with acute liver failure demonstrate clinical and/or radiographic evidence of pulmonary edema,[70] which is higher than has been observed in children with ALF. It may be due to vasodilation and loss of vascular integrity and can respond to diuretics and correction of plasma oncotic pressure.

Pulmonary infection from *Staphylococcus aureus*, Gram-negative bacteria, *Pseudomonas*, and *Candida* often complicates the course. Risk factors include pulmonary edema, intubation, mechanical ventilation, and immunodeficiency. Prophylactic antibiotics should not be used, and positive endotracheal tube cultures should not be treated unless accompanied by clinical or radiographic evidence of pulmonary infection. Other complications include aspiration pneumonia and pleural effusions. Pulmonary hemorrhage is a terminal event.

Secondary bacterial and fungal infections

The majority of adults and 50% of children will develop significant infection,[71] which may be related to impairment of cellular and humoral immune systems. The organisms most often implicated are Gram-positive (*S. aureus*, *S. epidermidis*, and streptococci), presumably of skin origin. Occasionally, Gram-negative bacteria or fungal infection are observed. Urinary tract infections from indwelling catheters and pulmonary infection, particularly in ventilated children, are common.

Management includes surveillance cultures from indwelling catheters, urine cultures, and surface swabs. Broad-spectrum antibiotics should be started with the suspicion of sepsis, as the signs may be subtle. For example, a rise in heart rate, the difference in the core/toe temperature gradient, a fall in blood pressure or urine output, the rapid development of hypoglycemia, hypothermia, or a deterioration in the mental state. Amoxicillin (25 mg/kg/dose t.d.s.), cefuroxime (20 mg/kg/dose t.d.s.), and/or metronidazole (8 mg/kg/dose t.d.s.), if there is a suspicion of anaerobic infection, are reasonable first-line medications. Prophylactic antifungals such as liposomal amphotericin (3–5 mg/kg/day) or fluconazole (3–6 mg/kg/day) may be effective, although potentially nephrotoxic. Positive cultures in the absence of clinical infection should result in removal or replacement of the infected catheter and administration of the appropriate antimicrobials, with close attention to the possibility of additional, perhaps opportunistic infection. Aminoglycoside antibiotics should be avoided, if possible, because they can contribute to renal failure.

Pancreatitis

Pancreatic lesions consistent with acute pancreatitis have been found at autopsy in a significant proportion of adults with ALF, but this is rarely clinically evident. Children with valproic acid toxicity may have significant pancreatic lesions, with pain, hypotension, and disturbed calcium homeostasis.

Aplastic anemia

Bone-marrow failure is a potentially fatal complication of sporadic non-A–G hepatitis,[2,72] parvovirus B19, and HSV-VI acute liver failure. It may not be evident before transplantation and carries a high mortality. Bone-marrow transplantation, administration of granulocyte colony-stimulating factor, or granulocyte/macrophage-stimulating factor may be therapeutic options.

Specific therapies

Acetaminophen ingestion

The standard emergency management methods for ingested poison (gastric lavage, forced diuresis, etc.) are no longer used. Early detection of acetaminophen toxicity by estimating levels and/or metabolites is important. Treatment with *N*-acetylcysteine (140 mg/kg initially with 70 mg/kg 4-hourly) should start within 24 h of ingestion and then continue for at least 72 h or until liver failure has resolved and coagulation parameters are back to normal (see Chapter 9).

Amanita phalloides poisoning

Benzylpenicillin (10 000 000 U/kg/day) may reduce hepatic uptake of amatoxin, whilst thioctic acid (300 mg/kg/day i.v. infusion) may reduce hepatic damage. Hemodialysis or hemofiltration or the molecular adsorbent recirculating system (MARS) may also remove the amatoxin (see below).

Hepatic support

Many different measures have been used to support the liver while awaiting regeneration or transplantation, including a variety of experimental drugs such as prostaglandin E, insulin, or glucagon, which have not been shown to be effective.

Methods for removing potential neuroactive toxins include double-volume exchange transfusion, plasmapheresis, charcoal hemoperfusion, liver-assist devices containing chemical scrubbers or cultured hepatocytes,[73] extracorporeal perfusion through human or animal livers,[74] and cross-circulation with animals. Although these therapeutic maneuvers may provide support during liver regeneration or while awaiting a donor, none has been shown to have any benefit with regard to survival.

Double-volume exchange transfusion (in children < 15 kg) and plasmapheresis in older children may produce a transient improvement in coagulopathy and neurological state, but may contribute to hemodynamic instability.[75]

Artificial liver support, using either porcine hepatocytes or a hepatoma cell line, has shown some benefit in improving coagulopathy and reducing encephalopathy in adults, acting as a bridge to transplantation, although the long-term outcome and survival were not affected.[76] There is limited anecdotal experience in children.[77,78]

Molecular Adsorbent Recirculating System (MARS)

MARS is an alternative form of hemodialysis that uses a specific filter to remove toxic products, but not albumin. It has a role in the management of both acute liver failure and acute-on-chronic liver failure in adults.[79,80] Its use in the management of children is anecdotal, but it may have a role to play in creating a bridge to transplantation,[81] or in the setting of drug-induced liver failure or toxic mushroom poisoning.[82]

Hepatocyte transplantation

Hepatocyte transplantation, as a treatment for acute liver failure using cell suspensions or synthetic constructs, is at an early stage of research, but has shown promise in animal models.[83] There have been anecdotal reports that it is effective in mushroom poisoning.[84]

Liver transplantation

Liver transplantation should be considered in all children who develop stage III or IV hepatic coma, as the mortality in this group exceeds 70%.[85] Transplantation is indicated for ALF caused by viral hepatitis (including hepatitis B), acetaminophen overdose, halothane hepatitis, and mushroom poisoning, as well as those with an indeterminate cause. It is also appropriate for certain forms of inborn errors of metabolism—for example, Wilson's disease and tyrosinemia type I, although it is contraindicated in children with multisystem disease or mitochondrial deletions.[33]

As a successful outcome following liver transplantation is less likely than with other forms of liver disease,[86,87] selection is critical,[88] and is based on previous experience of mortality in the pretransplant era.[85] Transplantation using a living donor can accelerate the process and is associated with a better outcome in the setting of ALF.[89–91]

The etiology of ALF is an important factor in determining whether transplantation is appropriate. The highest mortality is seen in children with hepatitis of indeterminate cause, particularly those with a delayed onset of coma and rapid progression to stage III or IV hepatic coma, a shrinking liver and falling transaminases associated with an increase in bilirubin, and coagulopathy.[6,21,92] These children should be immediately considered for transplantation. Children with fulminant Wilson's disease are unlikely to recover with medical treatment and require transplantation.

In contrast, children with hepatitis A and children with drug-induced liver disease, particularly acetaminophen poisoning, may make a complete recovery with intensive medical therapy. Careful monitoring for poor prognostic factors is thus required before selection.

In practical terms, it is appropriate to list for emergency liver transplantation all children who have reached stage III hepatic coma, as the shortage of donor organs may mean a considerable wait for transplantation or death on the waiting list.

As the development of irreversible brain damage is a major contraindication to transplantation, it is essential to be certain that brain damage has not occurred prior to the operation. Current techniques are inadequate, but include monitoring ICP, the identification of cerebral infarction or intracranial hemorrhage by cerebral CT or MRI scans, and looking for evidence of midbrain coning, such as fixed, dilated pupils.

Auxiliary transplantation, in which the recipient liver is left in situ to regenerate, is a controversial treatment for ALF, but may have the benefit that the graft may be removed if the original liver regenerates.[93,94] It is not suitable for transplantation for acute liver failure secondary to metabolic liver disease, as there is no potential for these livers to recover and there may be a risk of hepatoma in the cirrhotic liver.

Family support

Families of children with ALF are naturally devastated by the development of potentially fatal acute liver failure in their child. These families require a considerable amount of psychological support and counseling, particularly as many families will not be able to grasp the seriousness of their child's condition and the complications of liver transplantation. Psychological problems in both the family and the recipient of the liver transplant are common and will need addressing following the operation. The particular problems of self-poisoning in adolescents may need additional psychiatric help.

Prognosis

There are few reliable criteria that determine the prognosis in a child with ALF, despite attempts to correlate clinical variables and laboratory data with outcome.[95–97]

Children under 10 years and adults over 40 years of age have been reported to have the worst overall prognosis,[85,98] which varied depending on the etiology. Both adults and children with fulminant hepatitis A had the best overall survival at 68%, while survival rates for other etiologies in descending order were: acetaminophen overdose 53%, hepatitis B 39%, indeterminate hepatitis 20%, with halothane and other drug toxicities having the poorest survival at 12%.[98] The absence of an obvious etiology in a child with severe hepatitis with encephalopathy (a presumed diagnosis of sporadic indeterminate hepatitis) is an indicator of a poor outcome, since the recovery rate in such cases is less than 10%.

A recent study of 97 children in the United Kingdom confirmed the improved prognosis for recovery following acetaminophen poisoning (50%) and hepatitis A (44%) in comparison with indeterminate hepatitis (20%).[6] Another pediatric study in the United States has also confirmed these findings.[99] In the PALF series, spontaneous recovery occurred in 94% of patients with acetaminophen toxicity versus 47% of all other diagnoses.[8]

Infants under the age of 1 year with severe coagulopathy secondary to metabolic liver disease or familial erythrophagocytosis have a particularly poor prognosis,[100] as they often present as neonates and the diagnosis may not be established soon enough. Although liver transplantation is a viable option in children of any age, the difficulty of obtaining suitable donor organs in time means that many infants die without transplantation.

In acetaminophen poisoning, acid–base status, and renal function at presentation correlate with the prognosis,[66,85] while other studies have indicated that factor V levels of < 20% are associated with a high mortality and requirement for rapid transplantation.[11,101] In a large British study, children who presented late to hospital for treatment after acetaminophen poisoning, those with progressive hepatotoxicity with prothrombin time > 100 s, hypoglycemia, serum creatinine > 200 μmol/L, acidosis (pH < 7.3), and those who developed encephalopathy grade III, had a poor prognosis and required liver transplantation or died[24] (see also Chapter 9).

As in adults, the duration of illness before the onset of encephalopathy at the time of presentation may have prognostic significance in children.[92] There does not appear to be any significant difference in the survival rate between patients who present with late-onset hepatic failure and those with acute fulminant hepatitis.

Survival does correlate with the degree of severity of encephalopathy, as survival was 18% for patients with stage IV hepatic coma, 48% for those with grade III coma, and 66% for those with grade II coma. The development of cerebral edema and renal failure—particularly in association with shrinking liver (collapsing liver mass)—is associated with a grave prognosis. Clinical experience indicates that patients showing signs of stabilization and improved coagulation parameters have a better outlook for spontaneous recovery.[88]

A prothrombin time > 50 s, which correlates with the degree of necrosis, is a bad prognostic sign, but does not necessarily indicate a fatal outcome. Increased concentrations of α-fetoprotein as an index of regeneration do not necessarily predict survival, and some patients recover without developing detectable α-fetoprotein levels.

Although the mortality tends to be greater with more extensive histological necrosis and complete absence of regenerative activity, attempts to correlate the potential survival with assessment of histological damage have not been helpful and do not justify performing a liver biopsy.[88] Spontaneous recovery from ALF is associated with complete histological recovery, even when extensive necrosis is present.

Outcome

The mortality without treatment for ALF is in excess of 70%. The major causes of death in children before viable liver transplantation were: sepsis, 15%; hemorrhage, 50%; renal failure, 30%; and cerebral edema, 56%;[6] these continue to be the main causes of death.[88] Only liver transplantation has an appreciable effect on the mortality, although the long-term survival is lower than with transplantation for other forms of liver disease. A recent analysis of data from the Studies of Pediatric Liver Transplantation (SPLIT) Registry revealed a 4-year post-transplant patient survival rate of 69% for children with acute liver failure, in comparison with 86% for all other patients.[102] Cerebral dysfunction or brain death following transplantation was an important cause of death in all of the above series, indicating the importance of not transplanting patients with irreversible brain damage.

In patients with spontaneous regeneration of the liver, the long-term outlook is excellent. Complete clinical and biochemical resolution occurs, and the liver recovers completely,[103] although postnecrotic cirrhosis may develop in some survivors.

Case study

A 5-year-old boy presented with a 3-day history of jaundice and fatigue. His parents denied other symptoms, and there was no significant travel or exposure history. He had not taken any medications or nutritional supplements within the previous 6 weeks.

The physical examination revealed a well-developed, jaundiced boy who was uncooperative during the examination, but was oriented and alert. The cardiopulmonary examination was normal and there was no significant lymphadenopathy. The liver was enlarged and palpable 4 cm below the right coastal margin. A spleen tip was palpable in the left upper quadrant. There were no physical signs of chronic liver disease.

At presentation, the total/direct bilirubin value was 166 μmol/L (normal > 20), the alanine aminotransferase level was 3335 IU/L (normal < 40), γ-glutamyltransferase was 217 U/L (normal < 40), and the international normalized ratio was 2 (normal 1.0). Work-up for viral hepatitis, autoimmune disease, Wilson's disease, and fatty acid oxidation defects was negative. Liver biopsy revealed severe hepatitis with minimal inflammatory changes (Figure 7.5A). Over the following 6 days, the coagulation status became increasingly worse, and the patient became more lethargic and was no longer responding to verbal commands. On physical examination, his liver remained large and he developed hyperreflexia and clonus. He was admitted to intensive care for management of his encephalopathy and was listed for a super-urgent liver transplant. On the seventh day of his illness, he received a deceased-donor segmental liver graft. Histological examination of the explant demonstrated severe panacinar hepatic necrosis with some evidence of regeneration, but little inflammation. The appearance was compatible with indeterminate hepatitis (Figure 7.5B). Early liver function was excellent, and the patient was discharged on the tenth postoperative day. At a 6-month follow-up examination, he had returned to school and there was no indication of any developmental delay or intellectual deficits.

A

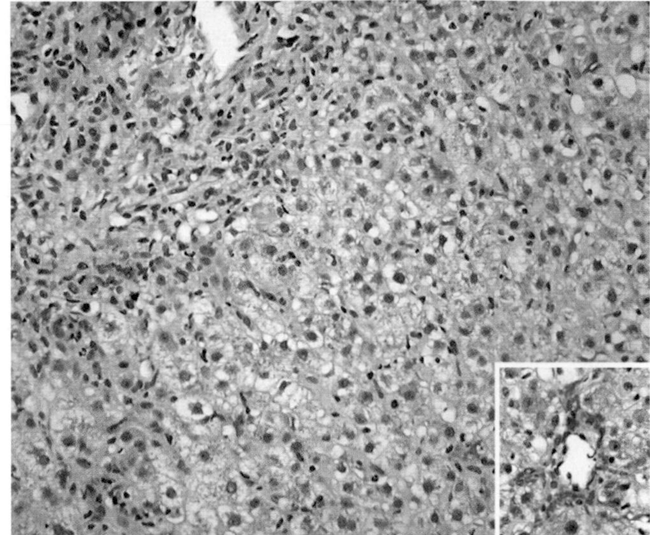

B

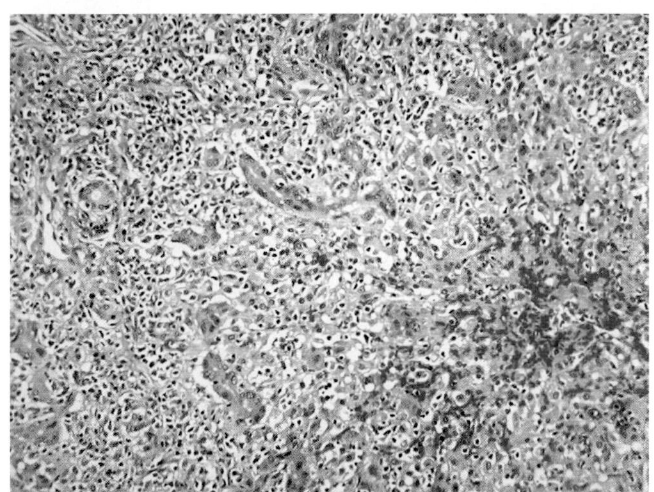

Figure 7.5 A Liver biopsy. Part of a portal tract is present on the upper left of the image. There is no significant portal inflammation, except for a minimal mixed infiltrate at the edge of the portal tract, which accompanies a mild ductular reaction (not well-defined in this image). Hepatocytes are moderately swollen and pleomorphic, with scattered individually necrotic hepatocytes ("acidophilic bodies"). There is a mild sprinkling of inflammatory cells throughout the lobule. The inset (lower right) shows a central vein, which is surrounded by hemorrhage due to mild centrilobular hepatocyte dropout (hematoxylin–eosin, original magnification in both images 100 ×). **B** The explant. Part of a portal tract is present on the left, and there is a centrilobular area on the right. The edge of the portal tract is poorly defined due to extensive hepatocellular necrosis, with prominent proliferation of reactive ductular structures, which involve the edge of the portal tract. There is a moderate lymphocytic inflammatory infiltrate involving the portal tracts and the parenchyma. There is prominent centrilobular hepatocyte dropout and hemorrhage (hematoxylin–eosin, original magnification 100 ×). (Photomicrograph courtesy of Dr. Hector Melin-Aldana).

Comment. Acute liver failure is a rare but often fatal disease. It is a heterogeneous condition with many different etiologies in which the pathophysiology is unclear, preventing substantial therapeutic advances. Therapy consists of supportive measures, with a focus on the prevention or treatment of complications and early consideration for liver transplantation and referral to a suitable center. Transplantation is indicated when there is progression of liver disease and no sign of irreversible brain injury. The prognosis for recovery is poor if there is no clear cause for the liver failure (indeterminate hepatitis), as in this case, and early consideration for liver transplantation is essential.

This young boy made a good recovery without long-term sequelae.

References

1 Sanyal AJ, Stravitz RT. Acute liver failure. In: Zakim D, Boyer TD, eds. *Hepatology*, 4th ed. Philadelphia: Saunders, 2003: 445–96.

2 Whitington PF, Alonso EM. Fulminant hepatitis in children: evidence for an unidentified hepatitis virus. *J Pediatr Gastroenterol Nutr* 2001;**33**:529–36.

3 Williams R. Classification, etiology, and considerations of outcome in acute liver failure. *Semin Liver Dis* 1996;**16**:343–8.

4 Trey C, Davidson CS. The management of fulminant hepatic failure. *Prog Liver Dis* 1970;**2**:282–98.

5 Durand P, Debray D, Mandel R, *et al.* Acute liver failure in infancy: a 14-year experience of a pediatric liver transplantation center. *J Pediatr* 2001;**139**:871–6.

6 Psacharopoulos HT, Mowat AP, Davies M, Portmann B, Silk DBA, Williams R. Fulminant hepatic failure in childhood: an analysis of 31 cases. *Arch Dis Child* 1980;**55**:252–8.

7 Saunders SJ, Hickman R, MacDonald R, Terblanche J. The treatment of acute liver failure. *Prog Liver Dis* 1972;**3**:333–44.

8 Lee WS, McKiernan P, Kelly DA. Etiology, outcome and prognostic indicators of childhood fulminant hepatic failure in the United Kingdom. *J Pediatr Gastroenterol Nutr* 2005;**40**:575–81.

9 Squires RH Jr, Shneider BL, Bucuvalas J, *et al.* Acute liver failure in children: the first 348 patients in the pediatric acute liver failure study group. *J Pediatr* 2006;**148**:652–8.

10 Debray D, Cullufi P, Devictor D, Fabre M, Bernard O. Liver failure in children with hepatitis A. *Hepatology* 1997;**26**:1018–22.

11 Averhoff F, Shapiro CN, Bell BP, *et al.* Control of hepatitis A through routine vaccination of children. *JAMA* 2001;**286**: 2968–73.

12 Bernuau J, Goudeau A, Poynard T, *et al.* Multivariate analysis of prognostic factors in fulminant hepatitis B. *Hepatology* 1986;**6**: 648–51.

13 Schiodt FV, Atillasoy E, Shakil AO, *et al.* Etiology and outcome for 295 patients with acute liver failure in the United States. *Liver Transpl Surg* 1999;**5**:29–34.

14 Teo EK, Ostapowicz G, Hussain M, Lee WM, Fontana RJ, Lok AS. Hepatitis B infection in patients with acute liver failure in the United States. *Hepatology* 2001;**33**:972–6.

15 Chang MH, Lee CY, Chen DS, Hsu HC, Lai MY. Fulminant hepatitis in children in Taiwan: the important role of hepatitis B virus. *J Pediatr* 1986;**3**:34–8.

16 Gimson AES, White YS, Eddleston WF, Williams R. Clinical and prognostic differences in fulminant hepatitis type A, B and non-A, non-B. *Gut* 1983;**24**:1194–8.

17 Kao J, Hsu H, Shau W, Chang M, Chen D. Universal hepatitis B vaccination and the decreased mortality from fulminant hepatitis in infants in Taiwan. *J Pediatr* 2001;**139**:349–52.

18 Farci P, Alter HJ, Shimoda A, *et al.* Hepatitis C virus-associated fulminant hepatic failure. *N Engl J Med* 1996;**335**:631–4.

19 Feranchak AP, Tyson RW, Narkewicz MR, Karrer FM, Sokol RJ. Fulminant Epstein–Barr viral hepatitis: orthotopic liver transplantation and review of the literature. *Liver Transpl Surg* 1998;**4**:469–76.

20 Dirix L, Polson RJ, Richardson A, Williams R. Primary sepsis presenting as fulminant hepatic failure. *QJM* 1989;**271**:1037–4.

21 Whitington PF, Soriano HE, Alonso EM. Fulminant hepatic failure in children. In: Suchy FJ, Sokol RJ, Balistreri WF, eds. *Liver Disease in Children*, 2nd ed. Philadelphia: Lippincott, Williams and Wilkins, 2001: 63–88.

22 Russo MW, Galanko JA, Shrestha R, Fried MW, Watkins P. Liver transplantation for acute liver failure from drug induced liver injury in the United States. *Liver Transpl* 2004;**10**:1018–23.

23 Arundel C, Lewis JH. Drug-induced liver disease in 2006. *Curr Opin Gastroenterol* 2007;**23**:244–54.

24 Mahadevan SBK, McKiernan PJ, Davies P, Kelly DA. Acetaminophen-induced hepatotoxicity in children. *Arch Dis Child* 2006;**91**:598–603.

25 Lee WM. Acetaminophen and the U.S. Acute Liver Failure Study Group: lowering the risks of hepatic failure. *Hepatology* 2004;**40**:6–9.

26 Davern TJ 2nd, James LP, Hinson JA, *et al.* Measurement of serum acetaminophen-protein adducts in patients with acute liver failure. *Gastroenterology* 2006;**130**:687–94.

27 Mutimer DJ, Ayres RC, Neuberger JM, *et al.* Serious acetaminophen poisoning and the results of liver transplantation. *Gut* 1994;**35**:809–14.

28 Bernal W, Wendon J, Rela M, Heaton N, Williams R. Use and outcome of liver transplantation in acetaminophen-induced acute liver failure. *Hepatology* 1998;**27**:1050–5.

29 Reich DJ, Fiel I, Guarrera JV, *et al.* Liver transplantation for autoimmune hepatitis. *Hepatology* 2000;**32**(4 Pt 1):693–700.

30 Maggiore G, Porta G, Bernard O, *et al.* Autoimmune hepatitis with initial presentation as acute hepatic failure in young children. *J Pediatr* 1990;**116**:280–2.

31 Gregorio GV, Portmann B, Reid F, *et al.* Autoimmune hepatitis in childhood: a 20-year experience. *Hepatology* 1997;**25**:541–7.

32 Whitington PF. Metabolic liver disease in childhood. In: Kaplowitz N, ed. *Liver and Biliary Diseases*, 2nd ed. Baltimore: Williams and Wilkins, 1996: 511–34.

33 Thomson M, McKiernan P, Buckels J, Mayer D, Kelly D. Generalised mitochondrial cytopathy is an absolute contraindication to orthotopic liver transplant in childhood. *J Pediatr Gastroenterol Nutr* 1998;**26**:478–81.

34 Sokal EM, Sokol R, Cormier V, *et al.* Liver transplantation in mitochondrial respiratory chain disorders. *Eur J Pediatr* 1999; **158**(Suppl 2):S81–4.

35 Sussman NB. Fulminant hepatic failure. In: Zakim D, Boyer TD, eds. *Hepatology*, 3rd ed. Philadelphia: Saunders, 1996: 618–50.

36 Gazzard BG, Portmann B, Murray-Lyon IM, Williams R. Causes of death in fulminant hepatic failure and relationship to quantitative histological assessment of parenchymal damage. *QJM* 1975;**44**:615–26.

37 Portmann B, Talbot IC, Day DW, Davidson AR, Murray-Lyon IM, Williams R. Histopathological changes in the liver following a acetaminophen overdose: correlation with clinical and biochemical parameters. *J Pathol* 1975;**117**:169–81.

38 Horney JT, Galambos JT. The liver during and after fulminant hepatitis. *Gastroenterology* 1977;**73**:639–45.

39 Benjamin SB, Goodman ZD, Ishak KG, Zimmerman HJ, Irey NS. The morphologic spectrum of halothane-induced hepatic injury: analysis of 77 cases. *Hepatology* 1985;**5**:1163–71.

40 Dupuy JM, Dulac O, Dupuy C, Alagille's D. Severe hyporegenerative viral hepatitis in children. *Proc R Soc Med* 1977;**70**:228–32.

41 Odaib AA, Shneider BL, Bennett MJ, *et al.* A defect in the transport of long-chain fatty acids associated with acute liver failure. *N Engl J Med* 1998;**339**:1752–7.

42 Davis MA, Peters RL, Redeker AG, Reynolds TB. Appraisal of the mortality in acute fulminant viral hepatitis. *N Engl J Med* 1968;**278**:1248–53.

43 Sawhey VK, Knauer CM, Gregory PB. Rapid reduction of transaminase levels in fulminant hepatitis. *N Engl J Med* 1980; **302**:970.

44 Berk PD, Popper H. Fulminant hepatic failure. Annotated abstracts of a workshop held at the National Institutes of Health, 1977. *Am J Gastroenterol* 1978;**69**:349–400.

45 Basile AS, Jones EA. Ammonia and GABA-ergic neurotransmission: interrelated factors in the pathogenesis of hepatic encephalopathy. *Hepatology* 1997;**25**:1303–5.

46 Blei AT. Brain edema and portal-systemic encephalopathy. *Liver Transpl* 2000;**6**(4 Suppl 1):S14–20.

47 Ferenci P, Lockwood A, Mullen K, Tarter R, Weissenborn K, Blei AT. Hepatic encephalopathy—definition, nomenclature, diagnosis, and quantification: final report of the working party at the 11th World Congresses of Gastroenterology, Vienna, 1998. *Hepatology* 2002;**35**:716–21.

48 Alonso EM, Sokol RJ, Hart J, Tyson RW, Narkewicz MR, Whitington PF. Fulminant hepatitis associated with centrilobular necrosis in young children. *J Pediatr* 1995;**127**:888–94.

49 Devictor D, Tahiri C, Rousset A, Massenavette B, Russo M, Huault G. Management of fulminant hepatic failure in children—an analysis of 56 cases. *Crit Care Med* 1993;**21**(9 Suppl):S348–9.

50 Kucharski SA. Fulminant hepatic failure. *Crit Care Nurs Clin North Am* 1993;**5**:141–51.

51 Munoz SJ. Difficult management problems in fulminant hepatic failure. *Semin Liv Dis* 1993;**13**:395–413.

52 Larcher VF, Wyke RJ, Mowat AP, Williams R. Bacterial and fungal infection in children with fulminant hepatic failure: possible role of opsonisation and complement deficiency. *Gut* 1982;**23**:1037–43.

53 Vilstrup H, Iversen J, Tygstrup N. Glucoregulation in acute liver failure. *Eur J Clin Invest* 1986;**16**:193–7.

54 Walsh TS, Wigmore SJ, Hopton P, Richardson R, Lee A. Energy expenditure in acetaminophen-induced fulminant hepatic failure. *Crit Care Med* 2000;**28**:649–54.

55 Clark SJ, Shojaee-Moradie F, Croos P, *et al.* Temporal changes in insulin sensitivity following the development of acute liver failure secondary to acetaminophen. *Hepatology* 2001;**34**:109–15.

56 Harry R, Auzinger G, Wendon J. The clinical importance of adrenal insufficiency in acute hepatic dysfunction. *Hepatology* 2002;**36**:395–402.

57 Teasdale G, Jennett B. Assessment of coma and impaired consciousness. A practical scale. *Lancet* 1974;**2**:81–3.

58 Bansky G, Meier PJ, Riederer E, Walser H, Ziegler WH, Schmid M. Effects of the benzodiazepine receptor antagonist flumazenil in hepatic encephalopathy in humans. *Gastroenterology* 1989; **97**:744–50.

59 O'Brien CJ, Wise RJS, O'Grady JG, Williams R. Neurological sequelae in patients recovered from fulminant hepatic failure. *Gut* 1987;**28**:93–5.

60 Lidofsky SD, Bass NL, Prager MC, *et al.* Intracranial pressure monitoring and liver transplantation for fulminant hepatic failure. *Hepatology* 1992;**16**:1–7.

61 Keays R, Potter D, O'Grady J, Peachey T, Alexander G, Williams R. Intracranial and cerebral perfusion pressure changes before, during, and immediately after orthotopic liver transplantation for fulminant hepatic failure. *QJM* 1991;**79**:425–33.

62 Jalan R, Olde Damink SW, Deutz NE, *et al.* Moderate hypothermia prevents cerebral hyperemia and increase in intracranial pressure in patients undergoing liver transplantation for acute liver failure. *Transplantation* 2003;**75**:2034–9.

63 Belanger M, Desjardins P, Chatauret N, Rose C, Butterworth RF. Mild hypothermia prevents brain edema and attenuates upregulation of the astrocytic benzodiazepine receptor in experimental acute liver failure. *J Hepatol* 2005;**42**:694–9.

64 Keays RT, Alexander GJ, Williams R. The safety and value of extradural intracranial pressure monitors in fulminant hepatic failure. *J Hepatol* 1993;**18**:205–9.

65 Record CO, Iles RA, Cohen RD, Williams R. Acid–base and metabolic disturbances in fulminant hepatic failure. *Gut* 1975; **16**:144–9.

66 Bernal W, Donaldson N, Wyncoll D, Wendon J. Blood lactate as an early predictor of outcome in acetaminophen-induced acute liver failure: a cohort study. *Lancet* 2002;**359**:558–63.

67 Wilkinson SP, Hurst D, Portmann B, Williams R. Pathogenesis of renal failure in cirrhosis and fulminant hepatic failure. *Postgrad Med J* 1975;**51**:503–5.

68 Bihari DJ, Gimson AE, Williams R. Cardiovascular, pulmonary and renal complications of fulminant hepatic failure. *Semin Liver Dis* 1986;**6**:119–28.

69 Brown RS Jr, Lombardero M, Lake JR. Outcome of patients with renal insufficiency undergoing liver or liver–kidney transplantation. *Transplantation* 1996;**62**:1788–93.

70 Warren R, Trewby JW, Laws JW, Williams R. Pulmonary complications in fulminant hepatic failure: analysis of serial radiographs from 100 consecutive patients. *Clin Radiol* 1978; **29**:363–9.

71 Rolando N, Harvey F, Brahm J, *et al.* Prospective study of bacterial infection in acute liver failure: an analysis of fifty patients. *Hepatology* 1990;**11**:49–53.

72 Tzakis AG, Arditi M, Whitington PF, *et al.* Aplastic anemia complicating orthotopic liver transplantation for non-A, non-B hepatitis. *N Engl J Med* 1988;**319**:393–6.

73 Sussman NL, Chong MG, Koussayer T, *et al.* Reversal of fulminant hepatic failure using an extracorporeal liver assist device. *Hepatology* 1992;**16**:60–5.

74 Horslen SP, Hammel JM, Fristoe LW, *et al.* Extracorporeal liver perfusion using human and pig livers for acute liver failure. *Transplantation* 2000;**70**:1472–8.

75 Singer AL, Olthoff KM, Kim H, Rand E, Zamir G, Shaked A. Role of plasmapheresis in the management of acute hepatic failure in children. *Ann Surg* 2001;**234**:418–24.

76 Hughes RD, Williams R. Use of bioartificial and artificial liver support devices. *Semin Liver Dis* 1996;**16**:435–44.

77 LePage EB, Rozga J, Rosenthal P, *et al.* A bioartificial liver used as a bridge to liver transplantation in a 10-year-old boy. *Am J Crit Care* 1994;**3**:224–7.

78 Okamoto K, Kurose M, Ikuta Y, *et al.* Prolonged artificial liver support in a child with fulminant hepatic failure. *ASAIO J* 1996;**42**:233–5.

79 Nadalin S, Heuer M, Wallot M, *et al.* Paediatric acute liver failure and transplantation: the University of Essen experience. *Transpl Int* 2007;**20**:519–27.

80 Tissieres P, Sasbon JS, Devictor D. Liver support for fulminant hepatic failure: is it time to use the molecular adsorbents recycling system in children? *Pediatr Crit Care Med* 2005;**6**:585–91.

81 Hommann M, Kasakow LB, Geoghegan J, *et al.* Application of MARS artificial liver support as bridging therapy before split liver retransplantation in a 15-month-old child *Pediatr Transplant* 2002;**6**:340–3.

82 Covic A, Goldsmith DJA, Gusbeth-Tatomir P, *et al.* Successful use of Molecular Absorbent Regenerating System (MARS) dialysis for the treatment of fulminant hepatic failure in children accidentally poisoned by toxic mushroom ingestion. *Liver Int* 2003;**23**(Suppl 3):21–7.

83 Nussler A, Konig S, Ott M, *et al.* Present status and perspectives of cell-based therapies for liver diseases. *J Hepatol* 2006;**45**: 144–59.

84 Schneider A, Attaran M, Meier PN, *et al.* Hepatocyte transplantation in an acute liver failure due to mushroom poisoning. *Transplantation* 2006;**82**:1115–6.

85 O'Grady JG, Alexander GJM, Hayllar KM, Williams R. Early indicators of prognosis in fulminant hepatic failure. *Gastroenterology* 1989;**97**:439–45.

86 Brems JJ, Hiatt JR, Ramming KP, Quinones-Baldrich WJ, Busuttil RW. Fulminant hepatic failure: the role of liver transplantation as primary therapy. *Am J Surg* 1987;**154**:137–41.

87 Superina RA, Pearl RH, Roberts EA, *et al.* Liver transplantation in children: the initial Toronto experience. *J Pediatr Surg* 1989; **24**:1013–9.

88 Emond JC, Aran PP, Whitington PF, Broelsch CE, Baker AL. Liver transplantation in the management of fulminant hepatic failure. *Gastroenterology* 1989;**96**:1583–8.

89 Emre S, Schwartz ME, Shneider B, *et al.* Living related liver transplantation for acute liver failure in children. *Liver Transpl Surg* 1999;**5**:161–5.

90 Miwa S, Hashikura Y, Mita A, *et al.* Living-related liver transplantation for patients with fulminant and subfulminant hepatic failure. *Hepatology* 1999;**30**:1521–6.

91 Mack CL, Ferrario M, Abecassis M, Whitington PF, Superina RA, Alonso EM. Living donor liver transplantation for children

with liver failure and concurrent multiple organ system failure. *Liver Transpl* 2001;**7**:890–5.
92 Rivera-Penera T, Moreno J, Skaff C, McDiarmid S, Vargas J, Ament ME. Delayed encephalopathy in fulminant hepatic failure in the pediatric population and the role of liver transplantation. *J Pediatr Gastroenterol Nutr* 1997;**24**:128–34.
93 Jaeck D, Pessaux P, Wolf P. Which types of graft to use in patients with acute liver failure? (A) Auxiliary liver transplant (B) Living donor liver transplantation (C) The whole liver. (A) I prefer auxiliary liver transplant. *J Hepatol* 2007;**46**:570–3.
94 Kato T, Selvaggi G, Levi D, *et al.* Routine use of auxiliary partial orthotopic liver transplantation for children with fulminant hepatic failure: preliminary report. *Transplant Proc* 2006;**38**: 3607–8.
95 Trey C, Lipworth L, Davidson CS. Parameters influencing survival in the first 318 patients report to the fulminant hepatic failure surveillance study [abstract]. *Gastroenterology* 1970;**58**:306.
96 Tygstrup N, Ranek L. Assessment of prognosis in fulminant hepatic failure. *Semin Liver Dis* 1986;**6**:129–37.
97 Shakil AO, Kramer D, Mazariegos GV, Fung JJ, Rakela J. Acute liver failure: clinical features, outcome analysis, and applicability of prognostic criteria. *Liver Transpl* 2000;**6**:163–9.
98 O'Grady JG, Gimson AES, O'Brien CJ, Pucknell A, Hughes RD, Williams R. Controlled trials of charcoal hemoperfusion and prognostic factors in fulminant hepatic failure. *Gastroenterology* 1988;**94**:1186–92.
99 Ee LC, Shepherd RW, Cleghorn GJ, *et al.* Acute liver failure in children: a regional experience. *J Paediatr Child Health* 2003;**39**:107–10.
100 Bhaduri BR, Mieli-Vergani G. Fulminant hepatic failure: pediatric aspects. *Semin Liv Dis* 1996;**16**:349–55.
101 Pereira SP, Langley PG, Williams R. The management of abnormalities of hemostasis in acute liver failure. *Semin Liver Dis* 1996;**16**:403–14.
102 Baliga P, Alvarez S, Lindblad A, Zeng L. Posttransplant survival in pediatric fulminant hepatic failure: the SPLIT Experience. *Liver Transplantation* 2004;**10**:1364–71.
103 Karvountzis GG, Redeker AG, Peters RL. Long term follow-up studies of patients surviving fulminant viral hepatitis. *Gastroenterology* 1974;**67**:870–7.

6 Liver Disease in Older Children

8 Autoimmune Liver Disease

Giorgina Mieli-Vergani and Diego Vergani

Definition

Autoimmune liver diseases are characterized histologically by a dense mononuclear cell infiltrate in the portal tract (interface hepatitis; Figure 8.1) and serologically by high levels of transaminases and immunoglobulin G (IgG) and positive autoantibodies, in the absence of a known etiology. These disorders typically respond to immunosuppressive treatment, which should be instituted as soon as a diagnosis is made.

In pediatrics, there are three liver disorders in which liver damage is likely to arise from an autoimmune attack: autoimmune hepatitis (AIH); autoimmune sclerosing cholangitis (ASC); and de novo autoimmune hepatitis after liver transplantation.

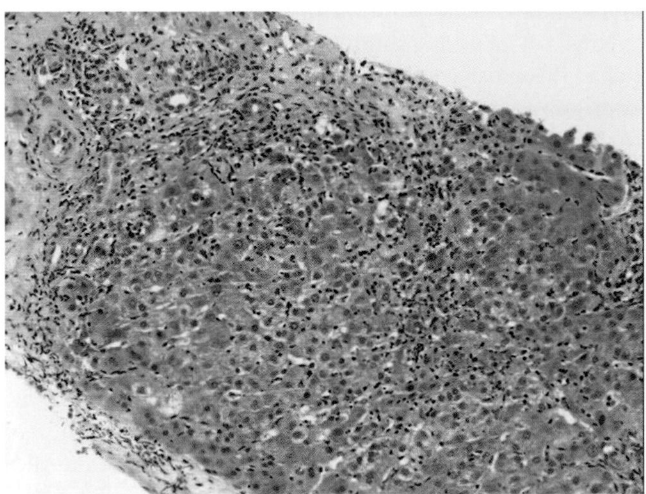

Figure 8.1 Portal and periportal lymphocyte and plasma cell infiltrate, extending to and disrupting the parenchymal limiting plate (interface hepatitis). Swollen hepatocytes, pyknotic necroses, and acinar inflammation are present (hematoxylin–eosin, original magnification 40×). (Image kindly provided by Dr. Alberto Quaglia.)

Diseases of the Liver and Biliary System in Children, 3rd edition. Edited by Deirdre Kelly. ISBN: 978-1-4051-6334-7.

Autoimmune hepatitis

History and epidemiology

AIH is a recently recognized disease, which was described for the first time by Waldenström in 1950.[1] Seropositivity for antinuclear antibody (ANA), the hallmark of systemic lupus erythematosus, led Mackay *et al.* to call it "lupoid hepatitis,"[2] a term that is no longer used. As the disease frequently presents acutely, the term "chronic active hepatitis," which implied that the disease should be chronic—i.e., of at least 6 months' duration—before institution of treatment, is similarly obsolete. Before the efficacy of immunosuppression was established, untreated severe AIH had a mortality of 50% at 5 years and 90% at 10 years.[3,4] The prevalence of AIH is unknown. Reported prevalences vary from one in 200 000 in the general population in the United States[5] to 20 in 100 000 in females over 14 years of age in Spain,[6] although probably both figures are underestimates. Data collected at our tertiary center suggest that there is an increasing annual incidence of both AIH and ASC in childhood. In the 1990s, these conditions represented 2.3% of children older than 4 months referred to the King's Paediatric Liver Service during one year, whereas in the 2000s, their incidence has increased to 12%.

Etiology and pathogenesis

The etiology of AIH is unknown, although both genetic and environmental factors are involved in its expression.

Genetics. AIH is a "complex-trait" disease—i.e., a condition not inherited in a Mendelian autosomal-dominant, autosomal-recessive, or sex-linked fashion. The mode of inheritance of a complex-trait disorder is unknown and involves one or more genes operating alone or in concert to increase or reduce the risk of the trait, and interacting with environmental factors.

Susceptibility to AIH is imparted by genes in the histocompatibility leukocyte antigen (HLA) region on the short arm of chromosome 6, especially those encoding DRB1 alleles. These class II major histocompatibility complex (MHC) molecules are involved in peptide antigen presentation to CD4 T cells, suggesting the involvement of MHC class II antigen presentation and T-cell activation in the pathogenesis of AIH.

In Europe and North America, susceptibility to AIH type 1 is conferred by the possession of HLA DR3 (*DRB1*0301*) and DR4 (*DRB1*0401*), both heterodimers containing a lysine residue at position 71 of the DRB1 polypeptide and the hexameric amino acid sequence LLEQKR at positions 67–72.[7–9] In Japan, Argentina, and Mexico, susceptibility is linked to *DRB1*0405* and *DRB1*0404*, alleles encoding arginine rather than lysine at position 71, but sharing the motif LLEQ-R with *DRB1*0401* and *DRB1*0301*.[10] Thus, K or R at position 71 in the context of LLEQ-R may be critical for susceptibility to AIH, favoring the binding of autoantigenic peptides, complementary to this hexameric sequence.

The lysine-71 and other models for AIH type 1 cannot explain the disease completely, since in European and North American patients, for example, the presence of lysine-71 is associated with a severe and mainly juvenile disease in those who are positive for *DRB1*0301*, but to a mild and adult-onset disease in those who are positive for *DRB1*0401*. Other genes inside and/or outside the MHC are therefore likely to be involved in determining the phenotype. Possible candidates are the MHC-encoded complement and tumor necrosis factor-α genes, mapping to the class III MHC region, and the MHC class I chain-related A and B genes. Patients with AIH, whether positive for anti-liver–kidney microsomal antibody type 1 (anti-LKM-1) or ANA/SMA, have isolated partial deficiency of the HLA class III complement component C4, which is genetically determined.[11,12]

Susceptibility to AIH type 2 is conferred by the possession of HLA DR7 (*DRB1*0701*) and DR3 (*DRB1*0301*), and patients who are positive for *DRB1*0701* have a more aggressive disease and a more severe prognosis.[13]

A form of AIH resembling AIH type 2 affects some 20% of patients with autoimmune polyendocrinopathy–candidiasis–ectodermal dystrophy (APECED), a condition also known as autoimmune polyendocrine syndrome 1. APECED is a monogenic autosomal-recessive disorder caused by homozygous mutations in the *AIRE1* gene and characterized by a variety of organ-specific autoimmune diseases, the most common of which are hypoparathyroidism and primary adrenocortical failure, accompanied by chronic mucocutaneous candidiasis.[14,15] The *AIRE1* gene sequence consists of 14 exons containing 45 different mutations, with a 13-base pair deletion at nucleotide 964 in exon 8 accounting for more than 70% of APECED alleles in the United Kingdom.[14] The protein predicted to be encoded by *AIRE1* is a transcription factor. *AIRE1* is highly expressed in medullary epithelial cells and other stromal cells in the thymus that are involved in clonal deletion of self-reactive T cells. Studies in a murine model indicate that the gene inhibits organ-specific autoimmunity by inducing thymic expression of peripheral antigens in the medulla, leading to central deletion of autoreactive T cells. Interestingly, APECED has a high level of variability in symptoms, especially between populations. Since various gene mutations have the same effect on thymic transcription of ectopic genes in animal models, it is likely that the clinical variability across human populations is related to environmental or genetic modifiers. Of the various genetic modifiers, perhaps the most likely to synergize with *AIRE* mutations are polymorphisms in the HLA region. HLA molecules are not only highly variable and strongly associated with multiple autoimmune diseases, but are also able to affect thymic repertoire selection of autoreactive T-cell clones. Carriers of a single *AIRE* mutation do not develop APECED. However, although the inheritance pattern of APECED indicates a strictly recessive disorder, there are anecdotal reports of mutations in a single copy of *AIRE* being associated with human autoimmunity of a less severe form than classically defined APECED.[14,15] The role of the *AIRE1* heterozygote state in the development of AIH remains to be established.

Immune mechanisms. Immunohistochemical studies have identified the phenotype of the cells infiltrating the portal tract and invading the parenchyma in the typical AIH histological picture of interface hepatitis. T lymphocytes mounting the α/β T-cell receptor predominate. Among the T cells, the majority are positive for the CD4 helper/inducer phenotype, and a sizable minority are positive for the CD8 cytotoxic phenotype. Lymphocytes of non–T-cell lineage are fewer and include (in decreasing order of frequency) natural killer cells (CD16/CD56-positive), macrophages, and B lymphocytes.[16] The recently described natural killer T cells, which simultaneously express markers of both natural killer (CD56) and T cells (CD3), were found to be involved in liver damage in an animal model of autoimmune hepatitis.[17]

Powerful recruiting stimuli must be promoting the formation of the massive inflammatory cell infiltrate that is present at diagnosis. Whatever the initial trigger, it is most probable that such a high number of activated inflammatory cells cause liver damage.

There are different possible pathways that an autoimmune attack can follow to inflict damage on hepatocytes (Figure 8.2). It is believed that liver damage is orchestrated by $CD4^+$ T lymphocytes recognizing a self-antigenic peptide on hepatocytes. To trigger an autoimmune response, the peptide has to be embraced by an HLA class II molecule and presented to uncommitted (naïve) $CD4^+$ T helper (Th0) cells by professional antigen-presenting cells (APC), with the co-stimulation of ligand–ligand ($CD28^+$ on Th0, $CD80^+$ on APC) fostering interaction between the two cells. Th0 cells become activated, differentiate into functional phenotypes according to the cytokines prevailing in the microenvironment and the nature of the antigen, and initiate a cascade of immune reactions determined by the cytokines these activated T cells produce. Th1 cells, arising in the presence of the macrophage-produced interleukin 12 (IL-12), secrete mainly IL-2 and interferon gamma (IFN-γ), which activate macrophages, enhance expression of HLA class I (increasing liver cell vulnerability to a $CD8^+$ T-cell cytotoxic attack) and induce

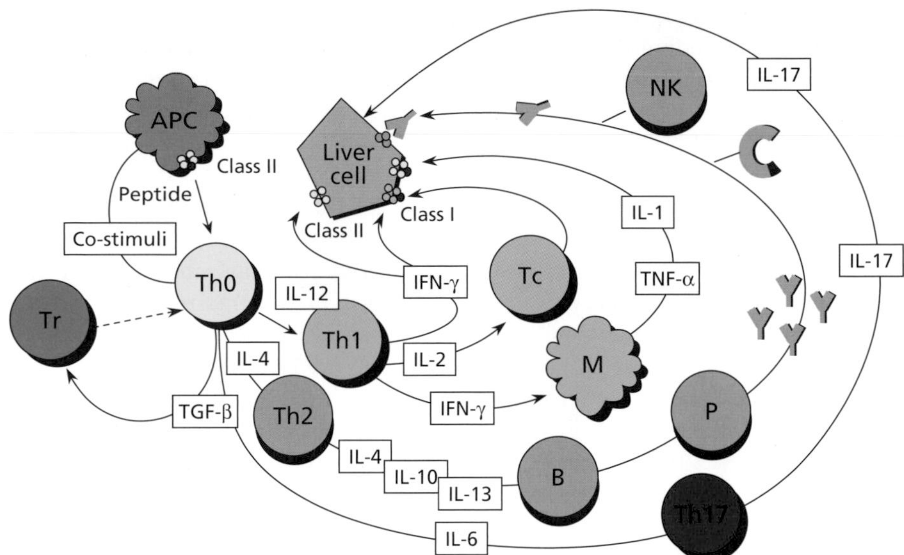

Figure 8.2 Autoimmune attack on the liver cell. A specific autoantigenic peptide is presented to an uncommitted T helper (T_H0) lymphocyte within the HLA class II molecule of an antigen-presenting cell (APC). T_H0 cells become activated and, depending on the presence in the microenvironment of interleukin-12 (IL-12) or IL-4 and the nature of the antigen, differentiate into T_H1 or T_H2 and initiate a series of immune reactions determined by the cytokines they produce. T_H2 cells mainly secrete IL-4, IL-10, and IL-13, and direct autoantibody production by B lymphocytes. T_H1 cells secrete IL-2 and interferon gamma (IFN-γ), which stimulate T cytotoxic (Tc) lymphocytes, enhance expression of class I, and induce expression of class II HLA molecules on hepatocytes and activate macrophages. Activated macrophages release IL-1 and tumor necrosis factor alpha (TNF-α). If regulatory T cells (Tr) do not oppose, a variety of effector mechanisms are triggered: liver cell destruction could result from the action of Tc lymphocytes; cytokines released by T_H1 and recruited macrophages; complement activation or engagement of Fc receptor–bearing cells such as natural killer (NK) lymphocytes by the autoantibody bound to the hepatocyte surface. The role of the recently described Th17 cells, which arise in the presence of tissue growth factor beta (TGF-β) and IL-6 is under investigation.

expression of HLA class II molecules on hepatocytes. Th2 cells, which differentiate from Th0 if the microenvironment is rich in IL-4, mainly produce IL-4, IL-10, and IL-13, which favor autoantibody production by B lymphocytes. Physiologically, Th1 and Th2 antagonize each other. Th17 cells, a recently described population,[18,19] arise in the presence of transforming growth factor-β (TGF-β) and IL-6 and appear to have an important effector role in inflammation and autoimmunity. The process of autoantigen recognition is strictly controlled by regulatory mechanisms, such as those exerted by $CD4^+CD25^+$ regulatory T cells, which are derived from Th0 in the presence of TGF-β, but in the absence of IL-6. If regulatory mechanisms fail, the autoimmune attack develops and persists.

Various aspects of the above pathogenic scenario have been investigated during the last 30 years:

• *Regulatory T cells.* Autoimmunity arises against a background of defective immunoregulation, and this has been repeatedly reported in AIH. Early studies showed that patients with AIH have low levels of circulating T cells expressing the $CD8^+$ marker, and impaired suppressor cell function, which segregates with the possession of the disease-predisposing HLA haplotype *B*08/DRB1*03* (formerly B8/DR3) and is correctable by therapeutic doses of corticosteroids.[20,21] It is possible, although not formally tested, that these early characterized $CD8^+$ T cells with a suppressor function represent the recently defined $CD8^+CD28^-$ suppressor T cells.[22] Furthermore, patients with AIH have been shown to have a defect in a subpopulation of T cells controlling the immune response to liver-specific membrane antigens.[23] Novel experimental evidence confirms an impairment of the immunoregulatory function in AIH. Amongst recently defined T-cell subsets with potential immunosuppressive function, $CD4^+$ T cells constitutively expressing the IL-2 receptor α chain (CD25; T regulatory cells, T-regs) have emerged as the dominant immunoregulatory subset of lymphocytes.[24] These cells, which represent some 5% of the total population of peripheral $CD4^+$ T cells in health, control innate and adaptive immune responses by preventing proliferation and effector function of autoreactive T cells. In patients with AIH, T-regs are defective in number and function in comparison with normal controls, and this impairment relates to the stage of disease, being more evident at diagnosis than during drug-induced remission.[25–27] The percentage of T-regs inversely correlates with markers of disease severity, such as anti-SLA and anti-LKM1 autoantibody titers, suggesting that a reduction in regulatory T cells favors the serological expression of autoimmune liver disease. If loss of immunoregulation is central to the pathogenesis of AIH, treatment should concentrate on restoring the T-regs' ability to expand, with a consequent increase in their number and function. This is at least partially achieved by standard immunosuppression, since numbers of T-regs increase during remission.[25–27]

• *Autoreactive T cells.* As mentioned above, to trigger an autoimmune response, a peptide embraced by an HLA class II molecule has to be presented to uncommitted T-helper (Th0) cells by professional APCs (Figure 8.2). Given the impaired regulatory function described above, it is suspected that in AIH, an autoantigenic peptide is indeed presented to the helper/inducer T cells, leading to their sustained activation. There is direct, albeit limited, evidence that an autoantigenic peptide is presented and recognized in AIH type 2.[13] Activation of T helper cells has been documented in earlier studies on AIH, both in the liver and in the peripheral blood.[16,28] These activated cells are mainly of the CD4 phenotype, and their numbers are highest in the most active stages of the disease.

Major advances in the study of T cells have occurred in AIH type 2, since the knowledge that CYP2D6 is the main autoantigen has made it possible to characterize both CD4 and CD8 T cells targeting this cytochrome. One study has shown that CD4 T cells from patients with type 2 AIH who are positive for the predisposing HLA allele *DRB1*0701* recognize seven regions of CYP2D6,[13] five of which have later been shown to be also recognized by CD8 T cells.[29] High numbers of antigen-specific interferon gamma–producing CD4 and CD8 T cells are associated with biochemical evidence of liver damage, suggesting a combined cellular immune attack.

What triggers the immune system to react to an autoantigen is unknown. A lesson may be learned by the study of humoral autoimmune responses during viral infections. Thus, recent studies aimed at determining the specificity of the LKM-1 antibody—present in both the juvenile form of AIH and in some patients with chronic hepatitis C virus (HCV) infection—have shown a high amino acid sequence homology between the HCV polyprotein and CYP2D6, the molecular target of LKM-1, implicating a mechanism of molecular mimicry as a trigger for the production of anti-LKM-1 in HCV infection.[30–32] It is therefore conceivable that an as yet unknown virus infection may be at the origin of the autoimmune attack in AIH.

Titers of antibodies to liver-specific lipoprotein, a macromolecular complex present on the hepatocyte membrane, and to its well-characterized component asialoglycoprotein receptor, correlate with the biochemical and histologic severity of AIH.[33,34] Immunofluorescence studies of monodispersed suspensions of liver cells obtained from patients with AIH have shown that these cells are coated with antibodies in vivo.[35] A pathogenic role for these autoantibodies has been indicated by cytotoxicity assays showing that autoantibody-coated hepatocytes from patients with AIH are killed when incubated with autologous[36] lymphocytes. The effector cell was identified as an Fc receptor–positive mononuclear cell.[36] T-cell clones obtained from liver biopsies of patients with AIH and expressing the γ/δ T-cell receptor have been shown to be cytotoxic to a variety of targets, but to preferentially kill liver-derived cells as opposed to cell lines derived from other organs.[37]

The establishment of cell lines and clones enabled Wen and colleagues[37,38] and Löhr and colleagues[39,40] to show that the majority of T-cell clones obtained from the peripheral blood and a proportion of those from the liver of patients with AIH are CD4-positive and use the conventional α/β T-cell receptor. Some of these CD4-positive clones were further characterized and were found to react with partially purified antigens, such as crude preparations of liver cell membrane or liver-specific lipoprotein,[38] and with purified asialoglycoprotein receptor[38,40] or recombinant CYP2D6,[39] and to be restricted by HLA class II molecules in their response. Because CD4 is the phenotype of Th cells, both Wen and colleagues[38] and Löhr and colleagues[40] investigated whether these clones were able to help autologous B lymphocytes in the production of immunoglobulin in vitro and found that their coculture with B lymphocytes resulted in a dramatic increase in autoantibody production. All of the above experimental evidence suggests that cellular immune responses are involved in the liver damage that occurs in AIH, although the evidence that the trigger is an autoantigen is still incomplete.

Clinical features

AIH affects mainly females and is divided into two main types according to the autoantibody profile: type 1 is positive for ANA and/or anti-smooth muscle (SMA) antibody, type 2 is positive for anti-liver–kidney microsomal antibody type 1 (anti-LKM-1). Pediatric series, including the King's one, have reported a similarly severe disease in ANA/SMA-positive and anti-LKM-1–positive patients.[41,42] We reviewed the clinical, biochemical, and histological features and outcomes of type 1 and type 2 AIH in 52 children referred between 1973 and 1993 (Table 8.1).[8,42,43] Thirty-two patients were positive for ANA and/or SMA, and 20 were positive for anti-LKM-1.

The clinical features included:

• 75% female preponderance
• Variable age at onset (median of 10 years in type 1 and 7.4 years in type 2), with occasional presentation in infancy
• Other autoimmune disorders affecting patients in 20% and a first-degree relative in 40% of cases
• Similar severity and outcome

The mode of presentation was variable, with the following predominant types emerging:

• Acute presentation resembling that of viral hepatitis (in 50% of patients with type 1 and 65% of patients with type 2 AIH) with nonspecific symptoms of malaise, nausea/vomiting, anorexia, and abdominal pain, followed by jaundice, dark urine, and pale stools.
• Fulminant hepatic failure (in 11%, five out of six of these patients having type 2); with grade II to IV hepatic

Table 8.1 Autoimmune hepatitis type 1, autoimmune hepatitis type 2, and autoimmune sclerosing cholangitis: clinical, laboratory and histological features at presentation.[8,43]

	Type 1 AIH	Type 2 AIH	ASC
Median age in years	11	7	12
Females (%)	75	75	55
Mode of presentation (%)			
Acute hepatitis	47	40	37
Acute liver failure	3	25	0
Insidious onset	38	25	37
Complication of portal hypertension	12	10	26
Associated autoimmune diseases (%)	22	20	48
Inflammatory bowel disease (%)	20	12	44
Family history of autoimmune disease (%)	43	40	37
Abnormal cholangiogram (%)	0	0	100
Interface hepatitis (%)	66	72	35
Biliary features (%)	28	6	31
Cirrhosis (%)	69	38	15
Remission after immunosuppressive treatment (%)	97	87	89
Increased frequency of HLA *DR*0301*	Yes	No*	No
Increased frequency of HLA *DR*0701*	No	Yes	No
Increased frequency of HLA *DR*1301*	No	No	Yes
ANA/SMA (%)	100	25	96
Anti-LKM-1 (%)	0	100	4
pANCA (%)	45	11	74
Anti-SLA (%)†	58	58	41
Increased IgG level (%)	84	75	89
Partial IgA deficiency (%)	9	45	5
Low C4 level (%)	89	83	70

AIH, autoimmune hepatitis; ANA, anti-nuclear antibodies; ASC, autoimmune sclerosing cholangitis; C4, C4 component of complement; HLA, human leukocyte antigen; IgA, immunoglobulin A; IgG, immunoglobulin G; LKM-1, liver–kidney microsomal type 1 antibody; pANCA, perinuclear anti-neutrophil cytoplasmic antibody; SLA, soluble liver antigen; SMA, anti-smooth muscle antibody.
* Increased in patients who are negative for HLA *DR*0701*.
† Measured by radioligand assay.

encephalopathy developing 2 weeks to 2 months (median 1 month) after the onset of symptoms.

- Insidious onset, characterized by progressive fatigue, relapsing jaundice, headache, anorexia, and weight loss, lasting from 6 months to 2 years (median 9 months) before diagnosis (25% of patients with type 2 and 38% of patients with type 1 AIH).
- Complications of cirrhosis and portal hypertension. In six patients (two of whom were positive for anti-LKM-1), there was no history of jaundice, and the diagnosis followed presentation with complications of portal hypertension, such as hematemesis from esophageal varices, bleeding diathesis, chronic diarrhea, weight loss, and vomiting.
- Incidental finding of raised hepatic aminotransferases.

Associated disorders

There was also no significant difference in the frequency of associated autoimmune disorders and a family history of autoimmune disease. Associated autoimmune disorders included:

- Behçet disease
- Insulin-dependent diabetes
- Graves disease
- Celiac disease
- Inflammatory bowel disease
- Sjögren syndrome
- Hemolytic anemia
- Glomerulonephritis
- Idiopathic thrombocytopenia
- Urticaria pigmentosa in type 1 AIH
- Thyroiditis, vitiligo, hypoparathyroidism, and Addison disease in type 2 AIH

Autoimmune hepatitis may also occur in 10–20% of patients with autoimmune polyglandular syndrome type 1 (autoimmune polyendocrinopathy–candidosis–ectodermal dystrophy, APECED).

The mode of presentation of AIH in childhood is therefore variable, and the disease should be suspected and excluded in all children presenting with symptoms and signs of prolonged or severe liver disease.

Differential diagnosis

The differential diagnosis, depending on presentation, includes:

- Autoimmune hepatitis
- Sclerosing cholangitis
- Chronic viral hepatitis
- Acute infective hepatitis
- Drug-induced liver disease
- Metabolic liver disease
- Cystic fibrosis
- α_1-Antitrypsin deficiency
- Wilson's disease

A careful history is invaluable in considering this wide range of disorders.

Diagnosis and laboratory findings

These should include the following: elevated serum transaminase and IgG/γ-globulin levels, and presence of ANA, SMA, or anti-LKM-autoimmune markers.[44,45]

Biochemistry

Biochemical abnormalities in AIH hepatitis are nonspecific:

- Serum aminotransferases—alanine aminotransferase (ALT) and aspartate aminotransferase (AST)—are usually raised.
- Serum alkaline phosphatase and γ-glutamyltransferase (GGT) are usually normal or mildly elevated.
- Serum bilirubin is variable.
- Albumin may be low.
- Coagulation may be abnormal, particularly in chronic disease or fulminant hepatitis.

Overall, anti-LKM-1–positive patients had higher median levels of bilirubin and aspartate aminotransferase than those who were ANA/SMA-positive, but if the six patients presenting with acute hepatic failure are excluded, the differences for these two parameters are not significant. Severely impaired hepatic synthetic function, as assessed by prolonged prothrombin time and hypoalbuminemia, tended to be more common in patients with type 1 AIH (53%) than in those with type 2 AIH (30%).

Immunoglobulins

The majority (80%) of the patients had increased levels of IgG, but 10 (five of whom were positive for anti-LKM-1) had a normal serum IgG level for age, including three patients who presented with acute hepatic failure—indicating that normal IgG values do not exclude the diagnosis of AIH. As previously reported, we found that partial IgA deficiency is significantly more common in type 2 than in type 1 AIH (45% versus 9%).[46]

Histology

Liver biopsy is necessary to establish the diagnosis. The typical histological picture includes:

- A dense mononuclear and plasma cell infiltration of the portal areas, which expands into the liver lobule
- Destruction of the hepatocytes at the periphery of the lobule, with erosion of the limiting plate ("interface hepatitis"; Figure 8.1)
- Connective-tissue collapse resulting from hepatocyte death and expanding from the portal area into the lobule ("bridging collapse")
- Hepatic regeneration with "rosette" formation
- Cirrhosis

The severity of interface hepatitis is similar in both type 1 and 2 at diagnosis. Cirrhosis on initial biopsy was more frequent in ANA/SMA-positive patients (69%) than in anti-LKM-1–positive patients (38%). Fifty-seven percent of patients who were already cirrhotic at diagnosis presented with a clinical picture reminiscent of that of prolonged acute virus-like hepatitis. Multiacinar or panacinar collapse, which suggests an acute liver injury, was present in eight patients (15%, five of whom were anti-LKM-1–positive), six of whom had acute liver failure. In these patients, it was not possible to ascertain the degree of fibrosis or the presence or absence of cirrhosis. The question of whether the acute presentation in these patients represented a sudden deterioration of an underlying unrecognized chronic process or a genuinely acute liver damage remains open.

The diagnosis of AIH has been advanced by the criteria developed by the International Autoimmune Hepatitis Group (IAIHG),[44,47] in which negative criteria such as evidence of infection with hepatitis B or C virus or Wilson's disease are taken into account in addition to the positive criteria mentioned above. The IAIHG has provided a scoring system for the diagnosis of AIH, mainly used for research purposes.

Autoantibodies. Autoantibody detection by immunofluorescence (Figure 8.3) not only assists in the diagnosis, but also allows differentiation of AIH types. ANA and SMA, which characterize type 1 AIH, and anti-LKM-1, which defines type 2 AIH, are practically mutually exclusive. In the rare instances in which they are present simultaneously, the disease is classified as type 2 AIH. Recognition and interpretation of the immunofluorescence patterns is not always simple.[47] The operator dependency of the technique and the relative rarity of AIH explain the not infrequent occurrence of errors in reporting, particularly of less frequent findings such as anti-LKM-1. There are problems between laboratory reporting and the clinical interpretation of the results, which are partly dependent on insufficient standardization of the tests, but also partly dependent on a degree of unfamiliarity of some clinicians with the disease spectrum of AIH. With regard to standardization, guidelines have been provided by the IAIHG serology committee.[47] The basic technique for the

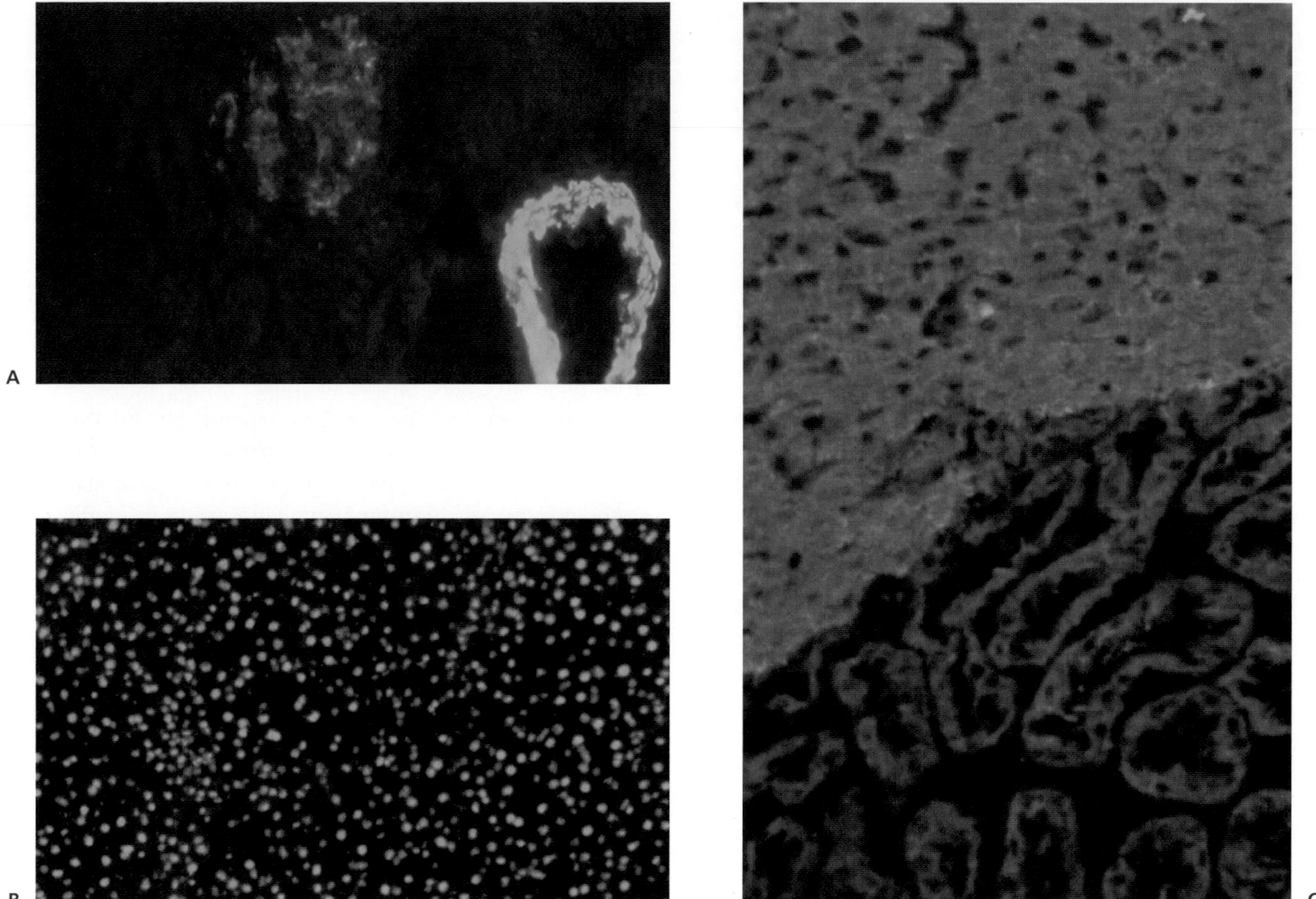

Figure 8.3 Immunofluorescence appearance of smooth muscle (SMA), antinuclear (ANA) and liver–kidney microsomal type 1 (LKM-1) autoantibodies on renal and liver rodent sections. SMA stains the small artery and the glomerulus in a renal section (**A**), ANA the nuclei in a liver section (**B**), and LKM-1 the cytoplasm of hepatocytes and proximal renal tubules (**C**). SMA and/or ANA are the markers of autoimmune hepatitis type 1; their molecular targets are still unknown. LKM-1 characterizes autoimmune hepatitis type 2, and its target is cytochrome P4502D6.

routine testing of autoantibodies relevant to AIH is indirect immunofluorescence on a freshly prepared rodent substrate, which should include kidney, liver, and stomach, to allow the detection of ANA, SMA, anti-LKM-1 as well as anti-liver cytosol type 1 (anti-LC-1), but also of antimitochondrial antibody (AMA), the serological hallmark of primary biliary cirrhosis. Commercially available sections are of variable quality because, in order to lengthen their shelf-life, they are treated with fixatives (acetone, ethanol, or methanol), which readily result in enhanced background staining that may hinder the recognition of diagnostic autoantibodies, especially when these are present at low titer. In healthy children, autoantibody reactivity is infrequent, so that titers of 1/20 for ANA and SMA and 1/10 for anti-LKM-1 are clinically relevant. Positive sera should be titrated to extinction. The laboratory should report any level of positivity from 1/10 in children and 1/40 in adults, and the attending physician should interpret the result within the clinical context.

ANA is readily detectable as a nuclear stain in kidney, stomach, and liver. On the latter in particular, the ANA pattern may be detected as homogeneous, or coarsely or finely speckled. In most cases of AIH, but not in all, the pattern is homogeneous. To obtain a much clearer and easier definition of the nuclear pattern, HEp2 cells that have prominent nuclei should be used. However, HEp2 cells, derived from a laryngeal carcinoma, should not be used for screening purposes, because nuclear reactivity to these cells is frequent at a low serum dilution (1/40) in the normal population.[48] For ANA, likely molecular targets include nuclear chromatin and histones, akin to lupus, but there are probably several others.

SMA is detected on kidney, stomach, and liver, where it stains the walls of the arteries. In the stomach, it also stains the muscularis mucosa and the lamina propria. On the renal substrate, it is possible to visualize the V, G, and T patterns; V refers to vessels, G to glomeruli, and T to tubules.[49] The V pattern is present also in non-autoimmune inflammatory liver disease, in autoimmune diseases not affecting the liver, and in viral infections, but the VG and VGT patterns are more specific for AIH. The VGT pattern corresponds to the so-called "F actin" or microfilament (MF) pattern observed using cultured fibroblasts as substrate. However, neither the VGT nor the anti-MF patterns are entirely specific for the diagnosis of AIH type 1 Although it has been suggested that the VGT–MF pattern is due to a specific antibody uniquely found in AIH type 1, it probably just reflects high-titer SMA. The molecular target of the microfilament reactivity that is observed in AIH type 1 has yet to be identified. Although "anti-actin" reactivity is strongly associated with AIH type 1, some 20% of SMA-positive AIH type 1 patients do not have the F-actin/VGT pattern. The absence of anti-actin SMA therefore does not exclude the diagnosis of AIH.[50]

Anti-LKM-1 brightly stains the liver cell cytoplasm and the P3 portion of the renal tubules, but does not stain gastric parietal cells. Anti-LKM-1 is often confused with AMA, since both autoantibodies stain liver and kidney. In comparison with anti-LKM-1, AMA stains the liver more faintly and the renal tubules more diffusely, with an accentuation of the small distal ones. In contrast to anti-LKM-1, AMA also stains the gastric parietal cells. AMA positivity in childhood AIH is exceedingly rare.[51] The identification of the molecular targets of anti-LKM-1, i.e., cytochrome P4502D6 (CYP2D6), and of AMA, i.e., enzymes of the 2-oxo-acid dehydrogenase complexes, has led to the establishment of immunoassays based on the use of the recombinant or purified antigens.[47] Commercially available enzyme-linked immunosorbent assays (ELISAs) are accurate for detecting anti-LKM-1, at least in the context of AIH type 2, and reasonably accurate for the detection of AMA. Therefore, if any doubt remains after immunofluorescence examination, it can be resolved by using molecular-based immunoassays.

Other autoantibodies less commonly tested, but of diagnostic importance, include those to liver cytosol type 1 (LC-1), antineutrophil cytoplasm (ANCA), and soluble liver antigen (SLA). Anti-LC-1, which may be present on its own but frequently occurs in association with anti-LKM-1, is an additional marker for AIH type 2 and targets formiminotransferase cyclodeaminase (FTCD).[52] Antineutrophil cytoplasmic antibody (ANCA) can also be positive in AIH.[42,47] There are three types of ANCA—namely, cytoplasmic (cANCA), perinuclear (pANCA), and atypical perinuclear, the target of which is a peripheral nuclear and not cytoplasmic perinuclear antigen (hence the suggested term "pANNA"—i.e., peripheral antinuclear neutrophil antibody). The type found in AIH type 1 is pANNA, which is also found in inflammatory bowel disease and sclerosing cholangitis, while it is virtually absent in type 2 AIH. Anti-SLA, which was originally described as the hallmark of a third type of AIH,[53] is also found in some 50% of patients with type 1 and type 2 AIH, in whom it defines a more severe course.[54] Screening of cDNA expression libraries using high-titer anti-SLA serum has made it possible to identify the molecular target antigen as UGA tRNA suppressor–associated antigenic protein (tRNP(Ser)Sec).[7,55]

After assessment of all the specific findings described above, there is still a small proportion of patients with AIH who do not have detectable autoantibodies. This condition, which responds to immunosuppression in the same way as the seropositive form, represents seronegative AIH, and its prevalence and clinical characteristics have yet to be defined.

Management and prognosis

AIH is exquisitely responsive to immunosuppression. The rapidity and degree of the response depends on the disease severity at presentation. All types of presentation, with the exception of fulminant hepatic failure with encephalopathy, respond to standard treatment with prednisolone with or without azathioprine.

Standard treatment for AIH consists of prednisolone 2 mg/kg/day (maximum 40–60 mg/day), which is gradually decreased over a period of 4–8 weeks in parallel to the decline of transaminase levels. Once normal liver function tests are obtained, which may take several weeks or even a few months, the patient is maintained on the minimal dosage that is capable of sustaining normal transaminase levels—usually 5 mg/day.[42] During the first 6–8 weeks of treatment, liver function tests are checked weekly to allow frequent fine-tuning, avoiding severe steroid side effects. If progressive normalization of the liver function tests is not obtained over this period of time, or if too high a dose of prednisolone is required to maintain normal transaminases, azathioprine is added at a starting dose of 0.5 mg/kg/day, which—in the absence of signs of toxicity—is increased up to a maximum of 2.0–2.5 mg/kg/day until biochemical control is achieved. Azathioprine is not recommended as first-line treatment because of its hepatotoxicity in severely jaundiced patients, but 85% of the patients will eventually require the addition of azathioprine.

Children who present with acute hepatic failure pose a particularly difficult therapeutic problem. If not encephalopathic, they usually benefit from conventional immunosuppressive therapy, but only one of the six children with acute liver failure and encephalopathy in the King's series responded to immunosuppression and survived without transplantation.[42]

A preliminary report in a cohort of 30 children with AIH suggests that the measurements of the azathioprine metabolites 6-thioguanine and 6-methylmercaptopurine are useful in identifying drug toxicity and nonadherence and in achieving a level of 6-thioguanine considered therapeutic for inflammatory bowel disease[56]—although an ideal therapeutic level for AIH has not been determined. Although an 80% decrease in the initial transaminase levels is obtained within 6 weeks of the start of treatment in most patients, complete normalization of liver function may take several months. In the King's series, normalization of transaminase levels occurred at median of 6 months in children who were positive for ANA/SMA and 9 months in children who were positive for LKM-1.[42]

Withdrawal of treatment

Cessation of treatment is considered if a liver biopsy shows minimal or no inflammatory changes after 1 year of normal liver function tests. However, it is advisable not to attempt to withdraw treatment within 3 years of diagnosis or during or immediately before puberty, when relapses are more common. In the King's experience, successful long-term withdrawal of treatment was achieved in 20% of patients with AIH type 1, but in none with AIH type 2.[42]

In pediatric care, an important role in monitoring the response to treatment is the measurement of autoantibody titers and IgG levels, the fluctuation of which correlates with disease activity.[57]

Outcome

Progression to cirrhosis was more common in type 1 than in type 2 AIH. Overall, 74% of ANA/SMA-positive and 44% of anti-LKM-1–positive patients showed evidence of cirrhosis on initial or follow-up histological assessment, indicating that, apart from the higher tendency to present with acute liver failure, the severity of type 1 and type 2 AIH is similar. Recently, we have demonstrated that a more severe disease and a higher tendency to relapse are associated with the possession of antibodies to soluble liver antigen (SLA), which are present in about half of patients with AIH type 1 or 2 at diagnosis.[54]

Side effects of steroid treatment were mild, the only serious complication being psychosis during induction of remission in 4%, which resolved after withdrawal of prednisolone. All patients developed a transient increase in appetite and mild cushingoid features during the first few weeks of treatment. After 5 years of treatment, 56% of the patients maintained the baseline centile for height or went up across a centile line, 38% dropped across one centile line, and only 6% dropped across two centile lines.[58] In addition, it has recently been shown that long-term daily treatment with prednisolone in children with autoimmune liver disease does not affect their expected final adult height relative to parental stature.[59]

Sustained remission, achieved with prednisolone and azathioprine, has been maintained with azathioprine alone in some patients with AIH type 1, akin to the experience in adults,[60] but not in AIH type 2.

Relapse during treatment is common, occurring in about 40% of patients and requiring a temporary increase in the steroid dose. An important role in relapse is played by nonadherence, which is common, particularly in adolescents and young adults.[61] The risk of relapse may also be higher if steroids are administered on an alternate-day schedule, which is often instituted because it may have a less negative effect on the child's growth. Small daily doses are more effective in maintaining disease control and minimize the need for high-dose steroid pulses during relapses (with the consequent more severe side effects).

Treatment can be safely continued during pregnancy. Although the experience is limited, there do not appear to be any adverse events for mother and baby.[62] In particular, no teratogenic effects have been described with azathioprine in humans, although for women who are concerned about its use, treatment with steroids alone can be considered.

Despite the efficacy of standard immunosuppressive treatment, severe hepatic decompensation may develop even after many years of apparently good biochemical control, leading to transplantation 10–15 years after diagnosis in 10% of the patients. Overall, in the King's series, over 97% of patients treated with standard immunosuppression were alive between 0.3 and 19 years (median 5 years) after diagnosis, including 8% after liver transplantation.

Other immunosuppressive agents

Mycophenolate mofetil

Mycophenolate mofetil (MMF) is the prodrug of mycophenolic acid. Its effect on purine synthesis leads to decreased T and B lymphocyte proliferation. In patients (up to 10%) in whom standard immunosuppression is unable to induce stable remission, or who are intolerant to azathioprine, mycophenolate mofetil at a dose of 20 mg/kg twice daily, together with prednisolone, is successfully used.[58] If there is a persistent absence of response or if there is intolerance for mycophenolate mofetil (headache, diarrhea, nausea, dizziness, hair loss, and neutropenia), the use of calcineurin inhibitors (cyclosporine A or tacrolimus) should be considered.

Cyclosporine

Induction of remission has been obtained in 71% of treatment-naïve children with AIH using cyclosporine A alone for 6 months, followed by maintenance with low-dose prednisone and azathioprine.[63] Whether this mode of induction has any advantage over the standard treatment has yet to be evaluated in controlled studies in specialized centers. However, as the side effects of cyclosporine—including renal impairment, gingival hyperplasia, and hirsutism—may cause more significant morbidity than those of prednisolone, it has not become established as a first-line treatment.

Cyclosporine has been shown to be effective in patients with AIH type 1 and 2 who are resistant to prednisolone/azathioprine, and it is well tolerated.[63]

Tacrolimus

Tacrolimus is a more potent immunosuppressive agent than cyclosporine, but it also has significant toxicity. There is limited evidence supporting its role in the treatment of AIH apart from anecdotal evidence, but it may be useful in combination with prednisolone as second-line therapy.

Indications for liver transplantation

Despite an apparent initial response to immunosuppression, gradual histological progression may occur over a period of years. Failure of medical treatment is more likely when established cirrhosis is present at diagnosis, or if there is a long history before the start of treatment.

Approximately 10–20% of children with AIH require liver transplantation for the following indications:

- Fulminant hepatic failure
- Complications of cirrhosis
- Failure of medical therapy

AIH recurs in approximately 25%, and this needs to be included in pretransplantation counseling, as does the need for lifelong steroid therapy.

Autoimmune hepatitis/sclerosing cholangitis overlap syndrome

Sclerosing cholangitis

Sclerosing cholangitis is a chronic inflammatory disorder that may affect both the intrahepatic and extrahepatic bile ducts and may lead to fibrosis. The diagnosis is based on typical bile duct lesions being visualized on cholangiography. The increasing recognition of this disease in children—rising from five cases before 1987 to almost 200 reported since—reflects the introduction of percutaneous and endoscopic cholangiography into pediatric practice, rather than an actual increase in the prevalence of the condition.

Autoimmune hepatitis/sclerosing cholangitis overlap syndrome (autoimmune sclerosing cholangitis, ASC) has the same prevalence as AIH type 1 in childhood.[43] This has been shown in a prospective study conducted over a period of 16 years, in which all children with serological features (i.e., autoantibodies, high IgG levels) and histological features (i.e., interface hepatitis) of autoimmune liver disease underwent cholangiography at the time of presentation. Approximately 50% of these patients had alterations in the bile ducts characteristic of sclerosing cholangitis, although the changes were generally less advanced than those observed in adult primary sclerosing cholangitis (Figure 8.4). A quarter of the children with ASC, despite abnormal cholangiograms, had no histological features suggesting bile duct involvement, and the diagnosis of sclerosing cholangitis was only possible because of the cholangiographic studies. Susceptibility to ASC in children is conferred by the possession of HLA *DRB1*1301*.[64] The clinical, laboratory, and histological features of type 1 and 2 AIH and ASC are compared in Table 8.1.

Clinical features of ASC include:

- 50% of the patients are female.

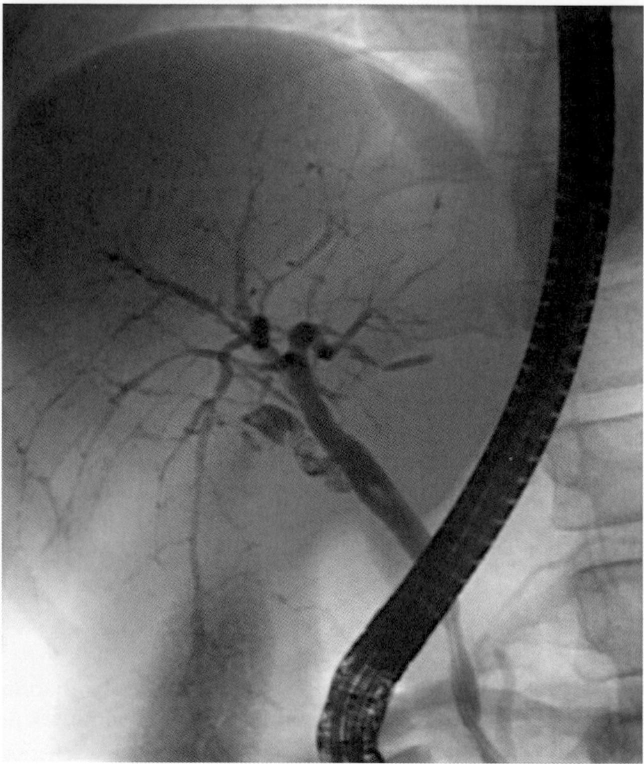

Figure 8.4 Endoscopic retrograde cholangiopancreatography (ERCP) of a child with autoimmune sclerosing cholangitis, demonstrating cholangiopathy with strictures and dilations affecting the intrahepatic and extrahepatic bile ducts.

- Abdominal pain, weight loss, and intermittent jaundice, resembling AIH type 1.
- Inflammatory bowel disease is present in about 45% of children with ASC, in comparison with about 20% of those with classical AIH.
- Virtually all patients are seropositive for ANA and/or SMA.
- 90% of children with ASC have greatly increased serum IgG levels.
- Standard liver function tests do not help in discriminating between AIH and ASC (Table 8.2).[8,43]
- pANCA was present in 74% of patients with ASC, in comparison with 45% of patients with AIH type 1 and 11% of those with AIH type 2.

Laboratory investigation

Elevated alkaline phosphatase and γ-glutamyltransferase (GGT) may be the most consistent biochemical abnormalities, except in early disease.

- *Alkaline phosphatase.* Although occasionally normal at presentation, it subsequently becomes elevated during the course of the disease.
- *GGT.* This is elevated if the diagnosis is made late.

Table 8.2 Autoimmune hepatitis and autoimmune sclerosing cholangitis: liver function tests at presentation.[8,43]

	AIH (n = 28)	ASC (n = 27)
Bilirubin (normal < 20 μmol/L)	35 (4–306)	20 (4–179)
AST (normal < 50 IU/L)	333 (24–4830)	102 (18–1215)
GGT (normal < 50 IU/L)	76 (29–383)	129 (13–948)
AP (normal < 350 IU/L)	356 (131–878)	303 (104–1710)
AP/AST ratio	1.14 (0.05–14.75)	3.96 (0.20–14.20)
Albumin (normal > 35 g/L)	35 (25–47)	39 (27–54)
INR (< 1.2)	1.2 (0.96–2.5)	1.1 (0.9–1.6)

Results are presented as medians (range). AP, alkaline phosphatase; AST, aspartate aminotransferase; GGT, γ-glutamyltransferase; INR, international normalized ratio (prothrombin).

• *Bilirubin*. The bilirubin level in serum may be normal at presentation in at least 50% of cases, contributing to the diagnostic delay. It may be intermittently elevated during the course of disease, with persistent elevation (see above) being associated with a poorer prognosis.

• *Hepatic transaminases*. These are moderately elevated in the majority of cases, and may be raised to 50 times the upper limit of normal.

• *Prothrombin time and albumin*. Hepatic synthetic function is usually preserved unless decompensation has occurred following progression to cirrhosis. An elevated prothrombin time may occur due to fat-soluble vitamin deficiency and may therefore be responsive to vitamin K.

Diagnostic imaging

Ultrasound

Ultrasonography may reveal intrahepatic and extrahepatic bile duct dilation, a heterogeneous or nodular echotexture characteristic of cirrhosis, or the manifestations of portal hypertension—including splenomegaly, ascites, and varices. However, the appearance may be normal in up to 50% of cases, particularly in early cases.

Cholangiography

The diagnosis of sclerosing cholangitis is confirmed by cholangiography (Figure 8.4), which reveals lesions typical of:

• Irregular intrahepatic ducts
• Focal saccular dilation
• Intervening short annular strictures (producing a beaded appearance)
• An abnormally large gallbladder
• Increased diameter of the common bile duct
• Extrahepatic ductal irregularity

Cholangiography can be carried out either using a direct intraoperative approach, a percutaneous transhepatic route, or with endoscopic retrograde cholangiopancreatography (ERCP). Although ERCP is technically feasible in children, it is associated with a risk of pancreatitis. More recently, the development of magnetic resonance cholangiopancreatography (MRCP) has provided a noninvasive method of diagnosis. Experience with this in children is increasing (Figure 8.5), although ERCP has proved to be much more accurate than MRI in early disease.

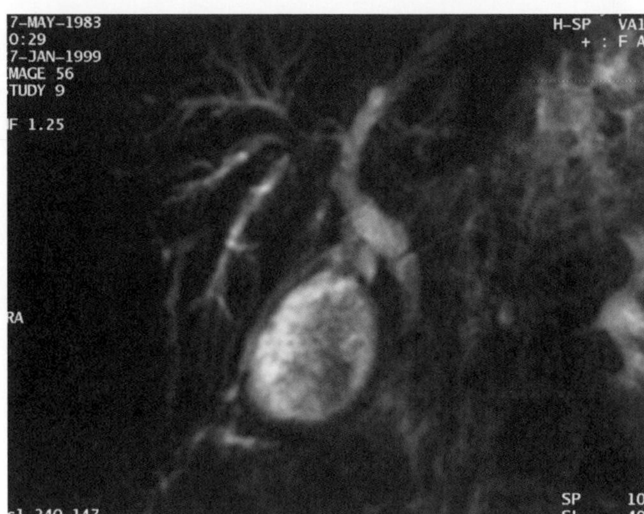

Figure 8.5 Magnetic resonance imaging is less invasive than endoscopic retrograde cholangiopancreatography and demonstrates the characteristic features of an enlarged gallbladder, with irregularity of the intrahepatic ducts due to septal dilation and short strictures.

Histology

The pathognomonic feature of sclerosing cholangitis—i.e., fibrous obliterative cholangitis with periductular fibrosis—is rarely seen in early cases, in which the patients mostly show inflammatory changes similar to those in AIH (Figure 8.6).

Treatment and prognosis

Children with ASC respond to the same immunosuppressive treatment described above for AIH.[25] Liver test abnormalities resolve in most patients within a few months after treatment has been started. However, although steroids and azathioprine are beneficial in abating the parenchymal inflammatory lesion, they appear to be less effective in controlling the bile duct disease. Following favorable reports in adult primary sclerosing cholangitis,[65,66] ursodeoxycholic acid is usually added at a dosage of 20–30 mg/kg/day, although there is no information on whether it is helpful in arresting the progression of ASC. Fat-soluble vitamin supplements are required if cholestasis develops. As in AIH, measurement of autoantibody titers and IgG levels is useful in monitoring disease activity and the response to treatment.[57] The medium term prognosis is good, with a reported 7-year survival of 100%, although 15% of the patients required

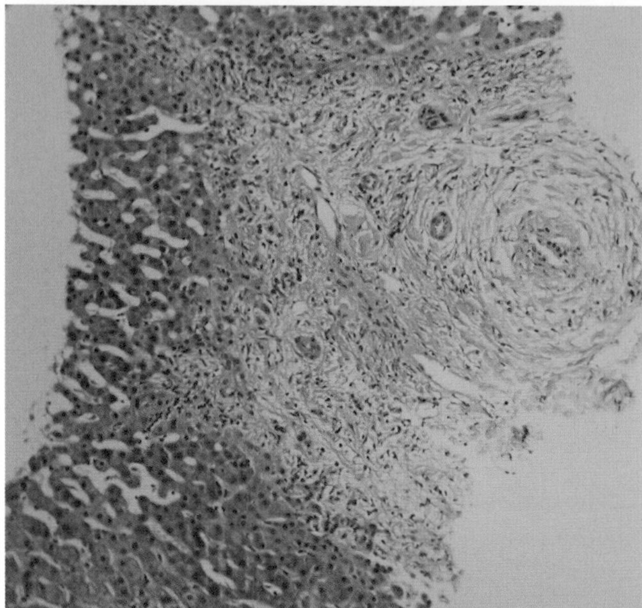

Figure 8.6 Liver histology in autoimmune sclerosing cholangitis may demonstrate the characteristic "onion-skin" appearance of the bile ducts secondary to fibrosis, in association with an inflammatory infiltrate, usually at an advanced stage of the disease.

liver transplantation during this follow-up period.[43] Evolution from AIH to ASC has been documented, suggesting that AIH and ASC may be part of the same pathogenic process.[43]

Recurrence of autoimmune liver disease after transplantation

Recurrence of AIH after liver transplantation has been reported in several studies.[67] The diagnosis is based on the reappearance of clinical symptoms and signs, histological features of periportal hepatitis, elevation of transaminases, circulating autoantibodies, and elevated IgG, associated with a response to steroids and azathioprine. Possession of the HLA DR3 allele appears to confer a predisposition to disease recurrence, as it does to the original AIH, although this has not been universally confirmed. Recurrence has been noted in both adult and pediatric series, and although the rate of this complication increases with the post-transplantation interval, it may appear as early as 1 month after surgery. Most transplant recipients with recurrent AIH respond to an increase in the dosage of corticosteroids and azathioprine, but in a few cases, recurrence can lead to graft failure and to a need for retransplantation. Caution should be exercised in weaning immunosuppression in patients who undergo transplantation for AIH, since discontinuation of corticosteroid therapy may increase the risk for recurrent disease.

ASC also recurs after liver transplantation—probably more frequently and with more severe consequences than AIH. Of six patients with ASC who underwent transplantation in our own series, three developed recurrent disease, with two requiring retransplantation, one of whom had a further recurrence, leading to a further transplantation (unpublished data; see also Chapter 21).

De novo AIH after transplantation

Tissue autoantibodies after liver transplantation—particularly ANA and SMA—are also common in patients who undergo transplantation for non-autoimmune liver disease.[67] Anti-LKM-1 is the third most frequently reported antibody, but its fluorescence pattern is at times atypical, staining the renal tubules preferentially and sparing the liver. The reported prevalence of post–liver transplantation autoantibodies is variable—probably reflecting the different techniques used for detecting them, the cut-off point above which the autoantibodies are considered positive, the time after transplantation at which they are tested, the nature of the clinical condition leading to transplantation, and the presence or absence of post-transplantation complications. In the late 1990s, it was observed that AIH can arise de novo after liver transplantation in children who had not undergone transplantation for autoimmune liver disease.[68] After the original report, de novo AIH after liver transplantation has been confirmed by several studies, both in adult and pediatric patients.[67,69] Importantly, treatment with prednisolone and azathioprine, using the same schedule for classical AIH, is also effective in de novo AIH, leading to excellent graft and patient survival. It is of interest that these patients do not respond satisfactorily to standard antirejection treatment, making it essential to reach an early diagnosis in order to avoid graft loss. It was recently reported, in a cohort of patients who underwent transplantation during childhood, that progressive liver damage over a 10-year follow-up period was associated with serological features of autoimmunity and a histological picture of chronic hepatitis[70] (see also Chapter 21).

The recurrence of AIH after transplantation can be readily explained. The recipient's immune system is sensitized to species-specific antigens and has a pool of memory cells, which are restimulated and reexpanded when the target antigens, "autoantigens," are presented to the recipient's immune system either by the recipient's APC repopulating the grafted liver, or by the donor's APC sharing histocompatibility antigens with the recipient. In contrast, akin to autoimmune liver disease outside the context of transplantation, the pathogenesis of post-transplantation de novo AIH remains to be defined. There are several possible explanations, which are not mutually exclusive. In addition to the release of autoantigens from damaged tissue, one possible mechanism is molecular mimicry, in which exposure to viruses that share amino acid sequences with autoantigens leads to cross-reactive immunity.[71] Viral infections, which are frequent after transplantation, may also lead to autoimmunity through other mechanisms, including polyclonal stimulation, enhancement and induction of membrane expression of MHC class I and II antigens, and/or interference with immunoregulatory cells. Another possible mechanism has been suggested by animal experiments showing that the use of calcineurin inhibitors predisposes to autoimmunity and autoimmune disease, possibly by interfering with the maturation of T lymphocytes or with the function of regulatory T cells, with the consequent emergence and activation of autoaggressive T-cell clones.[69] Another proposed mechanism stems from observations by Aguilera *et al.*,[72] who reported that an antibody directed to glutathione-S-transferase T1 (GSTT1) was characteristic in their patients with de novo AIH.[72–74] Since the gene encoding this protein is defective in a fifth of Caucasoid individuals and the encoded enzyme was absent in patients experiencing de novo AIH, the authors speculated that graft dysfunction resulted from the recognition as foreign of GSTT1 acquired with the graft. However, we have been unable to confirm this observation, having investigated reactivity against GSTT1 sequentially on 60 occasions in 20 patients with post-transplantation de novo AIH (Komorowski *et al.*, unpublished data).

It has been unequivocally demonstrated in a murine model of heart allograft that allogeneic transplantation of a solid organ can lead to the development of autoimmunity;[75,76] heart transplantation from an allogeneic donor resulted not only in signs of rejection, but also in the production of antibodies and $CD4^+$ T cells directed against cardiac myosin in the recipient. The relative importance of autoantigenic and allogeneic stimuli in the development of de novo AIH after liver transplantation remains to be elucidated.

Conclusions

Autoimmunity is an important cause of liver disease in childhood—autoimmune liver diseases being quite frequent and severe, but eminently treatable. The prognosis with immunosuppression treatment is excellent, with symptom-free long-term survival in the majority of patients. However, a failure to diagnose and promptly treat these conditions can have severe consequences, including cirrhosis, end-stage liver disease, transplantation, or death. During the past 30 years, several pathogenic aspects of liver autoimmunity have been elucidated, including predisposing genetic factors and disease-specific humoral and cellular immune responses. Research tasks for the future include further elucidation of the pathogenesis and the establishment of novel treatments aimed at specifically arresting liver autoaggression or, ideally, at reinstating tolerance to liver antigens.

Case study

Presentation. A 3-year-old girl presented with a 2-day history of jaundice, fatigue, and mild drowsiness. Blood tests at her local hospital showed: AST 2700 IU/L, bilirubin 150 μmol/L, and INR 2.2.

Her *medical history* was negative; the girl had been born following a normal pregnancy with a normal, spontaneous delivery.

Her *family history* included a maternal aunt with autoimmune thyroiditis and an identical twin sister who had been diagnosed with type 1 diabetes (insulin-dependent) 1 week before the onset of her symptoms.

She was referred to the pediatric liver center at King's College Hospital, where blood tests confirmed an AST in the thousands and a deteriorating INR (3.2). Albumin was 32 g/L (normal value > 35 g/L). A full blood count and electrolytes were normal, but blood sugar was high, with glycosuria and ketotic acidosis. Immunological tests showed positive anti-LKM-1 (titer 1 : 1280) and anti-islet cell antibodies, with normal IgG levels. A diagnosis of AIH type 2 in association with type 1 diabetes was made. Genetic tests excluded APECED.

Management. The girl was started on prednisolone at a dosage of 2 mg/kg/day despite her diabetes, due to the severity of the liver failure. Over the next few weeks, a rapid improvement in both liver function tests and insulin requirements was observed, suggesting that immunosuppression was abating the autoimmune process that was affecting not only the liver but also the pancreatic beta cells. After 6 weeks of treatment, during which liver function was monitored weekly and the steroid dosage was steadily reduced to 10 mg daily because of stabilization of the AST levels, and in an attempt to further reduce the steroid dosage, azathioprine was added at a starting dose of 0.5 mg/kg/day, to be increased by 0.5 mg/kg/day at weekly intervals after a review of the blood tests. Within 3 months, the girl had normal liver function tests and INR, the anti-LKM-1 titer decreased to 1 : 160, and she was clinically well, taking prednisolone 5 mg/day and azathioprine 1.5 mg/kg/day, with minimal insulin requirements. A liver biopsy performed 3 months after presentation, when the INR had normalized, showed a picture of interface hepatitis.

During the follow-up period, she had several relapse episodes, mainly due to her parents attempting alternative medicines, but always responded well to the reintroduction of immunosuppressive treatment. Her thyroid function, checked every 6 months, remained normal. Her diabetes remained easily controlled and she required lower doses of insulin than her twin sister. Ten years after the diagnosis of AIH type 2, she is still receiving prednisolone 5 mg/day and azathioprine 1.5 mg/kg/day, has no signs of portal hypertension, is living a normal life and is only 1 cm shorter than her twin sister, with both sisters at the 75th centile for height.

References

1 Waldenstrom J. Leber, Blutproteine und Nahrungseiweiss. *Dtsch Z Verdauung Stoffwechselkr* 1950;**15**:113–9.

2 Mackay IR, Taft LI, Cowling DC. Lupoid hepatitis. *Lancet* 1956;ii: 1323–6.

3 Soloway RD, Summerskill WH, Baggenstoss AH, *et al.* Clinical, biochemical, and histological remission of severe chronic active liver disease: a controlled study of treatments and early prognosis. *Gastroenterology* 1972;**63**:820–33.

4 Murray-Lyon IM, Stern RB, Williams R. Controlled trial of prednisone and azathioprine in active chronic hepatitis. *Lancet* 1973;**i**:735–7.

5 Manns MP, Luttig B, Obermayer-Straub P. Autoimmune hepatitis. In: Rose NR, Mackay IR, eds. *The Autoimmune Diseases,* 3rd ed. San Diego: Academic Press, 1998: 511–25.

6 Primo J, Merino C, Fernandez J, Moles JR, Llorca P, Hinojosa J. [Incidence and prevalence of autoimmune hepatitis in the area of the Hospital de Sagunto (Spain)]. *Gastroenterol Hepatol* 2004; **27**:239–43.

7 Costa M, Rodriguez-Sanchez JL, Czaja AJ, Gelpi C. Isolation and characterization of cDNA encoding the antigenic protein of the human tRNP(Ser)Sec complex recognized by autoantibodies from patients with type-1 autoimmune hepatitis. *Clin Exp Immunol* 2000;**121**:364–74.

8 Donaldson PT. Genetics in autoimmune hepatitis. *Semin Liver Dis* 2002;**22**:353–64.

9 Donaldson PT. Genetics of autoimmune and viral liver diseases; understanding the issues. *J Hepatol* 2004;**41**:327–32.

10 Czaja AJ, Donaldson PT. Genetic susceptibilities for immune expression and liver cell injury in autoimmune hepatitis. *Immunol Rev* 2000;**174**:250–9.

11 Vergani D, Wells L, Larcher VF, *et al.* Genetically determined low C4: a predisposing factor to autoimmune chronic active hepatitis. *Lancet* 1985;**ii**:294–8.

12 Doherty DG, Underhill JA, Donaldson PT, *et al.* Polymorphism in the human complement C4 genes and genetic susceptibility to autoimmune hepatitis. *Autoimmunity* 1994;**18**:243–9.

13 Ma Y, Bogdanos DP, Hussain MJ, *et al.* Polyclonal T-cell responses to cytochrome P450IID6 are associated with disease activity in autoimmune hepatitis type 2. *Gastroenterology* 2006;**130**:868–82.

14 Simmonds MJ, Gough SC. Genetic insights into disease mechanisms of autoimmunity. *Br Med Bull* 2004;**71**:93–113.

15 Liston A, Lesage S, Gray DH, Boyd RL, Goodnow CC. Genetic lesions in T-cell tolerance and thresholds for autoimmunity. *Immunol Rev* 2005;**204**:87–101.

16 Senaldi G, Portmann B, Mowat AP, Mieli-Vergani G, Vergani D. Immunohistochemical features of the portal tract mononuclear cell infiltrate in chronic aggressive hepatitis. *Arch Dis Child* 1992; **67**:1447–53.

17 Takeda K, Hayakawa Y, Van Kaer L, Matsuda H, Yagita H, Okumura K. Critical contribution of liver natural killer T cells to a murine model of hepatitis. *Proc Natl Acad Sci U S A* 2000;**97**: 5498–503.

18 Weaver CT, Harrington LE, Mangan PR, Gavrieli M, Murphy KM. Th17: an effector CD4 T cell lineage with regulatory T cell ties. *Immunity* 2006;**24**:677–88.

19 Steinman L. A brief history of T(H)17, the first major revision in the T(H)1/T(H)2 hypothesis of T cell-mediated tissue damage. *Nat Med* 2007;**13**:139–45.

20 Nouri-Aria KT, Donaldson PT, Hegarty JE, Eddleston AL, Williams R. HLA A1-B8-DR3 and suppressor cell function in first-degree relatives of patients with autoimmune chronic active hepatitis. *J Hepatol* 1985;**1**:235–41.

21 Nouri-Aria KT, Hegarty JE, Alexander GJ, Eddleston AL, Williams R. Effect of corticosteroids on suppressor-cell activity in "autoimmune" and viral chronic active hepatitis. *N Engl J Med* 1982;**307**:1301–4.

22 Cortesini R, LeMaoult J, Ciubotariu R, Cortesini NS. $CD8^+CD28^-$ T suppressor cells and the induction of antigen-specific, antigen-presenting cell-mediated suppression of Th reactivity. *Immunol Rev* 2001;**182**:201–6.

23 Vento S, Hegarty JE, Bottazzo G, Macchia E, Williams R, Eddleston AL. Antigen specific suppressor cell function in autoimmune chronic active hepatitis. *Lancet* 1984;**i**:1200–4.

24 Shevach EM, McHugh RS, Piccirillo CA, Thornton AM. Control of T-cell activation by $CD4^+$ $CD25^+$ suppressor T cells. *Immunol Rev* 2001;**182**:58–67.

25 Longhi MS, Ma Y, Bogdanos DP, Cheeseman P, Mieli-Vergani G, Vergani D. Impairment of CD4(+)CD25(+) regulatory T-cells in autoimmune liver disease. *J Hepatol* 2004;**41**:31–7.

26 Longhi MS, Ma Y, Mitry RR, *et al.* Effect of $CD4^+$ $CD25^+$ regulatory T-cells on CD8 T-cell function in patients with autoimmune hepatitis. *J Autoimmun* 2005;**25**:63–71.

27 Longhi MS, Hussain MJ, Mitry RR, *et al.* Functional study of $CD4^+CD25^+$ regulatory T cells in health and autoimmune hepatitis. *J Immunol* 2006;**176**:4484–91.

28 Lobo-Yeo A, Alviggi L, Mieli-Vergani G, Portmann B, Mowat AP, Vergani D. Preferential activation of helper/inducer T lymphocytes in autoimmune chronic active hepatitis. *Clin Exp Immunol* 1987;**67**:95–104.

29 Longhi MS, Hussain MJ, Bogdanos DP, *et al.* Cytochrome P450IID6-specific CD8 T cell immune responses mirror disease activity in autoimmune hepatitis type 2 *Hepatology* 2007;**46**:472–84.

30 Manns MP, Griffin KJ, Sullivan KF, Johnson EF. LKM-1 autoantibodies recognize a short linear sequence in P450IID6, a cytochrome P-450 monooxygenase. *J Clin Invest* 1991;**88**:1370–8.

31 Vento S, Cainelli F, Renzini C, Concia E. Autoimmune hepatitis type 2 induced by HCV and persisting after viral clearance [letter]. Lancet 1997;**350**:1298–9.

32 Kerkar N, Choudhuri K, Ma Y, *et al.* Cytochrome P4502D6(193-212): a new immunodominant epitope and target of virus/self cross-reactivity in liver kidney microsomal autoantibody type 1-positive liver disease. *J Immunol* 2003;**170**:1481–9.

33 Jensen DM, McFarlane IG, Portmann BS, Eddleston AL, Williams R. Detection of antibodies directed against a liver-specific membrane lipoprotein in patients with acute and chronic active hepatitis. *N Engl J Med* 1978;**299**:1–7.

34 McFarlane BM, McSorley CG, Vergani D, McFarlane IG, Williams R. Serum autoantibodies reacting with the hepatic asialoglycoprotein receptor protein (hepatic lectin) in acute and chronic liver disorders. *J Hepatol* 1986;**3**:196–205.

35 Vergani D, Mieli-Vergani G, Mondelli M, Portmann B, Eddleston AL. Immunoglobulin on the surface of isolated hepatocytes is

associated with antibody-dependent cell-mediated cytotoxicity and liver damage. *Liver* 1987;**7**:307–15.

36 Mieli-Vergani G, Vergani D, Jenkins PJ, *et al.* Lymphocyte cytotoxicity to autologous hepatocytes in HB_sAg-negative chronic active hepatitis. *Clin Exp Immunol* 1979;**38**:16–21.

37 Wen L, Ma Y, Bogdanos DP, *et al.* Pediatric autoimmune liver diseases: the molecular basis of humoral and cellular immunity. *Curr Mol Med* 2001;**1**:379–89.

38 Wen L, Peakman M, Lobo-Yeo A, *et al.* T-cell-directed hepatocyte damage in autoimmune chronic active hepatitis. *Lancet* 1990; **336**:1527–30.

39 Löhr H, Manns M, Kyriatsoulis A, *et al.* Clonal analysis of liver-infiltrating T cells in patients with LKM-1 antibody-positive autoimmune chronic active hepatitis. *Clin Exp Immunol* 1991;**84**: 297–302.

40 Löhr H, Treichel U, Poralla T, Manns M, Meyer zum Buschenfelde KH. Liver-infiltrating T helper cells in autoimmune chronic active hepatitis stimulate the production of autoantibodies against the human asialoglycoprotein receptor in vitro. *Clin Exp Immunol* 1992;**88**:45–9.

41 Maggiore G, Veber F, Bernard O, *et al.* Autoimmune hepatitis associated with anti-actin antibodies in children and adolescents. *J Pediatr Gastroenterol Nutr* 1993;**17**:376–81.

42 Gregorio GV, Portmann B, Reid F, *et al.* Autoimmune hepatitis in childhood: a 20-year experience. *Hepatology* 1997;**25**:541–7.

43 Gregorio GV, Portmann B, Karani J, *et al.* Autoimmune hepatitis/sclerosing cholangitis overlap syndrome in childhood: a 16-year prospective study. *Hepatology* 2001;**33**:544–53.

44 Johnson PJ, McFarlane IG. Meeting report: International Autoimmune Hepatitis Group. *Hepatology* 1993;**18**:998–1005.

45 Alvarez F, Berg PA, Bianchi FB, *et al.* International Autoimmune Hepatitis Group Report: review of criteria for diagnosis of autoimmune hepatitis. *J Hepatol* 1999;**31**:929–38.

46 Homberg JC, Abuaf N, Bernard O, *et al.* Chronic active hepatitis associated with antiliver/kidney microsome antibody type 1: a second type of "autoimmune" hepatitis. *Hepatology* 1987;**7**: 1333–9.

47 Vergani D, Alvarez F, Bianchi FB, *et al.* Liver autoimmune serology: a consensus statement from the committee for autoimmune serology of the International Autoimmune Hepatitis Group. *J Hepatol* 2004;**41**:677–83.

48 Tan EM, Feltkamp TE, Smolen JS, *et al.* Range of antinuclear antibodies in "healthy" individuals. *Arthritis Rheum* 1997;**40**: 1601–11.

49 Bottazzo GF, Florin-Christensen A, Fairfax A, Swana G, Doniach D, Groeschel-Stewart U. Classification of smooth muscle autoantibodies detected by immunofluorescence. *J Clin Pathol* 1976; **29**:403–10.

50 Muratori P, Muratori L, Agostinelli D, *et al.* Smooth muscle antibodies and type 1 autoimmune hepatitis. *Autoimmunity* 2002; **35**:497–500.

51 Gregorio GV, Portmann B, Mowat AP, Vergani D, Mieli-Vergani G. A 12-year-old girl with antimitochondrial antibody-positive autoimmune hepatitis. *J Hepatol* 1997;**27**:751–4.

52 Lapierre P, Hajoui O, Homberg JC, Alvarez F. Formiminotransferase cyclodeaminase is an organ-specific autoantigen recognized by sera of patients with autoimmune hepatitis. *Gastroenterology* 1999;**116**:643–9.

53 Manns M, Gerken G, Kyriatsoulis A, Staritz M, Meyer zum Buschenfelde KH. Characterisation of a new subgroup of autoimmune chronic active hepatitis by autoantibodies against a soluble liver antigen. *Lancet* 1987;**i**:292–4.

54 Ma Y, Okamoto M, Thomas MG, *et al.* Antibodies to conformational epitopes of soluble liver antigen define a severe form of autoimmune liver disease. *Hepatology* 2002;**35**:658–64.

55 Wies I, Brunner S, Henninger J, *et al.* Identification of target antigen for SLA/LP autoantibodies in autoimmune hepatitis. *Lancet* 2000;**355**:1510–5.

56 Rumbo C, Emerick KM, Emre S, Shneider BL. Azathioprine metabolite measurements in the treatment of autoimmune hepatitis in pediatric patients: a preliminary report. *J Pediatr Gastroenterol Nutr* 2002;**35**:391–8.

57 Gregorio GV, McFarlane B, Bracken P, Vergani D, Mieli-Vergani G. Organ and non-organ specific autoantibody titres and IgG levels as markers of disease activity: a longitudinal study in childhood autoimmune liver disease. *Autoimmunity* 2002;**35**:515–9.

58 Mieli-Vergani G, Bargiota K, Samyn M, Vergani D. Therapeutic aspects of autoimmune liver disease in children. In: Dienes HP, Leuschner U, Lohse AW, Manns MP, eds. *Autoimmune Liver Diseases: Falk Symposium.* Dordrecht: Springer, 2005: 278–82.

59 Samaroo B, Samyn M, Buchanan C, Mieli-Vergani G. Long-term daily oral treatment with prednisolone in children with autoimmune liver disease does not affect final adult height. *Hepatology* 2006;**44**:438A.

60 Johnson PJ, McFarlane IG, Williams R. Azathioprine for long-term maintenance of remission in autoimmune hepatitis. *N Engl J Med* 1995;**333**:958–63.

61 Kerkar N, Annunziato RA, Foley L, *et al.* Prospective analysis of nonadherence in autoimmune hepatitis: a common problem. *J Pediatr Gastroenterol Nutr* 2006;**43**:629–34.

62 Heneghan MA, Norris SM, O'Grady JG, Harrison PM, McFarlane IG. Management and outcome of pregnancy in autoimmune hepatitis. *Gut* 2001;**48**:97–102.

63 Alvarez F, Ciocca M, Canero-Velasco C, *et al.* Short-term cyclosporine induces a remission of autoimmune hepatitis in children. *J Hepatol* 1999;**30**:222–7.

64 Underhill J, Ma Y, Bogdanos DP, Cheeseman P, Mieli-Vergani G, Vergani D. Different immunogenetic background in autoimmune hepatitis type 1, type and autoimmune sclerosing cholangitis. *J Hepatol* 2002;**36**(Suppl 1):156A.

65 Lindor KD. Ursodiol for primary sclerosing cholangitis. Mayo Primary Sclerosing Cholangitis-Ursodeoxycholic Acid Study Group. *N Engl J Med* 1997;**336**:691–5.

66 Mitchell SA, Bansi DS, Hunt N, Von Bergmann K, Fleming KA, Chapman RW. A preliminary trial of high-dose ursodeoxycholic acid in primary sclerosing cholangitis. *Gastroenterology* 2001;**121**: 900–7.

67 Vergani D, Mieli-Vergani G. Autoimmunity after liver transplantation. *Hepatology* 2002;**36**:271–6.

68 Kerkar N, Hadzic N, Davies ET, *et al.* De-novo autoimmune hepatitis after liver transplantation. *Lancet* 1998;**351**:409–13.

69 Mieli-Vergani G, Vergani D. De novo autoimmune hepatitis after liver transplantation. *J Hepatol* 2004;**40**:3–7.

70 Evans HM, Kelly DA, McKiernan PJ, Hubscher S. Progressive histological damage in liver allografts following pediatric liver transplantation. *Hepatology* 2006;**43**:1109–17.

71 Vergani D, Choudhuri K, Bogdanos DP, Mieli-Vergani G. Pathogenesis of autoimmune hepatitis. *Clin Liver Dis* 2002;**6**:439–49.

72 Aguilera I, Wichmann I, Sousa JM, *et al.* Antibodies against glutathione S-transferase T1 (GSTT1) in patients with de novo immune hepatitis following liver transplantation. *Clin Exp Immunol* 2001;**126**:535–9.

73 Aguilera I, Sousa JM, Gavilan F, Bernardos A, Wichmann I, Nunez-Roldan A. Glutathione S-transferase T1 mismatch constitutes a risk factor for de novo immune hepatitis after liver transplantation. *Liver Transpl* 2004;**10**:1166–72.

74 Aguilera I, Wichmann I, Gentil MA, Gonzalez-Escribano F, Nunez-Roldan A. Alloimmune response against donor glutathione S-transferase T1 antigen in renal transplant recipients. *Am J Kidney Dis* 2005;**46**:345–50.

75 Fedoseyeva EV, Tam RC, Popov IA, Orr PL, Garovoy MR, Benichou G. Induction of T cell responses to a self-antigen following allotransplantation. *Transplantation* 1996;**61**:679–83.

76 Fedoseyeva EV, Zhang F, Orr PL, Levin D, Buncke HJ, Benichou G. De novo autoimmunity to cardiac myosin after heart transplantation and its contribution to the rejection process. *J Immunol* 1999;**162**:6836–42.

9 Drug-Induced Liver Disease

Karen F. Murray

Introduction

In modern society, exposure to synthesized pharmacological agents or herbal medications in the treatment of disease is widespread. In addition, children and young people use recreational drugs for pleasure or as self-prescribed remedies. For most medications, the benefits outweigh the risks of toxicity. Nevertheless, many of these "safe" compounds are potentially hepatotoxic, and awareness of this allows early recognition and prevention of severe toxicity. As will be discussed under the individual drug headings below, some drugs clearly have a dose-dependent toxicity, whereas others cause hepatotoxicity with a seemingly idiosyncratic pattern (Table 9.1). With medications that have dose-dependent toxicity—e.g., acetaminophen and minocycline—the toxicity becomes apparent after an overdose or prolonged exposure. With acetaminophen, both acute overdose and accumulated toxicity with chronic use result in hepatotoxicity. Minocycline, on the other hand, can cause both an acute reaction and an autoimmune reaction, which only becomes apparent months to years after the exposure. Medications that have an idiosyncratic pattern exhibit a less predictable pattern of toxicity. In either case, the drug toxicity diagnosis may be complicated by the disease state for which the medication is being used, and consequently a high index of suspicion is required for accurate diagnosis.

Table 9.1 Exposure pattern of hepatotoxicity.

Dose-dependent	Idiosyncratic
Acetaminophen	Antiepileptic medications
Isoniazid	Antibiotics other than those listed at left
Tetracyclines	
Oxypenicillins	
Ureidopenicillins	

Diseases of the Liver and Biliary System in Children, 3rd edition. Edited by Deirdre Kelly. © 2008 Blackwell Publishing, ISBN: 978-1-4051-6334-7.

Role of the liver in drug metabolism

The liver plays a crucial role in the metabolism of virtually all drugs.[1] Most drugs are lipophilic, and thus to be detoxified and excreted in bile or filtered by the renal glomerulus they must be rendered hydrophilic. This is achieved in the liver by two predominant mechanisms: firstly, oxidation or demethylation by the cytochrome P450 enzyme system (see below), and secondly conjugation by glucuronidation or sulfation by specific transferases. In addition, other enzymes—for example, alcohol dehydrogenase—are required for the metabolism of certain drugs. Electrophilic intermediate metabolites generated during these reactions are potentially harmful: binding of glutathione, catalyzed by glutathione *S*-transferase, provides a mechanism for detoxification of these reactive species.

Mechanisms of drug-induced liver disease

The term "drug-induced liver disease" (DILD) encompasses liver dysfunction caused by two distinct mechanisms: direct hepatotoxicity and adverse drug reaction. The distinction lies in the predictability of the toxic effect:

- Direct hepatotoxicity arises from the administration of a drug with intrinsic toxicity to the liver and is usually dose-dependent (e.g., acetaminophen, aspirin).
- Adverse drug reactions comprise the majority of DILDs. An adverse drug reaction is unpredictable and idiosyncratic, and may occur despite recommended treatment regimens being prescribed. This type of reaction occurs with a low frequency in the population exposed to the drug, is variable in presentation, is dose-independent, and may result in diverse pathology. Host factors may be of particular importance (see below).

Pathogenesis

Drug-induced injury most commonly arises in the hepatocyte, due to its central role in drug metabolism—although biliary cells, Ito cells, and sinusoidal endothelium may also be targets. A drug itself or an intermediate metabolite may:

- Impair cell structure
- Inhibit enzyme activity
- Overwhelm glutathione cytoprotection
- Provide an antigenic determinant on the cell surface, provoking an inflammatory response
- Evoke a type IV systemic hypersensitivity reaction

These mechanisms may occur in combination, and for many drugs, the precise mechanism remains unknown. The outcome for a given agent may be largely determined by host factors.

Host factors

DILD may be regarded as the end result of an interaction between a pharmacologically active compound after host metabolism, in the presence of environmental influences. Consideration of factors that can affect drug metabolism is crucial if inappropriate prescribing and the risk of DILD are to be minimized.

Factors affecting enzyme activity

Genetic factors. The cytochrome P450 system is composed of a family of almost 300 genes that code for P450 enzymes. These genes are distributed among several chromosomes, and the encoded enzymes are thus susceptible to considerable polymorphism. Genetic variation in these enzymes influences drug metabolism and may contribute to DILD, either by excess toxic metabolite production or deficient precursor metabolism.

Other hepatic enzymes are also polymorphic: genetic variation in *N*-acetyltransferase-2 activity is expressed phenotypically as a slow or fast acetylator and is relevant to isoniazid toxicity.

Age. Full activity of an enzyme system may not be present in the first few years of life, as it may be subject to developmental regulation. These developmental deficiencies may be of clinical significance. The rate of cytochrome P450 activity may also be influenced by age. In children, a relative decrease in metabolism by glucuronidation, in comparison with sulfation, may be responsible for their decreased susceptibility to acetaminophen hepatotoxicity.

Concomitant drug therapy. Enzyme activity, especially of cytochrome P450, may be enhanced or inhibited by other drugs. Induction (e.g., by ethanol, phenobarbitone, phenytoin, carbamazepine, rifampicin, isoniazid, omeprazole) may increase the rate of generation of toxic metabolites, increasing the susceptibility to DILD.

Factors affecting glutathione cytoprotection

Alcohol and starvation may lead to glutathione depletion, and thus diminished cytoprotection, especially relevant in acetaminophen toxicity. Replenishing with *N*-acetylcysteine reestablishes protection. Drugs that induce enzyme activity may also lead to glutathione depletion, because of the increased generation of metabolites requiring conjugation.

Other risk factors

There is an increased risk of adverse drug reactions with age, which may reflect polypharmacy or an increased likelihood of concurrent disease. There is, however, an increased risk of valproate hepatotoxicity in children less than 3 years of age (see also Chapter 5). For unknown reasons, many forms of DILD—especially acute and chronic hepatitis—are more common in women. Individuals with a history of an adverse drug reaction are also more likely to experience a reaction to another agent.

Clinicopathological spectrum

DILD may be associated with a wide spectrum of severity of liver injury and can resemble all other forms of liver disease. There is considerable overlap in the type of disease produced, and many drugs may produce more than one syndrome. Early symptoms are nonspecific, although fever, rash, and eosinophilia may be present in hypersensitivity reactions. A particular feature of DILD is significant biochemical and histological abnormality occurring with few symptoms (Table 9.2). The histological features of drug-induced hepatotoxicity are frequently nonspecific, but the patients can be categorized into those with primarily acute inflammatory hepatocellular injury, those with prominent cholestasis, and those with vanishing bile duct syndrome (Table 9.3). The predominant clinicopathological manifestations of DILD are outlined below.

Enzyme induction without disease

Induction of hepatic enzymes may be of no clinical significance and not associated with hepatic disease or dysfunction —for example, γ-glutamyltransferase (GGT) induction by phenytoin/phenobarbitone.

Acute hepatitis/hepatocellular necrosis/acute liver failure

This is the most common manifestation of DILD. The clinical presentation may be similar to those in:

- Acute viral hepatitis, with fever, anorexia, nausea, or vomiting, followed by right upper quadrant tenderness with variable jaundice.
- Allergic hepatitis, presenting with fever, rash, eosinophilia, and lymphadenopathy, which may resemble infectious mononucleosis. Drug rash with eosinophilia and systemic symptoms (DRESS) is a term applied when the clinical presentation is that of a cutaneous eruption, fever, multiple peripheral ganglions, and potentially life-threatening multiorgan failure.
- Acute liver failure (Figures 9.1, 9.2).

Table 9.2 Clinical category and timing after exposure of drug toxicity.

Drug	Hepatitis	Jaundice	Hypersensitivity
Acetaminophen	1–2 days	3–5 days	
Halothane	7–13 days	10–28 days	7–13 days
Isoniazid	< 2 months (50%) 2–14 months (50%)	2–15 months	
Rifampicin		Weeks	
Amoxicillin–clavulanic acid		Days–2 months	
Flucloxacillin		2–5 weeks	
Tetracycline	4–6 days		
Minocycline	Months		Days–weeks
Erythromycin	1–3 weeks		
Trimethoprim–sulfamethoxazole	2–3 weeks	2–3 weeks	2–3 weeks
Ketoconazole	2–3 weeks		
Carbamazepine	2–3 weeks	2–3 weeks	Weeks
Phenytoin	1–3 weeks	1–3 weeks	Weeks

Table 9.3 General histological categories of drug-induced hepatotoxicity.

Hepatocellular inflammation	Cholestasis	Vanishing bile duct syndrome
Acetaminophen	Amoxicillin–clavulanic acid	Flucloxacillin
Halothane	Erythromycin	Tetracycline
Isoniazid	Sulfonamides	Ampicillin/amoxicillin
Cephalosporins	Ketoconazole	Amoxicillin–clavulanic acid
Tetracyclines (steatosis)	Carbamazepine	
Erythromycin		
Ketoconazole		
Carbamazepine		
Phenytoin		
Cannabis		
Amphetamines		

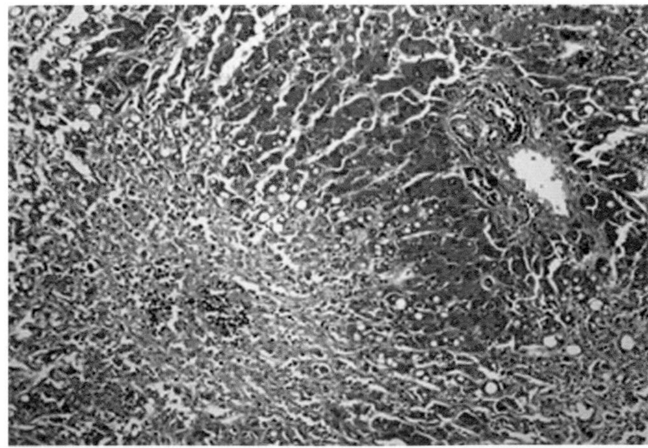

Figure 9.1 Acetaminophen-induced liver disease, showing pericentrivenular necrosis (hematoxylin–eosin, original magnification × 200).

Drug-induced acute liver failure (ALF) represents approximately 20% of pediatric cases of ALF. Of the initial 348 children enrolled in the Pediatric Acute Liver Failure Study Group, a clinical research network established by the National Institutes of Health in the United States (including 21 sites in the U.S., one in Canada, and two in the United Kingdom), 5% of cases of ALF were due to an identifiable drug other than acetaminophen, 14% to acetaminophen, and 48% were indeterminate; some of the latter may have been drug-related. The prognosis in the drug-induced ALF population depends on the cause. Survival without liver transplantation following acetaminophen poisoning has been reported as 94%, but only 41% in children who developed ALF due to other drugs.[2]

Histological changes in acute hepatitis reflect hepatocellular damage with degeneration and necrosis, accompanied by an inflammatory cell infiltrate, with a variable degree of acute hepatic necrosis (Figures 9.1–9.3).

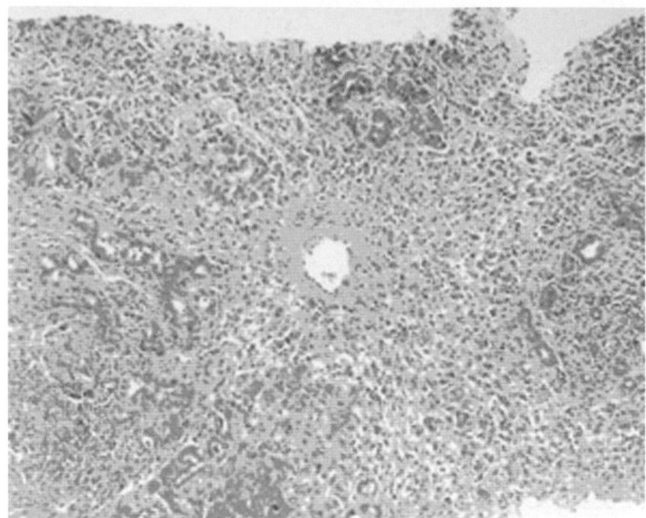

Figure 9.2 Acute liver failure secondary to halothane exposure. Postnecrotic confluent cell loss with inflammation, including pigmented macrophages, periportal ductular reaction, and only a few islands of surviving hepatocytes.

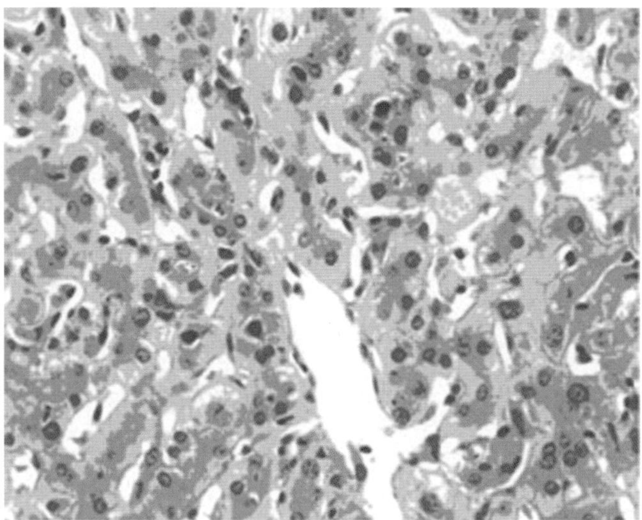

Figure 9.3 Minocycline-induced hepatitis. Portal inflammation with mononucleated cells, plasma cells, and eosinophils spilling over the parenchymal limiting plates, resembling an autoimmune hepatitis.

Cholestasis

Acute cholestasis manifests with a rapid onset of jaundice and pruritus. Causes include co-trimoxazole and erythromycin estolate. Without hepatitis, recovery is usually rapid and complete, but with hepatitis there may be a more prolonged course. Histological features include inspissated bile within the canaliculi and bile pigment in hepatocytes and Kupffer cells. Significant bile duct injury may occur (e.g., with flucloxacillin) and lead to more severe and chronic symptoms and resemble sclerosing cholangitis or vanishing bile duct syndrome. Cholestasis may be accompanied by mild or moderate hepatocellular necrosis (Figure 9.4).

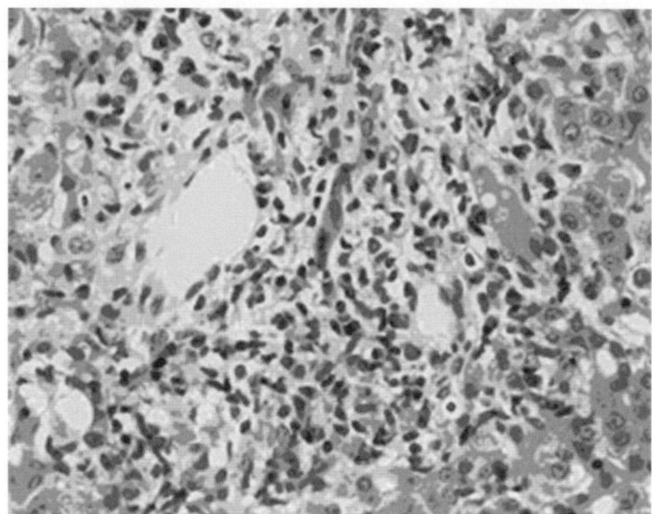

Figure 9.4 Clavulanic acid-related cholestasis. Liver biopsy specimen, showing severe canalicular bile plugging with only minimal necroinflammatory activity.

Granulomatous hepatitis

A wide variety of drugs may be responsible, although the most frequent cause is carbamazepine (Figures 9.5, 9.6). Clinical features include fever and malaise. The associated degree of hepatitis and cholestasis is variable.

Drug-induced chronic hepatitis

This is one of the least common forms of DILD, but it is important, as prevention is possible. Examples of responsible agents include methyldopa, nitrofurantoin, minocycline, and chronic acetaminophen ingestion.

Clinical features

Drug-induced chronic hepatitis may resemble autoimmune hepatitis, with either an acute hepatitic onset or a more insidious onset of tiredness, lethargy, anorexia, weight loss, and hepatic discomfort. Jaundice and pruritus are unusual at presentation. A prolonged course is usually due to continued ingestion, as there is rarely perpetuation of the hepatic injury after withdrawal of the drug. Signs of liver disease are more likely than in acute hepatitis.

Histological features

These are often nonspecific and resemble those of autoimmune hepatitis. The severity of the histological changes is the most important factor predicting the outcome (Figure 9.3).

Fatty liver. Microvesicular fat within hepatocytes is associated with cellular dysfunction, and is typical of Reye syndrome, and valproic acid and tetracycline hepatotoxicity. Macrovesicular

A

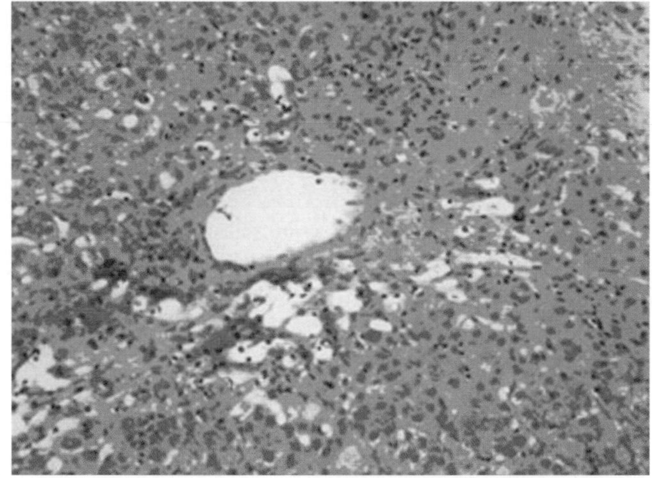

B

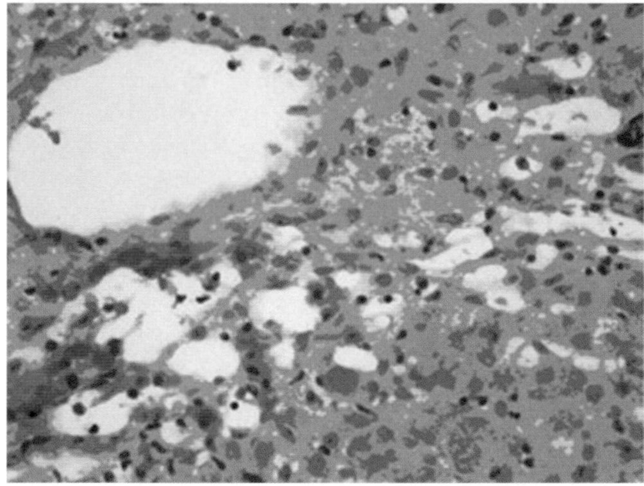

Figure 9.5 Carbamazepine-induced cholestatic liver disease, with perivenular necroinflammation and cholestasis shown (hematoxylin–eosin, original magnification **A** × 200, **B** × 400).

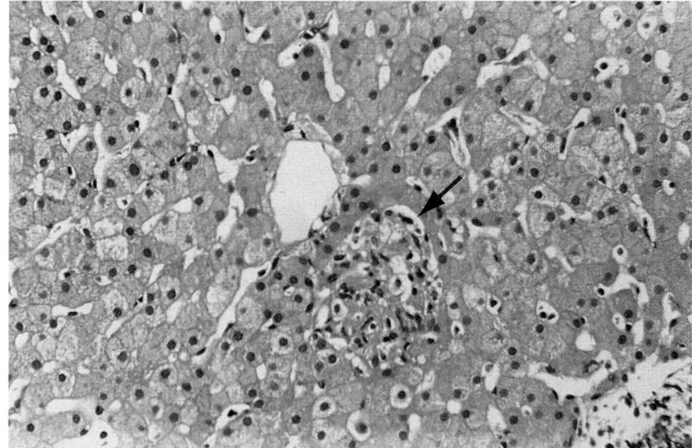

Figure 9.6 Carbamazepine may also cause granulomatous hepatitis or acute liver failure.

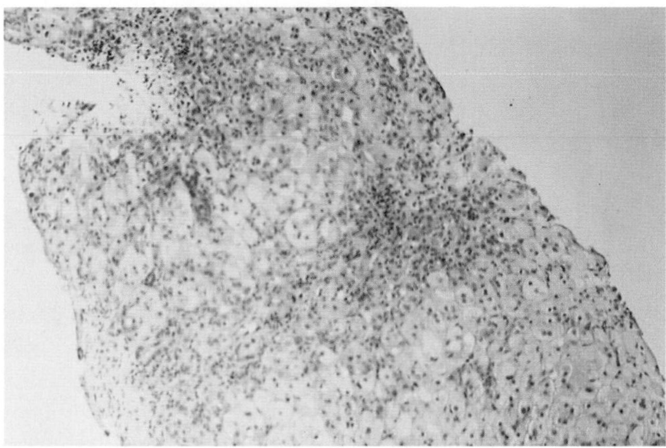

Figure 9.7 Sodium valproate and tetracycline both cause fatty liver, with microvesicular fat in the hepatocytes, which is associated with hepatocellular dysfunction and may progress to acute liver failure.

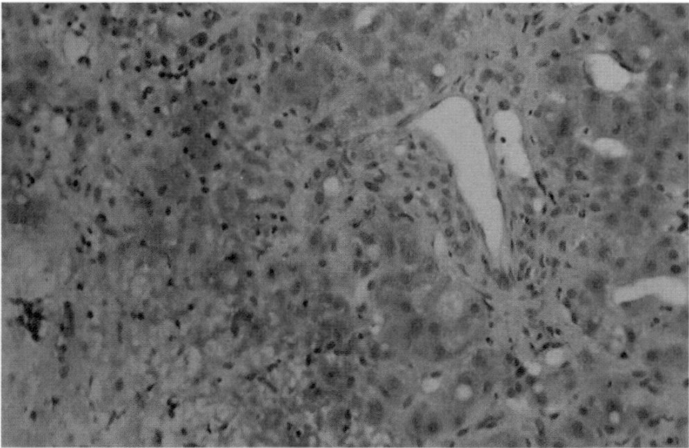

Figure 9.8 Actinomycin and other forms of chemotherapy for malignancy may cause hepatocellular necrosis and acute liver failure.

fat may be seen with amiodarone and may lead to rapid progression to cirrhosis (Figure 9.7).

Fibrosis. Progressive fibrosis without clinical manifestations may occur—for example, due to methotrexate, vitamin A, actinomycin D (Figure 9.8).

Vascular disorders

These range from sinusoidal dilation (with estrogens) to veno-occlusive disease (with cytotoxic chemotherapy—e.g., thioguanine).[3] Anabolic steroids and cytotoxic chemotherapy have been implicated in peliosis hepatitis, in which hepatic sinusoids are destroyed, forming blood-filled lakes or lacunae within the liver, which may rupture spontaneously.

Hepatic tumors

These are the least common form of DILD, accounting for < 1%, with oral contraceptive steroids being the most commonly implicated agent.

Natural history

Resolution of histological and biochemical changes is the usual outcome following withdrawal of the agent causing DILD. The time for recovery is variable, depending on the type of hepatic injury. However, there is evidence to suggest that full recovery is not invariable. Of 33 adults reevaluated 1–19 years after a definite diagnosis of DILD, 13 (39%) had abnormal liver enzymes, abnormal imaging (ultrasound or isotope scan) or both, and three of five repeat liver biopsies showed significant abnormality. Factors predicting persistence or development of chronic liver disease were fibrosis at the original biopsy and continued exposure to the drug. The drugs most commonly implicated in this series were antibiotics, nonsteroidal anti-inflammatory drugs (NSAIDs), and psychotropic drugs.

Diagnosis of suspected DILD

History

The diagnosis of DILD rests predominantly on an accurate history, which should cover the following aspects:

- All drugs ingested in at least the 3 months before the symptoms, including those bought over the counter and those accidentally ingested.
- Total dosage given and previous courses (e.g., methotrexate):
  —Timing of symptoms in relation to drug administration.
  —Symptomatology: presence of fever, rash, etc.
- Risk factors: previous drug reaction, family history, alcohol intake, concomitant drug therapy, underlying disease.
- Exclusion of other causes of the symptoms and biochemical/histological pattern: risk factors for other diseases should be considered (e.g., hepatitis A/B, autoimmune disease, etc.).
- Resolution after drug withdrawal (recurrence after a challenge may be confirmatory, but is usually contraindicated).

Laboratory investigation

The diagnosis of DILD is usually based on circumstantial evidence and exclusion of other causes. In instances of dose-dependent direct hepatotoxicity, a specific diagnosis or likely diagnosis may be achieved by:

- Drug levels (aspirin, acetaminophen)
- Specific antibodies (halothane)
- Eosinophilia

If no biochemical or clinical improvement is seen after withdrawal, the diagnosis of DILD should be reconsidered.

Histology

Liver biopsy is of value unless rapid resolution of liver function occurs following drug withdrawal. Histological assessment makes it possible to establish the severity of the condition, as well as supporting causation and excluding differential diagnoses (Figures 9.1–9.9).

Prevention

The risk of DILD can be minimized by careful prescribing: the specific risk factors in an individual patient (see the section on host factors, above) have to be considered, as well as the indications for a drug with known hepatotoxic effects (e.g., flucloxacillin). Continued prescribing of drugs with a dose-dependent effect or toxic threshold (e.g., methotrexate) requires careful monitoring of levels and of liver function.

Treatment

Early detection and withdrawal of the causative drug is the most effective and important step in minimizing hepatic disease and allowing prompt recovery. Specific treatment is rarely necessary. Two exceptions are acetaminophen toxicity, in which the provision of *N*-acetylcysteine is of benefit (see below), and sodium valproate toxicity, in which carnitine may be of benefit. Repeat exposure to some drugs can be life-threatening, whereas others may be used with care and expectant monitoring for any recurrent toxicity. Supportive treatment for acute liver failure is detailed in Chapter 7.

Analgesic medications

The most common analgesic medications associated with hepatotoxicity are acetaminophen and nonsteroidal anti-inflammatory drugs.

Acetaminophen

Acetaminophen hepatotoxicity results when the normal toxin scavenger mechanisms are overwhelmed. It has a bimodal presentation. Although acetaminophen overdose occurs most commonly following suicide (in adolescents) or accidental acute poisoning (in children aged 1–4 years), deliberate poisoning by care providers is a possibility. Toxin accumulation may also occur with chronic acetaminophen use, due to the inadvertent depletion of glutathione, especially if other hepatotoxins such as alcohol or recreational drugs are present.[4]

Pathogenesis

Acetaminophen metabolism is predominantly via conjugation by sulfation or glucuronidation. A small amount is normally oxidized by cytochrome P450 proteins to NAPQI (*N*-acetyl-*p*-benzoquinone imine), however. NAPQI is a highly reactive species and readily binds covalently to hepatic proteins, causing hepatocellular necrosis—the basis for acetaminophen-induced hepatotoxicity. NAPQI is removed via conjugation with glutathione. In the setting of

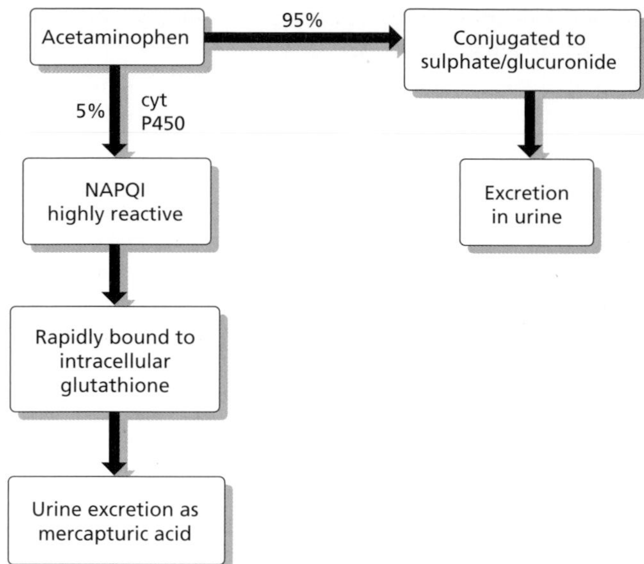

Figure 9.9 Metabolism of acetaminophen.

acetaminophen overdose, glutathione stores are depleted, NAPQI builds up, and hepatocellular necrosis and hence hepatotoxicity result (Figure 9.9).[5–7] Histologically, this is seen as pericentrivenular necrosis (Figure 9.1).

The development of liver failure is dose-dependent, with hepatic failure more likely with ingested doses over 150 mg/kg. Children have a lower incidence of liver failure from acetaminophen overdose than adults, however, perhaps because of the effect of age on glutathione stores and production.[4,8]

The risk of hepatoxicity with acetaminophen ingestion is increased depending on the age of the child, the dose ingested, whether there is a delay before treatment is started, concomitant ingestion of enzyme inducers—e.g., antituberculous or anticonvulsant therapy—and glutathione depletion (associated with alcohol or starvation).[4]

Prevention

Rates of acetaminophen-related hepatotoxicity correlate loosely with the potential for exposure. In the United States, the ability to purchase acetaminophen in bulk allows easy access for both accidental and nonaccidental overdose. In the United Kingdom, the issue of preventing accidental and deliberate overdose from acetaminophen has recently been addressed by limiting the pack size available for purchase to 16 tablets from supermarkets and 32 tablets from pharmacies. This change in packaging has led to a 22% reduction in suicide deaths and a 30% reduction in admissions to liver units for ALF in the United Kingdom.[9,10]

Clinical presentation and prognosis

Initial symptoms of acetaminophen-induced toxicity include:

- *First 24 hours:* anorexia, nausea, and vomiting. In very severe ingestions, this early phase may be complicated by hypoglycemia and lactic acidosis.
- *24–48 hours:* minimal symptoms; hepatic enlargement and right upper quadrant tenderness.
- *Days 2–4:* overt hepatic injury; marked elevation of hepatic transaminases, jaundice, coagulopathy out of proportion to the rise in bilirubin.
- *Days 3–5:* jaundice and encephalopathy, associated with renal failure due to acute tubular necrosis, with oliguria or anuria with metabolic acidosis in 25–30%.[4,9,11]
- *Days 4–5:* recovery may occur.

The development of lactic acidosis or renal or other organ failure, as well as cerebral edema, are poor prognostic signs that should prompt early evaluation for liver transplantation.

Treatment and outcome

Acetaminophen levels in plasma, measured at least 4 h after ingestion, are of value in determining the need for treatment, but treatment should not be delayed to await acetaminophen levels. As metabolism of acetaminophen leads to a progressive reduction in measured levels following ingestion, the diagnosis may not be confirmed if a prolonged interval has lapsed prior to assay. The estimation in the serum of the adduct formed by NAPQI binding to cellular proteins, 3-(cysteine-*S*-yl)-acetaminophen, may be of value in confirming the suspected diagnosis.[12]

Although exogenously administered glutathione cannot gain entry into the hepatocyte, *N*-acetylcysteine is able to substitute for glutathione in conjugation with NAPQI. Studies have indicated that treatment with intravenous *N*-acetylcysteine 150 mg/kg in reducing dosages, if instituted early, is effective treatment, as it repletes glutathione, thereby preventing further hepatocellular injury—particularly if begun 12–24 hours after ingestion. Treatment within 15 h of ingestion is beneficial in preventing massive hepatic necrosis, but later administration, even up to 36 h after ingestion, may also have a beneficial effect on survival.[4]

Careful monitoring of coagulation, glucose, acid–base, and renal function is essential (Chapter 7). Fluid intake should be restricted to at most 60% of maintenance requirements, to protect against cerebral edema, and vitamin K should be administered (5–10 mg, by slow intravenous infusion, daily for 3 days) to support coagulation factor synthesis. It is important to continue *N*-acetylcysteine until coagulation parameters return to normal.[4,6,11,13,14]

Most children (94%) spontaneously recover from acetaminophen toxicity, with only 6% of children and adolescents dying or requiring transplantation.[1] The likelihood of a worse prognosis increases with increased acetaminophen dose, or with the concomitant use of another hepatotoxin such as alcohol, antiepileptic medications, antituberculous drugs, or recreational drugs.[4,7]

Children who develop severe hepatotoxicity need to be admitted to a specialist unit for management of acute liver and renal failure and consideration for liver transplantation.[4]

The likelihood of spontaneous recovery or the need for transplantation is dependent on the severity of hepatic failure: prognostic factors and further management are detailed in Chapter 7. Despite the relatively infrequent requirement for liver transplantation among children with acetaminophen toxicity, however, the post-transplant survival is only 50%, due to the associated complications.[2,4,15]

Nonsteroidal anti-inflammatory drugs

Although a structurally heterogeneous group, most nonsteroidal anti-inflammatory drugs (NSAIDs) not only share similar therapeutic anti-inflammatory and antipyretic effects, but also adverse effects. Although toxicity is rare with individual agents, together they cause a significant proportion of DILD, reflecting their widespread use. Appreciation of their toxicity in children, particularly with over-the-counter medications and in children with chronic rheumatic conditions, is increasing.[16]

Most NSAID-associated liver disease occurs within the first 2 months of commencing treatment and is due to hepatocellular injury, although cholestasis may also occur. For some agents, features of hypersensitivity are characteristic. Clinically insignificant elevation of hepatic aminotransferases is common, occurring in up to 15%. Severe and fulminant hepatitis has been reported. In patients with elevated baseline aminotransferase activity, the more frequently hepatotoxic NSAIDs should be avoided. Serum aminotransferase activity should be monitored monthly for the first 6 months, and more frequently if they become elevated. At systemic signs of hypersensitivity (fever, rash, eosinophilia), the NSAID should be discontinued and one of a different chemical group instituted.

Aspirin

In the majority of cases, aspirin hepatotoxicity is mild, asymptomatic, and reversible. Aspirin gives rise to dose-dependent hepatotoxicity when its metabolic pathway becomes saturated. The precise hepatotoxic mechanism of the salicylic metabolite is not known.

Salicylate levels are useful in establishing a likely diagnosis. Adverse effects are associated with levels exceeding 15 mg/dL in 90% of those affected (levels that are regularly achieved in children treated for juvenile chronic arthritis), and exceeding 25 mg/dL in 70%, and relate to both the dose and duration of treatment. An asymptomatic elevation in transaminases (usually < 500 IU/L) with a normal bilirubin level is usual, the onset occurring at least 6 days after initiation of treatment. Rarely, severe hepatocellular injury may ensue, with prompt recovery on withdrawal of treatment. Clinical features of hypersensitivity do not normally occur.

Aspirin and Reye syndrome. Reye syndrome may be defined as an acute noninflammatory encephalopathy with hepatic injury (at least a threefold rise in hepatic transaminases and ammonia or microvesicular steatosis on biopsy) occurring without a recognized cause. Reye syndrome in children is associated with ingestion of aspirin in 90% of cases, especially in those with chickenpox or influenza. Its pathogenesis is multifactorial, and may reflect a genetic predisposition and mitochondrial enzyme abnormality, in which the viral infection or the aspirin ingestion may promote the hepatocellular insult. There is, however, no relationship between the salicylate level and the severity of hepatic dysfunction, and Reye syndrome may occur in the absence of aspirin ingestion (Chapters 4 and 13).

Histological changes are characteristic: there is diffuse microvesicular fatty change without an inflammatory reaction or significant hepatocellular necrosis (Figure 9.7). Electron microscopy reveals abnormal, enlarged mitochondria with disrupted cristae. Treatment is supportive.

Other NSAID-associated liver dysfunction

Toxicity is rare, especially in childhood, and is idiosyncratic and dose-independent. With some agents, there is a female preponderance. Table 9.4 lists the typical manifestations of commonly used NSAIDs.

Anesthetic agents

Halothane

Liver damage following halothane anesthesia is rare and usually mild. As the use of halothane has decreased over the decades, so has the incidence of hepatotoxicity. The risk of hepatitis increases with repeat exposures, particularly within 1 month, and in obese females.[17] The risk of developing ALF in adults has been calculated as between one in 8000 and one in 36 000 exposures.[18]

Although hepatotoxicity from halothane in children is relatively uncommon (an incidence of one in 82 000 exposures has been suggested)[19] there are reports of serious hepatitis and liver failure, and the same increased risk exists when the halothane is administered with multiple other anesthetics, and after multiple exposures within a short period of time.[20–23] Consequently, the Committee on Safety of Medicine in the United Kingdom has produced guidelines for the usage of halothane discouraging its use if there have been prior episodes of pyrexia or jaundice after halothane administration, and warning against repeating the drug within 3 months in any patient.[24]

Pathogenesis

Halothane is stored in adipose tissue and subsequently released, which may contribute to the higher risk of toxicity among the obese and those who have repeated exposures within a short period of time.[17] The underlying mechanism for liver damage is the formation of trifluoroacetylated proteins by cytochrome P450 (CYP 450). Approximately 20% of halothane is metabolized by CYP 450, predominantly CYP 2E1, to the unstable intermediate trifluoroacetyl chloride.[24]

Table 9.4 Liver dysfunction associated with nonsteroidal anti-inflammatory drugs (NSAIDs).

NSAID	Type	Manifestations	Onset	Additional
Indomethacin	Indole acetic acid derivative	Hepatocellular dysfunction Variable cholestasis Occasional microvesicular fat	1–7 months	Severe toxicity reported in patients with JCA also receiving diclofenac
Sulindac	Indole acetic acid derivative	Cholestasis May have hepatocellular damage Hypersensitivity with fever, rash, facial edema	Within 4 weeks	Low incidence of gastrointestinal side effects, therefore wide use, higher risk of DILD than other NSAIDs
Ibuprofen	Propionic acid Derivative	Hepatocellular dysfunction Occasionally cholestasis Fever, Stevens–Johnson syndrome	Within 3 weeks	Rare cause, sporadic reports of DILD
Naproxen	Propionic acid derivative	Mixed hepatocellular damage/cholestasis	Within 12 weeks	Widespread use, but only very occasional DILD
Piroxicam	Oxicam	Massive hepatocellular necrosis Prolonged cholestatic hepatitis	Within 3 months	Rare, but high mortality
Diclofenac	Phenylacetic acid derivative	Hepatocellular injury Occasional mixed hepatitis/cholestasis	Within 3 months	Commonly raised AST

AST, aspartate aminotransferase; DILD, drug-induced liver damage; JCA, juvenile chronic arthritis; NSAID, nonsteroidal anti-inflammatory drug.

This intermediate binds to liver proteins, causing hepatocellular necrosis.[25–27] In some patients, there is an immune response with antibody production against CYP 2E1. Although these antibodies may further damage the hepatocytes, their presence also serves as a diagnostic tool in the diagnosis of halothane-induced hepatitis.[26]

Clinical presentation and prognosis

The clinical features include an allergic-type reaction with pyrexia, associated with rigors, approximately 1–2 weeks after the first exposure to halothane. Symptoms such as malaise and right hypochondrial abdominal pain have been described. Jaundice appears within 10–28 days. These symptoms are commonly accentuated and hastened when the halothane exposure is in combination with other anesthetics.[22]

The laboratory profile reveals elevated transaminases and frequently an elevated eosinophil count. Histologically, the liver is comparable with the findings in viral hepatitis, with leukocyte infiltration of the sinusoids, fatty changes, and granulomas, but extensive hepatocellular necrosis is seen in severe toxicity (Figure 9.2).

Halothane-induced acute liver failure carries a poor prognosis, but those who only have mild hepatitis recover spontaneously and do well as long as repeat exposure is prevented. In one report of seven children who developed halothane-induced hepatitis and antibodies, six survived. The child who died had developed ALF from the drug.[24] Similarly, 11 of 15 adults who suffered halothane-induced ALF required liver transplantation for survival.[23]

Enflurane, isoflurane, desflurane

As with halothane, hepatotoxicity has been reported with comparable anesthetics, although usually to a less severe extent. The clinical presentation is similar, and the pathogenesis is also due to an immune response directed against the P450-created trifluoroacetylated proteins.[28]

Antimicrobial medications

Antimycobacterial medications

Current treatment for tuberculosis (TB) includes isoniazid (INH), rifampicin, ethambutol or streptomycin, and pyrazinamide for the first 3 months, followed by either INH or rifampicin for the next 6 months. Adverse events with these medications can involve nearly all body systems, but the most common and important is hepatotoxicity, which accounted for nearly half of the 23% rate of therapy-terminating side effects in 519 patients treated and studied in one series. Also, patients who received high-dose pyrazinamide had more severe side effects (15%) in comparison with those who received either INH (7%) or rifampicin (1.5%).[29]

The overall risk of hepatotoxicity from anti-TB therapy is believed to be between 2.5% and 35%, but the risk is highest in individuals who are over the age of 50, have chronic liver disease, especially chronic hepatitis B or C, abuse alcohol, are malnourished, or are infected with human immunodeficiency virus (HIV).[30–32] Reflecting on this observation of increased toxicity, the American Thoracic Society (ATS) recommends that alanine aminotransferase (ALT) levels should be monitored during treatment of TB infection in those who chronically consume alcohol, are taking other potentially hepatotoxic drugs, have viral hepatitis or other persistent hepatopathy, have experienced prior INH hepatitis, are infected with HIV, or are pregnant or within 3 months postpartum. Treatment should be interrupted in any patient who has an asymptomatic rise in ALT above five times the upper limit of normal, or a rise of greater than three times the upper level of normal in conjunction with symptoms of hepatitis or jaundice.[33]

In comparison with the incidence of hepatotoxicity to these medications in adults, children are believed to develop hepatotoxicity in less than 0.3% of cases.[34] One study of children under 16 years of age found that 8% of 99 children evaluated developed elevation of their transaminases to five times the upper limit of normal. The two factors that most correlated with the development of this toxicity were age under 5 years and treatment with pyrazinamide.[35]

Isoniazid

INH is by far the most effective and commonly used antimycobacterial medication. Although asymptomatic elevation of transaminases has been documented in 10–20% of individuals treated,[36] the rates of symptomatic hepatotoxicity are only 0.1–0.3%.[37–40]

Pathogenesis

INH is converted to monoacetylhydrazine, most of which is further metabolized and excreted by the kidneys. Some of the monoacetylhydrazine is converted via the P450 enzymes to reactive electrophilic intermediates, however, which are hepatotoxic. There is an increased risk of isoniazid-induced hepatotoxicity with age, and with concomitant medication that increases the activity of the P450 system, such as rifampicin (by enzyme induction) and pyrazinamide therapy. A genetic predisposition has been suggested, due to specific polymorphisms of *N*-acetyltransferase leading to differing rates of activity. "Rapid acetylators" may have an increased risk of toxicity due to an increased rate of production of monoacetylhydrazine. "Slow acetylators" may also be at risk, however, due to longer exposure to monoacetylhydrazine before its subsequent detoxification, or due to the generation of an alternative hepatotoxic metabolite. Alone, rifampicin rarely causes severe hepatotoxicity, but in combination with INH, the rate of hepatotoxicity is 5–8% more frequent than with either of the medications alone.[41]

Clinical presentation and prognosis

- The most usual presentation is characterized by an asymptomatic mild elevation of the hepatic transaminases. Histology reveals only minor and focal hepatocellular damage.[42] Although ongoing monitoring is recommended in this situation, changes in or termination of the therapy are not usually required.
- Hepatitis develops in either the first 2 months of therapy (50%) or with a delayed onset (50%), with symptoms commencing as long as 14 months into therapy.[38,43,44] The symptoms are similar to those with viral hepatitis, with fatigue, anorexia and nausea, malaise, and sometimes vomiting. Ten percent of patients will subsequently develop jaundice, usually days to weeks after the onset of the initial symptoms.[38,44,45] Histology shows inflammatory infiltrates with prominent eosinophils, hepatocyte necrosis, and ballooning degeneration.

Once the medication has been discontinued, most individuals experience gradual resolution of the hepatitis over 1–4 weeks. In general, patients who develop delayed-onset hepatitis (> 2 months) have a worse prognosis,[44,46] with a case fatality rate of approximately 10%.[44,47] On the other hand, if the INH is continued despite symptomatic hepatitis, patients may develop life-threatening hepatitis.[48,49] In this situation, liver transplantation has been life-saving in both adults and children.[43,50–55]

Rifampicin

Rifampicin is relatively safe when used alone. Although asymptomatic elevation of transaminases is more common, symptomatic hepatitis has been noted in only 0.6–2.7% (meta-analysis mean of 1.1%) of treated individuals.[41,56,57] Liver disease and concomitant isoniazid therapy increase the half-life, and thus more toxicity occurs in patients receiving both isoniazid and rifampicin than with rifampicin alone.

Pathogenesis

Rifampicin is rapidly eliminated in bile, undergoes enterohepatic circulation, and progressively undergoes deacetylation in the liver. It impairs bilirubin uptake and may elevate serum bilirubin. It also induces cytochrome P450 and thus enhances its own metabolism. Some 1–3% of the reactions are thought to be predominantly allergic, whereas the majority are thought to result from the rifampicin competing with bilirubin uptake at the plasma membrane of the hepatocyte.[58,59]

Clinical presentation and prognosis

The vast majority of patients who develop asymptomatic elevation of transaminases will have complete recovery upon discontinuation of the medication. For those who develop symptomatic hepatitis, the symptoms may be akin to those of viral hepatitis, but jaundice is usually prominent. The histopathology is patchy and generally shows less periportal inflammation than is seen with INH hepatitis.

Pyrazinamide

Pyrazinamide may lead to dose-related hepatotoxicity. Previous high-dose regimens were associated with liver injury in 15% of cases, whereas current lower-dose regimens carry a lower risk. When used alone, pyrazinamide, like rifampicin, is safe, but in combination with either rifampicin or INH, hepatotoxicity may be serious. For instance, when pyrazinamide and rifampicin are used together for only 2 months, there is more severe hepatotoxicity (7.7%) than with INH for 6 months (1%).[60] Because of this relatively high rate of hepatotoxicity with pyrazinamide and rifampicin, this combination therapy is now not recommended.[61]

Antibiotics

Antibiotics are commonly prescribed in pediatric practice, but hepatotoxicity is rare. Drug reactions are idiosyncratic and dose-unrelated, often with features of hypersensitivity such as fever, rash, and eosinophilia. It may be difficult to differentiate manifestations of drug toxicity from the underlying illness, as it may be complicated by multiple antibiotic exposures and other medications. Erythromycin, flucloxacillin, and tetracycline have most clearly been implicated in DILD (see below). Table 9.5 lists those antimicrobials in widespread use in pediatric practice in which DILD has been described.

There is no specific therapy other than immediate discontinuation of the offending medication, supportive care of the patient, and monitoring of the laboratory values.

β-Lactam antibiotics

Amoxicillin and amoxicillin–clavulanic acid

The synthetic penicillins cause a subclinical cytolytic hepatocellular injury, whereas the natural penicillins do so less commonly.[62,63] Some of the most commonly prescribed antibiotics in pediatrics, amoxicillin and ampicillin, cause hepatotoxicity in 0.3 cases per 10 000 prescriptions,[64] presenting most commonly as vanishing bile duct syndrome with cholestasis (Table 9.3) and less commonly as acute granulomatous hepatitis.[65–67] Similarly, amoxicillin–clavulanic acid (ACA) has been associated with hepatotoxicity, although at a higher rate (1.7 per 10 000 prescriptions), with the relative risk increasing with patient age and length of medication exposure (Figure 9.4).[64]

Pathogenesis

Amoxicillin rarely causes hepatotoxicity, unless combined with clavulanic acid. Patients with previous hepatotoxicity with ACA have successfully been treated with amoxicillin alone without ill effect. In contrast, rechallenge with ACA usually results in recurrent hepatotoxicity. It is therefore believed that the clavulanic acid component is the primary cause of the liver toxicity.[68,69] This concept is further supported by a comparison of 93 433 recipients of ACA with 360 333 recipients of amoxicillin alone, in which the incidence rate ratios were heavily weighted towards ACA causing more acute liver injury (6.3; 95% CI, 3.2 to 12.7) and jaundice (8.4; 95% CI, 3.6 to 20.8).[64]

The frequent features of a hypersensitivity reaction suggest an immunoallergic mechanism of the drug reaction, possibly affected by histocompatibility leukocyte antigen (HLA) haplotypes. A study of 35 biopsy-documented patients with ACA-induced hepatitis in comparison with a group of control

Table 9.5 Antimicrobial-associated drug-induced liver damage (DILD).

Drug	DILD reported
Antibacterial	
Amoxycillin/ampicillin	Increased transaminases rarely clinically significant, case reports of more severe injury Anecdotal granulomatous hepatitis
Augmentin (amoxycillin/clavulanic acid)	Cholestatic hepatitis within 1–6 weeks, rare in children, usually mild but may be protracted Accelerated onset with subsequent exposure
Cephalosporins	Rare and usually not significant; mild abnormality of aminotransferases or mild, reversible cholestasis
Co-trimoxazole	Acute and cholestatic hepatitis, vanishing bile duct syndrome, increased risk with human immunodeficiency virus (HIV) infection
Erythromycin	Cholestatic hepatitis
Flucloxacillin	Cholestasis
Imipenem	Minor liver injury and cholestasis
Quinolones	Cholestasis, mild hepatitis, reports of severe liver injury
Sulfonamides	Hepatitic, cholestatic or mixed hepatic injury, occurs within 4 weeks with features of hypersensitivity
Tetracycline	Microvesicular steatosis
Antifungals	
Ketoconazole	Rare, range from mild hepatitis to fulminant hepatic failure
Itraconazole	Rare, occasional hepatitis
Fluconazole	No hepatic injury
Antiviral agents	Liver toxicity not a major problem, but may be unrecognized due to underlying viral dysfunction

individuals showed a significant increase in the ACA toxicity group (57% versus 11.7%) of the DRB1*1501–DRB5*0101–DQB1*0602 haplotype. In addition, individuals with this haplotype were more likely to have a cholestatic (70% versus 60%) or mixed (30% versus 13%) pattern of hepatitis, and less likely to have a hepatocellular pattern (0% versus 27%) in comparison with those without this haplotype.[70] This haplotype association is clearly not the only factor, however, as it is present in 11.7% of people, whereas hepatotoxicity results from ACA treatment in only one in 1000–10 000 individuals treated.[64,69]

Clinical presentation and prognosis

A meta-analysis of the hepatotoxicity from ACA in 153 patients of all ages illustrates the variability of the clinical presentation:[71]

- 23% had hepatocellular injury.
- 16% were cholestatic.
- 54% had evidence of both hepatitis and cholestasis.
- 30–60% experienced systemic symptoms consistent with a hypersensitivity reaction (rash, fever, arthralgias, and elevated serum eosinophils).
- Jaundice may develop after cessation of the medication (days to 2 months).[68,71–73]
- Lacrimal gland inflammation, acute interstitial nephritis, and sialadenitis were rarely associated.[74]

Liver histology demonstrates predominant bile duct damage and biliary proliferation,[75] with less specific features of centrilobular canalicular cholestasis (Figure 9.4), eosinophil, neutrophil, and lymphocyte-rich inflammatory infiltrates, and portal edema. In those who develop chronic liver disease, focal destruction of the bile ducts with extensive inflammatory infiltrates and associated bile ductular wall necrosis is found, similar to primary sclerosing cholangitis.[68]

Most patients do well; jaundice resolves within 1–8 weeks and hepatic transaminases return to normal in 1–4 months.[62] However, in a meta-analysis of the hepatotoxicity from ACA, three of 153 of patients died from liver failure, while a 3-year-old required liver transplantation for vanishing bile duct syndrome after a 10-day course of ACA for the treatment of otitis media.[71,72]

Other penicillins

The semisynthetic penicillinase-resistant oxypenicillins, such as flucloxacillin and oxacillin, are well known to cause hepatotoxicity. The risk of hepatotoxicity with flucloxacillin ranges from one in 10 000 to one in 30 000.[76–78] The risk factors are: older age, treatment longer than 14 days, and higher daily dosage. In this case, gender was also important, with women being twice as likely as men to develop toxicity.[76,79] The clinical presentation and timing relative to therapy is similar to that of ACA. Histologically, the bile ducts may be reduced in number and size, the epithelium shows degeneration, and cholestasis is dominant.[62] In contrast to ACA hepatotoxicity, however, the jaundice tends to be prolonged, with 10–30% of individuals experiencing jaundice for more than 6 months. In these cases, the histological findings are more typical of paucity of the smaller bile ducts, with portal tract inflammation centered around the bile ducts, progressing to vanishing bile duct syndrome.[76,80,81] Cases of ALF secondary to flucloxacillin exposure have been reported.[82]

The other oxypenicillins, such as oxacillin, have a risk of cholestatic hepatotoxicity approximately half of that of flucloxacillin. The jaundice typically appears after 1–4 weeks of therapy or within 1 week of discontinuing the drug. Spontaneous recovery occurs within 3 months.[76]

The ureidopenicillins (mezlocillin, azlocillin, piperacillin) cause a twofold to threefold increase in serum aminotransferase levels in 19.3% of patients given the drug for prolonged periods of time (e.g., in the treatment of osteomyelitis).[83] The severity of the reaction appears to correlate with the cumulative dose and/or duration of therapy.[62]

Cephalosporins

The cephalosporins are commonly associated (in 0.7–11% of cases) with transient serum aminotransferase and alkaline phosphatase elevations.[84,85] In infants, ceftriaxone especially is associated with a transient cholestasis.[86] Spontaneous resolution is expected after cephalosporin-induced hepatotoxicity.

Tetracycline antibiotics

Dose-related hepatotoxicity can result from tetracycline usage, especially in women, during pregnancy, and in individuals with renal insufficiency.[62] The incidences of hepatotoxicity, expressed in exposed person-months, for oxytetracycline/tetracycline and minocycline are 0.69 per 10 000 and 1.04 per 10 000, respectively. This results in odds ratios, in comparison with those not taking the medications, of 1.46 for oxytetracycline/tetracycline and 2.1 for minocycline.[87]

Pathogenesis

The tetracyclines interfere with the mitochondrial oxidation of fatty acids, which results in an increased concentration of precursor free fatty acids in the liver. It is thought that both of these precursor free fatty acids and their oxidation metabolites are mitochondrial toxins, ultimately resulting in hepatocellular damage and the hepatotoxicity observed.[88]

Clinical presentation and prognosis

With tetracycline-induced hepatotoxicity, typical clinical features of acute hepatitis are experienced. Some 4–6 days into therapy, the patient experiences nausea, vomiting, abdominal pain, and mild jaundice. The laboratory profile reveals:

- Aminotransferase levels as high as 10 times the upper limit of normal.
- A significantly elevated amylase level.

• Histological features demonstrate microvesicular steatosis, minimal portal mononuclear inflammation, and hepatocellular necrosis (Figure 9.7).[88] Although chronic cholestasis is far less common, there have been reports of tetracycline-associated and doxycycline-associated vanishing bile duct syndrome.[89]

The clinical presentation of minocycline-induced hepatotoxicity deserves special mention, as three unique presentations can occur with this medication:

• An acute hypersensitivity reaction within days to weeks of starting the medication, characterized by fever, rash, lymphadenopathy, and associated peripheral eosinophilia with evidence of hepatocellular hepatitis. Rarely, acute liver failure has resulted from this reaction.[90–92]

• Hepatitis resembling autoimmune hepatitis (Figure 9.3). This is more common in young women; the onset is usually within months, but may be years after starting the medication, and may be complicated by polyarthritis, drug-induced systemic lupus erythematosus, rash, and hypergammaglobulinemia. Laboratory evaluation reveals elevated serum transaminases 2–15 times the upper limits of normal, a positive antinuclear antibody, but negative anti–smooth muscle and liver–kidney microsomal antibodies. Once the medication has been discontinued, the symptoms and hepatitis usually resolve within 3 months.

• Chronic hepatitis resulting in cirrhosis has been reported,[93,94] as have cases in the pediatric population.[90,95,96]

Macrolide antibiotics

The class of macrolide antibiotics includes erythromycin, roxithromycin, and clarithromycin. The incidence of hepatotoxicity is 2.28 per million to 3.6 per 100 000 patients treated for at least 10 days with erythromycin, which is low in comparison with many other medications.[97–99] Hepatotoxicity with roxithromycin is uncommon, with 0.7% of 2917 treated individuals reported in one study developing hepatitis by laboratory measures.[100] Clarithromycin leads to serum transaminase elevation in as many as 5% of individuals treated,[101] but more severe reactions of cholestatic hepatotoxicity have been observed, most commonly in elderly patients with a low body mass receiving high doses of the medication.[102]

Pathogenesis

The pathogenesis of hepatotoxicity with macrolide exposure involves both a direct cytotoxic affect as well as an immunoallergic reaction. In favor of the former is the observation that erythromycin is directly cytotoxic to cultured hepatocytes.[103] In contrast, the clinical presentation of a delayed onset of hepatotoxicity with peripheral eosinophilia, rash and fever, and prompt recurrence on rechallenge, favors an immunoallergic pathogenesis.[104–107] Erythromycin increases the activity of cytochrome P450 3A, and is metabolized via demethylation and oxidation into unstable intermediates.[103,108] These unstable intermediate metabolites in turn bind to the P450 3A protein and other hepatocellular proteins, thereby inhibiting them and causing cellular injury.[105,109]

Clinical presentation and prognosis

The onset of symptoms is usually 1–3 weeks after the medication is started, but reexposure may lead to a more rapid onset within 12 h, irrespective of the interval since the initial reaction. Symptoms are typical of hepatitis, including right upper quadrant pain, fever, nausea, and jaundice.[97,105] Laboratory evaluation reveals a peripheral eosinophilia in half of patients, elevated alkaline phosphatase and bilirubin levels, and hepatic transaminases are elevated up to 10 times the upper limit of normal. The histological features typically show centrilobular cholestasis with mild hepatocellular necrosis, in conjunction with intense portal and lobular inflammatory infiltrates, predominantly eosinophils.[106,110]

Most patients recover completely within weeks of discontinuation of the macrolide antibiotic. There have been reports of fatal liver injury, or injury requiring liver transplantation, in both children and adults, accentuating the potential severity of the hepatotoxicity.[110,111] As the onset of hepatotoxicity is rapid and more severe with reexposure, recognition of the causal relationship between the macrolide antibiotic and hepatotoxicity is essential to prevent reuse of that antibiotic.

Sulfonamide antibiotics

The most common hepatotoxicity experienced with sulfonamides is asymptomatic transient elevation of the transaminases (as high as 10% of patients), which is only detected by laboratory profiling.[112] Clinically apparent hepatitis requiring hospitalization is less common, but is estimated to occur in the range of one in 100 000–280 000 prescriptions.[97,113] Patients infected with HIV, however, are at higher risk, as use of the sulfonamide antibiotics results in hepatotoxicity in 20% of patients.[114,115] This is thought to be due to HIV-induced increased oxidation by their P450 enzymes, and hence increased production of the toxic hydroxylamine metabolite.[116]

Pathogenesis

Excretion of sulfonamides is predominantly via the kidneys after *N*-acetylation.[62] A small percentage of the drug is oxidized via the P450 enzymes in the liver, resulting in a reactive hydroxylamine species that is potentially toxic. If the normal detoxification mechanisms are insufficient for the load of hydroxylamine, this metabolite causes direct cytotoxicity against hepatocytes, and binds to cellular macromolecules, creating haptens. These haptens elicit an immune response, which contributes to the idiosyncratic hypersensitivity reaction and enhanced hepatitis seen in some patients.[62,117]

Clinical presentation and prognosis

Symptoms of a hypersensitivity DRESS reaction (fever, rash, peripheral eosinophilia), usually become apparent within days to 4 weeks of the medication being started. This reaction is sometimes associated with jaundice, pancreatitis, renal insufficiency, and lymphadenopathy.[62,118,119]

Centrilobular cholestasis usually dominates the histological findings, with only mild to moderate lymphocytic portal inflammation and minimal eosinophils and neutrophils.[118,120,121] Although less common, it should be noted that granulomatous hepatitis and massive hepatocellular necrosis have been reported.[120,122–124]

Once the medication is discontinued, the systemic and hepatic illness resolve within 3 months. Persistent cholestasis[125] and hepatic-related deaths have been reported.[119,120,126] It is important to prevent reexposure to the offending medication, as this may lead to a rapid onset of fatal hepatotoxicity.[126,127]

Quinolone antibiotics

The quinolones include ciprofloxacin, norfloxacin, ofloxacin, levofloxacin, trovafloxacin, and nalidixic acid. Overall, these medications are safe and rarely cause hepatotoxicity; however, individual reports of hepatoxicity have been associated with most of these medications.

The drug most commonly implicated with hepatotoxicity among the quinolones is ciprofloxacin. One database report of oral ciprofloxacin, including a wide range of doses (200–2000 mg/day) and treatment duration (2 days to over 90 days), revealed a rate of asymptomatic elevation in the serum aminotransferases or alkaline phosphatase of 3.6%. Spontaneous resolution of the hepatotoxicity was observed in all cases.[128] Another report, however, observed only three cases of hepatotoxicity among 37 000 recipients of the drug.[129] Intravenous ciprofloxacin has been linked to cholestasis, or elevation of alkaline phosphatase or the serum aminotransferases, in 0.1–2.1% of drug recipients.[129,130] Despite the relatively low incidence of hepatotoxicity, cases of ALF due to ciprofloxacin have been reported, all within days of the medication being initiated in older adults.[131,132]

The incidence of hepatotoxicity with trovafloxacin is 0.0056% (140 per 2.5 million prescriptions).[62,133] Among the 140 adult patients who developed hepatotoxicity, however, 14 advanced to liver failure, resulting in four patients undergoing transplantation and five deaths. The hepatotoxicity occurred 1–60 days after initiation of the therapy, resembled a hypersensitivity-type reaction, and clearly correlated with therapy of 14 days' duration or longer. On the basis of these findings, the Food and Drug Administration (Public Health Advisory, June 9, 1999) recommended limiting the use of trovafloxacin to hospitalized patients with serious infections, and that the liver enzymes should be closely monitored.[62,133]

Clindamycin

Clindamycin causes an asymptomatic rise in serum aminotransferases in as many as 50% of recipients.[134,135] However, symptomatic hepatitis or cholestasis is limited to individual case reports.[136,137]

Antifungal medications

The most commonly used antifungal medications include amphotericin B, ketoconazole, fluconazole, and itraconazole. Overall, these medications are relatively safe with regard to hepatotoxicity. However, patients who are immunosuppressed and systemically ill are at risk for hepatotoxicity.

Ketoconazole

Ketoconazole carries the highest risk for hepatotoxicity, with an incidence of between 1.3 per 1000 and one in 3000, and a relative risk compared to individuals not taking the medication of 228 (95% CI, 33.9 to 993).[62,138,139]

Pathogenesis

Although the mechanism for ketoconazole-induced hepatitis is not fully understood, the drug's extensive metabolism in the liver would suggest either the development of toxic metabolites or direct toxicity. Although recurrence of hepatotoxicity with reexposure is common, the symptoms are neither consistent nor immediate, arguing against an immunoallergic mechanism of injury.[62]

Clinical presentation and prognosis

Asymptomatic elevation of the transaminases will develop in 2–17% of users after weeks of therapy,[140,141] but most cases will resolve spontaneously despite continued use.[141,142] Approximately 3% of patients receiving ketoconazole will develop symptomatic hepatitis.[141] In this situation, recovery is expected approximately 3 months after medication is discontinued. However, fatal hepatitis and ALF have been reported.[139,143–145]

Liver histology shows patchy and centrilobular necrosis, with portal mononuclear cellular infiltration. The laboratory abnormalities suggest a hepatocellular pattern in more than half of the cases (54%), and a cholestatic (16%) or mixed pattern (25%) in the rest.[138,141,142,145]

Although it is not possible to predict the development of toxicity, the likelihood increases with prolonged use. Consequently, 2-weekly laboratory monitoring of biochemical liver function is suggested in patients on medication for longer than 10 days. Asymptomatic laboratory elevation should be rechecked 1 week later, and the development of significant laboratory elevation or symptoms should precipitate immediate discontinuation of the medication.[62,142]

Amphotericin B, itraconazole, fluconazole

Significant liver toxicity from these commonly prescribed antifungal agents is uncommon. In the case of amphotericin

B, there are only individual cases of hepatotoxicity in adults,[140,146–148] and no fatal cases in children. In reported cases, an asymptomatic elevation of transaminases and alkaline phosphatase occurred 10 days to 3 weeks into therapy, and all laboratory values returned to normal after discontinuation of the medication. The most prominent histological finding in the liver was centrilobular focal fatty infiltration.

The relative risk of developing acute hepatitis due to itraconazole is 17.7 (95% CI, 2.6 to 72.6), with asymptomatic elevation of biochemical liver function tests occurring in 1–7% of patients.[138,149,150] The pattern is usually hepatocellular, but cholestasis is also observed.[151] As with amphotericin B, laboratory abnormalities resolve after cessation of the medication, although ALF has been reported with itraconazole.[151–153]

Fluconazole is a commonly used antifungal, and transient mild elevation of hepatic enzymes is observed in 5% of patients.[154] Symptomatic hepatitis and ALF are rare.[155–157] Histological findings with fluconazole-induced serious hepatotoxicity ranges from a mixed hepatocellular–cholestatic pattern to diffuse necrosis.[62]

Flucytosine is associated with hepatotoxicity in 5–15% of patients treated, with most remaining asymptomatic.[140] Elevation of the serum aminotransferases, with or without elevation of the alkaline phosphatase and bilirubin, is the most common presentation. Hepatic necrosis has been reported.

Antiepileptic medications

Abnormal serum liver enzyme values are commonly associated with the antiepileptic medications, but as children on these medications frequently have underlying metabolic conditions or serious seizures, it is important to distinguish whether the enzyme elevations are due to drug toxicity or underlying disease, a "tolerable" side effect, or progressive liver insufficiency.[158] Prolonged convulsions may lead to hypoxic/ischemic liver damage and must be considered in the differential diagnosis of liver dysfunction.

Although elevation of liver laboratory values has been reported with many antiepileptic medications (chloral hydrate, clonazepam, diazepam, mephenytoin, primidone and sultiame), significant hepatotoxicity has only been reported for phenobarbital, carbamazepine, phenytoin, lamotrigine, vigabatrin, felbamate, valproate, and oxcarbazepine.[159–162]

The risk of a fatal outcome due to anticonvulsant therapy in children is low. Surveillance for fatal suspected adverse drug events, performed in the United Kingdom from 1964 to 2000, identified 65 deaths in association with anticonvulsants, of which 31 were related to sodium valproate.[163]

The most common clinical presentations include hepatocellular cytotoxicity or DRESS, the hypersensitivity reaction.[164,165]

Phenobarbital

Although phenobarbital is one of the most commonly used antiepileptic medications, with nearly half of a century of use experience, there have been relatively few reports of significant hepatotoxicity. Hepatocellular, cholestatic, and DRESS hepatoxicity have been observed.[161,164]

Carbamazepine

Hepatotoxicity from carbamazepine and related drugs (e.g., oxcarbazepine) is due to disturbance of glutathione metabolism. Carbamazepine toxicity resembles that of phenytoin, with both hepatocellular and cholestatic features and evidence of hypersensitivity (DRESS). Typically, the onset of symptoms occurs after 4 weeks, with high fever, rigors, weakness, jaundice, and hepatic discomfort, resembling cholangitis. There may be a skin rash and peripheral edema. Serum immunoglobulins, especially immunoglobulin E (IgE), may be raised, while complement levels may be decreased. Eosinophilia is usually present. Clinical deterioration may continue despite medication being stopped.[166,167]

Histological changes reflect both hepatocellular damage and cholestasis, and granulomas may be seen (Figures 9.5 and 9.6). In children, fatal hepatocellular necrosis has also been described.[166]

Phenytoin

Hepatotoxicity from phenytoin is uncommon, but benign elevation of GGT and alkaline phosphatase as a result of hepatic enzyme induction is not uncommon. Acute or cholestatic hepatitis with features of allergy—including fever, rash, and eosinophilia, and a high frequency of lymphadenopathy and splenomegaly—may occur within the first weeks of starting the medication. Histology may reveal the presence of granulomas. Recovery is expected after discontinuation of the drug, but fatal outcomes have been reported when the drug is continued despite the onset of hepatotoxicity.[168,169]

Lamotrigine

Although there is relatively limited experience with lamotrigine, hepatotoxicity from this medication appears to be relatively uncommon. The risk increases in combination with other antiepileptic or psychotic medications, and cases of fatal hepatotoxicity have been reported in both adults and children.[170]

Felbamate

Felbamate is an effective treatment for Lennox–Gastaut syndrome. The drug causes aplastic anemia and ALF in a significant proportion of patients. The risk of ALF is between one in 10 000 and one in 20 000 patients treated, of whom 60% will have a fatal outcome. Due to this substantial risk, frequent monitoring of the biochemical liver laboratory values before and during therapy is recommended. Therapy should be discontinued at the first sign of transaminase elevation.[171,172]

Valproate

Valproate is an effective antiepileptic medication that is usually well tolerated. Asymptomatic elevation of liver-associated laboratory values may be observed in 20% of patients on this medication. The estimated risk for liver failure, however, increases in combination with other antiepileptic medications, and inversely with age. In children under 2 years of age, the risk of liver failure is one in 8000 in children treated with valproate alone and increases to one in 550 when combined with other antiepileptic medications. The risk decreases to one in 6000–12 000 for children aged 3–10 years and to less than one in 50 000 in children older than 10 years.[173,174] Apart from age, other risk factors include fatty acid oxidation defects, urea cycle disorders, and mitochondrial diseases. Patients with Alpers disease, chronic progressive external ophthalmoplegia, and carnitine palmitoyltransferase type II deficiency have developed significant deterioration of liver function with the introduction of valproate therapy.[175–178]

Pathogenesis

Valproate is synthesized by medium-chain acyl-CoA synthetase in the mitochondrial matrix into valproyl–adenosine monophosphate and valproyl-CoA. During its metabolism, the intramitochondrial pool of the CoA cofactor is potentially depleted, impairing or inactivating the mitochondrial enzymes involved in β-oxidation of long-, medium-, and short-chain fatty acids[179]—hence the reaction in children with mitochondrial disease.

Clinical presentation and prognosis

Although asymptomatic laboratory elevation is common, the onset of hepatitis is a sign of potentially serious hepatotoxicity. Routine monitoring of liver function may not distinguish those with impending liver failure from those with minor enzyme elevation: fulminant failure can occur without any preceding biochemical abnormality and may progress despite discontinuation of valproate.

The onset of hepatotoxicity is typically within 5 months of the start of treatment, and manifests as acute liver failure due to hepatocellular necrosis, usually with macrovesicular and sometimes extensive microvesicular fatty change in the liver.

The most common presenting symptoms in patients with fatal valproate hepatotoxicity are:

- Diminished conscious level
- Jaundice
- Vomiting
- Bleeding
- Increased frequency of convulsions
- Anorexia
- Edema
- Mild pancreatitis

If symptoms do develop, the drug should be immediately discontinued. The early administration of intravenous L-carnitine is associated with improved hepatic survival.[173,174] Treatment is otherwise supportive, as for fulminant hepatic failure. The role of transplantation is controversial: the presence of an underlying metabolic or mitochondrial disorder with likely progressive multisystem manifestations, not reversible by liver transplantation, should be sought. Transplantation is contraindicated in this situation (see Chapter 21).

Herbal medications

Herbal medications are increasingly used in the United States and Europe by consumers who are under the misconception that they are natural and hence must be safe. In fact, these products are commonly unpurified extracts from plants and do not fall under the normal oversight and regulatory systems used to scrutinize allopathic pharmacologic products.[180–182] The herbal medications that have been reported to cause hepatotoxicity are listed in Table 9.6.

Pathogenesis

The pathogenesis of liver toxicity in most of the herbal medications is unknown. This is in large part because they are actually mixtures of multiple compounds, not all known. In addition, their wide availability over the counter allows for unregulated usage and potentially harmful medication combinations. For instance, as some of these herbal remedies induce the P450 enzyme system, they could enhance the hepatotoxicity of conventional medications.[183]

Clinical presentation and prognosis

The first step in identifying an herbal medication as etiological in the development of hepatotoxicity is obtaining an exposure history. Many patients do not volunteer the information that they are taking herbal preparations. Furthermore, like many allopathic medications, significant indirect exposure is possible. For instance, exposure to an infant transplacentally or via breast milk has been reported with pyrrolizidine alkaloids and other compounds, causing fatal fetal veno-occlusive disease or obstructive jaundice.[184,185]

Many of the herbal medications have been described as causing liver damage with characteristic histological features.[186,187] These patterns are the same as seen with conventional medication toxicity, but may help differentiate between herbal causes when there are multiple exposures. For instance, the pyrrolizidine alkaloids cause veno-occlusive disease, *Chelidonium majus* causes a cholestatic hepatitis,[188] *Larrea tridentata* and pennyroyal result in hepatocyte necrosis in zone 3,[186] and kava can induce a nonspecific hepatitis.[189]

When it is suspected that hepatotoxicity is the result of herbal exposure, immediate withdrawal of that medication is recommended. Subsequent resolution of the hepatotoxicity strengthens the causal suspicion, and reexposure is then contraindicated.

Table 9.6 Herbal medications reported to cause hepatotoxicity.

Amanita phalloides
Pyrrolizidine alkaloids
Crotalaria
Heliotropium
Senecio
Symphytum officinale
Symphytum longilobus
Mate ("Paraguay tea")
Chinese herbal medicines
Jin bu huan (*Lycopodium serratum*)
Ma huang (ephedra alkaloid)
Sho-saiko-to
Paeonia spp.
Dictamnus spp.
Lingzhi (*Ganoderma lucidum*)
Shou-wu-pian (*Polygonum multiflorum*)
Germander
Teucrium chamaedrys
Teucrium polium
Atractylosides
Atractylis gummifera
Callilepsis laureola
Chaparral
Larrea tridentata
Anthraquinones
Senna (*Cassia angustifolia*)
Cascara sagrada
Noni (*Morinda citrifolia*)
Miscellaneous
Mistletoe (*Viscum album*)
Valerian (*Valeriana officinalis*)
Skullcap (*Scutellaria* spp.)
Pennyroyal (*Mentha pulegium*)
Margosa oil (*Azadirachta indica*)
Sassafras (*Sassafras albidum*)
Kava (*Piper methysticum*)
Greater celandine (*Chelidonium majus*)

Recreational drugs

Cannabis, cocaine, and heroin have been used for medicinal and illicit purposes for centuries, and continue to be commonly used for recreational purposes. The amphetamine derivatives (ecstasy and others) have become increasingly popular, and the relative ease of home preparation has both facilitated their use and increased the potential for toxic contamination.[190] Finally, the obesity epidemic that is affecting many Westernized societies and the social pressure to be fit and have a slim figure has increased the use of medications intended to aid with weight loss, many times without physician supervision. As with the herbal medications discussed above, these recreational drugs are frequently impure or contaminated with other potential toxins and are not regulated to control their concentration and contents and to document toxicities. Consequently, the rates of hepatotoxicity with these drugs are all subject to inaccuracy.

Cannabis

Cannabis (*C. sativa:* marijuana; *C. indica:* hashish) are plants with more than 400 chemical compounds, including the Δ-9-tetrahydrocannabinol that leads to the attractiveness of this drug for its analgesic and recreational affects.[191] An association with hepatotoxicity is uncommon,[191,192] but a clear toxicity analysis is difficult given the high frequency with which these drugs are used in association with alcohol or other drugs, and the rate of viral hepatitis that is common among parenteral drug users who also frequently use cannabis. A Brazilian community-based study evaluated the rates of aspartate aminotransferase (AST), alanine aminotransferase (ALT), and alkaline phosphatase elevation among nonparenteral seronegative illicit drug users.[193] In the group using marijuana alone, AST, ALT, and alkaline phosphatase were elevated in 42.3%, 34.6%, and 53.8% of users, respectively. Another investigator found AST elevation in 66% of users of nonparenteral drugs, with acute hepatitis (53%) and nonspecific hepatitis (44%) found in those who had liver biopsies.[194]

Amphetamines

The amphetamines and their derivatives can cause neurotoxicity and hepatotoxicity. The clinical presentation typically resembles viral hepatitis,[195] and histological features similarly resemble acute viral hepatitis.[196,197] Cases of ALF have also been described, resulting in a fatal outcome or a need for transplantation.[198,199]

Slimming agents

As the obesity epidemic has worsened, the use of some herbal weight-loss agents and formulated chemical mixture compounds to affect weight loss has increased. As the use of these agents is commonly in the setting of obesity, and hence frequently with underlying fatty liver disease, the potential for hepatotoxicity is enhanced. ALF has been described with the use of *ma huang* (ephedra alkaloid), usnic acid (lichen alkaloid), *chaso*, and *onshido*.[200,201] In addition, a series of six patients suffered acute hepatitis, with one developing ALF, while using LipoKinetix (norephedrine, sodium usniate, diiodothyronine, yohimbine, and caffeine).[202]

Pathogenesis

Although the exact mechanism for hepatotoxicity is unknown, these slimming medications and herbal remedies result in hepatotoxicity in part by causing oxidative stress-related mitochondrial injury, especially in the setting of obesity-related liver disease.[203]

Drugs used in gastrointestinal disorders

H_2-antagonists and proton-pump inhibitors

Both cimetidine and ranitidine are associated with raised aminotransferase activity, which is common, transient, and may reverse while therapy is continued. Significant hepatocellular or cholestatic injury is rare in children. Hypersensitivity reactions are unusual.

Cimetidine is a reversible inhibitor of cytochrome P450, depending on host variation and other drugs, which has a theoretical but unproven beneficial effect in acetaminophen toxicity. Other drug effects may be potentiated (e.g., warfarin) and the dose should be reduced accordingly. Ranitidine has a lower affinity for cytochrome P450, and interaction with other drugs is less marked or significant.

Omeprazole has similar adverse effects to H_2-blockers in type and frequency, with reversible elevation in aminotransferase levels reported.[204] Other proton-pump inhibitors, including lansoprazole and pantoprazole, are structurally very similar and considered likely to have similar pharmacokinetics, metabolism, and interactions.[205]

Sulfasalazine and related compounds

Liver injury associated with sulfasalazine is uncommon, and relates to a hypersensitivity reaction to the sulfapyridine moiety. Fever, rash, lymphadenopathy, and eosinophilia may occur within 2–3 weeks of treatment, but massive hepatic necrosis, although documented, is rare.

Olsalazine and mesalazine lack the sulfapyridine moiety, and were initially considered to be less hepatotoxic. However, mesalazine associated hepatotoxicity including cholestasis, chronic hepatitis, and granulomatous hepatitis, is becoming more apparent.[206]

Immunosuppressive drugs

Azathioprine

Azathioprine can give rise to a broad spectrum of liver dysfunction:

- Asymptomatic liver enzyme elevation
- Hepatitis and/or cholestasis and bile duct injury
- Vascular injury (especially after renal transplantation)
- Sinusoidal dilation, perisinusoidal fibrosis
- Peliosis (blood-filled cavities without endothelial lining)
- Veno-occlusive disease

As indications for azathioprine include organ transplantation, chronic inflammatory disorders, and autoimmune disease, liver damage may occur in a complex setting, and azathioprine may not be considered as the potential cause. The onset may be months to years after the start of treatment, although the hepatitic and cholestatic features may manifest earlier. Disease progression occurs with continued treatment. A therapeutic trial of azathioprine withdrawal may be necessary to establish or exclude its role.

Cyclosporine

Cyclosporine may rarely be associated with hyperbilirubinemia, cholestasis, and cholelithiasis.

Methotrexate

Methotrexate is a folic acid antagonist and has an expanding therapeutic role, including leukemia, solid tumors, psoriasis, and rheumatoid arthritis. It is a dose-dependent hepatotoxin, which has a fibrogenic effect, possibly by activation of hepatic Ito cells. The total dose administered is the most important predictor of fibrosis, although the dose schedule used may be relevant: low-dose, weekly pulsed therapy appears to carry a lower risk of significant fibrosis.

Other risk factors for methotrexate toxicity include alcohol ingestion and preexisting liver disease. In addition, as methotrexate is renally excreted, impairment of renal function (including decreased renal blood flow due to NSAID administration) will contribute to the risk of toxicity.

Hepatic fibrosis is usually asymptomatic, unless accompanied by manifestations of portal hypertension. Extensive fibrosis may be present with normal liver function, but serial monitoring is recommended. Minor enzyme abnormalities are common, especially with high doses, and do not correlate with significant hepatic damage. Liver biopsy should be performed to assess hepatic fibrosis if liver enzymes are persistently abnormal, or after 4 g or 2 years of treatment.

In the presence of fibrosis, the risks and benefits of continued treatment have to be considered, as there may be some reversal of fibrosis after stopping treatment.

Cytotoxic therapy

Cytotoxic chemotherapy and veno-occlusive disease are discussed in Chapter 16.

Case study

A 16-year-old Caucasian female presents to the hepatology clinic with a 3-month history of dizziness, fatigue, ankle swelling and discomfort, and elevated transaminases, after returning from a trip to a developing country. She had been a previously well child and was only taking minocycline for the treatment of acne; she had been on this medication for 1.5 years at the time of presentation.

Her physical examination was normal, with the exception of a body mass index of 25 and mild swelling of her ankles bilaterally without erythema.

Two months into these symptoms, she had a laboratory profile that revealed an AST of 65 U/L (normal = 5–41 U/L) and ALT of 150 U/L (normal = 5–40 U/L). The complete blood count, serum albumin level, thyroid function testing, prothrombin time, immunoglobulins, and serum chemistry tests were otherwise normal. Epstein–Barr virus IgM and stool for ova and parasites and bacterial pathogens were negative. Screening tests for hepatitis

A–C were negative. Hepatic ultrasound was normal. Three months into her symptoms, her AST had increased to 150 U/L and ALT to 230 U/L. Further screening at that time revealed a negative cytomegalovirus IgM, normal ceruloplasmin level, and quantitative urine copper. Her α_1-antitrypsin level and phenotype were normal. Her antinuclear antibody was positive, with a titer of 1 : 640–5120, but anti–smooth muscle and anti-liver–kidney microsomal antibodies were negative. HLA-B27 was undetectable.

The differential diagnosis of chronic hepatitis in this age group includes:

- Autoimmune hepatitis type 1 or 2
- Wilson's disease
- α_1-Antitrypsin deficiency
- Drug-induced liver disease
- Chronic viral hepatitis

On the basis of the laboratory profile and symptoms suggestive of possible minocycline-induced hepatitis, the medication was discontinued and follow-up laboratory evaluations planned. Two weeks after the medication had been discontinued, her transaminases had decreased to an AST of 75 U/L and an ALT of 100 U/L. One month after discontinuation of the medications, her ankle swelling and discomfort had resolved and transaminases and autoimmune markers normalized. Over the next month, the dizziness and fatigue also resolved.

Comment: Autoimmune hepatitis is a common cause of chronic liver disease in this age group and must form part of the differential diagnosis. Although the immunoglobulins were normal, this can occur in 25% of patients at presentation (see Chapter 8). Wilson's disease is excluded by the normal copper evaluation and α_1-antitrypsin deficiency by the normal levels and phenotype. The resolution of all clinical and laboratory markers following discontinuation of minocycline indicates the etiology in this case.

Acknowledgments

The author acknowledges the contributions of Dr. Stefan Wirth and Dr. Nedim Hadzic for their intellectual contribution to this chapter and assistance in gathering histology figures. Figures 9.2–9.4 were provided by Professor Bernard Portmann, Institute of Liver Studies, King's College Hospital, London.

References

1 Farrell GC, Liddle C. Drugs and the liver updated, 2002. *Semin Liver Dis* 2002;**22**:109–13.
2 Squires RH Jr, Shneider BL, Bucuvalas J, *et al.* Acute liver failure in children: the first 348 patients in the pediatric acute liver failure study group. *J Pediatr* 2006;**148**:652–8.
3 Ravikumara M, Hill FG, Wilson's DC, *et al.* 6-Thioguanine-related chronic hepatotoxicity and variceal haemorrhage in children treated for acute lymphoblastic leukaemia—a dual-centre experience. *J Pediatr Gastroenterol Nutr* 2006;**42**:535–8.
4 Mahadevan SB, McKiernan PJ, Davies P, Kelly DA. Acetaminophen induced hepatotoxicity. *Arch Dis Child* 2006;**91**:598–603.
5 Murray KF, Messner DJ, Kowdley KV. Mechanism of hepatocyte detoxification. In: Johnson LR, ed. *Physiology of the Gastrointestinal Tract,* 4th ed. Burlington, MA: Elsevier Academic Press, 2006: 1483–504.
6 Bromer MW, Black M. Acetaminophen hepatoxicity. *Clin Liver Dis* 2003;**7**:351–67.
7 Rivera-Penera T, Gugig R, Davis J, *et al.* Outcome of acetaminophen overdose in pediatric patients and factors contributing to hepatotoxicity. *J Pediatr* 1997;**130**:300–4.
8 Lauterburg BH, Vaishnav Y, Stillwell WG, Mitchell JR. The effects of age and glutathione depletion on hepatic glutathione turnover in vivo determined by acetaminophen probe analysis. *J Pharmacol Exp Ther* 1980;**213**:54–8.
9 Morgan O, Majeed A. Restricting acetaminophen in the United Kingdom to reduce poisoning: a systematic review. *J Public Health (Oxf)* 2005;**27**:12–8.
10 Hawton K, Simkin S, Deeks J, *et al.* UK legislation on analgesic packs: before and after study of long term effect on poisonings. *BMJ* 2004;**329**:1076.
11 Rumack BH. Acetaminophen overdose in children and adolescents. *Pediatr Clin N Am* 1986;**33**:691–701.
12 Heubi JE. Measurement of serum acetaminophen-protein adducts in patients with acute liver failure. *J Pediatr Gastroenterol Nutr* 2007;**44**:513–5.
13 Sztajnkerycer MJ, Bond GR. Chronic acetaminophen overdosing in children: risk assessment and management. *Curr Opin Pediatr* 2001;**13**:177–82.
14 Kozer E, Koren G. Management of acetaminophen overdose: current controversies. *Drug Saf* 2001;**24**:503–12.
15 Lee WS, McKiernan P, Kelly DA. Etiology, outcome and prognostic indicators of childhood fulminant hepatic failure in the United Kingdom. *J Pediatr Gastroenterol Nutr* 2005;**40**:575–81.
16 Teoh NC, Farrell GC. Hepatotoxicity associated with non-steroidal anti-inflammatory drugs. *Clin Liver Dis* 2003;**7**:401–13.
17 Voigt MD, Workman B, Lombard C, Kirsch RE. Halothane hepatitis in a South African population—frequency and the influence of gender and ethnicity. *S Afr Med J* 1997;**87**:882–5.
18 Weber P, Scheurlen M, Irkin I, *et al.* [Liver transplantation in halothane-induced liver necrosis; in German.] *Zentralbl Chir* 1994;**119**:305–8.
19 Wark HJ. Postoperative jaundice in children. The influence of halothane. *Anaesthesia* 1983;**38**:237–42.
20 Pratilas V, Pratila MG. Multiple halothane anesthesias in a child: a case report. *Mt Sinai J Med* 1978;**45**:480–3.
21 Hassall E, Israel DM, Gunasekaran T, Steward D. Halothane hepatitis in children. *J Pediatr Gastroenterol Nutr* 1990;**11**:553–7.
22 Kenna JG, Neuberger J, Mieli-Vergani G, Mowat AP, Williams R. Halothane hepatitis in children. *Br Med J (Clin Res Ed)* 1987;**294**:1209–11.
23 Lo SK, Wendon J, Mieli-Vergani G, Williams R. Halothane-induced acute liver failure: continuing occurrence and use of liver transplantation. *Eur J Gastroenterol Hepatol* 1998;**10**:635–9.
24 Committee on Safety of Medicines. *Current Problems.* London: Committee on Safety of Medicines, 1986.

25 Kharasch ED, Hankins D, Mautz D, Thummel KE. Identification of the enzyme responsible for oxidative halothane metabolism: implications for prevention of halothane hepatitis. *Lancet* 1996; **347**:1367–71.

26 Eliasson E, Kenna JG. Cytochrome P450 2E1 is a cell surface autoantigen in halothane hepatitis. *Mol Pharmacol* 1996;**50**: 573–82.

27 Bourdi M, Chen W, Peter RM, *et al.* Human cytochrome P450 2E1 is a major autoantigen associated with halothane hepatitis. *Chem Res Toxicol* 1996;**9**:1159–66.

28 Njoku D, Laster MJ, Gong DH, Eger EI 2nd, Reed GF, Martin JL. Biotransformation of halothane, enflurane, isoflurane, and desflurane to trifluoroacetylated liver proteins: association between protein acylation and hepatic injury. *Anesth Analg* 1997;**84**:173–8.

29 Schaberg T, Rebhan K, Lode H. Risk factors for side-effects of isoniazid, rifampin and pyrazinamide in patients hospitalized for pulmonary tuberculosis. *Eur Respir J* 1996;**9**:2026–30.

30 Fernández-Villar A, Sopeña B, Fernández-Villar J, *et al.* The influence of risk factors on the severity of anti-tuberculosis drug-induced hepatotoxicity. *Int J Tuberc Lung Dis* 2004;**8**:1499–505.

31 Ungo JR, Jones D, Ashkin D, *et al.* Antituberculosis drug-induced hepatotoxicity. The role of hepatitis C virus and the human immunodeficiency virus. *Am J Respir Crit Care Med* 1998;**157**:1871–6.

32 Wong WM, Wu PC, Yuen MF, *et al.* Antituberculosis drug-related liver dysfunction in chronic hepatitis B infection. *Hepatology* 2000;**31**:201–6.

33 Saukkonen JJ, Cohn DL, Jasmer RM, *et al.* An official ATS statement: hepatotoxicity of antituberculosis therapy. *Am J Respir Crit Care Med* 2006;**174**:935–52.

34 [No authors listed.] National American College of Chest Physicians consensus conference on tuberculosis. *Chest* 1985; **87**(2 Suppl):115S–149S.

35 Ohkawa K, Hashiguchi M, Ohno K, *et al.* Risk factors for anti-tuberculosis chemotherapy-induced hepatotoxicity in Japanese pediatric patients. *Clin Pharmacol Ther* 2002;**72**:220–6.

36 Brummer DL. Isoniazid and liver disease. *Ann Intern Med* 1971;**75**:643–4.

37 LoBue PA, Moser KS. Use of isoniazid for latent tuberculosis infection in a public health clinic. *Am J Respir Crit Care Med* 2003;**168**:443–7.

38 Larson AM, Graziani AL. *Isoniazid Hepatoxicity*. In: Up to Date, Rose, BD, ed., 2007; Up to Date, Wellesley, MA.

39 Nolan CM, Goldberg SV, Buskin SE. Hepatotoxicity associated with isoniazid preventive therapy: a 7-year survey from a public health tuberculosis clinic. *JAMA* 1999;**281**:1014–8.

40 Kopanoff DE, Sinder DE, Caras GH. Isoniazid-related hepatitis A. U.S. Public Health Service cooperative surveillance study. *Am Rev Respir Dis* 1978;**117**:991–1001.

41 Steele MA, Burk RF, DesPrez RM. Toxic hepatitis with isoniazid and rifampin—a meta-analysis. *Chest* 1991;**99**:465–71.

42 Scharer L, Smith JP. Serum transaminase elevations and other hepatic abnormalities in patients receiving isoniazid. *Ann Intern Med* 1969;**71**:113–20.

43 Centers for Disease Control and Prevention (CDC). Severe isoniazid-associated hepatitis—New York, 1991–1993. *MMWR Morb Mortal Wkly Rep* 1993;**42**:545–7.

44 Black M, Mitchell JR, Zimmerman HJ, Ishak KG, Epler GR. Liver physiology and disease: isoniazid-associated hepatitis in 114 patients. *Gastroenterology* 1975;**69**:289–302.

45 Maddrey WC, Boitnott JK. Isoniazid hepatitis. *Ann Intern Med* 1973;**79**:1–12.

46 Girling DJ. The hepatic toxicity of antituberculosis regimens containing isoniazid, rifampicin and pyrazinamide. *Tubercle* 1978;**59**:13–32.

47 Bass NM, Ockner RK. Drug-induced liver disease. In: Zakim D, Boyer TD, eds. *Hepatopathology*. Philadelphia: Saunders, 1996: 962–1017.

48 Snider DE Jr, Caras GJ. Isoniazid-associated hepatitis deaths: a review of available information. *Am Rev Respir Dis* 1992;**145**: 494–7.

49 Cohen R, Kalser MH, Thompson RV. Fatal hepatic necrosis secondary to isoniazid therapy. *JAMA* 1961;**176**:877–9.

50 Farrell FJ, Keeffe EB, Man KM, Imperial JC, Esquivel CO. Treatment of hepatic failure secondary to isoniazid hepatitis with liver transplantation. *Dig Dis Sci* 1994;**39**:2255–9.

51 Cillo U, Bassanello M, Vitale A, *et al.* Isoniazid-related fulminant hepatic failure in a child: assessment of the native liver's early regeneration after auxiliary partial orthotopic liver transplantation. *Transpl Int* **2005**;17:713–6.

52 Vanderhoof JA, Ament ME. Fatal hepatic necrosis due to isoniazid chemoprophylaxis in a 15-year-old girl. *J Pediatr* 1976;**88**:867–8.

53 Berkowitz FE, Henderson SL, Fajman N, Schoen B, Naughton M. Acute liver failure caused by isoniazid in a child receiving carbamazepine. *Int J Tuberc Lung Dis* 1998;**2**:603–6.

54 Casteels-Van Daele M, Igodt-Ameye L, Corbeel L, Eeckels R. Hepatoxicity of rifampicin and isoniazid in children. *J Pediatr* 1975;**86**:739–41.

55 Hasagawa T, Reyes J, Nour B, *et al.* Successful liver transplantation for isoniazid-induced hepatic failure—a case report. *Transplantation* 1994;**57**:1274–7.

56 Raleigh JW. Rifampin in treatment of advanced pulmonary tuberculosis. Report of a VA cooperative pilot study. *Am Rev Respir Dis* 1972;**105**:397–409.

57 Lees AW, Allan GW, Smith J. Toxicity from rifampin plus isoniazid and rifampin plus ethambutol therapy. *Tubercle* 1971; **52**:182–90.

58 Kenwright S, Levi AJ. Sites of competition in the selective hepatic uptake of rifampicin-SV, flavaspidic acid, bilirubin, and bromsulphthalein. *Gut* 1974;**15**:220–6.

59 Mulder DJ, Mulder RJ. Drugs used in the treatment of tuberculosis and leprosy. In: Dukes MUG, ed. *Meyler's Side Effects of Drugs*. Oxford: Excerpta Medica, 1977: 676–89.

60 Jasmer RM, Saukkonen JJ, Blumberg HM, *et al.* Short-course rifampin and pyrazinamide compared with isoniazid for latent tuberculosis infection: a multicenter clinical trial. *Ann Intern Med* 2002;**137**:640–7.

61 Centers for Disease Control and Prevention (CDC); American Thoracic Society. Update: adverse event data and revised American Thoracic Society/CDC recommendations against the use of rifampin and pyrazinamide for treatment of latent tuberculosis infection—United States, 2003. *MMWR Morb Mortal Wkly Rep* 2003;**52**:735–9.

62 Westphal JF, Brogard JM. Antibacterials and antifungal agents. In: Kaplowitz N, DeLeve LD, eds. *Drug-Induced Liver Disease*. New York: Marcel-Dekker, 2003: 471–504.

63 Olsson R, Wiholm BE, Sand C, Zettergren L, Hultcrantz R, Myrhed M. Liver damage from flucloxacillin, cloxacillin and dicloxacillin. *J Hepatol* 1992;**15**:154–61.

64 Parry MF. The penicillins. *Med Clin North Am* 1987;**71**:1093–112.

65 Garcia Rodriguez LA, Stricker BH, Zimmerman HJ. Risk of acute liver injury associated with the combination of amoxicillin and clavulanic acid. *Arch Intern Med* 1996;**156**:1327–32.

66 Anderson CS, Nicholls J, Rowland R, LaBrooy JT. Hepatic granulomas: a 15-year experience in the Royal Adelaide Hospital. *Med J Aust* 1988;**148**:71–4.

67 Cavanzo FJ, Garcia CF, Botero RC. Chronic cholestasis, paucity of the bile ducts, red cell aplasia and the Stevens–Johnson syndrome: an ampicillin-associated case. *Gastroenterology* 1990;**99**: 854–6.

68 Nathani MG, Mutchnick MG, Tynes DJ, Ehrinpreis MN. An unusual case of amoxicillin/clavulanic acid-related hepatotoxicity. *Am J Gastroenterol* 1998;**93**:1363–5.

69 Stiegbauer KT, Smith C, Snoyer DC. The histological features of amoxicillin/clavulanic acid-induced hepatotoxicity. *Hepatology* 1994;**20**:190A.

70 Larrey D, Vial T, Micaleff A, *et al.* Hepatitis associated with amoxycillin–clavulanic acid combination: report of 15 cases. *Gut* 1992;**33**:368–71.

71 Davies MH, Harrison RF, Elias E, Hübscher SG. Antibiotic-associated acute vanishing bile duct syndrome: a pattern associated with severe, prolonged, intrahepatic cholestasis. *J Hepatol* 1994;**20**:112–6.

72 Gresser U. Amoxicillin–clavulanic acid therapy may be associated with severe side effects—review of the literature. *Eur J Med Res* 2001;**6**:139–49.

73 Chawla A, Kahn E, Yunis EJ, Daum F. Rapidly progressive cholestasis: an unusual reaction to amoxicillin/clavulanic acid therapy in a child. *J Pediatr* 2000;**136**:121–3.

74 Ryley NG, Fleming KA, Chapman RW. Focal destructive cholangiopathy associated with amoxycillin/clavulanic acid (Augmentin). *J Hepatol* 1995;**23**:278–82.

75 Hautekeete ML, Brenard R, Horsmans Y, *et al.* Liver injury related to amoxicillin–clavulanic acid: interlobular bile-duct lesions and extrahepatic manifestations. *J Hepatol* 1995;**22**:71–7.

76 Mollison LC, Angus P, Richards M, Jones RM, Ireton J. Hepatitis due to nitrofurantoin. *Med J Aust* 1992;**156**:347–9.

77 Hautekeete ML, Horsmans Y, Van Waeyenberge C, *et al.* HLA association of amoxicillin-clavulanate–induced hepatitis. *Gastroenterology* 1999;**117**:1181–6.

78 George DK, Crawford DH. Antibacterial-induced hepatotoxicity. Incidence, prevention and management. *Drug Saf* 1996;**15**: 79–85.

79 Derby LE, Jick H, Henry DA, Dean AD. Cholestatic hepatitis associated with flucloxacillin. *Med J Aust* 1993;**158**:596–600.

80 Fairley CK, McNeil JJ, Desmond P, *et al.* Risk factors for development of flucloxacillin-associated jaundice. *BMJ* 1993;**306**: 233–5.

81 Miros M, Kerlin P, Walker N, Harris O. Flucloxacillin-induced delayed cholestatic hepatitis. *Aust N Z J Med* 1990;**20**:251–3.

82 Easton-Carter KL, Hardikar W, Smith AL. Possible roxithromycin-induced fulminant hepatic failure in a child. *Pharmacotherapy* 2001;**21**:867–70.

83 Turner IB, Eckstein RP, Riley JW, Lunzer MR. Prolonged hepatic cholestasis after flucloxacillin therapy. *Med J Aust* 1989;**151**:701–5.

84 Lang R, Lishner M, Ravid M. Adverse reactions to prolonged treatment with high doses of carbenicillins and ureidopenicillins. *Rev Infect Dis* 1991;**13**:68–72.

85 Thompson JW, Jacobs RF. Adverse effects of newer cephalosporins: an update. *Drug Saf* 1993;**9**:132–42.

86 Fekety FR. Safety of parenteral third-generation cephalosporins. *Am J Med* 1990;**88**(Suppl 4A):38S–44S.

87 Kiessling S, Forrest K, Moscow J, *et al.* Interstitial nephritis, hepatic failure, and systemic eosinophilia after minocycline treatment. *Am J Kidney Dis* 2001;**38**:E36.

88 Fréneaux E, Labbe G, Letteron P, *et al.* Inhibition of the mitochondrial oxidation of fatty acids by tetracycline in mice and in man: possible role in microvesicular steatosis induced by this antibiotic. *Hepatology* 1988;**8**:1056–62.

89 Combes B, Whalley PJ, Adams RH. Tetracycline and the liver. *Prog Liver Dis* 1972;**4**:589–96.

90 Pohle T, Menzel J, Domschke W. Minocycline and fulminant hepatic failure necessitating liver transplantation. *Am J Gastroenterol* 2000;**95**:560–1.

91 Hunt CM, Washington K. Tetracycline-induced bile duct paucity and prolonged cholestasis. *Gastroenterology* 1994;**107**:1844–7.

92 Davies MG, Kersey PJ. Acute hepatitis and exfoliative dermatitis associated with minocycline. *BMJ* 1989;**298**:1523–4.

93 Min DI, Burke PA, Lewis WD, Jenkins RL. Acute hepatic failure associated with oral minocycline: a case report. *Pharmacotherapy* 1992;**12**:68–71.

94 Seaman HE, Lawrenson RA, Williams TJ, MacRae KD, Farmer RD. The risk of liver damage associated with minocycline: a comparative study. *J Clin Pharmacol* 2001;**41**:852–60.

95 Bhat G, Jordan J Jr, Sokalski S, Bajaj V, Marshall R, Berkelhammer C. Minocycline-induced hepatitis with autoimmune features and neutropenia. *J Clin Gastroenterol* 1998;**27**: 74–5.

96 Chamberlain MC, Schwarzenberg SJ, Akin EU, Kurth MH. Minocycline-induced autoimmune hepatitis with subsequent cirrhosis. *J Pediatr Gastroenterol Nutr* 2006;**42**:232–5.

97 Carson JL, Strom BL, Duff A, *et al.* Acute liver disease with erythromycins, sulfonamides, and tetracyclines. *Ann Intern Med* 1993;**119**:576–83.

98 Derby LE, Jick H, Henry DA, Dean AD. Erythromycin-associated cholestatic hepatitis. *Med J Aust* 1993;**158**:600–2.

99 Avila P, Capellà D, Laporte JR, Moreno V. Which salt of erythromycin is most hepatotoxic? *Lancet* 1988;**i**:1104.

100 Young RA, Gonzales JP, Sorkin EM. Roxithromycin: a review of its antibacterial activity, pharmacokinetic properties and clinical efficacy. *Drugs* 1989;**37**:8–41.

101 Peters DH, Clissold SP. Clarithromycin. A review of its antimicrobial activity, pharmacokinetic properties and therapeutic potential. *Drugs* 1992;**44**:117–64.

102 Yew WW, Chau CH, Lee J, Leung CW. Cholestatic hepatitis in a patient who received clarithromycin therapy for a *Mycobacterium chelonae* lung infection [letter]. *Clin Infect Dis* 1994;**18**:1025–6.

103 Dujovne CA. Hepatotoxic and cellular uptake interactions among surface active components of erythromycin preparations. *Biochem Pharmacol* 1978;**27**:1925–30.

104 Pessayre D, Larrey D, Funck-Brentano C, Benhamou JP. Drug interactions and hepatitis produced by some macrolide antibiotics. *J Antimicrob Chemother* 1985;**16**(Suppl A):181–94.

105 Braun P. Hepatotoxicity of erythromycin. *J Infect Dis* 1973;**119**: 300–6.

106 Diehl AM, Latham P, Boitnott JK, Mann J, Maddrey WC. Cholestatic hepatitis from erythromycin ethylsuccinate. *Am J Med* 1984;**76**:931–4.

107 Zimmerman HJ, Maddrey WC. Drug-induced hepatotoxicity. In: Schiff L, Schiff ER, eds. *Diseases of the Liver*. Philadelphia: Lippincott, 1987: 707–783.

108 Zhang XJ, Thomas PE. Erythromycin as a specific substrate for cytochrome P450 3A isoenzymes and identification of a high affinity erythromycin *N*-demethylase in adult female rats. *Drug Metab Dispos* 1996;**24**:23–7.

109 Larrey D, Funck-Brentano C, Breil P, *et al.* Effects of erythromycin on hepatic drug-metabolizing enzymes in humans. *Biochem Pharmacol* 1983;**32**:1063–8.

110 Zafrani ES, Ishak KG, Rudzki C. Cholestatic and hepatocellular injury associated with erythromycin esters: report of nine cases. *Dig Dis Sci* 1979;**24**:385–96.

111 Gholson CF, Warren CH. Fulminant hepatic failure associated with intravenous erythromycin lactobionate. *Arch Intern Med* 1990;**150**:215–6.

112 Farrell GC. *Drug-Induced Liver Disease*. Edinburgh: Churchill Livingstone, 1994.

113 Beard K, Belic L, Aselton P, Perera DR, Jick H. Outpatient drug-induced parenchymal liver disease requiring hospitalization. *J Clin Pharmacol* 1986;**26**:633–7.

114 Gordin FM, Simon GL, Wofsy CB, Mills J. Adverse reactions to trimethoprim-sulfamethoxazole in patients with the acquired immunodeficiency syndrome. *Ann Intern Med* 1984;**100**:495–9.

115 Sattler FR, Cowan R, Nielsen DM, Ruskin J. Trimethoprim-sulfamethoxazole compared with pentamidine for treatment of *Pneumocystis carinii* pneumonia in the acquired immunodeficiency syndrome: a prospective, noncrossover study. *Ann Intern Med* 1988;**109**:280–7.

116 Droge W. Cysteine and glutathione deficiency in AIDS patients: a rationale for the treatment with *N*-acetylcysteine. *Pharmacology* 1993;**46**:61–5.

117 Rieder MJ. Mechanisms of unpredictable adverse drug reactions. *Drug Saf* 1994;**11**:196–212.

118 Dujovne CA, Chan CH, Zimmerman HJ. Sulfonamide hepatic injury. Review of the literature and report of a case due to sulfamethoxazole. *N Engl J Med* 1967;**277**:785–8.

119 Fatal multisystemic toxicity after co-trimoxazole. *Lancet* 1978;**i**: 831.

120 Colucci CF, Cicero ML. Hepatic necrosis and trimethoprim-sulfamethoxazole. *JAMA* 1975;**233**:952–3.

121 Tonder M, Nordoy A, Elgjo K. Sulfonamide-induced chronic liver disease. *Scand J Gastroenterol* 1974;**9**:93–6.

122 Lazar HP, Murphy RL, Phair JP. Fansidar and hepatic granulomas. *Ann Intern Med* 1985;**102**:722.

123 Callen JP, Soderstrom RM. Granulomatous hepatitis associated with salicylazosulfapyridine therapy. *South Med J* 1978;**71**: 1159–60.

124 Steward DL, Johnson RC. Acute hepatitis caused by sulfamethoxazole-trimethoprim. *Gastroenterology* 1980;**78**:1323.

125 Kowdley KV, Keeffe EB, Fawaz KA. Prolonged cholestasis due to trimethoprim-sulfamethoxazole. *Gastroenterology* 1992;**102**: 2148–50.

126 Ransohoff DF, Jacobs G. Terminal hepatic failure following a small dose of sulfamethoxazole-trimethoprim. *Gastroenterology* 1981;**80**:816–9.

127 Thies PW, Dull WL. Trimethoprim-sulfamethoxazole-induced cholestatic hepatitis: inadvertent rechallenge. *Arch Intern Med* 1984;**144**:1691–2.

128 Schacht P, Hullmann R. Safety of oral ciprofloxacin: an update based on clinical trial results. *Am J Med* 1989;**87**(Suppl 5A): 98S–102S.

129 Jick SS, Jick HJ, Dean AD. A follow-up safety study of ciprofloxacin users. *Pharmacotherapy* 1993;**13**:461–4.

130 Arcieri GM, Becker N, Esposito B, *et al.* Safety of intravenous ciprofloxacin: a review. *Am J Med* 1989;**87**(Suppl 5A):92S–97S.

131 Fuchs S, Simon Z, Brezin M. Fatal hepatic failure associated with ciprofloxacin. *Lancet* 1994;**343**:738–9.

132 Grassmick BK, Lehr VT, Sundareson AS. Fulminant hepatic failure possibly related to ciprofloxacin. *Ann Pharmacother* 1992; **26**:636–9.

133 Dembry LM, Farrington JM, Andriole VT. Fluoroquinolone antibiotics: adverse effects and safety profile. *Infect Dis Clin Pract* 1999;**8**:421–8.

134 Stricker BH. *Drug-Induced Hepatic Injury*, 2nd ed. Amsterdam: Elsevier, 1992.

135 Fass RJ, Saslaw S. Clindamycin: clinical and laboratory evaluation of parenteral therapy. *Am J Med Sci* 1972;**263**:369–82.

136 Elmore M, Rissing JP, Rink L, Brooks GF. Clindamycin-associated hepatotoxicity. *Am J Med* 1974;**57**:627–30.

137 Altraif I, Lilly L, Wanless IR, Heathcote J. Cholestatic liver disease with ductopenia (vanishing bile duct syndrome) after administration of clindamycin and trimethoprim-sufamethoxazole. *Am J Gastroenterol* 1994;**89**:1230–4.

138 García Rodríguez LA, Duque A, Castellsague J, Pérez-Gutthann S, Stricker BH. A cohort study on the risk of acute liver injury among users of ketoconazole and other antifungal drugs. *Br J Clin Pharmacol* 1999;**48**:847–52.

139 Stricker BH, Blok AP, Bronkhorst FB, Van Parys GE, Desmet VJ. Ketoconazole-associated hepatic injury: a clinicopathological study of 55 cases. *J Hepatol* 1986;**3**:399–406.

140 Perfect JR, Lindsay MH, Drew RH. Adverse drug reactions to systemic antifungals: prevention and management. *Drug Saf* 1992;**7**:323–63.

141 Chien RN, Yang LJ, Lin PY, Liaw YF. Hepatic injury during ketoconazole therapy in patients with onychomycosis: a controlled cohort study. *Hepatology* 1997;**25**:103–7.

142 Rollman O, Loof L. Hepatic toxicity of ketoconazole. *Br J Dermatol* 1983;**143**:376–8.

143 Lake-Bakaar G, Scheuer PJ, Sherlock S. Hepatic reactions associated with ketoconazole in the United Kingdom. *BMJ* 1987;**294**:419–22.

144 Zollner E, Delport S, Bonnici F. Fatal liver failure due to ketoconazole treatment of a girl with Cushing's syndrome. *J Pediatr Endocrinol* 2001;**14**:335–8.

145 Findor JA, Sorda JA, Igartua EB, Avagnina A. Ketoconazole-induced liver damage. *Medicina* 1998;**58**:277–81.

146 Gill J, Sprenger HR, Ralph ED, Sharpe MD. Hepatotoxicity possibly caused by amphotericin B. *Ann Pharmacother* 1999;**33**:683–5.

147 Gallis HA, Drew RH, Pickard WW. Amphotericin B: 30 years of clinical experience. *Rev Infect Dis* 1990;**12**:308–29.

148 Miller MA. Reversible hepatotoxicity related to amphotericin B. *Can Med Assoc J* 1984;**131**:1245–47.

149 Grant SM, Clissold SP. Itraconazole. A review of its pharmacodynamic and pharmacokinetic properties, and therapeutic use in superficial and systemic mycoses. *Drugs* 1989;**37**:310–44.

150 Tucker RM, Haq Y, Denning DW, Stevens DA. Adverse events associated with itraconazole in 189 patients on chronic therapy. *J Antimicrob Chemother* 1990;**26**:561–6.

151 Srebrnik A, Levtov S, Ben-Ami R, Brenner S. Liver failure and transplantation after itraconazole treatment for toenail onychomycosis. *J Eur Acad Dermatol Venereol* 2005;**19**:205–7.

152 Lavrijsen AP, Balmus KJ, Nugteren-Huying WM, Roldaan AC, van't Wout JW, Stricker BH. Hepatic injury associated with itraconazole. *Lancet* 1992;**340**:251–2.

153 Gallardo-Quesada S, Luelmo-Aguilar J. Hepatotoxicity associated with itraconazole. *Int J Dermatol* 1995;**34**:589.

154 Hay RJ. Risk/benefit ratio of modern antifungal therapy: focus on hepatic reactions. *J Am Acad Dermatol* 1993;**29**:S50–S54.

155 Bronstein JA, Gros P, Hernandez E, Larroque P, Molinié C. Fatal acute hepatic necrosis due to dose-dependent fluconazole hepatotoxicity. *Clin Infect Dis* 1997;**25**:1266–7.

156 Crerar-Gilbert A, Boots R, Fraenkel D, MacDonald GA. Survival following fulminant hepatic failure from fluconazole induced hepatitis. *Anaesth Intensive Care* 1999;**27**:650–2.

157 Jacobson MA, Hanks DK, Ferrell LD. Fatal acute hepatic necrosis due to fluconazole. *Am J Med* 1994;**96**:188–90.

158 Anderson GD. Children versus adults: pharmacokinetic and adverse-effect differences. *Epilepsia* 2002;**43**:53–9.

159 Wallace SJ. A comparative review of the adverse effects of anticonvulsants in children with epilepsy. *Drug Saf* 1996;**15**:378–93.

160 Tidwell A, Swims M. Review of the newer antiepileptic drugs. *Am J Manag Care* 2003;**9**:253–76.

161 Swann AC. Major system toxicities and side effects of anticonvulsants. *J Clin Psychiatry* 2001;**62**(Suppl 14):16–21.

162 Chitturi S, George J. Hepatotoxicity of commonly used drugs: nonsteroidal anti-inflammatory drugs, antihypertensives, antidiabetic agents, anticonvulsants, lipid-lowering agents, psychotropic drugs. *Semin Liver Dis* 2002;**22**:169–83.

163 Clarkson A, Choonara I. Surveillance for fatal suspected adverse drug reactions in the UK. *Arch Dis Child* 2002;**87**:462–6.

164 Li AM, Nelson EA, Hon EK, *et al.* Hepatic failure in a child with anti-epileptic hypersensitivity syndrome. *J Paediatr Child Health* 2005;**41**:218–20.

165 Licata AL, Louis ED. Anticonvulsant hypersensitivity syndrome. *Compr Ther* 1996;**22**:152–5.

166 Hadzić N, Portmann B, Davies ET, Mowat AP, Mieli-Vergani G. Acute liver failure induced by carbamazepine. *Arch Dis Child* 1990;**65**:315–7.

167 Bosdure E, Cano A, Roquelaure B, *et al.* [Oxcarbazepine and DRESS syndrome: a paediatric cause of acute liver failure; in French.] *Arch Pediatr* 2004;**11**:10737.

168 Mitchell AA, Lacouture PG, Sheehan JE, Kauffman RE, Shapiro S. Adverse drug reactions in children leading to hospital admission. *Pediatrics* 1988;**82**:24–9.

169 Powers NG, Carson SH. Idiosyncratic reactions to phenytoin. *Clin Pediatr* 1987;**26**:120–4.

170 Overstreet K, Costanza C, Behling C, Hassanin T, Masliah E. Fatal progressive hepatic necrosis associated with lamotrigine treatment: a case report and literature review. *Dig Dis Sci* 2002;**47**:1921–5.

171 Wallace SJ. Newer antiepileptic drugs: advantages and disadvantages. *Brain Dev* 2001;**23**:277–83.

172 Onat F, Ozkara C. Adverse effects of new antiepileptic drugs. *Drugs Today (Barc)* 2004;**40**:325–42.

173 Verrotti A, Greco R, Latini G, Chiarelli F. Endocrine and metabolic changes in epileptic patients receiving valproic acid. *J Pediatr Endocrinol Metab* 2005;**18**:423–30.

174 Sztajnkrycer MD. Valproic acid toxicity: overview and management. *J Toxicol Clin Toxicol* 2002;**40**:789–801.

175 Narkewicz MR, Sokol RJ, Beckwith B, Sondheimer J, Silverman A. Liver involvement in Alpers disease. *J Pediatr* 1991;**119**: 260–7.

176 Kottlors M, Jaksch M, Ketelsen UP, Weiner S, Glocker FX, Lücking CH. Valproic acid triggers acute rhabdomyolysis in a patient with carnitine palmitoyltransferase type II deficiency. *Neuromuscul Disord* 2001;**11**:757–9.

177 Krähenbühl S, Brandner S, Kleinle S, Liechti S, Straumann D. Mitochondrial diseases represent a risk factor for valproate-induced fulminant liver failure. *Liver* 2000;**20**:346–8.

178 Lam CW, Lau CH, Williams JC, Chan YW, Wong LJ. Mitochondrial myopathy, encephalopathy, lactic acidosis and stroke-like episodes (MELAS) triggered by valproate therapy. Eur *J Pediatr* 1997;**156**:562–4.

179 Fromenty C, Pessayre D. Impaired mitochondrial function in microvesicular steatosis. *J Hepatol* 1997;**26**(Suppl 2):43–53.

180 Stedman C. Herbal hepatotoxicity. *Semin Liver Dis* 2002;**22**:195–206.

181 Schuppan D, Jia JD, Brinkhaus B, Hahn EG. Herbal products for liver disease: a therapeutic challenge for the new millennium. *Hepatology* 1999;**30**:1099–104.

182 Larrey D. Hepatotoxicity of herbal remedies. *J Hepatol* 1997; **26**(Suppl 1):47–51.

183 Abebe W. Herbal medication: potential for adverse interactions with analgesic drugs. *J Clin Pharm Ther* 2002;**27**:391–401.

184 Bagnell PC, Ellenberg HA. Obstructive jaundice due to a chlorinated carbon in breast milk. *Can Med Assoc J* 1977;**117**:1047–8.

185 Rasenack R, Müller C, Kleinschmidt M, Rasenack J, Wiedenfeld H. Veno-occlusive disease in a fetus caused by pyrrolizidine alkaloids of food origin. *Fetal Diagn Ther* 2003;**18**:223–5.

186 Seeff LB, Lindsay KL, Bacon BR, Kresina TF, Hoofnagle JH. Complementary and alternative medicine in chronic liver disease. *Hepatology* 2001;**34**:595–603.

187 Aithal GP. When is a herb a drug? *Eur J Gastroenterol Hepatol* 2005;**17**:391–3.

188 Stickel F, Pöschl G, Seitz HK, Waldherr R, Hahn EG, Schuppan D. Acute hepatitis induced by Greater Celandine (*Chelidonium majus*). *Scand J Gastroenterol* 2003;**38**:565–8.

189 Stickel F, Baumüller HM, Seitz K, *et al.* Hepatitis induced by Kava (*Piper methysticum rhizoma*). *J Hepatol* 2003;**9**:62–7.

190 Maurer HH, Kraemer T, Springer D, Staack RF. Chemistry, pharmacology, toxicology and hepatic metabolism of designer drugs of the amphetamine (ecstasy), piperazine and pyrrolidinophenone types: a synopsis. *Ther Drug Monit* 2004;**26**:127–31.

191 Kew MC, Bersohn I, Siew S. Possible hepatotoxicity of cannabis. *Lancet* 1969;**i**:578–9.

192 Hochman JS, Brill NQ. Chronic marihuana usage and liver function. *Lancet* 1971;**ii**:818–9.

193 Borini P, Guimares RC, Borini SB. Possible hepatotoxicity of chronic marijuana usage. *Sao Paulo Med J* 2004;**122**:110–6.

194 Cooper AD, Niejadlik D, Huston K. Liver disease in nonparenteral drug abusers. *JAMA* 1975;**233**:964–6.

195 Andreu V, Mas A, Bruguera M, *et al.* Ecstasy: a common cause of severe hepatic hepatoxicity. *J Hepatol* 1998;**29**:394–7.

196 Fidler H, Dhillon A, Gertner D, Burroughs A. Chronic ecstasy (3,4-methylenedioxymetamphetamine) abuse: a recurrent and unpredictable cause of severe acute hepatitis. *J Hepatol* 1996;**2**: 563–6.

197 Dykhuizen RS, Brunt PW, Atkinson P, Simpson JG, Smith CC. Ecstasy induced hepatitis mimicking viral hepatitis. *Gut* 1995; **36**:939–41.

198 Ellis AJ, Wendon JA, Williams R. Acute liver damage and ecstasy ingestion. *Gut* 1996;**38**:454–8.

199 Lange-Brock N, Berg T, Müller AR, *et al.* [Acute liver failure following the use of ecstasy (MDMA); in German.] *J Gastroenterol* 2002;**40**:581–6.

200 Neff GW, Reddy KR, Durazo FA, Meyer D, Marrero R, Kaplowitz N. Severe hepatotoxicity associated with the use of weight loss diet supplements containing ma huang or usnic acid. *J Hepatol* 2004;**41**:1062–4.

201 Adachi M, Saito H, Kobayashi H, *et al.* Hepatic injury in 12 patients taking the herbal weight loss aids chaso or onshido. *Ann Intern Med* 2003;**139**:488–92.

202 Favreau JT, Ryu ML, Braunstein G, *et al.* Severe hepatotoxicity associated with the dietary supplement LipoKinetix. *Ann Intern Med* 2002;**136**:590–5.

203 Han D, Matsumaru K, Rettori D, Kaplowitz N. Usnic acid-induced necrosis of cultured mouse hepatocytes: inhibition of mitochondrial function and oxidative stress. *Biochem Pharmacol* 2004;**67**:439–51.

204 Koury SI, Stone CK, La Charite DD. Omeprazole and the development of acute hepatitis. *Eur J Emerg Med* 1998;**5**:467–9.

205 Andersson T. Pharmacokinetics, metabolism and interactions of acid pump inhibitors. Focus on omeprazole, lansoprazole and pantoprazole. *Clin Pharmacokinet* 1996;**31**:9–28.

206 Braun M, Fraser GM, Kunin M, Salamon F, Kaspa RT. Mesalamine-induced granulomatous hepatitis. *Am J Gastroenterol* 1999;**94**:1973–4.

10 Congenital and Structural Abnormalities of the Liver

Jaime Liou Wolfe and Kathleen B. Schwarz

This chapter provides a comprehensive overview and problem-orientated approach to the diagnosis and management of intrahepatic congenital and structural abnormalities, with particular emphasis on two major categories—fibropolycystic disease and vascular anomalies.

The hereditary fibropolycystic diseases are a heterogeneous group of conditions in which there is increased hepatic fibrosis in association with cysts lined with biliary epithelium. These conditions include solitary cysts, autosomal-dominant polycystic kidney disease (ADPKD), autosomal-recessive polycystic kidney disease (ARPKD), congenital hepatic fibrosis (CHF), Caroli disease, and Caroli syndrome. The clinical presentation varies from asymptomatic hepatomegaly, as in the case of solitary cysts, to portal hypertension, renal failure, and rarely liver failure.

The majority of vascular anomalies of the liver are hemangiomas, which—like solitary cysts—may present as incidental findings or as asymptomatic hepatomegaly; giant cavernous hemangiomas may be complicated by symptoms related to the massive hepatomegaly and compression of abdominal viscera and/or by the consequences of arteriovenous shunting, such as congestive heart failure and pulmonary edema. In pediatrics, innovative imaging methods such as computed tomography (CT), magnetic resonance imaging (MRI), magnetic resonance cholangiopancreatography (MRCP), and color Doppler ultrasonography have enhanced the noninvasive diagnosis of these abnormalities.

Fibropolycystic disease

Polycystic disease was first described by Bristowe.[1] The term "fibropolycystic disease" is a general term used to describe several conditions with a variable degree of intrahepatic biliary duct (IHBD) dilation and associated periportal fibrosis. Polycystic disease is usually not confined to the liver, and other organs may be affected. In particular, as the cystic lesions most severely affect the kidneys, the severity of the renal lesions determines the clinical presentation and the long-term prognosis of polycystic disease.

Diseases of the Liver and Biliary System in Children, 3rd edition. Edited by Deirdre Kelly. © 2008 Blackwell Publishing, ISBN: 978-1-4051-6334-7.

Embryology of the IHBDs, ductal plate, and ductal plate malformation

The pathogenesis of congenital fibrocystic diseases of the liver is linked with the embryonic development of the IHBDs. It is thought that the IHBDs develop from the hepatocyte precursor cells, which lie in contact with the mesenchyme surrounding the portal vein. This process starts during the third month of gestation with the formation of the larger IHBDs at the level of the hilum and proceeds distally to the smaller terminal portal branches, which are completed in the first month of the postnatal period.[2] The basic lesion in all variants of fibropolycystic disease is ductal plate malformation, which affects all levels of the intrahepatic biliary tree, such as the segmental, septal, and interlobular ducts and the ducts of the terminal portal tracts (Figure 10.1). The ductal plate is a structure corresponding to the most immature state of the bile duct and is characterized by an interrupted cylindrical layer of cells around the future portal tract, which is later doubled by a second layer of keratin-rich bile duct epithelium over several segments of its circumference. Around the 12th week of gestation, the ductal plate is remodeled in response to unknown signals induced by epithelial–mesenchyme interactions, which result in the incorporation of dilated parts of the double epithelial layer into the portal mesenchyme. The unincorporated epithelial layer then disappears. The normal development of IHBDs requires progressive remodeling of the ductal plate, involving precisely tuned interactions between the mesenchyme and the ductal plate epithelia. Any interruption in the remodeling of the ductal plate may result in persistence of the excess embryonic epithelial duct structures, termed ductal plate malformation (DPM).[3]

The exact biochemical defect that leads to the formation of cysts remains unknown. DPM is often associated with abnormalities in the ramification pattern of the portal vein, giving rise to smaller, more closely spaced branches, termed "pollard willow formation."[4,5] DPM involving all segments

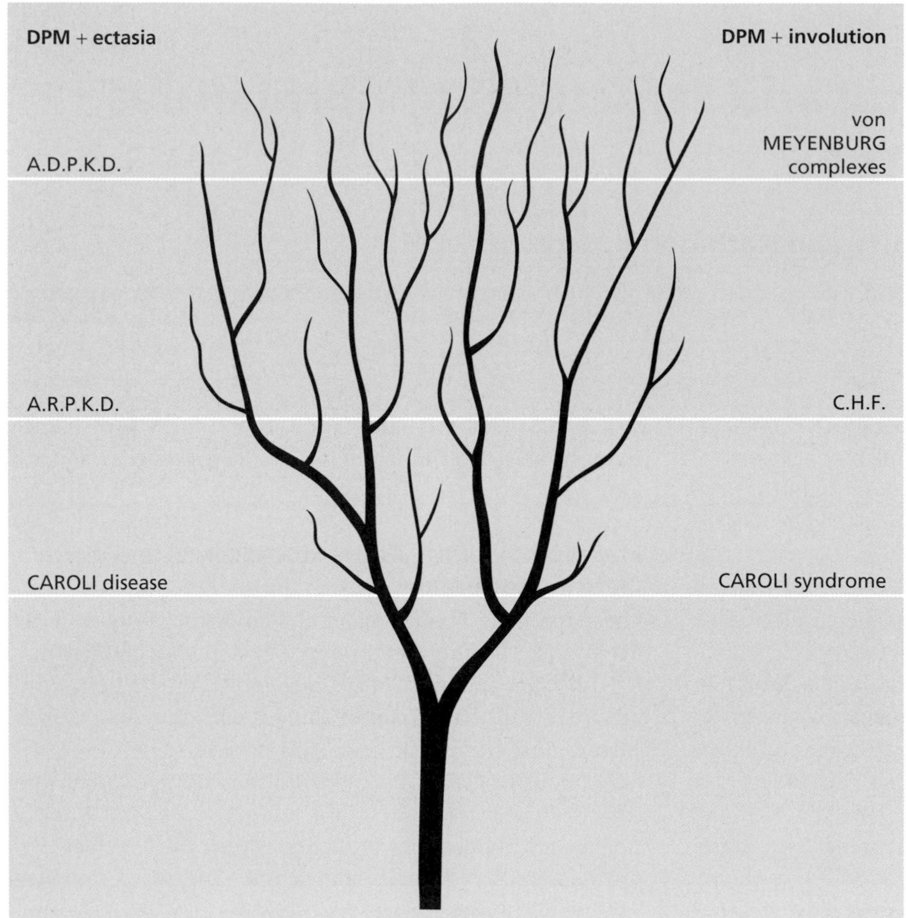

Figure 10.1 Schematic representation of the biliary tree and the diseases discussed in this chapter. The placement of diseases at different levels of the tree indicates the approximate size of the bile ducts affected by ductal plate malformation (DPM) in a particular disorder. The disorders mentioned on the left are characterized by mild or marked dilation of the bile duct structures, whereas the entities listed on the right develop with a variable degree of involution ("destructive cholangitis") of the ductal plate remnants associated with fibrosis. (Reproduced with permission from Desmet.[2])

of the IHBDs results in a combination of anatomical clinical entities including CHF–ARPKD, ARPKD–Caroli, CHF–Caroli, and CHF–Meyenburg complex.[2,6,7]

Classification

Cystic diseases of the liver may be parasitic or nonparasitic. Typically, nonparasitic cystic lesions are solitary or multiple (sporadic), or polycystic (hereditary). The older literature is confusing, and many changes in the classification of fibropolycystic diseases of the liver and kidneys have been proposed, primarily due to changes in the classification of cystic renal lesions.[8] The basis of the modern classification is shown in Table 10.1.

The intrahepatic bile duct cysts may be connected to the biliary tree (communicating or noncommunicating). Communicating ductal cysts have more clinical significance, as they tend to present with medical complications such as cholangitis and biliary calculi. Desmet divided the congenital diseases of the IHBDs, as illustrated in Figure 10.1, into two main groups:[2]

• Diseases characterized by necroinflammatory destruction of the IHBDs

• Diseases characterized by a degree of dilation of IHBDs, also associated with a variable degree of fibrosis

Disorders associated with dilation of the bile ducts include ADPKD, ARPKD, and Caroli disease, whereas disorders that develop with involution or destructive cholangitis include Meyenburg complexes (or microhamartomas), CHF, and Caroli syndrome. The cause of involution of the bile ducts and renal epithelia remains unknown.

Solitary cysts

Solitary simple cysts occur at all ages, without symptoms (Figure 10.2). They may be discovered incidentally by antenatal ultrasound or radiographic studies, or at autopsy. They most frequently involve the right lobe of the liver. The cysts usually contain serous fluid and are lined by atrophic biliary epithelium. Multiple cysts develop with potassium deficiency, toxic renal injury, metabolic disease, and congenital disorders. Management is usually conservative. Observation alone is recommended unless there are symptoms such as abdominal pain from bleeding into the cyst, or rapid

Table 10.1 Classification of fibropolycystic lesions of the liver.

Parasitic
Nonparasitic
Solitary/multiple—sporadic
Polycystic—hereditary
Not communicating with the biliary system
Autosomal-dominant polycystic kidney disease (ADPKD)
Communicating with the biliary system
Autosomal-dominant polycystic kidney disease (ARPKD)
Congenital hepatic fibrosis (CHF)
ARPKD or ADPKD
Caroli disease (Caroli syndrome)
Nephronophthisis
Tuberous sclerosis
Vaginal atresia
Malformations
Meckel–Gruber syndrome, Jeune syndrome
Ivemark syndrome, Laurence–Moon–Biedl
Caroli disease
Polycystic liver disease—isolated
Miscellaneous
Traumatic, infarction, neoplastic

enlargement. Radiographic or surgical aspiration is rarely required. If the cysts become infected, antibiotic therapy is recommended, with lipid-soluble antibiotics such as trimethoprim-sulfamethoxazole or ciprofloxacin.[9,10]

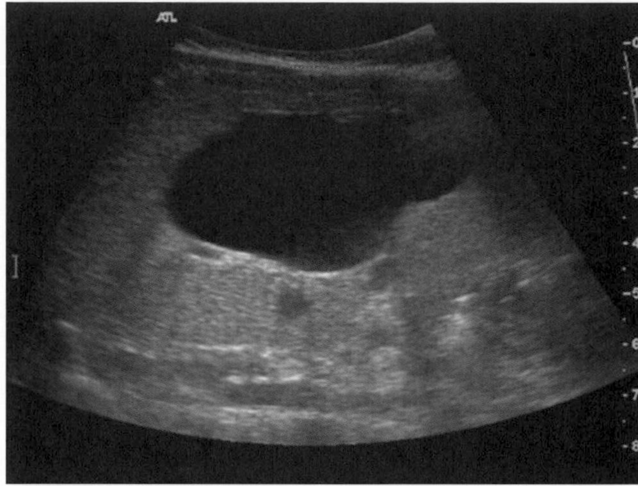

A

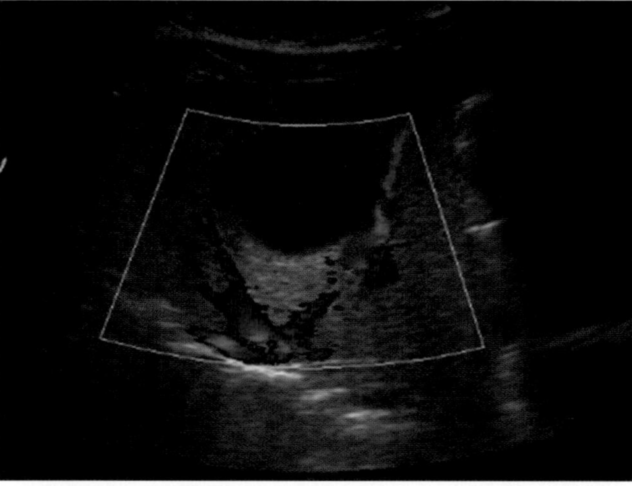

B

Figure 10.2 **A** Abdominal ultrasound, showing a single hepatic cyst with an irregular border. **B** Using Doppler ultrasound, the medial hepatic vein can be seen on the lateral border and the portal vein and hepatic artery are seen on the medial border. These cysts are often asymptomatic, but can be aspirated under imaging guidance if symptoms arise.

Autosomal-dominant polycystic kidney disease

This was the first fibropolycystic liver disease to be described as a heritable trait.[11] Although it was previously referred to as adult polycystic kidney disease (APKD), the nomenclature has changed, since the disease may present in early infancy and childhood and is now more correctly termed ADPKD. This disease results in cyst formation in the kidneys, liver, pancreas, spleen, thyroid, endometrium, ovaries, seminal vesicles, and epididymis, and it is associated with intracranial aneurysms.[12,13] The disease is inherited as an autosomal-dominant trait, and each offspring of an affected person runs a 50% risk of acquiring the disease. Both sexes are affected equally.

Molecular genetics and pathogenesis

ADPKD is one of the most common genetic disorders worldwide, with an estimated prevalence of one in 400–1000 people.[14] It accounts for 12% of patients with end-stage renal disease (ESRD) in the United States.[15] Fifty percent of affected individuals have renal failure by the age of 50.[16]

At least two causal genes are thought to be responsible for ADPKD: *PKD1* and *PKD2*, which code for polycystin 1 and 2, respectively. *PKD1* is located on chromosome 16p13.3 and is responsible for 85% of families with ADPKD, whereas *PKD2* is mapped on chromosome 4q21-23 and causes approximately 15% of cases of familial ADPKD.[17–21] There is now a mutation database with information about germ-line and somatic disease-causing variants and polymorphisms.[22] Germ-line mutations in both genes and the somatic mutations identified from individual *PKD1* or *PKD2* cysts indicate that loss of function of either *PKD1* or *PKD2* is the mechanism for cyst formation.[21]

Pathology

Macroscopically, large asymmetric hepatic cysts are visualized throughout the liver and tend to increase with age. The cysts are lined with biliary epithelium, which secretes a serous fluid that fills the cavity.[23] They are surrounded by a fibrous capsule and do not communicate with the biliary tree. They are frequently associated with Meyenburg complexes or microhamartomas, which are rounded nodules, 1 cm in diameter, closely related to the portal tracts, and are scattered through the entire liver parenchyma.[23] The microhamartomas are usually discovered at autopsy, as they are asymptomatic. In contrast, the renal cysts are irregular in size and have an uneven distribution, affecting the collecting system, tubules, and glomeruli, and progressively replace the parenchyma, leading to renal failure.[24] Asymptomatic pancreatic cysts occur in 5–10% of patients.[25]

Clinical features

ADPKD presents with abdominal distension due to bilaterally enlarged kidneys and hepatomegaly, abdominal pain, hematuria, hypertension, renal infection, nephrolithiasis, and renal insufficiency.[24] Loss of renal concentrating ability and hypertension are early signs of the disease. Sixteen percent of children under the age of 18 have systolic blood pressures in the 95th percentile for their age.[25] Flank pain, renal cyst hemorrhage, infection, or nephrolithiasis most commonly occur after the fourth decade of life.[9]

Hepatic cysts are the most common extrarenal manifestation of ADPKD and appear more frequently with increasing age and declining renal function. Although liver cysts are uncommon in pediatric patients with ADPKD, they are found in 30% of adult patients with ADPKD under the age of 40 and in 77% of patients over 60 years of age.[26–28] Approximately 25% of ADPKD-affected individuals do not develop liver cysts.[28] Hepatic cysts have been diagnosed by biopsy as early as 8 months of age.[29] Both sexes are affected equally, although women tend to have more extensive liver cysts, correlating directly with the number of pregnancies.[30]

Patients with *PKD2* mutations have a typically milder course than those with *PKD1* mutations.[31] The median age of death or onset of ESRD is 53 years in individuals with *PKD1* and 69 years in those with *PKD2*. *PKD1* patients are four times more likely to have hypertension than *PKD2* patients. The overall survival is significantly higher in women than men with *PKD2*, but this difference is not observed with *PKD1*.

Other associations with ADPKD include intracranial aneurysms,[32,33] cardiac disease,[34] and inguinal and abdominal hernias.[35]

Hepatic cysts tend to have fewer complications, such as bleeding and infection, than renal cysts, but may result in massive hepatomegaly and chronic abdominal pain. Complications noted in adults include ascites and esophageal varices, secondary to noncirrhotic portal hypertension,[36] and obstructive jaundice, secondary to biliary obstruction, cholangitis, Caroli syndrome,[37] or gallbladder involvement. Biliary colic has been associated with an intraluminal cyst in the cystic duct, resulting in hydrops of the gallbladder.[38] Gallbladder disease is more common with symptomatic liver disease.[39] Hepatic cysts may result in compression of the pancreas, displacement of other organs, and elevation of the diaphragm, leading to dyspnea.[40] Rare complications include Budd–Chiari syndrome secondary to anatomical obstruction of the inferior vena cava from enlarged liver cysts, which has been reported in adults, particularly after nephrectomy.[41] Despite the presence of multiple cysts, the liver parenchyma remains intact. Serum aminotransferases, albumin, and prothrombin time are normal, although γ-glutamyltransferase (GGT) may be mildly elevated in symptomatic liver disease.

Diagnosis

The diagnosis is primarily obtained on abdominal ultrasonography of the liver and kidneys. ADPKD should be considered in any child with a renal cyst, whereas the presence of more than three cysts in both kidneys in a patient with a positive family history strongly suggests ADPKD.[42] False-negative ultrasound examinations in patients under the age of 30 may be more common in families with the *PKD2* gene mutations, as renal cysts develop later in life.[43] CT with contrast enhancement is slightly more sensitive than ultrasound for detecting cysts and is particularly useful in identifying cyst hemorrhage. The combination of MRI and ultrasound may demonstrate the internal morphology of a cyst and distinguish a simple hepatic cyst from other hepatic cystic lesions. MRI is particularly helpful in displaying the relationship of the cyst to the hepatic vascular structures.[44] The diagnosis can be confirmed by hepatic and renal histology. Prenatal diagnosis of ADPKD is possible using a linked DNA probe derived from the α-globin region.[45] On prenatal ultrasound, affected kidneys may appear enlarged and hyperechogenic, but fetal presentation of ADPKD is not common and ultrasound alone is not used in the prenatal diagnosis of ADPKD.

Management and outcome

Management is directed toward treatment of both renal and liver disease. Treatment for renal disease is supportive and includes standard therapy with nutritional support, a low-sodium and low-protein diet, antihypertensive medication and dialysis, and/or renal transplantation for ESRD.

Treatment for liver disease is directed toward the prevention and management of complications. Families should be reassured that despite abdominal distension, hepatic function remains normal for many years. Recurrent cholangitis should be managed with lipid-soluble antibiotics such as trimethoprim-sulfamethoxazole, chloramphenicol, or ciprofloxacin, which penetrate cyst walls, and with prophylactic antibiotics.[9]

Pain from cyst hemorrhage is usually self-limited and may be treated with mild analgesics and bed rest.[12] Percutaneous or surgical decompression of the cysts should be reserved for severe, unmanageable pain. Somatostatin has been used in reducing ascites by inhibiting bile secretion after surgical fenestration of cysts.[36] Cholecystectomy should be considered in patients with severe hepatic involvement.[39] Initial treatment of portal hypertension should be conservative in the first instance, although occasionally portal-systemic shunting may be appropriate.

Successful liver–kidney transplantation has been performed for severe complications of liver disease, with up to 60 months' survival and normal hepatic function.[46,47]

Prophylactic screening of all patients with ADPKD for intracranial aneurysms is mandatory, with surgery as indicated by a neurosurgeon. As intracranial arachnoid cysts are asymptomatic and do not enlarge with age, surgery is not required.[48]

Autosomal-recessive polycystic kidney disease (ARPKD)

The term "ARPKD" has replaced the older term "infantile polycystic disease," as the disease also presents in adults. ARPKD is characterized by the association of renal cysts arising from dilated collecting ducts, and biliary dysgenesis known as congenital hepatic fibrosis. It has an incidence of one in 6000, and one in 40 000 births.[49] Intrafamilial variation of the disease has been reported, which implies different expression of the same gene complex.[13]

Molecular genetics

The gene responsible for ARPKD, *PKHD1*, has been mapped to 6p21.1-p12.[50–53] Two groups simultaneously reported that *PKHD1* is a large gene, encoding a 4074 amino-acid protein, called fibrocystin by one group[54] and polyductin by another group.[55] The function of fibrocystin is not yet known, but it may act as a receptor with critical roles in the development of collecting ducts and biliary ducts.[54] Interestingly, polyductin shares the general structural features of hepatocyte growth-factor receptor and plexin, which belong to a superfamily of proteins involved in the regulation of cell proliferation and of cellular adhesion and repulsion.[55] A recent mouse model of ARPKD in which there was no functional fibrocystin/polyductin demonstrated hepatic, pancreatic, and renal abnormalities with progressive bile duct dilation, cyst formation, and fibrotic livers. The primary cilia in the bile ducts of these mutant mice had structural abnormalities, suggesting that this disease could be classified as a ciliopathy.[56]

Pathology

In ARPKD, there is both renal and hepatic enlargement. The kidneys are symmetrically affected. The renal cysts develop at the terminal collecting tubules in association with interstitial fibrosis, which leads to the appearance of medullary sponge kidney or even ADPKD. Hepatic lesions are uniform and are not seen macroscopically, although macroscopic cysts may be present in more severe forms. The portal tracts are filled with connective tissue and abnormal bile ducts, which are dilated and communicate with the rest of the biliary system.[57] With increasing age, a decrease in the number of ductular structures and an increase in portal fibrosis are noted. If the immature bile ducts undergo necroinflammatory changes resulting in fibrosis, ARPKD is associated with CHF. If incomplete remodeling of the ductal plate occurs earlier in development, when the larger segmental ducts begin to form, ARPKD is associated with Caroli disease.[2]

Clinical features

The main clinical features are renal. Blyth and Ockenden[24] assigned patients with ARPKD to four groups according to the age of presentation—perinatal, neonatal, infantile, and juvenile groups.

In the perinatal group, infants are born with large renal masses, resulting in abdominal distension, uremia, hypertension, and metabolic acidosis and die shortly after birth, secondary to renal failure and respiratory distress. The respiratory failure is caused by compression of the thoracic viscera, atelectasis, congestive heart failure, or even pneumomediastinum. Mechanical ventilation and management of hypertension may prolong life beyond the first month of life. The majority of renal tubules are dilated at autopsy, whereas there is only minimal periportal hepatic fibrosis.

In the neonatal group, children present in the first few months of life with bilaterally enlarged kidneys, and progressively develop renal failure. Death occurs within weeks to a few months after presentation. All have dilated IHBDs, with minimal periportal fibrosis.

In the infantile group, children present with enlarged kidneys and hepatosplenomegaly at between 3 and 6 months of age. Chronic renal failure with hypertension and portal hypertension ensues. Without medical intervention, death may occur before the age of 10. All have dilated IHBDs, with moderate periportal fibrosis.

In the juvenile form, children present between 6 weeks and 1–5 years, mainly with hepatomegaly, which later may progress to portal hypertension, often necessitating a portocaval shunt. They have the mildest renal disease in comparison with the other groups, as they have fewer renal cysts. However, all have dilated IHBDs, with gross periportal fibrosis.

Diagnosis

The diagnosis is established by ultrasonography, CT, MRI, MRCP, intravenous pyelography, and percutaneous liver and kidney biopsies. Liver function may be normal.

Haplotype-based prenatal diagnosis is feasible and reliable in pregnancies at risk for ARPKD,[58] provided an accurate diagnosis of ARPKD has been made in a previously affected sibling.

Management

Currently, treatment consists of symptomatic management of the sequelae of the disease. This includes: control of hypertension, which is the major cause of morbidity in the neonatal period; and treatment of renal failure with dialysis and renal transplantation. Treatment of the hepatobiliary disease consists of controlling variceal bleeding, either with sclerotherapy[59,60] or banding. Occasionally, portosystemic shunts are necessary to reduce bleeding if hepatic function remains normal. Transjugular intrahepatic portosystemic stent shunting (TIPSS) has been successful in one patient with ARPKD and portal hypertension.[61] The long-term outcome depends on the severity of the renal disease.

Congenital hepatic fibrosis

CHF was first reported by Kerr *et al.*[62] and is an autosomal-recessive disorder that is characterized by hepatomegaly and portal hypertension with intact lobular architecture but with superimposed periportal fibrosis and dilated IHBDs. Renal cystic disease is present in the medulla and cortex in most patients and most closely corresponds to ARPKD. Because CHF is most commonly associated with ARPKD, many authorities suggest that the juvenile form of the ARPKD is synonymous with CHF, based on the similar clinical presentation and pathology findings.[10] The exact incidence of the disease is not known.

Pathology

CHF results from ductal plate malformation of the intrahepatic bile ducts.[6] Macroscopically, the hepatic cysts may or may not be visible, or may be confined to one lobe.[63] As discussed above, a process of destructive cholangitis and involution occurs, resulting in periportal fibrosis. The rate of bile duct destruction and fibrosis differs from patient to patient, and may remain unchanged in some.[64] The liver contains broad bands of fibrous tissue, which are separate from the hepatic parenchyma and contain irregular cysts lined by biliary epithelial cells. The portal tracts are enlarged and are linked by the bands of fibrous tissue. The biliary cysts are numerous and may communicate with the rest of the biliary system. The portal vein branches are often hypoplastic and the hepatic artery branches are supernumerous.[65] There is little inflammatory infiltrate unless there is coexistent cholangitis. The hepatic parenchyma is normal (Figure 10.3).

In the kidneys, the cystic dilation affects the collecting ducts and distal tubules, and is less frequent than in ARPKD. The renal cysts develop from involution of the abnormal tubules. Progressive involution leads to nephronophthisis.[66]

Other associations

CHF has been associated with the following conditions:

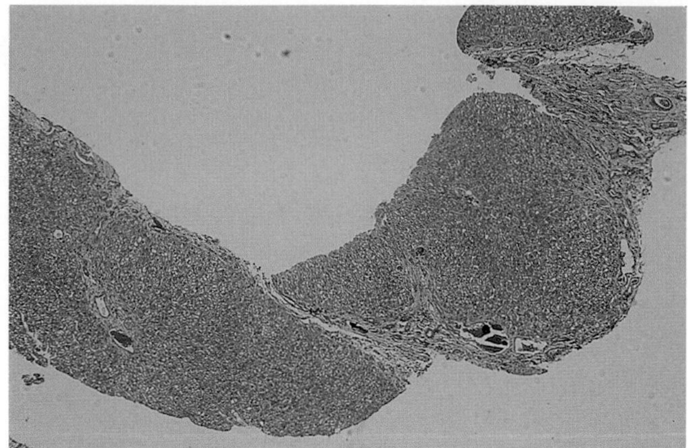

Figure 10.3 Histology of congenital hepatic fibrosis demonstrates widened portal tracts, which are linked by broad bands of fibrous tissue. The bile ducts are prominent, dilated, and abnormal. Recurrent cholangitis may lead to biliary cirrhosis.

- Medullary cystic kidney disease (MCKD), juvenile nephronophthisis (NPHP), renal dysplasia,[67] and ADPKD.[68]
- Meckel–Gruber syndrome of encephalocele, polydactyly, and hepatosplenomegaly is an autosomal-recessive disorder that presents at birth with massive renal lesions and severe hepatic cystic disease.[69]
- Jeune syndrome is an autosomal-recessive disorder with typical radiological features of pulmonary hypoplasia due to underdevelopment of the thoracic cage. Other common features include renal, hepatic, and pancreatic abnormalities. It is characterized by less severe hepatic cystic disease than CHF or Meckel–Gruber syndrome, and later-onset renal cystic disease.[69]
- Ivemark familial dysplasia includes CHF with localized renal dysplasia, with severe interstitial fibrosis leading to renal failure in infancy.[69]
- CHF is also seen in combination with Meyenburg complexes, Caroli disease, and choledochal cysts.[70]
- Other associated malformations include the Lawrence–Moon–Biedl syndrome,[71] hypoplasia of the musculus depressor anguli oris,[72] arteriovenous pulmonary fistula,[73] pulmonary fibrosis and emphysema,[74] vaginal atresia, and tuberous sclerosis.[69]
- CHF has been associated with increased copper deposition, which exceeded 500 μg/g of dry liver.[75]
- Intestinal lymphangiectasia and gluten-sensitive enteropathy have been reported in two children.[76] Pelletier *et al.*[77] described a new syndrome with intestinal lymphangiectasia, secretory diarrhea, enterocolitis cystica superficialis, and CHF.
- Cavernous transformation of the portal vein is significantly increased in CHF.[78]

Clinical features. Clinical symptomatology varies, and different forms of CHF have been described, such as portal hypertensive CHF, cholangitic CHF, and latent forms of CHF.[79]

Symptoms may manifest early in life, in childhood, or in adult life, and include:

- Upper gastrointestinal hemorrhage from ruptured esophageal varices[62] secondary to portal hypertension, which is caused by presinusoidal block. Gastrointestinal bleeding has been reported as early as 19 months of age.[80] The course of the disease is dominated by recurrent gastrointestinal bleeding, which is well tolerated and not associated with encephalopathy.[63,76]
- Recurrent episodes of cholangitis from associated anomalies of the IHBDs, Caroli disease, choledochal cyst, and gallstones may lead to septicemia.
- Arterial hypertension, proteinuria, and microscopic hematuria.
- Failure to thrive in patients with significant renal involvement.
- Renal failure may occur due to associated polycystic kidneys.

On physical examination, abdominal distension is present due to hepatosplenomegaly. The liver is firm, with a prominent left lobe.

Diagnosis

Ultrasonography of the liver and kidneys will provide information about the extent of renal cystic involvement and associated choledochal cysts or Caroli disease (described below). The liver appears hyperechoic secondary to fibrosis and ductular proliferation. Concomitant liver Doppler flow studies may detect portal hypertension. Liver function tests, including serum aminotransferases, bilirubin, cholesterol, albumin, ammonia, and prothrombin time are all normal. Serum alkaline phosphatase and GGT levels may be normal or mildly elevated, especially if there is recurrent cholangitis.[62] Thrombocytopenia, either isolated or associated with neutropenia, is seen in patients with hypersplenism. The diagnosis is made by percutaneous liver biopsy, but since a large number of portal tracts is needed, a surgical biopsy may be more helpful.

Renal function abnormalities are less frequent than in ARPKD and include a decreased glomerular filtration rate, a reduced ability to concentrate the urine, and decreased acidification. Plasma urea and creatinine may be elevated.

Upper gastrointestinal endoscopy will identify esophageal or gastric varices and is indicated when gastrointestinal bleeding occurs. Splenoportography may demonstrate elevated portal and splenic pressures, portal thrombosis, splenic occlusion, duplication of the intrahepatic branches of the portal vein, or even natural splenorenal or gastrorenal shunts.[63] MRI and hepatic angiography are helpful for visualizing the vascular anatomy.

Management

Management is aimed at preventing the sequelae of portal hypertension. Prompt intervention and management of acute variceal bleeding with sclerotherapy or banding via upper endoscopy is required. H_2-receptor antagonist therapy may be started to avoid bleeding episodes from coexisting peptic ulcer disease. Early surgical intervention with portocaval, splenorenal, or meso-Rex shunting should be considered, particularly in patients with recurrent bleeding despite optimal medical management and trials of variceal ablation. Careful selection of the shunt operation is required in order not to impair the feasibility of liver or renal transplantation if required subsequently.[63] Splenectomy at the time of the shunt operation may facilitate renal transplantation, but is associated with an increased risk of bacterial infection and requires preoperative pneumococcal vaccination and lifelong prophylactic penicillin.[81] Ascending cholangitis should be treated aggressively with antibiotics after the responsible organism is identified by blood culture or liver-tissue culture, in order to avoid worsening liver function.

Prognosis and outcome

The prognosis depends on the extent of hepatic and renal disease. Liver disease usually does not progress in childhood, but in the past, before the advent of liver–kidney transplantation, some patients died of complications of portal hypertension, hypersplenism, and renal failure. If required, portosystemic shunting reduces portal hypertension and is well tolerated,[62,63] but it may now be replaced with a meso-Rex shunt if this is technically possible.[82] Unless kidney failure is present, patients can have a normal diet and lead a normal life. Recurrent uncontrolled cholangitis is an indication for liver transplantation.[83] Cholangiocarcinoma and amyloidosis may develop in adulthood.

Caroli disease and Caroli syndrome

Caroli disease was first described by Caroli[84] as an entity characterized by segmental or saccular dilation of the IHBDs, associated with renal tubular ectasia or medullary sponge kidney and pancreatic cysts. Subsequently, a second entity was described that was seen in children and was characterized by dilation of the larger IHBDs, periportal fibrosis, cirrhosis, and portal hypertension, corresponding to CHF. This second entity has been termed Caroli syndrome, and is more frequently encountered than Caroli disease. The two varieties may be autosomal-recessive and are associated with renal lesions closely related to ARPKD.[8]

Pathology

Caroli disease represents ductal plate malformation of the larger IHBDs. In the simple variety, there is saccular dilation of the right and left hepatic ducts, with predominant involvement of the segmental ducts. Intraluminal polypoid projections and crossbridges have been seen within the saccular dilations of the IHBDs. The ectatic ducts communicate with the rest of the biliary system and contain bile. Stagnant bile sludge contained within the dilated ducts is prone to infection and stone formation. Percutaneous liver biopsy reveals centrilobular cholestasis and bile ductule proliferation, with polymorphonuclear cell infiltration of the portal tracts. Caroli syndrome involves ductal plate malformation of the large intrahepatic and interlobular bile ducts, which undergo involution, resulting in the formation of the typical CHF lesion.[2] There is associated periportal fibrosis, as seen in CHF. Macroscopically, the liver contains multiple cysts up to 1 cm in diameter and dilated IHBDs with inspissated bile and calculi, and the parenchyma is nodular. The common bile duct and right and left hepatic ducts may be dilated. Many authorities now believe that Caroli disease is an unfortunate term, as it describes a large spectrum of clinically different cystic diseases such as any radiographically evident communication of the biliary tree, isolated dilation without ductal plate malformation, intrahepatic dilation with associated choledochal cyst (types IV and V), Caroli disease associated with CHF, and others. In addition, a variety of renal lesions (ADPKD, ARPKD) have been associated with the two entities, which differ from the original lesion first described by Caroli.[10,85,86]

Clinical features

The clinical symptoms of Caroli disease are repeated episodes of cholangitis, biliary cholelithiasis, and hepatic abscesses leading to septicemia.[84] The disease presents at any age but usually manifests in young adults, with fever and with or without jaundice. Patients with Caroli syndrome display symptoms of Caroli disease and CHF—i.e., cholangitis and the sequelae of portal hypertension. In both entities, patients are anicteric and have firm hepatomegaly.

Diagnosis

The ultrasound findings include anechoic, ovoid structures with irregular margins, suggesting communication between the lesions (Figure 10.4).[87] Occasionally, the intrahepatic cystic dilations may be confused with multiple hepatic abscesses, but concurrent gallium citrate Ga 67 scintigraphy may be helpful in distinguishing between the two entities. CT scanning demonstrates low-density, branching, tubular structures, which may help distinguish it from polycystic disease. CT scanning with contrast, showing retention of contrast in the dilated bile ducts, may further increase the sensitivity of the study. Hepatic scintigraphy using derivatives of ^{99m}Tc iminodiacetic acid cannot distinguish biliary dilation due to Caroli disease from dilation due to obstruction. More invasive procedures, such as endoscopic retrograde cholangiography or percutaneous transhepatic cholangiography, may differentiate intrahepatic or extrahepatic dilations and identify biliary stones (Figure 10.5). The diagnosis may be confirmed by histology,[88] which demonstrates centrilobular cholestasis and bile ductule proliferation, with polymorphonuclear cell infiltration of the portal tracts.[89]

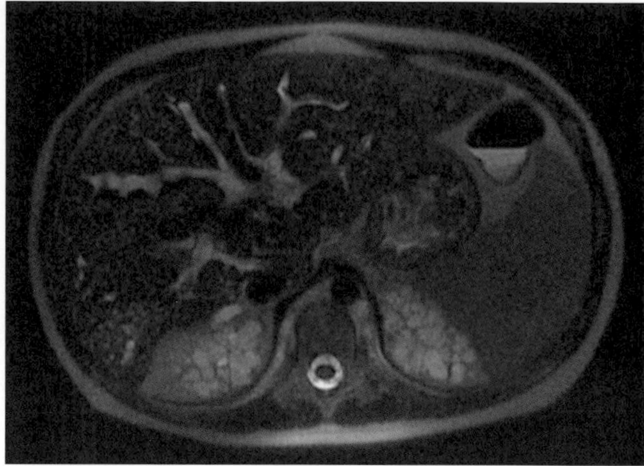

Figure 10.4 Magnetic resonance cholangiopancreatogram, demonstrating multiple, tiny intrahepatic cysts, consistent with Caroli disease and hepatic fibrosis.

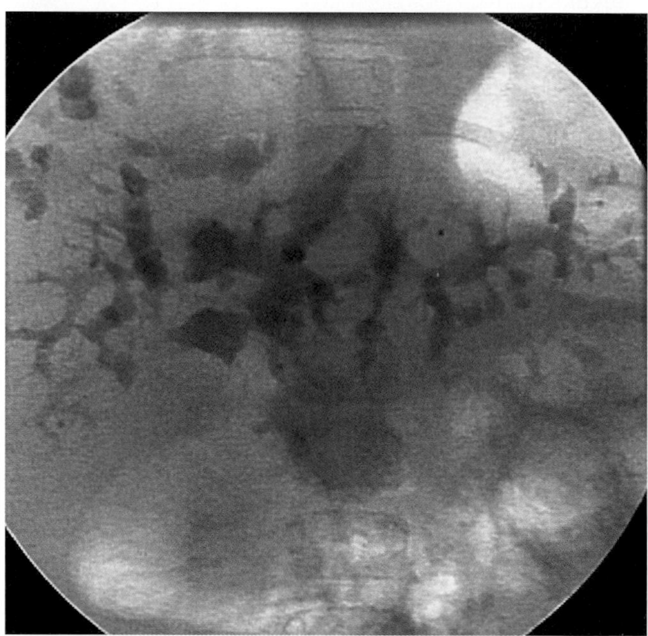

Figure 10.5 Endoscopic retrograde cholangiography in a patient with Caroli disease, congenital hepatic fibrosis, and minimal polycystic renal disease. The image demonstrates gross abnormalities of the intrahepatic biliary tree, which communicates with hepatic cysts.

Serum aminotransferases, alkaline phosphatase, and serum bilirubin levels are usually normal unless the patient has active cholangitis.

Management and prognosis

Management includes antibiotics either for prophylaxis or treatment of cholangitis. The role of surgery is limited unless there is mechanical obstruction due to biliary calculi, and may cause worsening of cholangitis. The long-term prognosis in the disease depends on the severity of the renal lesions and the degree of periportal fibrosis and hepatic dysfunction. Cholangiocarcinoma and amyloidosis are long-term sequelae of the disease.

Polycystic liver disease

Autosomal-dominant polycystic liver disease (ADPLD) has recently been described as a separate entity genetically distinct from ADPKD and Caroli disease.[90–92] It includes the development of multiple cysts in the liver, and rarely in other organs. Cysts are thought to originate from dilation of biliary microhamartomas and peribiliary glands. In 2000, a genetic locus for isolated polycystic liver disease (PCLD) was mapped to chromosome 19p13.2-13.1.[93] In 2003, protein kinase C substrate 80K-H (*PRKCSH*) was reported as the gene mutated in ADPLD, encoding for a protein of 527 amino acids and 59 kDa called hepatocystin.[94,95] The exact intracellular location and function remain unclear, but it may be related to regulation of cell proliferation.[96] Mutations in *SEC63* have also been linked to ADPLD.[97] In an autopsy series, the incidence of isolated hepatic disease was 0.05%, and Meyenburg complexes were microscopically present in all cases of PCLD.[98]

Clinical features and diagnosis

The majority of patients with hepatic cysts related to ADPLD are asymptomatic. Hepatic involvement is associated with abdominal discomfort secondary to hepatomegaly. Signs of cyst infection such as fever, leukocytosis, and right upper quadrant abdominal pain must also be monitored. In most patients, liver tissue is intact; there is no fibrosis, and liver function remains normal.[99] Portal hypertension is a rare complication. One study has focused solely on the manifestations of PCLD; 3.6% of the 117 patients studied had intracranial aneurysms, and 20.4% had structural mitral valve leaflet abnormalities.[100] The diagnosis is suggested by ultrasound or CT scanning and may be confirmed by histology or family history.

Management

Management includes renal support and/or transplantation, or control of portal hypertension. Occasionally, large cysts require aspiration or drainage into the peritoneal cavity.

Traumatic cysts

Traumatic cysts are thought to occur after intrahepatic hemorrhage from abdominal trauma. The blood is resorbed and bile fills the space, creating a cyst. They are asymptomatic, but may occasionally present with anorexia or abdominal pain due to distension or rupture of the cyst. Rarely, they may become infected. Treatment includes antibiotics, and aspiration or drainage of the cysts if symptoms are severe.

Cysts secondary to infarction

These cysts occur after focal vascular insufficiency of the liver and have been observed in liver transplant recipients following occlusion of the hepatic artery. They are lined by endothelium and contain bile. They are asymptomatic, but may occasionally become infected. They are usually discovered incidentally on CT or ultrasound.

Differential diagnosis of fibropolycystic disease of the liver

An algorithm for the evaluation of a child with fibropolycystic disease detected by ultrasound of the liver is shown in Figure 10.6. In order to distinguish between the different forms of fibropolycystic disease in a child with hepatomegaly, a thorough medical history must be taken. Patients with a positive family history of cystic diseases, especially among first-degree relatives, are particularly at risk for having polycystic disease. A history of previous fever, chills, jaundice, hematemesis, melena, hematuria, and abdominal pain or trauma should be sought.

On physical examination, the liver and kidneys should be carefully palpated. Typically, hepatomegaly is obvious. When present, splenomegaly and prominent superficial abdominal veins suggest portal hypertension, which is the presenting sign of CHF in childhood. Bilateral abdominal masses represent markedly enlarged kidneys, which are easier to palpate in neonates and infants with ARPKD. Flank tenderness secondary to pyelonephritis may be present in patients with significant renal involvement. If there is significant renal involvement, then either ADPKD or ARPKD is likely. The blood pressure may be at or above the 95th percentile for age. More subtle signs of renal tubular disease—particularly loss of concentrating ability, microscopic hematuria, and proteinuria—may be detected by urinalysis.

If portal hypertension is prominent, then CHF is likely. Laboratory tests, including serum aspartate aminotransferase (AST), alanine aminotransferase (ALT), alkaline phosphatase, GGT, prothrombin time, albumin, and conjugated and unconjugated bilirubin are normal, as the liver parenchyma is intact. Thrombocytopenia or leukopenia suggests hypersplenism. Elevated liver enzymes suggest cholangitis or another liver disease. Occasionally, there is cholestasis with mild elevations in GGT if there is sludge formation from stagnant bile in Caroli disease and choledochal cyst. The erythrocyte sedimentation rate (ESR) is elevated in cholangitis, which may occur with the cholangitic type of CHF, Caroli disease, and Caroli syndrome.

Ultrasound of the abdomen is helpful in differentiating between the different forms of polycystic disease.

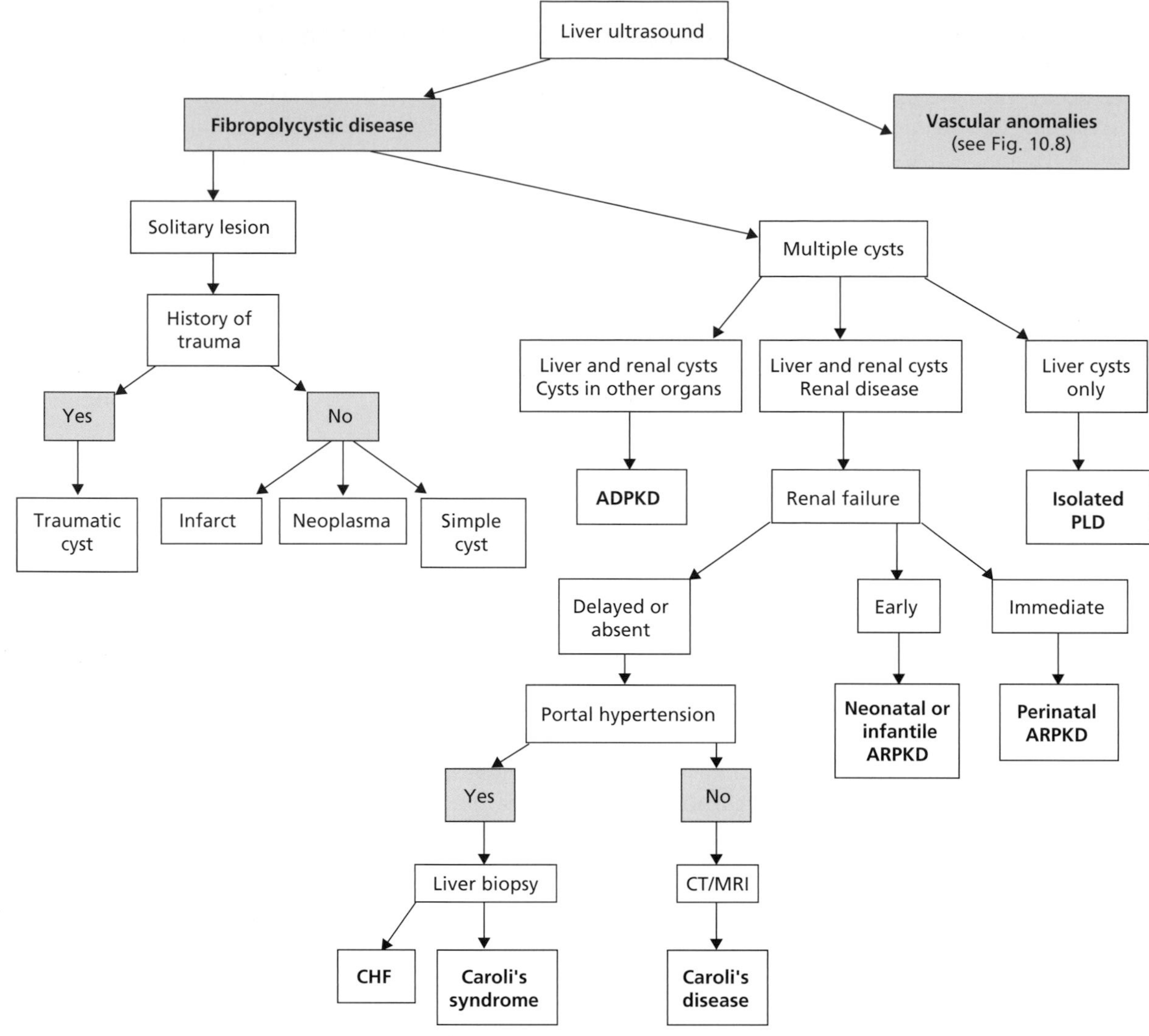

Figure 10.6 Algorithm for the diagnosis of fibrocystic diseases of the liver.

- A single hepatic cyst may be solitary, traumatic, neoplastic, or secondary to infarction.
- Multiple cysts affecting the liver, kidneys, pancreas, ovaries, and other organs suggest ADPKD.
- Cysts confined to the liver may represent PCLD or perhaps variable expression of ADPKD, and these patients should be followed up over time.
- Patients with combined hepatic and renal cysts may have either ARPKD or CHF. If renal failure is prominent within the first days or months of life, ARPKD is likely, although CHF is also associated with a variety of renal disorders, which may mimic ARPKD. The presence of portal hypertension suggests CHF.

Percutaneous renal biopsy will help distinguish between ADPKD, ARPKD, and other lesions associated with the polycystic diseases.

Management issues

Transjugular intrahepatic portosystemic stent shunts

TIPSS is a percutaneously created shunt through the liver parenchyma connecting an intrahepatic branch of the portal vein to a main hepatic vein.[101,102] The TIPSS procedure was designed to decompress the portal circulation in patients with portal hypertension and is similar to a surgical side-to-side portocaval shunt, but it avoids the need for general anesthesia and laparotomy. It has been used increasingly to treat complications of portal hypertension such as variceal bleeding, refractory ascites, hepatic hydrothorax, and hepatorenal syndrome.[103,104] This procedure has been successfully used in the pediatric population.[105–108]

TIPSS have been successfully placed in the setting of polycystic liver disease[109–111] and ARPKD prior to renal transplantation.[61]

Although multiple prospective randomized clinical trials have shown that TIPSS is significantly more effective in reducing variceal rebleeding from portal hypertension of diverse etiology in adults in comparison with endoscopic sclerotherapy or band ligation,[104] the survival rates are comparable. Since TIPSS may be complicated by shunt stenosis or occlusion rates of up to 87% in the first year,[104] it is unlikely that this procedure will be useful in the long-term management of a child with portal hypertension secondary to ARPKD and/or CHF; however, it may serve as a bridge to transplantation.

Indications for liver transplantation

In most patients with fibropolycystic disease of the liver, hepatic function remains normal, but portal hypertension is a major problem. The indications for liver transplantation are related to the development of hepatic dysfunction, which may occur secondary to recurrent cholangitis, extensive biliary disease, increasing hepatic fibrosis, or gross abdominal distension with respiratory embarrassment. Combined liver and kidney transplantation may be required for both renal and hepatic dysfunction.

Future research

- The functions of polycystin-1 and -2 and their interactions with various signaling molecules are not entirely clear. Studies investigating the effects of various cytokines and growth factors on cyst proliferation, and the role of cilia in renal and liver cyst formation, would significantly advance our understanding of ADPKD. It is known that the protein products of *PKD1*, *PKD2*, and *PKHD1* localize to the primary cilia of renal tubules.[112,113] Studies in mouse models are investigating the role of cilia in liver cysts as well.[114]
- Another promising area of research is the role of signal transduction modulators, such as transforming growth factor-α (TGF-α), ErbB2, and Ras inhibitors, in renal and liver cyst formation. TGF-α is overexpressed in transgenic mice with ADPKD.[115] Increased activity of the epidermal growth factor receptor (EGFR) in the affected kidneys has been consistently observed. Interestingly, a mutant EGFR with decreased tyrosine kinase activity in a murine model of ARPKD is correlated with an improvement in kidney function and a substantial decrease in cyst formation in the collecting ducts.[116] Therefore, approaches to target TGF-α, tyrosine kinase,[117] and EGFR would have the potential to decrease cyst formation. Other promising signal-transduction modulators include ErbB TK inhibitors, Ras inhibitors, and PKA type 1 inhibitors.[118] Another promising mode of treatment for renal disease is the use of vasopressin V2-receptor antagonists, which reduce renal cyclic adenosine monophosphate (cAMP), which is involved in cystic fluid secretion and cell proliferation.[119] The relevance of this for cystic disease of the liver has not yet been explored.
- Since somatic mutations are important for cyst development, it is conceivable that any treatment capable of reducing the rate of somatic mutations would slow down the progression of ADPKD. These may include antimutagens (inhibitors of phase 1 enzymes or inducers of phase 2 enzymes) and antioxidants.
- The long-term goal would be gene therapy to express the respective wild-type polycystin protein or replace the mutated gene with the normal *PKD* gene.

Hepatic vascular anomalies

The great majority of vascular anomalies of the liver in infancy and childhood are hemangiomas.[120–123] The utility of histology will be reviewed in detail.

Classification

Vascular anomalies can be classified clinically by symptoms (Table 10.2). Although cystic mesenchymal hamartomas are usually avascular at angiography,[124] they are included

Table 10.2 Classification of vascular malformations of the liver.

Asymptomatic
Incidental
Solitary hemangioma
Multiple hemangiomas
Hepatomegaly
Cystic mesenchymal hamartoma
Extramedullary hematopoiesis
Focal nodular hyperplasia
Symptomatic
Congestive heart failure/hepatomegaly
Infantile hemangioendothelioma
Giant cavernous hemangioma
Arteriovenous malformation
Arterioportal fistula
Portovenous fistula
Other extrahepatic conditions
Syndromes
Klippel–Trenaunay–Weber
Rendu–Osler–Weber
Miscellaneous
Systemic cystic angiomatosis
Angiosarcoma
Bacillary angiomatosis
Peliosis hepatis

in the list of vascular anomalies because they may contain areas of vascular connective tissue. Rarely, infantile hemangioendothelioma and mesenchymal hamartoma may coexist in the same patient.[125] Focal nodular hyperplasia is a disorder in which a benign single or multifocal lesion of the liver occurs, which is characterized by a firm, irregular mass with a central scar supplied by single or multiple large "feeder arteries."[126]

Symptomatic hemangiomas of the liver in childhood fall into two types: infantile hemangioendotheliomas, seen principally in the first year of life,[127] which tend to be solid; and cavernous hemangiomas, which tend to be cystic. Both forms may be found in the same lesion. By convention, cystic hemangiomas larger than 4 cm in diameter have been referred to as "giant cavernous hemangiomas." Hemangioendotheliomas are mesenchymal tumors with interconnecting small-diameter vascular channels. Type I lesions will typically involute and regress, whereas type II lesions are more aggressive and can even metastasize.[128] In some classifications, but not in others, type II hemangioendothelioma is synonymous with hepatic angiosarcoma. Some authors describe a variant called epithelioid hemangioendothelioma that can develop in different tissues, including the liver.[129]

Kassarjian *et al.*[123] proposed a classification system for hepatic hemangioma based on angiographic findings and classified lesions into five types. Type 1 lesions were the classic hemangiomas, with early filling of abnormal vascular channels and with stagnation and pooling of contrast material. They did not have any early filling of hepatic veins or an arteriovenous or portovenous shunt. Type 2 lesions contained focal high-flow nodules, with early filling of veins and with no visible direct shunts. Type 3 lesions contained angiographically visible direct arteriovenous (including arterioportal) shunts, whereas type 4 lesions contained direct portovenous shunts. Type 5 lesions contained both direct arteriovenous and portovenous shunts.

Basic mechanisms and pathophysiology

Hepatic hemangiomas are not usually thought of as genetic disorders in the conventional sense, although one family in which several members developed giant cavernous hepatic hemangiomas exhibited selective inhibition of natural killer cell activity.[130] The fact that there are rare reports of familial hepatic hemangiomas does lend credence to the notion of genetic modifiers of the disease.[131] Possible candidates include vascular endothelial growth factor (VEGF); Derlin-1, a factor known to be implicated in the retro-translocation of misfolded proteins from ER to cytoplasm; and the von Hippel–Lindau (VHL) gene.

Recent evidence has implicated high levels of VEGF in the pathogenesis of hemangiomas. Kitajima *et al.* created a transgenic rabbit model with increased hepatic expression of the human VEGF 165 transgene under the control of the human α-antitrypsin promotor.[132] The rabbits showed marked hepatomegaly and several features of diffuse hemangiomas, including prominent dilation of the sinusoids and various-sized networks of blood vessels. The rabbits also suffered from hemolytic anemia, thrombocytopenia, and splenomegaly in association with marked extramedullary hematopoiesis—features that may be seen in Kasabach–Merritt syndrome. This model may prove useful for investigation of the therapeutic effect of anti-VEGF inhibitors of angiogenesis.

In addition to the above research on vascular growth factors, another insight into the pathogenesis of human hepatic cavernous hemangiomas has come from ultrastructural investigations demonstrating that the endoplasmic reticulum (ER) in hepatic cavernous hemangiomas is enlarged. In studies by Hu *et al.*,[133] Derlin-1 was down-regulated in endothelial cells derived from hepatic cavernous hemangiomas. There was activation of the unfolded protein response (UPR), with increased expression of the immunoglobulin heavy chain-binding protein and UPR-specific splicing of X-box DNA binding protein 1 mRNA. Overexpression of Derlin-1 induced the dilated ER to return to normal size and was associated with reversal of the UPR.

Another insight into the pathogenesis of hepatic vascular tumors has come from mice with conditional inactivation of the VHL gene.[134] These mice develop multiple hepatic hemangiomas. While such tumors are rare in patients with VHL, Takahashi *et al.*[135] have recently identified a novel mutation in the VHL gene in a Japanese family with pheochromocytoma, one member of which has hepatic hemangiomas.

Clinical features

The most common vascular anomalies in childhood are hemangiomas (Figure 10.7). In a series of 43 children with hepatic vascular anomalies in infancy, 90% had hemangiomas and 10% had arteriovenous malformations.[121]

- *Hemangioma.* Solitary or multiple hemangiomas are asymptomatic and may be an incidental finding at any age. These benign tumors may present with asymptomatic hepatomegaly, which may be associated with a systolic bruit. Almost all patients with symptomatic hepatic hemangiomas present before 6 months of age and most present within the first 2 months.[136] In one series, about 80% of infants with multiple hepatic hemangiomas had the classic triad of hepatomegaly, congestive heart failure, and anemia.[121] Sudden infant death secondary to tumor rupture has been reported.[137] Diffuse neonatal hemangiomatosis is a rare disease in which hepatic involvement may be prominent.[138] Rarely, hepatic hemangiomas can present as hydrops fetalis. Morimura *et al.* reported fetal hepatic hemangioma presenting as a nonreassuring pattern in fetal heart rate monitoring leading to fetal loss from tumor hemorrhage, despite emergency cesarean section.[139] Hemangioendotheliomas have fairly high morbidity and mortality rates; in a recent series of 13 cases there were four deaths, due to sepsis, hepatic failure, disseminated

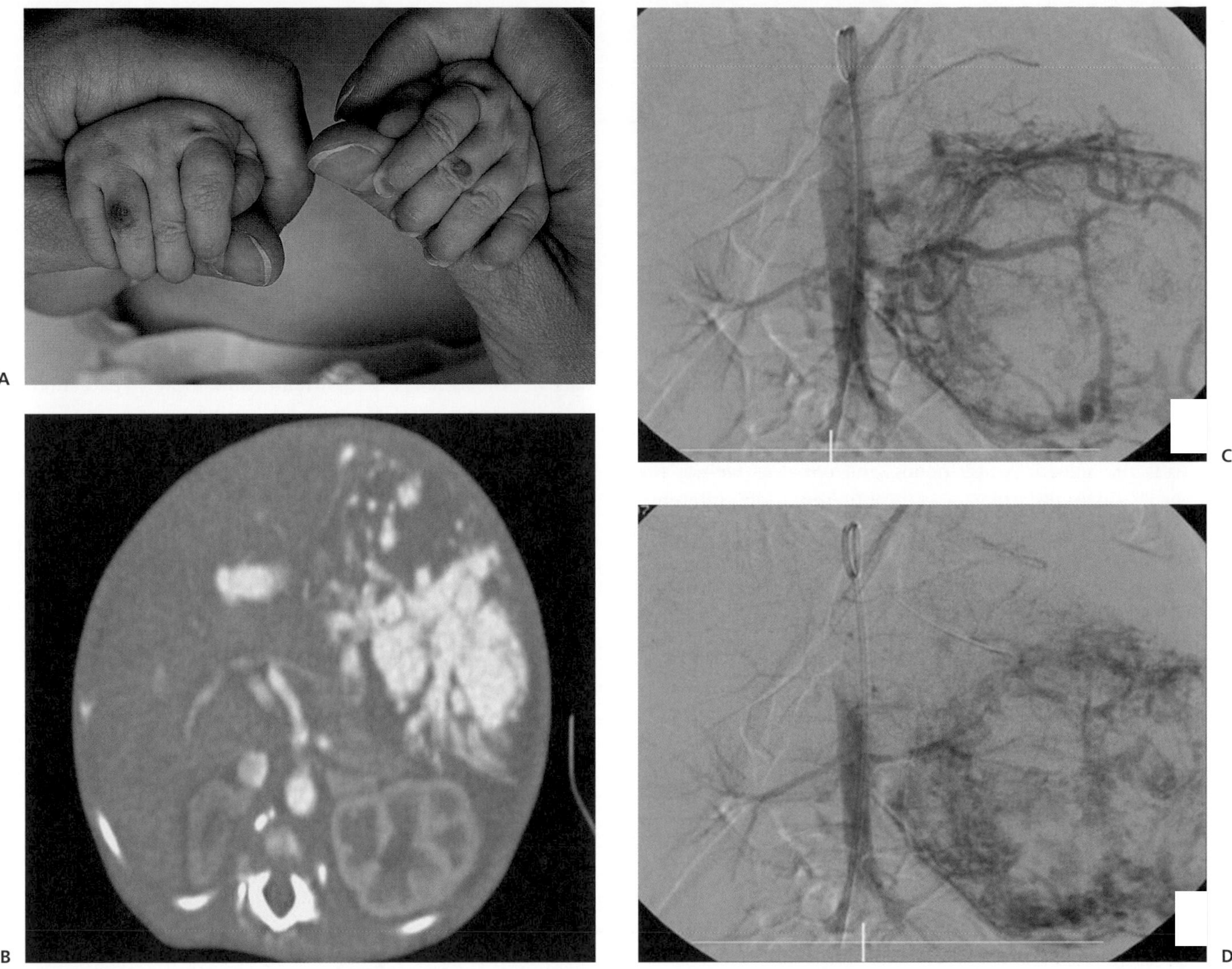

Figure 10.7 **A** Cutaneous hemangiomas are common and usually regress within 6 months. They may be associated with multiple hemangiomas, leading to high output cardiac failure. **B** This computed-tomographic angiogram in a 12-week-old infant demonstrates a large hepatic hemangioma. **C, D** Treatment includes cyanoacrylate glue embolization using a pigtail catheter in the lower thoracic aorta, showing intense hypervascularity of the hepatic hemangioma before (**C**) and a reduction in blood flow after (**D**) successful embolization. Hepatic artery ligation or liver transplantation are alternative treatments.

intravascular coagulopathy, or tumor rupture with hemorrhagic shock.[140]

• *Arteriovenous malformations* (AVMs) are much less common than hemangiomas. In the neonatal period, AVMs usually present as congestive heart failure. Later in childhood, most hepatic AVMs are seen in patients with hereditary hemorrhagic telangiectasia and result in congestive heart failure, hepatic ischemia, and portal hypertension.[122]

• *Arterioportal fistula* usually occurs as an isolated congenital anomaly and can be seen in patients with hereditary hemorrhagic telangiectasia, Ehlers–Danlos syndrome, trauma, and iatrogenic procedures such as liver biopsy.[141] The main symptoms at presentation are symptoms of portal hypertension with associated ascites, malabsorption, gastrointestinal bleeding, and abdominal pain. A small percentage of patients present with high-output congestive heart failure.

• *Intrahepatic portovenous fistulas* (PVFs) are very rare and usually seen in infants with hepatic hemangioma, although isolated cases are reported.[142]

• *Klippel–Trenaunay–Weber syndrome* is a nonhereditary congenital condition characterized by hemihypertrophy, capillary malformations, and venous stasis, with or without arteriovenous malformations.[143] Hepatic hemangiomas and focal nodular hyperplasia, presumably secondary to an abnormal hepatic vascular supply, have been associated with this syndrome.[144]

• *Osler–Weber–Rendu disease,* or hereditary hemorrhagic telangiectasia, is an autosomal-dominant condition in which the vascular lesions can involve the liver in addition to the gut and the skin.[145]

- *Systemic cystic angiomatosis* is a congenital vascular malformation involving multiple organ systems, particularly the liver, spleen, kidney, and colon.[146] The clinical presentation is determined by the organ(s) involved.
- *Hepatic angiosarcomas* are rare, highly vascular malignant tumors in children[147] sometimes associated with cutaneous hemangiomas, exposure to arsenicals or neurofibromatosis. Patients usually present with jaundice and a rapidly enlarging abdomen and may rarely have multiple cutaneous hemangiomata prognosis is extremely poor.[148]
- *Bacillary angiomatosis* (BA) is caused by a rickettsial organism, *Bartonella henselae*. The patient may present with chills, headaches, fever, and malaise, and typical cutaneous lesions appear as bright-red, round papules or nodules. The lesion affects the spleen, lymph nodes, and bone, as well as the liver.[149] Given the dramatic clinical presentation, differentiation of the hepatic BA lesion from other vascular malformations is not difficult.
- Peliosis hepatitis is a rare lesion characterized by blood-filled cavities, which are scattered throughout the liver. Medications such as androgen-anabolic steroids, estrogens, oral contraceptives, and azathioprine have been implicated.[150]

Diagnosis

A diagnostic algorithm for vascular anomalies of the liver is shown in Figure 10.8. Vascular abnormalities of the liver are usually discovered in an infant or child when hepatomegaly and/or right upper quadrant pain lead to the performance of an ultrasound scan. Ultrasound of a hemangioma typically detects a heterogeneous, septated, space-occupying lesion with a mixture of hypoechoic, isoechoic, and hyperreflective areas.[151] The diagnosis of fetal hepatic hemangioma can be made by prenatal sonography.[152] It is important to differentiate neuroblastomas, which tend to be more hyperechoic, from hemangiomas in the neonatal period.

Cavernous hemangiomas can be differentiated from malignant neoplasms ultrasonographically, as the hemangiomas usually exhibit signs of increased blood flow such as enlarged upper abdominal aorta, celiac, and hepatic arteries and veins, combined with a smaller aorta inferiorly. Differentiation of a cavernous hemangioma from a malignant neoplasm can be difficult, and referral to a specialized unit is recommended.

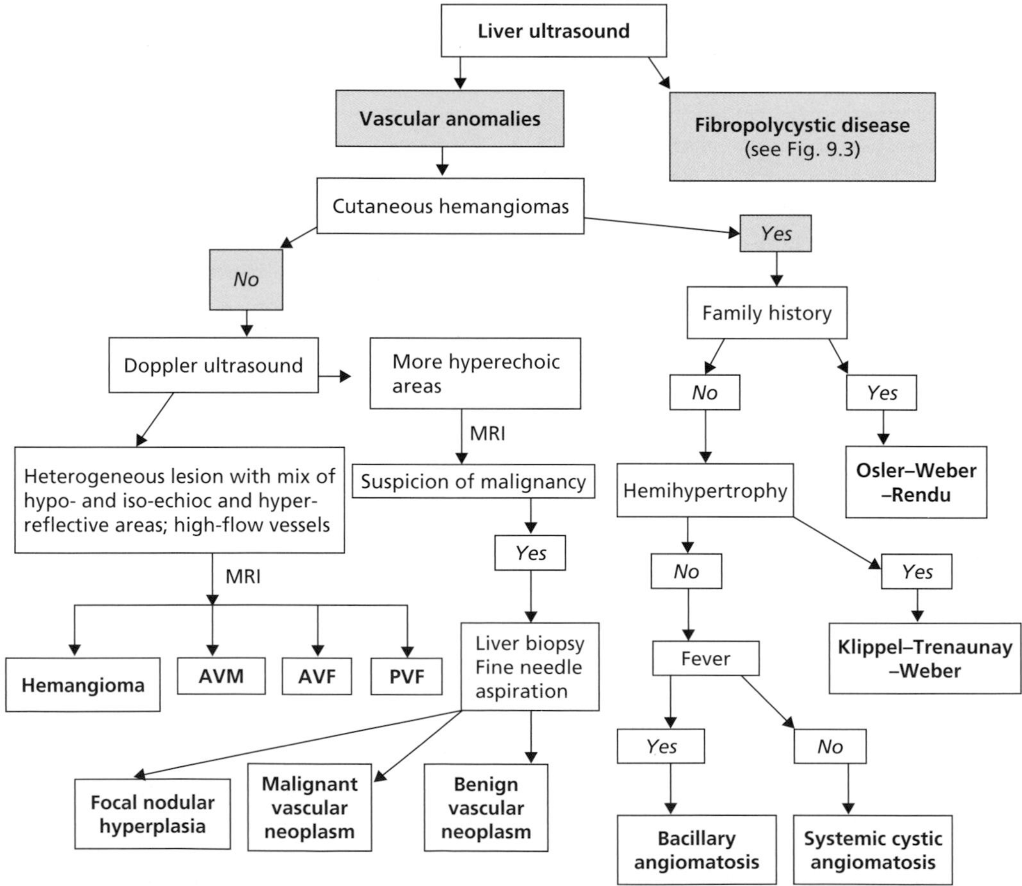

Figure 10.8 Diagnostic algorithm for vascular anomalies of the liver. APF, arterioportal fistula; AVM, arteriovenous malformation; PVF, portovenous fistula.

Color Doppler techniques demonstrate a variety of flow patterns, which may overlap with patterns described for malignant tumors but only hemangiomas or arteriovenous malformations exhibit blood velocities faster than the aorta.[153] This technique may also demonstrate low-resistance flow in the hepatic artery, or reverse flow in the distal aorta characteristic of a "steal" to the low-resistance bed of the hemangioma during the diastolic phase. The combination of color Doppler ultrasound and the contrast agent Levovist may be useful in difficult cases, as there is no signal enhancement in the center of the hemangioma.[154] Further confirmation can be obtained with contrast CT, in which the characteristic finding is initial peripheral and septal enhancement of contrast with delayed partial centripetal filling. However, this appearance has also been seen with cystic mesenchymal hamartoma.[155] Using a galactose-palmitic acid contrast agent, Numata *et al.*[156] showed that the sensitivity and specificity for hepatic hemangioma were 96% and 94%, respectively.

Magnetic resonance imaging (MRI) is the most useful single modality in the diagnosis of hepatic hemangiomas.[157] MRI can show the extent of hepatic hemangioma, as well as its characteristics and structure. It has a sensitivity of 90% and a specificity of 92% for the diagnosis of hemangiomas, and the technique has been useful in evaluation of premature newborns.[158] Intravenous gadolinium and a gradient-recalled echo sequence are extremely helpful, especially in the focal lesions, to distinguish hemangioma from malignant tumors or AVMs[122] and from mesenchymal hamartoma, a cystic benign liver mass occurring in children.[159] Quantitative analysis of diffusion-weighted MRI can distinguish between hepatocellular carcinoma, hepatic metastases, cavernous hemangioma, and hepatic cysts.[160] Ferucarbotran-enhanced dynamic MRI imaging has a high sensitivity and specificity for distinguishing these types of lesions.[161] Using this technique, Schmitz *et al.* reported that the tumor-to-vessel ratio is an extremely reliable way of differentiating hemangioma from metastases.[162]

Hepatic angiography is generally reserved for patients with congestive heart failure, for whom therapeutic embolization is considered.[122] It helps classify the lesion on the basis of the variable angioarchitecture of the hepatic hemangioma, and it can demonstrate any direct arteriovenous, arterioportal, and portovenous shunts within the hemangioma.[123]

Laboratory findings in children with hemangioma include anemia, increased aminotransferase levels, and hyperbilirubinemia. Although high serum AFP levels up to 35 000 ng/mL have been reported, the AFP level is not usually elevated and may differentiate malignant vascular lesions from benign lesions.[163] Many angiogenesis-related markers, such as vascular endothelial growth factor (VEGF) and basic fibroblast growth factor (bFGF) in body fluids (particularly blood and urine) are of prognostic significance.[164] Hypothyroidism may be associated with infantile hepatic hemangiomas, perhaps because bFGF or other growth factors induce type 3 iodothyronine deiodinase expression in hemangiomas. It requires very high doses of levothyroxine treatment to reduce serum thyrotropin concentrations to normal.[165] Therefore, thyroid function should be assessed in children with large hemangiomas.

If diagnosis is not possible using noninvasive techniques, CT or ultrasound-guided percutaneous liver biopsy can be used to establish the diagnosis, although there is a high risk of hemorrhage.[166] Reports in adults suggest that fine-needle aspiration under ultrasound guidance can be performed with minimal risk to the patient.[167] No large series of infants or children undergoing percutaneous liver biopsy or fine-needle aspiration to establish the diagnosis of cavernous hemangioma of the liver have been reported to date. If this type of technique is contemplated, it should be performed only in a clinical setting of optimum safety, including back-up by pediatric surgeons and a pediatric intensive-care unit, and with appropriate blood products (fresh frozen plasma, platelets, and packed red blood cells) available in case of hemorrhage.

Pathology

Angiomas can be differentiated from other liver neoplasms by immunohistochemistry using stains for factor VIII and basement membrane protein, which are negative in tumors such as fibrosarcomas.[168] Cytokeratin 7 is typical of the mature biliary tract, and cytokeratin 19 is typical of embryonic and fetal hepatocytes. Hemangiomas typically are positive for cytokeratin 7, whereas hepatoblastomas exhibit cytokeratin 19.[169] Ultrastructural analysis of hemangiomas reveals capillaries and stromal cells, including typical smooth-muscle cells, modified smooth-muscle cells, and fibroblast-like cells. Mo *et al.* recently demonstrated that Glut1 endothelial reactivity can be used to differentiate hepatic infantile hemangioma from congenital hepatic vascular malformation with associated capillary proliferation.[170] Arteriovascular malformations can be distinguished from hemangiomas by the use of Movat pentachrome vascular staining to identify elastic vessels and S100 immunostaining to identify nerves in the neurovascular bundles.[171] Frischer *et al.* have shown that angiogenic factors can be useful for differentiating vascular anomalies with different clinical behaviors.[172]

Management and outcome

Therapy is determined by the severity of symptoms and the size of the tumor. Most lesions continue to grow during the first year of life, and then spontaneously regress. Complications such as congestive heart failure, arteriovenous shunting, and coagulopathy often dictate earlier therapeutic intervention. Asymptomatic hemangiomas and giant cavernous hemangiomas require no treatment except careful observation for the known complications. Indications for treatment include: rapid enlargement of the tumor with respiratory embarrassment, cardiac failure, or abdominal pain; and large solitary tumors which may rupture—particularly giant cavernous hemangiomas, which can lead to spontaneous hemoperitoneum and progressive portal hypertension from arterioportal venous shunting.[173] Kassarjian *et al.*[157] found that MRI findings were useful in predicting the clinical outcome of children with infantile hepatic hemangiomas. Patients with focal lesions without high flow needed no treatment, whereas those with a central varix and direct shunt usually developed severe high-output heart failure, which responded quickly to embolization. If the liver showed massive replacement by hemangioma, this condition was associated with hypothyroidism, abdominal compartment syndrome, and a high mortality rate.

Systemic or intralesional corticosteroids may encourage resolution in symptomatic hemangiomas,[174] particularly prior to surgery. In the past, interferon-α (IFN-α) was tried, with some success.[175] However, spastic diplegia has been reported as a severe complication of IFN-α treatment of hemangiomas in infancy, and IFN-α is therefore no longer indicated.[176] Vincristine was also reported as an effective treatment of corticoid-resistant life-threatening infantile hemangiomas.[177] Radiotherapy is controversial and probably ineffective. Hepatic artery embolization may be effective, particularly to stabilize patients before elective hepatic resection, or as an alternative to hepatic artery ligation.[178] Success has been reported with a Lipiodol–Histoacryl mix,[179] endovascular coil occlusion,[180] and Amplatzer vascular plugs.[181] Surgical ligation of the hepatic artery may not provide sufficient control of cardiac failure, as portohepatic shunts (between the portal and hepatic veins) as well as arteriovenous shunts (between the hepatic artery and hepatic veins) can occur[123] and embolization may be needed.

Solitary symptomatic hemangiomas should be removed surgically, while surgical management of cavernous hemangiomas should be reserved for progressive tumor enlargement and subcapsular bleeding. Congestive heart failure should be managed in the conventional way.

In a series of 16 infants and children with hepatic hemangiomas, high-output cardiac failure was present in 58% of newborns, and seven hemangiomas were resected; the outcome was excellent.[182] Successful liver transplantation has been reported for giant cavernous hemangiomas complicated by consumption coagulopathy (Kasabach–Merritt syndrome) and for infantile hepatic hemangioendothelioma type II.[183]

Although Subramanyan *et al.*[184] recently reported a successful transcatheter coil occlusion of hepatic arteriovenous malformation in a neonate, embolization is not usually a good option for AVMs, because of their diffuse nature and the risk of causing further hepatic ischemia and necrosis, and liver transplantation may be required.[122]

Intrahepatic PVFs may involute spontaneously before 1 year of age[185] or may be cured by embolization.[141]

Sharif *et al.*[186] recently reviewed the management and outcome of hepatic epithelioid hemangioendotheliomas in children. Of the five children identified, four had unresectable tumors. Two underwent transplantation and died of tumor recurrence or sepsis. Ifosfamide-based chemotherapy failed in two of the children, but they were stabilized on platinum-based chemotherapy. Cyclophosphamide has been used successfully to treat infants with life-threatening diffuse neonatal hemangiomatosis.[187]

Promising lines of research

- The natural history and effectiveness of treatment options for vascular anomalies are unclear. Due to the rarity of these lesions, multicenter cooperative studies are needed to clarify the role of corticosteroids and IFN-α for hemangiomas, cyclophosphamide, endovascular embolization, surgical resection, and liver transplantation.
- Accurate diagnosis of vascular anomalies is essential for any new treatment protocol. The angiographic classification by Kassarjian *et al.*[123] provides the best angioarchitecture description for hemangioma, but it is invasive and not practical for all patients. Noninvasive vascular imaging techniques such as MRI with intravenous gadolinium should be applied to the classification system.
- The role of vascular growth factors, abnormalities in protein unfolding, and genetic factors in the pathogenesis of hepatic vascular tumors should be explored further and may lead to promising antiangiogenic therapies.

Case study

The patient is a boy, now aged 11, who first presented at the age of 8 months with a palpable abdominal mass. Ultrasound examination of the abdomen revealed bilaterally enlarged kidneys with diffuse echogenicity, suggestive of diffuse microcysts, consistent with autosomal-recessive polycystic kidney disease (ARPKD). Intravenous pyelography confirmed the diagnosis of ARPKD. Ultrasound also showed a diffusely coarse liver with a heterogenous echotexture, consistent with hepatic fibrosis. The common bile duct appeared minimally prominent; however, there was no intrahepatic biliary ductal dilation. The patient developed hypertension, but renal function was normal. He was followed with annual renal ultrasound examinations and biannual renal laboratory assessments. Normal values included blood urea nitrogen 17 mmol/L (normal range 7–22), creatinine 0.5 μmol/L (normal range 0.6–1.3), ALT 16 U/L (normal range 0–40), and bilirubin 0.7 μmol/L (normal range 0.2–1.2). Serum markers of liver function, such as prothrombin time 11.4 seconds (normal 11.5–13.5) and albumin 4.0 g/L (normal 3.5–5.3), were also normal. AST was only mildly elevated at 44 U/L (normal 0–35).

When he was aged 33 months, a clinical examination revealed marked hepatosplenomegaly. At this time, the patient was also anemic and thrombocytopenic, presumably secondary to hypersplenism. Liver biopsy showed marked periportal fibrosis and bile duct dilation, consistent with congenital hepatic fibrosis. Upper endoscopy at that time revealed grade 1 gastric varices, and due to signs of portal hypertension, the patient was placed on the liver transplant list. However, liver synthetic function remained adequate, and he did therefore did not undergo transplantation. He was treated supportively with ursodeoxycholic acid, H_2-receptor antagonists, and antihypertensives.

At the age of 6 years, the patient was admitted to the hospital secondary to fever and abdominal pain. Magnetic resonance cholangiopancreatography (MRCP) demonstrated marked, nonobstructive, intrahepatic and extrahepatic biliary ductal dilation, consistent with Caroli disease. He was diagnosed with cholangitis and treated with a third-generation cephalosporin and metronidazole. A few months later, he had a recurrence of fever and abdominal pain. Percutaneous transhepatic cholangiography and liver biopsy were performed, which demonstrated multiple microabscesses, and culture of aspirated bile grew methicillin-resistant *Staphylococcus aureus* (MRSA). He was treated with vancomycin and ampicillin. Repeat percutaneous transhepatic cholangiography and liver biopsy 1 month later showed resolution of the MRSA and microabscesses following a course of antibiotics.

Over the course of the next few years, the patient developed chronic renal insufficiency, and at age 10 he underwent a living related donor kidney transplant. Before the transplantation, upper endoscopy was performed to evaluate for and potentially sclerose or band esophageal varices, of which none were found. MRCP 1 year later showed diffuse biliary ductal dilation, mildly increased from the previous examination, as well as multiple, tiny intrahepatic cysts, consistent with Caroli disease and hepatic fibrosis (Figure 10.4).

This case demonstrates a typical presentation of autosomal-recessive polycystic kidney disease, with the initial detection of enlarged kidneys, followed by imaging revealing multiple small cysts and associated cystic liver disease. Congenital hepatic fibrosis is always present in ARPKD,[99] but hepatic function and liver synthetic dysfunction are rare. This patient's illness represents the infantile type of ARPKD, with late development of intrahepatic biliary ductal dilation. He demonstrated several of the potential complications of portal hypertension and renal failure, and was treated with supportive care until decompensation necessitated renal transplantation. When he presented, it was debatable whether or not he would undergo renal transplantation or combined or sequential liver–kidney transplantation. As his hepatic synthetic function has remained normal, liver transplantation has not been necessary.

Surgical treatment may be indicated in symptomatic Caroli disease. Isolated disease may be treated with focal resection, and more extensive resection with hepaticojejunostomy or liver transplantation may be warranted in more diffuse disease or cirrhosis. Cholangiocarcinoma is the most common neoplasm associated with Caroli disease, with an incidence of 7–14%. This association, and the risk of disease progression in the remaining liver, should be considered when deciding on surgical management. Unfortunately, there are no definitive methods for detecting early cholangiocarcinoma. Serial CA 19-9 may be helpful.

References

1 Bristowe F. Cystic disease of the liver associated with similar disease of the kidneys. *Trans Pathol Soc London* 1856;**7**:229–34.

2 Desmet V. Congenital diseases of intrahepatic bile ducts: variations on the theme "ductal plate malformation." *Hepatology* 1992;**16**:1069–83.

3 Jørgensen MJ. The ductal plate malformation. *Acta Pathol Microbiol Scand Suppl* 1977;(**257**):1–87.

4 Desmet VJ. Intrahepatic bile ducts under the lens. *J Hepatol* 1985;**1**:545–59.

5 Desmet V, Callea F. Cholestatic syndromes of infancy and childhood. In: Zakim D, Boyer T, eds. *Hepatology: a Textbook of Liver Disease*, 2nd ed., vol. 2. Philadelphia: Saunders, 1990: 1355–95.

6 Desmet V. What is congenital hepatic fibrosis? *Histopathology* 1992;**20**:465–77.

7 Sung J, Huang X, Lin M, Ruaan C, Lin C, Chang T. Caroli's disease and congenital hepatic fibrosis associated with polycystic kidney disease. *Clin Nephrol* 1991;**38**:324–28.

8 Welling LW, Grantham JJ. Cystic disease of the kidney. In: Tisher CC, Brenner BM, eds. *Renal Pathology, with Clinical and Functional Correlations*. Philadelphia: Lippincott, 1989: 1233–75.

9 Gabow P, Bennett W. Renal manifestations: complications of management and long-term outcome of autosomal dominant polycystic kidney disease. *Semin Nephrol* 1991;**11**:643–52.

10 Piccoli D, Witzleben C. Disorders of the intrahepatic bile ducts. In: Walker W, Durie P, Hamilton J, Walker-Smith J, Watkins J, eds. *Pediatric Gastrointestinal Disease: Pathophysiology, Diagnosis, Management*. Philadelphia: Dekker, 1991: 1124–40.

11 Steiner D. Über grosscystische Degeneration der Nieren und der Leber. *Dtsch Med Wochenschr* 1899;**25**:677–8.

12 Fick G, Gabow P. The urgent complications of autosomal dominant polycystic kidney disease. *J Crit Illn* 1992;**7**:1905–20.

13 Martinez JR, Grantham JJ. Polycystic kidney disease: etiology, pathogenesis, and treatment. *Dis Mon* 1995;**41**:693–765.

14 Gabow PA. Autosomal dominant polycystic kidney disease. *N Engl J Med* 1993;**329**:332–42.

15 Vollmer W, Wahl P, Blagg C. Survival with dialysis and transplantation in patients with end-stage renal disease. *N Engl J Med* 1983;**308**:1553–58.

16 Low SH, Vasanth S, Larson CH, *et al.* Polycystin-1, STAT6 and P100 function in a pathway that transudes ciliary mechanosensation and is activated in polycystic kidney disease. *Dev Cell* 2006;**10**:57–69.

17 Reeders ST, Zerres K, Gal A, *et al.* Prenatal diagnosis of autosomal dominant polycystic kidney disease with a DNA probe. *Lancet* 1986;**ii**:6–8.

18 Kimberling WJ, Kumar S, Gabow PA, Kenyon JB, Connolly CJ, Somlo S. Autosomal dominant polycystic kidney disease: localization of the second gene to chromosome 4q13-q23. *Genomics* 1993;**18**:467–72.

19 Mochizuki T, Wu G, Hayashi T, Xenophontos SL, Veldhuisen B, Saris JJ. *PKD2*, a gene for polycystic kidney disease that encodes an integral membrane protein. *Science* 1996;**272**:1339–42.

20 Arnaout MA. Molecular genetics and pathogenesis of autosomal dominant polycystic kidney disease. *Ann Rev Med* 2001;**52**:93–123.

21 Wu G. Current advances in molecular genetics of autosomal-dominant polycystic kidney disease. *Curr Opin Nephrol Hypertens* 2001;**10**:23–31.

22 Gout AM, Martin NC, Brown AF, Ravine D. PKDB: Polycystic Kidney Disease Mutation Database—a gene variant database for autosomal dominant polycystic kidney disease. *Hum Mutat* 2007;**28**:654–9.

23 Grunfeld JP, Albouze G, Junger P. Liver changes and complications in adult polycystic kidney disease. *Adv Nephrol Necker Hosp* 1985;**14**:1–20.

24 Blyth H, Ockenden BG. Polycystic disease of kidney and liver presenting in childhood. *J Med Genet* 1971;**8**:257–84.

25 Fick G, Gabow P. Natural history of autosomal dominant polycystic kidney disease. *Ann Rev Med* 1994;**45**:23–9.

26 Milutinovic J, Fialkow P, Rudd T, Agodoa LY, Phillips LA, Bryant JI. Liver cysts in patients with autosomal dominant polycystic kidney disease. *Am J Med* 1980;**68**:741–4.

27 Gabow P, Johnson A, Kaehny W, Manco-Johnson ML, Duley IT, Everson GT. Risk factors for the development of hepatic cysts in autosomal dominant polycystic kidney disease. *Hepatology* 1990;**11**:1033–7.

28 Torres VE. Extrarenal manifestations of autosomal dominant polycystic kidney disease. *Am J Kidney Dis* 1999;**34**:45–8.

29 Milutinovic J, Schabel S, Ainsworth S. Autosomal dominant polycystic kidney disease with liver and pancreatic involvement in early childhood. *Am J Kidney Dis* 1989;**13**:334–44.

30 Everson G, Scherzinger A, Berger-Leff N, Juerg D, Manco-Johnson M, Gabow P. Polycystic liver disease: quantitation of parenchymal and cyst volumes from computed tomography images and clinical correlates of hepatic cysts. *Hepatology* 1988;**8**:1627–34.

31 Hateboer N, Lazarou LP, Williams AJ, Holmans P, Ravine D. Familial phenotype differences in PKD1. *Kidney Int* 1999;**56**:34–40.

32 Chapman AB, Rubinstein D, Hughes R, *et al.* Intracranial aneurysms in autosomal dominant polycystic kidney disease. *N Engl J Med* 1992;**327**:916–20.

33 Chauveau D, Pirson Y, Verelloen-Dumoulin C, Grunfeld J. Ruptured intracranial aneurysms in autosomal dominant polycystic kidney disease [abstract]. *J Am Soc Nephrol* 1992;**3**:293.

34 Hossack K, Leddy C, Johnson A, Schrier R, Gabow P. Echocardiographic findings in autosomal dominant polycystic kidney disease. *N Engl J Med* 1988;**319**:907–12.

35 Scheff R, Zuckerman G, Harter H, *et al.* Diverticular disease in patients with chronic renal failure due to polycystic kidney disease. *Ann Intern Med* 1980;**92**:202–4.

36 Vauthey J, Maddern G, Kolbinger P, Bae H. Clinical experience with adult polycystic liver disease. *Br J Surg* 1992;**79**:562–5.

37 Shedda S, Robertson A. Caroli's syndrome and adult polycystic kidney disease. *Aust N Z J Surg* 2007;**77**:292–4.

38 Hollingsworth A. The gallbladder in polycystic liver disease [letter]. *JAMA* 1982;**247**:462.

39 Harris R, Gray D, Britton J, Toogood G, Morris P. Hepatic cystic disease in an adult polycystic kidney disease transplant population. *Aust N Z J Surg* 1996;**66**:166–8.

40 Wallach PM, O'Donnell L, Leibowitz A, Adelman H, Flannery M. Symptomatic adult polycystic liver disease in a young woman. *J Fla Med Assoc* 1991;**78**:637–40.

41 Clive D, Davidoff A, Schweizer R. Budd–Chiari syndrome in autosomal dominant polycystic kidney disease: a complication of nephrectomy in patients with liver cysts. *Am J Kidney Dis* 1993;**21**:202–5.

42 Parfrey P, Bear J, Morgan J, *et al.* The diagnosis and prognosis of autosomal dominant polycystic kidney disease. *N Engl J Med* 1990;**323**:1085–90.

43 Bear J, Parfrey P, Morgan J, Martin CJ, Cramer BC. Autosomal dominant polycystic kidney disease: new information for genetic counseling. *Am J Med Genet* 1992;**43**:548–53.

44 Wilcox D, Weinreb J, Lesh P. MR imaging of a hemorrhagic hepatic cyst in a patient with polycystic liver disease. *J Comput Assist Tomogr* 1985;**9**:183–5.

45 Reeders S, Breuning M, Davies K. A highly polymorphic DNA marker linked to adult polycystic kidney disease on chromosome 16. *Nature* 1985;**317**:542–4.

46 Starzl T, Reyes J, Tzakis A, Mieles L, Todo S, Gordon R. Liver transplantation for polycystic liver disease. *Arch Surg* 1990;**125**:575–7.

47 Rogers J, Bueno B, Shapiro R, *et al.* Results of simultaneous and sequential pediatric liver and kidney transplantation. *Transplantation* 2001;**27**:1666–70.

48 Raffel C, McComb J. Arachnoid cysts. In: Cheek W, ed. *Pediatric Neurosurgery: Surgery of the Developing Nervous System*, vol. 3. Philadelphia: Saunders, 1994: 104–10.

49 Cole B. Autosomal recessive polycystic kidney disease. In: Gardner K, Bernstein J, eds. *The Cystic Kidney*. Dordrecht: Kluwer Academic, 1990: 327–50.

50 Zerres K, Mucher G, Bachner L, *et al.* Mapping of the gene for autosomal recessive polycystic kidney disease (ARPKD) to chromosome 6p21-cen. *Nat Genet* 1994;**7**:429–32.

51 Guay-Woodford LM, Muecher G, Hopkins SD, *et al.* The severe perinatal form of autosomal recessive polycystic kidney disease maps to chromosome 6p21.1-p12: implications for genetic counseling. *Am J Hum Genet* 1995;**56**:1101–7.

52 Lens XM, Onuchic LF, Wu G, *et al.* An integrated genetic and physical map of the autosomal recessive polycystic kidney disease region. *Genomics* 1997;**41**;463–6.

53 Mücher G, Becker J, Knapp M, *et al.* Fine mapping of the autosomal recessive polycystic kidney disease locus (PKHD1) and the genes MUT, RDS, CSNK2b, and GSTA1 at 6p21.2-p12. *Genomics* 1998;**48**:40–5.

54 Ward CJ, Hogan MC, Rossetti S, *et al.* The gene mutated in autosomal recessive polycystic kidney disease encodes a large, receptor-like protein. *Nat Genet* 2002;**30**:259–69.

55 Onuchic LF, Furu L, Nagasawa Y, *et al.* PKHD1, the polycystic kidney and hepatic disease 1 gene, encodes a novel large protein containing multiple immunoglobulin-like plexin-transcription-factor domains and parallel beta-helix 1 repeats. *Am J Hum Genet* 2002;**70**:1305–17.

56 Woollard JR, Punyashtiti R, Richardson S, *et al.* A mouse model of autosomal recessive polycystic kidney disease with biliary duct and proximal tubule dilatation. *Kidney Int* 2007;**72**:328–36.

57 Witzleben C. Cystic diseases of the liver. In: Zakim D, Boyer T. *Hepatology: a Textbook of Liver Disease*. Philadelphia: Saunders, 1990: 1395–11.
58 Zerres K, Mucher G, Becker J, *et al*. Prenatal diagnosis of autosomal recessive polycystic kidney disease (ARPKD): molecular genetics, clinical experience, and fetal morphology. *Am J Med Genet* 1998;**76**:137–44.
59 Roy S, Dillon MJ, Trompeter RS, Barratt TM. Autosomal recessive polycystic kidney disease: long-term outcome of neonatal survivors. *Pediatr Nephrol* 1997;**11**:302–6.
60 Jamil B, McMahon LP, Savige JA, Wang YY, Walker RG. A study of long-term morbidity associated with autosomal recessive polycystic kidney disease. *Nephrol Dial Transplant* 1999;**14**:205–9.
61 Benador N, Grimm P, Lavine J, Rosenthal P, Reznik V, Lemire J. Transjugular intrahepatic portosystemic shunt prior to renal transplantation in a child with autosomal-recessive polycystic kidney disease and portal hypertension: a case report. *Pediatr Transplant* 2001;**5**:210–4.
62 Kerr D, Okonkwo S, Choa R. Congenital hepatic fibrosis: the long-term prognosis. *Gut* 1978;**19**:514–20.
63 Alvarez F, Bernard O, Brunelle F, *et al*. Congenital hepatic fibrosis in children. *J Pediatr* 1981;**99**:370–5.
64 Bernstein J, Stickler GB, Neel IV. Congenital hepatic fibrosis: evolving morphology. *APMIS Suppl* 1988;**4**:17–26.
65 Fauvert R, Benhamou J. Congenital hepatic fibrosis. In: Schaffner F, Sherlock S, Leevy C, eds. *The Liver and its Diseases*. New York: Intercontinental Medical Book Corporation, 1974: 283–8.
66 Witzleben C, Sharp A. "Nephronophthisis—congenital hepatic fibrosis": an additional hepatorenal disorder. *Hum Pathol* 1982; **13**:728–33.
67 Proesmans W, Moerman P, De Praetere M, Van Damme B. Association of bilateral renal dysplasia and congenital hepatic fibrosis. *In J Pediatr Nephrol* 1986;**7**:113–6.
68 Tazelaar H, Payne J, Patel S. Congenital hepatic fibrosis and asymptomatic familial adult-type polycystic disease in a 19-year old woman. *Gastroenterology* 1984;**86**:757–60.
69 Landing BH, Wells TR, Claireaux AE. Morphometric analysis of liver lesions in cystic diseases of childhood. *Hum Pathol* 1980;**11**(5 Suppl):549–60.
70 Buts J, Otte J, Claus D, Van Craynest MP, De Meyer R. [Choledochus cyst: a case with dilatation of the intrahepatic bile ducts and congenital liver fibrosis; in French.] *Helv Paediatr Acta* 1980;**35**:289–95.
71 Nakamura F, Sasak, H, Kajihara H, Yamanoue M. Laurence–Moon–Biedl syndrome accompanied by congenital hepatic fibrosis. *J Gastroenterol Hepatol* 1990;**5**:206–10.
72 Thapa B, Sahni A, Mehta S. Familial congenital hypoplasia of depressor anguli oris muscle with congenital hepatic fibrosis. *Indian Pediatr* 1989;**26**:82–5.
73 Maggiore G, Borgna-Pignatti C, Marni E, *et al*. Pulmonary arteriovenous fistula: an unusual complication of congenital hepatic fibrosis. *J Pediatr Gastroenterol Nutr* 1983;**2**:183–6.
74 Williams R, Scheuer P, Heard B. Congenital hepatic fibrosis with an unusual pulmonary lesion. *J Clin Pathol* 1964;**17**:135–42.
75 Evans J, Harris O, VanDeth A. Congenital hepatic fibrosis associated with Mallory bodies and copper retention. *Aust N Z J Med* 1984;**14**:500–3.
76 Abdullah A, Nazer H, Atiyeh M, Ali M. Congenital hepatic fibrosis in Saudi Arabia. *J Trop Pediatr* 1991;**37**:240–3.
77 Pelletier V, Galeano N, Brochu P, *et al*. Secretory diarrhea with protein-losing enteropathy, intestinal lymphangiectasia and congenital hepatic fibrosis. *J Pediatr* 1986;**108**:61–5.
78 Bayraktar Y, Balkanci F, Kayhan B. *et al*. Congenital hepatic fibrosis associated with cavernous transformation of the portal vein. *Hepatogastroenterology* 1997;**44**:1588–94.
79 Murray-Lyon I, Ockenden B, Williams R. Congenital hepatic fibrosis—is it a single clinical entity? *Gastroenterology* 1978;**64**: 653–6.
80 Fiorillo A, Migliorati R, Varo P, Caldore M, Vecchione R. Congenital hepatic fibrosis with gastrointestinal bleeding in early infancy. *Clin Pediatr* 1982;**21**:183–4.
81 McGonigle RJS, Mowat AP, Bewick M, *et al*. Congenital hepatic fibrosis and IPCD: role of portocaval shunting and transplantation in 3 patients. *QJM* 1981;**199**:269–72.
82 De Ville de Goyet, J, Alberti D, Falchetti D, *et al*. Treatment of extrahepatic portal hypertension in children by mesenteric-to-left portal vein bypass: a new physiological procedure. *Eur J Surg* 1999;**165**:777–81.
83 De Vos M, Barbier F, Cuvenlier C. Congenital hepatic fibrosis. *J Hepatol* 1988;**6**:222–8.
84 Caroli J, Couinaud C, Soupault R, Porcher P, Eteve J. [A new disease, undoubtedly congenital, of the bile ducts: unilobar cystic dilation of the hepatic ducts; in French.] *Sem Hop* 1958;**34**:496–502.
85 Mall J, Chahreman, G, Boyer J. Caroli's disease associated with congenital hepatic fibrosis and renal tubular ectasia. *Gastroenterology* 1974;**66**;1029–53.
86 Jordan D, Harpaz N, Thung S. Caroli's disease and adult polycystic kidney disease: a rarely recognized association. *Liver* 1989;**9**:30–5.
87 Bass EM, Funston MR, Shaff MI. Caroli's disease: an ultrasonic diagnosis. *Br J Radiol* 1977;**50**:366–9.
88 Hermansen M, Starshak R, Werlin S. Caroli disease: the diagnostic approach. *J Pediatr* 1979;**94**:879–82.
89 Moreno AJ, Parker AL, Spice MJ, Brown TJ. Scintigraphic and radiographic findings in Caroli's disease. *Am J Gastroenterol* 1984;**79**:299–303.
90 Berrebi G, Erickson R, Marks, B. Autosomal dominant polycystic liver disease: a second family. *Clin Genet* 1982;**21**:342–7.
91 Simon P, Ang K, Charasse C, Ghali N, Catroux B, Houitte H. [Hepatic polycystic disease is not always associated with polycystic kidney: epidemiological data; in French.] *Rev Med Interne* 1993;**14**:1037.
92 Pirson Y, Lannoy N, Peters D, Geubel A, Gigot J, Breuning M. Isolated polycystic liver disease as a distinct genetic disease, unlinked to polycystic kidney disease 1 and polycystic kidney disease 2. *Hepatology* 1996;**23**:249–52.
93 Reynolds DM, Falk CT, Li A, *et al*. Identification of a locus for autosomal dominant polycystic liver disease, on chromosome 19p13.2-13.1. *Am J Hum Genet* 2000;**67**:1598–604.
94 Drenth JP, Te Morsche RH, Smink R, Bonifacino JS, Jansen JB. Germline mutations in PRKSCSH are associated with autosomal dominant polycystic liver disease. *Nat Genet* 2003;**33**:345–7.
95 Li A, Tian X, Sung SW, Somio S. Identification of two novel polycystic kidney disease-1-like genes in human and mouse genomes. *Genomics* 2003;**81**:596–608.

96 Drenth JP, Martina JA, Te Morsche RH, Jansen JB, Bonifacino JS. Molecular characterization of hepatocystin, the protein that is defective in autosomal dominant polycystic liver disease. *Gastroenterology* 2004;**126**:1819–27.
97 Davila S, Furu L, Gharavi AG, *et al.* Mutations in *SEC63* cause autosomal dominant polycystic liver disease. *Nat Genet* 2004;**36**: 575–7.
98 Karhunen P, Tenhu M. Adult polycystic liver and kidney disease are separate entities. *Clin Genet* 1986;**30**:29–37.
99 Tahvanainen E, Tahvanainen P, Kaariainen H, Hockerstedt K. Polycystic liver and kidney diseases. *Ann Med* 2005;**37**:546–55.
100 Qian Q, Li A, King BF, *et al.* Clinical profile of autosomal dominant polycystic liver disease. *Hepatology* 2003;**37**:164–71.
101 Richter GM, Noeldge G, Palmaz JC, *et al.* Transjugular intrahepatic portacaval stent shunt: preliminary clinical results. *Radiology* 1990;**174**:1027–30.
102 Zemel, G, Katzen BT, Becker GJ, Benenati JF, Sallee DS. Percutaneous transjugular portosystemic shunt. *JAMA* 1991; **266**:390–3.
103 Jalan R, Lui HF, Redhead DN, Hayes PC. TIPS 10 years on. *Gut* 2000;**46**:578–81.
104 Ong JP, Sands M, Younossi ZM. Transjugular intrahepatic portosystemic shunts (TIPS): a decade later. *J Clin Gastroenterol* 2000;**30**:14–28.
105 Johnson SP, Leyendecker JR, Joseph FB, *et al.* Transjugular portosystemic shunts in pediatric patients awaiting liver transplantation. *Transplantation* 1996;**62**:1178–81.
106 Heyman MB, LaBerge JM, Somberg KA, *et al.* Transjugular intrahepatic portosystemic shunts (TIPS) in children. *J Pediatr* 1997;**131**:914–9.
107 Hackworth CA, Leef JA, Rosenblum JD, Whitington PF, Millis JM, Alonso EM. Transjugular intrahepatic portosystemic shunt creation in children: initial clinical experience. *Radiology* 1998; **206**:109–14.
108 Kimura BT, Hasegawa T, Oue T, *et al.* Transjugular intrahepatic portosystemic shunt performed in a 2-year-old infant with uncontrollable intestinal bleeding. *J Pediatr Surg* 2000;**35**:1597–9.
109 Spillane RM, Kaufman JA, Powelson J, Geller SC, Waltman AC. Successful transjugular intrahepatic portosystemic shunt creation in a patient with polycystic liver disease. *AJR Am J Roentgenol* 1997;**169**:1542–4.
110 Bahramipour PF, Festa S, Biswal R, Wachsberg RH. Transjugular intrahepatic portosystemic shunt for the treatment of intractable ascites in a patient with polycystic liver disease. *Cardiovasc Intervent Radiol* 2000;**23**:232–4.
111 Shin ES, Darcy MD. Transjugular intrahepatic portosystemic shunt placement in the setting of polycystic liver disease: questioning the contraindication. *J Vasc Intervent Radiol* 2001;**12**: 1099–2002.
112 Wang S, Luo Y, Wilson's PD, Witman GB, Zhou J. The autosomal recessive polycystic kidney disease protein is localized to primary cilia, with concentration in the basal body area. *J Am Soc Nephrol* 2004;**15**:592–602.
113 Ward CJ, Yuan D, Masyuk TV, *et al.* Cellular and subcellular localization of the ARPKD protein; fibrocystin is expressed on primary cilia. *Hum Molec Genet* 2003;**12**:2703–10.
114 Davenport JR, Toder BK. An incredible decade for the primary cilium: a look at a once-forgotten organelle. *Am J Physiol Renal Physiol* 2005;**289**:F1159–69.
115 Lowden DA, Lindemann, GW, Merlino G, Barash BD, Calvet JP, Gattone VH. Renal cysts in transgenic mice expressing transforming growth factor-alpha. *J Lab Clin Med* 1994;**124**:386–94.
116 Richards WG, Sweeney WE, Yoder BK, Wilkinson JE, Woychik RP, Avner ED. Epidermal growth factor receptor activity mediates renal cyst formation in polycystic kidney disease. *J Clin Invest* 1998;**101**:935–9.
117 Sweeney WE, Futey L, Frost P, Avner ED. In vitro modulation of cyst formation by a novel tyrosine kinase inhibitor. *Kidney Int* 1999;**56**:406–13.
118 Qian Q, Harris PC, Torres VE. Treatment prospects for autosomal-dominant polycystic kidney disease. *Kidney Int* 2001;**59**:2005–22.
119 Torres VE. Vasopressin antagonists in polycystic kidney disease. *Kidney Int* 2005;**68**:2405–18.
120 Ehren H. Benign liver tumors in infancy and childhood. Report of 48 cases. *Am J Surg* 1983;**145**:325–9.
121 Boon LM, Burrows PE, Paltiel HJ, *et al.* Hepatic vascular anomalies in infancy: a twenty-seven-year experience. *J Pediatr* 1996;**129**:346–54.
122 Burrows PE, Dubois J, Kassarjian A. Pediatric hepatic vascular anomalies. *Pediatr Radiol* 2001;**31**:533–45.
123 Kassarjian A, Dubois J, Burrows PE. Angiographic classification of hepatic hemangiomas in infants. *Radiology* 2002;**222**:693–98.
124 Stocker J, Ishak K. Mesenchymal hamartoma of the liver. A 35-year review. *Arch Surg* 1990;**125**:598–600.
125 Bejarano PA, Serrano MF, Casillas J, *et al.* Concurrent infantile hemangioendothelioma and mesenchymal hamartoma in a developmentally arrested liver of an infant requiring hepatic transplantation. *Pediatr Dev Pathol* 2003;**6**:552–7.
126 Stocker J, Ishak K. Focal nodular hyperplasia of the liver: a study of 21 pediatric cases. *Cancer* 1981;**48**:336–45.
127 Dehner L. Hepatic tumors in the pediatric age group. In: Rosenberg H, Bolande R, eds. *Perspectives in Pediatric Pathology*, vol. 4. Chicago: Year Book Medical, 1978: 241–251.
128 Emre S, McKenna GJ. Liver tumors in children. *Pediatr Transplant* 2004:**8**:632–8.
129 Mehrabi A, Kashfi A, Schemmer P, *et al.* Surgical treatment of primary hepatic epithelioid hemangioendothelioma. *Transplantation* 2005;**80**(1 Suppl):S109–12.
130 Tomiyama T, Uchida K, Yoshida K, *et al.* Giant cavernous hemangioma of the liver and multiple primary malignant tumors in a patient with suspected familial inhibition of natural killer cell activity—a case report. *Jpn J Surg* 1989;**19**:216–22.
131 Diez Redondo P, Velicia Llames R, Caro-Paton A. Familial hepatic hemangiomas. *Gastroenterol Hepatol* 2004;**27**:314–6.
132 Kitajima S, Lio E, Morimoto M, *et al.* Transgenic rabbits with increased VEGF expression develop hemangiomas in the liver: a new model for Kasabach–Merritt syndrome. *Lab Invest* 2005; **85**:1517–27.
133 Hu D, Ran YL, Zhong X, *et al.* Overexpressed Derlin-1 inhibits ER expansion in the endothelial cells derived from human hepatic cavernous hemangioma. *Biochem Mol Biol* 2006;**39**:677–85.
134 Ma W, Tessarollo L, Hong SB, *et al.* Hepatic vascular tumors, angiectasis in multiple organs, and impaired spermatogenesis in mice with conditional inactivation of the VHL gene. *Cancer Res* 2003;**63**:5320–8.
135 Takahashi K, Iida K, Okimura Y, *et al.* A novel mutation in the von Hippel–Lindau tumor suppressor gene identified in a

Japanese family with pheochromocytoma and hepatic hemangioma. *Intern Med* 2006;**45**:265–9.

136 Iyer CP, Stanley P, Mahour GH. Hepatic hemangiomas in infants and children: a review of 30 cases. *Am Surg* 1996;**62**: 356–60.

137 Lunetta P, Karikoski R, Penttila A, Sajantila A. Sudden death associated with a multifocal type II hemangioendothelioma of the liver in a 3-month-old infant. *Am J Forensic Med Pathol* 2004;**25**:56–9.

138 Wananukul S, Voramethkul W, Nuchprayoon I, Seksarn P. Diffuse neonatal hemangiomatosis: report of 5 cases. *J Med Assoc Thai* 2006;**89**:1297–303.

139 Morimura Y, Fujimori K, Ishida T, Ito A, Nomura Y, Sato A. Fetal hepatic hemangioma representing non-reassuring pattern in fetal heart rate monitoring. *J Obstet Gynaecol Res* 2003;**29**: 347–50.

140 Chen CC, Kong MS, Yang CP, Hung IJ. Hepatic hemangioendothelioma in children: analysis of thirteen cases. *Acta Paediatr Taiwan* 2003;**44**:8–13.

141 Vauthey JN, Tomczak RJ, Helmberger T, *et al.* The arterioportal fistula syndrome: clinicopathologic features, diagnosis, and therapy. *Gastroenterology* 1997;**113**:1390–1.

142 Kim IO, Cheon JE, Kim WS, *et al.* Congenital intrahepatic portohepatic venous shunt: treatment with coil embolisation. *Pediatr Radiol* 2000;**30**:336–8.

143 Alpay F, Kurekci A, Gunesli S, Gokcay E. Klippel–Trenaunay–Weber syndrome with hemimegalencephaly. Report of a case. *Turkish J Pediatr* 1996;**38**:277–80.

144 Haber M, Reuben A, Burrell M, Oliverio P, Salem R, West B. Multiple focal nodular hyperplasia of the liver associated with hemihypertrophy and vascular malformations. *Gastroenterology* 1995;**108**:1256–62.

145 Vase P, Grove O. Gastrointestinal lesions in hereditary hemorrhagic telangiectasis. *Gastroenterology* 1986;**91**:1079–83.

146 Bardequez A, Chatterjee M, Tepedino M, Sicuranza B. Systemic cystic angiomatosis in pregnancy: a case presentation and review of the literature. *Am J Obstet Gynecol* 1990;**163**:42–5.

147 Alt B, Hafez GR, Trigg M, Shahidi NT, Gilbert EF. Angiosarcoma of the liver and spleen in an infant. *Pediatr Pathol* 1985;**4**:331–9.

148 Nord KM, Kandel J, Lefkowitch JH, *et al.* Multiple cutaneous infantile hemangiomas associated with hepatic angiosarcoma: case report and review of the literature. *Pediatrics* 2006;**118**; e907–13.

149 Ramírez Ramírez CR, Saavedra S, Ramírez Ronda C. Bacillary angiomatosis: microbiology, histopathology, clinical presentation, diagnosis and management. *Bol Asoc Med P R* 1995;**87**:140–6.

150 Herrera LO, Glassman CI, Teixido RA, Oglesby JT 2nd, Andrade EL, Rodrigue RB. Peliosis hepatis associated with cavernous hemangioma and hepatocarcinoma. *Am Surg* 1981;**47**:502–6.

151 Samad S, Maimunah A, Zulfiqar A, Zaharah M. Ultrasound (US) and computed tomographic (CT) appearances of large (giant) hepatic cavernous hemangiomas. *Med J Malaysia* 1995; **50**:82–6.

152 Sepulveda W, Donetch G, Giuliano A. Prenatal sonographic diagnosis of fetal hepatic hemangioma. *Eur J Obstet* 1993;**48**: 73–6.

153 Paltiel H, Patriquin H, Keller M, Babcock D, Leithiser R. Infantile hepatic hemangioma: Doppler US. *Radiology* 1992;**182**: 735–42.

154 Ernst H, Hahn E, Balzer T, Schlief R, Heyder N. Color Doppler ultrasound of liver lesions: signal enhancement after intravenous injection of the ultrasound contrast agent Levovist. *J Clin Ultrasound* 1996;**24**:31–5.

155 Kaufman R. Is cystic mesenchymal hamartoma of the liver similar to infantile hemangioendothelioma and cavernous hemangioma on dynamic computed tomography? *Pediatr Radiol* 1992;**22**:582–3.

156 Numata K, Isozaki T, Morimoto M, Sugimori K, Kunisake R, Tanaka K. Prospective study of differential diagnosis of hepatic tumors by pattern-based classification of contrast-enhanced sonography. *World J Gastroenterol* 2006;**12**:6290–8.

157 Kassarjian A, Zurakowski D, Dubois J, Paltiel HJ, Fishman SJ, Burrows PE. Infantile hepatic hemangiomas: clinical and imaging findings and their correlation with therapy. *AJR Am J Roentgenol* 2004;**182**:785–95.

158 Rodríguez-Balderrama I, Rodríguez-Juárez DA, Rodríguez-Bonito R, Quiroga-Garza A. [Hepatic hemangioma in a premature newborn. The magnetic resonance images; in Spanish.] *Bol Med Hosp Infant Mex* 1993;**50**:121–4.

159 Andronikou S, Soin S, Nafoos O, Platt K, Lakhoo K. Hepatic mesenchymal hamartoma mimicking hemangioma on multiple-phase gadolinium-enhanced MRI. *J Pediatr Hematol Oncol* 200;**28**:322–4.

160 Sun XJ, Quan XY, Huang FH, Xu YK. Quantitative evaluation of diffusion-weighted resonance imaging of focal hepatic lesions. *World J Gastroenterol* 2005;**11**:6535–7.

161 Hori M, Murakami T, Kim T, *et al.* Hemodynamic characterization of focal hepatic lesions: role of ferucarbotran-entranced dynamic MR imaging using T2-weighted multishot spin-echo-planar sequence. *J Magn Reson Imaging* 2006;**23**:509–19.

162 Schmitz SA, Nikolova A, O'Regan D, Albrecht T, Hohmann J. Quantitative assessment of iron-oxide-enhanced magnetic resonance imaging of the liver: vessel isointensity is a potential characteristic of liver hemangiomas on late T1-weighted images. *Acta Radiol* 2006;**47**:634–42.

163 Mhanni AA, Chodirker BN, Evans JA, *et al.* Fetal hepatic haemangioendothelioma: a new association with elevated maternal serum alpha-fetoprotein. *Prenat Diagn* 2000;**20**:432–5.

164 Qin LX, Tang ZY. The prognostic molecular markers in hepatocellular carcinoma. *World J Gastroenterol* 2002;**8**:385–92.

165 Huang SA, Tu HM, Harney JW, *et al.* Severe hypothyroidism caused by type 3 iodothyronine deiodinase in infantile hemangiomas. *N Engl J Med* 2000;**34**:185–9.

166 Tung G, Cronan J. Percutaneous needle biopsy of hepatic cavernous hemangioma. J Clin Gastroenterol 1993;**16**:117–22.

167 Kaw Y, Esparza A. Cytologic diagnosis of cavernous hemangioma of the liver with fine-needle biopsy. *Diagn Cytopathol* 1991;**7**:628–30.

168 Saeger W. [Vascular tumors of the liver. Morphology, differential diagnosis, prognosis; in German.] *Fortschr Med* 1990;**108**: 329–33.

169 Pontisso P, Barzon M, Basso G, Cedchetto G, Perilongo G, Alberti A. Cytokeratin patterns in childhood primary liver tumors. Int J Clin Lab Res 1993;**23**:225–7.

170 Mo JQ, Dimashkieh H, Bove KE. GLUT1 endothelial reactivity distinguishes hepatic infantile hemangioma from congenital hepatic vascular malformation with associated capillary proliferation. *Hum Pathol* 2004;**35**:200–9.

171 Adegboyega PA, Qiu S. Hemangioma versus vascular malformation. Presence of nerve bundle is a diagnostic clue for vascular malformation. *Arch Pathol Lab Med* 2005;**129**:772–5.

172 Frischer JS, Huang J, Serur A, Kadenhe A, Yamashiro DJ, Kandel JJ. Biomolecular Markers and Involution of Hemangiomas. *J Pediatr Surg* 2004;**39**:400–4.

173 Shimada M, Matsumata T, Ikeda Y, *et al.* Multiple hepatic hemangiomas with significant arterioportal venous shunting. *Cancer* 1994;**73**:304–7.

174 Lemarchand-Venencie F. [Management of hemangioma in the infant; in French.] *J Malad Vasc* 1992;**17**:33–40.

175 Ezekowitz RA, Mulliken JB, Folkman J. Interferon alfa-2a therapy for life-threatening hemangiomas of infancy. *N Engl J Med* 1992;**326**:1456–63.

176 Wörle H, Maass E, Köhler B, Treuner J. Interferon alpha-2a therapy in haemangiomas of infancy: spastic diplegia as a severe complication. *Eur J Pediatr* 1999;**158**:344.

177 Perez J, Pardo J, Gomez C. Vincristine—an effective treatment of corticoid-resistant life-threatening infantile hemangiomas. *Acta Oncol* 2002;**41**:197–9.

178 Yamamoto T, Kawarada Y, Yano T, Noguchi T, Mizumoto R. Spontaneous rupture of hemangioma of the liver: treatment with transcatheter hepatic arterial embolization. *Am J Gastroenterol* 1991;**86**:1645–9.

179 Kullendorff CM, Cwikiel W, Sandstrom S. Embolization of hepatic hemangiomas in infants. *Eur J Pediatr Surg* 2002;**12**:348–52.

180 Warmann S, Bertram H, Kardorff R, Sasse M, Hausdorf G, Fuchs J. Interventional treatment of infantile hepatic hemangioendothelioma. *J Pediatr Surg* 2003;**38**:1177–81.

181 Kretschmar O, Knirsch W, Bernet V. Interventional treatment of a symptomatic neonatal hepatic cavernous hemangioma using the Amplatzer vascular plug. *Cardiovasc Intervent Radiol* 2006 Oct 6 [Epub ahead of print].

182 Luks F, Yazbeck S, Brandt M, Bensoussan A, Brouchu P, Blanchard H. Benign liver tumors in children: a 25-year experience. *J Pediatr Surg* 1991;**26**:1326–30.

183 Walsh R, Harrington J, Beneck D, Ozkaynak MF. Congenital infantile hepatic hemangioendothelioma type II treated with orthotopic liver transplantation. *J Pediatr Hematol Oncol* 2004; **26**:121–3.

184 Subramanyan R, Narayan R, Costa DD, Derweesh A, Khusaiby SM. Transcatheter coil occlusion of hepatic arteriovenous malformation in a neonate. *Indian Heart J* 2001;**3**:782–4.

185 Ono H, Mawatari H, Mizoguchi N, Eguch T, Sakura N. Clinical features and outcome of eight infants with intrahepatic portovenous shunts detected in neonatal screening for galactosaemia. *Acta Paediatr* 1998;**87**:631–4.

186 Sharif K, English M, Ramani P, *et al.* Management of hepatic epithelioid haemangio-endothelioma in children: what option? *Br J Cancer* 2004;**90**:1498–501.

187 Gottschling S, Schneider G, Myer S, Reinhard H, Dill-Mueller D, Graf N. Two infants with life-threatening diffuse neonatal hemangiomatosis treated with cyclophosphamide. *Pediatr Blood Cancer* 2006;**46**:239–42.

11 Nonalcoholic Steatosis

Eve A. Roberts

Introduction

Steatosis—the accumulation of fat in hepatocytes—is a feature of many liver diseases. Steatosis is categorized as "large-droplet" (macrovesicular) when one or a few fat droplets nearly fill the hepatocyte, or as "small-droplet" (microvesicular) when numerous tiny droplets are found, giving the hepatocyte a somewhat foamy appearance. Inflammation may also be present. In adults, alcoholic liver disease is a common cause of steatosis. Although alcoholic liver disease may occur in adolescents, it is rare in younger children. In children, the causes of steatosis include certain drugs, such as methotrexate, various inherited metabolic disorders, and liver disease associated with obesity and/or disordered action of insulin, known as nonalcoholic fatty liver disease (NAFLD), which has become very common and is the major focus of this chapter. Microvesicular steatosis, associated with mitochondrial dysfunction or sodium valproate toxicity, is discussed in detail in Chapters 5, 9, and 13.

NAFLD in adults

Childhood NAFLD must be considered in the context of the disease in adults. In the late 1970s, chronic liver disease associated with obesity (with or without hyperlipidemia and with or without non–insulin-dependent diabetes mellitus) was described as a new and separate disease entity.[1,2] This condition was originally called "nonalcoholic steatohepatitis" (NASH), because it resembled alcoholic hepatitis histologically but was not due to ethanol abuse. Recently, the more inclusive term "nonalcoholic fatty liver disease" (NAFLD) has come into general use, as it includes the entire spectrum—simple hepatic steatosis without inflammation, NASH, and the resulting cirrhosis in which steatosis may no longer be prominent. NAFLD is highly prevalent in adult populations.[3]

Diseases of the Liver and Biliary System in Children, 3rd edition. Edited by Deirdre Kelly. © 2008 Blackwell Publishing, ISBN: 978-1-4051-6334-7.

NAFLD occurs in both men and women, and although most adult patients with NAFLD are obese (with a body mass index > 30) and many have type 2 diabetes mellitus, not all affected patients are obese.[4] They may be entirely asymptomatic or have only nonspecific constitutional symptoms. Serum aminotransferases are modestly elevated, but serum bilirubin is normal or near-normal and biochemical features of cholestasis are not present. Findings suggestive of an autoimmune process may be present, such as increased serum immunoglobulin G (IgG) and nonspecific tissue autoantibodies detectable in low titer. Hyperlipidemia is usually due to hypertriglyceridemia.

Hepatic histology is required for defining the NAFLD lesion rigorously.[5] In adults, there is a broad spectrum of findings: macrovesicular steatosis without or with active inflammation; mild to moderate fibrosis; or cirrhosis. If there is no inflammation, then the condition is considered to be simple steatosis, since by definition NASH involves inflammation and/or fibrosis (Figure 11.1). Signs of inflammation include ballooning degeneration of hepatocytes or focal hepatocyte drop-out. In typical adult-pattern NASH, neutrophils are usually found adjacent to degenerating hepatocytes, and Mallory bodies may be found in hepatocytes. If these are not obvious, histological staining for ubiquitin may reveal this feature.[6] Inflammation and fibrosis, often pericellular, are typically most severe in the perivenular zone. This histological pattern is now called type 1 NASH. In adults, these histological findings can be associated with other disease processes, notably Wilson's disease, and medications/herbs causing a "pseudo-alcoholic hepatitis" lesion. Chronic hepatitis C, particularly with genotype 3 infection, may be associated with steatosis and metabolic syndrome.[7] How much alcohol can be consumed by an individual before hepatic steatosis should be attributed to alcohol excess rather than to NAFLD remains somewhat controversial, but it is generally put at < 20 g per day.

NAFLD in adults is no longer regarded as a trivial disorder. Its increasing prevalence and the accumulating evidence for severe outcomes have reversed this assessment. Most adults with pure steatosis do not have progressive liver disease,[8] and weight reduction generally leads to improvement in serum aminotransferases.[9] In a prospective, relatively

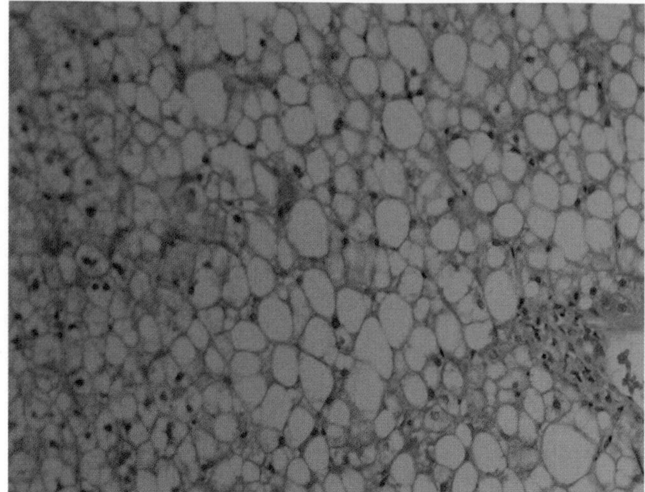
A

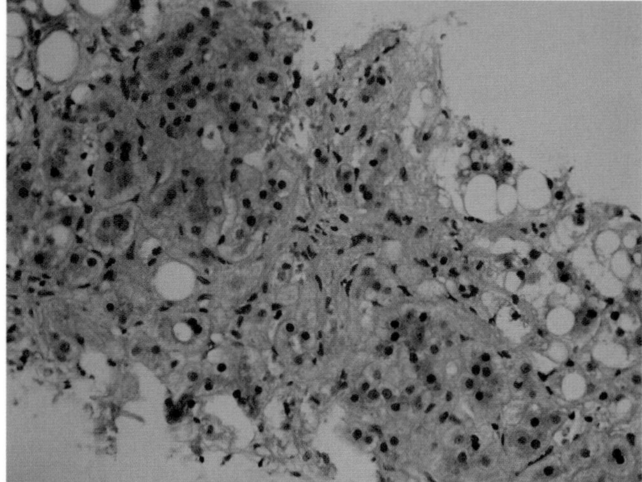
B

Figure 11.1 The liver biopsy in nonalcoholic fatty liver disease may demonstrate a spectrum of histological changes, which include macrovesicular steatosis, inflammation, Mallory bodies, and fibrosis, which sometimes develops into cirrhosis. Severe steatosis and inflammation (**A**) can progress to fibrosis (**B**).

unselected, study in the United States of 420 adult Minnesotan patients with NAFLD, the overall survival was less than that predicted for the general population, and approximately 5% of these patients developed cirrhosis and chronic liver failure.[10] In another study of adults with an average follow-up of 6.5 years, Kaplan–Meier analysis showed that the 5-year probability of survival in NAFLD was 67% and the 10-year survival was 59%.[11] Serial biopsy studies in adults NAFLD suggest that in many, fibrosis is slowly progressive.[12,13] Other studies suggest that 8–17% of adults with NASH ultimately develop cirrhosis.[3,14,15] Some adult patients with NAFLD eventually require liver transplantation; unfortunately, NAFLD may recur after liver transplantation.[16–18] Hepatocellular carcinoma can complicate NAFLD in adults.[19–22]

Pathogenesis of NAFLD

Hyperinsulinemia

Although NAFLD is a complex and possibly heterogeneous disorder, certain features of its pathogenesis have become clear (Figure 11.2). Hyperinsulinemia, in association with insulin resistance, is an essential component of the disease mechanism.[23–26] In many adult patients, NAFLD appears to be the hepatic manifestation of the metabolic syndrome. Differences between insulin resistance in the liver and peripheral tissues may account for some of the features of NAFLD. The greater insulin resistance in muscles and adipose tissue in comparison with the liver leads to mobilization of free fatty acids and hepatocellular deposition of free fatty acids. Equally, the hepatic response to insulin appears to be more disordered for lipid handling than for glucose metabolism. Moreover, hyperinsulinemia leads to mobilization of stored lipid (and adipocytokines) from adipose tissue and promotes hepatic steatosis. Increased plasma free fatty acids (FFAs; also known as nonesterified fatty acids) play an important role in the development of steatosis and inflammation.[27–31] FFAs are highly destructive in tissues and damage intracellular membranes through lipid peroxidation; FFA injury to mitochondria results in decreased β-oxidation of hepatic FFAs. Insulin inhibits oxidation of free fatty acids, and thus hyperinsulinemia may enhance free fatty acid hepatotoxicity. FFAs also activate hepatocellular signaling pathways related to inflammation and apoptosis.[32–34] Hyperinsulinemia may affect other pathways such as suppressors of cytokine signaling (SOCS)[35] and sterol response-element binding protein-1c (SREBP-1c),[36,37] which regulates hepatocellular glucose, triglyceride synthesis, and fat metabolism. Insulin up-regulates hepatocellular SOCS-3, which in turn down-regulates hepatocellular insulin receptors, and thus is potentially capable of promoting acquired insulin resistance in the liver. Both insulin and certain SOCS proteins upregulate SREBP-1c. With the abundance of available FFAs, up-regulation of SREBP-1c probably accounts for increased hepatocellular production of triglycerides and very-low-density lipoproteins, and thus the hypertriglyceridemia, which is characteristic of NAFLD. Recent reports suggest that other hepatocellular transcription factors, such as LXR, may play a role in the development of steatosis.[38,39]

The notion of a "two-hit" pathogenesis for NASH holds that hepatic steatosis occurs first, and then the transition to steatosis with inflammation/fibrosis requires further injurious factor(s).[40] It is possible that such injury stems directly from FFA toxicity to hepatocellular organelles and inflammatory or fibrogenic pathways that FFA can activate.[29,41,42] More often, this injury is categorized as oxidant stress or systemic inflammation. Candidate factors include mitochondrial dysfunction, functional changes due to cytokines such as tumor necrosis factor-α (TNF-α), increased toxification by

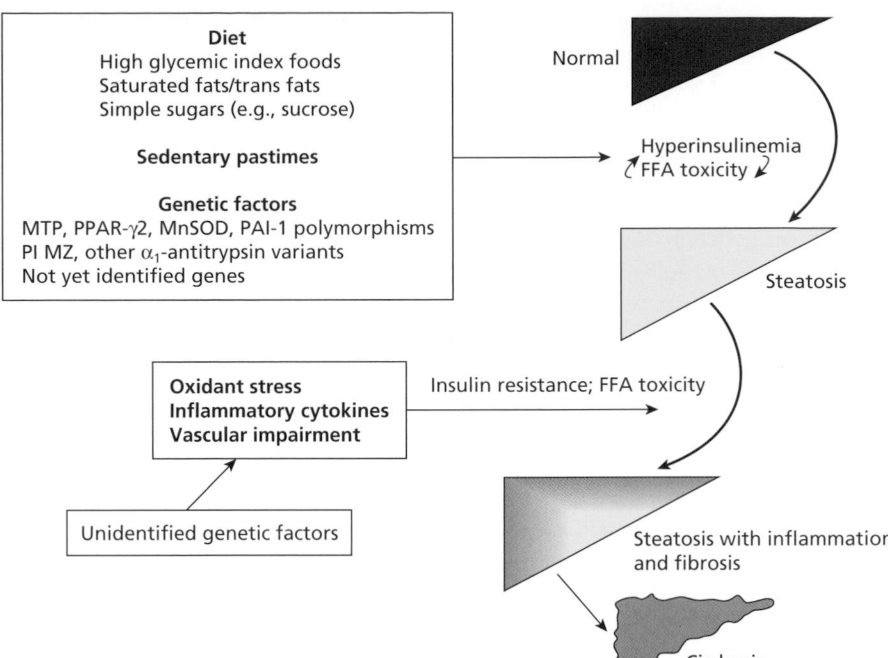

Figure 11.2 Elements in the pathogenesis of nonalcoholic fatty liver disease (NAFLD). NAFLD is typical of a polygenic disorder with a complex interaction between the environment (increased carbohydrate and fat intake, increased sedentary pastimes) and host characteristics, including genetic factors. Contributors to the pathogenesis of NAFLD may differ from patient to patient. Hyperinsulinemia (later, insulin resistance) and free fatty acid (FFA) toxicity are self-reinforcing. Many details of this disease mechanism are still unknown, including how it may vary in children in comparison with adults.

cytochromes P450 such as CYP2E1,[43,44] or by peroxisomes, or decreased cytoprotection in hepatocytes. Ongoing low-grade inflammation has been documented in obese adults, mainly with C-reactive protein and serum fibrinogen as sensitive markers for systemic inflammation.[45–47] Inflammatory factors can promote the hepatic metabolic disorder: specifically, increased hepatic levels of TNF-α enhance insulin resistance and mitochondrial production of reactive oxygen species.[48]

Recent studies indicate that similar mechanisms operate in children with NAFLD. An early clue to the importance of hyperinsulinemia/insulin resistance in childhood NAFLD was the finding of acanthosis nigricans, which is associated with hyperinsulinemia and is due to hyperplasia of pigmented skin cells bearing receptors for insulin and insulin-like growth factors,[49] in 30–50% of affected children (Figure 11.3).[50] Direct measurement of serum insulin and use of validated surrogate markers for insulin resistance such as the Homeostasis Model Assessment of Insulin Resistance (HOMA-IR) have shown that most children with NAFLD have hyperinsulinemia and insulin resistance.[51–53] Whether children with NAFLD have the "metabolic syndrome" is a difficult question, because of the lack of a consensus definition for metabolic syndrome in childhood. Children with acanthosis nigricans and obesity early in life may have the earliest clinical features of the metabolic syndrome.[54] Obese children have been found to have increased levels of circulating inflammatory factors[55,56] and decreased levels of antioxidants.[57,58]

A current concept for the development of NAFLD in children postulates that overnutrition and inadequate physical exercise lead to critical metabolic changes that involve sustained hyperinsulinemia and consequently hepatic steatosis. Currently, children typically eat energy-rich, palatable, and often nonsatiating foods; these foods contain a large proportion

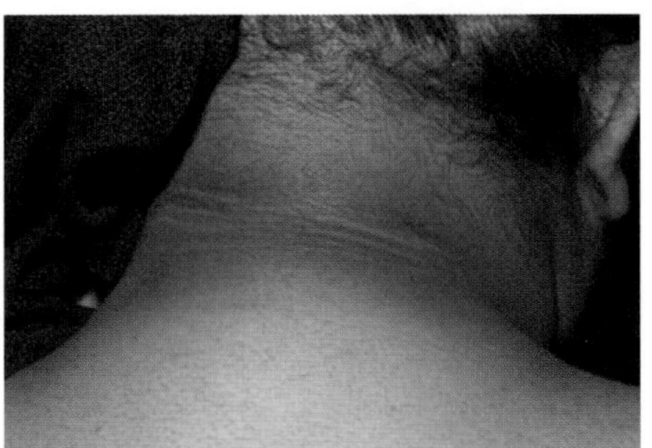

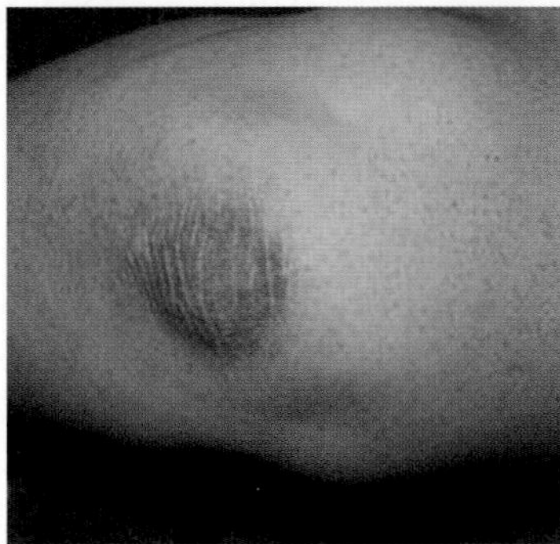

Figure 11.3 Acanthosis nigricans is a bluish-black pigmentation of the skin that is characteristic of insulin resistance from any cause. This young girl has grade 4 acanthosis nigricans in association with obesity, polycystic ovary syndrome, and nonalcoholic fatty liver disease.

of sugars (such as sucrose and high-density fructose) and saturated and/or *trans*-fats, but relatively little fiber. This type of diet can lead to hyperinsulinemia, provide exogenous FFAs, and drive the liver toward lipogenesis.[59,60] If energy intake exceeds energy utilization, excess weight or obesity will develop. Emerging data suggest that mechanisms in the central nervous system relating to satiety and peripheral metabolism may enhance peripheral hyperinsulinemia.[61–63] Thus, a complex, self-reinforcing metabolic disorder may develop. NAFLD represents only the hepatic manifestation of this disordered metabolism, and obviously other organ systems can be adversely affected.

Adipocytokines

Adipose tissue is hormonally active, not just a repository of fat. The metabolically active proteins it produces are known as adipocytokines. Some of these (TNF-α, adiponectin, and resistin) affect insulin action. Of these, adiponectin may be the most important. Adiponectin interferes with insulin action by modifying insulin receptor function and altering hepatocellular FFA metabolism. It has potent anti-inflammatory effects.[34,64] In addition to hyperinsulinemia, adult and pediatric NAFLD patients have decreased plasma levels of adiponectin.[65–67]Childhood obesity is associated with low serum adiponectin concentrations,[68,69] and the severity of insulin resistance in obese children is inversely correlated with the serum adiponectin concentration.[70,71] In adult NAFLD, histological abnormalities on liver biopsy are more severe in patients with lower serum adiponectin concentrations.[72] Resistin is an adipocytokine that has been linked to insulin resistance and obesity in animal and human studies;[73,74] however, the data for resistin's role in NAFLD are more convincing in animal models than in human disease and are not very strong in childhood obesity.

Leptin, a satiety factor synthesized in white adipose tissue, binds to hypothalamic receptors to reduce appetite and increase energy expenditure.[75,76] Genetically obese, diabetic mice (*ob/ob* mice) have a mutation that prevents the synthesis of leptin and thus they overeat, becoming obese. They also have insulin resistance, hyperlipidemia, and fatty livers.[77] Paradoxically, in NAFLD there is leptin resistance, with elevated plasma levels of leptin. Leptin resistance has also been identified as a feature of the metabolic syndrome.[78] Treatment of childhood NAFLD with leptin is thus unlikely to be of benefit. The exception is patients with lipodystrophy syndromes, in whom leptin deficiency is found.[79]

Genetic factors

Attempts to identify a genetic basis include examining the genes involved in the formation of adipose tissue and the development of insulin resistance, alcoholic liver disease, or related metabolic diseases. For example, the gene encoding 11β-hydroxysteroid dehydrogenase 1, which converts cortisone to cortisol, may be important in predisposing to the metabolic syndrome.[80] Validation of candidate genes can be difficult. Diverse genes have been implicated: a low-activity promoter polymorphism in the *MTP* gene,[81] mitochondrial manganese superoxide dismutase (MnSOD)—a polymorphism in the promoter region of the TNF-α gene—has been identified in association with NAFLD, but its mechanistic role requires further clarification.[82,83] Candidate polymorphisms relevant to childhood obesity and insulin resistance include the PPAR-γ2 Pro12Ala polymorphism,[84] PAI-1 6754G/5G polymorphism,[85] and variable repeats in the insulin gene.[86] Apolipoprotein E, which is polymorphic and functions as a modifier protein for other hepatic disorders, may function as a modifier gene in NAFLD.[87] Partial deficiency of α_1-antitrypsin is prevalent among patients with NAFLD, but whether this increases disease severity is unclear.[88,89]

What has become evident is that children from certain ethnic backgrounds are predisposed to NAFLD. These include Hispanics, mainly non-Cuban; Asians, specifically from China, the Philippines, and Japan; and indigenous peoples of North and South America.[90–92] Afro-Americans are less often affected.[93] Similar patterns of incidence have been described in adults.[91]

Childhood obesity

Childhood obesity has become a major public health problem.[94] Current estimates of the prevalence of excess weight and obesity in children depend on the definitions used. Definitions may use absolute weight, percentage of ideal weight-for-height, or age- and gender-normative data for body mass index (BMI), in which it is accepted that a BMI of > 25 is considered to represent excess weight and a BMI of > 30 is considered as obesity.[95,96] These definitions hold only for adolescents over the age of 18 and have to be redefined on an age-related basis for younger children. The multicultural analysis by the International Obesity Task Force provides a definitional strategy for BMI,[97] which is slightly different from that of the American Centers for Disease Control (CDC). Recent estimates for the worldwide incidence of childhood obesity are that 7–8% of children and adolescents in the 5–17-year-old age bracket are overweight and 2–3% of them are obese.[98] In general, the incidence of childhood obesity has doubled or tripled in the past 20 years in most economically advantaged countries.[99–103] In addition to diet, decreased physical activity, with more time spent watching television or working at a computer, is an important factor for this epidemic of childhood obesity. Other factors in early childhood, including disordered sleep patterns (with too little sleep), may play a role.[104] Although the exact relationship between childhood obesity and type 2 diabetes mellitus is uncertain, the incidence of both primary hypertension and type 2 diabetes mellitus has risen dramatically in children in the past decade.[95,105]

Epidemiology of NAFLD in children

Numerous large series of childhood NAFLD have now been reported. The initial reports included comparatively few patients and were subject to selection bias; since key definitional issues had not yet been sorted out, interpretation is difficult. The continuing lack of large prospective surveys of children for NAFLD makes it difficult to determine the prevalence of NAFLD in children, especially as this may vary in different populations. A broad cross-sectional study in California that looked at NAFLD in children who had died accidentally and were subject to examination by the coroner (742 children) found significant steatosis in 13%.[92] An ultrasonographic study of 810 schoolchildren from northern Japan demonstrated an overall prevalence of fatty liver in 2.6%, which had a strong correlation with indices of obesity such as BMI.[106] In the National Health and Examination Survey, cycle III (NHANES III) in the USA, serum alanine aminotransferase (ALT) and γ-glutamyltransferase (GGT) were measured in 2450 children aged 12–18 years, who were classified as "obese" if the BMI was above the 95th percentile for age and gender or as "overweight" if it was between the 85th and 95th percentiles. In this relatively unselected study, 6% of the overweight and 10% of the obese adolescents had an elevated ALT, but alcohol use could not be excluded.[107] The incidence of NAFLD among overweight/obese children is also not certain. In an Italian study, 42% of 375 morbidly obese children aged 9–16 were found to have hepatic steatosis on sonography.[108] In a Hong Kong study, 77% of 84 obese children had hepatic steatosis on sonography and 24% had sonographic evidence of hepatic steatosis plus elevated serum ALT.[109]

The first reports of childhood NASH appeared in the 1980s. Moran and colleagues reported three obese American children with fatty liver and steatohepatitis.[110] Other small studies documented the relationship between childhood obesity, elevated serum aminotransferases, hypertriglyceridemia, hyperlipidemia, and ultrasonographic evidence of steatosis,[111–113] while others confirmed the presence on liver biopsy of steatohepatitis,[114] fibrosis, and even cirrhosis.[115]

The first large clinical series of pediatric NAFLD included 36 patients from a variety of ethnic backgrounds collected prospectively between 1985 and 1995 at the Hospital for Sick Children in Toronto.[50] The male–female ratio was 3 : 2, and the patients were 4–16 years old at the time of diagnosis; 20% of whom were under the age of 10 at diagnosis. Most patients were obese (weight > 20% above ideal weight for height); the range was 114–192% of ideal weight for height. Approximately 30% of the cohort had acanthosis nigricans. Two brothers had Bardet–Biedl syndrome; one adolescent female had polycystic ovary syndrome. Nonspecific autoantibodies—most often low-titer anti-smooth muscle antibodies—were present in a few patients. Four children developed diabetes mellitus after the diagnosis of NAFLD had been established. Liver biopsy was performed in 24 patients, 71% of whom had some fibrosis. One child had cirrhosis at the age of 9. Weight loss was associated with improvement in serum aminotransferases.

A series of 17 patients, including one child with Alström syndrome, reported from Adelaide,[116] and a series of 27 in Montreal[117] had similar findings. Most of the children were obese and asymptomatic, although some had either abdominal pain or fatigue. Hypertriglyceridemia was found in 56% of the patients and hyperuricemia in 18%.[117] In the Adelaide series, one child was cirrhotic, three had simple steatosis, and the rest had NASH.[116] Thirty-nine children, predominantly male, with NAFLD have been described in Texas (R.H. Squires Jr. and M.J. Lopez, personal communication). This report highlighted the importance of ethnicity: 20 were Hispanic, 14 Caucasian, four Asian, and one Afro-American. Five children had recovered from childhood cancer. Acanthosis nigricans was present in more than 40%, and fasting serum insulin was three times the upper limit of normal in 17 patients. Thirty-one children underwent liver biopsy, which revealed steatohepatitis in all 31, fibrosis in 21, and cirrhosis in two children. Familial clustering of NAFLD was prominent in a large American study,[118] which highlighted a 14-year-old male with cirrhosis whose mother also had NAFLD with less severe fibrosis.

Large prospective series in San Diego[119] and Rome[52] have established the importance of hyperinsulinemia and/or insulin resistance in pediatric NAFLD. The San Diego study included 100 children ranging in age from 2–18 (mean age 12), of whom 65 were male, two-thirds were Hispanic, and 92% were obese. Laboratory findings included a mean ALT 104 U/L, mean aspartate aminotransferase (AST) 65 U/L, mean serum triglycerides 181 mg/dL, and a mean HOMA-IR of 11. Most children (84%) had NASH, but none had cirrhosis. The Rome study included 84 children, of whom 59 were male; the mean age was 11.7 years (range 3–18.8 years. In this study, 40% of the children included were obese and 51% were overweight. Liver test abnormalities were milder than in the San Diego study (mean ALT 76, mean AST 35). Although the mean HOMA-IR was 2.7 (range 0.7–6.7), 61% of these children had a HOMA-IR > 2). Liver biopsy revealed simple steatosis in 14 and NASH in the rest. Another American study limited to adolescents with morbid obesity (n = 41; BMI range 42–88) found modest elevations in serum aminotransferases (mean ALT 38, mean AST 35) and insulin resistance in every patient, with a mean HOMA-IR of 10.9 (range 2.5–27.1). On liver biopsy, performed at the time of gastric bypass surgery, there was simple steatosis in 10 and NASH in the rest; none of the patients had cirrhosis.[120]

Clinical features

The most common clinical presentation is the incidental finding of isolated hepatomegaly or slightly elevated serum aminotransferases in a child who may have:

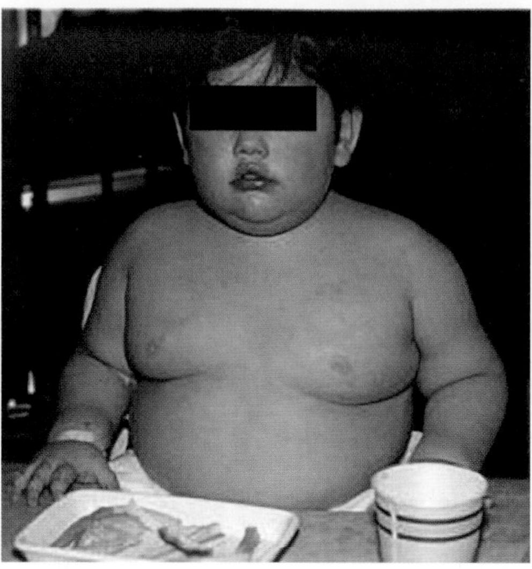

Figure 11.4 Nonalcoholic fatty liver disease (NAFLD) is a common disease in children with obesity, type 2 diabetes mellitus, and a number of inherited metabolic conditions. This boy developed hyperphagia, excessive weight gain, and fatty liver after hypothalamic surgery. Three years later, he developed splenomegaly and was found to have cirrhosis and portal hypertension.

- Excess weight or obesity (Figure 11.4). It is essential to use an age- and gender-adjusted guide to BMI for children, since the adult thresholds for excess weight (BMI 25) and obesity (BMI 30) only apply to individuals over 18 years old. Either the CDC tables or the boundary data for the International Obesity Task Force[97] can be used. Otherwise, the degree of adiposity may be greatly underestimated in young children. Recent reports suggest that measuring waist circumference can be useful for screening children for risk for NAFLD, but extensive data are not yet available. Waist circumference reflects abdominal adiposity. The waist–height ratio may also be a simple and relevant anthropometric measurement.[121] It has the advantage of being easy to calculate.
- Type 1 or 2 diabetes mellitus. The association of fatty liver and insulin resistance in adults with type 2 diabetes has been well defined and occurs in 10–75%. It is now thought to be a significant factor for mortality.[122] Fatty liver has also been described in children with type 1 diabetes mellitus, particularly if it is not well controlled (Mauriac syndrome). The typical child with NAFLD, however, has hyperinsulinemia with insulin resistance but is euglycemic.
- Acanthosis nigricans is associated with insulin resistance and is an important physical sign. It is graded 1–4, depending on severity (Figure 11.3).
- Previous chemotherapy. Obesity with or without the metabolic syndrome of obesity, hyperinsulinemia, and hyperlipidemia[123,124] in survivors of childhood neoplasia is a well-recognized problem, particularly following acute lymphoblastic leukemia.[124–128] This may explain a higher incidence of NAFLD, although other factors such as the drug treatment for childhood neoplasia may play a role.

Hypothalamic dysfunction or surgery

Children with congenital or postsurgical hypothalamic dysfunction—for example, after resection of a craniopharyngioma—may be hyperphagic and obese. Recent reports suggest that they are at risk for NAFLD with rapid development of cirrhosis.[129–135] NAFLD has been found in patients with Prader–Willi syndrome (PWS).

Metabolic disease

Fatty liver closely resembling NAFLD is associated with a number of metabolic or genetic diseases, which include the following.

Alström syndrome. Alström syndrome is a rare autosomal recessive disorder which is similar to Bardet–Biedl syndrome. It is characterized by pigmentary retinopathy with infantile cone–rod dystrophy, obesity, sensorineural deafness, dilated cardiomyopathy, diabetes mellitus with insulin resistance, and normal intelligence.[136,137] The genetic basis of Alström syndrome is mutations in the gene *ALMS1*.[138–140] There are numerous reports of associated hepatic dysfunction with Alström syndrome: the liver disease includes a spectrum from mild steatosis, portal inflammation, and moderate fibrosis[141] to hepatic steatosis with cirrhosis.[142,143] An 8-year-old girl with Alström syndrome who was obese with hyperinsulinemia with type 2 diabetes mellitus developed rapidly progressive NAFLD with decompensated cirrhosis at the age of 8.[144]

Bardet–Biedl syndrome. Bardet–Biedl syndrome is characterized by progressive loss of visual acuity due to retinal dystrophy, central obesity, renal dysgenesis leading to progressive renal insufficiency, and male hypogonadism. Polydactyly or other abnormalities of the extremities are variable features, and mental retardation appears to occur in only a few patients.[145] Type 2 diabetes mellitus may develop in these patients because of defective insulin receptor function.[145–147] Bardet–Biedl syndrome is genetically heterogeneous, with at least six different loci associated with the phenotype;[148,149] candidate gene products may be responsible for the functional disorder or may act as gene modifiers.[150,151] Cirrhosis has been reported in one patient previously.[152]

Polycystic ovary syndrome (PCOS). PCOS is a multisystem endocrine disorder of adolescent[153] and young adult women, characterized mainly by disorders of ovulation with menstrual disorders, features of androgen excess including hirsutism and acne, and structurally abnormal ovaries. Central obesity occurs in half of the patients. Acanthosis nigricans is frequently present (Figure 11.3).[154] Insulin resistance appears to be due to insulin receptor dysfunction or to postreceptor mechanisms.[155,156] Hyperinsulinemia intensifies the adverse effects of androgen excess. Hypertriglyceridemia is often present. Recent reports confirm that NAFLD occurs in PCOS.[157–159] Modest weight loss (5–10% overall) or metformin improves ovarian function and diminishes other features of androgen excess.[160–162]

Turner syndrome. Girls with Turner syndrome (XO) are often obese. Abnormal liver biochemistry has been attributed to hormonal treatment, including administration of growth hormone and estrogen, as in two girls aged 13 and 14 who had steatosis and fibrosis on liver biopsy.[163] Another 4-year-old with Turner syndrome and severe obesity (body weight 159% of ideal weight) had elevated ALT years prior to hormone treatment.[164]

Lipodystrophy. Lipodystrophy/lipoatrophy syndromes are primary disorders of insulin action, and hyperinsulinemia is associated with relative insulin resistance.[165] They are genetically heterogeneous. *AGPAT2* is mutated in congenital generalized lipodystrophy.[166] The gene product, 1-acylglycerol-3-phosphate *O*-acyltransferase, is involved in the synthesis of triacylglycerol and glycerophospholipids. In a different form of congenital generalized lipodystrophy, mutations are found in *BSCL2*, the gene product of which is a novel human protein called seipin, a protein of unknown function, although it is homologous to G-protein.[167] Some autosomal familial partial lipodystrophies are associated with mutations in *LMNA*, which encodes lamin A/C, a nuclear envelope protein.[168,169] Lamin A has been shown to interact with SREBP-1 and -2, which is at least a candidate mechanism for fatty liver.[170] Other autosomal familial partial lipodystrophies are associated with mutations in *PPARG*, which encodes the peroxisome proliferator-activated receptor-γ.[171] These observations in the lipodystrophy syndromes not only support the contention that hyperinsulinemia associated with insulin resistance is critical in the pathogenesis of NAFLD but also indicate some genes and gene products that may be important in the disease mechanism of NAFLD.

Patients with lipodystrophy/lipoatrophy syndromes have a complete or partial lack of adipose tissue, elevated insulin and low leptin levels. The most severely affected patients develop diabetes mellitus. NAFLD has been detected in patients with congenital forms of lipodystrophy, including one patient who later underwent liver transplantation.[172–174] The severity of the hepatic steatosis is proportional to the extent of extrahepatic fat loss.

Miscellaneous disorders. Typical features of NAFLD have been described in patients with mulibrey (muscle, liver, brain, eye) nanism, which is due to mutations in the *TRIM37* gene, which encodes a peroxisomal protein acting as a ubiquitin ligase.[175] NAFLD cirrhosis has been reported in both a child and an adult with Dorfman–Chanarin syndrome (ichthyotic neutral lipid storage disease).[176,177] In this disorder, *ABHD5* is mutated; its gene product is an enzyme with an esterase/lipase/thioesterase subfamily that serves as a cofactor to adipose triglyceride lipase and thus helps regulate lipolysis.[178] The significance of NAFLD in a 16-year-old male with a distal 1p36 deletion and clinical features of Cantu syndrome is not evident.[179]

Diagnostic approach

It is important to consider and exclude alternative etiologies for hepatic steatosis in any child who appears to have NAFLD[180] (Table 11.1). Many metabolic diseases can be eliminated on the basis of medical history. Competing diagnoses that require specific evaluation include:

- Chronic hepatitis C, which should be excluded by serology (anti-hepatitis C virus antibodies and hepatitis C virus RNA).
- Wilson's disease (Chapter 14), which may present with prominent hepatic steatosis. Serum ceruloplasmin and 24-h basal urinary copper excretion should be measured; doubtful cases require liver biopsy for histology and parenchymal copper determination.
- Cystic fibrosis (CF). Hepatic steatosis is a very common liver abnormality that affects 30–40% of CF patients[181] (Chapter 12). It should be excluded by sweat testing; in difficult cases, mutation analysis is advisable.
- Drug hepatotoxicity, especially methotrexate.

The main investigations are listed in Table 11.2 but should include:

- Routine hematology and liver function tests. Laboratory studies show that serum ALT is more elevated than serum AST.
- Urea and electrolytes
- Thyroid function tests
- Fasting (or 9 a.m.) cortisol
- Hemoglobin A_{1c}
- Fasting lipids. Hypertriglyceridemia is the typical blood lipid abnormality.
- Autoantibodies, immunoglobulins, and relevant metabolic investigations. Liver biopsy may be required to distinguish between NAFLD and autoimmune hepatitis in an overweight/obese child.
- Viral serology for hepatitis B and hepatitis C viruses, cytomegalovirus, Epstein–Barr virus (see also Chapter 6).
- Abdominal ultrasound. Studies in adults show that imaging can identify patients with hepatic steatosis quite accurately, especially if the steatosis is moderately severe, but does not distinguish simple steatosis from NASH[182] (Figure 11.5). Microvesicular steatosis due to inherited mitochondrial disorders, urea cycle disorders, and valproic acid hepatotoxicity may occasionally be severe enough to be identified by liver sonography and should be excluded by a careful history and/or relevant metabolic testing (see Chapters 5, 9, and 14).
- Liver biopsy is important for the diagnosis of NAFLD and may distinguish between NASH and other possible diagnoses. The optimal timing of liver biopsy has not been determined.

Table 11.1 Differential diagnosis of fatty liver in children with macrovesicular steatosis.

Nutritional
Nonalcoholic fatty liver disease
Hyperphagic disorders (congenital or acquired disorders of hypothalamus)
Jejuno-ileal bypass; gastric reduction operations
Dehydration, severe infection
Acute starvation
Protein-calorie malnutrition (kwashiorkor)
Total parenteral nutrition

Systemic disease
Chronic hepatitis C
Celiac disease
Inflammatory bowel disease
Diabetes mellitus
Nephrotic syndrome

Drugs
Amiodarone
Methotrexate
Prednisone/glucocorticoids
L-Asparaginase
Vitamin A
Ethanol

Inherited metabolic disorders with dysregulated insulin action
Bardet–Biedl syndrome
Alström syndrome
Polycystic ovary syndrome
Lipodystrophy syndromes

Inherited metabolic disorders
Cystic fibrosis
Wilson's disease
α_1-Antitrypsin deficiency
Hereditary tyrosinemia, type I
Homocystinuria
Galactosemia
Hereditary fructose intolerance
Glycogen storage diseases (mainly types I, VI)
Sialidosis, mannosidosis, fucosidosis
Refsum disease
Abeta- or hypobetalipoproteinemia
Neutral lipid storage disease
Cholesterol ester storage disease
Dorfman–Chanarin syndrome
Tangier disease
Familial hyperlipoproteinemias
Citrullinemia, argininemia, arginosuccinic aciduria (ornithine transcarbamylase deficiency; mainly microvesicular fat)
Systemic carnitine deficiency (usually microvesicular fat)
Weber–Christian disease
Chronic granulomatous disease
Porphyria cutanea tarda
Shwachman syndrome (pancreatic insufficiency)

Table 11.2 Diagnostic approach to the investigation of nonalcoholic fatty liver disease/nonalcoholic steatohepatitis.

Groups to be investigated
All children with:
- Simple obesity or excess weight, especially those with increased waist circumference
- Acanthosis nigricans
- history of certain interventions—e.g., cranial surgery and bone-marrow transplantation in whom ALT and/or AST have been raised at least twice in a 6-month period
- Type 2 diabetes mellitus

Routine blood tests
Full blood count and coagulation
Urea and electrolytes, uric acid
Liver function tests: bilirubin, AST, ALT, ALP, GGT, albumin; the ALT/AST ratio should be documented

Tests to exclude other causes of liver disease
Autoantibodies, immunoglobulins, and complement C3, C4
Copper and ceruloplasmin
α_1-Antitrypsin level and PI type
Amino and organic acids
Iron, ferritin
Thyroid function tests
Serology for CMV, EBV, HBV and HCV
Sweat chloride

Fasting lipids
Cholesterol
Triglycerides
HDL-cholesterol
Low-density lipoprotein

Fasting metabolic tests (possibly useful; † mainly research)*
Glucose
Insulin
Adiponectin*
C-peptide†
Leptin†
Lactate†
Free fatty acids*
3-hydroxybutyrate†

Ultrasonography of the abdomen (and ovaries if female)
Liver biopsy for histopathology and frozen specimen
DEXA scan for body fat composition and distribution

ALP, alkaline phosphatase; ALT, alanine aminotransferase; AST, aspartate aminotransferase; CMV, cytomegalovirus; DEXA, dual-energy x-ray absorptiometry; EBV, Epstein–Barr virus; GGT, γ-glutamyltransferase; HBV, hepatitis B virus; HCV, hepatitis C virus; HDL, high-density lipoprotein; PI, protease inhibitor.

Some have advocated deferring liver biopsy in children with possible NASH until after a trial of weight loss for 3–6 months; if weight loss is not achieved and serum aminotransferases remain elevated, a liver biopsy is performed. Early

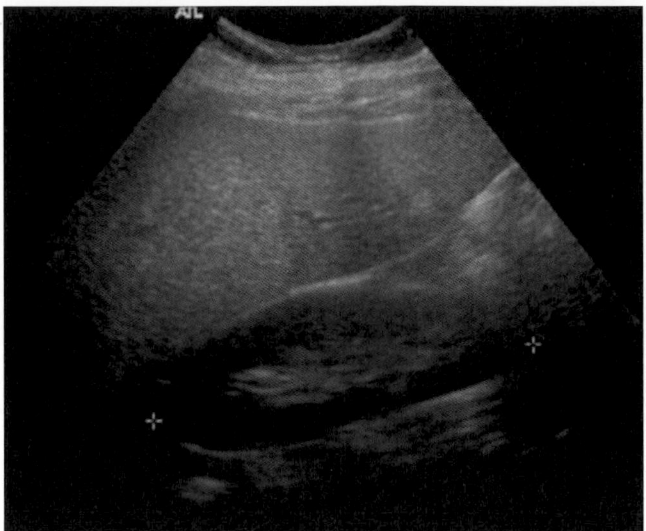

Figure 11.5 Sonogram of the liver in nonalcoholic fatty liver disease (NAFLD) demonstrates hyperreflectivity, suggestive of fatty infiltration. It should be noted how bright the liver is in comparison with the kidney. This is not specific for NAFLD, as similar appearances may be found in cystic fibrosis. Serial liver ultrasound examinations may demonstrate progression (or regression) of the disease.

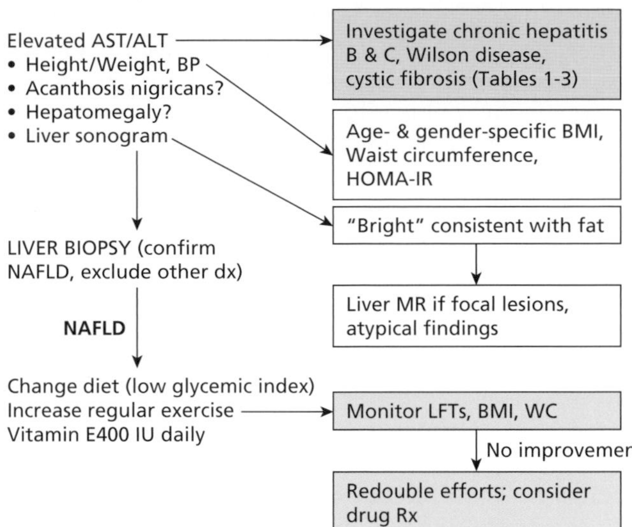

Figure 11.6 The approach to diagnosis and treatment. Most patients are asymptomatic and are referred because of elevated serum aminotransferases or findings on liver sonography consistent with steatosis. The timing of liver biopsy remains somewhat controversial, but it is required in order to confirm the diagnosis of nonalcoholic fatty liver disease (NAFLD) and assess inflammatory activity and the extent of fibrosis. Thus, liver biopsy should not be unduly delayed. Treatment modalities are not yet defined for children; clinical trials are in progress. HOMA-IR, Homeostasis Model Assessment of Insulin Resistance; NAFLD, nonalcoholic fatty liver disease; WC, waist circumference.

biopsy for younger children or those with acanthosis nigricans is reasonable, but insufficient data are available to evaluate these criteria systematically. Liver biopsy is essential when entities in the differential diagnosis cannot be excluded on clinical grounds. Histological findings in childhood NASH may be slightly different from those in adults with NASH,[183,184] but the essential findings of macrovesicular steatosis, inflammation or its residua, and fibrosis are present in the majority of cases.[50] Both the histological scoring and the histological features of NAFLD in children require further precision (Figure 11.1).

• Measurement of insulin resistance. These include fasting insulin and glucose. A formula for estimating insulin resistance, namely HOMA-IR,[185] has been validated for use in children.[186] The cut-off for insulin resistance is higher in children than in adults.[187] Its use is mainly limited to the research setting; however, it probably has clinical utility.

It is important to have a consistent approach to evaluating children with hepatic steatosis, which expedites the diagnostic process and facilitates treatment. A model based on current practice is shown in Figure 11.6.

Treatment

The approach to treatment is best within a multidisciplinary management team to deal with the diverse aspects of this disorder (medical, endocrinological, dietary, psychosocial). Treatment is directed towards management of obesity and insulin resistance or reducing oxidative stress. The usual reported end points for judging efficacy are normalization of serum aminotransferases or loss of steatosis on sonographic examination; histological improvement on liver biopsy has been reported only infrequently.

Obesity

The only treatment so far shown to be convincingly effective in childhood NAFLD is the treatment of obesity by weight loss. Reduction in body weight has led to normalization of serum aminotransferases in several clinical series,[50,111,116,188] while substantial improvement in liver histology was reported in one pediatric patient.[111] Although it has not been established how much weight must be lost to achieve improvement, the usual strategy is to reduce caloric intake and increase moderately intense aerobic exercise. Achieving and maintaining weight loss in children is difficult, especially as nutrition must be maintained for general growth. Well-designed studies examining treatment of childhood obesity have shown that a specific diet designed to minimize hyperinsulinemia may be more effective than the conventional low-calorie diet.[189–191] This low glycemic index diet may be easier to maintain over the long term than a calorie-restricted diet and consists of comparatively straightforward food inclusions/restrictions: inclusion of fruits, vegetables, legumes, whole-grain or high-fiber or traditionally processed grains and pasta, and exclusion or limited consumption of white potatoes, sugar (sucrose), and highly refined white flour.[192] Portion sizes should be rationalized. Complementing the child's weight-reduction regimen with family-based behavioral intervention may also enhance success.[193–195] Instituting a regimen of regular physical exercise is important, as exercise also reduces hyperinsulinemia.

Drug treatment of insulin resistance/ oxidative stress

Few pharmacological treatments have been investigated in either children or adults. Treatment directed towards reducing insulin resistance includes weight loss, but some drugs have been used:

• Metformin, which appears to act directly on SREBP-1c,[196,197] has been used for the treatment of NASH in adults.[198] In a 24-week, open clinical trial of metformin (500 mg twice daily) in 10 pediatric patients with biopsy-proven NASH, significant improvements in mean serum ALT were found. After treatment, ALT was normal in 40% of the patients; moreover, steatosis, measured by magnetic resonance spectroscopy, showed a mean reduction of 23% in 90% of the patients.[199] Metformin has been used effectively in children with obesity and evidence of insulin resistance.[200,201] It has also been used effectively for the treatment of children with type 2 diabetes mellitus,[202,203] polycystic ovary syndrome,[162,204] and Prader–Willi syndrome.[205] Favorable results with metformin as a treatment for NASH in adults have been reported.[206] A multicenter randomized controlled trial in pediatric NAFLD is being conducted.[207]

• Thiazolidinediones. Studies have been performed only in adults with NAFLD. Rosiglitazone treatment for 48 weeks decreased insulin resistance, serum ALT, and fibrosis.[208] The findings were similar with pioglitazone, but the drug was tolerated better.[209] Pioglitazone combined with vitamin E was more effective than vitamin E by itself in improving histological abnormalities.[210] Most patients experience weight gain despite hepatic improvement; anxiety about potential adverse effects of this class of drugs (for example, the cardiovascular risk with rosiglitazone) restrains enthusiasm about their use in NAFLD.

Drugs used to reduce or prevent lipid peroxidation or oxidative stress include *N*-acetylcysteine (used in the treatment of acetaminophen toxicity and acute liver failure), for which there are no specific data in NASH. The role of probiotics has hardly been explored. Others include:

• Ursodeoxycholic acid. A small randomized controlled trial of ursodeoxycholic acid (10.0–12.5 mg/kg/day was conducted, including 31 children with NAFLD diagnosed by sonography. There was no additional benefit over weight reduction and diet, and ursodeoxycholic acid alone was ineffective in improving liver biochemistries and the sonographic appearance.[211]

• Vitamin E (400–1200 IU/day orally), in an open-label pilot study in 11 children with NASH, was associated with improvements in serum aminotransferases, but there was no major change in BMI or in the sonographic appearance of the liver. Biochemical relapse occurred in two children who discontinued vitamin E.[212] In a small randomized controlled trial in children, vitamin E treatment showed some improvement in serum aminotransferases, but no change in apparent steatosis.[213] Studies in adult patients have also been inconsistent.[214,215]

Since hyperleptinemia and leptin resistance occur in NAFLD, simple supplementation along this regulatory pathway is unlikely to be effective. By contrast, in generalized lipodystrophy syndromes characterized by defective expression of leptin, leptin supplementation has improved hepatic steatosis.[216]

Standards of care for bariatric surgery in children and adolescents have not been established,[217,218] and the role of such surgery for the typical child with NAFLD remains uncertain. Its use in children with hyperphagic disorders and severe NAFLD merits investigation.

Outcome

The majority of children with nonalcoholic steatosis have childhood NAFLD. Simple hepatic steatosis appears to be benign, but there have been no long-term studies as yet to determine the outcome in children, and there are no data regarding long-term extrahepatic disease.

NASH may be more severe in certain ethnic groups, including Hispanics and Asians, or in association with metabolic disorders characterized by abnormalities in insulin-receptor signaling, such as lipodystrophy syndromes. Progression to cirrhosis has been reported but appears to be rare in children. Cirrhosis in childhood NAFLD may not be detected as often as it occurs; the prevalence might be as high as 1–2%.[92] Hepatocellular carcinoma may develop; however, screening strategies in childhood NAFLD have not been established. Adult studies demonstrate that the more severe forms of NAFLD may progress to chronic liver failure, necessitating liver transplantation. NASH recurs after liver transplantation.[17] The role of therapy is undetermined, as only weight loss has had a significant effect on histology.

Conclusion

NAFLD/NASH is due to disordered insulin action, with hyperinsulinemia and relative insulin resistance. Like type 2 diabetes in children, it is likely to become an important liver disease among children as the prevalence of childhood obesity continues to increase. It occurs in young children, and there is no female predominance in the pediatric age bracket. Most children are either asymptomatic or present with vague abdominal pain. Severe outcomes may occur, including cirrhosis. Weight loss through dietary redesign, with a low-glycemic-index diet and a regimen of regular exercise, is the current mainstay of treatment. The efficacy of vitamin E supplementation in children is unclear, although other drug treatments such as metformin may be shown to be effective in the near future. Likewise, the role of bariatric surgery in children is undefined. Since the outcomes may be severe and treatment may prove relatively ineffective, primary prevention of NAFLD should be a priority in the pediatric age bracket.

Case study

An 11-year-old boy complained of vague abdominal pain and was evaluated by his family doctor, who found evidence of hepatic steatosis on ultrasound examination of the liver (Figure 11.5). The child was otherwise well. The bowel habit was entirely normal, screening for celiac disease was negative, and the patient had no food aversions. A dietary history revealed that he liked a sugar-coated cereal for breakfast, had a sandwich and cookies for lunch, snacked constantly between coming home from school and dinner, rarely ate vegetables except for chips, and preferred apple juice over intact fruit. He generally watched television for 2–3 hours per day and admitted to playing computer games at least 1 hour daily.

The family history was positive for type 2 diabetes in an uncle and obesity in both his parents. Physical examination revealed a well-appearing male who looked obese. His height was 142 cm, his weight was 66 kg (BMI 32.7), and his waist circumference was 80 cm.

Acanthosis nigricans was obvious around the neck. Apart from abdominal striae, the abdominal examination was normal.

Laboratory tests showed: ALT 92 IU/L (normal < 40); AST 76 IU/L (normal < 40); normal bilirubin, albumin, and international normalized ratio (INR); serum ceruloplasmin 190 mg/L; serum copper within the normal range; and 24-h basal urinary copper excretion was 0.3 μmol. Anti–smooth muscle antibody was positive at a titer of 1 : 40; hemoglobin A_{1c} was normal, but HOMA indicated insulin resistance. Triglycerides were elevated. All other investigations were normal.

Liver biopsy showed > 90% hepatocytes with large-droplet steatosis, scattered chronic inflammatory cell infiltrate, and moderately severe periportal fibrosis, with septa occasionally connecting portal tracts.

A diagnosis of NAFLD was made. He was given advice about lifestyle, exercise, and diet, and the whole family were encouraged to take part in the regimen. Six months later, his weight had increased to 72 kg despite an increase in his physical exercise and a reduction in his carbohydrate intake. He was started on metformin (500 mg twice daily). There has since been an improvement in his hepatic aminotransferases and possibly in the ultrasound findings, but he is continuing to gain weight, although at a slower rate.

Comment. NAFLD is becoming the commonest cause of referral for abnormal aminotransferases in older children. Although metabolic disorders or polycystic ovary disease may account for some of these (see above), it is related to obesity and insulin resistance in the majority of cases. Diet and exercise may not be effective, and further therapy is required. Although metformin may play a role in improving the prognosis and reducing the progression of liver disease, this has not yet been established. As metformin may be hepatotoxic, it is essential to monitor liver function tests and discontinue the drug at any sign of toxicity.

References

1 Adler M, Schaffner F. Fatty liver hepatitis and cirrhosis in obese patients. *Am J Med* 1979;**67**:811–6.

2 Ludwig J, Viggiano TR, McGill DB, Ott BJ. Nonalcoholic steatohepatitis: Mayo Clinic experience with a hitherto unnamed disease. *Mayo Clin Proc* 1980;**55**:434–8.

3 Wanless IR, Lentz JS. Fatty liver hepatitis (steatohepatitis) and obesity: an autopsy study with analysis of risk factors. *Hepatology* 1990;**12**:1106–10.

4 Bacon BR, Farahwash MJ, Lanney CG, Neuschwander-Tetri BA. Nonalcoholic steatohepatitis: an expanded clinical entity. *Gastroenterology* 1994;**107**:1103–9.

5 Kleiner DE, Brunt EM, Van Natta M, *et al.* Design and validation of a histological scoring system for nonalcoholic fatty liver disease. *Hepatology* 2005;**41**:1313–21.

6 Banner BF, Savas L, Zivny J, Tortorelli K, Bonkovsky HL. Ubiquitin as a marker of cell injury in nonalcoholic steatohepatitis. *Am J Clin Pathol* 2000;**114**:860–6.

7 Adinolfi LE, Durante-Mangoni E, Zampino R, Ruggiero G. Review article: hepatitis C virus-associated steatosis—pathogenic mechanisms and clinical implications. *Aliment Pharmacol Ther* 2005;**22**(Suppl 2):52–5.

8 Teli MR, James OF, Burt AD, Bennett MK, Day CP. The natural history of nonalcoholic fatty liver: a follow-up study. *Hepatology* 1995;**22**:1714–9.

9 Palmer M, Schaffner F. Effect of weight reduction on hepatic abnormalities in overweight patients. *Gastroenterology* 1990;**99**: 1408–13.

10 Adams LA, Lymp JF, St. Sauver J, *et al.* The natural history of nonalcoholic fatty liver disease: a population-based cohort study. *Gastroenterology* 2005;**129**:113–21.

11 Propst A, Propst T, Judmaier G, Vogel W. Prognosis in nonalcoholic steatohepatitis. *Gastroenterology* 1995;**108**:1607.

12 Fassio E, Alvarez E, Dominguez N, Landeira G, Longo C. Natural history of nonalcoholic steatohepatitis: a longitudinal study of repeat liver biopsies. *Hepatology* 2004;**40**:820–6.

13 Adams LA, Sanderson S, Lindor KD, Angulo P. The histological course of nonalcoholic fatty liver disease: a longitudinal study of 103 patients with sequential liver biopsies. *J Hepatol* 2005;**42**: 132–8.

14 Lee RG. Nonalcoholic steatohepatitis: a study of 49 patients. *Hum Pathol* 1989;**20**:594–8.

15 Powell EE, Cooksley WGE, Hanson R, Searle J, Halliday JW, Powell LW. The natural history of nonalcoholic steatohepatitis:

a follow-up study of forty-two patients for up to 21 years. *Hepatology* 1990;**11**:74–80.
16 Charlton M, Kasparova P, Weston S, *et al.* Frequency of nonalcoholic steatohepatitis as a cause of advanced liver disease. *Liver Transpl* 2001;**7**:608–14.
17 Contos MJ, Cales W, Sterling RK, *et al.* Development of nonalcoholic fatty liver disease after orthotopic liver transplantation for cryptogenic cirrhosis. *Liver Transpl* 2001;**7**:363–73.
18 Ong J, Younossi ZM, Reddy V, *et al.* Cryptogenic cirrhosis and posttransplantation nonalcoholic fatty liver disease. *Liver Transpl* 2001;**7**:797–801.
19 Zen Y, Katayanagi K, Tsuneyama K, Harada K, Araki I, Nakanuma Y. Hepatocellular carcinoma arising in non-alcoholic steatohepatitis. *Pathol Int* 2001;**51**:127–31.
20 Ratziu V, Bonyhay L, Di Martino V, *et al.* Survival, liver failure, and hepatocellular carcinoma in obesity-related cryptogenic cirrhosis. *Hepatology* 2002;**35**:1485–93.
21 Shimada M, Hashimoto E, Taniai M, *et al.* Hepatocellular carcinoma in patients with non-alcoholic steatohepatitis. *J Hepatol* 2002;**37**:154–60.
22 Caldwell SH, Crespo DM, Kang HS, Al-Osaimi AM. Obesity and hepatocellular carcinoma. *Gastroenterology* 2004;**127**:S97–103.
23 Marchesini G, Brizi M, Morselli-Labate AM, *et al.* Association of nonalcoholic fatty liver disease with insulin resistance. *Am J Med* 1999;**107**:450–5.
24 Cortez-Pinto H, Camilo ME, Baptista A, De Oliveira AG, De Moura MC. Non-alcoholic fatty liver: another feature of the metabolic syndrome? *Clin Nutr* 1999;**18**:353–8.
25 Sanyal AJ, Campbell-Sargent C, Mirshahi F, *et al.* Nonalcoholic steatohepatitis: association of insulin resistance and mitochondrial abnormalities. *Gastroenterology* 2001;**120**:1183–92.
26 Pagano G, Pacini G, Musso G, *et al.* Nonalcoholic steatohepatitis, insulin resistance, and metabolic syndrome: further evidence for an etiologic association. *Hepatology* 2002;**35**:367–72.
27 Wanless IR, Bargman JM, Oreopoulos DG, Vas SI. Subcapsular steatonecrosis in response to peritoneal insulin delivery: a clue to the pathogenesis of steatonecrosis in obesity. *Mod Pathol* 1989;**2**:69–74.
28 de Almeida IT, Cortez-Pinto H, Figaldo G, Rodrigues D, Camilo ME. Plasma total and free fatty acids composition in human non-alcoholic steatohepatitis. *Clin Nutr* 2002;**21**:219–23.
29 Day CP. Pathogenesis of steatohepatitis. *Best Pract Res Clin Gastroenterol* 2002;**16**:663–78.
30 Feldstein AE, Werneburg NW, Canbay A, *et al.* Free fatty acids promote hepatic lipotoxicity by stimulating TNF-alpha expression via a lysosomal pathway. *Hepatology* 2004;**40**:185–94.
31 Boden G, She P, Mozzoli M, *et al.* Free fatty acids produce insulin resistance and activate the proinflammatory nuclear factor-kB pathway in rat liver. *Diabetes* 2005;**54**:3458–65.
32 Malhi H, Bronk SF, Werneburg NW, Gores GJ. Free fatty acids induce JNK-dependent hepatocyte lipoapoptosis. *J Biol Chem* 2006;**281**:12093–101.
33 Schattenberg JM, Singh R, Wang Y, *et al.* JNK1 but not JNK2 promotes the development of steatohepatitis in mice. *Hepatology* 2006;**43**:163–72.
34 Tilg H, Hotamisligil GS. Nonalcoholic fatty liver disease: Cytokine–adipokine interplay and regulation of insulin resistance. *Gastroenterology* 2006;**131**:934–45.
35 Ueki K, Kadowaki T, Kahn CR. Role of suppressors of cytokine signaling SOCS-1 and SOCS-3 in hepatic steatosis and the metabolic syndrome. *Hepatol Res* 2005;**33**:185–92.
36 Foufelle F, Ferre P. New perspectives in the regulation of hepatic glycolytic and lipogenic genes by insulin and glucose: a role for the transcription factor sterol regulatory element binding protein-1c. *Biochem J* 2002;**366**:377–91.
37 Horton JD, Goldstein JL, Brown MS. SREBPs: activators of the complete program of cholesterol and fatty acid synthesis in the liver. *J Clin Invest* 2002;**109**:1125–31.
38 Deng QG, She H, Cheng JH, *et al.* Steatohepatitis induced by intragastric overfeeding in mice. *Hepatology* 2005;**42**:905–14.
39 Larter CZ, Farrell GC. Insulin resistance, adiponectin, cytokines in NASH: Which is the best target to treat? *J Hepatol* 2006;**44**:253–61.
40 Day CP, James OFW. Steatohepatitis: a tale of two "hits." *Gastroenterology* 1998;**114**:842–5.
41 Paradis V, Perlemuter G, Bonvoust F, *et al.* High glucose and hyperinsulinemia stimulate connective tissue growth factor expression: a potential mechanism involved in progression to fibrosis in nonalcoholic steatohepatitis. *Hepatology* 2001;**34**:738–44.
42 Wanless IR, Shiota K. The pathogenesis of nonalcoholic steatohepatitis and other fatty liver diseases: a four-step model including the role of lipid release and hepatic venular obstruction in the progression to cirrhosis. *Semin Liver Dis* 2004;**24**:99–106.
43 Schattenberg JM, Wang Y, Singh R, Rigoli RM, Czaja MJ. Hepatocyte CYP2E1 overexpression and steatohepatitis lead to impaired hepatic insulin signaling. *J Biol Chem* 2005;**280**:9887–94.
44 Orellana M, Rodrigo R, Varela N, *et al.* Relationship between in vivo chlorzoxazone hydroxylation, hepatic cytochrome P450 2E1 content and liver injury in obese non-alcoholic fatty liver disease patients. *Hepatol Res* 2005;**34**:57–63.
45 Visser M, Bouter LM, McQuillan GM, Wener MH, Harris TB. Elevated C-reactive protein levels in overweight and obese adults. *JAMA* 1999;**282**:2131–5.
46 Festa A, D'Agostino R Jr, Williams K, *et al.* The relation of body fat mass and distribution to markers of chronic inflammation. *Int J Obes Relat Metab Disord* 2001;**25**:1407–15.
47 Pannacciulli N, Cantatore FP, Minenna A, Bellacicco M, Giorgino R, De Pergola G. C-reactive protein is independently associated with total body fat, central fat, and insulin resistance in adult women. *Int J Obes Relat Metab Disord* 2001;**25**:1416–20.
48 Pessayre D, Mansouri A, Fromenty B. Mitochondrial dysfunction in steatohepatitis. *Am J Physiol Gastrointest Liver Physiol* 2002;**282**:G193–199.
49 Torley D, Munro CS. Genes, growth factors and acanthosis nigricans. *Br J Dermatol* 2002;**147**:1096–101.
50 Rashid M, Roberts EA. Nonalcoholic steatohepatitis in children. *J Pediatr Gastroenterol Nutr* 2000;**30**:48–53.
51 Pacifico L, Di Renzo L, Anania C, *et al.* Increased T-helper interferon-gamma-secreting cells in obese children. *Eur J Endocrinol* 2006;**154**:691–7.
52 Nobili V, Marcellini M, Devito R, *et al.* NAFLD in children: a prospective clinical-pathological study and effect of lifestyle advice. *Hepatology* 2006;**44**:458–65.

53 Mager DR, Ling S, Roberts EA. *Paediatr Child Health* 2007;**13**: 111–117.

54 Kerem N, Guttmann H, Hochberg Z. The autosomal dominant trait of obesity, acanthosis nigricans, hypertension, ischemic heart disease and diabetes type 2. *Horm Res* 2001;**55**:298–304.

55 Visser M, Bouter LM, McQuillan GM, Wener MH, Harris TB. Low-grade systemic inflammation in overweight children. *Pediatrics* 2001;**107**:E13.

56 de Ferranti SD, Gauvreau K, Ludwig DS, Newburger JW, Rifai N. Inflammation and changes in metabolic syndrome abnormalities in US adolescents: findings from the 1988–1994 and 1999–2000 National Health and Nutrition Examination Surveys. *Clin Chem* 2006;**52**:1325–30.

57 Decsi T, Molnar D, Koletzko B. Reduced plasma concentrations of alpha-tocopherol and beta-carotene in obese boys. *J Pediatr* 1997;**130**:653–5.

58 Strauss RS. Comparison of serum concentrations of alpha-tocopherol and beta-carotene in a cross-sectional sample of obese and nonobese children (NHANES III). *J Pediatr* 1999;**134**: 160–5.

59 Isganaitis E, Lustig RH. Fast food, central nervous system insulin resistance, and obesity. *Arterioscler Thromb Vasc Biol* 2005;**25**:2451–62.

60 Pereira MA, Kartashov AI, Ebbeling CB, *et al.* Fast-food habits, weight gain, and insulin resistance (the CARDIA study): 15-year prospective analysis. *Lancet* 2005;**365**:36–42.

61 Lam TK, Schwartz GJ, Rossetti L. Hypothalamic sensing of fatty acids. *Nat Neurosci* 2005;**8**:579–84.

62 Lustig RH. Childhood obesity: behavioral aberration or biochemical drive? Reinterpreting the First Law of Thermodynamics. *Nat Clin Pract Endocrinol Metab* 2006;**2**:447–58.

63 Anthony K, Reed LJ, Dunn JT, *et al.* Attenuation of insulin-evoked responses in brain networks controlling appetite and reward in insulin resistance: the cerebral basis for impaired control of food intake in metabolic syndrome? *Diabetes* 2006;**55**: 2986–92.

64 Gil-Campos M, Canete RR, Gil A. Adiponectin, the missing link in insulin resistance and obesity. *Clin Nutr* 2004;**23**:963–74.

65 Bugianesi E, Pagotto U, Manini R, *et al.* Plasma adiponectin in nonalcoholic fatty liver is related to hepatic insulin resistance and hepatic fat content, not to liver disease severity. *J Clin Endocrinol Metab* 2005;**90**:3498–504.

66 Pagano C, Soardo G, Esposito W, *et al.* Plasma adiponectin is decreased in nonalcoholic fatty liver disease. *Eur J Endocrinol* 2005;**152**:113–8.

67 Louthan MV, Barve S, McClain CJ, Joshi-Barve S. Decreased serum adiponectin: an early event in pediatric nonalcoholic fatty liver disease. *J Pediatr* 2005;**147**:835–8.

68 Asayama K, Hayashibe H, Dobashi K, *et al.* Decrease in serum adiponectin level due to obesity and visceral fat accumulation in children. *Obes Res* 2003;**11**:1072–9.

69 Diamond FB Jr, Cuthbertson D, Hanna S, Eichler D. Correlates of adiponectin and the leptin/adiponectin ratio in obese and non-obese children. *J Pediatr Endocrinol Metab* 2004;**17**:1069–75.

70 Weiss R, Dziura J, Burgert TS, *et al.* Obesity and the metabolic syndrome in children and adolescents. *N Engl J Med* 2004;**350**: 2362–74.

71 Bacha F, Saad R, Gungor N, Arslanian SA. Adiponectin in youth: relationship to visceral adiposity, insulin sensitivity, and beta-cell function. *Diabetes Care* 2004;**27**:547–52.

72 Targher G, Bertolini L, Rodella S, *et al.* Associations between plasma adiponectin concentrations and liver histology in patients with nonalcoholic fatty liver disease. *Clin Endocrinol (Oxf)* 2006;**64**:679–83.

73 Farvid MS, Ng TW, Chan DC, Barrett PH, Watts GF. Association of adiponectin and resistin with adipose tissue compartments, insulin resistance and dyslipidaemia. *Diabetes Obes Metab* 2005;**7**: 406–13.

74 Gerber M, Boettner A, Seidel B, *et al.* Serum resistin levels of obese and lean children and adolescents: biochemical analysis and clinical relevance. *J Clin Endocrinol Metab* 2005;**90**: 4503–9.

75 Uygun A, Kadayifci A, Yesilova Z, *et al.* Serum leptin levels in patients with nonalcoholic steatohepatitis. *Am J Gastroenterol* 2000;**95**:3584–9.

76 Wang J, Obici S, Morgan K, Barzilai N, Feng Z, Rossetti L. Overfeeding rapidly induces leptin and insulin resistance. *Diabetes* 2001;**50**:2786–91.

77 Pelleymounter MA, Cullen MJ, Baker MB, *et al.* Effects of the obese gene product on body weight regulation in *ob/ob* mice. *Science* 1995;**269**:540–3.

78 Kennedy A, Gettys TW, Watson P, *et al.* The metabolic significance of leptin in humans: gender-based differences in relationship to adiposity, insulin sensitivity, and energy expenditure. *J Clin Endocrinol Metab* 1997;**82**:1293–300.

79 Oral EA, Simha V, Ruiz E, *et al.* Leptin-replacement therapy for lipodystrophy. *N Engl J Med* 2002;**346**:570–8.

80 Masuzaki H, Paterson J, Shinyama H, *et al.* A transgenic model of visceral obesity and the metabolic syndrome. *Science* 2001;**294**:2166–70.

81 Bernard S, Touzet S, Personne I, *et al.* Association between microsomal triglyceride transfer protein gene polymorphism and the biological features of liver steatosis in patients with type II diabetes. *Diabetologia* 2000;**43**:995–9.

82 Grove J, Daly AK, Bassendine MF, Day CP. Association of a tumor necrosis factor promoter polymorphism with susceptibility to alcoholic steatohepatitis. *Hepatology* 1997;**26**:143–6.

83 Valenti L, Fracanzani AL, Dongiovanni P, *et al.* Tumor necrosis factor alpha promoter polymorphisms and insulin resistance in nonalcoholic fatty liver disease. *Gastroenterology* 2002;**122**:274–80.

84 Scaglioni S, Verduci E, Salvioni M, *et al.* PPAR-gamma2 Pro12Ala variant, insulin resistance and plasma long-chain polyunsaturated fatty acids in childhood obesity. *Pediatr Res* 2006;**60**:485–9.

85 Berberoglu M, Evliyaoglu O, Adiyaman P, *et al.* Plasminogen activator inhibitor-1 (PAI-1) gene polymorphism (-675 4G/5G) associated with obesity and vascular risk in children. *J Pediatr Endocrinol Metab* 2006;**19**:741–8.

86 Heude B, Petry CJ, Pembrey M, Dunger DB, Ong KK. The insulin gene variable number of tandem repeat: associations and interactions with childhood body fat mass and insulin secretion in normal children. *J Clin Endocrinol Metab* 2006;**91**: 2770–5.

87 Mensenkamp AR, van Luyn MJ, van Goor H, *et al.* Hepatic lipid accumulation, altered very low density lipoprotein formation

and apolipoprotein E deposition in apolipoprotein E3-Leiden transgenic mice. *J Hepatol* 2000;**33**:189–98.

88 Valenti L, Dongiovanni P, Piperno A, *et al.* Alpha 1-antitrypsin mutations in NAFLD: high prevalence and association with altered iron metabolism but not with liver damage. *Hepatology* 2006;**44**:857–64.

89 Regev A, Guaqueta C, Molina EG, *et al.* Does the heterozygous state of alpha-1 antitrypsin deficiency have a role in chronic liver diseases? Interim results of a large case-control study. *J Pediatr Gastroenterol Nutr* 2006;**43**(Suppl 1):S30–5.

90 Schwimmer JB, McGreal N, Deutsch R, Finegold MJ, Lavine JE. Influence of gender, race, and ethnicity on suspected fatty liver in obese adolescents. *Pediatrics* 2005;**115**:e561–5.

91 Weston SR, Leyden W, Murphy R, *et al.* Racial and ethnic distribution of nonalcoholic fatty liver in persons with newly diagnosed chronic liver disease. *Hepatology* 2005;**41**:372–9.

92 Schwimmer JB, Deutsch R, Kahen T, Lavine JE, Stanley C, Behling C. Prevalence of fatty liver in children and adolescents. *Pediatrics* 2006;**118**:1388–93.

93 Louthan MV, Theriot JA, Zimmerman E, Stutts JT, McClain CJ. Decreased prevalence of nonalcoholic fatty liver disease in black obese children. *J Pediatr Gastroenterol Nutr* 2005;**41**:426–9.

94 Strauss RS, Pollack HA. Epidemic increase in childhood overweight, 1986–1998. *JAMA* 2001;**286**:2845–8.

95 Power C, Lake JK, Cole T. Measurement and long-term health risks of child and adolescent fatness. *Int J Obes Relat Metab Disord* 1997;**21**:507–26.

96 Kiess W, Reich A, Muller G, *et al.* Clinical aspects of obesity in childhood and adolescence-diagnosis, treatment and prevention. *Int J Obes Relat Metab Disord* 2001;**25**(Suppl 1):S75–9.

97 Cole TJ, Bellizzi MC, Flegal KM, Dietz WH. Establishing a standard definition for child overweight and obesity worldwide: international survey. *BMJ* 2000;**320**:1240–3.

98 Lobstein T, Baur L, Uauy R. Obesity in children and young people: a crisis in public health. *Obes Rev* 2004;**5**(Suppl 1):4–104.

99 Ogden CL, Carroll MD, Curtin LR, McDowell MA, Tabak CJ, Flegal KM. Prevalence of overweight and obesity in the United States, 1999–2004. *JAMA* 2006;**295**:1549–55.

100 James PT, Rigby N, Leach R. The obesity epidemic, metabolic syndrome and future prevention strategies. *Eur J Cardiovasc Prev Rehabil* 2004;**11**:3–8.

101 Cecil JE, Watt P, Murrie IS, *et al.* Childhood obesity and socioeconomic status: a novel role for height growth limitation. *Int J Obes (Lond)* 2005;**29**:1199–203.

102 Willms JD, Tremblay MS, Katzmarzyk PT. Geographic and demographic variation in the prevalence of overweight Canadian children. *Obes Res* 2003;**11**:668–73.

103 Magarey AM, Daniels LA, Boulton TJ. Prevalence of overweight and obesity in Australian children and adolescents: reassessment of 1985 and 1995 data against new standard international definitions. *Med J Aust* 2001;**174**:561–4.

104 Reilly JJ, Armstrong J, Dorosty AR, *et al.* Early life risk factors for obesity in childhood: cohort study. *BMJ* 2005;**330**:1357.

105 Fagot-Campagna A, Pettitt DJ, Engelgau MM, *et al.* Type 2 diabetes among North American children and adolescents: an epidemiologic review and a public health perspective. *J Pediatr* 2000;**136**:664–72.

106 Tominaga K, Kurata JH, Chen YK, *et al.* Prevalence of fatty liver in Japanese children and relationship to obesity. An epidemiological ultrasonographic survey. *Dig Dis Sci* 1995;**40**: 2002–9.

107 Strauss RS, Barlow SE, Dietz WH. Prevalence of abnormal serum aminotransferase values in overweight and obese adolescents. *J Pediatr* 2000;**136**:727–33.

108 Guzzaloni G, Grugni G, Minocci A, Moro D, Morabito F. Liver steatosis in juvenile obesity: correlations with lipid profile, hepatic biochemical parameters and glycemic and insulinemic responses to an oral glucose tolerance test. *Int J Obes Relat Metab Disord* 2000;**24**:772–6.

109 Chan DF, Li AM, Chu WC, *et al.* Hepatic steatosis in obese Chinese children. *Int J Obes Relat Metab Disord* 2004;**28**:1257–63.

110 Moran JR, Ghishan FK, Halter SA, Greene HL. Steatohepatitis in obese children: a cause of chronic liver dysfunction. *Am J Gastroenterol* 1983;**78**:374–7.

111 Vajro P, Fontanella A, Perna C, Orso G, Tedesco M, De Vincenzo A. Persistent hypertransaminasemia resolving after weight reduction in obese children. *J Pediatr* 1994;**125**:239–41.

112 Kocak N, Yuce A, Gurakan F, Ozen H. Obesity: a cause of steatohepatitis in children. *Am J Gastroenterol* 2000;**95**:1099–1100.

113 Tazawa Y, Noguchi H, Nishinomiya F, Takada G. Effect of weight changes on serum transaminase activities in obese children. *Acta Paediatr Jpn* 1997;**39**:210–4.

114 Baldridge AD, Perez-Atayde AR, Graeme-Cooke F, Higgins L, Lavine JE. Idiopathic steatohepatitis in childhood: a multicenter retrospective study. *J Pediatr* 1995;**127**:700–4.

115 Kinugasa A, Tsunamoto K, Furukawa N, Sawada T, Kusunoki T, Shimada N. Fatty liver and its fibrous changes found in simple obesity of children. *J Pediatr Gastroenterol Nutr* 1984;**3**:408–14.

116 Manton ND, Lipsett J, Moore DJ, Davidson GP, Bourne AJ, Couper RT. Non-alcoholic steatohepatitis in children and adolescents. *Med J Aust* 2000;**173**:476–9.

117 Sathya P, Martin S, Alvarez F. Nonalcoholic fatty liver disease (NAFLD) in children. *Curr Opin Pediatr* 2002;**14**:593–600.

118 Willner IR, Waters B, Patil SR, Reuben A, Morelli J, Riely CA. Ninety patients with nonalcoholic steatohepatitis: insulin resistance, familial tendency, and severity of disease. *Am J Gastroenterol* 2001;**96**:2957–61.

119 Schwimmer JB, Behling C, Newbury R, *et al.* Histopathology of pediatric nonalcoholic fatty liver disease. *Hepatology* 2005;**42**: 641–9.

120 Xanthakos S, Miles L, Bucuvalas J, Daniels S, Garcia V, Inge T. Histologic spectrum of nonalcoholic fatty liver disease in morbidly obese adolescents. *Clin Gastroenterol Hepatol* 2006;**4**:226–32.

121 McCarthy HD, Ashwell M. A study of central fatness using waist-to-height ratios in UK children and adolescents over two decades supports the simple message—"keep your waist circumference to less than half your height." *Int J Obes (Lond)* 2006;**30**: 988–92.

122 de Marco R, Loentelli F, Zoppini G, Verlate G, Bonora E, Muggeo M. Cause-specific mortality in type 2 diabetes. The Verona Diabetes Study. *Diabetes Care* 1999;**22**:756–61.

123 Talvensaari KK, Knip M, Lanning P, Lanning M. Clinical characteristics and factors affecting growth in long-term survivors of cancer. *Med Pediatr Oncol* 1996;**26**:166–72.

124 Talvensaari KK, Lanning M, Tapanainen P, Knip M. Long-term survivors of childhood cancer have an increased risk of

manifesting the metabolic syndrome. *J Clin Endocrinol Metab* 1996;**81**:3051–5.

125 Reilly JJ, Ventham JC, Newell J, Aitchison T, Wallace WH, Gibson BE. Risk factors for excess weight gain in children treated for acute lymphoblastic leukaemia. *Int J Obes Relat Metab Disord* 2000;**24**:1537–41.

126 Jarfelt M, Lannering B, Bosaeus I, Johannsson G, Bjarnason R. Body composition in young adult survivors of childhood acute lymphoblastic leukaemia. *Eur J Endocrinol* 2005;**153**:81–9.

127 Kourti M, Tragiannidis A, Makedou A, Papageorgiou T, Rousso I, Athanassiadou F. Metabolic syndrome in children and adolescents with acute lymphoblastic leukemia after the completion of chemotherapy. *J Pediatr Hematol Oncol* 2005;**27**:499–501.

128 Ness KK, Oakes JM, Punyko JA, Baker KS, Gurney JG. Prevalence of the metabolic syndrome in relation to self-reported cancer history. *Ann Epidemiol* 2005;**15**:202–6.

129 Molleston JP, White F, Teckman J, Fitzgerald JF. Obese children with steatohepatitis can develop cirrhosis in childhood. *Am J Gastroenterol* 2002;**97**:2460–2.

130 Adams LA, Feldstein A, Lindor KD, Angulo P. Nonalcoholic fatty liver disease among patients with hypothalamic and pituitary dysfunction. *Hepatology* 2004;**39**:909–14.

131 Basenau D, Stehphani U, Fischer G. [Development of complete liver cirrhosis in hyperphagia-induced fatty liver; in German.] *Klin Pädiatr* 1994;**206**:62–4.

132 Altuntas B, Ozcakar B, Bideci A, Cinaz P. Cirrhotic outcome in patients with craniopharyngioma. *J Pediatr Endocrinol Metab* 2002;**15**:1057–8.

133 Brunt EM, Neuschwander-Tetri BA, Oliver D, Wehmeier KR, Bacon BR. Nonalcoholic steatohepatitis: histologic features and clinical correlations with 30 blinded biopsy specimens. *Hum Pathol* 2004;**35**:1070–82.

134 Evans HM, Shaikh MG, McKiernan PJ, *et al.* Acute fatty liver disease after suprasellar tumor resection. *J Pediatr Gastroenterol Nutr* 2004;**39**:288–91.

135 Nakajima K, Hashimoto E, Kaneda H, *et al.* Pediatric nonalcoholic steatohepatitis associated with hypopituitarism. *J Gastroenterol* 2005;**40**:312–5.

136 Michaud JL, Heon E, Guilbert F, *et al.* Natural history of Alström syndrome in early childhood: onset with dilated cardiomyopathy. *J Pediatr* 1996;**128**:225–9.

137 Russell-Eggitt IM, Clayton PT, Coffey R, Kriss A, Taylor DS, Taylor JF. Alström syndrome. Report of 22 cases and literature review. *Ophthalmology* 1998;**105**:1274–80.

138 Collin GB, Marshall JD, Ikeda A, *et al.* Mutations in *ALMS1* cause obesity, type 2 diabetes and neurosensory degeneration in Alström syndrome. *Nat Genet* 2002;**31**:74–8.

139 Hearn T, Renforth GL, Spalluto C, *et al.* Mutation of *ALMS1*, a large gene with a tandem repeat encoding 47 amino acids, causes Alström syndrome. *Nat Genet* 2002;**31**:79–83.

140 Titomanlio L, De Brasi D, Buoninconti A, *et al.* Alström syndrome: intrafamilial phenotypic variability in sibs with a novel nonsense mutation of the *ALMS1* gene. *Clin Genet* 2004;**65**:156–7.

141 Connolly MB, Jan JE, Couch RM, Wong LT, Dimmick JE, Rigg JM. Hepatic dysfunction in Alström disease. *Am J Med Genet* 1991;**40**:421–4.

142 Awazu M, Tanaka T, Yamazaki K, Kato S, Higuchi M, Matsuo N. A 27-year-old woman with Alström syndrome who had liver cirrhosis. *Keio J Med* 1995;**44**:67–73.

143 Awazu M, Tanaka T, Sato S, *et al.* Hepatic dysfunction in two sibs with Alström syndrome: case report and review of the literature. *Am J Med Genet* 1997;**69**:13–6.

144 Quiros-Tejeira RE, Vargas J, Ament ME. Early-onset liver disease complicated with acute liver failure in Alström syndrome. *Am J Med Genet* 2001;**101**:9–11.

145 Green JS, Parfrey PS, Harnett JD, *et al.* The cardinal manifestations of Bardet–Biedl syndrome, a form of Laurence–Moon–Biedl syndrome. *N Engl J Med* 1989;**321**:1002–9.

146 Escallon F, Traboulsi EI, Infante R. A family with the Bardet–Biedl syndrome and diabetes mellitus. *Arch Ophthalmol* 1989; **107**:855–7.

147 Iannello S, Bosco P, Camuto M, Cavaleri A, Milazzo P, Belfiore F. A mild form of Alström disease associated with metabolic syndrome and very high fasting serum free fatty acids: two cases diagnosed in adult age. *Am J Med Sci* 2004;**327**:284–8.

148 Katsanis N, Ansley SJ, Badano JL, *et al.* Triallelic inheritance in Bardet–Biedl syndrome, a Mendelian recessive disorder. *Science* 2001;**293**:2256–9.

149 Katsanis N, Lupski JR, Beales PL. Exploring the molecular basis of Bardet–Biedl syndrome. *Hum Mol Genet* 2001;**10**: 2293–9.

150 Hamacher M, Pippirs U, Köhler A, Müller HW, Bosse F. Plasmolipin: genomic structure, chromosomal localization, protein expression pattern, and putative association with Bardet–Biedl syndrome. *Mamm Genome* 2001;**12**:933–7.

151 Mykytyn K, Braun T, Carmi R, *et al.* Identification of the gene that, when mutated, causes the human obesity syndrome BBS4. *Nat Genet* 2001;**28**:188–91.

152 Pagon RA, Haas JE, Bunt AH, Rodaway KA. Hepatic involvement in the Bardet–Biedl syndrome. *Am J Med* Genet 1982;**13**: 373–81.

153 Lewy VD, Danadian K, Witchel SF, Arslanian S. Early metabolic abnormalities in adolescent girls with polycystic ovarian syndrome. *J Pediatr* 2001;**138**:38–44.

154 Conway GS, Jacobs HS. Acanthosis nigricans in obese women with the polycystic ovary syndrome: disease spectrum not distinct entity. *Postgrad Med J* 1990;**66**:536–8.

155 Dunaif A. Insulin resistance and the polycystic ovary syndrome: mechanism and implications for pathogenesis. *Endocr Rev* 1997; **18**:774–800.

156 Parsanezhad ME, Alborzi S, Zarei A, Dehbashi S, Omrani G. Insulin resistance in clomiphene responders and non-responders with polycystic ovarian disease and therapeutic effects of metformin. *Int J Gynaecol Obstet* 2001;**75**:43–50.

157 Setji TL, Holland ND, Sanders LL, Pereira KC, Diehl AM, Brown AJ. Nonalcoholic steatohepatitis and nonalcoholic fatty liver disease in young women with polycystic ovary syndrome. *J Clin Endocrinol Metab* 2006; **91**:1741–7.

158 Schwimmer JB, Khorram O, Chiu V, Schwimmer WB. Abnormal aminotransferase activity in women with polycystic ovary syndrome. *Fertil Steril* 2005;**83**:494–7.

159 Brown AJ, Tendler DA, McMurray RG, Setji TL. Polycystic ovary syndrome and severe nonalcoholic steatohepatitis: beneficial effect of modest weight loss and exercise on liver biopsy findings. *Endocr Pract* 2005;**11**:319–24.

160 Batukan C, Baysal B. Metformin improves ovulation and pregnancy rates in patients with polycystic ovary syndrome. *Arch Gynecol Obstet* 2001;**265**:124–7.

161 De Conciliis B, Passannanti G, Romano L, Santarpia R. Effects of metformin on the insulin resistance and on ovarian steroidogenesis in women with polycystic ovary syndrome. *Minerva Ginecol* 2001;**53**:239–50.

162 Nardo LG, Rai R. Metformin therapy in the management of polycystic ovary syndrome: endocrine, metabolic and reproductive effects. *Gynecol Endocrinol* 2001;**15**:373–80.

163 Salerno M, DiMaio S, Gasparini N, Rizzo M, Ferri P, Vajro P. Liver abnormalities in Turner syndrome. *Eur J Pediatr* 1999;**158**: 618–23.

164 Sato H, Miyamoto S, Sasaki N. Liver abnormality in Turner syndrome. *Eur J Pediatr* 2001;**160**:59.

165 Simha V, Garg A. Lipodystrophy: lessons in lipid and energy metabolism. *Curr Opin Lipidol* 2006;**17**:162–9.

166 Agarwal AK, Arioglu E, de Almeida S, *et al. AGPAT2* is mutated in congenital generalized lipodystrophy linked to chromosome 9q34. *Nat Genet* 2002;**31**:21–3.

167 Magre J, Delepine M, Khallouf E, *et al.* Identification of the gene altered in Berardinelli–Seip congenital lipodystrophy on chromosome 11q13. *Nat Genet* 2001;**28**:365–70.

168 Shackleton S, Lloyd DJ, Jackson SN, *et al. LMNA*, encoding lamin A/C, is mutated in partial lipodystrophy. *Nat Genet* 2000;**24**:153–6.

169 De Sandre-Giovannoli A, Chaouch M, Kozlov S, *et al.* Homozygous defects in LMNA, encoding lamin A/C nuclear-envelope proteins, cause autosomal recessive axonal neuropathy in human (Charcot– Marie–Tooth disorder type 2) and mouse. *Am J Hum Genet* 2002;**70**:726–36.

170 Lloyd DJ, Trembath RC, Shackleton S. A novel interaction between lamin A and SREBP1: implications for partial lipodystrophy and other laminopathies. *Hum Molec Genet* 2002;**11**:769–77.

171 Agarwal AK, Garg A. A novel heterozygous mutation in peroxisome proliferator-activated receptor-gamma gene in a patient with familial partial lipodystrophy. *J Clin Endocrinol Metab* 2002; **87**:408–11.

172 Powell EE, Searle J, Mortimer R. Steatohepatitis associated with limb lipodystrophy. *Gastroenterology* 1989;**97**:1022–4.

173 Cauble MS, Gilroy R, Sorrell MF, *et al.* Lipoatrophic diabetes and end-stage liver disease secondary to nonalcoholic steatohepatitis with recurrence after liver transplantation. *Transplantation* 2001; **71**:892–5.

174 Ludtke A, Genschel J, Brabant G, *et al.* Hepatic steatosis in Dunnigan-type familial partial lipodystrophy. *Am J Gastroenterol* 2005;**100**:2218–24.

175 Karlberg N, Jalanko H, Kallijarvi J, Lehesjoki AE, Lipsanen-Nyman M. Insulin resistance syndrome in subjects with mutated RING finger protein TRIM37. *Diabetes* 2005;**54**:3577–81.

176 Srinivasan R, Hadzic N, Fischer J, Knisely AS. Steatohepatitis and unsuspected micronodular cirrhosis in Dorfman–Chanarin syndrome with documented *ABHD5* mutation. *J Pediatr* 2004; **144**:662–5.

177 Ciesek S, Hadem J, Fischer J, Manns MP, Strassburg CP. A rare cause of nonalcoholic fatty liver disease. *Ann Intern Med* 2006; **145**:154–5.

178 Yen CL, Farese RV Jr. Fat breakdown: a function for CGI-58 (*ABHD5*) provides a new piece of the puzzle. *Cell Metab* 2006;**3**: 305–7.

179 Tan TY, Bankier A, Slater HR, Northrop EL, Zacharin M, Savarirayan R. A patient with monosomy 1p36, atypical features and phenotypic similarities with Cantu syndrome. *Am J Med Genet A* 2005;**139A**:216–20.

180 Schwimmer JB. Definitive diagnosis and assessment of risk for nonalcoholic fatty liver disease in children and adolescents. *Semin Liver Dis* 2007;**27**:312–8.

181 Colombo C, Crosignani A, Battezzati PM. Liver involvement in cystic fibrosis. *J Hepatol* 1999;**31**:946–54.

182 Saadeh S, Younossi ZM, Remer EM, *et al.* The utility of radiological imaging in nonalcoholic fatty liver disease. *Gastroenterology* 2002;**123**:745–50.

183 Matteoni CA, Younossi ZM, Gramlich T, Boparai N, Liu YC, McCullough AJ. Nonalcoholic fatty liver disease: a spectrum of clinical and pathological severity. *Gastroenterology* 1999;**116**: 1413–9.

184 Brunt EM. Nonalcoholic steatohepatitis: definition and pathology. *Semin Liver Dis* 2001;**21**:3–16.

185 Matthews DR, Hosker JP, Rudenski AS, Naylor BA, Treacher DF, Turner RC. Homeostasis model assessment: insulin resistance and beta-cell function from fasting plasma glucose and insulin concentrations in man. *Diabetologia* 1985;**28**:412–9.

186 Gungor N, Saad R, Janosky J, Arslanian S. Validation of surrogate estimates of insulin sensitivity and insulin secretion in children and adolescents. *J Pediatr* 2004;**144**:47–55.

187 Keskin M, Kurtoglu S, Kendirci M, Atabek ME, Yazici C. Homeostasis model assessment is more reliable than the fasting glucose/insulin ratio and quantitative insulin sensitivity check index for assessing insulin resistance among obese children and adolescents. *Pediatrics* 2005;**115**:e500–3.

188 Vajro P, Fontanella A, Perna C, Orso G, Tedesco M, De Vincenzo A. Persistent hyperaminotransferasemia resolving after weight reduction in obese children. *J Pediatr* 1994;**125**:239–41.

189 Ludwig DS, Majzoub JA, Al-Zahrani A, Dallal GE, Blanco I, Roberts SB. High glycemic index foods, overeating, and obesity. *Pediatrics* 1999;**103**:E26.

190 Spieth LE, Harnish JD, Lenders CM, *et al.* A low-glycemic index diet in the treatment of pediatric obesity. *Arch Pediatr Adolesc Med* 2000;**154**:947–51.

191 Ebbeling CB, Leidig MM, Feldman HA, Lovesky MM, Ludwig DS. Effects of a low-glycemic load vs low-fat diet in obese young adults: a randomized trial. *JAMA* 2007;**297**:2092–102.

192 Ludwig DS. The glycemic index: physiological mechanisms relating to obesity, diabetes, and cardiovascular disease. *JAMA* 2002;**287**:2414–23.

193 Goldfield GS, Epstein LH, Kilanowski CK, Paluch RA, Kogut-Bossler B. Cost-effectiveness of group and mixed family-based treatment for childhood obesity. *Int J Obes Relat Metab Disord* 2001;**25**:1843–9.

194 Zametkin AJ, Zoon CK, Klein HW, Munson S. Psychiatric aspects of child and adolescent obesity: a review of the past 10 years. *J Am Acad Child Adolesc Psychiatry* 2004;**43**:134–50.

195 Golan M, Kaufman V, Shahar DR. Childhood obesity treatment: targeting parents exclusively v. parents and children. *Br J Nutr* 2006;**95**:1008–15.

196 Lin HZ, Yang SQ, Chuckaree C, Kuhajda F, Ronnet G, Diehl AM. Metformin reverses fatty liver disease in obese, leptin-deficient mice. *Nat Med* 2000;**6**:998–1003.

197 Zhou G, Myers R, Li Y, *et al.* Role of AMP-activated protein kinase in mechanism of metformin action. *J Clin Invest* 2001; **108**:1167–74.

198 Marchesini G, Brizi M, Bianchi G, Tomassetti S, Zoli M, Melchionda N. Metformin in non-alcoholic steatohepatitis. *Lancet* 2001;**358**:893–4.

199 Schwimmer JB, Middleton MS, Deutsch R, Lavine JE. A phase 2 clinical trial of metformin as a treatment for non-diabetic paediatric non-alcoholic steatohepatitis. *Aliment Pharmacol Ther* 2005;**21**:871–9.

200 Hermanns-Le T, Hermanns JF, Pierard GE. Juvenile acanthosis nigricans and insulin resistance. *Pediatr Dermatol* 2002;**19**:12–4.

201 Kay JP, Alemzadeh R, Langley G, D'Angelo L, Smith P, Holshouser S. Beneficial effects of metformin in normoglycemic morbidly obese adolescents. *Metabolism* 2001;**50**:1457–61.

202 Jones KL, Arslanian S, Peterokova VA, Park JS, Tomlinson MJ. Effect of metformin in pediatric patients with type 2 diabetes: a randomized controlled trial. *Diabetes Care* 2002;**25**:89–94.

203 Zuhri-Yafi MI, Brosnan PG, Hardin DS. Treatment of type 2 diabetes mellitus in children and adolescents. *J Pediatr Endocrinol Metab* 2002;**15**:541–6.

204 Arslanian SA, Lewy V, Danadian K, Saad R. Metformin therapy in obese adolescents with polycystic ovary syndrome and impaired glucose tolerance: amelioration of exaggerated adrenal response to adrenocorticotropin with reduction of insulinemia/insulin resistance. *J Clin Endocrinol Metab* 2002;**87**:1555–9.

205 Chan NN, Feher MD, Bridges NA. Metformin therapy for diabetes in Prader–Willi syndrome. *J R Soc Med* 1998;**91**:598.

206 Bugianesi E, Gentilcore E, Manini R, *et al.* A randomized controlled trial of metformin versus vitamin E or prescriptive diet in nonalcoholic fatty liver disease. *Am J Gastroenterol* 2005;**100**: 1082–90.

207 Lavine JE, Schwimmer JB. Clinical Research Network launches TONIC trial for treatment of nonalcoholic fatty liver disease in children. *J Pediatr Gastroenterol Nutr* 2006;**42**:129–30.

208 Neuschwander-Tetri BA, Brunt EM, Wehmeier KR, Oliver D, Bacon BR. Improved nonalcoholic steatohepatitis after 48 weeks of treatment with the PPAR-gamma ligand rosiglitazone. *Hepatology* 2003;**38**:1008–17.

209 Promrat K, Lutchman G, Uwaifo GI, *et al.* A pilot study of pioglitazone treatment for nonalcoholic steatohepatitis. *Hepatology* 2004;**39**:188–96.

210 Sanyal AJ, Mofrad PS, Contos MJ, *et al.* A pilot study of vitamin E versus vitamin E and pioglitazone for the treatment of nonalcoholic steatohepatitis. *Clin Gastroenterol Hepatol* 2004;**2**:1107–15.

211 Vajro P, Franzese A, Valerio G, Iannucci MP, Aragione N. Lack of efficacy of ursodeoxycholic acid for the treatment of liver abnormalities in obese children. *J Pediatr* 2000;**136**:739–43.

212 Lavine JE. Vitamin E treatment of nonalcoholic steatohepatitis in children: a pilot study. *J Pediatr* 2000;**136**:734–8.

213 Vajro P, Mandato C, Franzese A, *et al.* Vitamin E treatment in pediatric obesity-related liver disease: a randomized study. *J Pediatr Gastroenterol Nutr* 2004;**38**:48–55.

214 Harrison SA, Torgerson S, Hayashi P, Ward J, Schenker S. Vitamin E and vitamin C treatment improves fibrosis in patients with nonalcoholic steatohepatitis. *Am J Gastroenterol* 2003;**98**: 2485–90.

215 Kugelmas M, Hill DB, Vivian B, Marsano L, McClain CJ. Cytokines and NASH: a pilot study of the effects of lifestyle modification and vitamin E. *Hepatology* 2003;**38**:413–9.

216 Obici S, Wang J, Chowdury R, *et al.* Identification of a biochemical link between energy intake and energy expenditure. *J Clin Invest* 2002;**109**:1599–605.

217 Inge TH, Krebs NF, Garcia VF, *et al.* Bariatric surgery for severely overweight adolescents: concerns and recommendations. *Pediatrics* 2004;**114**:217–23.

218 Lawson ML, Kirk S, Mitchell T, *et al.* One-year outcomes of Roux-en-Y gastric bypass for morbidly obese adolescents: a multicenter study from the Pediatric Bariatric Study Group. *J Pediatr Surg* 2006;**41**:137–43.

12 Hepatobiliary Disease in Cystic Fibrosis

Carla Colombo

Introduction

Cystic fibrosis (CF) is the most common life-limiting autosomal recessive disease of the Caucasian population, with an incidence of approximately one in every 3000 live births worldwide.[1] It is a multiorgan disease, affecting more frequently the lungs, pancreas, sweat glands, and in males the wolffian ducts. Lung disease is the primary cause of morbidity and mortality and results from the combined and sustained effect of chronic infection from different respiratory pathogens and inflammation, leading to progressive damage and eventually to respiratory failure.

Other clinical manifestations include exocrine pancreatic insufficiency with intestinal malabsorption, intestinal obstruction in the neonatal period (meconium ileus) or later in life (distal intestinal obstructive syndrome), hepatobiliary disease, and elevated sweat electrolyte concentrations. An increasing proportion of patients develop diabetes mellitus in the second decade of life, and virtually all men with CF are infertile due to atresia or complete absence of the vas deferens. The phenotypic expression of CF disease is extremely heterogeneous in terms of the severity and type of organs involved. The major clinical manifestations of CF, the pathogenetic mechanism involved, and their relative frequencies are listed in Table 12.1.

When first described in 1938, the disease was almost invariably fatal during early childhood, and for many years the basic defect has remained unknown. At present, the median survival is approaching 40 years, but premature death due to respiratory failure is still a major problem.[2]

Potential contributors to the improved survival over the past two decades include centralized care in dedicated CF clinics[3] and advances in nutritional and respiratory treatment.[4]

In 1989, the discovery of the gene responsible for CF[5] led to recognition of the key role of the encoded protein—the cystic fibrosis transmembrane regulator (CFTR)—in maintaining fluid balance across epithelial cells. CFTR, a large protein of 1480 amino acids, belongs to the adenosine triphosphate (ATP)-binding cassette family and functions mainly as a low-conductance cyclic adenosine monophosphate (cAMP)-dependent chloride channel at the apical membrane of epithe lial cells, where it promotes transmembrane efflux of chloride ions.[6] The CF secretory defect leads to an inability to maintain the luminal hydration of ducts, leading to physicochemical abnormalities of secretions and duct obstruction.

CF is characterized by a striking genetic heterogeneity, with more than 1500 different disease-causing mutations identified to date.[7] Mutations have been grouped into six classes according to the known or presumed molecular mechanisms of dysfunction of the CFTR protein and the corresponding residual activity at the apical membrane of epithelial cells.[8] Class I, II, and III mutations are defined as severe and result in complete loss of chloride-channel function through different molecular mechanisms (lack of production, defect in protein packaging and transport, defect in chloride channel regulation); in contrast, class IV, V, and VI mutations are classified as mild mutations and are associated with altered conductance properties, reduced synthesis or defective stability of normal CFTR, and some residual CFTR membrane activity.[1]

This classification system based on functional classes of mutations allows evaluation of genotype/phenotype correlations, despite the wide genetic heterogeneity.[9] A good association has been established exclusively for the exocrine pancreas, patients with pancreatic insufficiency being generally homozygous or compound heterozygous for class I, II, and III mutations.[9–11] For other manifestations of CF, additional genetic factors (termed "modifier genes") and/or extrinsic factors (environmental, therapeutic, and iatrogenic) are probably important in determining disease heterogeneity.[12]

Using the same classification system, the genotype was found to be highly associated with outcome, with class I, II, and III mutations being associated with the highest mortality.[13]

On clinical grounds, the term "classic CF" refers to the more severe form of the disease, with multiorgan involvement and pancreatic insufficiency, and is associated with the presence of two severe mutations. Nonclassic forms of CF occur in around 10% of cases, are associated with mild mutations, and are characterized by residual pancreatic function

Diseases of the Liver and Biliary System in Children, 3rd edition. Edited by Deirdre Kelly. © 2008 Blackwell Publishing, ISBN: 978-1-4051-6334-7.

Table 12.1 Major clinical manifestations in cystic fibrosis.

Organ involved	Functional/structural abnormalities	Clinical manifestation	Frequency (%)
Sweat glands	Salt hyperconcentration	High sweat chloride concentrations	95–98%
		Salt loss syndrome	undefinined
Pancreas	Ducts obstruction with fibrocystic transformation	Pancreatic insufficiency	85%
	Inflammatory response in the surviving pancreatic tissue	Chronic /recurrent pancreatitis (if pancreatic sufficiency)	3–4%
	Islet cell strangulation	Diabetes mellitus	10–25%
Intestine	Thickened intestinal content	Meconium ileus	10–20%
		Distal intestinal obstruction	10%
		Rectal prolapse	1–2%
Liver and biliary tract	Thickened ductular secretions	Focal biliary cirrhosis	20–30%
		Multilobular biliary cirrhosis	10%
		Portal hypertension	2–5%
	Nutritional deficiencies	Liver steatosis	23–67%
		Microgallbladder	30%
	Lithogenic bile	Cholelithiasis	15%
Nose and paranasal	Mucus stagnation/infection	Sinusitis	90%
		Mucocele	16%
		Nasal polyps	15–26%
Lung	Defective mucus clearance	Chronic respiratory infections	97%
	obstruction-infection-inflammation	Pneumothorax	5–8%
		Massive hemoptysis	5%
		Allergic Broncopulmonary Aspergillosis	10%
Reproductive system			
-vas deferens	Atresia-azoospermia	Male sterility	98%
-uterine cervix	Cervical mucus abnormalities	Decreased female fertility	Undefined

and often single-organ disease (chronic bronchitis, sinusitis with nasal polyposis, pancreatitis, male infertility due to obstructive azoospermia).[14]

With the improved survival of CF patients, the clinical presentation of this complex, multisystem disease is continuing to evolve; epidemiologic studies have provided important insight into the disease's course, prognosis, and complications, including hepatobiliary disease.[15]

Spectrum of hepatobiliary manifestations of CF

Improved life expectancy and prolonged follow-up of CF patients have led to the recognition of the development of liver disease and a better understanding of the hepatobiliary manifestations of CF. There is now increased awareness of the wide spectrum of hepatic problems, which include specific alterations that can be ascribed to the underlying CFTR defect as well as lesions of iatrogenic origin or reflecting the effects of extrahepatic disease (Table 12.2).[16]

Liver disease (cholestasis/ focal biliary cirrhosis/ multilobular cirrhosis)

Involvement of the liver was described soon after CF was discovered,[17–19] and the disease was subsequently recognized as one of the relatively common causes of biliary cirrhosis in children.

Focal biliary cirrhosis is the classic and pathognomonic hepatic lesion of CF and is regarded as a direct consequence of the basic defect that results from biliary obstruction and progressive periportal fibrosis. This is the most clinically relevant CF-associated hepatic problem, since extension of the initially focal fibrogenic process may lead to multilobular biliary cirrhosis, portal hypertension, and related complications.[20]

Unlike pulmonary and pancreatic diseases that affect the majority of CF patients, liver disease develops in no more than one-third of patients. Nevertheless, liver disease and liver failure remain the single most important nonpulmonary cause of death, accounting for 2.5% of overall CF mortality.[21]

Pathogenesis

CF-associated liver disease represents the only inherited

Table 12.2 Hepatobiliary manifestations in cystic fibrosis.

Type of lesion	Clinical manifestation	Frequency (%)
Specific alterations ascribable to the underlying *CFTR* defect	Focal biliary cirrhosis	20–30
	Multilobular biliary cirrhosis	10
	Portal hypertension	2–5
	Neonatal cholestasis	Rare
	Sclerosing cholangitis	Rare
	Microgallbladder	30
	Cholelithiasis	15
Lesions of iatrogenic origin	Hepatic steatosis	23–67
	Drug hepatotoxicity	Undefined
Lesions reflecting the effects of a disease process that occurs outside the liver	Hepatic congestion	Rare
	Common bile duct stenosis	Rare

liver disease resulting from impaired secretory function of the biliary epithelium; it is currently classified among genetic cholangiopathies,[22] since it affects CFTR, one of the multiple cholangiocyte flux molecules that function as channels, exchangers, and transporters at the cholangiocyte plasma membrane.[23] In the hepatobiliary system, CFTR expression is indeed restricted to the apical membrane of cholangiocytes and gallbladder epithelial cells.[24] At this level, CFTR regulates the fluid and electrolyte content of bile and participates in the choleretic effect of secretin.[24]

In physiological conditions, cAMP-stimulated Cl^- secretion through low-conductance Cl^- channels imposes a negative luminal potential and an osmotic gradient that triggers passive secretion of Na^+ and water. The change in the apical Cl^- gradient facilitates HCO_3^- extrusion via Cl^-/HCO_3^- exchange, providing the biliary alkalization required for the digestive function and for the solubility of organic components of bile (Figure 12.1).

Lack of CFTR has a greater impact on cell function than could be predicted by its role as a cAMP-stimulated Cl^- channel.[6] CFTR plays an important role in the regulation of other membrane transport proteins, including Na^+ channels (EnaC), K^+ channels, outward rectifying Cl^- channels (ORCC) and Cl^-/HCO_3^- exchangers (AE2).[6,23] There is also evidence that CFTR regulates cellular secretion of ATP, intracellular vesicle acidification, and the processing and trafficking of certain proteins, including mucin secretion.

Ductal cholestasis due to reduced CFTR-related fluid and electrolyte transport by cholangiocytes is considered the central step in the pathogenetic sequence of CF-associated liver disease, and liver disease has been shown to occur in a long-living CFTR knockout murine mice model.[25]

In addition, a study in primary culture of human cholangiocytes has clearly documented that cAMP-stimulated Cl^- and HCO_3^- transport are both impaired in CF.[26] The resulting reduction in bile fluidity and alkalinity would lead to plugging of intrahepatic bile ducts by inspissated secretions. Quantitative and qualitative abnormality in mucin secretion may also contribute to abnormal bile viscosity in CF patients: secretion of chondroitin sulphate was shown to be markedly increased in CF biliary epithelium in vitro,[27] and its accumulation may well explain bile duct plugging by eosinophilic material, which is one of the early histological changes found in infants and children with CF.[28]

Cholangiocyte injury, with irregular shapes, reduced microvilli, necrosis, and periductular collagen deposition, was a consistent finding in asymptomatic CF patients well before the development of clinical evidence of liver disease,[29] suggesting that damage to the bile duct epithelium may be the primary event in the development of periportal fibrosis. These lesions may represent the anatomical expression of long-standing impairment in ductular bile flow, which may increase susceptibility of the biliary epithelium to damage by cytotoxic compounds excreted into bile and to aggression by microbial pathogens. In addition, retention of endogenous hydrophobic bile acids may be responsible for cell membrane injury also at the hepatocellular level[30] (Figure 12.2). Oxidative injury to the liver cell membrane may occur through increased free radical production favored by decreased lipid-soluble antioxidant activity.[31] Injured cholangiocytes may release proinflammatory cytokines and growth factors that would recruit and activate hepatic stellate cells for collagen synthesis (Figure 12.2).[32]

In CF, the biliary canaliculi and small bile ducts become focally obstructed with inspissated biliary secretions, gradually leading to the development of portal fibrosis, bridging, and eventually cirrhosis. This process begins focally in the liver, possibly because of interductal connections that allow adequate bile drainage from some areas.[33] The progression from cholestasis to focal biliary cirrhosis to multilobular cirrhosis is a slow process that should be viewed as a continuum.[20]

In summary, the current evidence suggests that liver disease in CF is related to the basic defect at the hepatobiliary

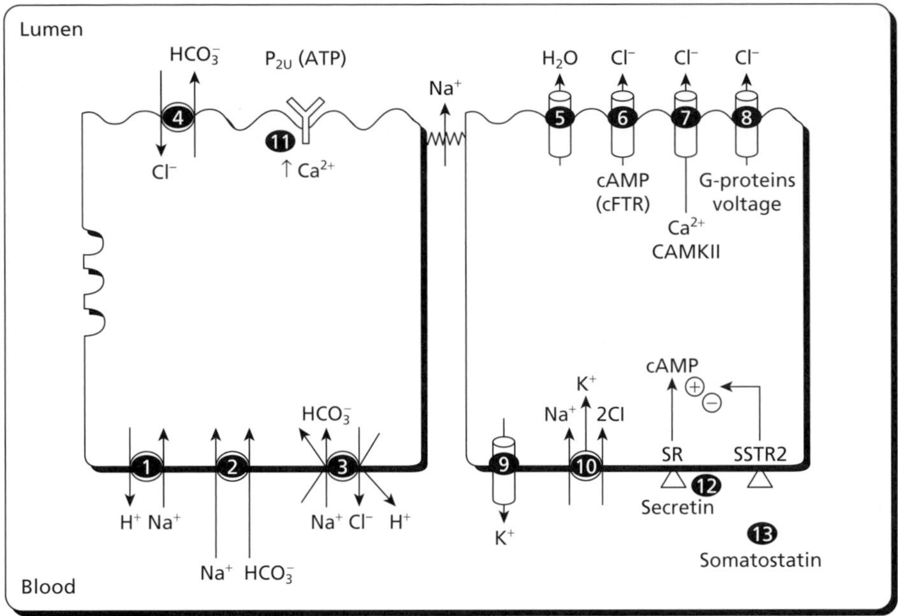

Figure 12.1 Model of cholangiocyte bile formation. Bile formation requires the coordinated function of two epithelial cell types that form a functional bile secretory unit. Hepatocytes secrete the major biliary osmolytes and constituents, such as bile acids, lipids, glutathione, organic cations, and anions, xenobiotics, proteins, and electrolytes. Cholangiocytes (represented in the figure) are located downstream, and are responsible for the rapid regulation of bile volume, fluidity, and alkalinity in response to a complex network of hormones, such as secretin (12) and somatostatin (13), and paracrine mediators, such as ATP (11). Their interplay results in net secretion or absorption of osmolytes, mainly Cl^- and HCO_3^-. Studies in isolated cholangiocyte preparations have recently elucidated the basic mechanisms involved in constitutive and stimulated Cl^- and HCO_3^- transport in the biliary epithelium. Basolateral Na^+/H^+ exchanger (1) and Na^+/HCO_3^- symporter (2)—Na^+-dependent Cl^-/HCO_3^- exchanger in humans (3)—mediates cellular HCO_3^- uptake. Bicarbonate is then secreted into the biliary lumen by a Cl^-/HCO_3^- exchanger (4) located at the apical membrane. Water channels (5) located at the apical and lateral membrane facilitate H_2O movements flowing across the established osmotic gradients. Basolateral Cl^- uptake involves a bumetanide-sensitive $Na^+/K^+/2Cl^-$ cotransporter (10), while apical Cl^- efflux is mainly mediated by a cAMP-activated Cl^- channel with electrophysiological features that are similar to CFTR (6). In addition to CFTR, a number of Cl^- conductive pathways, including a Ca^{2+}/CAMK II-activated Cl^- channel (7), and a G protein–regulated, voltage-dependent Cl^- channel (8), are located at the apical cell membrane of cholangiocytes. Basolateral K^+ channels (9) modulate the membrane potential difference. (Reproduced with permission from Colombo *et al., Semin Liver Dis* 1998;**18**:227–35.)

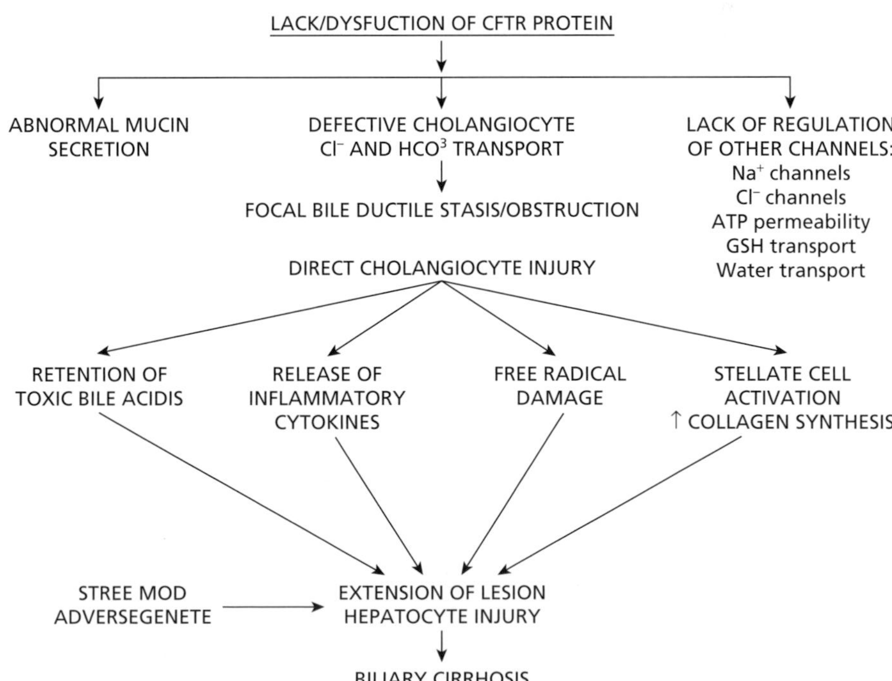

Figure 12.2 Proposed pathogenetic model for cystic fibrosis–associated liver disease.

level. However, it remains to be explained why only one-third of CF patients develop liver disease and why liver disease shows a great degree of variability in terms of its severity. It should be noted that, in addition to CFTR, a number of Cl^- conductive pathways, including a Ca^{2+}-activated Cl^- channel and a G protein–regulated voltage-dependent Cl^- channel, are located at the apical cell membrane of the cholangiocytes[34] and may partly compensate the CF secretory defect in the liver (Figure 12.1). Indeed, in human CF cholangiocytes, alternative Ca^{2+}-activated Cl^- channels have been shown to be able to support HCO_3^- secretion.[26]

The development of liver disease appears to be restricted to patients with a severe genotype, but no specific CFTR mutations have been associated with the presence and severity of liver disease,[35,36] suggesting a multifactorial pathogenesis. Although familial clustering of liver disease has occasionally been reported, the poor concordance of liver disease in sibling pairs appears to exclude a major role for environmental factors. On the other hand, a study of siblings with discordant liver expression has suggested that genetic factors inherited independently from the *CFTR* gene could modulate the clinical expression and severity of liver disease in CF.[37]

The role of modifier genes in CF is presently the object of much research interest and a genetic variation in the 5′ terminal of transforming growth factor-β1 (TGF-β1) has recently been shown to modify lung disease severity in CF patients.[38] With regard to liver disease, there is some evidence that polymorphisms in genes that up-regulate inflammation, fibrosis, or oxidative stress may confer increased susceptibility for its development. A complex multigenic inheritance may be present, with possible interaction of different genes (α_1-antitrypsin deficiency, TGF-β cytokine, mannose-binding lectin 2, and glutathione *S*-transferase).[39–41] Identification of genetic modifiers for liver disease is a research priority, as it may allow early identification of patients at risk who might benefit from prophylactic strategies.

Hepatic steatosis

The most common hepatic lesion associated with CF is steatosis, which does not appear to be directly related to the CF secretory defect (Table 12.2). Steatosis may be detected in a substantial proportion (23–67%) of CF patients of any age. The pathogenesis is still largely unknown, but it does not appear to be directly related to the basic CF defect. The available evidence suggests that it may well be because the liver is involved as an innocent bystander. Massive steatosis, once frequently observed in newly diagnosed patients with pancreatic insufficiency and severe malnutrition, has become infrequent due to earlier diagnosis and to more appropriate nutritional care. Mild steatosis is now more common and has been associated with selective nutritional deficiencies including essential fatty acids,[42] carnitine, choline, trace elements, mineral and altered phospholipid metabolism in CF;[43] it may be also a consequence of diabetes or long-term antibiotic therapy. Increasingly recognized in non-CF adult populations, steatosis may be a hepatic consequence of the metabolic syndrome and conditions associated with insulin resistance,[44] which is a common event in CF patients due to chronic infection and inflammation.[45] It has been suggested that in CF patients who are chronically colonized by respiratory pathogens, steatosis may result from the effect of circulating cytokines on hepatic fatty acid oxidation or mitochondrial function.[46] Steatosis has been regarded as a benign condition in CF, without a proven relationship to the subsequent development of cirrhosis. The available data on the role of nonalcoholic steatohepatitis as a cause of cirrhosis in adults[47,48] may lead to reconsideration of this issue in CF patients.

Prevalence of liver disease

There are marked differences in the reported prevalence of CF-associated liver disease, which can be explained by differences in the diagnostic criteria and in the populations studied. The highest figures have been provided by autopsy studies, which have also documented a progressive increase in the prevalence of liver disease with age, from 10% in infants[28] to 72% in adults.[49] However, autopsy data in CF may be affected by significant bias, since liver disease may have contributed to death or may have been the reason for postmortem evaluation. On the other hand, histological data obtained by means of liver biopsy during life are insufficient to provide reliable epidemiologic information.

Prevalence figures obtained by retrospective analyses in clinical settings are much lower, ranging between 4.2%[43] and 17%.[50] However, cross-sectional studies in which liver disease was actively searched for using biochemical and ultrasonographic assessment have provided higher prevalence figures (from 18% to 37%);[51] the prevalence appears to increase through childhood, with a peak in mid-adolescence and no increase in frequency thereafter.[52]

More recently, prospective studies have been carried out to assess the incidence and risk factors for the development of liver disease. Long-term follow-up of different cohorts of CF patients carefully monitored for hepatic status has indicated a cumulative incidence of liver disease ranging between 27% and 35%, without incident cases after the age of 18 years.[42,53,54]

Overall, these data suggest that, for CF patients who will develop liver disease, the mechanism and risk factors for liver damage are already present in early childhood.

Risk factors for liver disease in CF

Identification of CF patients at risk of developing liver disease is a major clinical issue, since therapeutic intervention are likely to be more effective in patients with early stage liver disease. Several factors have been recognized to be significantly associated with the development of CF liver disease, including pancreatic insufficiency, severe genotype, male sex, history of meconium ileus, and age at diagnosis of CF.[35,36,54–56]

There is general agreement that liver disease should be considered as part of the classic CF phenotype with pancreatic insufficiency,[14] and it has only been occasionally reported in pancreatic sufficient patients.[57]

Despite the lack of association between any specific CFTR mutation and the development of liver disease,[35,36] the incidence of liver disease is higher in patients with severe genotypes—i.e., carrying class I, II, or III mutations on both alleles,[54] suggesting that this is necessary but not sufficient for the development of liver disease in CF.

A preponderance of male subjects among CF patients with liver disease has been reported by several studies[52,50,54,58] and was recently confirmed by a survey of European CF patients who had undergone liver transplantation.[59] This gender difference suggests a possible role of endocrine factors in the development or recognition of this complication. In this respect, estrogens and their receptors have been shown to play a critical role in modulating proliferative and secretory activities of hepatocytes and intrahepatic biliary epithelium as a response to liver damage; female patients may therefore be protected from severe liver damage after puberty.[54]

A few studies have reported a significantly higher incidence of liver disease in CF patients with a positive history of meconium ileus.[54,55,58,60] This association, linking inspissated gut content and biliary secretions, was first described in a necropsy study,[61] but was not consistently found in cross-sectional studies involving different CF patient populations,[36,42] and a study recently reported that meconium ileus was associated with an absence of liver disease.[56] In patients with a positive history of meconium ileus, additional risk factors for the development of liver disease may include abdominal surgery with extensive small-bowel resection, poor nutrition in early life, and prolonged total parenteral nutrition. Alternatively, a number of unknown factors, including genetic modifiers associated with gender or ethnic group, may explain the different susceptibility to liver and intestinal involvement in CF patients.

Finally, one study from Ireland has recently reported that age at diagnosis of CF represents an important risk factor for the development of liver disease.[56] The finding that later diagnosis (with a poor nutritional status) may predispose children with CF to liver disease supports the newborn screening programs aimed at earlier diagnosis of CF.[62]

Clinical features

Liver disease associated with CF usually develops before puberty and is often asymptomatic and slowly progressive. Signs of chronic liver disease such as jaundice, palmar erythema, and spider hemangiomas are rarely present and generally limited to patients with end-stage liver disease.

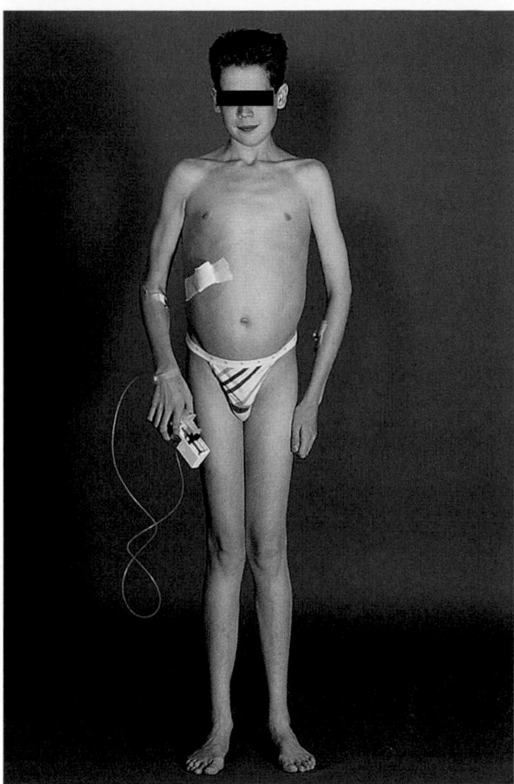

Figure 12.3 The commonest presentation of cystic fibrosis is with malnutrition, abdominal distension, and hepatosplenomegaly secondary to cirrhosis and portal hypertension.

The most common presentation is the occasional finding of hepatomegaly on routine physical examination, which may be associated with abnormalities in liver biochemistry (Figure 12.3), but the spectrum includes neonatal disease and gallbladder disease.

Neonatal cholestasis

Liver involvement as the direct consequence of the basic CF defect (Table 12.2) rarely presents with neonatal cholestasis, caused by obstruction of the extrahepatic bile ducts by viscous biliary secretions,[63] but it may be the presenting symptom of CF.

Infants may present with:

- Cholestatic neonatal hepatitis (see Chapter 4)
- Fat malabsorption and failure to thrive
- Vitamin K–responsive hemorrhagic disease
- Meconium ileus
- Recurrent chest infections
- Inspissated bile syndrome

Cholestasis may be complete, mimicking biliary atresia, but serum cholesterol concentrations are generally normal.[64] At greater risk are infants with meconium ileus, particularly those with other conditions enhancing the risk of cholestasis—i.e., total parenteral nutrition or abdominal surgery.

Although CF infants may require a much longer period to clear jaundice than infants with other medical disorders presenting with neonatal jaundice (median time in one study 7.36 months versus 2.5 months),[63] cholestasis generally resolves spontaneously over the first months of life, perhaps because of the resolution of physiologic cholestasis and the maturation of biliary secretion.[65] In addition, these infants do not have a higher risk of developing cirrhosis.

Hepatomegaly and portal hypertension

A more usual presentation in older children is with:

- Intermittent transaminitis and a raised alkaline phosphatase
- Asymptomatic hepatomegaly
- Hepatosplenomegaly
- Hypersplenism
- Variceal hemorrhage from portal hypertension
- Malnutrition
- Clubbing, which may be related to either liver or pulmonary disease
- Diabetes mellitus

Hepatomegaly may be due to steatosis, fibrosis, or right ventricular failure in severely ill children. The development of splenomegaly, palmar erythema, and telangiectasia suggests cirrhosis. Multilobular biliary cirrhosis is considered to develop sequentially from focal biliary cirrhosis in around 10% of patients,[42] but progression of liver disease from the early asymptomatic stage to liver failure remains unpredictable and may take years or even decades to occur;[9] in a minority of patients, often in the pediatric age group, liver disease may represent the dominant manifestation of CF and its progression may be unusually rapid, suggesting the role of adverse genetic modifiers.

As in other forms of liver disease characterized by initial involvement of bile ducts and not of hepatocytes, liver failure is a late event. In contrast, the hemodynamic consequences of cirrhosis are often prominent, favoring early development of portal hypertension and related complications.[58,66] The divergence in timing between presentation with portal hypertension and decompensation of hepatocellular function frequently reported in CF may be also explained by the characteristic focal distribution of hepatic lesions.[67]

Once cirrhosis is established, the risk of gastrointestinal bleeding from esophageal or gastric varices is high. Splenomegaly is often asymptomatic, but hypersplenism may develop, with thrombocytopenia and leukopenia; however, this is rarely clinically significant without portal hypertension. Massive splenic enlargement may cause abdominal discomfort or pain and deterioration of pulmonary function due to diaphragmatic splinting;[58] ascites, encephalopathy, fatigue, and coagulopathy occur later, when cirrhosis decompensates and there is an indication for transplantation.

Progress of liver disease

In a retrospective study spanning a 26-year period, of 44 children with CF investigated for liver cirrhosis at a tertiary referral pediatric hepatology center, esophageal varices developed in 38 (86%), and in half of these patients esophageal bleeding occurred early during the second decade of life; liver failure occurred in 15 patients (36%) at a mean age of 15 years.[58] Another study reported variceal bleeding in 1.6% of a large series of adult CF patients (18 of 1154) followed at a single center, at a median age of 20 years (range 9.7–30.9 y); bleeding was the only clinical consequence of liver disease in approximately one-third of the patients, in whom hepatic function was relatively well preserved;[66] the median survival after variceal bleeding was 8.4 years, in comparison with a 1-year survival of only 34% in the general cirrhotic population, suggesting that a history of bleeding in the absence of decompensated cirrhosis may not represent an indicator of a markedly adverse prognosis in CF.[66]

The natural history and outcome of liver disease in CF patients have also been evaluated in prospective studies.[42,54,55] Slow progression of liver disease was demonstrated in a histological study reported by Lindblad *et al.*[42] The incidence of cirrhosis was between 2.28[55] and 4.5 per 100 patient-years.[54] In the study carried out at the Milan CF Center, during more than 8 years from the diagnosis of liver disease, the incidence of major complications of cirrhosis (gastrointestinal bleeding, encephalopathy, ascites) was 0.4 cases per 100 cirrhotic patient-years (95% CI, 0 to 2.0) (Table 12.3),[54] in comparison with a hepatic decompensation rate of 10% in cirrhosis in adults.[68]

Finally, the current evidence suggests that the impact of liver disease on the outcome of CF is negligible in comparison with the general CF population until end-stage liver failure develops. There is no significant increase in the rate of respiratory failure, need for oxygen therapy, frequency of hospitalization, or mortality in CF patients with liver disease,[42,54] and a study has also suggested that children with CF-associated liver disease may have a better pulmonary

Table 12.3 Incidence of liver disease and its complications in cystic fibrosis.

	Incidence (n/100 patient-years) (95% CI)
Liver disease	
Overall	1.8 (1.3 to 2.4)
First 10 y of life	2.5 (1.8 to 3.3)
Cirrhosis, liver disease patients	4.5 (2.3 to 7.8)
Portal hypertension, cirrhotic patients	28.8 (15.4 to 49.3)
Liver decompensation, cirrhotic patients	0.4 (0 to 2.0)
Death of any cause, or orthotopic liver transplantation	
Liver disease patients	0.4 (0.1 to 1.2)
Cirrhotic patients	1.6 (0.3 to 4.7)

Reproduced with permission from Pinto *et al.*, *J Hepatol* 2006;**44**:197–208.[48]

prognosis than those without liver disease[69]—providing support for the old belief that "bad livers" are often associated with "good lungs."

Overall, the data suggest that liver disease does not expose CF patients to a higher risk of severe pulmonary disease, other negative outcome events, or mortality.

Impact of end-stage liver disease in CF

In contrast, the impact of advanced liver disease on the pulmonary function and the nutritional status of CF patients are becoming increasingly evident. During the progression of liver disease, CF patients are at risk of developing not only complications related to portal hypertension, but also several extrahepatic complications, including malnutrition and wasting, hepatic osteodystrophy, and deterioration of pulmonary status.

Malnutrition. Malnutrition is a common complication of cystic fibrosis in general, but may be exacerbated by the development of liver disease with an increase in fat malabsorption and protein wasting (Chapter 15; Figure 12.3).

The pathogenesis of malnutrition is multifactorial and involves the increase in resting energy expenditure (REE),[70] abnormalities in nutrient intake (due to anorexia and, in patients with encephalopathy, to protein restriction), malabsorption (due to the combined effect of cholestasis and pancreatic insufficiency), and abnormal metabolism of nutrients (Table 12.4).[70] Many CF patients develop decompensated liver disease as adolescents, when glucose intolerance or diabetes are more likely to develop;[71] in addition, advanced liver disease may induce insulin resistance and thus represent a major risk factor for the development of CF-related diabetes.[72]

End-stage liver disease may also induce significant changes in body composition, including osteoporosis and reduced fat and lean body mass. Severe osteopenia was documented in a group of CF patients with multilobular biliary cirrhosis and portal hypertension, which was significantly corrected after transplantation but not after conservative management.[73] The effect is presumably linked to the restoration of hepatic function and bile flow after transplantation.

With regard to pulmonary status, cirrhosis and portal hypertension can negatively affect respiratory function due to organomegaly, ascites-induced diaphragmatic splinting, and intrapulmonary shunting, leading to recurrent respiratory infections from multiresistant bacteria, frequent hospital admissions, and a significant deterioration in quality of life.

Hepatic congestion

Other conditions involving hepatic damage as the effect of a disease process occurring outside the liver include hepatic congestion from right-side heart failure, although this is confined to a relatively small group of older patients with advanced CF.

Gallbladder abnormalities

CFTR is expressed in the gallbladder epithelium;[24] this may explain the high frequency of gallbladder abnormalities observed in CF patients, although symptomatic biliary disease is uncommon. Symptoms and signs may include:

- Asymptomatic gallstones, which are found in 20–30% (Figure 12.4)
- Microgallbladder on ultrasound, which is present in 10–40% of the patients[74,75]
- Nonvisualized, nonfunctioning gallbladders on hepatobiliary scintigraphy in over 50%;[76] this does not need any therapeutic intervention
- Sclerosing cholangitis
- Biliary strictures

Submucosal cysts, septate gallbladders, and adenomyomas have also been described.[49]

Cholelithiasis is often an occasional finding in CF patients. Symptoms have been reported to occur in less than 4% of cases;[77] the prevalence appears to increase with age (from

Table 12.4 Causes of malnutrition in cystic fibrosis patients with liver disease.

Reduced caloric intake:
Anorexia
Protein restriction (if encephalopathy)
Malabsorption of lipid-soluble nutrients/vitamins:
Reduced bile flow
Pancreatic insufficiency
Abnormal metabolism of nutrients:
Carbohydrates: glucose intolerance/diabetes, reduced hepatic glycogen, insulin resistance
Protein: hypercatabolic state, increased tyrosine and phenylalanine, decreased branched amino acids
Lipids: essential fatty acid deficiency
Vitamin D: reduced 25-hydroxylation
Vitamin A: defective release from liver stores
Increased resting energy expenditure (REE)

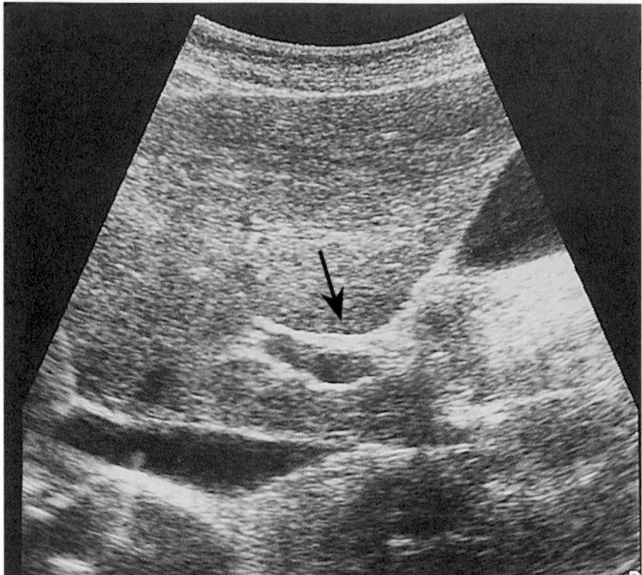

Figure 12.4 Ultrasound examination often demonstrates a coarse liver texture and a microgallbladder with gallstones.

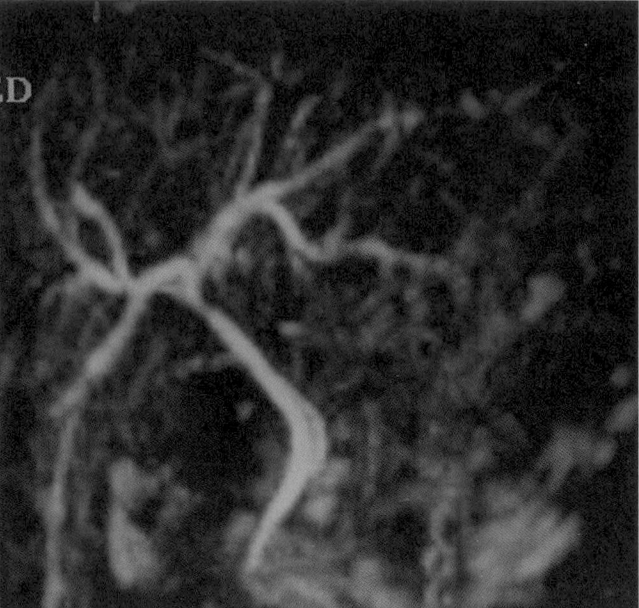

Figure 12.5 Magnetic resonance cholangiopancreatography is less invasive than endoscopic retrograde cholangiography and produces excellent imaging, demonstrating variable dilation of the bile ducts.

8–12% in late childhood, to more than 20% in adults), but the frequency of this complication may have decreased over the last decade due to better correction of pancreatic insufficiency and nutritional status of CF patients.[78] The pathogenesis of cholelithiasis was considered to be related to the production of lithogenic bile[79] as a result of bile acid malabsorption associated with steatorrhea,[80] but a subsequent study has indicated that the main component of CF gallstones is calcium bilirubinate, rather than cholesterol.[81] This finding is in agreement with the reported failure of ursodeoxycholic acid therapy to dissolve radiolucent gallstones in CF patients.[82] Bile stasis and abnormalities in biliary mucus may predispose to nidus formation.

Intrahepatic stones have been also observed.[83] Motor abnormalities of the extrahepatic biliary tree (dyskinesia) have also been reported, and these may be associated with gallbladder distension and biliary pain.[84]

Sclerosing cholangitis

Sclerosing cholangitis, with strictures and beads in the larger intrahepatic bile ducts, was initially reported in a few adult CF patients, sometimes in association with inflammatory bowel disease.[85] However, typical cholangiographic abnormalities of the intrahepatic bile ducts have been subsequently reported in the majority of adult patients with CF-associated liver disease,[84] suggesting that they may be related to the underlying CFTR defect. Such lesions have been considered to be the expression of an inflammatory process involving the bile ducts, accumulation of proteins and mucus, and compression of intrahepatic bile ducts induced by fibrosis, and they may be a marker of severe hepatic damage. More recently, using magnetic resonance cholangiography, cholangitic abnormalities have also been documented in a significant proportion of CF patients without clinically apparent liver disease, and may therefore reflect the presence of inspissated biliary secretions related to the CF secretory defect.[86] Interestingly, an increased prevalence of *CFTR* mutations has been reported in patients with primary sclerosing cholangitis,[87] suggesting that patients with inflammatory bowel disease who are heterozygous carriers of *CFTR* mutations may be at increased risk of developing sclerosing cholangitis (Figure 12.5).

Common bile duct stenosis

Stenosis of the intrapancreatic portion of the common bile duct due to pancreatic fibrosis is an example of hepatic damage secondary to a disease process occurring outside the liver. With the exception of one study that documented its presence in the vast majority of CF patients with liver disease,[76] common bile duct stenosis is a rare complication.[83,84] It may cause complete or partial biliary obstruction—often associated with jaundice, right upper quadrant pain, or excessive steatorrhea—and may respond to surgical decompression.[76] Biliary pain may be related to inflammation proximal to the stenosis or to a pressure effect, producing enlarged, distended gallbladders, which were seen in around 20% of the patients described by Gaskin *et al.*[76]

Diagnosis of CF-associated liver disease

Evidence of liver disease in CF patients is often subclinical, with normal biochemical liver function tests until pathological

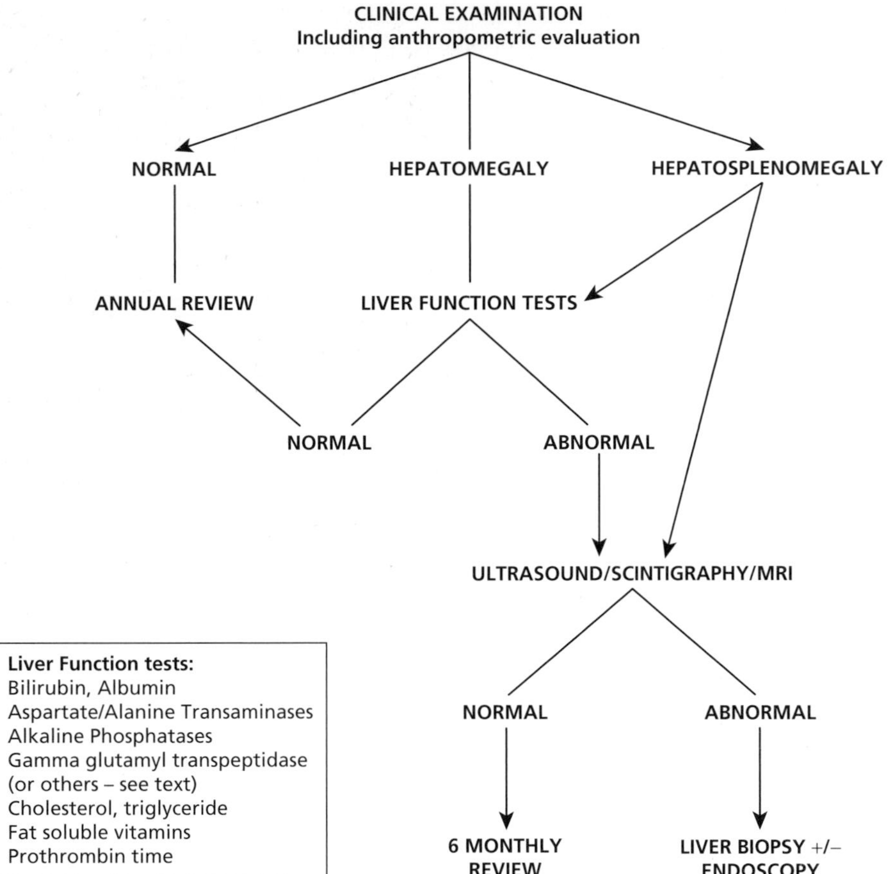

Figure 12.6 The algorithm for routine investigations for liver disease in cystic fibrosis.

changes are diffuse and advanced, and so it is often underdiagnosed. Early detection can be difficult but is essential, as early lesions are likely to be reversible. As there are no good tests for biliary cell dysfunction, the diagnosis of CF-associated liver disease is based on clinical examination and a combination of biochemical tests and imaging techniques (Figure 12.6).

Physical examination

Regular clinical examination is still of major importance for detecting and evaluating progression of liver disease in CF. The liver may be firm and nodular, often extending more than 3 cm below the right costal margin, and its enlargement may be limited to the right—or, more often, to the left lobe, which protrudes centrally. Since the liver is often pushed down as a result of pulmonary disease, it is important to measure the liver span at the right midclavicular line through percussion and palpation.[20,88] The presence of hepatomegaly correlated with the degree of liver fibrosis at the time of biliary tract surgery.[76]

Splenomegaly is the first sign of portal hypertension and requires close monitoring at every follow-up visit. Attention should be paid to the presence of peripheral signs of chronic liver disease, including spider nevi, palmar erythema, jaundice, edema, distension of abdominal wall veins, and eversion of the umbilicus (Figure 12.3).

Liver biochemistry

Biochemical abnormalities are frequently mild or only present intermittently and have shown low sensitivity and no correlation with the histologic findings;[89] not infrequently, CF patients with multilobular biliary cirrhosis have completely normal liver biochemistry. Nonspecific biochemical abnormalities have been documented in more than 50% of infants with CF, with complete normalization in most cases within 2–3 years of age and no impact on future development of liver disease.[42]

Common findings include:

• Intermittent rises in plasma transaminases—aspartate aminotransferase (AST) and alanine aminotransferase (ALT)—in 30% of patients.
• Serum levels of alkaline phosphatase may be elevated in 50% of children, but are difficult to evaluate in growing children.
• Serum levels of γ-glutamyltransferase (GGT), leucine aminopeptidase, and 5′ nucleotidase may be abnormal in those with more serious liver disease.

Occasional biochemical abnormalities occur as a result of drug treatment, infection, or malnutrition. It is therefore important to exclude other causes of acute or chronic elevation of hepatic aminotransferases (infectious and autoimmune hepatitis, metabolic disorders, drug hepatotoxicity).

Isolated elevation of serum transaminase levels, with normal concentrations of enzyme related to cholestasis (GGT and alkaline phosphatase) suggests the presence of steatosis, and requires correction of nutritional deficiencies, if present.

Ultrasonography

Ultrasonography of the hepatobiliary system is recommended as the most suitable initial noninvasive method of investigation. Ultrasound technology has improved in recent years and reliably distinguishes between normal parenchyma, steatosis, fibrosis, cirrhosis, portal hypertension, and ductal abnormalities. Abnormal echogenicity frequently precedes clinical and biochemical manifestations of liver disease, suggesting that routine ultrasonography may be a valuable marker of early liver disease in CF.[90,91] Doppler ultrasound can evaluate the flow patterns of hepatic vasculature: decreased portal venous flow velocities or reversal of flow (hepatofugal) in the portal vein are indicative of portal hypertension. Thrombosis of the portal or splenic veins as a cause of splenomegaly can also be documented.

To overcome the problem of interobserver and intraobserver variability, attempts have been made to standardize the method of assessment, and scoring systems have been developed. A simple echographic scoring system based on the coarseness of the liver parenchyma, nodularity of the liver edge, and increased periportal echogenicity was first proposed for the hepatic follow-up of these patients.[92] More recently, Stewart proposed an alternative, more complex scoring system that considers many different components of liver disease and is presently under evaluation.[93]

Hepatobiliary scintigraphy

Hepatobiliary scintigraphy with third-generation iminodiacetic acid derivative tracers (which concentrate well in the biliary tree) has been used to screen for biliary tract disease in CF patients.[76] Scintigraphy can document a typical picture of biliary drainage impairment, with dilation of the intrahepatic and extrahepatic bile ducts and delayed biliary excretion and intestinal appearance of the tracer; it also provides functional information.[94–96] In one study, it was used in association with percutaneous transhepatic cholangiography to identify the presence of true stenosis of the common bile duct, which was subsequently confirmed at surgery.[76]

Scintigraphy has also been used to document time-related progression of liver disease[95] and to monitor the response to treatment with ursodeoxycholic acid (Figure 12.7).[96]

Computed tomography

Computed tomography may be helpful in confirming the presence of multilobular biliary cirrhosis and portal hypertension, but it lacks both specificity and sensitivity in diagnosing focal biliary cirrhosis.

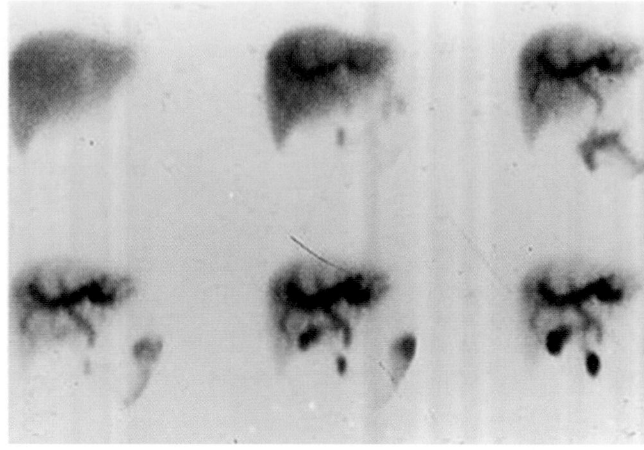

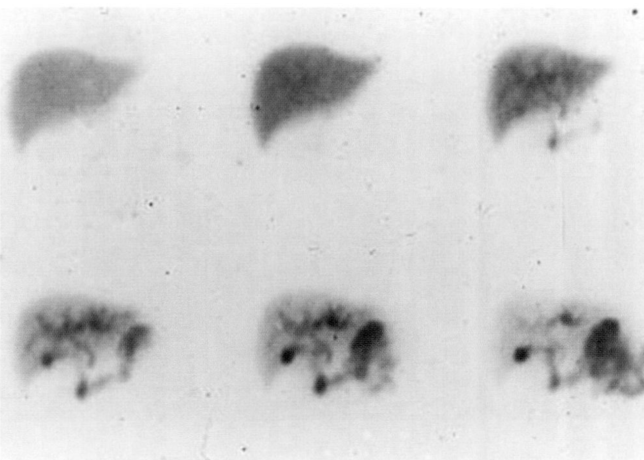

Figure 12.7 Hepatobiliary scintigraphy before (**A**) and after (**B**) ursodeoxycholic acid therapy, demonstrating improved biliary flow. (Reproduced with permission from Colombo *et al.*, *Hepatology* 1992;**15**:677–84.[96])

Cholangiography

Percutaneous transhepatic cholangiography and endoscopic retrograde cholangiography (ERCP) are invasive procedures (with considerable potential for complications) for the investigation of patients with symptoms and signs suggestive of sclerosing cholangitis[85] and distal stenosis of the common bile duct,[76] and for those with choledocholithiasis, for whom ERCP also provides a therapeutic option. For both procedures, oblique films may be required for visualization of the distal common bile duct, which is often displaced posteriorly to the duodenum.[76]

Magnetic resonance cholangiography

Magnetic resonance cholangiography imaging of the biliary tree in CF patients has revealed cholangitic lesions in all patients with liver disease and in half of those without clinically apparent liver disease, suggesting that this technique may be employed for early detection of intrahepatic biliary tract involvement, which cannot be achieved with other noninvasive methods (Figure 12.5).[86]

Liver pathology

Histological assessment, which represents the gold standard in the diagnostic work-up of many chronic liver diseases, is controversial in CF patients because of the potential risk of sampling error due to patchy distribution of lesions and underrepresentation of the extent of the disease.[76,88] Despite this, a good correlation between wedge biopsies and needle biopsies has been demonstrated.[89]

The indications for liver biopsy include:

- Persistent transaminitis
- Hepatic echogenicity on ultrasound
- Hepatomegaly and/or splenomegaly
- Evidence of hepatic dysfunction (falling albumin or abnormal coagulation)
- If there is any doubt about the diagnosis
- To stage the disease (e.g., to establish whether cirrhosis is present)
- Prior to medical treatment or liver transplantation

It is advisable to follow the general rules for liver biopsy (Chapter 2).

The histologic hallmark of CF-related liver disease is the deposition of inspissated bile (appearing as eosinophilic material with variable degrees of periodic acid–Schiff-positive reaction) in dilated cholangioles. There is focal periportal obstructive disease with bile duct proliferation and cholangitis, a variable combination of inspissation, inflammation around the portal tracts, fatty infiltration (hepatocyte vacuolization with micro and macrodroplet steatosis), and fibrosis (starting around the portal tracts and then extending intralobularly). Fibrosis and fatty infiltration are the most common features, whereas the presence of inspissated bile in cholangioles is infrequent.[89] Liver biopsy may provide important information on the type of predominant lesion (steatosis or focal biliary cirrhosis), the extent of portal fibrosis, the rate of progression of liver disease, and the response to treatment with ursodeoxycholic acid (Figure 12.8).

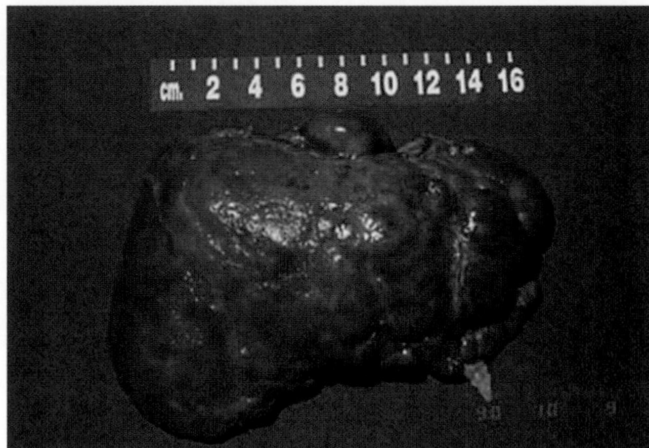

A

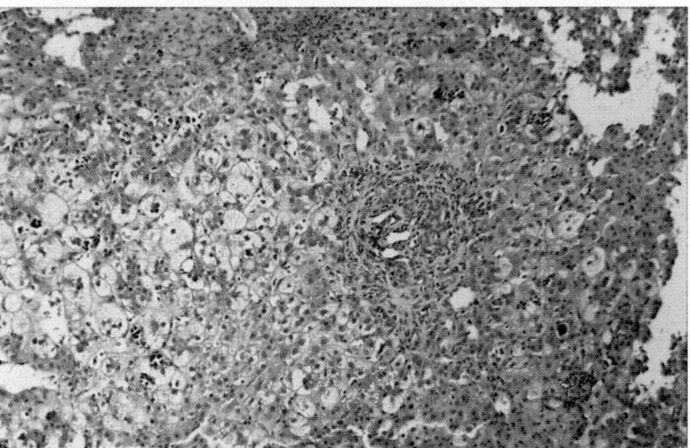

B

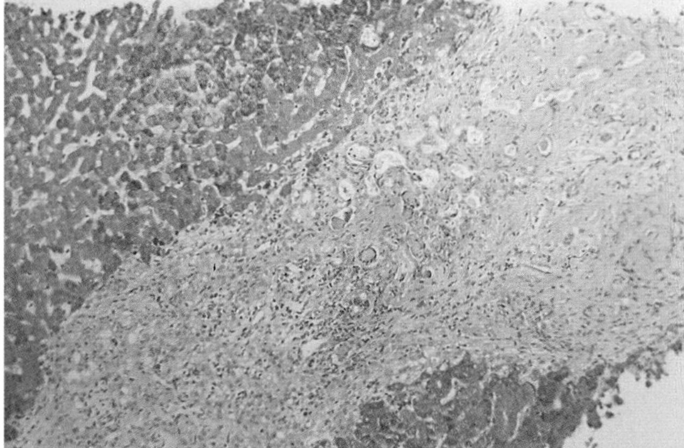

C

Figure 12.8 A Multilobular biliary cirrhosis a 9-year-old boy with cystic fibrosis. **B** Histology may also demonstrate steatosis and chemical cholangitis, or focal biliary fibrosis (**C**) with portal inflammation.

Hepatic follow-up of CF patients

Regular monitoring of hepatic status with liver biochemistry and ultrasound scanning is essential in all patients with CF and should be included in their routine annual schedule.

In patients with cirrhosis, α-fetoprotein levels should be measured annually to monitor the possible development of hepatocellular carcinoma.[97,98]

Upper gastrointestinal endoscopy is most useful in detecting the presence of esophageal varices and portal hypertensive gastropathy, and should be performed at least annually in patients with portal hypertension.

Treatment options for CF-associated liver disease

Because of the decreasing mortality from extrahepatic causes, the treatment of liver disease in CF patients is a relevant clinical issue. At present, management of CF-associated liver disease depends on the clinical manifestations. Oral bile acid therapy is generally started early in the course of the disease when the patient is asymptomatic, whereas end-stage liver disease often requires a complex and multidisciplinary approach, including a variety of surgical interventions.

Bile acid therapy

Oral bile acid therapy, aimed at improving biliary secretion in terms of bile viscosity and bile acid composition, is currently the only available therapeutic approach for CF-associated liver disease.

Ursodeoxycholic acid (UDCA) administration affects several of the mechanisms involved in cholestasis-induced liver injury.[99] The changes induced on bile acid composition through replacement and/or displacement of hydrophobic endogenous bile acids prevents perpetuation of liver damage caused by their retention within the hepatocyte during cholestasis.

Other mechanisms of action may be involved, including direct cytoprotection of biological membranes, a protective effect against apoptosis induced by endogenous hydrophobic bile acids, and stimulation of bile secretion by hepatocytes and bile duct epithelial cells.[99] Recent data indicate that the beneficial effects of UDCA in CF-associated liver disease may be mainly related to stimulation of Cl^- secretion through Ca^{2+}-dependent Cl^- conductance and to concomitant reduction in mucin secretion.[100] This may lead to improvement in biliary drainage, which has been documented on hepatobiliary scintigraphy (Figure 12.7).[96]

UDCA has been also administered in infants with CF-related neonatal cholestasis.[63]

The optimal daily dose of UDCA is 20 mg/kg body weight;[101] this dose is higher than that conventionally used in other cholestatic liver diseases to achieve comparable biliary enrichment, due to poor intestinal bile acid absorption in CF patients.[102]

The beneficial effects on liver biochemistry have been consistently documented in the context of randomized clinical trials.[103] There is evidence of improvement in liver histology[104] and in essential fatty acid status.[105] The latter may have potential extrahepatic implications, since essential fatty acid deficiency in CF occurs secondary to a specific defect in fatty acid metabolism, producing a membrane lipid imbalance, which in turn influences inflammatory status and the severity of pulmonary disease.[106] The beneficial effects of UDCA on hepatic excretory function, biliary drainage,[96] quantitative liver function, and nutritional status have been reported only in uncontrolled trials, while one study reported that UDCA led to normalization of early changes on ultrasonography.[107] UDCA is well tolerated, without significant side effects.

Despite the absence of evidence-based data on clinical outcome and survival,[108] UDCA is currently widely used for the treatment of CF-associated liver disease. Asymptomatic patients with early-stage liver disease are more likely to benefit from UDCA administration, but there are no long-term data. A prophylactic study evaluating the efficacy of UDCA in at-risk CF patients is required in order to establish its role in the prevention of liver disease.

Nutritional support

The recognition that malnutrition is an important complication of cystic fibrosis means that most children with CF are prescribed high-energy diets with pancreatic enzyme supplements. The development of liver disease may further exacerbate malnutrition by increasing fat malabsorption and protein loss (Chapter 15).

The following dietary management is recommended:

- An increase in energy intake to 120–150% of the estimated average requirement (EAR), which may be achieved by adding carbohydrate supplements such as glucose polymers and increasing the percentage of fat.
- Increasing the proportion of fat to 40–50% of the energy content of the feed or diet, with special attention to increased supplementation of polyunsaturated fatty acids.
- Providing protein supplements to ensure an intake of 3 g/kg/day.
- Ensuring that sufficient pancreatic enzymes are prescribed to allow optimal absorption of long-chain triglycerides and essential fatty acids.

In infants, these supplements may be added directly to the formula, although use of a modular feed may allow careful adjustment of the food constituents. In older children, supplementation of regular food with vegetable oils is preferable, but can be supplemented by high-energy carbohydrate and protein drinks. In children in whom anorexia is a problem, enteral nasogastric or gastrostomy feeding may be required to ensure adequate caloric intake. Gastrostomy feeding is not recommended in children with advanced liver disease, varices, or portal gastropathy, because of the risk of gastric hemorrhage.

Fat-soluble vitamin supplementation. It is justified to prescribe high oral doses of vitamin A (5000–15 000 international units daily), vitamin E (α-tocopherol 100–500 mg daily), and vitamin D (α-calcidiol 50 ng/kg to a maximum of 1 μg). Vitamin K is sometimes required (1–10 mg daily). In addition to their nutritional importance, supplementation of vitamins that are also antioxidants, such as α-tocopherol, β-carotene, and vitamin C, might reduce lipid peroxidation and tissue damage. Supplementation with vitamin A should be carefully monitored with plasma levels, to prevent toxicity.

Treatment of portal hypertension and end-stage of liver disease

The management of CF patients with advanced liver disease, severe portal hypertension, and hypersplenism is similar to that of other patients (Chapter 15). There are few data regarding prophylactic therapy for portal hypertension before the first episode of variceal bleeding; the efficacy of α-receptor blockade has not been evaluated in CF because of the adverse effects of alpha-blockers on airway reactivity. Although adult data demonstrate the efficacy of endoscopic variceal ligation in comparison with beta-blockers for primary prophylaxis of variceal bleeding,[109] there are no data in children with CF. It is important to treat the complications of portal hypertension effectively, as many CF patients with severe portal hypertension and hypersplenism may remain stable for years and long-term survival has been reported after variceal bleeding.[66]

Variceal bleeding may require sclerotherapy or preferably variceal ligation during the acute episode; vasopressin or octreotide can be used to control bleeding, but may cause systemic hypertension and splanchnic ischemia. Although endoscopic treatment is successful in most cases, in some patients gastric variceal bleeding or portal hypertensive gastropathy develop and may require additional therapeutic interventions (see Chapters 15 and 19).

There are no prospective studies to assess the indications, optimal timing, and actual benefits of different therapeutic interventions, including esophageal band ligation, intrahepatic transjugular portosystemic shunt (TIPSS), and surgical portosystemic shunts in CF. Esophageal band ligation is a preferable alternative to sclerotherapy and should be repeated until varices are eradicated, which has implications for children with CF who require repeated anesthetics and the necessary antibiotic prophylaxis.[20] Neither procedure addresses the clinical complications related to hypersplenism.

Alternatively, TIPSS has been employed for portal decompression in patients with recurrent bleeding, both as a long-term treatment for portal hypertension and as a bridge for liver transplantation.[110]

Elective surgical portosystemic shunting represents a more definitive treatment option for refractory bleeding in patients with preserved liver function and without severe pulmonary disease, allowing prolonged postoperative survival.[58,111] Potential complications include development or worsening of hepatic encephalopathy, shunt thrombosis, or occlusion, and these may make transplantation more hazardous.

Splenectomy has been performed, alone or in association with splenorenal shunt, in CF patients with hypersplenism showing an accelerated decline in lung function[112] and/or variceal bleeding.[113] It should be considered, however, that the beneficial effects that have been reported following this procedure (improvement in leukopenia, thrombocytopenia, and nutritional status) must be weighed against a mortality risk of up to 15% and a long-term postoperative risk of infection or fulminant sepsis. For these reasons, partial splenectomy with conservation of the upper pole of the spleen has been performed in patients with massive splenic enlargement,[114] in order to decrease the spleen's volume and blood supply while maintaining its immunological function. Information regarding the efficacy of these procedures is still very limited and they are generally not recommended, as transplantation may be a more effective strategy.[115]

Liver transplantation

Liver transplantation is an effective therapeutic option for CF patients with end-stage liver disease, but there is no general agreement on the precise indications, due to a lack of evidence-based specific guidelines. This is made more complex because liver failure is a late event, and biochemical parameters and classification systems used to monitor severe liver disease—such as the Child–Pugh score, Model for End-Stage Liver Disease (MELD), and Pediatric End-Stage Liver Disease (PELD)—are therefore less suitable for CF-associated liver disease, in which the complications of portal hypertension may occur with isolated hepatic fibrosis and good hepatic synthetic function.

Opinions vary between those who consider that transplantation should take place early in order to prevent progression of pulmonary disease,[50,116,117] and those who take the view that transplantation is only indicated if there is clear evidence of liver failure.[66,118,119]

Recently, a poll among European CF and transplantation centers was carried out in order to obtain information on current practices and outcomes for liver transplant in CF patients in Europe. In the majority of cases, the decision to transplant was based on the contemporary presence of various factors, and often transplantation was performed before the development of end-stage liver disease.[59]

Specific clinical scores that take into account not only features of portal hypertension, hepatocellular function, and hypersplenism, but also nutritional and pulmonary status, have been devised in order to evaluate the need for and timing of liver transplantation in CF patients; however, these need to be further evaluated.[117]

The agreed indications for liver transplantation in CF liver disease are:

- Progressive hepatic dysfunction (falling albumin < 30 g/L; increasing coagulopathy, not corrected by vitamin K)
- Development of ascites and jaundice
- Intractable variceal bleeding that is not controlled by conventional means
- Severe malnutrition, unresponsive to intensive nutritional support
- A deteriorating quality of life related to liver disease

In summary, although the ideal candidates for liver transplantation are CF patients who have clear evidence of hepatocellular failure, rather than CF patients with severe portal hypertension, adequate consideration should be given to the severity of the involvement of other organs as an indication for transplantation. In order to address this issue, exceptions to the MELD and PELD scores have been proposed for CF patients with severe pulmonary disease, in order to give them additional priority and improve their access to the few suitable donors of both liver and lung.[120]

The transplant assessment should evaluate pulmonary and cardiac function in order to establish whether liver transplantation alone is required, or whether a combined heart–lung–liver transplantation is more appropriate.[121] With increasing experience, early liver transplantation is recommended for children with deteriorating lung function (FEV_1 < 50%), as there is evidence that respiratory function improves after transplantation.[117]

Preoperative management includes adequate treatment of lung disease, such as vigorous physiotherapy, control of infection, and mucus-dissolving agents such as bromhexine and DNAse. It is essential to plan appropriate postoperative antibiotic therapy by ensuring that regular sputum cultures are performed in order to identify the antibiotic sensitivity of colonized organisms.

Preoperative information about pancreatic endocrine function is important, because the immunosuppressive drugs used after transplantation, such as steroids and tacrolimus (Chapter 21), have a diabetogenic effect. Hepatojejunostomy (Roux loop) may be routinely performed due to the high risk of biliary complications after liver transplantation.

Survival after liver transplantation is similar to that in other groups of children (Chapter 21). There is no increase in chest infections or other postoperative complications. Absorption of immunosuppressive drugs may be a problem, although this has been improved following the introduction of water-miscible forms of cyclosporine (Neoral) and tacrolimus, which is well absorbed. Higher doses may be required to obtain therapeutic levels, due to the abnormal pharmacokinetics in CF. Early deaths are related to pulmonary complications in patients below the 5% percentiles for height and weight.[122]

The 1-year survival rate after transplantation in CF patients is approximately 90%,[117] with beneficial effects on lung function, nutritional status, body composition, and quality of life in most cases;[73] a 5-year survival rate of 75% has been reported, with late mortality generally being related to progression of pulmonary disease.[116] The survival data for combined liver–lung transplantation are also comparable to those observed in other groups of patients receiving lung transplants, with reported 1-year and 5-year actuarial survival rates of 85.7% and 64.2%, respectively.[121]

Future treatment options

With better knowledge of the mechanisms involved in the pathogenesis of CF-associated liver disease, there is potential for several therapeutic strategies, including liver-targeted gene therapy and pharmacologic correction of the defective ion-transport function. None of these treatment options is yet available for clinical use.

Somatic gene therapy aimed at replacing the defective gene to the biliary epithelium has been shown to be feasible in the experimental animal[123] and may be curative, but cholangiocytes are less accessible to targeted drug and gene delivery than the airways epithelium, and the clinical application of this approach remains to be established.

Strategies aimed at stimulating fluid secretion by cholangiocytes may be easier to achieve and may represent a potential pharmacologic approach to CF-associated liver disease. Extracellular adenosine 5′-triphosphate (ATP) is known to be a potent Cl^- secretagogue and can activate the Ca^{2+}-dependent Cl^- channel in different cell types, including biliary epithelial cells.[124] Exogenous administration of nucleotide triphosphate may therefore correct the defective anion secretion in intrahepatic ducts.

The ability of glibenclamide, a sulfonylurea with known CFTR inhibitor activity, to paradoxically stimulate cholangiocyte secretion through exocytosis in CFTR-defective mice, has recently indicated that drugs with a similar mechanism of action may be designed for the treatment of CF-associated and other cholestatic liver diseases.[125]

Finally, docosahexaenoic acid (DHA) supplementation has been recently shown to induce a significant amelioration in the severity of liver disease in *CFTR* –/– mice, with a striking reduction in the degree of periportal inflammation.[126] The beneficial effect of DHA, which may be linked to its ability to inhibit cytokines and/or eicosanoid metabolism and to release endogenous inhibitors of inflammation, needs to be confirmed in CF patients.

Case study

MJ was admitted for further assessment of her liver disease. The diagnosis of cystic fibrosis had been made when she was 4½ months old, and she had relatively few problems with her chest. Abnormal liver function had first been noted 5 years earlier, when an ultrasound examination showed a diffusely abnormal liver and mild splenic enlargement. She had developed hepatosplenomegaly and had a variceal hemorrhage. Her esophageal varices were treated with a course of sclerotherapy. She also had intermittent abdominal pain related to meconium ileus.

Investigations: Bilirubin 3 μmol/L (normal < 20 μmol/L); alkaline phosphatase 555 U/L; AST 157 U/L (normal < 40 IU/L); ALT 151 U/L (normal < 40 IU/L); GGT 327 U/L (normal 35–40 IU/L); albumin 32 g/L (normal 35–52 g/L); hemoglobin 9.2 g/L; white blood count 5.0×10^9 g/L; platelets 133×10^9 g/L; prothrombin time 16 s (control 13 s); partial thromboplastin time 34 s (control 33 s).

Abdominal ultrasound. The liver parenchyma was diffusely heterogenous and echogenic, with increased periportal reflectivity. The appearances were in keeping with biliary cirrhosis. The gallbladder was not visualized. There was marked splenomegaly, with the spleen measuring 16 cm in length. There was moderate ascites in the pelvis.

Chest radiography. Hyperinflated, with perihilar bronchial wall thickening extending into all lobes, consistent with CF. No acute change demonstrated.

Upper gastrointestinal endoscopy and sclerotherapy. On esophagogastroduodenoscopy, several grade II varices were found, which were injected with ethanolamine 6 mL. One gastric varix was noted. The stomach and duodenum appeared otherwise normal.

Liver biopsy. This demonstrated biliary cirrhosis, compatible with CF.

Lung function. FEV_1 was 70%; forced vital capacity was 65%.

Further management. Following discussion with her family, the patient was listed for liver transplantation because of early decompensated liver disease, with gastric varices and good lung function. Before transplantation, she was managed with DNAse, chest physiotherapy, regular antibiotics, and standard liver-failure management.

She received a split liver (segments II, III, and IV) from a 60-kg donor. She made a good recovery, but had persistent ascites. Post-transplantation abdominal ultrasound showed normal flow in all vessels and considerable intra-abdominal fluid. The drain was removed on day 6, but the fluid continued to drain from the drain site and enterococcus was cultured from the abdominal drain fluid. After appropriate antibiotics, she was discharged on:

- Prednisolone 25 mg once a day
- Spironolactone 20 mg three times a day
- Omeprazole 10 mg twice a day
- Ursodeoxycholic acid 300 mg twice a day, to be reviewed in the clinic
- Azathioprine 23 mg once a day
- Cyclosporine 110 mg twice a day

One week later, she was admitted to the liver unit because of vomiting, weight loss of 3 kg, and lethargy. Her blood sugar was 39 mmol/L (normal < 4 mmol/L). She was not acidotic, potassium was normal, and there were no ketones in the urine. She was commenced on an insulin infusion, with intravenous fluids for correction of dehydration, and then on a combination of short-acting and medium-acting insulin. Five years later, she was well, but remains diabetic. She has successfully been transferred to the adult unit.

Comments. The timing and indications for liver transplantation in children with cystic fibrosis can be difficult. This girl had remained well for many years with liver disease, but underwent transplantation when her liver was beginning to decompensate and she still had good liver function. She developed well-recognized postoperative complications, persistent ascites due to peritoneal infection and post-transplantation diabetes. Her diabetes was due to the combination of high-dose steroids and cyclosporine, both of which can cause diabetes—especially in children with CF, who are likely to develop diabetes.

References

1 Rowe SM, Miller S, Sorscher EJ. Mechanisms of disease, cystic fibrosis. *N Engl J Med* 2005;**352**:1992–2001.

2 Davis PB. Cystic fibrosis since 1938. *Am J Respir Crit Care Med* 2006;**173**;475–82.

3 Mahadeva R, Webb K, Westerbeek RC, *et al.* Clinical outcome in relation to care in centres specialising in cystic fibrosis: cross sectional study. *BMJ* 1998;**316**:1771–5.

4 Kulich M, Gross CH, Rosenfeld M. Improved survival among young patients with cystic fibrosis. *J Pediatr* 2003;**142**:631–36.

5 Riordan JR, Rommens JM, Kerem B, *et al.* Identification of the cystic fibrosis gene: cloning and characterization of complementary DNA. *Science* 1989;**245**:1066–73.

6 Mehta A. CFTR: more than just a chloride channel. *Pediatr Pulmonol* 2005;**39**:292–8.

7 www.genet.sickkids.on.ca/cftr/app.

8 Kerem B, Kerem E. The molecular basis for disease variability in cystic fibrosis. *Eur J Hum Genet* 1996;**4**:65–73.

9 Wilschanski M, Durie P. Patterns of gastrointestinal disease in adulthood associated with mutations in the *CFTR* gene. *Gut* 2007;**56**:1153–63.

10 Kerem E, Kerem B. Genotype–phenotype correlations in cystic fibrosis. *Pediatr Pulmonol* 1996;**22**:387–95.

11 Kristidis P, Bozon D, Coorey M, *et al.* Genetic Determination of exocrine pancreatic function in cystic fibrosis. *Am J Hum Genet* 1992;**50**:1178–84.

12 Zielenski J. Genotype and phenotype in cystic fibrosis. *Respiration* 2000;**67**:117–33.

13 McKone EF, Emerson SS, Edwards KL, Aitken ML. Effect of genotype on phenotype and mortality in cystic fibrosis: a retrospective cohort study. *Lancet* 2003;**361**:1871–6.

14 Knowles MR, Durie PR. What is cystic fibrosis? *N Engl J Med* 2002;**347**:439–42.

15 Gross CH, Rosenfeld M. Update on cystic fibrosis epidemiology. *Curr Opin Pulm Med* 2004;**10**:510–4.

16 Colombo C, Battezzati PM. Liver involvement in cystic fibrosis: primary organ damage or innocent bystander? *J Hepatol* 2004; **41**:1041–4.

17 Bodian MM. *Fibrocystic Disease of the Pancreas.* London: Heinemann, 1952.

18 Di Sant'Agnese PA and Blanc WA. A distinctive type of biliary cirrhosis of the liver associated with cystic fibrosis of the pancreas. *Pediatrics* 1956;**18**:387–409.

19 Craig JM, Haddad H, Shwachman H. The pathological changes in the liver in cystic fibrosis of the pancreas. *Am J Dis Child* 1957;**93**:357–69.

20 Sokol RJ, Durie PR. Recommendations for management of liver and biliary tract disease in cystic fibrosis. Cystic Fibrosis Foundation Hepatobiliary Disease Consensus Group. *J Pediatr Gastroenterol Nutr* 1999:**28**(Suppl 1):1–13.

21 Cystic Fibrosis Foundation. *Patient Registry 2003: Annual Report to the Center Directors.* Bethesda, Maryland: Cystic Fibrosis Foundation, 2004.

22 Laazaridis KN, Strazzabosco M, Larusso N. The cholangiopathies: disorders of biliary epithelia. *Gastroenterology* 2004; **127**:1565–77.

23 Strazzabosco M, Spirli C, Okolicsany L. Pathophysiology of the intrahepatic biliary epithelium. *J Gastroenterol Hepatol* 2000;**15**: 244–53.

24 Cohn JA, Strong TV, Picciotto MR, Nairn AC, Collins FS, Fitz JG. Localization of the cystic fibrosis transmembrane conductance

regulator in human bile duct epithelial cells. *Gastroenterology* 1993;**105**:1857–64.

25 Durie PR, Kent G, Phillips MJ, Ackerley CA. Characteristic multi-organ pathology of cystic fibrosis in a long-living cystic fibrosis transmembrane regulator knockout murine model. *Am J Pathol* 2004;**164**:1481–93.

26 Zsembery A, Jessner W, Sitter G, Spirli C, Strazzabosco M, Graf J. Correction of CFTR malfunction and stimulation of Ca-activated Cl channels restore HCO_3^- secretion in cystic fibrosis bile ductular cells. *Hepatology* 2002;**35**:95–104.

27 Bhaskar KR, Turner BS, Grubman SA, Jefferson DM, LaMont JT. Dysregulation of proteoglycan production by intrahepatic biliary epithelial cells bearing defective (Delta-f508) cystic fibrosis transmembrane regulator. *Hepatology* 1998;**27**:54–61.

28 Oppenheimer EH, Esterly JR. Hepatic changes in young infants with cystic fibrosis: possible relation to focal biliary cirrhosis. *J Pediatr* 1975;**86**:683–9.

29 Lindblad A, Hultcrantz R, Strandvik B. Bile duct destruction and collagen deposition: a prominent ultrastructural feature of the liver in cystic fibrosis. *Hepatology* 1992;**16**:372–1.

30 Paumgartner G. Medical treatment of cholestatic liver diseases: from pathobiology to pharmacological targets. *World J Gastroenterol* 2006;**12**:4445–51.

31 Lagrange-Puget M, Durieu I, Ecochard R, *et al.* Longitudinal study of oxidative status in 312 cystic fibrosis patients in stable state and during bronchial exacerbation. *Pediatr Pulmonol* 2004; **38**:43–9.

32 Lewindon PJ, Pereira TN, Hoskins AC, *et al.* The role of hepatic stellate cells and transforming growth factor-beta(1) in cystic fibrosis liver disease. *Am Pathol* 2002;**160**:1705–15.

33 Sinaasappel M. Hepatobiliary pathology in patients with cystic fibrosis. *Acta Paediatr Scand Suppl* 1989;**363**:45–51.

34 McGill JM, Basavappa S, Fitz JG. Characterization of high conductance anion channels in rat bile duct epithelial cells. *Am J Physiol* 1992;**262**:G703–10.

35 Colombo C, Apostolo MG, Ferrari M, *et al.* Analysis of risk factors for the development of liver disease associated with cystic fibrosis. *J Pediatr* 1994;**124**:393–9.

36 Wilschanski M, Rivlin J, Cohen S, *et al.* Clinical and genetic risk factors for CF-related liver disease. *Pediatrics* 1999;**103**: 52–7.

37 Castaldo G, Fuccio A, Salvatore D, *et al.* Liver expression in cystic fibrosis could be modulated by genetic factors different from the cystic fibrosis transmembrane regulator genotype. *Am J Med Genet* 2001;**98**:294–7.

38 Knowles MR, Drumm ML, Konstan MW, *et al.* Genetic modifiers of lung disease in cystic fibrosis. *N Engl J Med* 2005; **353**:1443–53.

39 Friedman KJ, Ling SC, Lange EM, *et al.* Genetic modifiers of severe liver disease in cystic fibrosis [abstract]. *Pediatr Pulmonol* 2005;**40**(Suppl 28):247.

40 Henrion-Caude A, Flamant C, Roussey M, Housset C, *et al.* Liver disease in pediatric patients with cystic fibrosis is associated with glutathione *S*-transferase P1 polymorphism. *Hepatology* 2002;**36**:913–7.

41 Gabolde M, Hubert D, Guilloud-Bataille M, Lenaerts C, Feingold J, Besmond C. The mannose binding lectin gene influences the severity of chronic liver disease in cystic fibrosis. *J Med Genet* 2001;**38**:310–1.

42 Lindblad A, Glaumann H, Strandvik B. Natural history of liver disease in cystic fibrosis. *Hepatology* 1999;**30**:1151–8.

43 Chen AH, Innis SM, Davidson GF, Jill James S. Phosphatidylcholine and lysophosphatidylcholine excretion is increased in children with cystic fibrosis and is associated with plasma homocysteine, *S*-adenosylhomocysteine, and *S*-adenosylmethionine. *Am J Clin Nutr* 2005;**81**:686–91.

44 Chitturi S, Farrel GC. Etiopathogenesis of nonalcoholic steatohepatitis. *Semin Lever Dis* 2001;**21**:27–41.

45 Hardin DS, LeBlanc A, Para L, Seilheimer DK. Hepatic insulin resistance and defects in substrate utilization in cystic fibrosis. *Diabetes* 1999;**48**:1082–7.

46 Feranchak AP, Sokol RJ. Cholangiocyte biology and cystic fibrosis liver disease. *Semin Liver Dis* 2001;**21**:471–88.

47 Falck-Ytter Y, Younossi ZM, Marchesini G, McCullough AJ. Clinical features and natural history of nonalcoholic steatosis syndromes. *Semin Liver Dis* 2001;**21**:17–26.

48 Pinto HC, Carniero de Moura M, Day C P. Non-alcoholic steatohepatitis from cell biology to clinical practice. *J Hepatol* 2006;**44**:197–208.

49 Vawter GF, Shwachman H. Cystic fibrosis in adults: an autopsy study. *Pathol Ann* 1979;**14**:357–82.

50 Feigelson J, Anagnostopoulos C, Poquet M, Pecau Y, Munck A, Navarro J. Liver cirrhosis in cystic fibrosis. Therapeutic implications and long-term follow-up. *Arch Dis Child* 1993;**68**: 653–7.

51 Colombo C, Battezzati PM, Podda M. Hepatobiliary disease in cystic fibrosis. *Semin Liver Dis* 1994;**14**:259–69.

52 Scott-Jupp R, Lama M, Tanner MS. Prevalence of liver disease in cystic fibrosis. *Arch Dis Child* 1991;**66**:698–701.

53 Ling SC, Wilkinson JD, Hollman AS, McColl J, Evans TJ, Paton JY. The evolution of liver disease in cystic fibrosis. *Arch Dis Child* 1999;**81**:129–32.

54 Colombo C, Battezzati PM, Crosignani A, *et al.* Liver disease in cystic fibrosis: a prospective study on incidence, risk factors and outcome. *Hepatology* 2002;**36**:1374–82.

55 Lamireau T, Monnereau S, Martin S, *et al.* Epidemiology of liver disease in cystic fibrosis: a longitudinal study. *J Hepatol* 2004;**41**:920–5.

56 Corbett K, Kelleher S, Rowland M, *et al.* Cystic fibrosis-associated liver disease: a population-based study. *J Pediatr* 2004;**145**:327–32.

57 Waters DL, Dorney SFA, Gruca MA, *et al.* Hepatobiliary disease in pancreatic sufficient patients with cystic fibrosis. *Hepatology* 1995;**21**:963–9.

58 Debray D, Lykavieris P, Gauthier F, *et al.* Outcome of cystic fibrosis-associated liver cirrhosis: management of portal hypertension. *J Hepatol* 1999;**31**:77–83.

59 Melzi ML, Kelly D, Colombo C, *et al.* Liver transplant in cystic fibrosis: a pool among European centers. A study from the European Liver Transplant Registry. *Transplant Int* 2006;**19**: 726–31.

60 Psacharopoulos HT, Howard ER, Portmann B, Mowat AP, Williams R. Hepatic complications of cystic fibrosis. *Lancet* 1981;**ii**:78–80.

61 Maurage C, Lenaerts C, Weber AM, *et al.* Meconium ileus and its equivalent as a risk factor for the development of cirrhosis: an autopsy study in cystic fibrosis. *J Pediatr Gastroenterol Nutr* 1989;**9**:17–20.

62 Farrell MP. Guidelines for implementation of cystic fibrosis newborn screening programs: Cystic Fibrosis Foundation Workshop Report. *Pediatrics* 2007;**119**:e495–e518.

63 Gooding I, Dondis V, Gyi KM, Hodson M, Westaby D. Variceal hemorrhage and cystic fibrosis: outcomes and implications for liver transplantation. *Liver Transpl* 2005;**11**:1522–6.

64 Lykavieris P, Bernard O, Hadchouel M. Neonatal cholestasis as the presenting feature in cystic fibrosis. *Arch Dis Child* 1996;**75**: 67–70.

65 Balistreri WF, Heubi JE, Suchy FJ. Immaturity of the enterohepatic circulation in early life: factors predisposing to "physiologic" maldigestion and cholestasis. *J Pediatr Gastroenterol Nutr* 1983;**2**:346–54.

66 Shapira R, Hadzic R, Francavilla R, Koukulis G, Price GF, Mieli-Vergani G. Retrospective review of cystic fibrosis presenting as infantile liver disease. *Arch Dis Child* 1999;**81**:125–8.

67 Jonas MM. The role of liver transplantation in cystic fibrosis re-examined. *Liver Transpl* 2005;**11**:1463–5.

68 Sherlock S, Dooley J. Hepatic cirrhosis. In: Sherlock S, Dooley J. *Diseases of the Liver and Biliary System*, 10th ed. Oxford: Blackwell Science, 1997: 371–84.

69 Slieker MG, van der Doef HP, Deckers-Kocken JM, van der Ent CK, Houwen RHJ. Pulmonary prognosis in cystic fibrosis patients with liver disease. *J Pediatr* 2006;**149**:144.

70 Pencharz PB, Durie PR. Pathogenesis of malnutrition in cystic fibrosis, and its treatment. *Clin Nutr* 2000;**19**:387–94.

71 Marshall BC, Butler SM, Stoddard M, Moran AM, Liou TG, Morgan WJ. Epidemiology of cystic fibrosis-related diabetes. *J Pediatr* 2005;**146**:681–7.

72 Minicucci L, Lorini R, Giannattasio A, *et al.* Liver disease as risk factor for cystic fibrosis-related diabetes development. *Acta Paediatr* 2007;**96**:736–9.

73 Colombo C, Costantini D, Rocchi A, *et al.* Effects of liver transplantation on the nutritional status of patients with cystic fibrosis. *Transplant Int* 2005;**18**:246–55.

74 Feigelson J, Anagnostopoulos C, Poquet M, Pecau Y, Munck A, Navarro J. Liver cirrhosis in cystic fibrosis. Therapeutic implications and long-term follow-up. *Arch Dis Child* 1993;**68**:653–7.

75 O'Brien S, Keogan M, Casey M, *et al.* Biliary complications of cystic fibrosis. *Gut* 1992;**33**:387–91.

76 Gaskin KJ, Waters DLM, Howman-Giles R, *et al.* Liver disease and common bile-duct stenosis in cystic fibrosis. *N Engl J Med* 1988;**318**:340–6.

77 Stern RC, Rothstein FC, Doershuk CF. Treatment and prognosis of symptomatic gallbladder disease in patients with cystic fibrosis. *J Pediatr Gastroenterol Nutr* 1986;**5**:35–40.

78 Gaskin KJ. The liver and biliary tract in cystic fibrosis. In: Suchy FJ, Sokol RJ, Balistreri WF, eds. *Liver Disease in Children*, 2nd ed. Philadelphia: Lippincott Williams & Wilkins, 2001: 549–63.

79 Roy CC, Weber AM, Morin CL, *et al.* Abnormal biliary lipid composition in cystic fibrosis. Effect of pancreatic enzymes. *N Engl J Med* 1977;**297**:1301–5.

80 Weber AM, Roy CC, Morin CL, Lasalle R. Malabsorption of bile acids in children with cystic fibrosis. *N Engl J Med* 1973;**289**: 1001–5.

81 Angelico M, Gandin C, Canuzzi P, *et al.* Gallstones in cystic fibrosis: a critical reappraisal. *Hepatology* 1991;**14**:768–75.

82 Colombo C, Bertolini E, Assaisso ML, Bettinardi N, Giunta A, Podda M. Failure of ursodeoxycholic acid to dissolve radiolucent gallstones in patients with cystic fibrosis. *Acta Paediatr* 1993;**82**:562–5.

83 Bass S, Connon JJ, Ho CS. Biliary tree in cystic fibrosis. Biliary tract abnormalities in cystic fibrosis demonstrated by endoscopic retrograde cholangiography. *Gastroenterology* 1983;**84**: 1592–6.

84 Nagel RA, Westaby D, Javaid A, *et al.* Liver disease and bile duct abnormalities in adults with cystic fibrosis. *Lancet* 1989;**ii**: 1422–5.

85 Strandvik B, Hjelte L, Gabrielsson N, Glaumann H. Sclerosing cholangitis in cystic fibrosis. *Scand J Gastroenterol Suppl* 1988; **143**:121–4.

86 Durieu I, Pellet O, Simonot L, *et al.* Sclerosing cholangitis in adults with cystic fibrosis: a magnetic resonance cholangiographic prospective study. *J Hepatol* 1999;**30**:1052–6.

87 Sheth S, Shea JC, Bishop MD, *et al.* Increased prevalence of CFTR mutations and variants and decreased chloride secretion in primary sclerosing cholangitis. *Hum Genet* 2003;**113**:286–92.

88 Lawson EE, Grand RJ, Neff RK, Cohen LF. Clinical estimation of liver span in infants and children. *Am J Dis Child* 1978;**132**: 474–6.

89 Potter CJ, Fishbein M, Hammond S, *et al.* Can the histologic changes of cystic fibrosis-associated hepatobiliary disease be predicted by clinical criteria? *J Pediatr Gastroenterol Nutr* 1997; **25**:32–6.

90 Patriquin H, Lenaerts C, Smith L, *et al.* Liver disease in children with cystic fibrosis: US and biochemical comparison in 195 patients. *Radiology* 1999;**211**:229–32.

91 Lenaerts C, Lapierre C, Patriquin H, *et al.* Surveillance for cystic fibrosis-associated hepatobiliary disease: early ultrasound changes and predisposing factors. *J Pediatr* 2003;**143**:343–50.

92 Williams SGJ, Evanson JE, Barrett N, Hodson ME, Boultbee JE, Westaby D. An ultrasound scoring system for the diagnosis of liver disease in cystic fibrosis. *J Hepatol* 1995;**22**:513–21.

93 Stewart L. The role of abdominal ultrasound in the diagnosis, staging and management of cystic fibrosis liver disease. *J R Soc Med* 2005;**98**:17–27.

94 O'Connor PJ, Southern KW, Bowler IM. The role of hepatobiliary scintigraphy in cystic fibrosis. *Hepatology* 1996;**23**:281–7.

95 Foster JA, Ramsden WH, Conway SP, Taylor JM, Etherington C. The role of IDA scintigraphy in the follow-up of liver disease in patients with cystic fibrosis. *Nucl Med Commun* 2002;**23**:673–81.

96 Colombo C, Castellani MR, Balistreri WF, Seregni E, Assaisso ML, Giunta A. Scintigraphic documentation of an improvement in hepatobiliary excretory function after treatment with ursodeoxycholic acid in patients with cystic fibrosis and associated liver disease. *Hepatology* 1992;**15**:677–84.

97 McKeon D, Day A, Parmar J, Alexander G, Bilton D. Hepatocellular carcinoma in association with cirrhosis in a patient with cystic fibrosis. *J Cyst Fibros* 2004;**3**:193–5.

98 Kelleher T, Staunton M, O'Mahony S, McCormick PA. Advanced hepatocellular carcinoma associated with cystic fibrosis. *Eur J Gastroenterol Hepatol* 2005;**17**:1123–4.

99 Paumgartner G, Beuers U. Ursodeoxycholic acid in cholestatic liver disease: mechanisms of action and therapeutic use revisited. *Hepatology* 2002;**36**:525–31.

100 Chinet T, Fouassier L, Dray-Charier N, *et al.* Regulation of electrogenic anion secretion in normal and cystic fibrosis gallbladder mucosa. *Hepatology* 1999;**29**:5–13.

101 Colombo C, Crosignani A, Assaisso ML, *et al.* Ursodeoxycholic acid therapy in cystic fibrosis associated liver disease: a dose–response study. *Hepatology* 1992;**16**:924–30.

102 Colombo C, Roda A, Roda E, *et al.* Evaluation of an ursodeoxycholic acid oral load in the assessment of bile acid malabsorption in cystic fibrosis. *Dig Dis Sci* 1983;**28**:306–11.

103 Colombo C, Battezzati PM, Podda M, Bettinardi, Giunta A, Italian Group for the Study of Ursodeoxycholic Acid in Cystic Fibrosis. Ursodeoxycholic acid for liver disease associated with cystic fibrosis: a double-blind multicenter trial. *Hepatology* 1996;**23**:1484–90.

104 Lindblad A, Glaumann H, Strandvik B. A two-year prospective study of the effect of ursodeoxycholic acid on urinary bile acid excretion and liver morphology in cystic fibrosis. *Hepatology* 1998;**23**:166–74.

105 Lepage G, Paradis K, Lacaille F, *et al.* Ursodeoxycholic acid improves the hepatic metabolism of essential fatty acids and retinol in children with cystic fibrosis. *J Pediatr* 1997;**130**:52–8.

106 Freedman SD, Blanco PG, Zaman MM, *et al.* Association of cystic fibrosis with abnormalities in fatty acid metabolism. *N Engl J Med* 2004;**350**:560–9.

107 Nousia-Arvanitakis S, Futoulaki M, Economou H, *et al.* Long-term prospective study of the effect of ursodeoxycholic acid on cystic fibrosis-related liver disease. *J Clin Gastroenterol* 2001; **32**:324–8.

108 Cheng K, Ashby D, Smyth R. Ursodeoxycholic acid for cystic fibrosis-related liver disease. *Cochrane Database Syst Rev* 2000;(**2**): CD000222.

109 Khuroo MS, Khuroo NS, Farahat KL, Khuroo YS, Sofi AA, Dahab ST. Meta-analysis: endoscopic variceal ligation for primary prophylaxis of oesophageal variceal bleeding. *Aliment Pharmacol Ther* 2005;**21**:347–61.

110 Pozler O, Krajina A, Vanicek H, *et al.* Transjugular intrahepatic portosystemic shunt in five children with cystic fibrosis: long-term results. *Hepatogastroenterology* 2003;**50**:1111–4.

111 Efrati O, Barak A, Modan-Moses D, *et al.* Liver cirrhosis and portal hypertension in cystic fibrosis. *Eur J Gastroenterol Hepatol* 2003;**15**:1073–8.

112 Linnane B, Oliver MR, Robinson PJ. Does splenectomy in cystic fibrosis related liver disease improve lung function and nutritional status? A case series. *Arch Dis Child* 2006;**91**:771–3.

113 Robberecht E, Van Biervliet S, Vanrentergem K, Kerremans I. Outcome of total splenectomy with portosystemic shunt for massive splenomegaly and variceal bleeding in cystic fibrosis. *J Pediatr Surg* 2006;**41**:1561–5.

114 Thalhammer GH, Eber E, Uranus S, Pfeifer J, Zach MS. Partial splenectomy in cystic fibrosis patients with hypersplenism. *Arch Dis Child* 2003;**88**:143–6.

115 Noble-Jamieson G, Barnes N, Jamieson N, Friend P, Cain R. Liver transplantation for hepatic cirrhosis in cystic fibrosis. *J R Soc Med* 1996;**89**:31–7.

116 Fridell JA, Bond GJ, Mazariegos GV, *et al.* Liver transplantation in children with cystic fibrosis: a long-term longitudinal review of a single center's experience. *J Pediatr Surg* 2003;**38**:1152–6.

117 Milkiewicz P, Skiba G, Kelly D, *et al.* Transplantation for cystic fibrosis: outcome following early liver transplantation. *J Gastroenterol Hepatol* 2002;**17**:208–13.

118 Mack DR, Traystman MD, Colombo JL, *et al.* Clinical denouement and mutation analysis of patients with cystic fibrosis undergoing liver transplantation for biliary cirrhosis. *J Pediatr* 1995;**127**:881–7.

119 Sharp HL. Cystic fibrosis liver disease and transplantation. *J Pediatr* 1995;**127**:944–6.

120 Horslen S, Sweet S, Gish RG, Shepherd R. Model for end-stage liver disease (MELD). Exception for cystic fibrosis. *Liver Transpl* 2006;**12**:S98–9.

121 Couetil JP, Soubrane O, Houssin DP, *et al.* Combined heart–lung–liver, double lung–liver, and isolated liver transplantation for cystic fibrosis in children. *Transpl Int* 1997;**10**:33–9.

122 Molmenti E, Nagata D, Roden J, *et al.* Pediatric liver transplantation for cystic fibrosis. *Transplant Proc* 2001;**33**:1738.

123 Yang Y, Raper SE, Cohn JA, Engelhardt JF, Wilson's JM. An approach for treating the hepatobiliary disease of cystic fibrosis by somatic gene transfer. *Proc Natl Acad Sci* 1993;**90**:4601–5.

124 Roman RM, Feranchak AP, Salter KD, *et al.* Endogenous ATP regulates Cl^- secretion in cultured human and rat biliary epithelial cells. *Am J Physiol* 1999;**276**:G1391–400.

125 Spirli C, Fiorotto R, Song L, Santos-Sacchi J, Okolicsany L, Maser S. Glibenclamide stimulates fluid secretion in rodent cholangiocytes through a cystic fibrosis transmembrane conductance regulator-independent mechanism. *Gastroenterology* 2005;**129**:220–33.

126 Beharry S, Ackerley C, Corey M, *et al.* Long-term docosahexaenoic acid therapy in a congenic murine model of cystic fibrosis. *Am J Physiol Gastrointest Liver Physiol* 2007;**292**:G839–48.

7 Metabolic Liver Disease

13 Metabolic Liver Disease in the Infant and Older Child

Anupam Chakrapani and Anne Green

There are a large number of inborn errors of metabolism (IEMs), many of which present with liver disease. Although most patients present in the neonatal period with cholestasis or an acute illness (Chapters 4 and 5), for many the condition only becomes manifest later in infancy or childhood. Recognition of a specific diagnosis is important for appropriate management, for the prognosis, and for genetic counseling. Diagnosis of these disorders may be complicated, as nonspecific liver dysfunction may lead to secondary biochemical disturbances, which are suggestive of a metabolic disorder.

The differential diagnosis of metabolic liver disease presenting in infancy and in older children varies with the type of clinical presentation.

Etiology and presentation of liver dysfunction in IEM

Most inborn errors involve abnormalities in enzymes and transport proteins. In some disorders, the basic defect involves only one functional system such as the endocrine system, immune system, coagulation system, etc. Others involve a basic biochemical dysfunction that is common to many organs or tissues; this group includes disorders of energy metabolism and intermediary metabolism. The liver may often be involved together with other organ systems.

From a pathophysiological perspective, disorders can be classified into three groups:

- Firstly, those that involve the synthesis or catabolism of complex molecules, of which the lysosomal and peroxisomal disorders are examples (see pp. 301 and 312). The affected organs, including the liver, are those in which the partly degraded molecules accumulate and cause disruption to the organ function.
- A second group are due to the accumulation of "toxic" compounds arising as a consequence of the enzyme defect, as occurs in galactosemia and tyrosinemia type I.
- Inborn errors of intermediary metabolism are a third group, with symptoms partly due to a deficiency in energy production. Included in this group are the glycogen storage disorders, fat oxidation, and mitochondrial disorders.

For several IEMs, liver dysfunction therefore arises as a primary effect of the IEM itself. However, for some disorders, although the defect—e.g., enzyme deficiency—is expressed in the liver cells, the liver function is not affected and the clinical effect is elsewhere.

The different etiologies of IEM will determine the type of presentation, and the differential diagnosis of metabolic liver disease varies with the clinical presentation. The following categories of presentation can be considered.

Liver failure—with manifestations of hepatocellular necrosis, including jaundice, edema, ascites, and coagulopathy. The differential diagnosis includes galactosemia, tyrosinemia type I, hereditary fructose intolerance, respiratory-chain disorders, Wilson disease, and α_1-antitrypsin+deficiency. This presentation is common in neonates (Chapter 4) and is rare beyond early infancy.

Encephalopathy or Reye-like illness—with prominent neurological features including recurrent encephalopathy, hypoglycemia, hyperammonemia, and Reye-like episodes. Fatty acid oxidation disorders, urea cycle defects, organic acidemias, and respiratory-chain disorders may present in this manner. Of specific importance is the need to investigate the unconscious infant/child for a variety of possible conditions.[1]

Chronic cholestasis. The majority of these cases present in the neonatal period (Chapter 4), and the differential diagnosis includes α_1-antitrypsin deficiency, neonatal hemochromatosis, inborn errors of bile acid synthesis, Niemann–Pick disease type C, inborn errors of peroxisomal function, and congenital disorders of glycosylation.

A few other metabolic disorders can cause cholestasis or transient anicteric hepatitis in early infancy. With two such conditions—Niemann–Pick disease type C and cerebrotendinous xanthomatosis (a disorder of bile acid metabolism—the early hepatitis typically resolves by late infancy. No symptoms are apparent until late childhood, after which patients

Diseases of the Liver and Biliary System in Children, 3rd edition. Edited by Deirdre Kelly. © 2008 Blackwell Publishing, ISBN: 978-1-4051-6334-7.

follow a slowly progressive neurodegenerative course. Other disorders of bile acid metabolism can manifest as early cholestasis followed by progressive liver disease. Signs and symptoms related to fat and fat-soluble vitamin malabsorption (such as rickets) are often prominent by late infancy in patients with these disorders.

Citrin deficiency has been described in infants with unexplained and prolonged cholestasis that subsequently resolves. There is a variety of associated biochemical abnormalities, which are transient, and the patient may then present in later childhood/adulthood with a type of citrullinemia.[2,3]

Hepatomegaly or hepatosplenomegaly. A palpable liver with a firm or hard consistency may be indicative of cirrhosis, and conditions such as galactosemia, hereditary fructose intolerance, tyrosinemia type I, α_1-antitrypsin deficiency, Wilson disease, glycogenosis type IV, Niemann–Pick disease, and Gaucher disease should be considered in the differential diagnosis. When the consistency of the liver is soft or normal and there is associated splenomegaly, lysosomal storage disorders should be considered. Associated features such as a coarse facial appearance, joint stiffness, corneal opacities, skeletal deformities, cardiomyopathy, oculomotor apraxia, and neurodevelopmental regression may suggest an underlying lysosomal storage disorder. Glycogen storage disease, Fanconi–Bickel syndrome, or fructose-1,6-bisphosphatase deficiency are usually associated with hypoglycemia and lactic acidosis. Other conditions that may be associated with isolated hepatomegaly include argininosuccinic aciduria, cholesterol ester storage disease, and congenital disorders of glycosylation.

Investigation and diagnosis

Diagnostic evaluation should begin with a complete history and physical examination. An inborn error of metabolism is suggested in the following situations:

- A positive family history and/or parental consanguinity.
- Sudden, unexplained death in a previous sibling.
- Acute fatty liver of pregnancy and the hemolysis, elevated liver enzymes, and low platelet count (HELLP) syndrome during pregnancies with affected fetuses are associated with some fatty acid oxidation defects.
- Recurrent episodes of clinical disease at times of catabolic stress can occur with fatty acid oxidation defects, urea cycle defects, and organic acidemias.
- A history of specific food avoidance may be suggestive of fructose intolerance or a urea cycle defect.

It is important to be aware that some IEMs may be tested for as part of newborn screening programs. In the United Kingdom, this only applies to phenylketonuria (PKU) and medium-chain acyl-CoA dehydrogenase deficiency (MCADD; for parts of the UK since 2004). This differs from other parts of the world—particularly the United States, parts of Europe, and Australia, where many other disorders may be routinely tested for.

In the UK, some cases of galactosemia and tyrosinemia type I may be diagnosed as a result of an elevated phenylalanine being detected due to liver dysfunction at the time of PKU screening. Screening will not detect all cases, and it should never be assumed that a particular disorder has been excluded because of newborn screening.

The physical examination should include:

- Assessment of growth and development.
- Examination for dysmorphism, organomegaly, and neurological dysfunction.
- Detailed ophthalmologic evaluation, as specific eye signs may be present in the lysosomal, peroxisomal and respiratory-chain disorders.
- Cardiac and renal assessment to detect multisystem disease.
- Neurophysiological studies may be helpful in defining the presence of multisystem involvement.

Initial investigations for metabolic liver disease

Conventional liver function tests are usually unhelpful in the differential diagnosis of metabolic liver diseases. Occasionally, however, a result can be suggestive of a particular disease and guide further investigations—e.g., disproportionately elevated alkaline phosphatase in tyrosinemia type I, or low γ-glutamyltransferase (GGT) in bile acid synthesis disorders.

It is usually difficult to distinguish clearly between liver disease that is due to an underlying metabolic defect and liver disease that is due to other non-IEM causes; therefore, initial investigations for liver dysfunction due to any cause should include tests for the more common metabolic conditions. Clinical indications must be provided on the request forms, including feeding status/diet and drug and transfusion histories, as these may confound the results of some metabolic tests and give misleading results. More specific investigations such as enzyme assays on tissue biopsies and DNA mutation analysis are only indicated if the clinical features or the initial investigations point to a specific diagnosis or group of conditions. The molecular basis of many of the inborn errors is now well understood, with availability of mutation analysis for many of the disorders. The relationship between phenotype and genotype is not always clear, however, and many genotypes can show huge variation in clinical presentation. For some mutations, it is unclear whether there is a functional abnormality which is disease-causing. For these reasons, caution is needed for some disorders in the use of molecular tests as a first-line or only diagnostic test for IEM.

Laboratory investigations for metabolic disorders often require special methods of specimen collection, storage, and transport, and it is best to plan such investigations in consultation with a specialist metabolic laboratory before taking any specimens

Table 13.1 Initial investigations for inborn errors of metabolism.

Presenting feature	Investigations
Liver failure	Erythrocyte galactose-1-phosphate uridyltransferase (Beutler test) Plasma and urine amino acids Urine organic acids Urine succinylacetone Plasma α-fetoprotein Plasma lactate Plasma/blood spot acylcarnitines Plasma ferritin, TIBC Serum α_1-antitrypsin and phenotype
Encephalopathy or Reye-like illness	Plasma ammonia Plasma lactate Urine organic acids Plasma and urine amino acids Plasma/blood spot acylcarnitines
Cholestasis	As for liver failure, *plus:* Plasma very long-chain fatty acids Plasma transferrin isoforms Vacuolated lymphocytes in peripheral blood Storage cells in liver/bone-marrow biopsy Consider specific enzyme assay in leukocytes/fibroblasts Urine and plasma bile acids
Isolated hepatomegaly or hepatosplenomegaly	Plasma glucose, lactate Plasma urate Plasma lipids Urine oligosaccharides Urine glycosaminoglycans Liver histology Consider specific enzyme analysis on liver/leukocytes Vacuolated lymphocytes Storage cells in liver/bone marrow Plasma chitotriosidase Plasma transferrin isoforms

TIBC, total iron-binding capacity.

Initial investigations should include tests for the more common metabolic conditions according to the presenting features (Table 13.1); more specific tests for individual conditions are detailed in Table 13.2.

Disorders of carbohydrate metabolism

Glycogen storage diseases (GSDs)

Glycogen is the main storage form of carbohydrate in animals and is most abundant in liver and muscle. Liver glycogen controls the export of glucose, which maintains blood glucose concentrations between meals, and is almost completely depleted within a few hours of fasting. Muscle glycogen provides muscles with readily available energy via glycolysis. The synthesis (glycogenesis) and breakdown (glycogenolysis) of glycogen are catalyzed by a number of different enzymes, which in turn are activated or inactivated by hormones. The glycogen storage diseases are due to defects of glycogen synthesis or breakdown, each caused by a specific enzyme defect, and result in abnormal storage and/or deficient mobilization of glycogen. Some enzyme defects are confined to the liver and are associated with hepatomegaly and hypoglycemia, whereas others affect only muscle glycogen metabolism and result in muscle cramps, weakness, and myopathy. Traditionally, the glycogen storage diseases have been denoted by a number relating to the historical sequence in which they were described; nowadays, they are also

Table 13.2 Specific investigations for metabolic liver disease.

Presenting feature	Metabolic conditions	Investigations
Liver failure	Galactosemia	Erythrocyte galactose-1-phosphate uridyltransferase Erythrocyte galactose-1-phosphate DNA mutation analysis
	Tyrosinemia type 1	Plasma and urine amino acids Urine organic acids Urine succinylacetone Erythrocyte porphobilinogen synthetase α-Fetoprotein
	Hereditary fructose intolerance	Plasma lactate DNA mutation analysis Enzyme analysis on liver biopsy
	Mitochondrial respiratory-chain defects	Plasma and CSF lactate mtDNA analysis (blood) Muscle biopsy for DNA, histology, histochemistry and enzyme analysis
	Long-chain fatty acid oxidation defects (usually with associated hypoglycemia)	Urine organic acids Plasma/blood spot acylcarnitines DNA mutation analysis
	Neonatal hemochromatosis (see Chapter 5)	Plasma ferritin, TIBC Liver or lip biopsy
	α_1-Antitrypsin deficiency	Serum α_1-antitrypsin and phenotype
Encephalopathy or Reye-like illness	Fatty acid oxidation defect Organic acidemias Urea cycle defects	Plasma ammonia Plasma lactate Urine organic acids Plasma and urine amino acids Plasma/blood spot acylcarnitines Fibroblast enzymes DNA mutation analysis for MCADD and LCHAD deficiency
Cholestasis (neonatal or later)	Disorders mentioned under "liver failure" above, *plus:*	
	Peroxisomal disorders	Plasma very-long-chain fatty acids, DHAPAT, phytanic/pristanic acid, plasmalogens Peroxisomal morphology in liver/fibroblasts
	CDG syndrome	Plasma transferrin isoforms
	Lysosomal storage disorders	Vacuolated lymphocytes in peripheral blood Storage cells in liver/bone marrow biopsy or skin fibroblasts Specific enzyme assay in leukocytes/fibroblasts
	Niemann–Pick C disease	Storage cells in bone marrow/liver Filipin staining for unesterified cholesterol on skin fibroblasts Cholesterol esterification studies
	Bile acid synthesis defects	Urine and plasma bile acids
Isolated hepatomegaly or hepatosplenomegaly	Glycogen storage diseases	Plasma glucose, lactate Plasma urate Plasma lipids Urine oligosaccharides Liver histology Enzyme analysis on liver/muscle/skin fibroblasts
Lysosomal storage disorders		Urine oligosaccharides and mucopolysaccharides Vacuolated lymphocytes Storage cells in liver/bone marrow Skin biopsy for fibroblasts Plasma chitotriosidase Specific enzyme assay in leukocytes/fibroblasts
	CDG syndrome	Plasma transferrin isoforms

CDG, carbohydrate-deficient glycoprotein; CSF, cerebrospinal fluid; DHAPAT, dihydroxyacetone phosphate acyltransferase; LCHAD, long-chain 3-hydroxyacyl-coenzyme A dehydrogenase deficiency; MCADD, medium-chain acyl-CoA dehydrogenase deficiency; TIBC, total iron-binding capacity.

known by the specific enzyme deficiencies. The overall frequency of the combined group is believed to be around one in 20 000 to one in 25 000 live births.[4]

Glycogen storage disease type I

Glycogen storage disease type I (GSD I) is due to defective breakdown of glucose-6-phosphate, resulting in decreased hepatic production of glucose and accumulation of glycogen in liver, kidney, and intestine. Two subtypes of GSD I are currently recognized: GSD Ia, due to glucose-6-phosphatase deficiency, and GSD Ib, due to defects of the glucose-6-phosphatase transporter.

GSD Ia: glucose-6-phosphatase deficiency, von Gierke disease

GSD Ia is inherited as an autosomal-recessive trait. The glucose-6-phosphatase gene has been mapped to chromosome 17q21. Over 70 mutations have been identified (in the Human Gene Mutation Database), and a number of ethnic-specific mutations have described: R83C and Q347X in Caucasians; R83C in Jews; G727T in Chinese and Japanese; and V166G in Arabs.[4] The diagnosis of GSD Ia can be established by mutation analysis in some cases, as an alternative to liver enzyme analysis.

Presentation

Patients typically present in the neonatal period or early infancy with hepatomegaly, hypoglycemia, and tachypnea secondary to metabolic acidosis. Older children tend to have a doll-like face, thin extremities, short stature, and a protuberant abdomen due to massive hepatomegaly. The kidneys are also enlarged, but there is no cardiac involvement or splenomegaly. Recurrent vomiting, diarrhea, and skin xanthomas may also occur.

Children have a short tolerance to fasting and typically become hypoglycemic if a feed is delayed or if intake is reduced during intercurrent illness. Symptoms of hypoglycemia are usually accompanied by tachypnea secondary to metabolic acidosis (lactic acidosis). Exceptional patients are able to tolerate prolonged fasting without becoming hypoglycemic, possibly due to residual glucose-6-phosphatase activity.[5]

Biochemical abnormalities are characterized by:

- *Hypoglycemia*, which occurs soon after dietary sources of glucose are exhausted. The degradation of glycogen to pyruvate remains intact, with resultant increases of blood lactate and pyruvate concentrations.
- *Hyperlacticacidemia.* Lactate can serve as an alternative fuel for the brain, and its overproduction is helpful unless pathological metabolic acidosis develops. Osteopenia may result from chronic lactic acidosis, as bone is believed to play an important role in buffering chronic acidosis.
- *Hyperlipidemia.* Increased activity of the glycolytic pathway results in increased acetyl-CoA production. Excess acetyl-CoA that is not used for energy production is converted to malonyl-CoA, an inhibitor of fatty acid oxidation and a potent stimulant of fatty acid synthesis, resulting in increased plasma triglycerides and to a lesser extent cholesterol.
- Hyperuricemia is caused both by reduced clearance of urate by the kidneys, due to competition with lactic acid, and by increased production of uric acid from adenine nucleotide degradation.

Diagnosis

Characteristic laboratory findings are:

- Fasting hypoglycemia (< 2.5 mmol/L)
- Blood lactate > 5 mmol/L
- Hyperlipidemia (cholesterol > 6 mmol/L and triglycerides > 3 mmol/L)
- Hyperuricemia (> 350 µmol/L, age-dependent)
- Mildly elevated plasma aminotransferases
- Normal plasma bilirubin, albumin, coagulation

Liver histology demonstrates uniform distension of hepatocytes with glycogen and prominent lipid vacuoles. The glycogen content of the liver is raised (normal < 6%). Normal liver architecture may be obscured by the distended hepatocytes, but there is no fibrosis or cirrhosis (Figure 13.1). The stored material stains strongly positive on periodic acid–Schiff (PAS) and is digestible by diastase. Histochemical stains for glucose-6-phosphatase are negative.

The diagnosis can be confirmed either by mutation analysis of the *G6PC* gene in leukocytes or by enzyme analysis on a liver biopsy specimen.

Antenatal diagnosis by chorionic villus sampling is possible if the mutation has been identified; otherwise, enzyme analysis on fetal liver biopsy is the only option.[6]

Management and outcome

The main aim of therapy is to prevent hypoglycemia and

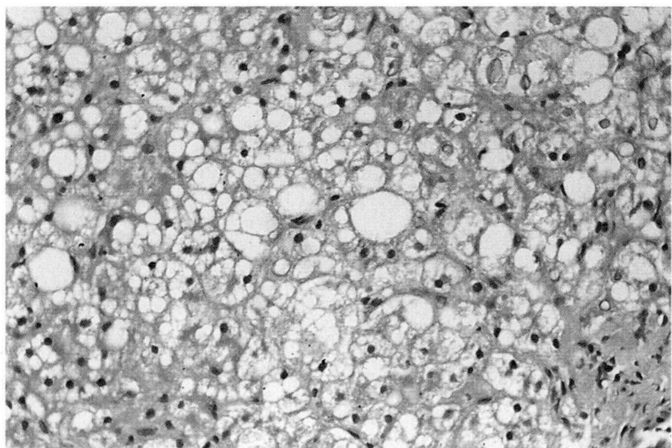

Figure 13.1 Glycogen storage disease types Ia and I non-a are characterized by increased glycogen storage. The hepatocytes are swollen with glycogen and steatosis is prominent. Glycogen-6-phosphatase is either deficient or functionally abnormal.

suppress the secondary metabolic derangements. This is achieved by providing a continuous supply of exogenous glucose, which maintains normal blood glucose concentrations and inhibits counter-regulatory responses. The glucose requirement has been estimated to be 8–10 mg/kg/min in infants and 5–7 mg/kg/min in older children.[4] In infants, this is best achieved by frequent daytime feeding. Continuous nocturnal enteral glucose feeds are usually required initially. In older children and adults, use of oral uncooked cornstarch, which is hydrolyzed in the gut to release glucose slowly over hours, may reduce the need for continuous or nocturnal feeding.[7] The dosage of cornstarch required to ensure metabolic stability varies greatly, but usually 1–2 g/kg/dose of cornstarch is given 4–12-hourly, depending on individual fasting tolerance. Tests to estimate fasting tolerance and monitoring of preprandial and postprandial glucose and lactate concentrations are useful in making decisions about dietary adjustments. With increasing age, the tendency towards hypoglycemia becomes less—perhaps as a result of the natural decrease in metabolic rate.[8]

Adequate dietary treatment can result in correction/reduced severity of many of the metabolic abnormalities and result in greatly reduced morbidity. Some long-term complications such as hypoglycemic brain damage and poor growth respond well to dietary management, although patients tend to be shorter than their peers.[9] The onset of puberty is often delayed. Most females have ultrasound evidence of polycystic ovaries, though other features of polycystic ovarian disease are rare[10] and the effects on fertility are unknown.

Chronic hyperuricemia can lead to gout, renal stones, and osteopenia, resulting in pathological fractures[11,12] and may require treatment with allopurinol. Early glomerular hyperfiltration slowly progresses to microalbuminuria, proteinuria, and eventually a reduced glomerular filtration rate secondary to focal glomerulosclerosis and interstitial fibrosis.[13] Declining renal function and hypertension eventually occur, and renal dialysis and transplantation may be necessary. Other renal abnormalities that have been described include a Fanconi-like syndrome, distal tubular dysfunction, kidney stones, and amyloidosis.[14,15] It is unclear whether dietary management can prevent long-term renal dysfunction and osteopenia,[16] but a recent study suggests that poor metabolic control results in reduced muscle strength and low bone mass.[17]

Atherosclerosis is rare, despite the atherogenic profile of plasma lipids.[18] There is an increased risk of pancreatitis secondary to the lipid abnormalities. Hypertriglyceridemia sometimes requires treatment; fish-oil supplements have been effective in lowering plasma triglycerides and cholesterol.[19]

Pulmonary hypertension is a rare fatal complication.[20,21] The exact cause is unknown, but vasoconstrictive stimuli such as severe metabolic acidosis, hypoxia, and abnormal hepatic clearance of circulating vasoactive agents have been proposed as possible mechanisms.[22]

Epistaxis and easy bruising following minor trauma are commonly observed; bleeding times are prolonged and associated with abnormal platelet adhesion and aggregation.[23] Surgical procedures should not be undertaken without first evaluating bleeding time and establishing good metabolic control. Intensive intravenous glucose therapy for 24–48 h before surgery can normalize abnormal bleeding times; 1-deamino-8-D-arginine vasopressin (DDAVP) has also been reported to reduce bleeding complications.[23] Successful pregnancies have been reported.[24]

Liver function is typically normal and cirrhosis does not develop. Hepatic adenomas are commonly present by the second or third decades of life, especially in suboptimally treated individuals.[25] The adenomas may be single or multiple, and have the potential for malignant transformation. Regular ultrasound examinations and serum α-fetoprotein determinations are therefore essential. Although hepatic adenomas have been shown to regress following intensive dietary treatment,[26] more recent long-term studies indicate that they may occur despite early continuous glucose therapy.[9]

Liver transplantation is rarely undertaken, as the disease should be adequately controlled with dietary management. However, liver transplantation may be indicated for symptomatic multiple hepatic adenomas, to prevent the development of hepatocellular carcinoma and/or poor metabolic control.[27–29] Successful liver transplantation restores normal metabolic balance, allows catch-up growth, and improves quality of life.[28,30] However, it may not prevent the development of renal dysfunction with focal segmental glomerulosclerosis,[27]and this needs to be considered when treating with nephrogenic immunosuppressive drugs. Successful hepatocyte transplantation has also been reported.[31]

Glycogen storage disease type I non-a (also known as GSD Ib, Ic, and Id)

Patients with GSD I non-a produce glucose-6-phosphatase but cannot transport it to its site of action at the inner wall of the endoplasmic reticulum (ER). The rest of the glycogenolytic enzymes are located in the cytoplasm, and glucose-6-phosphate has to be transported into the ER; the products of this reaction, glucose and phosphate, have to be transported out of the ER. It was originally believed that different proteins carried out these transport reactions, and the putative deficiencies of these transport proteins were labeled as GSD types Ib, Ic, and Id, respectively. Recent evidence suggests that GSD types Ic and Id do not differ from GSD Ib clinically, enzymatically, or genetically.[32] These conditions are therefore now categorized as GSD I non-a. The prevalence of GSD Ia relative to GSD I non-a is estimated to be around 5–10 to one.[33]

The glucose-6-phosphatase transporter gene has been localized to chromosome 11q23. Several mutations have been reported; G339C and 1211delCT appear to be common in Caucasian patients, while W118R appears to be common amongst Japanese patients.[34,35]

Presentation

The clinical presentation, metabolic derangements, and complications are the same as in GSD Ia, with the additional finding of neutropenia and impaired neutrophil function. Neutropenia becomes apparent in infancy or early childhood and is usually intermittent.[36] Inflammatory bowel disease resembling Crohn disease may also occur, often preceded or accompanied by oral, perioral, and perianal ulcers, infections, abscesses, and fistulas.

Diagnosis

Biochemical abnormalities and liver histology are indistinguishable from GSD Ia (Figure 13.1). Diagnosis requires DNA analysis or demonstration of deficient glucose-6-phosphatase activity in fresh liver biopsy tissue in which hepatocytes and microsomes are intact. When the cell is disrupted by freezing, measured glucose-6-phosphatase activity is normal, as the substrate has free access to the enzyme.

Antenatal diagnosis is possible by mutation analysis in chorionic villus tissue if the mutations are known; otherwise, fetal liver biopsy is required.

Management and outcome

Management of GSD I non-a patients is the same as in GSD Ia. Dietary metabolic control has no effect on neutropenia and neutrophil dysfunction, but treatment with granulocyte colony-stimulating factor (G-CSF) or granulocyte-macrophage colony-stimulating factor (GM-CSF) successfully corrects neutropenia, decreasing the frequency of bacterial infections and improving chronic inflammatory bowel disease in these patients.[37,38] Splenomegaly is an important short-term complication of G-CSF therapy in these patients, but usually does not result in clinically significant thrombocytopenia.[39] As Sweet syndrome (acute febrile neutrophilic dermatosis),[40] acute myelogenous leukemia,[41] and renal carcinoma[42] have been reported in patients receiving G-CSF treatment, close follow-up with annual bone-marrow aspiration and imaging studies is advisable. Prophylactic antibiotic therapy may be an option for patients with neutropenia who do not have inflammatory bowel disease. Liver transplantation has been successfully carried out in a few patients with GSD Ib.[28,43,44] Reported benefits include improved metabolic control and growth, as well as decreased hospitalization. However, improvement in neutropenia has been variable and patients have continued to require G-CSF treatment after hepatic transplantation. To date, we are aware of one patient with GSD Ib who has undergone bone-marrow transplantation for neutropenia and recurrent infections;[45] 1 year after transplantation, the patient demonstrated a markedly reduced rate of infection, improved growth, and reduced gastrointestinal symptoms and was able to stop G-CSF therapy, although he remained mildly neutropenic and his fasting intolerance persisted.

Glycogen storage disease type III

GSD type III is caused by deficiency of the debrancher enzyme amylo-1,6-glucosidase, resulting in accumulation of partially broken-down glycogen molecules (limit dextrin). Patients with liver and muscle involvement (GSD IIIa) have a generalized debrancher deficiency that affects liver, muscle, fibroblasts, cardiac muscle, and erythrocytes,[4] whereas patients with GSD IIIb have debrancher deficiency confined to the liver. Type IIIa is more common, occurring in about 80% of patients with GSD III.

The inheritance of GSD III is autosomal-recessive. The gene is located at chromosome 1p21 and several mutations have been reported. Muscle and liver isoforms of the enzyme are encoded by the same gene, although certain mutations (those associated with GSD IIIa) appear to be associated with retention of debrancher activity in muscle, but not in liver.[46]

Presentation

The presentation may be indistinguishable from that of GSD I, but milder. The main clinical features are hypoglycemia, hepatomegaly, short stature, skeletal myopathy, hyperlipidemia, and cardiomyopathy. There is wide variability in clinical and biochemical phenotypes, depending on the extent and localization of the enzyme defect.

In contrast to GSD I, however, renal enlargement is not present.

Patients who have muscle involvement often develop slowly progressive skeletal myopathy and wasting, progressing from minimal signs in childhood to severe muscle weakness by the third or fourth decade of life.[47,48] Muscular involvement can be very variable and range from mild to severe and life-threatening.[49] Left ventricular hypertrophy is common in patients with muscular involvement, and may lead to significant cardiac dysfunction in the long term.[49]

Diagnosis

Patients characteristically have:

- Fasting hypoglycemia with ketosis/ketonuria.
- Hyperlipidemia (cholesterol > 6 mmol/L with normal triglyceride < 3 mmol/L).
- Uric acid is usually normal.
- Lactate is moderately increased (2.5–5.0 mmol/L) or normal.
- Elevated hepatic aminotransferases.
- Increased creatine kinase (type IIIa); it should be noted that normal levels do not rule out muscle involvement.

Liver histology is similar to GSD I. Two distinguishing features in GSD III are the presence of fibrosis and a relative paucity of steatosis. The diagnosis is confirmed by identifying the deficient enzyme in leukocytes or hepatic tissue, or by DNA analysis.

Antenatal diagnosis is possible by enzyme assay in chorionic villus samples or cultured amniotic fluid cells, as well as by mutation analysis in informative families.

Management and outcome

The general principles of treatment and prevention of hypoglycemia are the same as for GSD I. Adequate dietary management is associated with catch-up growth, decreased liver size, and improved liver function. A high protein intake may help in improving glycemic control, as protein can be used for gluconeogenesis, a pathway that is intact in GSD III.[50]

With age, hepatomegaly, hepatic function, and fasting tolerance improve and may completely resolve after puberty.[51] However, progressive liver dysfunction and liver failure can occur. Hepatic adenomas have been reported in up to 25% of patients, but malignant transformation is rare. Hepatocellular carcinoma in association with advanced liver cirrhosis can occur.[28,52] Liver transplantation may be indicated for cirrhosis, end-stage liver failure, and/or hepatocellular carcinoma.[28]

The long-term outlook is favorable for patients without muscle involvement (GSD IIIb). For those with GSD IIIa, the prognosis depends on the severity of neuromuscular and cardiac disease. At present, there appears to be no satisfactory way of preventing progressive myopathy.[4]

Successful pregnancies have been reported.[53,54]

Glycogen storage disease type IV

This rare disease is due to a defect in the enzyme required for normal branching of the glycogen molecule (α1,4-glycan-6-glycosyltransferase). The glycogen that accumulates is abnormal and poorly soluble, with fewer branch points than normal glycogen. Accumulation is generalized and occurs in the liver, heart, muscle, skin, intestine, brain, and peripheral nervous system.

Inheritance is autosomal-recessive. The hepatic and neuromuscular forms of GSD IV are caused by mutations on the same gene, which has been localized to chromosome 3p12.[55]

Presentation

The most common presentation is in infancy, with liver dysfunction and failure to thrive. Initial hepatomegaly progresses to cirrhosis and portal hypertension with splenomegaly, ascites, and variceal bleeding, leading to death by the age of 5 years.[4] Hypoglycemia is rare, except as a feature of liver failure. Some patients appear to have nonprogressive liver disease,[56,57] and hepatocellular carcinoma has been reported in one such individual.[57]

Brancher enzyme deficiency may also present with neuromuscular symptoms without hepatic involvement. These individuals may present in the neonatal period with severe hypotonia and neurological involvement, leading to death in infancy, in late childhood with myopathy and/or cardiomyopathy, or in adulthood with diffuse central and peripheral neurological symptoms associated with polyglucosan body storage in the nervous system. In extreme cases, prenatal onset of symptoms may result in hydrops fetalis or fetal akinesia deformation sequence.[58,59]

Diagnosis

Clinical features of the hepatic form are indistinguishable from other causes of liver disease in infancy, and the diagnosis is usually suspected from liver histology. Pale, amphophilic hyaline deposits along with large lipid vacuoles are seen on light microscopy, with fibrosis or cirrhosis. The abnormal glycogen can be demonstrated as large PAS-positive, diastase-resistant deposits in hepatocytes (Figure 13.2) and with special stains such as Lugol's iodine or colloidal iron phosphate. Similar histological findings may be demonstrable on cardiac and skeletal muscle biopsy. Confirmation of the diagnosis requires enzyme assay in liver, muscle, leukocytes, or fibroblasts.

Antenatal diagnosis is possible by enzyme assay on cultured amniocytes or chorionic villus tissue, as well as by DNA analysis if the mutation(s) are known.

Management and outcome

Dietary management with continuous nasogastric feeding and/or cornstarch may help improve growth and muscle strength. Liver transplantation is an effective treatment for those patients who develop progressive liver failure. To date, 14 patients with GSD IV are reported to have undergone liver transplantation.[4,28,60,61] The nine survivors have not developed any neurological, muscular, or cardiac complications up to 13.5 years after transplantation, and some have had a progressive reduction in myocardial amylopectin storage.[62]

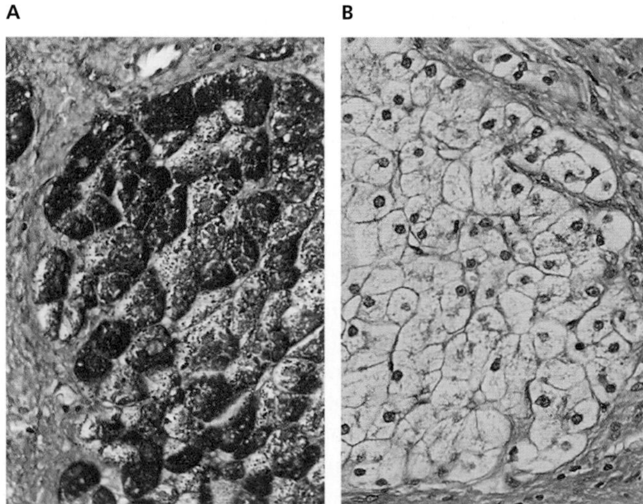

Figure 13.2 Glycogen storage type IV typically demonstrates cytoplasmic inclusions of the abnormal glycogen (amylopectin) (**A**), which is completely removed by diastase (**B**).

Deficiencies of the liver phosphorylase system: glycogen storage diseases types VI and IX

Defects of the phosphorylase system are either due to deficient phosphorylase enzymes or to defects of the phosphorylase-activating system. These systems are enzymatically distinct in the liver and skeletal muscles. Muscle phosphorylase deficiency (GSD VI) presents in adulthood with muscle cramps and exercise intolerance; it does not involve the liver and will not be discussed further. Of the liver phosphorylase system defects, phosphorylase kinase defects (GSD IX) are much more common than liver phosphorylase deficiency (GSD VI).

The liver phosphorylase gene is located on chromosome 14q21-22. The genetics of the phosphorylase kinase system is very complex, as the enzyme consists of four subunits encoded on different genes (X chromosome as well as autosomes), which are differentially expressed in different tissues. The clinical expression of individual enzyme deficiencies and isoforms is variable and depends on both the severity and the distribution of the enzyme defect.

Presentation

Patients with GSD VI usually present with hepatomegaly and growth failure in early childhood. Symptoms of hypoglycemia, hyperlipidemia, and hyperketosis are mild if present. Plasma lactate and urate concentrations are usually normal. There is no cardiac or skeletal muscle involvement, and the condition has a benign course, with a reduction in hepatomegaly after puberty.[63]

Phosphorylase kinase deficiency (GSD IX) is clinically and genetically more heterogeneous. Seventy-five percent of the patients have X-linked liver phosphorylase deficiency (type IXa), which manifests between the ages of 1 and 5 years with hepatomegaly, growth retardation, mild hypoglycemia, and mild elevation of hepatic transaminases, cholesterol, and triglycerides.[64] Hepatomegaly and growth retardation usually resolve after puberty.

Autosomal-recessive forms of phosphorylase kinase deficiency (GSD IXb, c) present with more severe liver disease, which may progress to cirrhosis,[65,66] with or without skeletal myopathy. Rare variants with isolated muscle and cardiac involvement have also been described.[67–69]

Diagnosis

Liver histology reveals nonuniform distension of hepatocytes with fibrosis and small fat droplets. On electron microscopy, the cytoplasmic glycogen particles are seen in rosette formation, less compact than normal, with a frayed pattern. Definitive diagnosis of phosphorylase and phosphorylase kinase deficiencies rely on specific enzyme assays in affected tissues—i.e., liver or muscle. Enzymes can be measured in leukocytes and erythrocytes, but the presence of different isoenzymes can make interpretation difficult. Genetic DNA analysis is increasingly possible for most defects.

Management and outcome

Treatment for these conditions is symptomatic. Frequent feeds and overnight feeding, with or without cornstarch,[70] may be necessary for more severely affected patients, but many do not require any specific intervention. The tendency to hypoglycemia diminishes with age, and catch-up growth usually occurs without any specific treatment.

Fanconi–Bickel syndrome (glycogen storage disease type XI)

This rare disorder is characterized metabolically by hepatorenal glycogen accumulation and fasting hypoglycemia, postprandial hyperglycemia, and hypergalactosemia. The disorder is due to defective function of the GLUT2 transporter, which is the most important glucose transporter in hepatocytes, pancreatic β-cells, enterocytes, and renal tubular cells.[71] Deficiency results in impaired import and export of glucose and galactose in affected tissues. Hypoglycemia is due to impaired glucose transport from the liver and defective renal reabsorption of glucose and galactose. Hepatic and renal glycogen accumulation results, leading to impaired tubular function, Fanconi nephropathy, and rickets.[72] Over 100 patients are currently known.[73]

GLUT2. The GLUT2 gene has been localized to chromosome 3q26.1-q26.3, and 34 different mutations have been reported.[73] Parental consanguinity is commonly observed.

Presentation

The main clinical features are hepatomegaly secondary to glycogen storage, and renal tubular dysfunction. Presentation in infancy includes recurrent vomiting, fever, failure to thrive, and hypophosphatemic rickets, while in early childhood, short stature, protuberant abdomen, hepatomegaly, moon-shaped facies, and fat deposition around the shoulders and abdomen is usual. Fasting hypoglycemia is a frequent finding, although symptomatic hypoglycemia is rare. Chronic diarrhea due to sugar malabsorption may occur. Rickets and osteoporosis lead to pathological fractures. Mild abnormalities of liver function are common, but hepatic adenomas and malignancies have not been reported.

Diagnosis

Characteristic findings on investigation include:

- Postprandial hyperglycemia and hypergalactosemia
- Fasting hypoglycemia
- Mildly abnormal liver function tests
- Generalized renal tubular reabsorption defects: glycosuria, galactosuria, generalized aminoaciduria, phosphaturia, hypercalciuria, hyperuricosuria, mild proteinuria
- Mild metabolic acidosis related to renal bicarbonate loss
- Increased liver glycogen content on biopsy specimens

The diagnosis can be confirmed by DNA mutation analysis. Antenatal diagnosis has not been reported.

Management and outcome

There is no definitive therapy available. Treatment is supportive, and includes replacement of water and electrolytes, alkalinization with bicarbonate solutions, vitamin D and phosphate supplementation, galactose restriction, and frequent small meals.[72] Uncooked cornstarch may be useful. Fructose may be used as an alternative carbohydrate source in patients with malabsorption, as its absorption is not mediated by GLUT2.

The prognosis is good, and many patients reach adulthood in a stable condition, including the original patient described by Fanconi and Bickel;[72] short stature appears to be the major subjective long-term problem.

Galactosemia

Galactosemia usually results in severe liver dysfunction in the neonatal period or early infancy, and is discussed in detail in Chapter 5.

Hereditary fructose intolerance

Fructose is an important dietary source of carbohydrate.[74] It is metabolized in the liver, renal cortex, and small intestine by three enzymes: fructokinase, aldolase B, and triokinase. Hereditary fructose intolerance (HFI) is caused by deficiency of aldolase B, resulting in an inability to convert fructose-1-phosphate into dihydroxyacetone phosphate and glyceraldehyde. Ingested fructose accumulates as fructose-1-phosphate, which has two major consequences:

- Hypoglycemia, resulting from inhibition of the glycogenolytic enzyme glycogen phosphorylase and impaired gluconeogenesis due to an inability to condense glyceraldehyde-3-phosphate and dihydroxyacetone phosphate.
- Depletion of the nucleotides adenosine triphosphate (ATP) and guanosine triphosphate (GTP), as a consequence of their high utilization and sequestration in the formation of large amounts of fructose-1-phosphate. ATP is believed to lead to impaired protein synthesis and ultimately to liver and renal dysfunction.

The incidence may be as high as one in 23 000 live births in the United Kingdom.[75] HFI is inherited as an autosomal-recessive trait. The gene for aldolase B has been mapped to chromosome 9q22.3. About 20 mutations are known; three common mutations are found in most patients of European origin. In Britain, the A149P mutation is common.[75] In southern Europe, the A174D mutation is most prevalent,[76] while in eastern Europe, N334K is the common mutation.[77]

Presentation

Infants and adults with HFI are asymptomatic until fructose, sucrose, or sorbitol is ingested. The age of presentation depends on the timing of the introduction of these sugars. Typically, the first symptoms occur during weaning when fruits and vegetables are introduced into the diet and include gastrointestinal discomfort and hypoglycemia following fructose-containing meals. Nausea, vomiting, pallor, sweating lethargy, tremors, and seizures may occur. If the condition remains unrecognized and fructose intake continues, failure to thrive, signs of liver disease (hepatomegaly, jaundice, coagulopathy) and proximal renal tubular dysfunction (renal tubular acidosis, hypophosphatemic rickets) develop. Younger infants and children may be at risk of death from liver and renal failure.

HFI patients who survive beyond infancy develop an aversion to sweet foods and self-select a low-fructose diet. School-age children may avoid social situations that require them to ingest sugar-containing foods, which can be misinterpreted as psychotic behavior. Characteristically, patients with HFI have caries-free teeth, and the diagnosis may be suspected by dentists.[78] Some individuals are diagnosed only during family testing or for investigation for growth retardation or isolated hepatomegaly; others are recognized only after receiving inadvertent fructose or sorbitol-containing infusions, sometimes with fatal results.[79]

Diagnosis

Characteristic findings are:

- Increased conjugated bilirubin.
- Hypoalbuminemia.
- Increased hepatic aminotransferases.
- Hypoglycemia.
- Lactic acidosis.
- Low plasma phosphate.
- Plasma tyrosine and methionine may be elevated secondary to liver dysfunction.
- Anemia, acanthocytosis and thrombocytosis.
- Positive urine-reducing substances, fructosuria, proteinuria, generalized aminoaciduria.
- Abnormal renal tubular function tests.

The diagnosis is confirmed by:

- Enzymatic deficiency (liver or intestinal mucosal biopsy)
- Mutation analysis

Hepatic pathology varies from hepatic necrosis in infants, who present with acute liver failure, to diffuse steatosis, periportal or lobular fibrosis, or cirrhosis (Figure 13.3). Electron microscopy demonstrates the pathognomonic punched-out areas between cytoplasmic organelles known as "fructose holes."[80]

Management and outcome

Management consists of eliminating fructose, sucrose, and sorbitol from the diet for life. Sucrose and sorbitol are frequently used as sweeteners in syrups and suspensions, as well as in tablet coatings and toothpaste; the suitability of all medications must be checked before prescribing. Fructose elimination usually results in a dramatic improvement in hepatic function, with regression of fibrosis and prevention of cirrhosis, as well as improvement in renal function. Provided liver and renal disease are not advanced, full restoration of normal health, growth, and development may be expected,

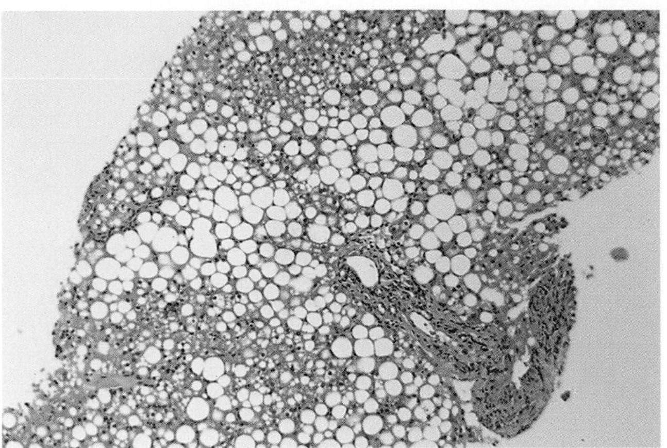

Figure 13.3 Hereditary fructose intolerance is associated with severe steatosis on liver histology. Persistent ingestion of fructose leads to cirrhosis.

although hepatomegaly may persist for years after adequate treatment.[81] Life-threatening fulminant hepatic failure may develop on the reintroduction of fructose, sucrose or sorbitol. The development of hepatoma has been reported.[82]

Fructose-1,6-bisphosphatase deficiency

Fructose-1,6-bisphosphatase deficiency results in impaired gluconeogenesis from all precursors, including fructose. Maintenance of normal glucose concentrations therefore depends on dietary glucose and galactose and on hepatic glycogenolysis. Hypoglycemia results when these sources of glucose are exhausted. Accumulation of the gluconeogenic precursors lactate, alanine, and glycerol occurs. It is a rare disorder and its incidence is unknown.

The condition is inherited as an autosomal-recessive trait. Liver and muscle express distinct enzymes, and the muscle enzyme is not involved in the disorder. The liver enzyme has been mapped to chromosome 9q22.2-22.3, and several mutations have been described.[83] In some patients, no mutations have been identified, suggesting the existence of unidentified mutations in the promoter region of the gene or mutations of other genes that regulate fructose-1,6-bisphosphatase activity.[84]

Presentation

Fructose-1,6-bisphosphatase deficiency is a life-threatening condition; about half of the affected patients become symptomatic in the newborn period, with lactic acidosis and hypoglycemia. Presenting symptoms include hyperventilation secondary to profound lactic acidosis, irritability, hypotonia, somnolence, apneic spells, coma, convulsions, and hepatomegaly. Other patients may present in infancy or early childhood with hypoglycemia and acidosis triggered by a febrile illness. Subsequent attacks may be triggered by intercurrent illnesses, though patients remain very well between attacks. Ingestion of large quantities of fructose or sucrose is known to precipitate acute decompensation, although in contrast to hereditary fructose intolerance, children do not avoid sweet foods.

Diagnosis

Characteristic findings are:
- Hypoglycemia
- Increased plasma lactate and ketones
- Metabolic acidosis
- Increased free fatty acids
- Hyperuricemia
- Normal liver and renal function

The diagnosis is confirmed by DNA mutation analysis or by demonstrating the enzyme deficiency in liver, renal cortex, or jejunum. The enzyme is also expressed at low levels in leukocytes, and diagnosis can be attempted in these cells; deficient leukocyte fructose-1,6-bisphosphatase activity is diagnostic, but normal activity does not rule out liver enzyme deficiency.[85] The enzyme is not expressed in skin fibroblasts or amniotic cells. Antenatal diagnosis is theoretically possible by mutation analysis, but has not yet been reported.

Management and outcome

Treatment of acute attacks consists of infusions of high-concentration glucose and bicarbonate to correct hypoglycemia and acidosis. The basic principle of long-term management is avoidance of fasting, particularly during intercurrent illnesses; overnight gastric drip feeding may be required in very young infants. Dietary fructose and sucrose may have to be restricted, particularly during febrile illnesses. After diagnosis and institution of adequate management, the condition follows a relatively benign course. Fasting tolerance improves with age, and may be normal in adults.[86]

Lysosomal storage disorders

The lysosomes are intracellular organelles containing a large number of different enzymes at acid pH whose main function is the degradation of macromolecules. The lysosomal storage disorders (LSDs) are each due to a specific enzyme deficiency resulting in abnormal storage of partially degraded macromolecules in the lysosomes. They can be considered as three groups (Table 13.3).

The clinical spectrum of the storage disorders is wide, ranging from prenatal hydrops fetalis to mild disease in adulthood.[87] Suggestive signs include coarsening of facial features, neurological deterioration, and hepatosplenomegaly. Patients with storage disorders often have a characteristic skeletal dysplasia (dysostosis multiplex), with a large skull, spinal deformities, and short, thick tubular bones. The liver and spleen are important sites for abnormal lysosomal storage, and hepatosplenomegaly is thus a frequent finding,

Table 13.3 Lysosomal storage disorders associated with hepatosplenomegaly.

Disorder	Enzyme defect	Clinical features	Hepatosplenomegaly (–, absent; +, mild; ++, moderate; +++, marked)	Outcome
I Sphingolipid and lipid storage disorders				
G_{M1} gangliosidosis	β-galactosidase	Neurodegeneration, dysostosis multiplex, coarse features, hepatosplenomegaly, cherry-red spot. Infantile, juvenile and adult forms recognized	Infantile form: ++ Juvenile forms – or + Adult form: –	Infantile: death by 2 y Juvenile: death 3–10 y Adult: onset 2nd-4th decade, slow neurodegeneration
Gaucher	β-glucosidase	Hepatosplenomegaly, bone and lung infiltration. Neurological (type II), nonneurological (type I) and intermediate (type III) forms	++ to +++	Type I (common): prolonged survival, death due to pulmonary or hematological complications Type II: death in infancy Type III: variable survival into childhood; enzyme replacement therapy available
Niemann–Pick A and B	Sphingomyelinase	Hepatosplenomegaly, lung infiltration, neurological (A) and nonneurological (B) types	++ to +++	Type A: death in infancy Type B: relatively normal lifespan
Niemann–Pick C	Cholesterol and lipid trafficking defect	Neonatal hepatitis, hepatospleno-megaly, vertical ophthalmoplegia, ataxia, later neurodegeneration	++ to +++	Death 1–3 decades after onset of neurodegeneration
Wolman disease and cholesterol ester storage disease	Acid esterase	Hepatosplenomegaly, steatorrhea, failure to thrive, adrenal calcification, neurodegeneration. Cholesterol ester storage disease a mild variant, causing hepatic fibrosis in adults	++	Wolman: death in infancy Cholesterol ester storage disease: death from liver failure in adulthood
Farber disease	Ceramidase	Psychomotor deterioration, subcutaneous nodules, painful and deformed joints	+ to ++	Death in infancy; late-onset variants known
II Mucolipidoses and glycoprotein storage disorders				
Mucolipidosis I (sialidosis)	α̃-Neuraminidase	Myotonic seizures, cherry-red spot, psychomotor retardation, hepatospleno-megaly, and dysostosis multiplex	– to ++	Severe cases: death in early childhood Milder cases: survival into adulthood, severely retarded
Mucolipidosis II (I-cell disease)	*N*-acetylglucosamine-1-phosphatase (defective enzyme transport into lysosomes)	Coarse facies, kyphoscoliosis, joint contractures, gingival hyperplasia, cardiomyopathy, dysostosis. Onset in infancy	++	Death by age 4–6 from cardiopulmonary disease
Mucolipidosis III	Same defect as mucolipidosis II	Stiff joints, kyphoscoliosis, short stature, low–normal intelligence. Presentation by 3–4 y	+ to ++	Usually survive into adulthood with severe orthopedic problems and mild cardiac involvement

Galactosialidosis	Neuraminidase and β-galactosidase	Combined features of mucolipidosis I and G_{M1} gangliosidosis, onset usually in late childhood	++	Survival into adulthood usual, with variable degree of mental retardation
Fucosidosis	α-Fucosidase	Psychomotor retardation, mild dysostosis multiplex, angiokeratoma, visceromegaly. Onset in early childhood	++	Severe form (type I): death by late childhood Mild form (type II): survival into adulthood, variable degree of mental retardation
α-Mannosidosis	α-Mannosidase	Deafness, mild Hurler phenotype, mental retardation. Onset in infancy or early childhood	++ to +++	Slow intellectual deterioration, eventual developmental level at 5–7 y. Survival into adulthood usual
Sialic acid storage disorder	Defective sialic acid transport out of lysosomes	Infantile form (infantile sialic acid storage disorder): psychomotor retardation, coarse facies, hepato-splenomegaly, cardiomyopathy, onset in first few months of life Late-onset form (Salla disease): ataxia, nystagmus, developmental delay in childhood; severe mental retardation in adulthood	Infantile form: ++ to +++ Late-onset form: –	Infantile form: rapid deterioration, death by 1–5 y Late-onset form: prolonged survival with slow neurodegeneration; average age at death 30–40 y
III Mucopolysaccharidoses				
MPS I (Hurler or Scheie)	α-Iduronidase	Hurler: psychomotor retardation, coarse facial features, growth retardation, dysostosis multiplex, corneal clouding, visceromegaly. Milder features in Scheie syndrome	Hurler: ++ Scheie: – to +	Hurler: psychomotor retardation and death by 8–10 y Scheie: normal intellect and lifespan; orthopedic problems common. Enzyme replacement therapy available
MPS II (Hunter)		Symptoms similar to Hurler syndrome, no corneal clouding. Rare milder variant with no mental retardation	Severe: ++ Mild: – to +	Death by mid-teens Milder variant: normal life span. Enzyme replacement therapy available
MPS III (Sanfilippo) Type A Type B Type C Type D		Commonest MPS disorder in United Kingdom, identical phenotype in all types. Marked mental retardation, severe behavioral and sleep disturbance. Mild somatic involvement, mild coarse features, no corneal clouding	All forms: – to +	Survival into late teens or adulthood with severe mental retardation
MPS IV (Morquio) Type A Type B		Both types phenotypically similar. No mental retardation, severe skeletal deformities and growth retardation, cervical myelopathy a potentially fatal hazard, mild corneal clouding	Both forms: +	Survival into adulthood common if death does not occur earlier due to cervical myelopathy. Cardiopulmonary compromise later due to thoracic deformity
MPS VI (Maroteaux–Lamy)		Skeletal deformities similar to Hurler syndrome, but no mental retardation. Variable cardiac involvement, mild corneal clouding	+	Severe forms: survival into late teens Mild form: normal lifespan. Enzyme replacement therapy available
MPS VII (Sly)		Variable phenotype ranging from hydrops fetalis to mild adult type similar to MPS I	++	Variable, depending on severity

MPS, mucopolysaccharidosis.

but the clinical picture is dominated by neurodevelopmental regression. Nevertheless, Gaucher disease, Niemann–Pick disease, Wolman disease and cholesterol ester storage disease have important hepatic manifestations. There have been major developments in treatment possibilities for LSD, especially enzyme replacement therapy.[88]

Gaucher disease

Gaucher disease is the commonest lysosomal storage disorder, with a global frequency of one in 200 000.[89] It is caused by deficiency of β-glucosidase (glucocerebrosidase), resulting in accumulation of glucosylceramide, a normal intermediate in the synthesis and catabolism of complex glycosphingolipids. Gaucher disease is classified according to the presence and severity of neurological manifestations:

- Type 1 (nonneuronopathic) Gaucher disease includes patients without neurological manifestations.
- Type 2 (acute neuronopathic) Gaucher disease includes patients with neurological involvement presenting in infancy.
- Type 3 (subacute neuronopathic) Gaucher disease presents in childhood and is associated with variable neurological manifestations.

Type 1 is the most common subtype; the relative frequencies of types 1, 2, and 3 Gaucher disease are 94%, 5%, and 1%, respectively.[90] The hallmark of this condition is the accumulation of characteristic tissue macrophages (Gaucher cells), which have a "crumpled-paper" appearance histologically, due to abnormal accumulation of phagocytosed glycosphingolipids. Gaucher cells are found in all tissues, and clinical manifestations reflect the sites and extent of abnormal glycosphingolipid storage.[91] The main storage sites are the liver, spleen, and bone marrow, although significant storage also occurs in the central nervous system, lymph nodes, lungs, and glomerular mesangium. Some of the pathological consequences in these tissues may relate to vascular blockage by the Gaucher cells. The major accumulating lipids, glucosylceramide and glucosylsphingosine, also induce the tissue macrophages to secrete a large number of proinflammatory cytokines, which are believed to mediate the acute inflammatory responses and tissue damage that underlie the clinical and biochemical manifestations.

The gene has been localized to chromosome 1q21 and over 160 mutations have been described. Six common mutations (N370S, 84GG, IVS2(+1), V394L, R496H and L444P) account for > 90% of Jewish and 60–70% of non-Jewish alleles.[92] Broad phenotype–genotype correlations exist, with the N370S allele generally associated with milder and nonneuronopathic disease, and the L444P allele strongly associated with neuronopathic disease.

Presentation

Clinical expression is heterogeneous, ranging from "congenital" Gaucher disease presenting with hydrops fetalis to asymptomatic glucocerebrosidase deficiency.

Type 1 Gaucher disease

The age at presentation varies from childhood to late adulthood. Presenting features are related to:

- Growth retardation
- Bone pain
- Hepatosplenomegaly
- Abdominal pain from hepatic or splenic Infarction
- Hypersplenism[93]

Without treatment, progressive splenomegaly leads to transfusion dependency, and the enlarged spleen may rupture with trauma. Liver fibrosis has been reported, but cirrhosis is rare.[94] Clinically, hepatic complications include portal hypertension, abnormal liver function, and liver infarction. The extent of bone involvement is a major determinant of long-term morbidity, and most adults with Gaucher disease develop complications including bone pain, osteoporosis, lytic lesions, pathological fractures and avascular necrosis.[95,96] Other significant complications include bone marrow failure,[96] pulmonary hypertension[97] and an increased risk of lymphoproliferative malignancy.[89]

Type 2 Gaucher disease

Type 2 differs from type 1 disease, as the presentation is in early infancy with:

- Marked hepatosplenomegaly
- Severe neurological involvement characterized by paralytic squint, dysphagia, persistent head hyperextension, trismus and generalized spasticity

Death occurs by 2 years of age, associated with progressive psychomotor regression and brainstem dysfunction.[98]

Exceptional patients have a prenatal onset with hydrops fetalis, or a later onset with similar but slower progression.

Type 3 Gaucher disease

Type 3 has intermediate severity between types 1 and 2. The main clinical features include:

- Severe visceromegaly, which can lead to death from liver disease and portal hypertension in the second to fourth decades.
- Characteristic oculomotor apraxia (horizontal supranuclear gaze palsy).
- Dementia, ataxia, spasticity, and epilepsy (myoclonic or complex partial seizures) develop over time and progress at variable rates.[98]
- Other patients have mild systemic manifestations, but severe progressive neurological involvement leads to death in childhood from neurological complications.

Diagnosis

Supportive tests include:

- Demonstration of Gaucher cells in bone-marrow aspirate or liver biopsy (Figure 13.4). Gaucher cells are not specific for Gaucher disease and have been described in leukemia, lymphoma, thalassemia, multiple myeloma, and acquired immune deficiency syndrome (AIDS) complicated by tuberculosis.

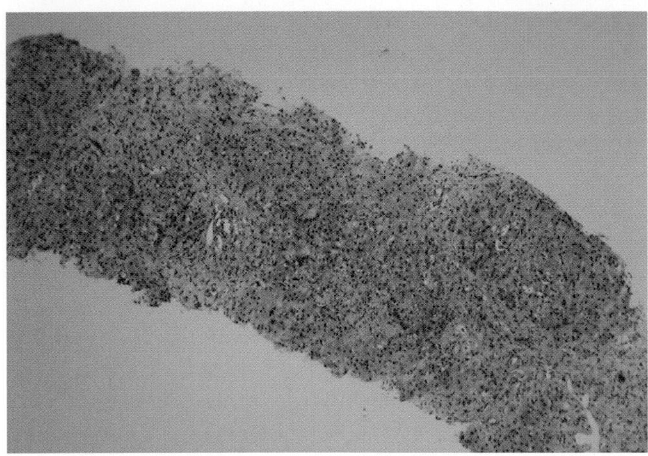

Figure 13.4 Gaucher disease affects reticuloendothelial cells in the liver, bone marrow, and lung. Liver histology shows fibrosis and Gaucher cells around the portal tract.

- Marked elevation of plasma angiotensin-converting enzyme (ACE), tartrate-resistant acid phosphatase (TRAP), and/or chitotriosidase or the chemokine CCL18/PARC.[99]

A number of *nonspecific* hematological and biochemical abnormalities may be present:

- Anemia, leukopenia, thrombocytopenia
- Abnormal hepatic transaminases
- Abnormal coagulation and fibrinolytic tests
- Increased ferritin and transcobalamin
- Polyclonal hypergammaglobulinemia

Specific diagnostic tests are:

- Glucocerebrosidase (leukocytes or cultured fibroblasts)
- Mutation analysis

Management and outcome

Recombinant enzyme therapy is the main treatment for types 1 and 3 disease,[100] allowing many individuals to live near-normal lives.

No satisfactory treatment is available for type 2 disease. Enzyme replacement therapy (ERT) results in rapid improvement of liver, splenic, and bone-marrow pathology, with corresponding clinical improvement, but skeletal disease is slow to respond and may be resistant to ERT. Advanced liver, splenic, and bone-marrow disease is not reversible by ERT. For children with type III disease, a higher dosage of 120 mg/kg every 2 weeks is recommended; bone-marrow transplantation should be considered if there is neurological deterioration.[101]

Substrate deprivation therapy is a recent development in the treatment of storage disorders. In lysosomal disorders, there is an imbalance between the rate of production of a particular substrate and its catabolism, leading to accumulation within the lysosome. Substrate deprivation therapy restores this balance by reducing the rate of synthesis of the substrate. Miglustat (*N*-butyldeoxynojirimycin) inhibits glucosyltransferase and impairs the synthesis of glycosphingolipids, which accumulate in a number of storage disorders. This product has been used in the treatment of nonneuronopathic Gaucher disease with favorable results and few side effects.[99,102,103]

Supportive and symptomatic treatment such as pain relief, bisphosphonates, calcium, vitamin D, steroids, bone-marrow transplantation, splenectomy, and liver transplantation are important in managing patients with Gaucher disease. Splenectomy is indicated only if severe hypersplenism is resistant to ERT or for splenic rupture, as acceleration of neurological, hepatic, and pulmonary disease has been reported following splenectomy.

Niemann–Pick disease (NPD)

Niemann–Pick disease is a group of storage disorders that are associated with a particular storage cell with a morphological appearance resembling "foamy" histiocytes, as a result of sphingomyelin storage. Currently, three forms of Niemann–Pick disease are recognized—types A, B, and C.

Types A and B

Types A and B disease are autosomal-recessive disorders caused by deficiency of the lysosomal enzyme sphingomyelinase. Niemann–Pick disease type A (NPA) is the infantile neurodegenerative phenotype, whereas type B (NPB) is defined by the absence of neurological involvement, with relatively late-onset hepatosplenomegaly and survival into adulthood. The sphingomyelinase gene has been localized to chromosome 11p15.4, and about 20 mutations are known. With Niemann–Pick A disease, three mutations (R496L, L302P and fsP330) account for > 95% of mutant alleles in the Ashkenazi Jewish population;[104] ΔR608 appears to be a relatively common type B mutation.[105] Several other "private" mutations have been identified in Jewish and non-Jewish families with Niemann–Pick disease types A and B.[106]

The spleen, lymph nodes, liver, bone marrow, kidneys, and lungs are the main sites of storage in both types A and B, while type A patients also accumulate sphingomyelin in the brain.

Presentation

Type A. The clinical presentation of type A is uniform and includes the following findings:

- A protuberant abdomen with massive liver and spleen enlargement becomes apparent in the first few months of life (usually by 3–4 months).
- Lymphadenopathy.
- Prolonged neonatal jaundice due to giant-cell transformation in some cases.
- Early neurological features include feeding difficulties, hypotonia and muscular weakness.
- Recurrent vomiting and constipation.

- Repeated chest infections and aspiration pneumonia; a chest radiograph often reveals alveolar infiltration with a diffuse reticular or finely nodular pattern of the lung fields.[107]
- A cherry-red macular spot is seen on ophthalmological examination in about 50% of patients.
- Psychomotor retardation becomes evident after 6 months, with progressive loss of developmental milestones; eventually, all motor and intellectual abilities are lost.
- Failure to thrive, spasticity, and rigidity are prominent features in the later stages.
- Cirrhosis and multiple hepatocellular adenomas have been described.[108]
- Death occurs by 2–3 years of age, usually from respiratory complications.

Type B. The clinical presentation of type B is more variable. Some individuals may not be diagnosed until adulthood, as there may be minimal clinical manifestations.[109,110] The features include the following findings:
- Hepatosplenomegaly, which may become less apparent as the child grows older. Progressive liver disease with biliary cirrhosis, portal hypertension, and ascites[111] has been reported. Hypersplenism may lead to pancytopenia or splenic rupture.[110]
- Pulmonary involvement, in the form of diffuse reticular or finely nodular infiltration on chest radiography. Lung disease may be progressive and lead to chronic hypoxia, dyspnea, recurrent bronchopneumonia, and in extreme cases, cor pulmonale.[112]
- The long-term natural history is characterized by hepatosplenomegaly with progressive hypersplenism, a worsening atherogenic profile, gradual deterioration in pulmonary function, and stable liver dysfunction.[113]
- Neurodevelopmental complications are rare, but neurological involvement such as cherry-red maculae, ataxia, parkinsonism, and mental retardation have been recorded; these patients are thought to have an intermediate phenotype between types A and B.[114–116]

Diagnosis
The diagnosis may be *suspected* when the characteristic Niemann–Pick "foam" cells are found on bone-marrow aspirate or on a liver biopsy. Niemann–Pick cells are not diagnostic of sphingomyelinase deficiency, as these cells may also be seen in other storage disorders, including Niemann–Pick C disease, cholesterol ester storage disease, Wolman disease, and G_{M1} gangliosidosis.

Specific diagnostic tests are:
- Sphingomyelinase (leukocytes, lymphocytes, or skin fibroblasts)
- Mutation analysis

Antenatal diagnosis is possible by assaying sphingomyelinase activity in chorionic villi or cultured amniocytes.[117,118] Theoretically, prenatal diagnosis should also be possible using mutation analysis.

Management and outcome
Currently, no specific treatment is available for Niemann–Pick disease A and B, and management is entirely supportive. Liver transplantation in an infant with NPA and amniotic cell transplantation in NPB patients have been attempted, with little success. One adult with NPB disease has had a liver transplant, with a subsequent reduction in hepatic cholesterol and sphingomyelin content, but long-term follow-up data are not available. Early bone-marrow transplantation failed to prevent progressive neurodegeneration in one infant; however, bone-marrow transplant was successful in reducing the size of the liver and spleen as well as improving the radiographic appearance of the lungs in one child with severe type B disease. Enzyme replacement therapy is potentially useful in type B disease, and clinical trials are planned; if these are successful, enzyme replacement therapy may become the treatment of choice for NPB disease in the near future. Developments with gene therapy are ongoing.

Type C
Niemann–Pick disease type C originally referred to a group of patients who had the classical histopathological findings of "foamy" histiocytes and increased tissue sphingomyelin, along with a slowly progressive neurological illness.[119] It is now known that NPC disease is clinically, biochemically, and genetically distinct form NPA and NPB; it is caused by a defect of intracellular lipid trafficking.

The estimated incidence of NPC is approximately one in 150 000, making it more common than NPA and NPB combined.[120] It is inherited in an autosomal-recessive manner. The defective gene (*NPC1*) has been localized to chromosome 18q11-12 in > 95% of patients. It codes for an endosomal membrane protein that plays an important role in intracellular cholesterol and glycosphingolipid trafficking,[121] resulting in impaired processing and accumulation. Over 100 mutations have been described, and three mutations (I1061T, P1007A, and G992W/G992R) are sufficiently common to justify diagnostic testing, especially in late-onset variants.[122] Genotype–phenotype correlation may be possible on the basis of the nature and location of the mutation within the NPC1 protein.[122] Less than 5% of patients with NPC have a defect in another gene, *NPC2*, which has been localized to chromosome 14q24.[123] The product of *NPC2* is a small (132 amino acid), soluble, ubiquitously expressed lysosomal protein that has a high affinity for unesterified cholesterol binding.[124,125] In vitro studies suggest that NPC1 and NPC2 act in concert to facilitate the intracellular transport of lysosomal lipids to other cellular sites. Broad genotype–phenotype correlations are possible, especially with *NPC2* mutations.[126]

Presentation
The manifestations of NPC disease are extremely heterogeneous, and presentation can be at any time from intrauterine

life to adulthood.[127] The most common ("classic") phenotype presents in childhood with:

- Neonatal cholestasis, which is self-limiting (Chapter 4).[128]
- Hepatosplenomegaly is prominent in childhood, but becomes less apparent with advancing age, although portal hypertension has been reported.[129]
- Clumsiness and ataxia.
- Early childhood development is usually normal, but behavioral problems may be noted as early as the preschool period.
- Supranuclear vertical gaze palsy, which is the neurologic hallmark of this disorder and is found in virtually all cases by adolescence; it may manifest in early childhood as eye blinking and head thrusting on attempted vertical gaze (Figure 13.5).

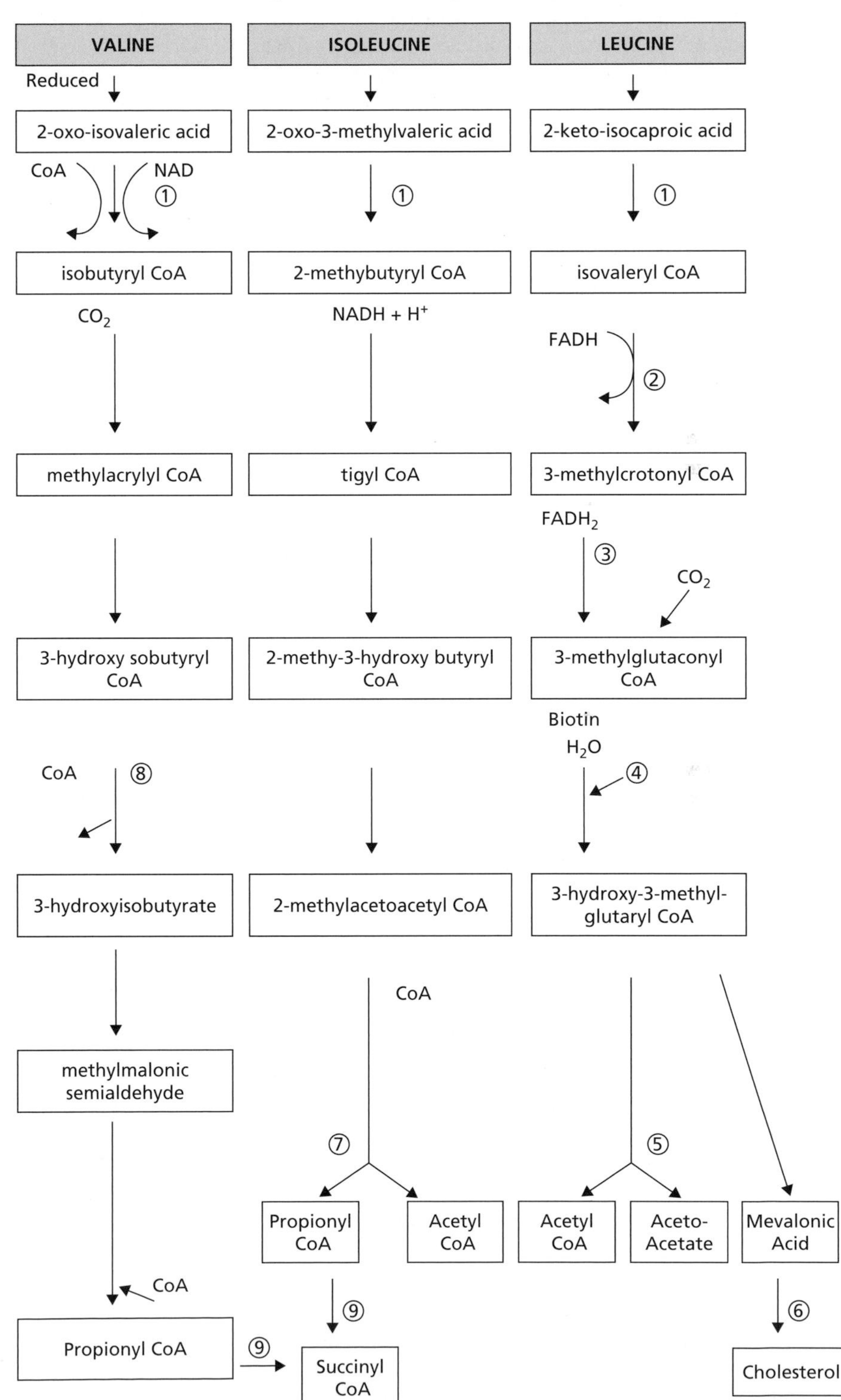

Figure 13.5 Disorders of branched amino acid metabolism. 1, Maple syrup urine disease; 2, isovaleric acidemia; 3, methylcrotonylglycinuria; 4, methylglutaconic aciduria; 5, 3-hydroxy 3-methylglutaric aciduria; 6, mevalonic aciduria; 7, beta-ketothidase deficiency; 8, 3-hydroxyisobutyric aciduria; 9, propionic and methylmalonic acidemia.

• Gelastic cataplexy (atonic seizures induced by emotional change).

A recently published natural-history study[119] divided the cohort into three groups based on the age of presentation. Approximately equal numbers of patients presented in each age group:

• *Neonatal-onset NPC.* Neonatal jaundice without other signs of liver disease may herald a more aggressive clinical course, with developmental delay, spasticity, and progressive liver disease appearing in infancy. These infants do not survive beyond 5 years, and vertical supranuclear gaze palsy is rarely seen. In patients who survive the neonatal liver disease, characteristic progressive neurological signs, including vertical supranuclear gaze palsy, ataxia, dementia, and spasticity appear over a variable time course over years to decades, similar to the childhood-onset form.

• *Childhood/juvenile onset NPC.* The onset is typically with mild learning difficulties in early childhood (4–9 years), followed by a slowly progressive onset of supranuclear gaze palsy, ataxia, and spasticity. Gelastic seizures, cataplexy, and other seizure types commonly occur. Dementia usually appears in the teenage years. Death, commonly from respiratory complications, may occur from the teenage years to adulthood.

• *Adolescent/adult onset NPC.* This presents with signs and symptoms similar to those of childhood-onset NPC, but in later life and with a more slowly progressive course.

A nonneuronopathic form of NPC has also been described in adults with isolated organomegaly.[130]

In addition, very severe variants of NPC may present with hydrops fetalis and liver and respiratory failure, leading to death in early infancy. Severe pulmonary involvement leading to early death from respiratory failure may be associated with mutations in the *NPC2* gene.

Diagnosis

The diagnosis is suggested by the finding of liver dysfunction in the neonatal period, associated with foam cells and sea-blue histiocytes in liver or bone-marrow histology (Figure 13.6).

Diagnostic tests are:

• Plasma chitotriosidase levels may be modestly elevated (20–30-fold) and can be a helpful clue to the diagnosis in a patient with a suggestive clinical picture.

• Accumulation of intracytoplasmic unesterified cholesterol in skin fibroblasts (by filipin staining).

• Defective cholesterol esterification (skin fibroblasts).

• Mutation analysis of the *NPC1* and *NPC2* genes.

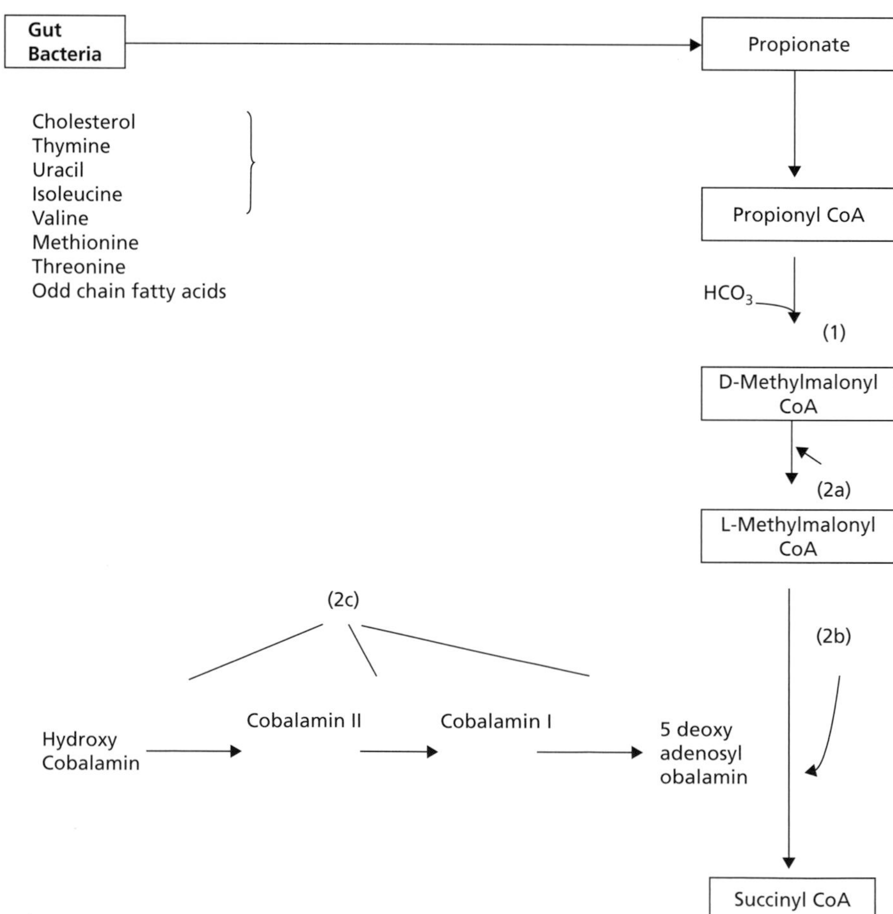

Figure 13.6 Disorders of propionate metabolism. 1, Propionic acidemia; 2a, 2b, methylmalonic acidemia due to mutase deficiency; 2c, methylmalonic acidemia due to defects in cobalamin metabolism.

Antenatal diagnosis is possible by filipin staining, cholesterol esterification studies, and/or mutation analysis of cultured chorionic villous cells or cultured amniocytes.

Management and outcome

Currently, there is no satisfactory treatment for NPC disease. Supportive and symptomatic management includes nutritional support for early liver disease, antiepileptic therapy and anticholinergics for dystonia and tremor. Multidisciplinary support is essential in the later stages, when there is significant neurological and psychomotor disability.

A number of different therapeutic approaches have failed to halt neurological progression. Liver transplantation in a 7-year-old girl with NPC disease and hepatocellular carcinoma[131] led to initial stabilization, but abnormal storage recurred in the transplanted liver and neurological deterioration continued. Similarly, bone-marrow transplantation in a 2-year-old resulted in regression of hepatosplenomegaly and decreased infiltration of foamy macrophages in the bone marrow and lung, but failed to prevent neurological deterioration.[132] Combinations of cholesterol-lowering agents have reduced hepatic cholesterol stores, but have not altered the long-term outcome.[120] As glycosphingolipid accumulation in the brain is thought to be the basis of the neuropathology of NPC disease, it is possible that inhibition of glycosphingolipid synthesis may be useful. OGT-918 (*N*-butyldeoxynojirimycin, miglustat) inhibits glucosyltransferase, impairs the synthesis of glycosphingolipids, and crosses the blood–brain barrier. It has been used in the treatment of nonneuronopathic Gaucher disease with favorable results and few side effects.[102] In animal models of NPC, *N*-butyldeoxynojirimycin has been shown to delay the onset of neurological symptoms, reduce glycosphingolipid accumulation, and increase the average lifespan.[133] An interim report from a recent randomized therapeutic trial of miglustat in 29 juvenile and adult NPC patients indicated improvement in several neurological parameters—including horizontal saccadic eye movements, swallowing capacity, and auditory acuity—in comparison with standard care in an untreated control population.[134] Additional benefits in terms of improvements in cognitive function and quality-of-life measures were also observed. Final results from this trial are awaited. Although rare, NPC disease due to *NPC2* mutations may be treatable with bone-marrow transplantation, as the NPC2 protein is a soluble molecule that is secreted by cells and is amenable to uptake into lysosomes via specific pathways.[126]

Wolman disease and cholesteryl ester storage disease

These two rare disorders are caused by a recessively inherited deficiency of lysosomal acid lipase resulting in accumulation of cholesterol esters and triglycerides in most body tissues. The disorders are allelic conditions that represent extreme variants of the same enzyme deficiency, with some residual enzyme activity in cholesteryl ester storage disease (CESD). A number of secondary changes occur, including increased cholesterol synthesis, up-regulation of low-density lipoprotein-receptor gene expression, and increased lipoprotein production. These changes are more pronounced in Wolman disease, which is associated with more severe acid lipase deficiency than in CESD.

Wolman disease and CESD are recessively inherited. The gene has been localized to chromosome 10q22.2-22.3, and over 20 mutations have been described.[135] There is some genotype–phenotype correlation for CESD, with a common splice junction mutation in exon 8 (called $\Delta 254\text{-}277_1$).[136,137] No common mutation has been described in Wolman disease.[138]

Presentation

Wolman disease. Patients usually present in the first few weeks of life with vomiting and diarrhea, malabsorption, failure to thrive, and hepatosplenomegaly.[138] Jaundice, low-grade pyrexia, anemia, abdominal distension, and leukopenia may be present initially. The most striking feature is adrenal calcification, which is demonstrable radiographically in most patients; other characteristic features are vacuolated lymphocytes in peripheral blood films and foam cells in bone-marrow aspirates. Neurological signs and symptoms are not prominent, although lipid storage in neurons, microglia and astrocytes, as well as delayed myelination may be found histologically. A rapid downhill course follows the initial presentation, and most patients die by 3–6 months of age.

CESD. The clinical manifestations are variable and less severe. The usual presenting feature is hepatomegaly in adult life, although liver enlargement is frequently detectable from early childhood.[138] Liver dysfunction, splenomegaly, hyperlipidemia, and xanthelasma are often present. Malabsorption and adrenal calcification are rare.[139] Hepatomegaly increases over time with fibrosis, and liver failure has been described. Although premature atherosclerosis and atheromas have been detected in autopsied patients, clinically significant coronary or systemic vascular atherosclerosis is rare.

Diagnosis

Suggestive abnormalities include:
- Adrenal calcification on abdominal radiography or ultrasound (decreased adrenal responsiveness may be found on provocative tests)
- Vacuolated lymphocytes on peripheral blood film
- Sea-blue histiocytes in bone-marrow aspirate
- Liver dysfunction
- Hypercholesterolemia and hypertriglyceridemia

Specific diagnosis:
- Acid lipase (leukocytes or cultured fibroblasts) and/or DNA sequencing

Liver histology in both conditions usually reveals enlarged and vacuolated hepatocytes and Kupffer cells, as well as large numbers of foamy histiocytes.[138] Periportal fibrosis may be prominent and cirrhosis may also be evident. Foam cells may also be seen in bone-marrow aspirates, spleen, and lymph nodes. In Wolman disease, small-intestinal biopsy usually reveals extensive infiltration of the lamina propria with foamy histiocytes.

Antenatal diagnosis is possible by direct enzyme assay in chorionic villus cells, or by mutation analysis.

Management and outcome

Treatment of Wolman disease with intravenous alimentation, plasma infusion, corticosteroids, and dietary supplements has been of limited benefit.[140] Bone-marrow transplantation has led to significant clinical and biochemical improvement for up to 4 years in some patients.[141,142] CESD responds to 3-hydroxy-3-methylglutaryl coenzyme A (HMG-CoA) reductase inhibitors, cholestyramine, a low-cholesterol diet, and fat-soluble vitamin supplements, with significant improvement in plasma lipoprotein abnormalities and possible improvement in organomegaly and adrenal dysfunction.[143,144] Successful liver transplantation for chronic liver failure has been reported.[143,145–147] Promising results have been reported with enzyme replacement therapy in a mouse model.[148]

Congenital disorders of glycosylation (carbohydrate-deficient glycoprotein syndrome)

Carbohydrate-deficient glycoprotein (CDG) syndrome is a group of metabolic disorders that arise from defective glycosylation of proteins. Almost all plasma proteins, many proteins of cellular membranes and connective tissues, blood group substances, immunoglobulins, and certain hormones are glycoproteins. The synthesis and function of glycoproteins are complex. The pathway involves at least 40 steps and the details are beyond the scope of this chapter, but excellent reviews of this process are available.[149,150] They are essential for many structural, transport, immunological, hormonal, cell–cell signaling, and enzymatic functions.[151,152] There are numerous defects in this pathway with severe multisystem clinical manifestations. Two main groups of CDG are recognized: disorders of *N*-glycosylation and disorders of *O*-glycosylation. The currently known disorders of *O*-glycosylation are mainly associated with musculoskeletal manifestations and will not be discussed further. The *N*-glycosylation disorders are classified into two broad biochemical categories: CDG I (types a–l, each associated with a distinct enzyme deficiency) is caused by defects of synthesis and transfer of the carbohydrate chain to the nascent protein molecule, whereas CDG II (types a–f) results from defective processing of the carbohydrate chains. The gene for phosphomannomutase (CDG Ia) has been localized and many mutations have been reported. The most frequent Caucasian mutation, R141H, is believed to be fatal in the homozygous state. Other mutations have been reported, such as F119L from Scandinavia, D188G from Belgium and the Netherlands, and F144L, R238P, and Y229S from Japan.[152] The genes for the other CDG subtypes are known.[135]

Presentation

The most common disorder is CDG Ia, which is caused by phosphomannomutase deficiency. Although neurological symptoms dominate the clinical picture in most cases, liver and gastrointestinal function pathology is common and is the predominant feature in CDG Ib. CDG syndrome should be considered in any patient with unexplained liver dysfunction, especially if there is multisystem disease.

CDG Ia. There are two groups:[153]

- *Neurological involvement.* The main neurological manifestations in both groups are neonatal hypotonia, ataxia, squint, cerebellar hypoplasia, and psychomotor retardation. Younger patients may have facial dysmorphism (almond-shaped, upslanting palpebral fissures, high forehead, and prominent maxilla), inverted nipples, and abnormal gluteal, perineal, or suprapubic pads of fat. Older children often have stroke-like episodes, retinitis pigmentosa, areflexia, spinal deformities, fixed flexion deformities, and in females, absent puberty.[153,154] They do not have progressive neurodegenerative disease, although the neurological signs become more prominent as children grow older.[153]
- *Multisystem disease.* The main clinical features include: failure to thrive, diarrhea, pericardial effusions, liver disease, and proximal tubulopathy. Hepatic involvement includes hepatomegaly, abnormal transaminases, hypoalbuminemia, coagulopathy, steatosis, fibrosis, and cirrhosis. Mortality is high in this group, and many patients do not survive beyond 2 years.

CDG Ib is caused by phosphomannose isomerase deficiency, and is phenotypically different from CDG Ia. Ten patients have been reported without neurological involvement, but with protein-losing enteropathy and congenital hepatic fibrosis. Infants present with diarrhea, vomiting, failure to thrive, hepatomegaly, edema due to severe hypoalbuminemia, coagulopathy, a thrombotic tendency, and hyperinsulinemic hypoglycemia.[152,155] Inverted nipples and abnormal fat pads have been reported, but not facial dysmorphism.[156]

CDG Ic–l and CDG IIa–f are rare. These patients have dysmorphism, epilepsy, psychomotor retardation, and peripheral neuropathy.[149] Some have hepatomegaly and liver dysfunction. Not all patients with CDG match known subtypes (CDG X). The clinical features of these patients include foetal hydrops, cataracts, psychomotor retardation, hypotonia, seizures, thrombocytopenia, diarrhea, vomiting, ascites, and renal tubulopathy.[157] A combined *N*- and *O*-glycosylation defect has recently been reported in a pair of siblings with dysmorphism, encephalopathy, and neonatal cholestatic liver disease.[158]

Diagnosis

Supportive findings are:

- Increased transaminases
- Hypoalbuminemia
- Coagulopathy

Histological examination of the liver usually reveals fibrosis, and jejunal biopsies may show villous atrophy and lymphangiectasis.

Separation of plasma transferrin isoforms usually reveals characteristic patterns, although not all cases are abnormal. Biochemical studies of other glycoproteins such as apolipoprotein C-III, α_1-antitrypsin, and α_1-antichymotrypsin may be helpful.[159,160] Confirmation of the diagnosis requires specific enzyme analysis in lymphoblasts or fibroblasts and mutation analysis.

Antenatal diagnosis is possible by a combination of enzyme analysis and mutation analysis in CDG Ia. Prenatal diagnosis has not been reported for the other CDG subtypes.

Management

Oral mannose supplementation is useful in treating CDG Ib, with improvement in gastrointestinal symptoms, hematological abnormalities, and growth.[156,161] It is unclear whether it will prevent progressive liver disease in CDG Ib. There is no therapy available for other forms of CDG, and treatment is supportive.

Mitochondrial respiratory-chain disorders

Disordered mitochondrial function leads to a wide variety of pathological and clinical manifestations. Hepatic and gastrointestinal diseases are often involved, and these disorders must be included in the differential diagnosis of liver disease in infancy and childhood. The clinical spectrum is very wide, and presentation may range from prenatal manifestation as hydrops fetalis, acute neonatal liver failure (Chapter 5) to mild myopathy in adulthood.

Inheritance is maternal or autosomal, depending on whether the defects are due to mitochondrial or nuclear DNA.

Presentation

Multisystem involvement is characteristic of respiratory-chain disorders, and the liver and gastrointestinal tract are important target organs. Liver disease in the neonatal period (see Chapters 4 and 5) or early childhood is a common presentation. Extrahepatic features are common and may include lethargy, hypotonia, vomiting, poor neonatal reflexes, seizures, recurrent apnea, and cardiomyopathy.[162–164] Intrauterine growth retardation, fetal hydrops, neonatal ascites, renal tubular disease, elevated α-fetoprotein, and hypoalbuminemia have also been described. Usually, progressive hepatic, neurological, and/or other systemic deterioration leads to death in infancy or early childhood. Occasionally, liver disease may be static or even resolve with time.[165] A syndrome of severe anorexia, diarrhea, vomiting, villous atrophy, and liver dysfunction in infancy associated with mtDNA rearrangements has been reported.[166] The diarrhea may improve or resolve by 5 years of age, but progressive neurological symptoms lead to rapid deterioration and death.

Pearson syndrome is a multisystem disorder of infancy that is characterized by exocrine pancreatic insufficiency and sideroblastic anemia.[165] Some patients develop progressive liver disease or renal Fanconi syndrome; those who survive may improve spontaneously but develop progressive external ophthalmoplegia (resembling Kearns–Sayre syndrome) in later life. Pearson syndrome is usually associated with mtDNA rearrangements.[167] mtDNA depletion syndrome—a relatively recently recognized condition that presents as hepatic failure, hypotonia, renal dysfunction, and lactic acidosis in the first few weeks of life—is associated with multiple respiratory-chain enzyme defects and is caused by a variety of nuclear DNA defects;[168] for a detailed discussion, see Chapter 5.

Diagnosis

Investigations for respiratory-chain disease include:

- Plasma lactate. Persistently elevated blood lactate concentrations are an important clue to respiratory-chain disease, but are not specific and may be found in any sick neonate or infant, especially with significant liver disease. Glucose loading tests and lactate–pyruvate ratios seldom add to the information provided by repeated lactate measurements.
- Increased cerebrospinal fluid lactate concentrations are more specific and must be compared to plasma lactate.
- Muscle biopsy for:
  - —Histology for evidence of steatosis, ragged red fibers (see Chapter 5).
  - —Histochemistry staining for cytochrome oxidase and succinate dehydrogenase.
  - —Electron microscopy for the number and morphology of mitochondria.
  - —Respiratory-chain enzyme analysis (complexes I–IV) usually confirms the diagnosis. Defects are often expressed in muscle, even in the absence of myopathy. Expression of results as ratios of activity improves discrimination.[169]
- Liver histology characteristically reveals a combination of steatosis, fibrosis, cholestasis, and necrosis,[165] and on electron microscopy there may be increased numbers of structurally abnormal mitochondria (see Chapter 5). Respiratory-chain enzyme analysis is possible on liver biopsy specimens, but the results may be difficult to interpret in the presence of liver failure.

- Mutation analysis for known mitochondrial and nuclear DNA defects.[168]
- Urine organic acid analysis may reveal abnormal but nonspecific findings.
- Evidence of multisystem involvement (echocardiography, neuroimaging, and neurophysiology).

When causative nuclear DNA mutations that underlie mitochondrial disease are known, antenatal diagnosis is readily available. For disorders caused by mitochondrial DNA mutations, if the respiratory-chain defect is expressed in skin fibroblasts from the index case, reliable biochemical diagnosis may be possible on chorionic villus cells.[170]

Management

Treatment includes cofactor therapy with riboflavin, artificial electron acceptors such as menadione and vitamin C, and a variety of free-radical scavengers such as coenzyme Q_{10} (ubiquinone), vitamin E, idebenone, carnitine, and methylene blue.[171] Experience is anecdotal and the results variable. A few of these medications have been evaluated in randomized controlled trials, which have not indicated reproducible clinical or biochemical improvement.[172]

Consideration of liver transplantation is a difficult management issue in an infant with liver failure due to suspected mitochondrial liver disease. In general, multisystem respiratory-chain disease is a contraindication to liver transplantation. In patients in whom the clinical disease appears to be confined to the liver, liver transplantation may be a therapeutic option. A few patients with isolated mitochondrial liver disease have undergone successful liver transplantation, with excellent long-term outcomes and no evidence of extrahepatic involvement.[173,174] However, other patients have developed progressive neurological disease after transplantation, even though they had no neurological involvement prior to transplantation.[175,176] The use of liver transplantation in treating progressive mitochondrial liver disease remains controversial (see also Chapter 5). In an acute situation, hepatocyte infusion may be considered in order to help control acute liver failure and to allow further evaluation of suitability for liver transplantation.[29]

Peroxisomal disorders

Peroxisomes are small, membrane-bound intracellular organelles that contain 40 different anabolic and catabolic enzymes. Their functions include:

- β-oxidation of very-long-chain fatty acids (VLCFAs)
- β-oxidation of phytanic acid, a dietary branched-chain fatty acid
- β-oxidation of dihydroxycholestanoic and trihydroxycholestanoic acids to chenodeoxycholic acid and cholic acid, which are bile acid precursors
- Conjugation of chenodeoxycholic acid and cholic acid with taurine and glycine to form the bile acids
- The initial reactions of isoprenoid (cholesterol, dolichol, and ubiquinone) biosynthesis, plasmalogen synthesis
- Lysine metabolism
- Glyoxylate metabolism
- Hydrogen peroxide metabolism
- Eicosanoid (prostaglandins, leukotrienes, thromboxane, prostacyclin) degradation

Peroxisomal disorders are classified into two main groups:

- Multiple-enzyme deficiencies (such as the "Zellweger spectrum" disorders and rhizomelic chondrodysplasia punctata), which arise from defective peroxisome synthesis, assembly and enzyme import.
- Genetic deficiency of a single peroxisomal enzyme (such as adrenoleukodystrophy, classical Refsum disease, and hyperoxaluria type I). Over 20 different disorders have been described. The overall prevalence has been estimated to be one in 25 000.[177]

The disorders of peroxisome biogenesis are genetically heterogeneous and belong to 11 different complementation groups, without any correlation between the complementation group and phenotype.[178] Mutations in the genes responsible for peroxisomal assembly (*PEX* genes) are known to be associated with Zellweger syndrome, neonatal adrenoleukodystrophy, infantile Refsum disease, and rhizomelic chondrodysplasia punctata.[179,180]

Presentation

Disorders with multiple-enzyme deficiencies. Patients who have a disorder of peroxisomal biogenesis lack normal peroxisomes. Four conditions are recognized: Zellweger syndrome (ZS; see also Chapter 4), neonatal adrenoleukodystrophy (NALD), infantile Refsum disease (IRD), and rhizomelic chondrodysplasia punctata (RCDP). They are all associated with severely deranged peroxisomal assembly, loss of multiple-enzyme activities, and multisystem involvement. Peroxisomes are absent or greatly reduced in number in skin fibroblasts and liver biopsy specimens. Zellweger syndrome is the most severe, infantile Refsum disease less so, and NALD is between the two.[181]

Infants with ZS present in the neonatal period with characteristic dysmorphic features (prominent forehead, large anterior fontanelle, broad nasal bridge, epicanthal folds, high arched palate, micrognathia, redundant neck skin folds, clinodactyly, and talipes equinovarus). Neurological abnormalities are prominent, including severe hypotonia, areflexia, poor suck reflex, and seizures. Neuronal migration defects may be observed on neuroimaging. Other features such as corneal clouding, cataracts, pigmentary retinopathy, polycystic kidneys, cryptorchidism, dislocated hips, and stippled epiphyses on radiographs (chondrodysplasia punctata) may be present. Liver disease is common and includes hepatomegaly, conjugated hyperbilirubinemia, progression to cirrhosis, and liver failure in the first few months of life, but the hepatic involvement is overshadowed by the neurological symptoms. Occasionally, the presentation resembles malabsorption, with hepatomegaly, prolonged jaundice, liver failure, anorexia, vomiting, and diarrhea leading to failure to thrive.[182] Failure of psychomotor development is evident in early infancy, and survival beyond 1 year is rare. Patients with NALD and IRD have the same features as in ZS, but a milder phenotype. Infants have hepatomegaly and neonatal cholestasis; progressive liver disease is only significant in children who survive the first decade.[181]

There is no hepatic involvement in "classic" rhizomelic chondrodysplasia punctata (RCDP), which presents with dysmorphism and psychomotor retardation.

Disorders due to single peroxisomal enzyme deficiencies. There are many isolated peroxisomal enzyme deficiencies (Table 13.4); hepatic involvement may be present. Intact peroxisomes are found in liver biopsy and skin fibroblast specimens, and the biochemical and clinical abnormalities relate to the individual pathway.

Diagnosis

For peroxisome biogenesis (with multiple-enzyme defects), initial investigations on plasma include:

- Very-long-chain fatty acids (VLCFAs)
- Dihydroxyacetone phosphate acyltransferase (DHPAT; blood)
- Phytanate/pristanate (plasma)
- Plasmalogens (plasma)

Morphological studies of liver/skin for fibroblasts may show a complete absence or a reduced or abnormal structure of peroxisomes. The diagnosis is confirmed by specific enzyme analysis in skin fibroblasts.

Antenatal diagnosis is possible by measurement of the VLCFA concentration and/or plasmalogen synthesis in cultured chorionic villus samples or amniocytes.

Management

There is no treatment for multiple-enzyme dysfunction, but supportive care with anticonvulsants, dietary supplements for the liver disease, and muscle relaxants is essential. Bile acid supplements have reduced cholestasis in a child with

Table 13.4 Disorders due to single peroxisomal enzyme deficiencies associated with liver disease.

Disorder/enzyme defect	Genetics	Clinical features	Biochemical features	Hepatic involvement	Outcome
Palmitoyl acyl-CoA oxidase deficiency	AR	Severe hypotonia, psychomotor retardation, seizures in infancy; no dysmorphism	Elevated plasma VLCFA	Hepatomegaly, fibrosis known to occur	Death by 2–4 y
Bifunctional protein deficiency (enoyl-CoA hydratase and hydroxyacyl-CoA dehydrogenase deficiency)	AR	Dysmorphism similar to Zellweger syndrome, severe hypotonia, intractable seizures, epiphyseal stippling	Elevated plasma VLCFA, DHCA, THCA, pristanic acid	Hepatomegaly, hepatic dysfunction, coagulopathy	Death by 6 months–2 years
Di- and trihydroxycholestanoic acidemia (unknown enzyme defects)	Unknown	Probably a group of heterogeneous disorders; mild dysmorphism, ataxia, psychomotor retardation reported	Elevated THCA, DHCA; normal VLCFA	Progressive liver dysfunction and failure known	Unknown
Mevalonic aciduria (mevalonate kinase deficiency)	AR	Severe deficiency: developmental delay, dysmorphism, cataracts, hepatosplenomegaly, lymphadeno-pathy Mild deficiency: hyperimmuno-globulinemia D and periodic fever syndrome (HIDS)	Mevalonic aciduria on urine organic acid analysis	Liver dysfunction common	Death in infancy or early childhood in severe deficiency

AR, autosomal-recessive; DHCA, dihydroxycholestanoic acid; HIDS, hyperimmunoglobulin D syndrome; THCA, α-trihydroxy-5-β-cholestannic acid; VLCFA, very-long-chain fatty acid.

ZS,[183] while docosahexanoic acid (DHA) has led to some clinical improvement in the "Zellweger spectrum."[181] Therapeutic options are available for some of the single-enzyme disorders.

Alper's–Huttenlocher syndrome (progressive infantile poliodystrophy, progressive neuronal degeneration of childhood)

Alper's–Huttenlocher or Alper's syndrome is a rapidly progressive early-childhood encephalopathy with intractable seizures and neuronal degeneration. The etiology of this disorder is unknown, and it may represent a heterogeneous group of disorders with common clinicopathological features.[157] In most cases, liver dysfunction is a prominent late feature. Historically, there has been much confusion about the nosology, pathogenesis, and diagnosis of the condition. Respiratory-chain abnormalities have been identified in a number of individuals who fulfill the diagnostic criteria,[184] including complex I defects,[185,186] partial complex IV deficiency,[157] mitochondrial DNA depletion,[187] decreased cytochrome aa_3,[188] decreased NADH utilization,[189] and citric acid cycle dysfunction.[186] More recently, a majority of patients with Alpers syndrome have been shown to have mitochondrial DNA depletion, decreased activity of mtDNA-encoded respiratory-chain complexes, and associated mutations in the mtDNA polymerase gamma (*POLG1*) gene, which plays an important role in mtDNA replication.[190,191] Two mutations, A467T and W748S, are particularly common, and screening for these has been proposed as the most rapid and sensitive test for Alpers syndrome.[192]

Alpers syndrome due to *POLG1* mutations has autosomal-recessive inheritance. Antenatal diagnosis has not been reported, but should be feasible if the causative mutations in the index case are known.

Presentation

Typically, the neonatal period is normal. Presentation is between 2 months and 2 years with physical and developmental delay, followed by the sudden onset of intractable epilepsy by 3 years. Rapid neurological deterioration and blindness usually follow the onset of seizures. Overt hepatic disease presents later, with jaundice, hepatomegaly, coagulopathy, and rapidly progressive liver failure,[193] although biochemical evidence of liver dysfunction may predate the seizures. The hepatic symptoms may be exacerbated by treatment with valproic acid.[194] Most patients do not survive beyond 3 years, but some may follow a protracted course.[184] A few patients may have typical neurological features of Alpers syndrome without liver disease; these infants follow an identical neurological course (see also Chapters 4 and 6).

Diagnosis

- Liver dysfunction may initially be mild, with elevation of transaminases and bilirubin, but later, synthetic function is impaired.
- Plasma carnitine concentrations may be low.
- Urinary organic acids are nonspecific, consistent with liver dysfunction.
- Electroencephalography demonstrates high-amplitude polyspikes.
- Visual evoked responses are reduced or absent.
- Electroretinograms are normal.
- Computed tomography (CT) or magnetic resonance imaging (MRI) scans show progressive cerebral atrophy with low-density areas in the occipital and posterior temporal areas; the white matter is usually spared.
- Liver histology reveals microvesicular fatty change, bile duct proliferation, and focal necrosis, leading to bridging fibrosis and cirrhosis (see Chapter 5). Neuropathology reveals cortical involvement, with neuronal cell loss and gliosis.[195]

There is no definitive metabolic test. Antenatal diagnosis has not been reported.

Management

There is no effective treatment. The condition is fatal, with most children dying before 3 years or within a few months of developing overt liver disease. Liver transplantation is contraindicated, as neurological progression continues after transplantation.[196]

Reye syndrome

Reye syndrome is an acute childhood illness characterized by encephalopathy and fatty degeneration of the liver. The definition of this disorder is nonspecific, and it is now recognized that a number of different conditions, especially some inborn errors of metabolism, can present as Reye syndrome. There has been a substantial decline in the number of cases of "classical" Reye syndrome,[197,198] attributed to public health campaigns warning against the use of salicylates in children with influenza-like illnesses,[198] the declining use of antiemetic medications in childhood illnesses,[199] and an increasing recognition that many patients previously diagnosed as having Reye syndrome have an underlying metabolic disorder.[197]

Presentation and definition

An internationally accepted epidemiological definition of Reye syndrome[197] is a child under 16 years of age with:

- Unexplained noninflammatory encephalopathy *and* one or more of:
- Serum hepatic transaminases elevated three or more times upper limit of normal

—*Or* plasma ammonia levels elevated three or more times upper limit of normal
—*Or* characteristic fatty infiltration of the liver

There are two major groups:

• *"Classic" or "idiopathic" Reye syndrome* typically occurs in children over 5 years of age, usually associated with an influenza or varicella-like prodrome with aspirin use in therapeutic dosage. There is a biphasic presentation—a viral prodrome (upper respiratory tract or gastrointestinal infection), followed several days later by the abrupt onset of encephalopathy heralded by profuse vomiting,[200] personality changes, and altered consciousness. Raised intracranial pressure may result in death or permanent neurological sequelae. The etiology of this form of Reye syndrome remains unclear, but epidemiological studies have suggested an association with aspirin exposure;[201,202] alternatively, the combination of a viral illness and the extrapyramidal reactions induced by antiemetics may result in a clinical syndrome indistinguishable from Reye syndrome.[199]
• *"Atypical" Reye syndrome or Reye-like illnesses* present in a similar manner to "classical" Reye syndrome, but in children less than 5 years of age. "Atypical" Reye syndrome is often associated with inherited metabolic disorders of fatty acid oxidation (such as MCADD), disorders of organic acid and amino acid metabolism, as well as urea cycle defects.[197,203,204] A number of patients previously diagnosed with Reye syndrome have had the diagnosis revised when a metabolic, toxic, or other cause has been identified on further investigation.[203,204] It is likely that the expansion of newborn screening programs for metabolic disorders will result in a decline in the numbers of children presenting with "atypical" Reye syndrome.

There is considerable overlap between these two groups, and all children with any form of Reye syndrome must undergo thorough investigation to rule out potential underlying causes.

Investigation of Reye syndrome and Reye-like illness

Typically, investigations demonstrate:

• Prolonged prothrombin time.
• Hepatic dysfunction with raised aminotransferases.
• Elevated ammonia.
• Hypoglycemia.
• CT scan may demonstrate cerebral edema.
• Electroencephalography demonstrates marked slowing.

Liver histology is not specific; the usual findings are a microvesicular steatosis with glycogen depletion and cytoplasmic swelling. Electron microscopy confirms a loss of glycogen and demonstrates proliferation of smooth endoplasmic reticulum and an increase in peroxisomes. Mitochondria may be pleomorphic. Skeletal muscle demonstrates glycogen deposition and fat deposition.

Etiological factors for treatable metabolic disorders include:

• Urine organic acids
• Urine amino acids
• Plasma amino acids
• Plasma and/or blood spot acylcarnitine profiles
• Screening for common MCADD and long-chain 3-hydroxyacyl-coenzyme A dehydrogenase deficiency (LCHAD) mutations

It is also important to rule out other causes of coma associated with abnormal biochemical liver function tests, including toxins, severe hypoxia, and infections such as hepatitis and septicemia.[1]

Management

The management of "classic" Reye syndrome is directed towards supportive treatment of acute cerebral edema, metabolic abnormalities, coagulopathy, and hepatic encephalopathy (Chapter 7). It is important to treat cerebral edema adequately in intensive-care units with full facilities for monitoring and controlling raised intracranial pressure (Chapter 7), as the prognosis depends on the prevention of irreversible brain damage. If an underlying cause such as a metabolic disorder or infection is identified, appropriate specific therapy is indicated. Liver transplantation is usually not necessary and may be contraindicated if there is severe multisystem involvement.

Disorders of intermediary metabolism

Metabolic defects in intermediary metabolism involve catabolic pathways of amino acids, organic acids, fatty acid oxidation, and the urea cycle. Some of these disorders can present with liver dysfunction, a Reye-like encephalopathy, a mild "biochemical" liver dysfunction or, more rarely, as acute liver failure.

Tyrosinemia type I

Amino acid disorders generally do not present with liver disease, with the exception of tyrosinemia type I (Tyr I), which is described in Chapter 5.

Organic acidemias

Organic acids are carboxylic acids of low molecular weight and are metabolites of amino acids, carbohydrates, and fats. Organic acid disorders are due to defects in the catabolism of the branched-chain amino acids, isoleucine, isoleucine and valine, and metabolism of propionate.[205] The accumulated organic acids exist as carnitine conjugates—e.g., propionyl carnitine and isovaleryl carnitine. Over 50 different disorders have been described, and their combined incidence is in the order of one in 5000–10 000. The commonest disorders are: methylmalonic acidemia (MMA), propionic acidemia (PA; see Chapter 4), and isovaleric acidemia (IVA).

Table 13.5 Organic acid disorders.

Conditions	Presentation/clinical features	Hepatic involvement
Propionic acidemia Methylmalonic acidemia	*Neonatal presentation:* acute encephalopathy, hyperammonemia, acidosis	Hepatomegaly, hyperammonemia, elevated transaminases, fatty infiltration on biopsy; pancreatitis has been described
Isovaleric acidemia	*Acute intermittent late-onset form:* recurrent encephalopathy or Reye-like illness in infancy *Chronic, progressive form:* anorexia, failure to thrive, gastrointestinal symptoms, psychomotor retardation	
Isolated 3-methylcrotonyl-CoA carboxylase deficiency	Reye-like illness in infancy or early childhood; recurrent acidosis, hypoglycemia, coma; chronic presentation with developmental delay has been described	Biochemical and histological features resembling Reye syndrome
3-methylglutaconyl-CoA hydratase deficiency	Variable presentation, including recurrent acidosis, hepatomegaly, Reye-like episodes, speech delay, hypotonia	Liver dysfunction and Reye-like features have been described
3-hydroxy-3-methylglutaryl-CoA lyase deficiency	Neonatal, infantile or childhood presentation with vomiting, lethargy, coma, hyperammonemia and hypoketotic hypoglycemia; Reye-like illness beyond the neonatal period	Biochemical and histological features resembling Reye syndrome
Mevalonate kinase deficiency (mevalonic aciduria)	Variable presentation with dysmorphism, failure to thrive, psychomotor retardation, ataxia, recurrent fever with rash, diarrhea and vomiting; milder variant with periodic fever and hyper-immunoglobulinemia D	Hepatosplenomegaly and cholestatic liver disease have been described
Mitochondrial acetoacetyl-CoA thiolase deficiency (β-ketothiolase deficiency)	Infantile presentation with ketoacidosis during acute infections; hyperglycemia and hyperammonemia may occur; asymptomatic between attacks	Fatty infiltration of the liver has been described
3-hydroxyisobutyric aciduria	Infantile presentation with dysmorphism, brain malformations, ketosis, acidosis, failure to thrive	Not described
Malonic aciduria	Presentation in infancy or early childhood with acidosis, hypoglycemia, developmental delay and cardiomyopathy	Not described

Presentation

All of these disorders have a neonatal presentation in first few days of life (see Chapter 5), but a less acute presentation in infancy or early childhood with developmental delay, failure to thrive, and metabolic acidoses secondary to episodic illness is common. A Reye-like encephalopathy also occurs. In these cases, there may be mild elevation of hepatic transaminases (Table 13.5).

Diagnosis

Characteristic features of these disorders include:

- Metabolic acidosis
- Hypoglycemia
- Hypocalcemia
- Ketonuria
- Neutropenia
- Hyperlacticacidemia
- Hyperuricemic
- Increased plasma and urine glycine

Diagnostic tests:

- Urine organic acids
- Acylcarnitine species (blood)
- Enzymes/substrate incorporation studies (fibroblasts)

DNA analysis is not usually required, as metabolite profiles (organic acids and acylcarnitines) are usually diagnostic.

Management

Whenever possible, specimens—blood (e.g., heparinized plasma) and urine (random)—should be collected when the infant is acutely ill—i.e., before treatment with a low-protein diet is started (Chapter 4). Liver transplantation has been reported in a few cases, but the outcome and long-term benefits are unclear.[29]

Urea cycle disorders

There are six disorders of the urea cycle. Most present with hyperammonemia in the neonatal period. The later-onset forms have variable presentations, which include

Table 13.6 Classification and genetics of porphyrias.

Condition	Deficient enzyme	Genetics	Porphyria types			
			Acute neurovisceral	Cutaneous	Hepatic	Erythropoietic
δ-ALA dehydratase deficiency	ALA dehydratase	AR	+		+	
Acute intermittent porphyria	PBG deaminase (hydoxymethylbilane synthase)	AD	+		+	
Congenital erythropoietic porphyria	Uroporphyrinogen cosynthase	AR		+		+
Porphyria cutanea tarda	Uroporphyrinogen decarboxylase	80% acquired 20% AD		+	+	
Hepatoerythropoietic porphyria	Uroporphyrinogen decarboxylase	*		+	+	+
Hereditary coproporphyria	Coproporphyrinogen oxidase	AD	+	+	+	
Variegate porphyria	Protoporphyrinogen oxidase	AD	+	+	+	
Erythropoietic protoporphyria	Ferrochelatase	Mainly AD		+		+

AD, autosomal-dominant; ALA, aminolevulinic acid; AR, autosomal-recessive; PBG, porphobilinogen.
* Considered to be the homozygous variant of porphyria cutanea tarda.

an encephalopathic (Reye-like) episode, anicteric hepatitis, and/or mild hepatomegaly (see Chapter 5). Liver transplantation or hepatocyte transplantation may be considered as a treatment option in selected cases.[29,31]

Fatty acid oxidation defects (see Chapter 5)

Mitochondrial β-oxidation of fatty acids plays a major role in energy production, especially during periods of fasting. It is a complex process that involves uptake of fatty acids into the cell, activation to acyl-CoA, and then transport into the mitochondria, which requires the carnitine transport cycle. Within the mitochondria, the β-oxidation spiral requires a series of enzymes with carbon chain length specificity.

These disorders can present as a Reye-like illness (e.g., MCADD) or with acute illness usually in early infancy, with hepatomegaly/liver dysfunction.

The porphyrias

The porphyrias are disorders of heme biosynthesis, which result in neurovisceral symptoms and/or cutaneous photosensitivity. They do not usually present as liver disease, but several forms can exhibit liver dysfunction. Most are caused by genetic deficiencies of the enzymes involved in heme biosynthesis, except for porphyria cutanea tarda, which is believed to be an acquired condition. Although porphyrias usually present in adulthood, symptoms can occasionally occur in childhood.

Heme is synthesized in the bone marrow for hemoglobin synthesis and in the liver for cytochrome P-450 enzymes. The liver and bone-marrow pathways are differently regulated, and drugs, hormones, and diet that can influence the pathway in the liver do not affect the bone marrow.

The porphyrias are classified[206] according to the primary tissue affected (hepatic or erythropoietic porphyrias), the specific enzyme deficiency, or the clinical presentation (acute neurovisceral or cutaneous) (Table 13.6).

Presentation

The symptoms may be nonspecific. Liver disease is not usually a presenting feature, although secondary liver disease may occur in some of the defects. Neurovisceral features are common if there is an accumulation of porphyrin precursors, especially δ-aminolevulinic acid.

Acute intermittent porphyria is the commonest of the acute porphyrias,[207,208] with an estimated prevalence of five per 100 000 in northern European populations. Symptoms rarely occur in childhood, and many adults with the genetic mutation remain asymptomatic. Acute attacks are precipitated by certain drugs, steroid hormones, and poor nutrition. Typical manifestations during an acute attack include abdominal pain, nausea, vomiting, limb and chest pain, muscle weakness, peripheral neuropathy, tachycardia, hypertension, tremors, and hypertension. Electrolyte imbalance, seizures, motor neuropathy, and death may occur if the porphyria is not recognized and treated. Attacks may last several days, and complete recovery follows appropriate treatment. There is an increased risk of hepatocellular carcinoma in acute intermittent porphyria, as well as in porphyria cutanea tarda (see below). Similar neurovisceral symptoms occur in other acute porphyrias (Table 13.7).

Table 13.7 Diagnosis, clinical features, and treatment of the porphyrias.

Condition	Diagnostic tests	Clinical features	Treatment
δ-ALA dehydratase deficiency	Increased urine δ-aminolevulinic acid and coproporphyrin, normal urine porphobilinogen; enzyme and DNA studies	Acute neurovisceral symptoms; anemia, failure to thrive; onset may be in childhood	Similar to acute intermittent porphyria (see below)
Acute intermittent porphyria	Increased urinary porphobilinogen, δ-aminolevulinic acid, and anduroporphyrin, normal fecal porphyrins; RBC enzyme assay and DNA studies	Acute neurovisceral symptoms; increased risk of hepatocellular carcinoma	Avoidance of precipitating factors; acute attacks: analgesia, i.v. heme infusion, oral or i.v. carbohydrate loading
Congenital erythropoietic porphyria	Increased urinary, fecal, and plasma porphyrins, especially uroporphyrin I; increased RBC zinc and free protoporphyrin enzyme and DNA studies	Severe cutaneous symptoms; onset in utero (fetal hydrops) or in neonatal period	Skin protection from sunlight; blood transfusion to suppress erythropoiesis; BMT
Porphyria cutanea tarda	Increased urinary, fecal, and plasma porphyrins with characteristic fecal porphyrin present	Cutaneous symptoms; onset in adulthood; risk of hepatocellular carcinoma	Avoidance of precipitating factors; skin protection; repeated phlebotomy; chloroquine
Hepatoerythropoietic porphyria	Increased urine, fecal, and plasma and urine porphyrins; increased RBC zinc and free protoporphyrin; enzyme assay and DNA studies	Cutaneous symptoms; onset variable: neonatal period to adulthood	Skin protection from sunlight
Hereditary coproporphyria and variegate porphyria	Increased urine δ-aminolevulinic acid, porphobilinogen, and coproporphyrin; increased plasma porphyrins with characteristic fluorescence spectra; VP: fecal porphyrin with characteristic pattern HCP: enzyme assay and DNA studies	Cutaneous and/or acute neurovisceral symptoms Onset after puberty	Combination of strategies used in acute intermittent porphyria and skin protection from sunlight
Erythropoietic protoporphyria	Increased plasma porphyrins and free erythrocyte protoporphyrin; increased fecal protoporphyrin	Cutaneous symptoms; onset usually early childhood; liver dysfunction and liver failure may occur	Skin protection from sunlight; oral β-carotene, cholestyramine; transfusion and heme therapy; monitoring of liver function; liver transplantation for liver failure

ALA, aminolevulinic acid; BMT, bone-marrow transplant; HCP, hereditary coproporphyria; RBC, red blood cell.

Porphyria cutanea tarda is the most common cutaneous porphyria[209] and presents with chronic, blistering skin lesions on sun-exposed parts of the skin, such as the hands, neck, face, and back. Hypertrichosis, hyperpigmentation, thickening, scarring, and calcification of affected skin may occur. Precipitating factors include alcohol intake, hepatitis C infection, and estrogen use.

Other forms. Patients with *congenital erythropoietic porphyria* may also have hemolytic anemia and discoloration of the teeth. *Erythropoietic protoporphyria* may be complicated by liver disease, gallstone, and rapidly progressive hepatic failure,[210] which may be related to protoporphyrin accumulation in the liver.

If liver dysfunction is associated with skin abnormalities or acute neurovisceral symptoms, then porphyria should be considered.

Diagnosis and genetics

The clinical presentation determines the relevant diagnostic tests. With acute neurovisceral symptoms, urinary δ-aminolevulinic acid, porphobilinogen, and total porphyrins are the most useful first-line tests, whereas with cutaneous symptoms, a plasma porphyrin fluorescence emission screen should be measured initially.[211] Detailed fecal and erythrocyte porphyrins, specific enzyme assays, and DNA analysis are necessary for confirmation of the specific diagnosis (Table 13.7).

Management

The management is complex and varies for different disorders and specific patients (Table 13.7). Liver function should be monitored where appropriate. In erythropoietic porphyria, blood transfusions or heme therapy may be indicated in acute failure. Bone-marrow transplantation and/or liver transplantation may be beneficial.[206]

Abetalipoproteinemia

Lipids are transported in plasma as soluble lipoproteins and are classified according to their density and electrophoretic mobility. The typical lipoprotein consists of a lipid core (cholesterol and triglycerides) surrounded by a layer of phospholipid and cholesterol molecules and protein moieties called apoproteins. There are two major lipoprotein transport pathways. The exogenous pathway involves the transfer of dietary lipids from the intestines to the liver as chylomicrons, whereas the endogenous pathway transports lipids from the liver to peripheral tissues as very-low-density lipoproteins (VLDLs). Apoprotein B is the major component apoprotein of chylomicrons and VLDL, and abnormalities of this protein result in significant disruption of the major lipid transport pathways, with potentially serious clinical consequences.

Abetalipoproteinemia is a rare, autosomal-recessive disorder that is associated with an absence of plasma β-lipoprotein and undetectable plasma chylomicrons, low-density lipoprotein (LDL) levels, and VLDL levels. It results in severe fat malabsorption and secondary deficiency of fat soluble vitamins.

There is defective processing of B apoproteins or defective assembly and/or secretion of VLDLs and chylomicrons. Microsomal triglyceride transfer protein (MTP) permits the transfer of lipid to apoprotein B, and several mutations in the gene controlling this protein have been reported in patients with abetalipoproteinemia.[127]

Presentation

The main clinical features include:[212]

- Presentation in early infancy with diarrhea, vomiting, and failure to thrive. The intestinal symptoms relate to the amount of fat in the diet, and many patients develop a striking aversion to dietary fat.
- Fat malabsorption with fat-soluble vitamin deficiency.
- Acanthocytosis occurs as a result of altered lipid composition of erythrocyte membranes and results in shortened erythrocyte survival, hyperbilirubinemia, erythroid hyperplasia, and reticulocytosis.
- Spinocerebellar degeneration begins in adolescence and consists of ataxia, dysmetria, dysarthria, and peripheral neuropathy.
- Pigmentary retinal degeneration develops in late childhood and may lead to progressive blindness.
- Anemia secondary to nutritional deficiency and/or hemolytic may be present.
- Fatty infiltration of the liver is common, and cirrhosis has been reported in a number of individuals, especially after medium-chain triglyceride (MCT) supplementation.

Diagnosis

The diagnosis is suspected from:

- Acanthocytosis
- Low plasma vitamin concentration
- Absence of B lipoprotein on electrophoresis
- Undetectable apolipoprotein B

Hypobetalipoproteinemia is a distinct group of conditions associated with mutations of the apoprotein B gene. Over 30 mutations are currently known.[135] The condition is dominantly inherited. Heterozygotes are asymptomatic. In the homozygous state, the clinical symptoms are indistinguishable from those of abetalipoproteinemia, and these patients can only be differentiated by demonstrating hypolipidemia in their parents. The approach to treating homozygotes is the same as for abetalipoproteinemia.

Management

The gastrointestinal symptoms respond to a low-fat diet (total fat intake > 15 g/day), with clinical improvement and accelerated growth. Essential fatty acid supplementation is important. Medium-chain triglycerides release fatty acids without the formation of chylomicrons for absorption, and could be used as a dietary energy source in abetalipoproteinemia, but there is a risk of hepatic fibrosis.[212] Nevertheless, short-term use of MCT feeds may be helpful for extremely malnourished individuals.

Fat-soluble vitamin supplementation, especially vitamin A and vitamin K, is necessary. Tocopherol (vitamin E) supplementation (150–200 mg/kg/day) inhibits the progression of neurological and retinal disease and may ameliorate these symptoms if started early.[213,214]

Case study

MJ was a female infant born normally to consanguineous parents at term, weighing 3.4 kg. The antenatal and perinatal histories were normal. She was bottle-fed and discharged home on the second day. Jaundice was noticed on day 7, for which she was admitted to hospital and then transferred to the local tertiary liver unit.

On examination, she was active, alert, and jaundiced with no other signs of liver failure. She had no dysmorphic features. Hepatosplenomegaly was noted on abdominal examination. Initial investigations revealed:

- Normal electrolytes and renal function
- Normal blood count

- Alanine aminotransferase (ALT) 135 IU/L (normal < 50 IU/L)
- Aspartate aminotransferase (AST) 208 IU/L (normal < 50 IU/L)
- GGT 773 IU/L (normal < 30 IU/L)
- Total bilirubin 238 μmol/L (normal < 20 μmol/L)
- Conjugated bilirubin 124 μmol/L (normal < 20 μmol/l)
- Alkaline phosphatase 1390 IU/L (normal < 600 IU/L)
- Albumin 36 g/L (normal 35–50 g/L)
- Prothrombin time 12 s (normal)
- Activated partial thromboplastin time (APTT) 25 s (normal)

Plasma thyroid function tests, virology, α-fetoprotein, α_1-antitrypsin, cholesterol, triglycerides, ammonia, glucose, and lactate were normal.

The initial work-up for metabolic disorders revealed:

- Negative screening tests for galactosemia and tyrosinemia type I
- Normal urine amino acids and organic acids
- Normal plasma amino acids, carnitine, and acylcarnitine profile
- Normal urine oligosaccharides and glycosaminoglycans
- Normal white cell enzymes for Niemann–Pick A/B disease, Gaucher disease, Wolman disease, G_{M1} gangliosidosis
- I-cell disease screen normal
- Plasma chitotriosidase moderately elevated: 25 IU/L (normal < 2.5 IU/L)

On histology, there was preserved architecture; the acini showed occasional apoptotic bodies. There was no cholestasis or giant-cell transformation. Kupffer cells and hepatocytes showed a vacuolated appearance. The portal tracts were normal (see Figure 4.14A).

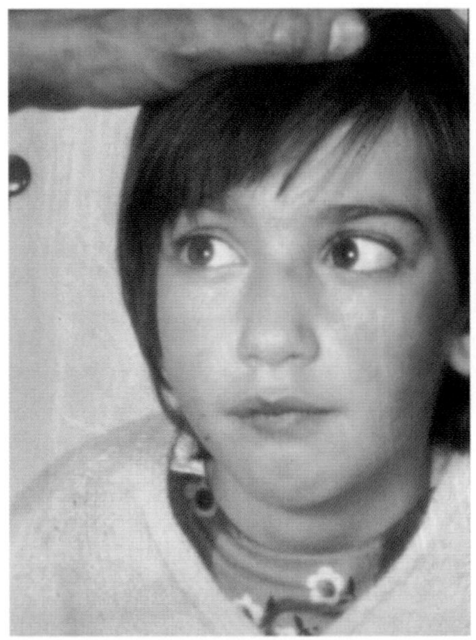
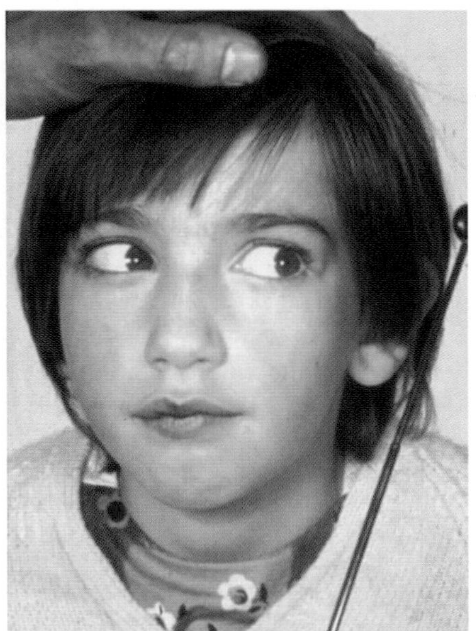

A

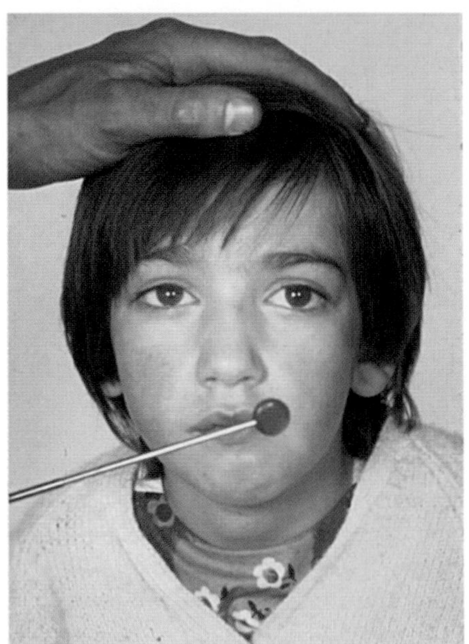
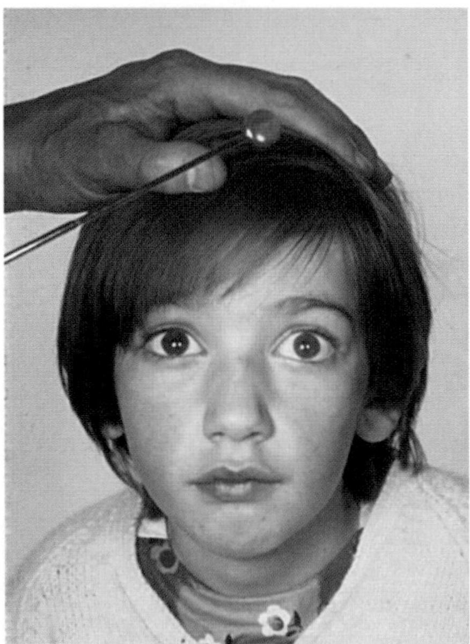

B

Figure 13.7 Vertical supranuclear gaze palsy in Niemann–Pick disease type C. **A** The patient has a normal horizontal gaze. **B** Paralysis of upward gaze when the patient attempts to look upwards.

Bone-marrow aspiration demonstrated foamy storage cells (see Figure 4.14B).

Treatment with fat-soluble vitamins was commenced, and further investigations (skin biopsy for fibroblast, filipin staining, and cholesterol esterification studies) were undertaken for Niemann–Pick disease type C.

Filipin staining and cholesterol esterification studies in skin fibroblasts were abnormal, confirming a diagnosis of Niemann–Pick disease type C. Mutation analysis of the *NPC1* gene revealed homozygosity for the P1007L mutation in exon 20, predicted to be disease-causing by destabilizing the NPC1 protein secondary structure in a transmembrane domain that is highly conserved.

Clinically, her cholestasis resolved after 4 months and she remained well for the first few years of her life.

Neurological signs first appeared when she was aged 5, with unsteadiness and frequent falls that prompted repeat referral. Examination at this stage revealed a slightly enlarged liver, with definite splenomegaly, hypotonia, and characteristic vertical supranuclear vertical gaze palsy (Figure 13.7). Subsequent developmental progress was slow. She developed ataxia, memory loss, and cataplexy by the age of 6.

By the age of 8, her speech was slurred and drooling became prominent. She developed generalized and myoclonic seizures, requiring treatment with multiple anticonvulsants. She had frequent episodes of respiratory infection and was treated with courses of antibiotics. Her motor and mental function deteriorated rapidly over the subsequent 6 months, and she was wheelchair-bound by 9 years of age.

Over the next 3 years, further loss of cognitive and fine motor skills occurred, with increasing spasticity, and she progressed to a near-vegetative state by the age of 13. She died from respiratory failure following a lower respiratory tract infection.

Comments. Niemann–Pick C is a fatal disease. In approximately 60% of children, it presents with neonatal jaundice, which resolves although splenomegaly persists. It is not curable by bone-marrow or liver transplantation, although recent experimental therapy with miglustat is encouraging. Most children die in adolescence from respiratory failure, as in this case. Parents and children need considerable support for this devastating condition.

References

1 Bowker R. *Management of the Child with a Decreased Conscious Level: an Evidence Based Guideline.* London: Royal College of Paediatrics and Child Health, 2005.

2 Saheki T, Kobayashi K, Iijima M, *et al.* Adult-onset type II citrullinemia and idiopathic neonatal hepatitis caused by citrin deficiency: involvement of the aspartate glutamate carrier for urea synthesis and maintenance of the urea cycle. *Mol Genet Metab* 2004;**81**(Suppl 1):S20–6.

3 Ohura T, Kobayashi K, Tazawa Y, *et al.* Clinical pictures of 75 patients with neonatal intrahepatic cholestasis caused by citrin deficiency (NICCD). *J Inherit Metab Dis* 2007;**30**:139–44.

4 Chen YT. Glycogen storage diseases. In: Scriver CR, Beaudet AL, Sly WS, Vall D, eds. *The Metabolic and Molecular Bases of Inherited Disease.* New York: McGraw-Hill, 2001: 1521–51.

5 Rother KI, Schwenk WF. Glucose production in glycogen storage disease I is not associated with increased cycling through hepatic glycogen. *Am J Physiol* 1995;**269**(4 Pt 1):E774–8.

6 Golbus MS, Simpson TJ, Koresawa M, Appelman Z, Alpers CE. The prenatal determination of glucose-6-phosphatase activity by fetal liver biopsy. *Prenat Diagn* 1988;**8**:401–4.

7 Chen YT, Bazzarre CH, Lee MM, Sidbury JB, Coleman RA. Type I glycogen storage disease: nine years of management with cornstarch. *Eur J Pediatr* 1993;**152**(Suppl 1):S56–9.

8 Smit GP. The long-term outcome of patients with glycogen storage disease type Ia. *Eur J Pediatr* 1993;**152**(Suppl 1):S52–5.

9 Wolfsdorf JI, Crigler JF Jr. Effect of continuous glucose therapy begun in infancy on the long-term clinical course of patients with type I glycogen storage disease. *J Pediatr Gastroenterol Nutr* 1999;**29**:136–43.

10 Lee PJ, Patel A, Hindmarsh PC, Mowat AP, Leonard JV. The prevalence of polycystic ovaries in the hepatic glycogen storage diseases: its association with hyperinsulinism. *Clin Endocrinol (Oxf)* 1995;**42**:601–6.

11 Talente GM, Coleman RA, Alter C, *et al.* Glycogen storage disease in adults. *Ann Intern Med* 1994;**120**:218–26.

12 Lee PJ, Patel JS, Fewtrell M, Leonard JV, Bishop NJ. Bone mineralisation in type 1 glycogen storage disease. *Eur J Pediatr* 1995;**154**:483–7.

13 Chen YT, Coleman RA, Scheinman JI, Kolbeck PC, Sidbury JB. Renal disease in type I glycogen storage disease. *N Engl J Med* 1988;**318**:7–11.

14 Kikuchi M, Haginoya K, Miyabayashi S, Igarashi Y, Narisawa K, Tada K. Secondary amyloidosis in glycogen storage disease type Ib. *Eur J Pediatr* 1990;**149**:344–5.

15 Restaino I, Kaplan BS, Stanley C, Baker L. Nephrolithiasis, hypocitraturia, and a distal renal tubular acidification defect in type 1 glycogen storage disease. *J Pediatr* 1993;**122**:392–6.

16 Wolfsdorf JI, Holm IA, Weinstein DA. Glycogen storage diseases. Phenotypic, genetic, and biochemical characteristics, and therapy. *Endocrinol Metab Clin North Am* 1999;**28**:801–23.

17 Schwahn B, Rauch F, Wendel U, Schonau E. Low bone mass in glycogen storage disease type 1 is associated with reduced muscle force and poor metabolic control. *J Pediatr* 2002;**141**:350–6.

18 Alaupovic P, Fernandes J. The serum apolipoprotein profile of patients with glucose-6-phosphatase deficiency. *Pediatr Res* 1985;**19**:380–4.

19 Levy E, Thibault L, Turgeon J, *et al.* Beneficial effects of fish-oil supplements on lipids, lipoproteins, and lipoprotein lipase in patients with glycogen storage disease type I. *Am J Clin Nutr* 1993;**57**:922–9.

20 Pizzo CJ. Type I glycogen storage disease with focal nodular hyperplasia of the liver and vasoconstrictive pulmonary hypertension. *Pediatrics* 1980;**65**:341–3.

21 Hamaoka K, Nakagawa M, Furukawa N, Sawada T. Pulmonary hypertension in type I glycogen storage disease. *Pediatr Cardiol* 1990;**11**:54–6.

22 Kishnani P, Bengur AR, Chen YT. Pulmonary hypertension in glycogen storage disease type I. *J Inherit Metab Dis* 1996;**19**:213–6.

23 Marti GE, Rick ME, Sidbury J, Gralnick HR. DDAVP infusion in five patients with type Ia glycogen storage disease and associated correction of prolonged bleeding times. *Blood* 1986;**68**: 180–4.

24 Ryan IP, Havel RJ, Laros RK Jr. Three consecutive pregnancies in a patient with glycogen storage disease type IA (von Gierke's disease). *Am J Obstet Gynecol* 1994;**170**:1687–90.

25 Howell RR, Stevenson RE, Ben Menachem Y, Phyliky RL, Berry DH. Hepatic adenomata with type 1 glycogen storage disease. *JAMA* 1976;**236**:1481–4.

26 Parker P, Burr I, Slonim A, Ghishan FK, Greene H. Regression of hepatic adenomas in type Ia glycogen storage disease with dietary therapy. *Gastroenterology* 1981;**81**:534–6.

27 Faivre L, Houssin D, Valayer J, Brouard J, Hadchouel M, Bernard O. Long-term outcome of liver transplantation in patients with glycogen storage disease type Ia. *J Inherit Metab Dis* 1999;**22**:723–32.

28 Matern D, Starzl TE, Arnaout W, *et al.* Liver transplantation for glycogen storage disease types I, III, and IV. *Eur J Pediatr* 1999;**158**(Suppl 2):S43–8.

29 Sokal EM. Liver transplantation for inborn errors of liver metabolism. *J Inherit Metab Dis* 2006;**29**:426–30.

30 Kirschner BS, Baker AL, Thorp FK. Growth in adulthood after liver transplantation for glycogen storage disease type I. *Gastroenterology* 1991;**101**:238–41.

31 Dhawan A, Mitry RR, Hughes RD. Hepatocyte transplantation for liver-based metabolic disorders. *J Inherit Metab Dis* 2006;**29**: 431–5.

32 Veiga-da-Cunha M, Gerin I, Van Schaftingen E. How many forms of glycogen storage disease type I? *Eur J Pediatr* 2000; **159**:314–8.

33 Rake JP, Visser G, Labrune P, Leonard JV, Ullrich K, Smit GP. Glycogen storage disease type I: diagnosis, management, clinical course and outcome. Results of the European Study on Glycogen Storage Disease Type I (ESGSD I). *Eur J Pediatr* 2002;**161**(Suppl 1):S20–34.

34 Veiga-da-Cunha M, Gerin I, Chen YT, *et al.* A gene on chromosome 11q23 coding for a putative glucose-6-phosphate translocase is mutated in glycogen-storage disease types Ib and Ic. *Am J Hum Genet* 1998;**63**:976–83.

35 Kure S, Suzuki Y, Matsubara Y, *et al.* Molecular analysis of glycogen storage disease type Ib: identification of a prevalent mutation among Japanese patients and assignment of a putative glucose-6-phosphate translocase gene to chromosome 11. *Biochem Biophys Res Commun* 1998;**248**:426–31.

36 Visser G, Rake JP, Fernandes J, *et al.* Neutropenia, neutrophil dysfunction, and inflammatory bowel disease in glycogen storage disease type Ib: results of the European Study on Glycogen Storage Disease type I. *J Pediatr* 2000;**137**:187–91.

37 Schroten H, Roesler J, Breidenbach T, *et al.* Granulocyte and granulocyte-macrophage colony-stimulating factors for treatment of neutropenia in glycogen storage disease type Ib. *J Pediatr* 1991;**119**:748–54.

38 Hoover EG, DuBois JJ, Samples TL, McCullough JS, Chenaille PJ, Montes RG. Treatment of chronic enteritis in glycogen storage disease type IB with granulocyte colony-stimulating factor. *J Pediatr Gastroenterol Nutr* 1996;**22**:346–50.

39 Calderwood S, Kilpatrick L, Douglas SD, *et al.* Recombinant human granulocyte colony-stimulating factor therapy for patients with neutropenia and/or neutrophil dysfunction secondary to glycogen storage disease type 1b. *Blood* 2001;**97**:376–82.

40 Garty BZ, Levy I, Nitzan M, Barak Y. Sweet syndrome associated with G-CSF treatment in a child with glycogen storage disease type Ib. *Pediatrics* 1996;**97**:401–3.

41 Pinsk M, Burzynski J, Yhap M, Fraser RB, Cummings B, Ste-Marie M. Acute myelogenous leukemia and glycogen storage disease 1b. *J Pediatr Hematol Oncol* 2002;**24**(9):756–758.

42 Donadieu J, Barkaoui M, Bezard F, Bertrand Y, Pondarre C, Guibaud P. Renal carcinoma in a patient with glycogen storage disease Ib receiving long-term granulocyte colony-stimulating factor therapy. *J Pediatr Hematol Oncol* 2000;**22**:188–9.

43 Bhattacharya N, Heaton N, Rela M, Walter JH, Lee PJ. The benefits of liver transplantation in glycogenosis type Ib. *J Inherit Metab Dis* 2004;**27**:539–40.

44 Martinez-Olmos MA, Lopez-Sanroman A, Martin-Vaquero P, *et al.* Liver transplantation for type Ib glycogenosis with reversal of cyclic neutropenia. *Clin Nutr* 2001;**20**:375–7.

45 Pierre G, Chakupurakal G, McKiernan P, Hendriksz C, Lawson S, Chakrapani A. Bone marrow transplantation in glycogen storage disease type 1b. *J Pediatr* 2008;**152**:286–8.

46 Shen J, Bao Y, Liu HM, Lee P, Leonard JV, Chen YT. Mutations in exon 3 of the glycogen debranching enzyme gene are associated with glycogen storage disease type III that is differentially expressed in liver and muscle. *J Clin Invest* 1996;**98**:352–7.

47 DiMauro S, Hartwig GB, Hays A, *et al.* Debrancher deficiency: neuromuscular disorder in 5 adults. *Ann Neurol* 1979;**5**:422–36.

48 Coleman RA, Winter HS, Wolf B, Gilchrist JM, Chen YT. Glycogen storage disease type III (glycogen debranching enzyme deficiency): correlation of biochemical defects with myopathy and cardiomyopathy. *Ann Intern Med* 1992;**116**:896–900.

49 Kiechl S, Kohlendorfer U, Thaler C, *et al.* Different clinical aspects of debrancher deficiency myopathy. *J Neurol Neurosurg Psychiatry* 1999;**67**:364–8.

50 Slonim AE, Coleman RA, Moses S, Bashan N, Shipp E, Mushlin P. Amino acid disturbances in type III glycogenosis: differences from type I glycogenosis. *Metabolism* 1983;**32**:70–4.

51 Coleman RA, Winter HS, Wolf B, Chen YT. Glycogen debranching enzyme deficiency: long-term study of serum enzyme activities and clinical features. *J Inherit Metab Dis* 1992;**15**:869–81.

52 Haagsma EB, Smit GP, Niezen-Koning KE, Gouw AS, Meerman L, Slooff MJ. Type IIIb glycogen storage disease associated with end-stage cirrhosis and hepatocellular carcinoma. The Liver Transplant Group. *Hepatology* 1997;**25**:537–40.

53 Lee P. Successful pregnancy in a patient with type III glycogen storage disease managed with cornstarch supplements. *Br J Obstet Gynaecol* 1999;**106**:181–2.

54 Mendoza A, Fisher NC, Duckett J, *et al.* Successful pregnancy in a patient with type III glycogen storage disease managed with cornstarch supplements. *Br J Obstet Gynaecol* 1998;**105**: 677–80.

55 Bao Y, Kishnani P, Wu JY, Chen YT. Hepatic and neuromuscular forms of glycogen storage disease type IV caused by mutations in the same glycogen-branching enzyme gene. *J Clin Invest* 1996;**97**:941–8.

56 McConkie-Rosell A, Wilson C, Piccoli DA, *et al.* Clinical and laboratory findings in four patients with the non-progressive hepatic form of type IV glycogen storage disease. *J Inherit Metab Dis* 1996;**19**:51–8.

57 de Moor RA, Schweizer JJ, van Hoek B, Wasser M, Vink R, Maaswinkel-Mooy PD. Hepatocellular carcinoma in glycogen storage disease type IV. *Arch Dis Child* 2000;**82**:479–80.

58 Alegria A, Martins E, Dias M, Cunha A, Cardoso ML, Maire I. Glycogen storage disease type IV presenting as hydrops fetalis. *J Inherit Metab Dis* 1999;**22**:330–2.

59 Bruno C, van Diggelen OP, Cassandrini D, *et al.* Clinical and genetic heterogeneity of branching enzyme deficiency (glycogenosis type IV). *Neurology* 2004;**63**:1053–8.

60 Sokal EM, Van Hoof F, Alberti D, de Ville DG, de Barsy T, Otte JB. Progressive cardiac failure following orthotopic liver transplantation for type IV glycogenosis. *Eur J Pediatr* 1992;**151**: 200–3.

61 Rosenthal P, Podesta L, Grier R, *et al.* Failure of liver transplantation to diminish cardiac deposits of amylopectin and leukocyte inclusions in type IV glycogen storage disease. *Liver Transpl Surg* 1995;**1**:373–6.

62 Selby R, Starzl TE, Yunis E, Brown BI, Kendall RS, Tzakis A. Liver transplantation for type IV glycogen storage disease. *N Engl J Med* 1991;**324**:39–42.

63 Fernandes J, Koster JF, Grose WF, Sorgedrager N. Hepatic phosphorylase deficiency: its differentiation from other hepatic glycogenoses. *Arch Dis Child* 1974;**49**:186–91.

64 Willems PJ, Gerver WJ, Berger R, Fernandes J. The natural history of liver glycogenosis due to phosphorylase kinase deficiency: a longitudinal study of 41 patients. *Eur J Pediatr* 1990;**149**:268–71.

65 van Beurden EA, de Graaf M, Wendel U, Gitzelmann R, Berger R, van den Berg IE. Autosomal recessive liver phosphorylase kinase deficiency caused by a novel splice-site mutation in the gene encoding the liver gamma subunit (*PHKG2*). *Biochem Biophys Res Commun* 1997;**236**:544–8.

66 Burwinkel B, Shiomi S, Al Zaben A, Kilimann MW. Liver glycogenosis due to phosphorylase kinase deficiency: *PHKG2* gene structure and mutations associated with cirrhosis. *Hum Mol Genet* 1998;**7**:149–54.

67 Eishi Y, Takemura T, Sone R, *et al.* Glycogen storage disease confined to the heart with deficient activity of cardiac phosphorylase kinase: a new type of glycogen storage disease. *Hum Pathol* 1985;**16**:193–7.

68 Servidei S, Metlay LA, Chodosh J, DiMauro S. Fatal infantile cardiopathy caused by phosphorylase b kinase deficiency. *J Pediatr* 1988;**113**:82–5.

69 Clemens PR, Yamamoto M, Engel AG. Adult phosphorylase b kinase deficiency. *Ann Neurol* 1990;**28**:529–38.

70 Nakai A, Shigematsu Y, Takano T, Kikawa Y, Sudo M. Uncooked cornstarch treatment for hepatic phosphorylase kinase deficiency. *Eur J Pediatr* 1994;**153**:581–3.

71 Brown GK. Glucose transporters: structure, function and consequences of deficiency. *J Inherit Metab Dis* 2000;**23**:237–46.

72 Santer R, Schneppenheim R, Suter D, Schaub J, Steinmann B. Fanconi–Bickel syndrome—the original patient and his natural history, historical steps leading to the primary defect, and a review of the literature. *Eur J Pediatr* 1998;**157**:783–97.

73 Santer R, Steinmann B, Schaub J. Fanconi–Bickel syndrome—a congenital defect of facilitative glucose transport. *Curr Mol Med* 2002;**2**:213–27.

74 Cox TM. The genetic consequences of our sweet tooth. *Nat Rev Genet* 2002;**3**:481–7.

75 James CL, Rellos P, Ali M, Heeley AF, Cox TM. Neonatal screening for hereditary fructose intolerance: frequency of the most common mutant aldolase B allele (A149P) in the British population. *J Med Genet* 1996;**33**:837–41.

76 Brooks CC, Tolan DR. Association of the widespread A149P hereditary fructose intolerance mutation with newly identified sequence polymorphisms in the aldolase B gene. *Am J Hum Genet* 1993;**52**:835–40.

77 Cross NC, de Franchis R, Sebastio G, *et al.* Molecular analysis of aldolase B genes in hereditary fructose intolerance. *Lancet* 1990;**335**:306–9.

78 Newbrun E, Hoover C, Mettraux G, Graf H. Comparison of dietary habits and dental health of subjects with hereditary fructose intolerance and control subjects. *J Am Dent Assoc* 1980; **101**:619–26.

79 Schulte MJ, Lenz W. Fatal sorbitol infusion in patient with fructose-sorbitol intolerance. *Lancet* 1977;**ii**:188.

80 Phillips MJ, Poucell M, Patterson J, Valencia P. *The Liver: an Atlas of Ultrastructural Pathology.* New York: Raven Press, 1987.

81 Odievre M, Gentil C, Gautier M, Alagille's D. Hereditary fructose intolerance in childhood. Diagnosis, management, and course in 55 patients. *Am J Dis Child* 1978;**132**:605–8.

82 See G, Marchal G, Odievre M. [Hepatocarcinoma in an adult with possible hereditary fructose intolerance; in French.] *Ann Pediatr (Paris)* 1984;**31**:49–51.

83 Kikawa Y, Inuzuka M, Jin BY, *et al.* Identification of genetic mutations in Japanese patients with fructose-1,6-bisphosphatase deficiency. *Am J Hum Genet* 1997;**61**:852–61.

84 Hers HG, van Schaftingen E. Fructose 2,6-bisphosphate 2 years after its discovery. *Biochem J* 1982;**206**:1–12.

85 Buhrdel P, Bohme HJ, Didt L. Biochemical and clinical observations in four patients with fructose-1,6-diphosphatase deficiency. *Eur J Pediatr* 1990;**149**:574–6.

86 Moses SW, Bashan N, Flasterstein BF, Rachmel A, Gutman A. Fructose-1,6-diphosphatase deficiency in Israel. *Isr J Med Sci* 1991;**27**:1–4.

87 Rapola J. Lysosomal storage diseases in adults. *Pathol Res Pract* 1994;**190**:759–66.

88 Brady RO. Enzyme replacement for lysosomal diseases. *Annu Rev Med* 2006;**57**:283–96.

89 Cox TM, Schofield JP. Gaucher's disease: clinical features and natural history. *Baillieres Clin Haematol* 1997;**10**:657–89.

90 Charrow J, Andersson HC, Kaplan P, *et al.* The Gaucher registry: demographics and disease characteristics of 1698 patients with Gaucher disease. *Arch Intern Med* 2000;**160**:2835–43.

91 Cox TM. Gaucher disease: understanding the molecular pathogenesis of sphingolipidoses. *J Inherit Metab Dis* 2001;**24**(Suppl 2):106–21.

92 Grabowski GA, Horowitz M. Gaucher's disease: molecular, genetic and enzymological aspects. *Baillieres Clin Haematol* 1997; **10**:635–56.

93 Zevin S, Abrahamov A, Hadas-Halpern I, *et al.* Adult-type Gaucher disease in children: genetics, clinical features and enzyme replacement therapy. *QJM* 1993;**86**:565–73.

94 James SP, Stromeyer FW, Chang C, Barranger JA. Liver abnormalities in patients with Gaucher's disease. *Gastroenterology* 1981;**80**:126–33.

95 Elstein D, Itzchaki M, Mankin HJ. Skeletal involvement in Gaucher's disease. *Baillieres Clin Haematol* 1997;**10**:793–816.

96 Wenstrup RJ, Roca-Espiau M, Weinreb NJ, Bembi B. Skeletal aspects of Gaucher disease: a review. *Br J Radiol* 2002;**75**(Suppl 1):A2–12.

97 Elstein D, Klutstein MW, Lahad A, Abrahamov A, Hadas-Halpern I, Zimran A. Echocardiographic assessment of pulmonary hypertension in Gaucher's disease. *Lancet* 1998;**351**:1544–6.

98 Erikson A, Bembi B, Schiffmann R. Neuronopathic forms of Gaucher's disease. *Baillieres Clin Haematol* 1997;**10**:711–23.

99 Deegan PB, Moran MT, McFarlane I, *et al.* Clinical evaluation of chemokine and enzymatic biomarkers of Gaucher disease. *Blood Cells Mol Dis* 2005;**35**:259–67.

100 Cox TM. Gaucher's disease—an exemplary monogenic disorder. *QJM* 2001;**94**:399–402.

101 Vellodi A, Wraith JE, McHugh K, Cooper A. *Guidelines for the Management of Paediatric Gaucher Disease in the United Kingdom.* London: Department of Health, United Kingdom, 2005. Available at: www.dh.gov.uk/en/Publicationsandstatistics/Publications/PublicationsPolicyAndGuidance/DH_4118403 (accessed 29 February 2008).

102 Cox T, Lachmann R, Hollak C, *et al.* Novel oral treatment of Gaucher's disease with *N*-butyldeoxynojirimycin (OGT 918) to decrease substrate biosynthesis. *Lancet* 2000;**355**:1481–5.

103 Aerts JM, Hollak CE, Boot RG, Groener JE, Maas M. Substrate reduction therapy of glycosphingolipid storage disorders. *J Inherit Metab Dis* 2006;**29**:449–56.

104 Schuchman EH, Miranda SR. Niemann–Pick disease: mutation update, genotype/phenotype correlations, and prospects for genetic testing. *Genet Test* 1997;**1**:13–9.

105 Vanier MT, Ferlinz K, Rousson R, *et al.* Deletion of arginine (608) in acid sphingomyelinase is the prevalent mutation among Niemann–Pick disease type B patients from northern Africa. *Hum Genet* 1993;**92**:325–30.

106 Schuchman EH, Desnick RJ. Niemann–Pick Diseases types A and B: acid sphingomyelinase deficiencies. In: Scriver CR, Beaudet AL, Sly WS, Vall D, eds. *The Metabolic and Molecular Bases of Inherited Disease.* New York: McGraw-Hill, 2001: 3589–609.

107 Grunebaum M. The roentgenographic findings in the acute neuronopathic form of Niemann–Pick disease. *Br J Radiol* 1976; **49**:1018–22.

108 Tamaru J, Iwasaki I, Horie H, *et al.* Niemann–Pick disease associated with liver disorders. *Acta Pathol Jpn* 1985;**35**:1267–72.

109 Chan WC, Lai KS, Todd D. Adult Niemann–Pick disease—a case report. *J Pathol* 1977;**121**:177–81.

110 Dawson PJ, Dawson G. Adult Niemann–Pick disease with sea-blue histiocytes in the spleen. *Hum Pathol* 1982;**13**:1115–20.

111 Tassoni JP Jr, Fawaz KA, Johnston DE. Cirrhosis and portal hypertension in a patient with adult Niemann–Pick disease. *Gastroenterology* 1991;**100**:567–9.

112 Lever AM, Ryder JB. Cor pulmonale in an adult secondary to Niemann–Pick disease. *Thorax* 1983;**38**):873–4.

113 Wasserstein MP, Desnick RJ, Schuchman EH, *et al.* The natural history of type B Niemann–Pick disease: results from a 10-year longitudinal study. *Pediatrics* 2004;**114**:e672–7.

114 Elleder M, Cihula J. Niemann–Pick disease (variation in the sphingomyelinase deficient group). Neurovisceral phenotype (A) with an abnormally protracted clinical course and variable expression of neurological symptomatology in three siblings. *Eur J Pediatr* 1983;**140**:323–8.

115 Lipson MH, O'Donnell J, Callahan JW, Wenger DA, Packman S. Ocular involvement in Niemann–Pick disease type B. *J Pediatr* 1986;**108**:582–4.

116 Takada G, Satoh W, Komatsu K, Konn Y, Miura Y, Uesaka Y. Transitory type of sphingomyelinase deficient Niemann–Pick disease: clinical and morphological studies and follow-up of two sisters. *Tohoku J Exp Med* 1987;**153**:27–36.

117 Maziere JC, Maziere C, Hosli P. An ultramicrochemical assay for sphingomyelinase: rapid prenatal diagnosis of a fetus at risk for Niemann–Pick disease. *Monogr Hum Genet* 1978;**9**:198–201.

118 Vanier MT, Boue J, Dumez Y. Niemann–Pick disease type B: first-trimester prenatal diagnosis on chorionic villi and biochemical study of a foetus at 12 weeks of development. *Clin Genet* 1985;**28**:348–54.

119 Crocker AC, Farber S. Niemann–Pick disease: a review of eighteen patients. *Medicine (Baltimore)* 1958;**37**:1–95.

120 Vanier MT. Disorders of sphingolipid metabolism. In: Fernandes J, Saudubray JM, van den Berghe G, Walter JH, eds. *Inborn Metabolic Diseases: Diagnosis and Treatment.* Heidelberg: Springer, 2006: 479–94.

121 Zhang M, Dwyer NK, Neufeld EB, *et al.* Sterol-modulated glycolipid sorting occurs in Niemann–Pick C1 late endosomes. *J Biol Chem* 2001;**276**:3417–25.

122 Millat G, Marcais C, Tomasetto C, *et al.* Niemann–Pick C1 disease: correlations between *NPC1* mutations, levels of NPC1 protein, and phenotypes emphasize the functional significance of the putative sterol-sensing domain and of the cysteine-rich luminal loop. *Am J Hum Genet* 2001;**68**:1373–85.

123 Millat G, Chikh K, Naureckiene S, *et al.* Niemann–Pick disease type C: spectrum of HE1 mutations and genotype/phenotype correlations in the NPC2 group. *Am J Hum Genet* 2001;**69**: 1013–21.

124 Cheruku SR, Xu Z, Dutia R, Lobel P, Storch J. Mechanism of cholesterol transfer from the Niemann–Pick type C2 protein to model membranes supports a role in lysosomal cholesterol transport. *J Biol Chem* 2006;**281**:31594–604.

125 Sleat DE, Wiseman JA, El Banna M, *et al.* Genetic evidence for nonredundant functional cooperativity between NPC1 and NPC2 in lipid transport. *Proc Natl Acad Sci U S A* 2004;**101**: 5886–91.

126 Verot L, Chikh K, Freydiere E, Honore R, Vanier MT, Millat G. Niemann–Pick C disease: functional characterization of three NPC2 mutations and clinical and molecular update on patients with NPC2. *Clin Genet* 2007;**71**:320–30.

127 Imrie J, Dasgupta S, Besley GT, *et al.* The natural history of Niemann–Pick disease type C in the UK. *J Inherit Metab Dis* 2007;**30**:51–9.

128 Vanier MT, Wenger DA, Comly ME, Rousson R, Brady RO, Pentchev PG. Niemann–Pick disease group C: clinical variability and diagnosis based on defective cholesterol esterification. A collaborative study on 70 patients. *Clin Genet* 1988;**33**:331–48.

129 Kelly DA, Portmann B, Mowat AP, Sherlock S, Lake BD. Niemann–Pick disease type C: diagnosis and outcome in children, with particular reference to liver disease. *J Pediatr* 1993;**123**:242–7.

130 Fensom AH, Grant AR, Steinberg SJ, *et al.* An adult with a non-neuronopathic form of Niemann–Pick C disease. *J Inherit Metab Dis* 1999;**22**:84–6.

131 Gartner JC Jr, Bergman I, Malatack JJ, *et al.* Progression of neurovisceral storage disease with supranuclear ophthalmoplegia following orthotopic liver transplantation. *Pediatrics* 1986;**77**:104–6.

132 Hsu YS, Hwu WL, Huang SF, *et al.* Niemann–Pick disease type C (a cellular cholesterol lipidosis) treated by bone marrow transplantation. *Bone Marrow Transplant* 1999;**24**:103–7.

133 Zervas M, Somers KL, Thrall MA, Walkley SU. Critical role for glycosphingolipids in Niemann–Pick disease type C. *Curr Biol* 2001;**11**:1283–7.

134 Patterson M, Vecchio D, Prady H, Abel L, Ait Aissa N, Wraith JE. Oral miglustat in adult and pediatric patients with Niemann–Pick type C (NPC) disease: rationale, methodology and interim analyses of a clinical study. [Paper presented at the 11th International Congress of Human Genetics, Brisbane, Queensland, 6–10 August 2006.]

135 Cooper DN, Ball EV, Stenson PD, Phillips AD, Howells K, Mort ME. Human gene mutation database at the Institute of Medical Genetics in Cardiff. Available at: www.uwcm.ac.uk/uwcm/mg/hgmd0.html (accessed 29 February 2008).

136 Aslanidis C, Ries S, Fehringer P, Buchler C, Klima H, Schmitz G. Genetic and biochemical evidence that CESD and Wolman disease are distinguished by residual lysosomal acid lipase activity. *Genomics* 1996;**33**:85–93.

137 Anderson RA, Bryson GM, Parks JS. Lysosomal acid lipase mutations that determine phenotype in Wolman and cholesterol ester storage disease. *Mol Genet Metab* 1999;**68**:333–45.

138 Assmann G, Seedorf U. Acid lipase deficiency: Wolman disease and cholesteryl ester storage disease. In: Scriver CR, Beaudet AL, Sly WS, Vall D, eds. *The Metabolic and Molecular Bases of Inherited Disease.* New York: McGraw-Hill, 2001: 3551–71.

139 Drebber U, Andersen M, Kasper HU, Lohse P, Stolte M, Dienes HP. Severe chronic diarrhea and weight loss in cholesteryl ester storage disease: a case report. *World J Gastroenterol* 2005;**11**:2364–6.

140 Wolman M. Wolman disease and its treatment. *Clin Pediatr (Phila)* 1995;**34**:207–12.

141 Krivit W, Peters C, Dusenbery K, *et al.* Wolman disease successfully treated by bone marrow transplantation. *Bone Marrow Transplant* 2000;**26**:567–70.

142 Stein J, Garty BZ, Dror Y, Fenig E, Zeigler M, Yaniv I. Successful treatment of Wolman disease by unrelated umbilical cord blood transplantation. *Eur J Pediatr* 2007;**166**:663–6.

143 Leone L, Ippoliti PF, Antonicelli R. Use of simvastatin plus cholestyramine in the treatment of lysosomal acid lipase deficiency. *J Pediatr* 1991;**119**:1008–9.

144 Rassoul F, Richter V, Lohse P, Naumann A, Purschwitz K, Keller E. Long-term administration of the HMG-CoA reductase inhibitor lovastatin in two patients with cholesteryl ester storage disease. *Int J Clin Pharmacol Ther* 2001;**39**:199–204.

145 Arterburn JN, Lee WM, Wood RP, Shaw BW, Markin RS. Orthotopic liver transplantation for cholesteryl ester storage disease. *J Clin Gastroenterol* 1991;**13**:482–5.

146 Ferry GD, Whisennand HH, Finegold MJ, Alpert E, Glombicki A. Liver transplantation for cholesteryl ester storage disease. *J Pediatr Gastroenterol Nutr* 1991;**12**:376–8.

147 Leone L, Ippoliti PF, Antonicelli R, Balli F, Gridelli B. Treatment and liver transplantation for cholesterol ester storage disease. *J Pediatr* 1995;**127**:509–10.

148 Du H, Schiavi S, Levine M, Mishra J, Heur M, Grabowski GA. Enzyme therapy for lysosomal acid lipase deficiency in the mouse. *Hum Mol Genet* 2001;**10**:1639–48.

149 Jaeken J, Carchon H. Congenital disorders of glycosylation: a booming chapter of pediatrics. *Curr Opin Pediatr* 2004;**16**:434–9.

150 Sparks SE. Inherited disorders of glycosylation. *Mol Genet Metab* 2006;**87**:1–7.

151 Keir G, Winchester BG, Clayton P. Carbohydrate-deficient glycoprotein syndromes: inborn errors of protein glycosylation. *Ann Clin Biochem* 1999;**36**:20–36.

152 Jaeken J, Matthijs G. Congenital disorders of glycosylation. *Annu Rev Genomics Hum Genet* 2001;**2**:129–51.

153 de Lonlay P, Seta N, Barrot S, *et al.* A broad spectrum of clinical presentations in congenital disorders of glycosylation I: a series of 26 cases. *J Med Genet* 2001;**38**:14–9.

154 Kjaergaard S, Schwartz M, Skovby F. Congenital disorder of glycosylation type Ia (CDG-Ia): phenotypic spectrum of the R141H/F119L genotype. *Arch Dis Child* 2001;**85**:236–9.

155 Babovic-Vuksanovic D, Patterson MC, Schwenk WF, *et al.* Severe hypoglycemia as a presenting symptom of carbohydrate-deficient glycoprotein syndrome. *J Pediatr* 1999;**135**:775–81.

156 Hendriksz CJ, McClean P, Henderson MJ, *et al.* Successful treatment of carbohydrate deficient glycoprotein syndrome type 1b with oral mannose. *Arch Dis Child* 2001;**85**:339–40.

157 Leonard J, Grunewald S, Clayton P. Diversity of congenital disorders of glycosylation. *Lancet* 2001;**357**:1382–3.

158 Spaapen LJ, Bakker JA, van der Meer SB, *et al.* Clinical and biochemical presentation of siblings with COG-7 deficiency, a lethal multiple *O*- and *N*-glycosylation disorder. *J Inherit Metab Dis* 2005;**28**:707–14.

159 Fang J, Peters V, Assmann B, Korner C, Hoffmann GF. Improvement of CDG diagnosis by combined examination of several glycoproteins. *J Inherit Metab Dis* 2004;**27**:581–90.

160 Wopereis S, Morava E, Grunewald S, *et al.* Patients with unsolved congenital disorders of glycosylation type II can be subdivided in six distinct biochemical groups. *Glycobiology* 2005;**15**:1312–9.

161 Niehues R, Hasilik M, Alton G, *et al.* Carbohydrate-deficient glycoprotein syndrome type Ib. Phosphomannose isomerase deficiency and mannose therapy. *J Clin Invest* 1998;**101**:1414–20.

162 Munnich A, Rotig A, Chretien D, *et al.* Clinical presentation of mitochondrial disorders in childhood. *J Inherit Metab Dis* 1996;**19**:521–7.

163 Cormier V, Rustin P, Bonnefont JP, *et al.* Hepatic failure in disorders of oxidative phosphorylation with neonatal onset. *J Pediatr* 1991;**119**:951–4.

164 Cormier-Daire V, Chretien D, Rustin P, *et al.* Neonatal and delayed-onset liver involvement in disorders of oxidative phosphorylation. *J Pediatr* 1997;**130**:817–22.

165 Morris AA. Mitochondrial respiratory chain disorders and the liver. *Liver* 1999;**19**:357–68.

166 Cormier-Daire V, Bonnefont JP, Rustin P, *et al.* Mitochondrial DNA rearrangements with onset as chronic diarrhea with villous atrophy. *J Pediatr* 1994;**124**:63–70.

167 Rotig A, Bourgeron T, Chretien D, Rustin P, Munnich A. Spectrum of mitochondrial DNA rearrangements in the Pearson marrow-pancreas syndrome. *Hum Mol Genet* 1995;**4**:1327–30.

168 Sarzi E, Bourdon A, Chretien D, *et al.* Mitochondrial DNA depletion is a prevalent cause of multiple respiratory chain deficiency in childhood. *J Pediatr* 2007;**150**:531–4.

169 Munnich A, Rotig A, Chretien D, Saudubray JM, Cormier V, Rustin P. Clinical presentations and laboratory investigations in respiratory chain deficiency. *Eur J Pediatr* 1996;**155**:262–74.

170 Wanders RJ, Ruiter JP, Wijburg FA, Zeman J, Klement P, Houstek J. Prenatal diagnosis of systemic disorders of the respiratory chain in cultured chorionic villus fibroblasts by study of ATP-synthesis in digitonin-permeabilized cells. *J Inherit Metab Dis* 1996;**19**:133–6.

171 Morris AA, Leonard JV. The treatment of congenital lactic acidoses. *J Inherit Metab Dis* 1996;**19**:573–80.

172 Chinnery P, Majamaa K, Turnbull D, Thorburn D. Treatment for mitochondrial disorders. *Cochrane Database Syst Rev* 2006;(**1**): CD004426.

173 Dubern B, Broue P, Dubuisson C, *et al.* Orthotopic liver transplantation for mitochondrial respiratory chain disorders: a study of 5 children. *Transplantation* 2001;**71**:633–7.

174 Rake JP, van Spronsen FJ, Visser G, *et al.* End-stage liver disease as the only consequence of a mitochondrial respiratory chain deficiency: no contra-indication for liver transplantation. *Eur J Pediatr* 2000;**159**:523–6.

175 Thomson M, McKiernan P, Buckels J, Mayer D, Kelly D. Generalised mitochondrial cytopathy is an absolute contraindication to orthotopic liver transplant in childhood. *J Pediatr Gastroenterol Nutr* 1998;**26**:478–81.

176 Sokal EM, Sokol R, Cormier V, *et al.* Liver transplantation in mitochondrial respiratory chain disorders. *Eur J Pediatr* 1999;**158(**Suppl 2):S81–4.

177 Roth KS. Peroxisomal disease—common ground for pediatrician, cell biologist, biochemist, pathologist, and neurologist. *Clin Pediatr (Phila)* 1999;**38**:73–5.

178 Moser AB, Rasmussen M, Naidu S, *et al.* Phenotype of patients with peroxisomal disorders subdivided into sixteen complementation groups. *J Pediatr* 1995;**127**:13–22.

179 Gartner J. Disorders related to peroxisomal membranes. *J Inherit Metab Dis* 2000;**23**:264–72.

180 Suzuki Y, Shimozawa N, Imamura A, *et al.* Clinical, biochemical and genetic aspects and neuronal migration in peroxisome biogenesis disorders. *J Inherit Metab Dis* 2001;**24**:151–65.

181 Poll-The BT, Auborg P, Wanders RJ. Peroxisomal disorders. In: Fernandes J, Saudubray JM, van den Berghe G, Walter JH, eds. *Inborn Metabolic Diseases: Diagnosis and Treatment.* Heidelberg: Springer, 2006: 509–22.

182 Poggi-Travert F, Fournier B, Poll-The BT, Saudubray JM. Clinical approach to inherited peroxisomal disorders. *J Inherit Metab Dis* 1995;**18**(Suppl 1):1–18.

183 Setchell KD, Bragetti P, Zimmer-Nechemias L, *et al.* Oral bile acid treatment and the patient with Zellweger syndrome. *Hepatology* 1992;**15**:198–207.

184 Harding BN. Progressive neuronal degeneration of childhood with liver disease (Alpers–Huttenlocher syndrome): a personal review. *J Child Neurol* 1990;**5**:273–87.

185 Tulinius MH, Holme E, Kristiansson B, Larsson NG, Oldfors A. Mitochondrial encephalomyopathies in childhood. I. Biochemical and morphologic investigations. *J Pediatr* 1991;**119**:242–50.

186 Tulinius MH, Holme E, Kristiansson B, Larsson NG, Oldfors A. Mitochondrial encephalomyopathies in childhood. II. Clinical manifestations and syndromes. *J Pediatr* 1991;**119**:251–9.

187 Naviaux RK, Nyhan WL, Barshop BA, *et al.* Mitochondrial DNA polymerase gamma deficiency and mtDNA depletion in a child with Alpers' syndrome. *Ann Neurol* 1999;**45**:54–8.

188 Prick MJ, Gabreels FJ, Trijbels JM, *et al.* Progressive poliodystrophy (Alpers' disease) with a defect in cytochrome aa3 in muscle: a report of two unrelated patients. *Clin Neurol Neurosurg* 1983; **85**:57–70.

189 Gabreels FJ, Prick MJ, Trijbels JM, *et al.* Defects in citric acid cycle and the electron transport chain in progressive poliodystrophy. *Acta Neurol Scand* 1984;**70**:145–54.

190 Nguyen KV, Ostergaard E, Ravn SH, *et al. POLG* mutations in Alpers syndrome. *Neurology* 2005;**65**:1493–5.

191 Kollberg G, Moslemi AR, Darin N, *et al. POLG1* mutations associated with progressive encephalopathy in childhood. *J Neuropathol Exp Neurol* 2006;**65**:758–68.

192 Nguyen KV, Sharief FS, Chan SS, Copeland WC, Naviaux RK. Molecular diagnosis of Alpers syndrome. *J Hepatol* 2006;**45**: 108–116.

193 Narkewicz MR, Sokol RJ, Beckwith B, Sondheimer J, Silverman A. Liver involvement in Alpers disease. *J Pediatr* 1991;**119**:260–7.

194 Zimmerman HJ, Ishak KG. Valproate-induced hepatic injury: analyses of 23 fatal cases. *Hepatology* 1982;**2**:591–7.

195 Harding BN, Egger J, Portmann B, Erdohazi M. Progressive neuronal degeneration of childhood with liver disease. A pathological study. *Brain* 1986;**109**:181–206.

196 Delarue A, Paut O, Guys JM, *et al.* Inappropriate liver transplantation in a child with Alpers–Huttenlocher syndrome misdiagnosed as valproate-induced acute liver failure. *Pediatr Transplant* 2000;**4**:67–71.

197 Hardie RM, Newton LH, Bruce JC, *et al.* The changing clinical pattern of Reye's syndrome 1982–1990. *Arch Dis Child* 1996;**74**: 400–5.

198 Belay ED, Bresee JS, Holman RC, Khan AS, Shahriari A, Schonberger LB. Reye's syndrome in the United States from 1981 through 1997. *N Engl J Med* 1999;**340**:1377–82.

199 Casteels-Van Daele M, Van Geet C, Wouters C, Eggermont E. Reye syndrome revisited: a descriptive term covering a group of heterogeneous disorders. *Eur J Pediatr* 2000;**159**:641–8.

200 Glasgow JF, Middleton B. Reye syndrome—insights on causation and prognosis. *Arch Dis Child* 2001;**85**:351–3.

201 Hall SM, Plaster PA, Glasgow JF, Hancock P. Preadmission antipyretics in Reye's syndrome. *Arch Dis Child* 1988;**63**:857–66.

202 Forsyth BW, Horwitz RI, Acampora D, *et al.* New epidemiologic evidence confirming that bias does not explain the aspirin/Reye's syndrome association. *JAMA* 1989;**261**:2517–24.

203 Rowe PC, Valle D, Brusilow SW. Inborn errors of metabolism in children referred with Reye's syndrome. A changing pattern. *JAMA* 1988;**260**:3167–70.

204 Porter JD, Robinson PH, Glasgow JF, Banks JH, Hall SM. Trends in the incidence of Reye's syndrome and the use of aspirin. *Arch Dis Child* 1990;**65**:826–9.

205 Wendel U, de Baulny HO. Branched-chain organic acidurias/acidemias. In: Fernandes J, Saudubray JM, van den Berghe G, Walter JH, eds. *Inborn Metabolic Diseases: Diagnosis and Treatment.* Heidelberg: Springer, 2006: 245–62.

206 Egger NG, Lee C, Anderson KE. Disorders of heme biosynthesis. In: Fernandes J, Saudubray JM, van den Berghe G, Walter JH, eds. *Inborn Metabolic Diseases: Diagnosis and Treatment.* Heidelberg: Springer, 2006: 451–64.

207 Grandchamp B. Acute intermittent porphyria. *Semin Liver Dis* 1998;**18**:17–24.

208 Kauppinen R, Mustajoki P. Prognosis of acute porphyria: occurrence of acute attacks, precipitating factors, and associated diseases. *Medicine (Baltimore)* 1992;**71**:1–13.

209 Elder GH. Porphyria cutanea tarda. *Semin Liver Dis* 1998; **18**:67–75.

210 Cox TM, Alexander GJ, Sarkany RP. Protoporphyria. *Semin Liver Dis* 1998;**18**:85–93.

211 Deacon AC, Elder GH. ACP Best Practice No 165: front line tests for the investigation of suspected porphyria. *J Clin Pathol* 2001;**54**:500–7.

212 Roderiguez-Oquendo A, Kwiterovich PO. Dyslipidemias. In: Fernandes J, Saudubray JM, van den Berghe G, Walter JH, eds. *Inborn Metabolic Diseases: Diagnosis and Treatment.* Heidelberg: Springer, 2006: 389–410.

213 Bishara S, Merin S, Cooper M, Azizi E, Delpre G, Deckelbaum RJ. Combined vitamin A and E therapy prevents retinal electrophysiological deterioration in abetalipoproteinaemia. *Br J Ophthalmol* 1982;**66**:767–70.

214 Chowers I, Banin E, Merin S, Cooper M, Granot E. Long-term assessment of combined vitamin A and E treatment for the prevention of retinal degeneration in abetalipoproteinaemia and hypobetalipoproteinaemia patients. *Eye* 2001;**15**:525–30.

14 Disorders of Copper Metabolism

Stuart Tanner

Copper—essential but toxic

Copper-containing enzymes are essential to life (Table 14.1). Copper deficiency in infancy causes anemia, neutropenia, and bone changes, but it is rare, as copper is freely available in the diet and drinking water. The effects of copper deficiency are demonstrated by Menkes syndrome, in which ATP7A deficiency prevents egress of copper from intestinal cells.

Copper is toxic. In the Fenton reaction, Cu^{1+} causes production of the highly reactive hydroxyl radical:

$$H_2O_2 + Cu^{1+} \rightarrow OH\cdot + Cu^{2+} + H_2O$$

Recent evidence implicates acid sphingomyelinase and ceramide in copper-induced apoptosis,[1] raising the possibility of pharmacological inhibition of acid sphingomyelinase as a potentially new approach to treatment. A further relationship between copper and cell death is that elevated cellular copper levels reduce levels of, and cause a conformational change in, the X-linked inhibitor of apoptosis (XIAP). XIAP suppresses apoptosis by binding to caspases. The copper-bound form of XIAP is unstable and impaired in its activity to inhibit caspase-3.[2] XIAP has a further role in copper homeostasis in binding COMMD1 (see below) and promoting its proteosomal degradation, so producing copper retention.[3]

Infantile copper toxicosis (Indian and Tyrolean childhood cirrhoses) and Wilson's disease (WD) result from copper overload of dietary and genetic causes, respectively (Table 14.2).

Copper metabolism

Body copper status is largely regulated by biliary excretion, whereas iron status is regulated by intestinal absorption. At every stage from intestinal absorption to excretion, copper is bound to a series of transporters and chaperones. There is less than one free Cu ion per cell.[4] Hepatocyte copper metabolism is shown in Figure 14.1. The proteins concerned with uptake (Ctr1), intracellular chaperoning (atox1, ccs, cox17), serum transport (ceruloplasmin), and the Wilson's disease protein ATP7B and its associated proteins are considered below. Within the enterocyte, copper is bound to metallothionein, a 10-kDa cytosolic cysteine-rich protein. Metallothionein synthesis is induced by zinc, causing copper to be bound in the enterocyte and lost as it is desquamated at the villous tip—a "mucosal block" to absorption. Copper is exported from the enterocyte to portal blood by the Menkes protein, ATP7A. Copper is carried in portal blood loosely bound to albumin and histidine.

Ctr1 is responsible for high-affinity Cu^{1+} uptake into human cells.[5] It is associated with a membrane metalloreductase, is demonstrable in many tissues, and shows changes with age and copper status.[6,7] A Ctr1 knockout mouse is not viable, whilst an intestinal epithelial cell-specific Ctr1 knockout mouse exhibits striking neonatal defects in Cu accumulation in peripheral tissues, hepatic iron overload, cardiac hypertrophy, and severe growth and viability defects and kinky whiskers, reminiscent of Menkes syndrome.[8,9] In the mammary gland, Cu transport is highest during early lactation, stimulated by suckling and hyperprolactinemia, which is associated with Ctr1 and Atp7A localization to the plasma membrane.[10] Ctr1 is involved in the uptake of platinum-containing drugs.[11] Theoretically, *CTR1* mutations might influence severity in WD.

Copper is carried to its various intracellular destinations by chaperones. Atox1, or HAH1 (human atx homolog-1) is a 68-amino-acid protein abundantly and ubiquitously expressed,[12] which carries Cu to the six Cu-binding sequences at the N-terminal end of ATP7A and ATP7B. These, like atox1, contain the common highly conserved metal-binding motif MXCXXC. Atox1 preferentially transfers Cu to metal-binding sites 2 and 4 in ATP7B.[13,14] Atox1 knockout mice pups usually die before weaning, and survivors show growth failure, skin laxity, hypopigmentation, and seizures because of perinatal copper deficiency. Atox1-deficient cells accumulate high levels of intracellular copper due to impaired cellular copper efflux.[15] Atox1 mutations have been sought unsuccessfully in WD patients without ATP7B mutations.[16] Defects in atox1 do not have a known role in copper storage disease in humans.

Diseases of the Liver and Biliary System in Children, 3rd edition. Edited by Deirdre Kelly. © 2008 Blackwell Publishing, ISBN: 978-1-4051-6334-7.

Table 14.1 Copper-containing enzymes.

Enzyme	Action	Function
Cytochrome c oxidase	Transfers 4 electrons to O_2 $O_2 + 4e^- + 4H^+ \rightarrow 2\ H_2O$	Cellular respiration
Superoxide dismutase	$2O_2^- \rightarrow H_2O_2 + O_2$	Free radical scavenging Antioxidant defence Dysfunction associated with amyotrophic lateral sclerosis
Lysyl oxidase	Oxidative deamination of lysine in newly formed collagen and tropoelastin	Connective-tissue synthesis
Tyrosinase	Monophenol monooxygenase	Melanin synthesis
Dopamine β-monooxygenase	Dopamine → norepinephrine	Catecholamine synthesis
Ceruloplasmin	Ferroxidase	Oxidizes Fe^{2+} to Fe^{3+}
Hephaestin	Ferroxidase in basolateral membrane of enterocyte	Fe egress from enterocyte
Clotting factors V and VIII	"A" domains homologous to ceruloplasmin	Blood clotting
Peptidylglycine monooxygenase	Neuropeptide processing	Neural function
Prion protein	$PrP^{(C)}$ binds Cu	Cell signaling

Table 14.2 Hepatic copper overload states in humans.

Clinical scenario	Cause	Animal model
Neonate	Physiological	Most mammals
Prolonged cholestasis (e.g., biliary atresia)	Impaired biliary Cu excretion	Bile duct ligation
Wilson's disease	Absent *trans*-Golgi Cu exporter	LEC rat Toxic milk mouse ATP7B knockout mice
Infantile copper toxicosis (e.g., ICC, Tyrolean childhood cirrhosis	Increased Cu ingestion, ? + other genetic or toxic factors	None
Sporadic copper-related cirrhosis	Unknown	
Human analogue not known	*MURR1* (*COMMD1*) mutations	Bedlington terrier disease
	Unknown	Physiologically and apparently harmless in some species (mute swan; white perch)[3]

ICC, Indian childhood cirrhosis; LEC, Long–Evans Cinnamon.

The copper chaperone for superoxide dismutase (CCS) carries copper to Cu,Zn-SOD, an important protector against cell injury by reactive oxygen species. Amyotrophic lateral sclerosis is a progressive lethal disorder of large motor neurons. In 20% of familial cases, it is due to a defect in Cu,Zn-SOD1. CCS interacts with and attempts to deliver copper to the defective SOD1, even when the enzyme cannot readily accept it, resulting in Cu-induced toxicity.[17]

Cox17p chaperones copper to the mitochondrion, where it is essential for the assembly of cytochrome *c* oxidase (COX), the terminal enzyme of the energy-transducing respiratory chain. COX has 13 subunits, and an additional 30 proteins

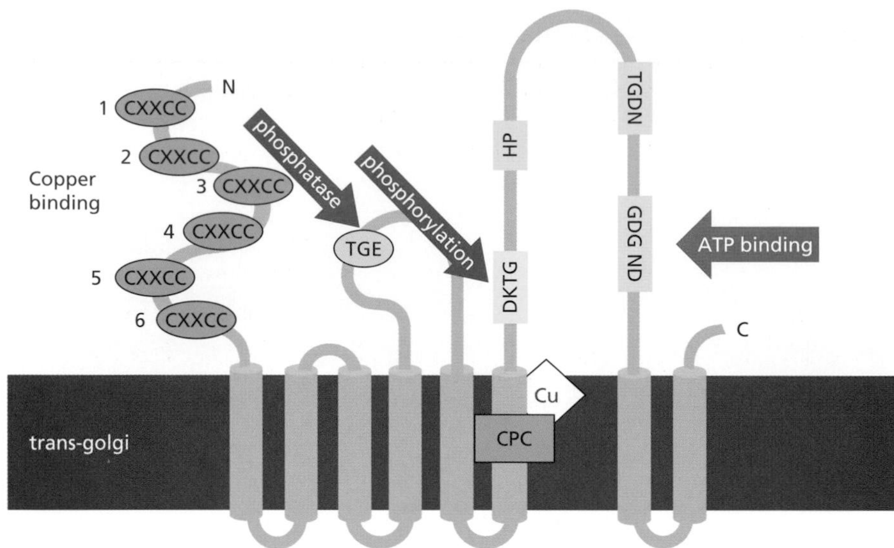

Figure 14.1 ATP7B has eight transmembrane domains that secure the protein in the *trans*-Golgi membrane. The $CPC_{983-985}$ motif in the sixth transmembrane domain reversibly binds copper to facilitate its translocation through the membrane. The ATP binding site G_{1266}DGVND, the phosphorylation domain D_{1027}KTG, and the phosphatase domainTGE$_{858-860}$ are invariant features of P-type ATPases. Six copper-binding sites (CXXC) lie in the N-terminal region.

are required for COX assembly. CoxI and CoxII contain copper. Five proteins (Cox11, Cox17, Cox19, Cox23, and Sco1/2) have been implicated in their synthesis and copper incorporation.[18] Cox17 (locus 3q) is a soluble metallochaperone localized both in the cytosol and in the mitochondrial intermembranous space. Cox17-null mouse embryos died between embryonic days 8.5 and 10.[19] Sco1/2 and Cox11 function downstream as membrane proteins in copper insertion into Cu_A and Cu_B, respectively. *SCO2* mutations are associated with neonatal encephalocardiomyopathy, and *SCO1* mutations with neonatal hepatic failure and ketoacidotic coma.[20] Cox19, also involved in yeast Cu insertion, has a human homolog,[21] but its function and that of Cox23 are less clear. A patient with features suggestive of mitochondrial cytopathy and repeatedly low copper and ceruloplasmin levels in whom no mutations were found, but in whom remarkable clinical and biochemical improvement followed copper histidinate supplementation, shows that there are other copper transport proteins yet to be discovered.[22]

The Wilson's disease protein, ATP7B

The Wilson's disease gene is on chromosome 13. It codes for a copper-transporting P-type ATPase, ATP7B, one of a family of transmembrane proteins[23] that mediate the translocation of cations across cellular membranes, often against concentration gradients. Mammals have two copper-translocating P-type ATPases, ATP7B and the Menkes disease protein ATP7A (Table 14.3). Common features are an ATP-binding site (GDGIND), a phosphorylation domain (DKTGT), a phosphatase domain (TGE), eight transmembrane regions, six Cu-binding sites in the N-terminal region, and a conserved Cys-Pro-X motif (X = Cys, His, or Ser) Cu-binding domain in the cation transduction channel in the sixth transmembrane domain (Figure 14.2). ATP7B is expressed predominantly in hepatocytes, but also in regions of the brain, breast, and placenta, while ATP7A is expressed in most extrahepatic tissues, but not the liver.

Function of ATP7B

ATP7B (reviewed in Bartee and Lutsenko[24]) has two functions: to translocate Cu into the *trans* Golgi for the synthesis of ceruloplasmin; and to export copper from the cell. Copper binding[14,25,26] stimulates ATP binding, phosphorylation of an aspartic acid at position 1027, copper translocation, and trafficking.[27] ATP binds via an adenosine buried in the cleft near residues H1069, R1151, and D1164 of ATP7B, which is brought into the vicinity of D1027 (asp 1027) by relative domain motions.[28,29] ATP binding and phosphorylation of the aspartic acid drives protein conformational changes, leading to the translocation of the bound cations across the lipid bilayer. The reaction cycle is completed with dephosphorylation by an intrinsic phosphatase activity (the TGE motif), returning the pump to its original conformation to allow further cation binding and translocation. In situations of low copper concentration, ATP7B resides in the membrane of the *trans*-Golgi. Copper loading causes it to migrate toward the canalicular membrane. This trafficking is correlated with the phosphorylation/dephosphorylation cycle. In the hepatocyte, ATP7B traffics to pericanalicular vesicles, which have not yet been characterized and are possibly novel compartments that sequester excess copper and undergo a mechanism similar to lysosomal exocytosis to expel their luminal contents into bile.[30] By contrast, the Menkes protein traffics to the basolateral membrane.

Ceruloplasmin

The blue copper-containing enzyme ceruloplasmin (Cp) is a ferroxidase, the function of which is best demonstrated by the effects of its deficiency in aceruloplasminemia (Table 14.4). The low plasma ceruloplasmin concentrations seen in WD

Table 14.3 Wilson's disease and Menkes disease.

	Wilson's disease	Menkes disease
Synonym	Hepatolenticular degeneration	Kinky hair, steely hair
Inheritance	Autosomal recessive	X-linked
Gene locus	13q14.3	Xq13.3
Gene	*ATP7B*	*ATP7A*
Tissue expression	Liver, kidney, placenta, brain	All tissues except liver
Cellular location of P-type ATPase	*trans*-Golgi, trafficking toward bile canalicular membrane	*trans*-Golgi, trafficking to plasma membrane
Biochemistry	Cu trapped in hepatocytes Impaired ceruloplasmin synthesis Basal ganglia Cu deposition Cu deposition in eye	Cu trapped in enterocytes Systemic Cu deficiency Impaired copper enzyme synthesis
Pathology	Hepatic damage Basal ganglia dysfunction Kayser–Fleischer rings	Abnormal connective tissue, and cerebral vasculature
Phenotypic variability		*Severe:* Menkes unresponsive to Cu-his treatment *Mild:* Occipital horn syndrome
Animal models	LEC rat Toxic milk mouse Knockout mouse	Mouse mutants (mottled, brindled)

LEC, Long–Evans Cinnamon.

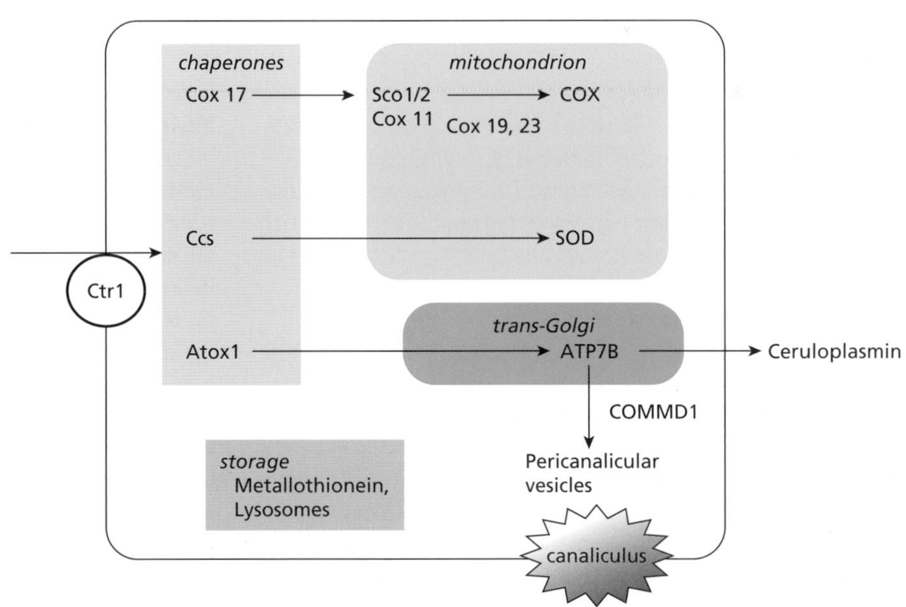

Figure 14.2 Pathways of copper through the hepatocyte. After uptake by Ctr1, copper is chaperoned to its sites of action: by cox17 to the mitochondrion for the synthesis of cytochrome oxidase (COX), with the participation of assembly proteins Sco1/2, cox11, cox19, cox23; by CCS (copper chaperone for superoxide dismutase) to superoxide dismutase; and by atox1 to the Wilson's disease protein ATP7B in the *trans*-Golgi. Copper loading of ATP7B induces trafficking to pericanalicular vesicles, with the participation of *COMMD1*. ATP7B passes copper to apoceruloplasmin for export. The tripeptide glutathione, the 10K protein metallothionein, and insoluble deposits in lysosomes store excess copper.

are not associated with an obvious disturbance of iron metabolism. In its synthesis, Cp is produced first as a precursor, which is glycosylated in the secretory compartment to the apoprotein, into which copper is introduced.[31] Apo-Cp has a short plasma half-life in humans, although it is readily detectable in the ATP7B knockout mouse. Cp is an "acute-phase reactant," in that its serum concentration rises in inflammatory states. The mechanism of this is not known,

Table 14.4 Aceruloplasminemia.

Inheritance	Autosomal-recessive
Clinical features	Dementia, dysarthria, dystonia, diabetes mellitus, onset age 40–60 y
Pathology	Iron deposition in liver, pancreas, and brain Neuronal loss, gliosis
Biochemistry	Plasma ceruloplasmin and Cu very low: hepatic Cu normal Plasma Fe low; hepatic Fe raised Basal ganglia Fe deposition shown on MRI
Cause	Failure of ceruloplasmin synthesis
Gene locus	3q25
Described mutations	5-bp insertion in exon 7 nt2389delG in exon 13
Treatment	None

MRI, magnetic resonance imaging.

but it might be important in increasing the delivery of copper to macrophages, where copper may participate in the generation of reactive oxygen species in phagosomes.

Most serum copper is in Cp. Non-Cp copper includes a fraction bound to albumin, and to a putative high-molecular-weight carrier, transcuprein. Canine albumen lacks a copper-binding site, and this may contribute to the copper-related liver disease in a number of breeds.

COMMD1

A mutation in the gene *COMMD1* (previously called *MURR1*) is responsible for the copper toxicosis of Bedlington terriers.[32] *COMMD1* interacts with ATP7B and may participate in the cellular copper excretion pathway.[33] Mutations in *COMMD1* have been sought but not found in WD.[34–36]

The cellular prion protein ($PrP^{(C)}$)

$PrP^{(C)}$ is a normal cell-surface glycoprotein, which in the prion diseases becomes an infectious, conformationally altered isoform ($PrP^{(Sc)}$). The physiological functions of $PrP^{(C)}$ include cellular uptake or binding of copper ions. $PrP^{(C)}$ is strongly expressed in the placenta in the first trimester, together with Ctr1, ATP7A, ATP7B, and COMMD1.[37] There is controversy as to whether copper-bound $PrP^{(C)}$ is an antioxidant supporting neuronal function or a pro-oxidant leading to neural damage.[38–40]

A $PrP^{(C)}$ polymorphism at codon 129 results in either methionine or valine. In one study of WD patients, homozygosity for the 129M allele was associated with later onset of neurological symptoms,[41] and in another with significantly more severe neurological symptoms in elderly patients.[42]

Table 14.5 Biochemical diagnosis of Wilson's disease.

	Normal	Wilson's disease
Plasma ceruloplasmin (mg/L)	> 200	< 200 in 85–90% of cases
Urine Cu pre-penicillamine		
μmol/24 h	< 1.25	> 1.25
μg/24 h	< 100	> 100
Urine Cu after penicillamine		
μmol/24 h	< 25	> 25
μg/24 h	< 1600	> 1600*
Liver copper (μg/g dry weight)	15–50	> 250
Serum copper (μM)	11–24	Low, normal or high
Free copper (μM)	< 1.6	> 7

* See text for discussion of the penicillamine challenge test.

Normal values

Normal values for copper-related parameters are shown in Table 14.5. The neonate differs from these values in having low plasma ceruloplasmin and copper, and a raised hepatic copper concentration, with values of up to 450 mg/g dry weight at birth, falling to adult values (< 50 mg/g) by 6 months. The newborn thus resembles the patient with Wilson's disease. This state presumably allows the fetus to store liver copper during gestation. It also makes a biochemical diagnosis of Wilson's disease impossible before 3 months of age.

Wilson's disease (OMIM 277900)

History[43]

Clinical descriptions of WD by Gowers, Strumpell, and Ormerod between 1888 and 1890 preceded Wilson's 1911 description of four patients with dysarthria, tremor, and progressive movement disorder who at postmortem had lenticular nucleus cavitation and cirrhosis. Kayser and Fleischer independently described a pigmented corneal ring in neurological patients in 1902–3. Excess hepatic copper was found by Rumpel in 1913, and Hall coined the term "hepatolenticular degeneration" in 1921 and described autosomal-recessive inheritance. In 1952, Scheinberg and Gitlin demonstrated low plasma levels of ceruloplasmin, but attempts to treat the disease with ceruloplasmin proved fruitless. Dimercaprol ("British anti-Lewisite,." BAL) was shown in the early 1950s to produce clinical improvement. In 1953, Walshe found dimethylcysteine (penicillamine) in the urine of a penicillin-treated liver patient, and 2 years later gave it to a patient with Wilson's disease to increase copper excretion after trying it on himself. Sheep were noted to be protected against copper toxicity by a high dietary molybdenum content, shown later to be due to the formation of ammonium tetrathiomolybdate in the rumen. Schouwink in 1961 noted evidence that zinc sulfate could induce copper deficiency in sheep and showed negative copper balance and clinical improvement in patients. Hoogenraad studied zinc treatment intensively, and in 1979[44] described resolution of Kayser–Fleischer (KF) rings with zinc. In 1969, Walshe gave triethylenetetramine hydrochloride to patients intolerant of penicillamine.[45] In 1986, Walshe suggested the use of ammonium tetrathiomolybdate in patients, and Brewer's subsequent studies have described its effect. The WD gene locus was shown to be linked to esterase D on chromosome 13 by a study of three kindreds in the Middle East.[46] January 1993 saw publication of the gene for Menkes disease, *ATP7A*,[47] and later in the same year three groups[48–51] published a homologous gene for Wilson's disease (*ATP7B*). Subsequent research has clarified the functions of ATP7B, intracellular copper chaperones, ceruloplasmin,[52] and COMMD1.[53] Animal models—both naturally occurring, such as the LEC rat[54] and the toxic milk mouse,[55] or created by gene knockout[56]—have been exploited. Genetic epidemiology has included identification of many mutations in large populations,[57] and the behavior of particular mutations in isolated communities such as Sardinia.[58]

Recent reviews of WD include Medici *et al.*[59] and Ala *et al.*[60]

Clinical features

The prevalence in Europe is reportedly 12–18 per million (approximately one in 50 000 to one in 80 000).[61] Wilson's disease may present in many different ways (Table 14.6). Adding together various series, the relative proportions of the four major presentations in 400 patients were: hepatic 20%; hepatic and neurological 20%; neurological or psychiatric 50%; and 10% other causes. However, since these surveys were from adult neurological units, they almost certainly underestimate the frequency of childhood hepatic cases—in particular failing to recognize cases of fulminant WD in childhood. The EuroWilson database will produce more accurate incidence figures.[62] WD may present at all ages—in infancy by the accidental discovery of abnormal liver function tests,[63] or as late as the eighth decade[64]—but the majority of patients present at the age of 6–12 years with liver disease, or during adolescence or early adult life with neurological or psychiatric manifestations.

Hepatic manifestations

The hepatic manifestations of Wilson's disease may be of any variety and severity (Table 14.6). The progression may be slow or very rapid. The important practical message therefore is: suspect Wilson's disease in any child with undiagnosed liver disease.

Table 14.6 Modes of presentation of Wilson's disease.

Asymptomatic	Detected during screening of family members
Hepatic (usually age 4–12 y)	Abnormal liver function tests, even as early as the first year of life Incidental finding of hepatomegaly Hepatomegaly or abnormal liver function tests identified during examination of a neurologically affected patient Insidious onset of vague symptoms followed by jaundice Acute hepatitis Chronic hepatitis Acute hepatic failure with hemolysis, with or without encephalopathy Portal hypertension: bleeding varices Decompensated cirrhosis
Neurological and psychiatric (in adolescents and adults)	Abnormalities of speech Mood/behavior changes Incoordination (handwriting deteriorates) Deteriorating school work Resting and intention tremors Dysarthria, excessive salivation Dysphagia, mask-like facies
Hematological	Acute hemolytic anemia
Renal	Renal tubular dysfunction (Fanconi, RTA, aminoaciduria) Renal calculi
Skeletal	Rickets/osteomalacia Arthropathy

RTA, renal tubular acidosis.

Acute liver failure in Wilson's disease (ALF-WD)

The first presentation in a previously apparently well child may be the appearance of jaundice and hepatitis, followed rapidly by coagulopathy (international normalized ratio ≥ 2) and encephalopathy. There may be a history of previous episodes of jaundice that resolved, or of a previous episode of hemolytic anemia.

There are some difficulties concerning the definition of acute liver failure (see Chapter 7). Children with WD and liver failure are often found to have cirrhosis in the explanted or postmortem liver. They have therefore had an acute deterioration in an already diseased liver, but because their liver disease was asymptomatic, they may fulfil the "adult" criteria for diagnosing fulminant liver failure: acute liver failure with coagulopathy and encephalopathy without preexisting liver disease and within 8 weeks of the onset of clinical liver disease. Secondly, encephalopathy may be difficult to diagnose or exclude in young children at an early stage. These difficulties are reflected in the slightly different definitions of acute liver failure used in different series. In the Birmingham series,[65] the criteria were prothrombin time (PT) ≥ 24 s prolonged or international normalized ratio (INR) ≥ 2.0 and hepatic encephalopathy without preexisting liver disease and within 8 weeks of the onset of clinical liver disease. WD was responsible for two of 97 cases. In the Pediatric Acute Liver Failure Group (PALF) registry, it was defined as biochemical evidence of acute liver injury with no known evidence of chronic liver disease and a coagulopathy of PT ≥ 15 s prolonged (INR ≥ 1.5) and encephalopathy, or a more severe coagulopathy (PT ≥ 20 s) without encephalopathy. Metabolic causes, mainly WD and mitochondrial, accounted for 22 of 348 children.[66]

There are reports of acute liver failure in WD being apparently precipitated by hepatitis E, hepatitis A, or measles, but in the majority no precipitant is recognized. Whilst adult series show a female preponderance, pediatric series do not,[67] probably because most cases are prepubertal.

Pointers to the diagnosis of WD in acute liver failure are:

- KF rings, which if present on slit-lamp examination make the diagnosis almost certain, but if absent do not exclude it; they are rare in childhood.
- A family history of WD, or parental consanguinity; again, this is unusual.
- Neurologic features of WD are rare in childhood, although slurred or slow speech may be a feature.
- Jaundice.
- Hemolysis.
- A high bilirubin (> 300 μmol/L) and relatively low transaminases (100–500 IU/L) and alkaline phosphatase (< 600 IU/L).[68]

A low alkaline phosphatase has been a frequent finding in adult and pediatric series of acute WD. A ratio of alkaline phosphatase (IU/L) to total bilirubin (mg/dL)[69] < 2 showed good discriminative power in some series,[70] although not all.[71] The poorer performance in pediatric series may be due to the contribution of the bone isoenzyme. The low alkaline phosphatase is unexplained.[72]

Without transplantation, survival from acute liver failure in WD with encephalopathy is extremely unlikely.[69] The diagnosis of WD may not be concluded before transplantation.[73]

Chronic hepatitis and WD

Children with a more insidious onset of liver disease may be difficult to distinguish from those with autoimmune hepatitis. The presence of low-titer autoantibodies, presumed to be secondary to exposure of antigens by hepatocyte necrosis, may cause confusion.[74] Cutaneous features of autoimmunity are usually absent, and plasma immunoglobulins are usually not raised. However, patients have been described in whom more convincing features of autoimmune hepatitis were present and an initial diagnosis of autoimmune disease led to treatment with steroids, with or without azathioprine, with initial improvement. In patients with autoimmune hepatitis, thorough screening for WD is therefore necessary.

Acute hepatitis

Patients diagnosed with WD may give a history of an "acute hepatitis"—an episode of jaundice and malaise from which they recovered. Whilst some of these may have been episodes of hemolysis or viral hepatitis, WD should always be excluded in the child with seronegative acute hepatitis.

Neurological presentation

In older children, the first symptoms may be neurological or psychiatric or both. They may develop insidiously or precipitously. Difficulty with speech is often reported. Movement disorders include tremors, poor coordination, and loss of fine-motor control, chorea, or choreoathetosis. The intention tremor may be initially unilateral, then becomes coarse, generalized, and incapacitating ("wing-beat" tremor). Spastic dystonia presents with a parkinsonian, mask-like facies, rigidity, and gait disturbance. Pseudobulbar involvement causes drooling and dysphagia. Features that are not usually present in WD are corticospinal or cerebellar signs, and abnormalities of the peripheral nerves, skeletal muscle, or cranial nerves. Neurologic WD patients have been classified into three groups:

- Pseudoparkinsonian, where bradykinesia predominates and cognitive impairment may occur.
- Pseudo-sclerotic—i.e., like multiple sclerosis, with prominent tremor.
- Dyskinetic.

The age of onset and the speed of progression are very variable, with some patients rapidly deteriorating to a chair-bound life with severe movement disorder while others continue with relatively mild symptoms.

The psychiatric disorders are also highly variable. Depression is common. Neurotic behavior includes phobias, compulsive behaviors, aggression, or antisocial behavior. Cognitive deterioration may also occur, with worsening school performance, poor memory, difficulty in abstract thinking, and shortened attention span. Pure psychotic disorders are uncommon.

The differential diagnosis of neuropsychiatric disease in the presence of liver disease includes: (i) late presentation of Niemann–Pick disease type C, particularly if splenomegaly is a feature; (ii) Lafora disease; and (iii) congenital disorders of glycosylation.

Hemolysis

Coombs-negative hemolysis may be the initial presentation, sometimes apparently precipitated by infection or drugs. There may be a history of a previous undiagnosed hemolytic episode in patients presenting with hepatic or neurological features, and hemolysis may be prominent in fulminant Wilson's disease.

Ophthalmic abnormalities

The KF ring is a gold or gray-brown opacity in the peripheral cornea (Figure 14.3). It first develops superiorly in the cornea (at the 12-o'clock position), then inferiorly, and finally in the horizontal meridian. It represents a deposit of copper and sulfur-rich granules in the Descemet membrane, and is reversible with treatment. Additional later ocular findings in Wilson's disease include sunflower cataracts, saccadic pursuit movements, loss of accommodation response, and apraxia of opening the eyelid.

Renal abnormalities

Renal tubular abnormalities are frequent and include glycosuria, aminoaciduria, renal tubular acidosis, impaired phosphate reabsorption, or a full-blown renal Fanconi syndrome. They are the presumed consequence of tubular copper deposition. Glomerular dysfunction is less frequent, but proteinuria may be exacerbated by penicillamine. Recurrent hypokalemic muscle weakness, hyperoxaluria, renal calculi, and nephrocalcinosis are uncommon features.

Skeletal manifestations

Copper-mediated oxidative damage to collagen probably underlies the arthritis that occurs in a small number of patients with Wilson's disease. The secondary effects of renal tubular phosphate leak and hepatic osteodystrophy are likely to be the cause of the radiological abnormalities, such as rickets or osteoporosis, that occur in a larger percentage. Skeletal complications appear to be more frequent in Asian/Indian patients.

Pathology

The earliest ultrastructural abnormalities are seen in mitochondria, which are pleomorphic and show increased matrix density, separation of the normally apposed inner and outer membranes, and widening of intercristal spaces. These changes are sufficiently specific to be of diagnostic value.

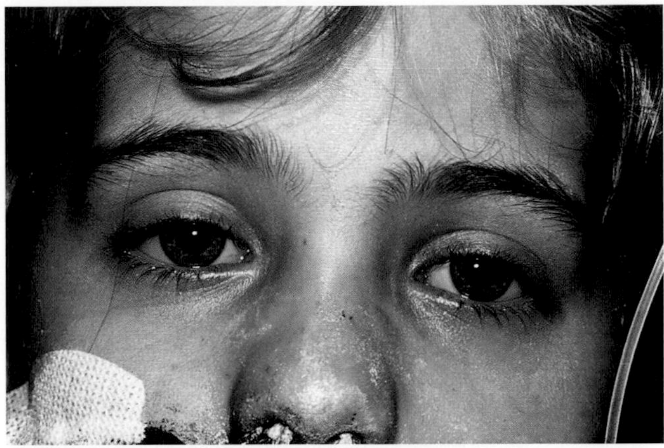

A

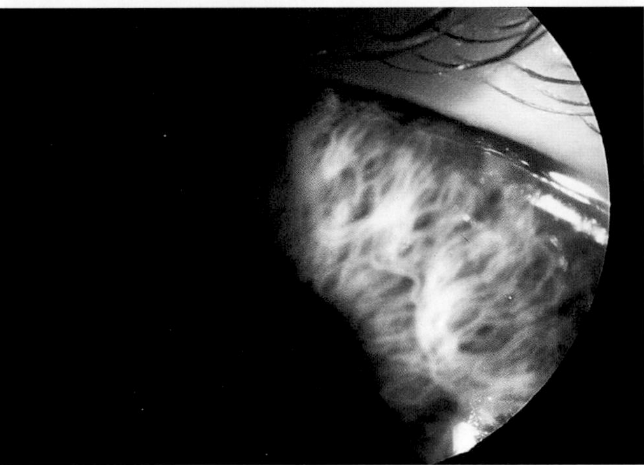

B

Figure 14.3 Wilson's disease may present with fulminant hepatitis (**A**), hemolysis, and low alkaline phosphatase. This young girl, who underwent successful transplantation, was found to have Kayser–Fleischer rings on slit-lamp examination (**B**).

The earliest histological changes comprise microvesicular and macrovesicular fatty deposition, glycogen-containing vacuoles in the nuclei of periportal hepatocytes, dense and enlarged peroxisomes. With progression, portal fibrosis and inflammation are seen. Children presenting with clinical liver disease may show a histological picture indistinguishable from autoimmune hepatitis with interportal fibrous bridging or frank cirrhosis (Figure 14.4). Features suggesting WD are:

- Fatty change
- Mallory bodies
- Glycogen-containing vacuoles in the nuclei
- Lipofuscin
- Copper staining
- Iron deposition in Kupffer cells in patients who have had hemolysis

Mallory bodies are irregularly shaped cytoplasmic inclusions comprising aggregated keratin 8, ubiquitin, heat-shock

A

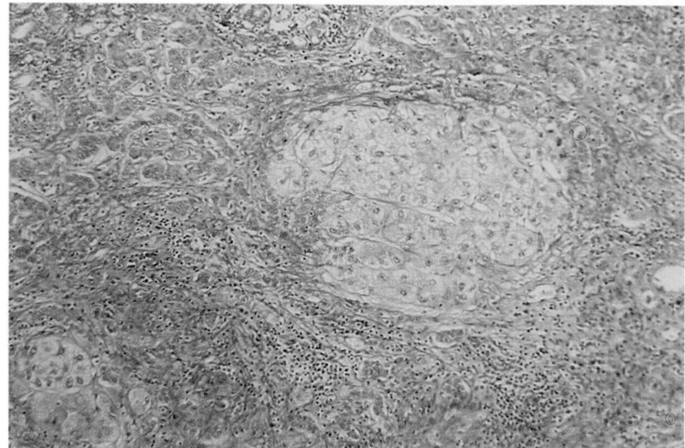

B

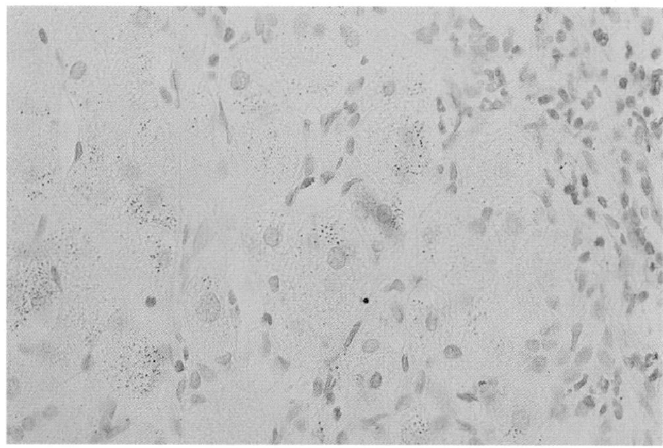

Figure 14.4 Liver biopsy demonstrated severe hepatitis and underlying cirrhosis (**A**). Copper storage was demonstrated using orcein staining (**B**).

proteins, and the stress protein p62, stabilized by transglutaminase cross-linking. Well-circumscribed homogeneous cytoplasmic eosinophilic globules lacking keratins also occur.[75]

In well-established liver disease, copper may be demonstrable by rhodanine or rubeanic staining. The elastin stains orcein and aldol fuchsin will then usually show granular staining, thought to represent lysosomal copper–protein polymer. It cannot be emphasized too strongly that these methods are negative in early cases, presumably because at that stage the copper is cytosolic and in low-molecular-weight complexes. The absence of histochemically demonstrable copper does not exclude a diagnosis of WD.

Liver copper in presymptomatic children is higher than in older symptomatic children.[76] This contradicts the common view that in WD, copper builds up in the liver to a level that causes damage, and suggests that some other factor initiates damage in the copper-laden liver. The relationship between copper and organelle damage remains unclear. In particular, it is unknown why some patients develop severe hepatic necrosis and others only minimal damage.

In contrast to hemochromatosis, WD is rarely associated with hepatoma.

WD heterozygotes may have a hepatic Cu of the order of 100–200 μg/g dry weight and mild histological portal tract changes, but there is no evidence of progression of liver disease.

Diagnosis

The first essential in making the diagnosis is to think of it. KF rings, if present, are highly suggestive, but:

- Are usually absent in children below 10 years with WD.
- At an early stage, will only be detected by slit-lamp examination (Figure 14.3B).
- Are difficult to see in brown or green eyes.
- Are not pathognomonic; they may rarely occur in copper overload due to chronic cholestasis.

Biochemical diagnosis

The biochemical diagnosis (Table 14.5) depends upon finding:

- A low plasma ceruloplasmin
- A raised urine copper, particularly after penicillamine
- A raised liver copper concentration

However, there are numerous pitfalls in these laboratory parameters, as outlined below.

Serum copper

Most plasma copper is within ceruloplasmin. In WD, serum copper may therefore be low because ceruloplasmin is low, or raised because hepatic necrosis releases "free" copper into the plasma, or somewhere in between. A normal plasma copper should never exclude a diagnosis of WD. In the patient treated with tetrathiomolybdate, serum copper remains high because complexed copper is retained.

Free (non-ceruloplasmin) serum copper is a theoretically attractive parameter, reflecting the portion of copper that is non–protein-bound, presumably released from the damaged liver, and presumably available to cause toxicity. It is calculated (in μmol/L) on the basis that 1 mg ceruloplasmin contains 3 μg or 3/63.5 μmol copper, and is approximately total Cu μM – (0.047 × ceruloplasmin mg/L). There are three major problems. First, it rests on the assumption that one molecule of ceruloplasmin contains six atoms of copper. Second, immunologically measured ceruloplasmin comprises both holo- and apoceruloplasmin, and the assumption that the amount of apoceruloplasmin is so small that it can be ignored is probably incorrect in WD. Third, it is calculated from two measured parameters and is thus subject to large error.

Ceruloplasmin

Various factors that may affect plasma ceruloplasmin have to be considered: plasma ceruloplasmin exceeds 200 mg/L in approximately 10% of WD cases. It is an acute-phase reactant, and will be elevated by hepatic or other inflammation. In cases with chronic histologically active hepatitis, ceruloplasmin may therefore initially be in the normal range, falling below 200 mg/L with treatment. Plasma ceruloplasmin may be low if overall hepatic protein synthesis is low, whether acutely as in fulminant failure, or in decompensated cirrhosis or in other situations of hypoproteinemia such as protein-losing enteropathy or severe malnutrition. A significant number of WD heterozygotes will have a plasma ceruloplasmin < 200 mg/L. Aceruloplasminemia may cause diagnostic confusion in neurological cases (Table 14.4), and an unknown percentage of normal individuals will be heterozygotes for aceruloplasminemia.

Urine copper

Urine copper may be raised in acute hepatitis, but is usually much higher in children with WD (Tables 14.5, 14.7). It is important to ensure an accurate 24-h urine collection of an uncontaminated sample. If the investigation is designed as a screen for WD, or as a basis for further testing, then 50 μg/24 h suggests WD, while a value of 100 μg/24 h, whilst less sensitive, carries a higher specificity.

A penicillamine challenge test gives greater discrimination. In the original description of this test in children with liver disease, penicillamine 0.5 g was given 12-hourly × 2. Urine copper exceeded 25 μmol/24 h in 15 of 17 patients with WD and one of 58 with other liver disorders.[77] A recent reevaluation confirms its usefulness in WD children with active liver disease, but shows very poor sensitivity in presymptomatic siblings. In the diagnostic scoring developed by an expert group, a postpenicillamine urine copper greater than five times the laboratory's normal upper limit is the stated cut-off (Table 14.7). In 24-h collections of urine during a second and third day of penicillamine treatment, the copper concentration may rise further, which is suggestive of the diagnosis, but this has not been formally evaluated. The penicillamine challenge has not been evaluated in neurologic cases. The difficulties in reliably collecting 24-h urines and the fact that the same dose is recommended for all ages are limitations to this test.

Liver copper

Copper may or may not be demonstrable in the liver. A liver copper > 250 μg/g dry weight (normal < 55 μg/g[78]) has been described as the gold standard diagnostic test, but it has limitations. Higher values are found in the newborn, settling to adult levels by 6 months. Prolonged cholestasis raises hepatic

Table 14.7 Diagnostic score in Wilson's disease, agreed at a consensus meeting.[144] In the EuroWilson database,[62] patients scoring ≥ 4 are accepted as having Wilson's disease.

Score	–1	0	1	2	4
Kayser–Fleischer rings		Absent		Present	
Neuropsychiatric symptoms suggestive of Wilson's disease (or typical brain MRI)		Absent		Present	
Coombs-negative hemolytic anemia + high serum Cu		Absent	Present		
Urinary copper (in the absence of acute hepatitis)		Normal	1–2 × ULN	> 2 × ULN, or > 5 × ULN 1 day after 2 × 0.5 g D-penicillamine	
Liver copper quantitative	Normal		< 5 × ULN	> 5 × ULN	
Rhodanine-positive hepatocytes (only if quantitative Cu measurement is not available)		Absent	Present		
Serum ceruloplasmin		> 0.2 g/L	0.1–0.2 g/L	< 0.1 g/L	
Disease-causing mutations detected		None	1		2

Assessment of the Wilson's disease diagnostic score:
0–1: unlikely
2–3: probable
4 or more: highly likely

MRI, magnetic resonance imaging; ULN, upper limit of normal.

copper by inhibiting its biliary excretion, and this may cause confusion in cases of autoimmune hepatitis with sclerosing cholangitis. In a study of adult liver biopsies, a value > 250 was found in only 95 of 114 patients with WD.[79] This may result from sampling error, particularly in the cirrhotic liver. Errors are reduced by providing a good-sized sample (1 cm of a biopsy core is desirable) and scrupulously preventing contamination.

Isotopic copper

Following an oral dose of labeled copper, two peaks in plasma activity are seen. The first, at around 4 h, represents newly absorbed copper, which is associated with albumin. The second, a slower rise, represents copper incorporation into ceruloplasmin. The radioisotopes ^{64}Cu or ^{67}Cu suffer from the disadvantages of a short half-life, limited availability, and radiation dosage. ^{65}Cu is infinitely stable and causes no radiation exposure, but requires the sophisticated technique of inductively coupled plasma mass spectrometry for analysis. This method is of some value in the diagnosis of the difficult case. Following a 3-mg dose of ^{65}Cu as copper sulfate in milk, blood samples are taken at 0, 4, 12, and 24 h. A 24 : 4-h activity ratio > 1 demonstrates normal ceruloplasmin synthesis and makes Wilson's disease unlikely. This test is now rarely performed.

Genetics

The WD gene, the *ATP7B* gene, comprises 80 000 base pairs on 21 protein-coding exons and 20 noncoding introns, plus an incompletely characterized promoter. It is transcribed and processed into a 7500-base mRNA, which is translated into the 1411 amino acid, 159 kDa ATPase. Many mutations have been found in WD patients, of which H1069Q (hist1069glu) is the commonest worldwide.

The H1069Q mutation (exon 14)

This is the most common mutation in patients from central, eastern, and northern Europe. Approximately 50–80% WD patients from these countries carry at least one allele with this mutation with an allele frequency of 30–70%.[57] Homozygote and heterozygote H1069Q frequencies are 39% and 48% in eastern Germany,[80] and 17% and 43% in Austria.[81] The H1069Q allele frequency is reported to be 57% in a Czech and Slovakian cohort,[82] 49% in Yugoslavia.[83] 35% in a largely neurologic series from Poland,[84] 38% in the United States,[85] and approximately 30% in the United Kingdom.[86] This distribution is consistent with the hypothesis that this mutation arose in eastern Europe. H1069Q is rare in Asian, Japanese, and Chinese patients.

The effect of the H1069Q sequence change is to prevent tight binding of ATP to the N domain of ATP7B. It does not alter the conformation of ATP7B. Structural studies of this domain show that residues H1069, G1099, G1101, I1102, G1149, and N1150 contribute to ATP binding,[29,87] and this area is the site of at least 30 known WD mutations affecting ATP binding or protein folding.[88]

H1069Q and genotype–phenotype correlation

Although it is common to find patients with the same genotype with different phenotypes, there is statistical evidence that H1069Q homozygotes are more likely to present at a later age and with neurological rather than hepatic disease. Amongst 70 Dutch patients, those who were homozygous or heterozygous for the H1069Q mutation presented more frequently with neurologic disease (63% and 43% vs. 15%), and at a later age (20.9 and 15.9 vs. 12.6 years) than patients without the H1069Q mutation. In a meta-analysis of 577 published patients, the odds ratio for neurologic presentation in homozygous or heterozygous H1069Q vs. non-H1069Q patients was 3.50 (95% CI, 2.01 to 6.09) and 2.13 (95% CI, 1.18 to 3.83), respectively, and the ages at presentation were 21.1, 19.2, and 16.5 years, respectively.[89] Some,[80,90] but not all,[82] other series support this association.

The Sardinian -441/-427del mutation

WD has an approximate incidence of one in 7000 live births in the Sardinian population. Molecular analysis of the WD chromosomes containing the most common haplotype showed a 15-nucleotide deletion in the promoter region.[58] Expression assays demonstrated a 75% reduction in the transcriptional activity of the mutated sequence in comparison with the normal control.[58] This -441/-427del mutation was found in 122 of 5290 neonatal blood spots in Sardinia.[91] This suggests a carrier frequency of 3.8%, which from the Hardy–Weinberg equation indicates a disease frequency of approximately one in 3000—at least twice the frequency of diagnosed cases. Because of wide confidence intervals, this must be interpreted cautiously, but it raises the important possibility of incomplete penetrance—i.e., that not all genotypically affected patients present with disease.

Other mutations

More than 300 mutations have been described.[92] Some are common in particular populations, such as Met645Arg in Spanish patients,[93] R778L in those from the Far East (China, South Korea, Japan, Taiwan[94]), and asp1279ser mutation in Costa Rican[85] patients. Many others are found at a low frequency.

Genetic testing strategy

A testing strategy must be developed for the population served. If one mutation is frequent, then direct testing is rapid and allows primary diagnosis. If there is a spectrum of mutations, then diagnosis is more challenging. Currently, most laboratories adopt a strategy of first sequencing the "hot-spot" exons for their population, which in the United Kingdom means exons 2, 8, 13–15, and 18–19. In a family in which it has not proved possible to identify mutations in a biochemically proven case, haplotype analysis makes it possible to determine with certainty whether the siblings are presymptomatic affected, heterozygote carriers, or unaffected.

Unlike Menkes syndrome, in which 22% of the mutations are sizable deletions, deletions are uncommon in WD. However, the possibility of a deletion must always be considered in apparent homozygotes; family studies should be performed to confirm that both parents are carriers.

Novel sequence changes may be disease-causing mutations or harmless polymorphisms. Approaches to distinguishing these are: seeking the sequence change in a panel of ethnically appropriate controls; species comparisons; toxicity testing in CHO cells using tetramethylbromide; transport complementation studies in yeast; and molecular modeling.

Diagnosis in practice

The diagnosis of Wilson's disease is difficult and depends on the clinical situation:

- In presymptomatic children, or neurological patients with mild abnormalities of liver function tests, ceruloplasmin will be low.
- In active liver disease, ceruloplasmin is less reliable, but postpenicillamine urine copper should be high.
- In acute liver failure, calculated serum free copper, baseline urine copper, and postpenicillamine copper should be high.

In all these situations, if a rapid test for H1069Q or the locally common mutation is available, a positive result supports the diagnosis and justifies starting treatment.

Treatment

Five drugs are available to treat the copper overload of WD: D-penicillamine, triethylenetetramine hydrochloride (trientine), zinc, ammonium tetrathiomolybdate, and BAL (Table 14.8). There are few randomized controlled clinical trials comparing agents.

Table 14.8 Drugs used in the treatment of Wilson's disease.

Drug	Dose
D-Penicillamine	20–35 mg/kg/day*
Triethylenetetramine dihydrochloride (trientine)†	2–12 y: 300 mg b.i.d. 12–18 years: 300–600 mg b.i.d.
Zinc acetate†	< 5 years: 25 mg b.i.d. 6–15 years: 25 mg t.d.s. > 16 y or if > 57 kg: 50 mg t.d.s.
Ammonium thiomolybdate	30 mg b.i.d.

* Should also have pyridoxine 50 mg/week.
† Should be administered 6 h apart to prevent chelation of zinc by trientine.

Penicillamine

Although "decoppering" was the rationale for initially using penicillamine, penicillamine treatment does not cause liver copper levels to fall to normal. It is therefore thought to "detoxify" the liver copper, by induction of metallothionein, favoring lysosomal sequestration (like zinc). Since the patient is not "decoppered," he or she remains at high risk of deterioration if treatment is discontinued. Numerous reports of rapid decline in hepatic function within 18–24 months of stopping penicillamine emphasize the need to maintain compliance.

DL-Penicillamine was associated with a high incidence of nephrotic syndrome and pyridoxine deficiency. D-Penicillamine is much less toxic, but nevertheless causes significant side effects in 5–10% of treated patients. These include:

- Skin rash, usually urticarial, occurring soon after commencing treatment, which usually responds to cessation of treatment and reintroduction gradually under steroid cover.
- Proteinuria, which is in most cases mild and does not require cessation of treatment. In a small number of patients, there may be an immune complex nephropathy leading to nephrotic syndrome.
- Marrow depression, particularly affecting platelet count.
- Systemic lupus erythematosus (SLE).
- Pyridoxine deficiency, particularly during growth or pregnancy.
- Effects on cutaneous collagen usually occurring after prolonged therapy, namely elastosis perforans serpiginosa and cutis laxa.

The most worrying adverse effect of penicillamine (and trientine) is the appearance of, or deterioration in, neurological dysfunction on starting treatment—well described in the patient with neurological features, and reported in cases without neurological signs.

Blood counts and urine testing for protein should be done fortnightly for the first 2 months then monthly for 6 months. Pyridoxine 50 mg/week should be given.

We have the longest clinical experience with penicillamine, but it is increasingly being replaced by trientine.

Trientine

Trientine was initially introduced as a second-line drug for patients intolerant of D-penicillamine. The majority of the above side effects do not occur with trientine, except for SLE. The most commonly reported side effect is sideroblastic anemia, particularly when given with zinc. Colitis, resolving on cessation of trientine, is also reported. Its introduction was initially limited by availability, licensing, and cost, but it is now an accessible and logical first-line treatment.

Zinc

The rationale for using zinc is that induction of metallothionein in intestinal cells will bind copper in the enterocyte and reduce absorption. Since zinc also powerfully induces hepatic metallothionein, like penicillamine, zinc is an attractive drug because it is more physiological than penicillamine or trientine, is of apparently low toxicity, and zinc sulfate is cheap. In high doses in animals it may cause pancreatic atrophy, but this has not been reported in humans. It may impair iron absorption. The principal practical problems are its unpalatability, and dyspeptic symptoms due to gastric irritation. Zinc acetate, which is less likely to cause these than zinc sulfate, is now commercially available and licensed (Wilzin), but is more expensive. Serum levels of amylase and lipase may rise because they are zinc-containing enzymes. Compliance can be checked by measuring the urinary zinc (> 2 mg/24 h). Overtreatment should be sought by monitoring urine copper and reducing the dose of zinc if it drops below 50 μg/24 h.

Tetrathiomolybdate (TM)

TM is a powerful copper chelator and became an effective veterinary therapy for ovine copper poisoning. Unlike the above drugs, it is able rapidly to bind copper already in tissues in an inert complex. Its clinical use is limited by toxicity—namely, marrow depression and, in growing animals, epiphyseal abnormalities. It may have a role in the initial treatment of neurological cases.

BAL

BAL (British anti-Lewisite, dimercaprol) was used for WD prior to the introduction of penicillamine. Given by intramuscular injection, it is painful and has many reported toxic side effects. Some authorities recommend its use in neurological cases refractory to other therapy.

Treatment regimens differ for the varying clinical scenarios described above.

Acute liver failure with encephalopathy

A child with acute liver failure and encephalopathy should be listed for urgent transplantation, and routine management of acute liver failure should be instituted (see Chapter 7). Trientine and zinc should be started, even if the diagnosis of WD is not certain, and be given 6 h apart to prevent chelation of zinc by trientine. If there is renal failure, excretion of the copper–drug complex will be impaired unless the child is dialyzed. There have been many attempts to remove copper from the WD-ALF patient. They depend on the hypothesis that nonceruloplasmin copper is largely albumin-bound and may be removed with consequent extraction of copper from the liver and reduced hepatic necrosis. There are reports of successful outcomes in teenage patients treated with plasmapheresis,[95] plasma exchange with continuous hemodiafiltration,[96] and albumen hemodialysis with continuous venovenous hemodiafiltration.[97] The Molecular Adsorbents Recirculating System (MARS) theoretically should remove albumin-bound copper by adsorption onto the MARSFlux membrane[98] and the toxins responsible for hepatic encephalopathy. There are anecdotal cases in which MARS alone or MARS with albumin–continuous venovenous hemofiltration (CVVH) have provided a successful bridge to transplantation.[98,99] Success is also reported for the Prometheus Fractionated Plasma Separation and Absorption (FPSA) system.[100] Given this evidence, it is reasonable to use MARS or Prometheus in a WD patient with ALF and encephalopathy if transplantation cannot be offered immediately, although randomized trials need to be carried out.

Liver failure without encephalopathy

The decision to list for transplant is more difficult if the child does not have encephalopathy, and it is necessary to balance the risk of rapid deterioration and encephalopathy, with the risk of removing a native liver which may recover with chelation therapy. The new Wilson's Predictive Index developed at King's College Hospital, London, is reported to be 93% sensitive and 98% specific, with a positive predictive value of 93% (Table 14.9).[67] If the score deteriorates, or is > 11, then the child should be listed urgently. A stable or improving score is an indication to continue with medical therapy.

Trientine and zinc should be started as above.[101]

Chronic hepatitis, acute hepatitis, cirrhosis with or without portal hypertension

Treatment regimens are based on single-center series rather than randomized controlled clinical trials[102–104] or agreed evidence-based guidelines. It is logical to use a combination of trientine and zinc acetate (Table 14.8). Once remission has been obtained, maintenance treatment with zinc acetate alone is possible.

Monitoring the effectiveness of and compliance with chelation therapy is difficult. Urine copper levels will rise to high values in the first 3 months, declining after 1 year of continued treatment. After this time, urine copper should be measured 6-monthly. A falling value suggests that patients may have discontinued the drug, whilst an unexpectedly very high value may suggest that they have restarted it recently in anticipation of the clinic visit. Effectiveness of therapy is monitored by biochemical liver function tests, which should show a steady improvement over the first months of treatment, and by serial liver biopsy. It is difficult to interpret liver copper levels in follow-up biopsies, since two effects are operative: (i) chelators remove that fraction of liver copper that is mobilizable, thus reducing liver copper; but (ii) both penicillamine and zinc induce metallothionein, which binds copper and may therefore cause liver copper concentration to rise. In interpreting serial liver copper levels, it is also important to remember that the right lobe tends to have higher values. For this reason, changes in hepatic inflammation are of more significance than changes

Table 14.9 Prognostic index in acute liver failure in Wilson's disease.

Score	Bilirubin (μmol/L)	INR	AST (IU/L)	WCC (× 10^9/L)	Albumin (g/L)
0	0–100	0–1.29	0–100	0–6.7	> 45
1	101–150	1.3–1.6	101–150	6.8–8.3	34–44
2	151–200	1.7–1.9	151–300	8.4–10.3	25–33
3	201–300	2.0–2.4	301–400	10.4–15.3	21–24
4	> 301	> 2.5	> 401	> 15.4	< 20

Sensitivity and specificity rates of 93% and 97%, and positive predictive value and negative predictive values of 92% and 97%, respectively, have been reported.[67]
A score > 11 indicates a need to list the patient for urgent liver transplantation.

in liver copper. Likewise, liver histology may rapidly decline despite no significant change in the hepatic copper concentration in the patient who discontinues treatment.

Neurological presentation

Neurological deterioration occurs in some patients at the start of treatment with penicillamine, trientine, or zinc.[105] This may be less likely using a regimen of 8 weeks of tetrathiomolybdate followed by zinc.[106,107] Given the lack of availability of tetrathiomolybdate and the lack of clinical experience other than in a research setting, patients will continue to receive zinc or a chelator. The practice of starting with a small dose of chelator and increasing slowly has logic, but there are no data to prove its benefit. Again, the choice between zinc and trientine lacks an evidence base.

Presymptomatic cases

With molecular methods, it is now easy to make the diagnosis of WD in unaffected siblings, even in the newborn period. It is believed that all genotypically affected patients are at risk of developing clinical disease at some time, though the evidence from Sardinia quoted above casts doubt on this assertion. The risk is difficult to quantify, because WD is so phenotypically variable, and some cases do not develop until late adult life. Even within sibships, there is phenotypic variability. Despite these caveats, treatment is currently to be recommended. Since clinically significant liver disease is not reported at ages < 3 years, treatment may logically begin at that age. Zinc, which is the least toxic and most physiological agent, is the treatment of choice. Presymptomatic treatment should prevent liver and neurological damage, but patients should be monitored for evidence of disease and for copper deficiency or pancreatic dysfunction.

Pregnancy

The danger of discontinuing treatment during pregnancy has been amply demonstrated. There are numerous reports of successful pregnancy in women treated with penicillamine. Early reports of unusual connective-tissue changes in babies born to women who were receiving penicillamine for cystinuria and rheumatoid arthritis suggest that zinc is a safer option during pregnancy.

Assuming no consanguinity, the fetus will be an obligate heterozygote. The risk that the baby will have WD is of the order of one in 300 for a population with a disease frequency of one in 100 000. It is recommended that the baby is allowed to breastfeed, but the full blood count and ceruloplasmin are followed to exclude hematological evidence of copper deficiency and confirm the physiological rise in ceruloplasmin.

Liver transplantation

Liver transplantation is indicated for those children who do not respond to therapy, or who have fulminant or advanced liver failure and/or portal hypertension (Chapter 21). The results of liver transplantation in WD are good. Following liver transplantation, the recipient takes on the biochemistry of the donor so far as plasma copper and ceruloplasmin are concerned. If a live related donor is a parent—i.e., an obligate heterozygote—this will be reflected in post-transplantation ceruloplasmin.[108–110] Since there is no evidence of morbidity in the heterozygote, this is not a concern.

If the neurologic abnormalities in WD are due to intrinsic abnormalities of copper metabolism in the brain, then liver transplantation will not improve them or alter the likelihood of their appearance or progression. If they are due to overspill of copper from a copper-laden liver, then liver transplantation should benefit the brain also. The neurologic outcome of liver transplant recipients is therefore of great scientific as well as clinical interest. Unfortunately, a clear picture does not appear from the literature.[111] Patients have been reported in whom transplantation has appeared to arrest neurologic deterioration or achieve improvement,[109,112–115] as well as others in whom it had the opposite effect.[108,116]

Likely explanations for this are that in the patient with liver failure, neurologic abnormalities may be contributed to by hepatic encephalopathy, whilst events surrounding transplant or subsequent immunosuppression may contribute to ongoing neurologic abnormality. Patients with WD may be more susceptible to the neurological side effects of tacrolimus.[117] The practical conclusion to be drawn is that neurologic abnormalities in a patient with severe liver disease are not a contraindication to liver transplantation, but that severe neurological disease in the absence of hepatopathy is not an indication for liver transplantation.

The future

WD should be an excellent candidate for correction by hepatocyte transplantation or gene therapy, because the normal or corrected hepatocytes should have a survival advantage over their copper-laden neighbors. Proof of this principle has been achieved in animal models, notably the Long–Evans Cinnamon (LEC) rat, in which a deletion of at least a 900-bp fragment in the 3′-terminal region of the rat homologue of *ATP7B* eliminates the normal gene product,[118] and the toxic milk mouse (tx),[119] which has a point mutation (A4066G).[55] Hepatocyte transplantation has shown encouraging results in the LEC rat[120–122] and the toxic milk mouse;[123,124] bone marrow stem cell in the tx mouse;[125] lentiviral gene transfer[126] and adenovirus-mediated transfer [127–129] in the LEC rat. A new approach may be to interfere with the mechanism by which copper causes cell damage.[1] Ribosomal read-through by PTC124 potentially allows "gene correction" for nonsense mutations.[130]

More immediate measures to improve patient outcomes include increasing awareness of WD, encouraging investigation for WD in patients with early symptoms possibly caused by WD, ensuring sibling screening is performed, mounting randomized treatment trials, and addressing compliance with therapy. A European clinical database[62] of WD patients may improve outcomes by evaluating the feasibility of setting up randomized trials.

Non-Wilsonian copper-related cirrhosis in childhood

Infantile copper toxicoses, in which in infants and young children developed rapidly progressive and fatal disorders caused by excessive copper ingestion, are now largely of historical interest, as the feeding patterns that produced them now rarely occur. They are therefore only described here briefly. These were:

- Indian childhood cirrhosis (ICC), in which copper was acquired from milk that had been heated in brass utensils.[131–134]
- Tyrolean childhood cirrhosis, in which copper was acquired from diluted sweetened milk that had been boiled in copper utensils, and for which a strong genetic susceptibility was demonstrated.[135–137]
- Sporadic childhood copper-related cirrhosis, in which copper was acquired from water used to make up infant feeds, that water having taken up copper from plumbing. Characteristic of this group was the use of a private well for water.

ICC

ICC had an incidence of one in 4000 rural live births, presenting at a mean age of 18 months. It affected boys more than girls, rural families more frequently than urban ones, middle-income families more frequently than very poor, and Hindus more frequently than Muslims. The onset was usually insidious, with abdominal distension, malaise, and irritability, progressing to jaundice, ascites, edema and respiratory distress, and death. The liver was large and very hard. The histology was characteristic, showing necrosis of hepatocytes with ballooning and Mallory hyaline; pericellular intralobular fibrosis; an inflammatory infiltrate; poor regenerative activity, to the extent that there was often little nodular change; absence of fatty change; absence of cholestasis until an advanced stage; and granular orcein staining. There was severe ultrastructural damage, with prominent end-stage copper-rich and sulfur-rich lysosomes, and severe morphological abnormalities of mitochondria. The etiology was shown to be the early introduction of cow or buffalo milk feeds contaminated with copper from untinned brass utensils. Penicillamine given early at a dosage of 20 mg/kg/day reduced the mortality from 92% to 53%. Resolution of liver disease, but the development of inactive micronodular cirrhosis, occurred. Liver copper concentrations fell to near normal levels. ICC was preventable by a change in infant feeding practice, and it has now virtually disappeared.

Tyrolean childhood cirrhosis

Between 1900 and 1974, 138 infants died in an area of the Austrian Tyrol[137] from an illness similar to ICC in its age of presentation, clinical features, short survival, and high mortality. Unlike ICC, the sexes were affected equally. These infants came from isolated farming households where the practice was to make up an infant feed from cows' milk, diluted and sweetened with sugar, and heated in a copper vessel. Siblings were often affected, parental consanguinity was common, and the segregation ratio was 0.2159. Since some infants fed in the same way escaped the disease, it was hypothesized that both genetic and environmental factors were involved.

Sporadic infantile copper toxicosis related to well water

Individual cases in Australia,[138] Germany,[139] and the United Kingdom[140] have resembled ICC. All of the patients affected have died or required transplantation, and all have been born in a rural household and have received milk made up with well water that has a low pH and has acquired high copper concentrations from copper plumbing or water heaters. In the well-documented cases, the water copper concentration has been hig. No cases occurred in houses receiving a regulated water supply.

Childhood copper toxicosis without excess copper ingestion

Histological features resembling ICC, and raised hepatic copper, were seen in four siblings aged 4.5–6 years who died with progressive liver disease.[141] Although these children were older than those with ICC, they had a similar clinical course and liver copper as high as 2083 mg/g dry weight. In these and in other reports of an ICC-like disorder,[142,143] there was no identifiable cause of excess copper ingestion. Amongst the small number of infants with ICC now being seen in India, are some with no history of exposure to copper-contaminated feeds.

Case study

An 11-year-old girl, Joanna, presented with jaundice and malaise for 1 week. A year earlier, she had had a transient illness with jaundice, but tests for hepatitis were negative. She was alert and had no neurological signs, KF rings, or hepatosplenomegaly. Her serum total bilirubin was 270 μmol/L, total conjugated bilirubin 132 μmol/L; aspartate aminotransferase (AST) 130 U/L, INR 2.8. The hemoglobin was 9 g/dL, with a film showing hemolysis and a negative Coombs test. The suspicion of WD was strengthened by finding a plasma ceruloplasmin of 0.08 g/L and a urine copper of 170 μg/24 h. Serum copper was 15 μmol/L (normal), so that calculated free copper was 11.2 μmol/L (high).

Penicillamine was given at 0 and 12 hours. At a second 24-h urine collection, the urine copper was 1700 μg/24 h (26.8 μmols/24 h). She therefore had a diagnostic score of 5 (WD highly likely). Treatment with zinc acetate and trientine was started.

Her prognostic score was 10, so she was not immediately listed for transplantation.

Calculation of free copper: free serum copper = total copper (μmol/L) – [ceruloplasmin (g/L) × 47.2] = 15 – [0.08 × 47.2] = 11.2 μmol/L.

Diagnostic score:

- Kayser–Fleischer rings: 0
- Neuropsychiatric symptoms: 0
- Coombs negative hemolytic anemia + high serum copper: 1
- Urinary copper (in the absence of acute hepatitis): 2
- Liver copper, quantitative: 0
- Rhodanine positive hepatocytes: 0
- Serum ceruloplasmin: 2
- Disease-causing mutations detected: 0
- *Total:* 5

Prognostic score:

- Bilirubin 270 μmol/L) 3
- INR 2.8 4
- AST 130 IU/L 1
- White cell count (WCC) 5.0 × 10^9/L 0
- Albumin 28 g/L 2
- *Total:* 10

Over the following week, her prognostic score deteriorated because her WCC and AST were rising. She became irritable, aggressive, and confused. She was listed urgently and received a liver. The explanted liver revealed cirrhosis, steatosis, necrosis, but no stainable copper; the liver copper measured by atomic absorption was 525 μg/g dry weight.

Genetic testing initially revealed one mutation, H1069Q. This was also present in three of her four siblings, who were well but in whom ceruloplasmin was 0.18 g/L (John), 0.13 g/L (George), and 0.06 g/L (Mary), respectively. Whilst awaiting further mutation data, zinc acetate treatment was started in Mary. Subsequently it was shown that Joanna and Mary are compound heterozygotes for H1069Q/c1568T>A mutations, whilst John, George, and both parents are carriers.

Two years later, the parents had another baby. Genetic testing showed that he had the same genotype as Joanna and Mary. He was followed up, and it was decided to start zinc acetate treatment at 2 years. He remains well.

References

1 Lang PA, Schenck M, Nicolay JP, *et al.* Liver cell death and anemia in Wilson's disease involve acid sphingomyelinase and ceramide. *Nat Med* 2007;**13**:164–70.

2 Mufti AR, Burstein E, Csomos RA, *et al.* XIAP is a copper binding protein deregulated in Wilson's disease and other copper toxicosis disorders. *Mol Cell* 2006;**21**:775–85.

3 Mufti AR, Burstein E, Duckett CS. XIAP: cell death regulation meets copper homeostasis. *Arch Biochem Biophys* 2007;**463**:168–74.

4 Rae TD, Schmidt PJ, Pufahl RA, Culotta VC, O'Halloran TV. Undetectable intracellular free copper: the requirement of a copper chaperone for superoxide dismutase. *Science* 1999;**284**:805–8.

5 Aller SG, Unger VM. Projection structure of the human copper transporter CTR1 at 6-A resolution reveals a compact trimer with a novel channel-like architecture. *Proc Natl Acad Sci U S A* 2006;**103**:3627–32.

6 Kuo YM, Gybina AA, Pyatskowit JW, Gitschier J, Prohaska JR. Copper transport protein (Ctr1) levels in mice are tissue specific and dependent on copper status. *J Nutr* 2006;**136**:21–6.

7 Kuo YM, Zhou B, Cosco D, Gitschier J. The copper transporter CTR1 provides an essential function in mammalian embryonic development. *Proc Natl Acad Sci U S A* 2001;**98**:6836–41.

8 Nose Y, Kim BE, Thiele DJ. Ctr1 drives intestinal copper absorption and is essential for growth, iron metabolism, and neonatal cardiac function. *Cell Metab* 2006;**4**:235–44.

9 Nose Y, Rees EM, Thiele DJ. Structure of the Ctr1 copper trans"PORE"ter reveals novel architecture. Trends Biochem Sci 2006;**31**:604–7.

10 Kelleher SL, Lonnerdal B. Mammary gland copper transport is stimulated by prolactin through alterations in Ctr1 and Atp7A localization. *Am J Physiol Regul Integr Comp Physiol* 2006;**291**: R1181–91.

11 Holzer AK, Manorek GH, Howell SB. Contribution of the major copper influx transporter CTR1 to the cellular accumulation of cisplatin, carboplatin, and oxaliplatin. *Mol Pharmacol* 2006;**70**: 1390–4.

12 Klomp LW, Lin SJ, Yuan DS, Klausner RD, Culotta VC, Gitlin JD. Identification and functional expression of HAH1, a novel human gene involved in copper homeostasis. *J Biol Chem* 1997;**272**:9221–6.

13 Walker JM, Tsivkovskii R, Lutsenko S. Metallochaperone Atox1 transfers copper to the NH2-terminal domain of the Wilson's disease protein and regulates its catalytic activity. *J Biol Chem* 2002;**277**:27953–9.

14 Bunce J, Achila D, Hetrick E, Lesley L, Huffman DL. Copper transfer studies between the N-terminal copper binding domains one and four of human Wilson's protein. *Biochim Biophys Acta* 2006;**1760**:907–12.

15 Hamza I, Faisst A, Prohaska J, Chen J, Gruss P, Gitlin JD. The metallochaperone Atox1 plays a critical role in perinatal copper homeostasis. *Proc Natl Acad Sci U S A* 2001;**98**:6848–52.

16 Moore SD, Helmle KE, Prat LM, Cox DW. Tissue localization of the copper chaperone ATOX1 and its potential role in disease. *Mamm Genome* 2002;**13**:563–8.

17 Casareno RL, Waggoner D, Gitlin JD. The copper chaperone CCS directly interacts with copper/zinc superoxide dismutase. *J Biol Chem* 1998;**273**:23625–8.

18 Cobine PA, Pierrel F, Winge DR. Copper trafficking to the mitochondrion and assembly of copper metalloenzymes. *Biochim Biophys Acta* 2006;**1763**:759–72.

19 Takahashi Y, Kako K, Kashiwabara S, *et al.* Mammalian copper chaperone Cox17p has an essential role in activation of cytochrome C oxidase and embryonic development. *Mol Cell* Biol 2002;**22**:7614–21.

20 Horng YC, Leary SC, Cobine PA, *et al.* Human Sco1 and Sco2 function as copper-binding proteins. *J Biol Chem* 2005;**280**: 34113–22.

21 Sacconi S, Trevisson E, Pistollato F, *et al.* hCOX18 and hCOX19: two human genes involved in cytochrome *c* oxidase assembly. *Biochem Biophys Res Commun* 2005;**337**:832–9.

22 Horvath R, Freisinger P, Rubio R, *et al.* Congenital cataract, muscular hypotonia, developmental delay and sensorineural hearing loss associated with a defect in copper metabolism. *J Inherit Metab Dis* 2005;**28**:479–92.

23 HUGO Gene Nomenclature Committee. ATPase superfamily. http://www.hugo-international.org/committeenomen.htm. Accessed April 2008.

24 Bartee MY, Lutsenko S. Hepatic copper-transporting ATPase ATP7B: function and inactivation at the molecular and cellular level. *Biometals* 2007;**20**:627–37.

25 Achila D, Banci L, Bertini I, Bunce J, Ciofi-Baffoni S, Huffman DL. Structure of human Wilson's protein domains 5 and 6 and their interplay with domain 4 and the copper chaperone HAH1 in copper uptake. *Proc Natl Acad Sci U S A* 2006;**103**:5729–34.

26 Lim CM, Cater MA, Mercer JF, La Fontaine S. Copper-dependent interaction of glutaredoxin with the N termini of the copper-ATPases (ATP7A and ATP7B) defective in Menkes and Wilson's diseases. *Biochem Biophys Res Commun* 2006;**348**:428–36.

27 Cater MA, La Fontaine S, Mercer JF. Copper binding to the N-terminal metal-binding sites or the CPC motif is not essential for copper-induced trafficking of the human Wilson's protein (ATP7B). *Biochem J* 2006;**401**:143–53.

28 Efremov RG, Kosinsky YA, Nolde DE, Tsivkovskii R, Arseniev AS, Lutsenko S. Molecular modelling of the nucleotide-binding domain of Wilson's disease protein: location of the ATP-binding site, domain dynamics and potential effects of the major disease mutations. *Biochem J* 2004;**382**:293–305.

29 Tsivkovskii R, Efremov RG, Lutsenko S. The role of the invariant His-1069 in folding and function of the Wilson's disease protein, the human copper-transporting ATPase ATP7B. *J Biol Chem* 2003;**278**:13302–8.

30 Cater MA, La Fontaine S, Shield K, Deal Y, Mercer JF. ATP7B mediates vesicular sequestration of copper: insight into biliary copper excretion. *Gastroenterology* 2006;**130**:493–506.

31 Harada M, Kawaguchi T, Kumemura H, *et al.* The Wilson's disease protein ATP7B resides in the late endosomes with Rab7 and the Niemann–Pick C1 protein. *Am J Pathol* 2005;**166**:499–510.

32 Klomp AE, van de Sluis B, Klomp LW, Wijmenga C. The ubiquitously expressed MURR1 protein is absent in canine copper toxicosis. *J Hepatol* 2003;**39**:703–9.

33 Tao TY, Liu F, Klomp L, Wijmenga C, Gitlin JD. The copper toxicosis gene product Murr1 directly interacts with the Wilson's disease protein. *J Biol Chem* 2003;**278**:41593–6.

34 Weiss KH, Merle U, Schaefer M, Ferenci P, Fullekrug J, Stremmel W. Copper toxicosis gene MURR1 is not changed in Wilson's disease patients with normal blood ceruloplasmin levels. *World J Gastroenterol* 2006;**12**:2239–42.

35 Wu ZY, Zhao GX, Chen WJ, *et al.* Mutation analysis of 218 Chinese patients with Wilson's disease revealed no correlation between the canine copper toxicosis gene MURR1 and Wilson's disease. *J Mol Med* 2006; **84**:438–42.

36 Lovicu M, Dessi V, Lepori MB, *et al.* The canine copper toxicosis gene MURR1 is not implicated in the pathogenesis of Wilson's disease. *J Gastroenterol* 2006;**41**:582–7.

37 Donadio S, Alfaidy N, De Keukeleire B, *et al.* Expression and localization of cellular prion and COMMD1 proteins in human placenta throughout pregnancy. *Placenta* 2007;**28**:907–11.

38 Westergard L, Christensen HM, Harris DA. The cellular prion protein (PrP(C)): its physiological function and role in disease. *Biochim Biophys Acta* 2007;**1772**:629–44.

39 Leach SP, Salman MD, Hamar D. Trace elements and prion diseases: a review of the interactions of copper, manganese and zinc with the prion protein. *Anim Health Res Rev* 2006;**7**:97–105.

40 Kawano T. Prion-derived copper-binding peptide fragments catalyze the generation of superoxide anion in the presence of aromatic monoamines. *Int J Biol Sci* 2007;**3**:57–63.

41 Merle U, Stremmel W, Gessner R. Influence of homozygosity for methionine at codon 129 of the human prion gene on the onset of neurological and hepatic symptoms in Wilson's disease. *Arch Neurol* 2006;**63**:982–5.

42 Grubenbecher S, Stuve O, Hefter H, Korth C. Prion protein gene codon 129 modulates clinical course of neurological Wilson's disease. *Neuroreport* 2006;**17**:549–52.

43 Warlow C, van Gijn J. The history of Wilson's disease. In: Hoogenraad TU, ed. *Wilson's disease*. London: Saunders, 1996: 1–13. (Major problems in neurology, 30.)

44 Hoogenraad TU, Koevoet R, de Ruyter Korver EG. Oral zinc sulphate as long-term treatment in Wilson's disease (hepatolenticular degeneration). *Eur Neurol* 1979;**18**:205–11.

45 Walshe JM. Management of penicillamine nephropathy in Wilson's disease: a new chelating agent. *Lancet* 1969;**ii**:1401–2.

46 Frydman M, Bonne-Tamir B, Farrer LA, *et al*. Assignment of the gene for Wilson's disease to chromosome 13: linkage to the esterase D locus. *Proc Natl Acad Sci U S A* 1985;**82**:1819–21.

47 Vulpe C, Levinson B, Whitney S, Packman S, Gitschier J. Isolation of a candidate gene for Menkes disease and evidence that it encodes a copper-transporting ATPase. *Nat Genet* 1993;**3**: 7–13.

48 Bull PC, Thomas GR, Rommens JM, Forbes JR, Cox DW. The Wilson's disease gene is a putative copper transporting P-type ATPase similar to the Menkes gene. *Nat Genet* 1993;**5**:327–37.

49 Petrukhin K, Lutsenko S, Chernov I, Ross BM, Kaplan JH, Gilliam TC. Characterization of the Wilson's disease gene encoding a P-type copper transporting ATPase: genomic organization, alternative splicing, and structure/function predictions. *Hum Mol Genet* 1994;**3**:1647–56.

50 Petrukhin K, Fischer SG, Pirastu M, *et al*. Mapping, cloning and genetic characterization of the region containing the Wilson's disease gene. *Nat Genet* 1993;**5**:338–43.

51 Tanzi RE, Petrukhin K, Chernov I, *et al*. The Wilson's disease gene is a copper transporting ATPase with homology to the Menkes disease gene. *Nat Genet* 1993;**5**:344–50.

52 Harris ZL, Takahashi Y, Miyajima H, Serizawa M, MacGillivray RT, Gitlin JD. Aceruloplasminemia: molecular characterization of this disorder of iron metabolism. *Proc Natl Acad Sci U S A* 1995;**92**:2539–43.

53 de Bie P, van de Sluis B, Klomp L, Wijmenga C. The many faces of the copper metabolism protein MURR1/COMMD1. *J Hered* 2005;**96**:803–11.

54 Mori M, Hattori A, Sawaki M, *et al*. The LEC rat: a model for human hepatitis, liver cancer, and much more. *Am J Pathol* 1994;**144**:200–4.

55 Theophilos MB, Cox DW, Mercer JF. The toxic milk mouse is a murine model of Wilson's disease. *Hum Mol Genet* 1996;**5**: 1619–24.

56 Huster D, Finegold MJ, Morgan CT, *et al*. Consequences of copper accumulation in the livers of the Atp7b–/– (Wilson's disease gene) knockout mice. *Am J Pathol* 2006;**168**:423–34.

57 Ferenci P. Regional distribution of mutations of the ATP7B gene in patients with Wilson's disease: impact on genetic testing. *Hum Genet* 2006;**120**:151–9.

58 Loudianos G, Dessi V, Lovicu M, *et al*. Molecular characterization of Wilson's disease in the Sardinian population—evidence of a founder effect. *Hum Mutat* 1999;**14**:294–303.

59 Medici V, Rossaro L, Sturniolo GC. Wilson's disease—a practical approach to diagnosis, treatment and follow-up. *Dig Liver Dis* 2007;**39**:601–9.

60 Ala A, Walker AP, Ashkan K, Dooley JS, Schilsky ML. Wilson's disease. *Lancet* 2007;**369**:397–408.

61 Hoogenraad TU, Houwen RHJ. Prevalence and genetics. In: Hoogenraad TU, ed. *Wilson's disease*. London: Saunders, 1996: 14–24. (Major problems in neurology, 30.)

62 Tanner S. Wilson's disease: creating a clinical database and designing clinical trials. *EuroWilson Newsl* 2007;**4** (www.eurowilson.org, accessed 8 March 2008).

63 Iorio R, D'Ambrosi M, Mazzarella G, Varrella F, Vecchione R, Vegnente A. Early occurrence of hypertransaminasemia in a 13-month-old child with Wilson's disease. *J Pediatr Gastroenterol Nutr* 2003;**36**:637–8.

64 Ala A, Borjigin J, Rochwarger A, Schilsky M. Wilson's disease in septuagenarian siblings: Raising the bar for diagnosis. *Hepatology* 2005;**41**:668–70.

65 Lee WS, McKiernan P, Kelly DA. Etiology, outcome and prognostic indicators of childhood fulminant hepatic failure in the United Kingdom. *J Pediatr Gastroenterol Nutr* 2005;**40**:575–81.

66 Squires RH Jr, Shneider BL, Bucuvalas J, *et al*. Acute liver failure in children: the first 348 patients in the pediatric acute liver failure study group. *J Pediatr* 2006;**148**:652–8.

67 Dhawan A, Taylor RM, Cheeseman P, De Silva P, Katsiyiannakis L, Mieli-Vergani G. Wilson's disease in children: 37-year experience and revised King's score for liver transplantation. *Liver Transpl* 2005;**11**:441–8.

68 Shaver WA, Bhatt H, Combes B. Low serum alkaline phosphatase activity in Wilson's disease. *Hepatology* 1986;**6**:859–63.

69 Berman DH, Leventhal RI, Gavaler JS, Cadoff EM, Van Thiel DH. Clinical differentiation of fulminant Wilsonian hepatitis from other causes of hepatic failure. *Gastroenterology* 1991;**100**: 1129–34.

70 Tissieres P, Chevret L, Debray D, Devictor D. Fulminant Wilson's disease in children: appraisal of a critical diagnosis. *Pediatr Crit Care Med* 2003;**4**:338–43.

71 Sallie R, Katsiyiannakis L, Baldwin D, *et al*. Failure of simple biochemical indexes to reliably differentiate fulminant Wilson's disease from other causes of fulminant liver failure. *Hepatology* 1992;**16**:1206–11.

72 Hoshino T, Kumasaka K, Kawano K, *et al*. Low serum alkaline phosphatase activity associated with severe Wilson's disease. Is the breakdown of alkaline phosphatase molecules caused by reactive oxygen species? *Clin Chim Acta* 1995;**238**:91–100.

73 Santos RG, Alissa F, Reyes J, Teot L, Ameen N. Fulminant hepatic failure: Wilson's disease or autoimmune hepatitis? Implications for transplantation. *Pediatr Transplant* 2005;**9**: 112–6.

74 Yener S, Akarsu M, Karacanci C, *et al*. Wilson's disease with coexisting autoimmune hepatitis. *J Gastroenterol Hepatol* 2004; **19**:114–6.

75 Denk H, Stumptner C, Fuchsbichler A, *et al*. Are the Mallory bodies and intracellular hyaline bodies in neoplastic and non-neoplastic hepatocytes related? *J Pathol* 2006;**208**:653–61.

76 Sternlieb I, Scheinberg IH. Prevention of Wilson's disease in asymptomatic patients. *N Engl J Med* 1968;**278**:352–9.

77 Martins da Costa C, Baldwin D, Portmann B, Lolin Y, Mowat AP, Mieli-Vergani G. Value of urinary copper excretion after penicillamine challenge in the diagnosis of Wilson's disease. *Hepatology* 1992;**15**:609–15.

78 Nuttall KL, Palaty J, Lockitch G. Reference limits for copper and iron in liver biopsies. *Ann Clin Lab Sci* 2003;**33**:443–50.

79 Ferenci P, Steindl-Munda P, Vogel W, *et al*. Diagnostic value of quantitative hepatic copper determination in patients with Wilson's Disease. *Clin Gastroenterol Hepatol* 2005;**3**:811–8.

80 Caca K, Ferenci P, Kuhn HJ, *et al.* High prevalence of the H1069Q mutation in East German patients with Wilson's disease: rapid detection of mutations by limited sequencing and phenotype-genotype analysis. *J Hepatol* 2001;**35**:575–81.
81 Cauza E, Ulrich-Pur H, Polli C, Gangl A, Ferenci P. Distribution of patients with Wilson's disease carrying the H1069Q mutation in Austria. *Wien Klin Wochenschr* 2000;**112**:576–9.
82 Vrabelova S, Letocha O, Borsky M, Kozak L. Mutation analysis of the ATP7B gene and genotype/phenotype correlation in 227 patients with Wilson's disease. *Mol Genet Metab* 2005;**86**:277–85.
83 Loudianos G, Kostic V, Solinas P, *et al.* Characterization of the molecular defect in the ATP7B gene in Wilson's disease patients from Yugoslavia. *Genet Test* 2003;**7**:107–12.
84 Panagiotakaki E, Tzetis M, Manolaki N, *et al.* Genotype-phenotype correlations for a wide spectrum of mutations in the Wilson's disease gene (ATP7B). *Am J Med Genet A* 2004;**131**:168–73.
85 Shah AB, Chernov I, Zhang HT, *et al.* Identification and analysis of mutations in the Wilson's disease gene (ATP7B): population frequencies, genotype-phenotype correlation, and functional analyses. *Am J Hum Genet* 1997;**61**:317–28.
86 Curtis D, Durkie M, Balac P, *et al.* A study of Wilson's disease mutations in Britain. *Hum Mutat* 1999;**14**:304–11.
87 Dmitriev O, Tsivkovskii R, Abildgaard F, Morgan CT, Markley JL, Lutsenko S. Solution structure of the N-domain of Wilson's disease protein: distinct nucleotide-binding environment and effects of disease mutations. *Proc Natl Acad Sci U S A* 2006;**103**:5302–7.
88 Morgan CT, Tsivkovskii R, Kosinsky YA, Efremov RG, Lutsenko S. The distinct functional properties of the nucleotide-binding domain of ATP7B, the human copper-transporting ATPase: analysis of the Wilson's disease mutations E1064A, H1069Q, R1151H, and C1104F. *J Biol Chem* 2004;**279**:36363–71.
89 Stapelbroek JM, Bollen CW, van Amstel JK, *et al.* The H1069Q mutation in ATP7B is associated with late and neurologic presentation in Wilson's disease: results of a meta-analysis. *J Hepatol* 2004;**41**:758–63.
90 Gromadzka G, Schmidt HH, Genschel J, *et al.* p.H1069Q mutation in ATP7B and biochemical parameters of copper metabolism and clinical manifestation of Wilson's disease. *Mov Disord* 2006;**21**:245–8.
91 Loudianos G. Wilson's disease. Genetic and metabolic liver disease in children. [Paper presented at the First International Meeting on Genetic and Metabolic Liver Disease in Children, Ischia, Italy, 7–9 October 2005].
92 Kenney S, Cox D. Wilson's Disease Mutation Database (http://www.medicalgenetics.med.ualberta.ca/wilson/index.php).
93 Margarit E, Bach V, Gomez D, *et al.* Mutation analysis of Wilson's disease in the Spanish population—identification of a prevalent substitution and eight novel mutations in the ATP7B gene. *Clin Genet* 2005;**68**:61–8.
94 Wan L, Tsai CH, Tsai Y, Hsu CM, Lee CC, Tsai FJ. Mutation analysis of Taiwanese Wilson's disease patients. *Biochem Biophys Res Commun* 2006;**345**:734–8.
95 Rodriguez Farina E, Tremosa Llurba G, Xiol Quingles X, *et al.* D-Penicillamine and plasmapheresis in acute liver failure secondary to Wilson's disease. *Rev Esp Enferm Dig* 2003;**95**:60–2, 63–5.
96 Nagata Y, Uto H, Hasuike S, *et al.* Bridging use of plasma exchange and continuous hemodiafiltration before living donor liver transplantation in fulminant Wilson's disease. *Intern Med* 2003;**42**:967–70.
97 Kreymann B, Seige M, Schweigart U, Kopp KF, Classen M. Albumin dialysis: effective removal of copper in a patient with fulminant Wilson's disease and successful bridging to liver transplantation: a new possibility for the elimination of protein-bound toxins. *J Hepatol* 1999;**31**:1080–5.
98 Sen S, Felldin M, Steiner C, *et al.* Albumin dialysis and Molecular Adsorbents Recirculating System (MARS) for acute Wilson's disease. *Liver Transpl* 2002;**8**:962–7.
99 Manz T, Ochs A, Bisse E, Strey C, Grotz W. Liver support—a task for nephrologists? Extracorporeal treatment of a patient with fulminant Wilson's crisis. *Blood Purif* 2003;**21**:232–6.
100 Skwarek A, Grodzicki M, Nyckowski P, *et al.* The use Prometheus FPSA system in the treatment of acute liver failure: preliminary results. *Transplant Proc* 2006;**38**:209–11.
101 Durand F, Bernuau J, Giostra E, *et al.* Wilson's disease with severe hepatic insufficiency: beneficial effects of early administration of D-penicillamine. *Gut* 2001;**48**:849–52.
102 LeWitt PA. Penicillamine as a controversial treatment for Wilson's disease. *Mov Disord* 1999;**14**:555–6.
103 Brewer GJ. Penicillamine should not be used as initial therapy in Wilson's disease. *Mov Disord* 1999;**14**:551–4.
104 Walshe JM. Penicillamine: the treatment of first choice for patients with Wilson's disease. *Mov Disord* 1999;**14**:545–50.
105 Merle U, Schaefer M, Ferenci P, Stremmel W. Clinical presentation, diagnosis and long-term outcome of Wilson's disease: a cohort study. *Gut* 2007;**56**:115–20.
106 Brewer GJ. The treatment of Wilson's disease. *Adv Exp Med Biol* 1999;**448**:115–26.
107 Brewer GJ, Askari F, Lorincz MT, *et al.* Treatment of Wilson's disease with ammonium tetrathiomolybdate, IV: comparison of tetrathiomolybdate and trientine in a double-blind study of treatment of the neurologic presentation of Wilson's disease. *Arch Neurol* 2006;**63**:521–7.
108 Tamura S, Sugawara Y, Kishi Y, Akamatsu N, Kaneko J, Makuuchi M. Living-related liver transplantation for Wilson's disease. *Clin Transplant* 2005;**19**:483–6.
109 Wang XH, Cheng F, Zhang F, *et al.* Living-related liver transplantation for Wilson's disease. *Transpl Int* 2005;**18**:651–6.
110 Podgaetz E, Chan C. Liver transplantation for Wilson's disease: our experience with review of the literature. *Ann Hepatol* 2003;**2**:131–4.
111 Senzolo M, Loreno M, Fagiuoli S, *et al.* Different neurological outcome of liver transplantation for Wilson's disease in two homozygotic twins. *Clin Neurol Neurosurg* 2007;**109**:71–5.
112 Medici V, Mirante VG, Fassati LR, *et al.* Liver transplantation for Wilson's disease: the burden of neurological and psychiatric disorders. *Liver Transpl* 2005;**11**:1056–63.
113 Geissler I, Heinemann K, Rohm S, Hauss J, Lamesch P. Liver transplantation for hepatic and neurological Wilson's disease. *Transplant Proc* 2003;**35**:1445–6.
114 Wu JC, Huang CC, Jeng LB, Chu NS. Correlation of neurological manifestations and MR images in a patient with Wilson's disease after liver transplantation. *Acta Neurol Scand* 2000;**102**:135–9.

115 Stracciari A, Tempestini A, Borghi A, Guarino M. Effect of liver transplantation on neurological manifestations in Wilson's disease. *Arch Neurol* 2000;**57**:384–6.

116 Kassam N, Witt N, Kneteman N, Bain VG. Liver transplantation for neuropsychiatric Wilson's disease. *Can J Gastroenterol* 1998; **12**:65–8.

117 Emiroglu R, Ayvaz I, Moray G, Karakayali H, Haberal M. Tacrolimus-related neurologic and renal complications in liver transplantation: a single-center experience. *Transplant Proc* 2006;**38**:619–21.

118 Wu J, Forbes JR, Chen HS, Cox DW. The LEC rat has a deletion in the copper transporting ATPase gene homologous to the Wilson's disease gene. *Nat Genet* 1994;**7**:541–5.

119 La Fontaine S, Theophilos MB, Firth SD, Gould R, Parton RG, Mercer JF. Effect of the toxic milk mutation (tx) on the function and intracellular localization of Wnd, the murine homologue of the Wilson's copper ATPase. *Hum Mol Genet* 2001;**10**:361–70.

120 Irani AN, Malhi H, Slehria S, *et al.* Correction of liver disease following transplantation of normal rat hepatocytes into Long-Evans Cinnamon rats modeling Wilson's disease. *Mol Ther* 2001;**3**:302–9.

121 Malhi H, Irani AN, Volenberg I, Schilsky ML, Gupta S. Early cell transplantation in LEC rats modeling Wilson's disease eliminates hepatic copper with reversal of liver disease. *Gastroenterology* 2002;**122**:438–47.

122 Park SM, Vo K, Lallier M, *et al.* Hepatocyte transplantation in the Long Evans Cinnamon rat model of Wilson's disease. *Cell Transplant* 2006;**15**:13–22.

123 Allen KJ, Cheah DM, Wright PF, *et al.* Liver cell transplantation leads to repopulation and functional correction in a mouse model of Wilson's disease. *J Gastroenterol Hepatol* 2004;**19**:1283–90.

124 Shi Z, Liang XL, Lu BX, *et al.* Diminution of toxic copper accumulation in toxic milk mice modeling Wilson's disease by embryonic hepatocyte intrasplenic transplantation. *World J Gastroenterol* 2005;**11**:3691–5.

125 Allen KJ, Cheah DM, Lee XL, *et al.* The potential of bone marrow stem cells to correct liver dysfunction in a mouse model of Wilson's disease. *Cell Transplant* 2004;**13**:765–73.

126 Merle U, Enckea J, Tuma S, Volkmann M, Naldini L, Stremmel W. Lentiviral gene transfer ameliorates disease progression in Long-Evans cinnamon rats: An animal model for Wilson's disease. *Scand J Gastroenterol* 2006;**41**:974–82.

127 Ha-Hao D, Merle U, Hofmann C, *et al.* Chances and shortcomings of adenovirus-mediated ATP7B gene transfer in Wilson's disease: proof of principle demonstrated in a pilot study with LEC rats. *Z Gastroenterol* 2002;**40**:209–16.

128 Terada K, Nakako T, Yang XL, *et al.* Restoration of holoceruloplasmin synthesis in LEC rat after infusion of recombinant adenovirus bearing WND cDNA. *J Biol Chem* 1998;**273**:1815–20.

129 Meng Y, Miyoshi I, Hirabayashi M, *et al.* Restoration of copper metabolism and rescue of hepatic abnormalities in LEC rats, an animal model of Wilson's disease, by expression of human ATP7B gene. *Biochim Biophys Acta* 2004;**1690**:208–19.

130 Welch EM, Barton ER, Zhuo J, *et al.* PTC124 targets genetic disorders caused by nonsense mutations. Nature 2007;**447**:87–91.

131 Tanner MS. Role of copper in Indian childhood cirrhosis. *Am J Clin Nutr* 1998;**67**:1074S–1081S.

132 Bavdekar AR, Bhave SA, Pradhan AM, Pandit AN, Tanner MS. Long term survival in Indian childhood cirrhosis treated with D-penicillamine. *Arch Dis Child* 1996;**74**:32–5.

133 Pradhan AM, Bhave SA, Joshi VV, Bavdekar AR, Pandit AN, Tanner MS. Reversal of Indian childhood cirrhosis by D-penicillamine therapy. *J Pediatr Gastroenterol Nutr* 1995;**20**:28–35.

134 Tanner MS, Bhave SA, Pradhan AM, Pandit AN. Clinical trials of penicillamine in Indian childhood cirrhosis. *Arch Dis Child* 1987;**62**:1118–24.

135 Tanner MS. Indian childhood cirrhosis and Tyrolean childhood cirrhosis. Disorders of a copper transport gene? *Adv Exp Med Biol* 1999;**448**:127–37.

136 Wijmenga C, Muller T, Murli IS, *et al.* Endemic Tyrolean infantile cirrhosis is not an allelic variant of Wilson's disease. *Eur J Hum Genet* 1998;**6**:624–8.

137 Muller T, Feichtinger H, Berger H, Muller W. Endemic Tyrolean infantile cirrhosis: an ecogenetic disorder. *Lancet* 1996;**347**: 877–80.

138 Walker-Smith J, Blomfield J. Wilson's disease or chronic copper poisoning? *Arch Dis Child* 1973;**48**:476–9.

139 Muller-Hocker J, Weiss M, Meyer U, *et al.* Fatal copper storage disease of the liver in a German infant resembling Indian childhood cirrhosis. *Virchows Arch A Pathol Anat Histopathol* 1987;**411**: 379–85.

140 Baker A, Gormally S, Saxena R, *et al.* Copper-associated liver disease in childhood. *J Hepatol* 1995;**23**:538–43.

141 Lefkowitch JH, Honig CL, King ME, Hagstrom JW. Hepatic copper overload and features of Indian childhood cirrhosis in an American sibship. *N Engl J Med* 1982;**307**:271–7.

142 Adamson M, Reiner B, Olson JL, *et al.* Indian childhood cirrhosis in an American child. *Gastroenterology* 1992;**102**:1771–7.

143 Hahn SH, Brantly ML, Oliver C, Adamson M, Kaler SG, Gahl WA. Metallothionein synthesis and degradation in Indian childhood cirrhosis fibroblasts. *Pediatr Res* 1994;**35**:197–204.

144 Ferenci P, Caca K, Loudianos G, *et al.* Diagnosis and phenotypic classification of Wilson's disease. *Liver Int* 2003;**23**:139–42.

8

Management of Chronic Liver Disease

15 Complications and Management of Chronic Liver Disease

Ross Shepherd

Mechanisms of chronic liver disease

Advances in the understanding of the basic mechanisms of liver injury are providing new insight into the complications of liver diseases in children, leading to new directions in the prevention and treatment of liver disease. An understanding of these mechanisms provides a useful conceptual framework for the clinician dealing with young patients with chronic liver diseases.

Cirrhosis

Most chronic liver diseases of childhood result in cirrhosis and/or cholestasis, from which the complications of chronic liver disease are derived. Cirrhosis (Greek *kirrhos*, or orange-yellow) is a chronic diffuse liver disease characterized by widespread hepatic fibrosis with regenerative nodule formation. Cholestasis, the accumulation of hydrophobic bile acids toxic to hepatocytes, may be either the cause or the effect of cirrhosis.[1] The liver appears to respond to injury in a stereotypic fashion with a complex but dynamic series of events (Figure 15.1) that includes programmed cell death (apoptosis), cell necrosis, and fibrogenesis. Hepatocyte injury leads to apoptosis by a number of pathways, including polarization of mitochondria, cytochrome *c* release, nuclear fragmentation, and formation of apoptotic bodies without inflammation. Necrosis involves depolarization of mitochondria, depletion of adenosine triphosphate (ATP), and cell lysis with inflammation. In response to any of these cellular events, there is oxidant stress and release of cytokines and other soluble growth factors. This cascade of signaling and transcriptional events results in the activation of a fibrogenic or wound-healing response, in which damaged areas of tissue are encapsulated by scarring, or extracellular matrix. Central to the development of hepatic fibrosis is widespread activation of extracellular matrix-producing cells, particularly hepatic stellate cells. The fibrotic and regenerative nodules that make up cirrhosis of the liver develop vascular anastomoses, which cause hemodynamic alterations, portosystemic shunting, and increased resistance to portal blood flow, which is a primary factor in the pathophysiology of portal hypertension. The diffuse pathology of cirrhosis superimposes on the primary liver disease, often obscuring the nature of the original insult. The major clinical consequences are the result of impaired hepatic function and portal hypertension.

Hepatic fibrogenesis

As indicated above, progressive liver fibrosis is the final common determinant of most forms of chronic liver diseases. Studies in animal models of chronic liver disease and pathological studies performed in human liver, including pediatric liver diseases,[2,3] demonstrate that fibrosis develops with different spatial patterns as a consequence of different mechanisms of parenchymal damage. For example, fibrosis observed as a consequence of chronic viral infection is initially periportal; fibrosis secondary to toxic/metabolic damage is located mainly in the centrilobular areas; and fibrosis in congenital hepatic fibrosis, and perhaps the embryonal forms of biliary atresia, is secondary to ductal plate malformation affecting the smallest intrahepatic bile ducts. In addition, it is increasingly evident that different cell types are involved in the deposition of fibrillar extracellular matrix during active hepatic fibrogenesis: hepatic stellate cells are mainly involved when hepatocellular damage is limited or concentrated within the liver lobule, whereas portal myofibroblasts and fibroblasts provide a predominant contribution when the damage is located in the proximity of the portal tracts. In the later stages of evolution (septal fibrosis and cirrhosis), it is likely that all extracellular matrix-producing cells contribute to fibrogenesis.

Extracellular matrix-producing cells are recruited to the site of tissue damage and activated by several different mechanisms:

- Firstly, there is accumulation of fibrillar extracellular matrix, with attempts at remodeling and regeneration by chronic activation of the tissue repair process after injury.
- Secondly, there is synthesis of fibrillar extracellular matrix as a result of oxidative stress, via reactive oxygen intermediates and reactive aldehydes, whose concentrations become critical in toxic/metabolic liver injury, even in the absence of significant hepatocyte damage and inflammation.

Diseases of the Liver and Biliary System in Children, 3rd edition. Edited by Deirdre Kelly. © 2008 Blackwell Publishing, ISBN: 978-1-4051-6334-7.

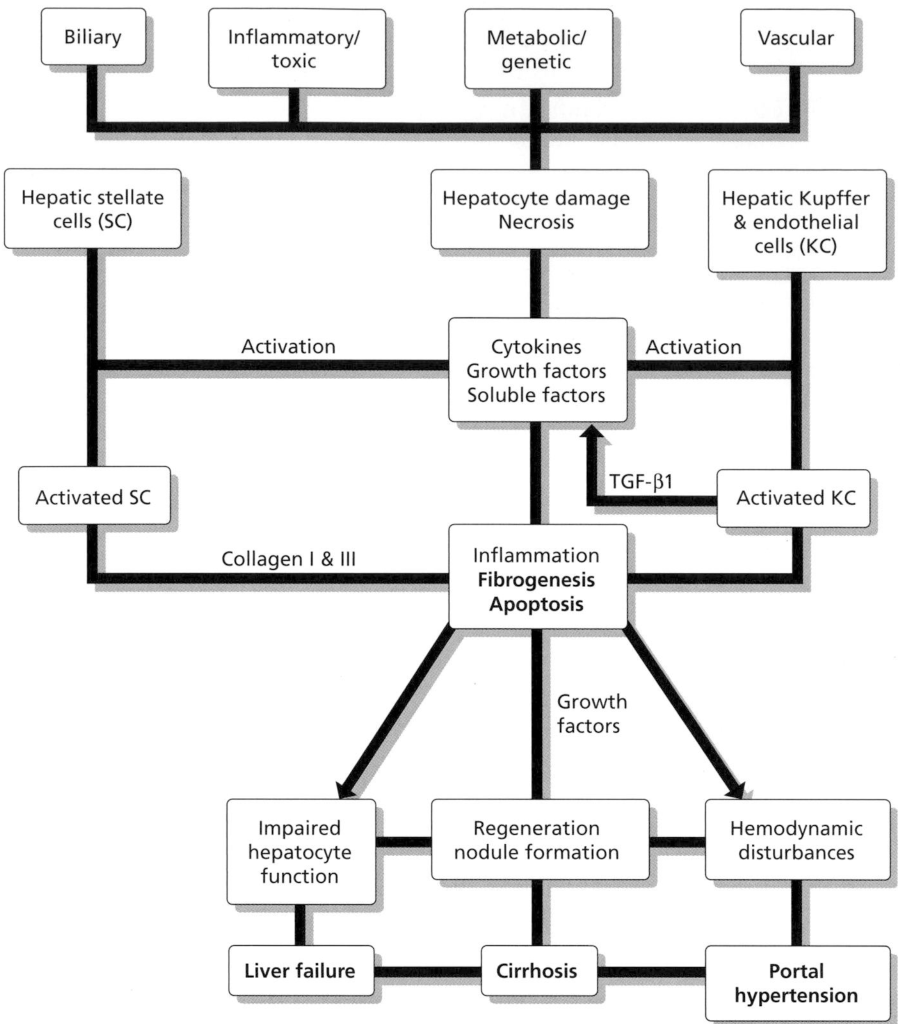

Figure 15.1 The pathogenesis of cirrhosis—a stereotypic response to liver injury.

- Thirdly, there is consensual proliferation of extracellular matrix-producing cells and progressive fibrogenesis when liver damage results in derangement of the normal epithelial/mesenchymal interaction, as typically occurs in conditions characterized by cholangiocyte apoptosis, damage, or proliferation.[4]
- Fourthly, fibrogenesis is stimulated by specific lymphocyte subsets.
- Fifthly, hepatocyte injury may be induced by accumulation of hydrophobic bile acids in cholestatic liver diseases,[1] causing oncotic necrosis or apoptosis.
- Finally, it is possible that dysregulation of apoptosis in both bile duct epithelial cells and hepatocytes may cause liver injury in many different liver diseases.[4]

Advances in our understanding of the molecular mechanisms of fibrogenesis is also derived from in-vitro studies investigating the biological role of growth factors/cytokines and other soluble factors and their intracellular signaling pathways. For example, all extracellular matrix-producing cells when activated express an intracellular microfilament protein, a smooth muscle actin (SMA), which can be used as a marker protein of the activated phenotype. They express a number of different cytokine receptors, such as transforming growth factor-β1 (TGF-β1) receptor. TGF-β is a cytokine involved in tissue growth, differentiation, and the immune response, and it appears to be a dominant stimulus to extracellular matrix production. Finally, liver fibrosis is a bidirectional process, and increasing data from laboratory and clinical studies demonstrate that even advanced fibrosis and cirrhosis are potentially reversible by clearance of hepatic stellate cells through apoptosis.

Exploration of the molecular mechanisms underlying this bidirectionality will hopefully lead to characterization of the essential attributes of antifibrotic therapies that hold promise for the future.

Portal hypertension

Portal hypertension is responsible for the more severe, potentially lethal complications of chronic liver disease requiring specific management, such as bleeding esophageal varices, renal dysfunction, encephalopathy, and, in part, ascites and nutritional disturbances. Splenomegaly and hypersplenism rarely require specific intervention, as they do not significantly affect morbidity or mortality. There is often (unfounded) concern about traumatic splenic rupture, but this is extremely rare. The pancytopenia due to sequestration in the spleen likewise causes little or no morbidity, as the blood cells present, although lower in number, are highly functional.

In general, portal hypertension is the result of a combination of increased portal blood flow and increased portal resistance, and occurs when portal pressure and the hepatic venous pressure gradient (the portal vein–vena cava pressure gradient) rises above 10–12 mmHg, a critical threshold for the development of complications. The effects of portal hypertension are primarily the result of decompression of elevated portal blood pressure through portosystemic collaterals. The physiological basis for maintenance of portal pressure[5,6] is in accordance with Ohm's law, where changes in portal pressure are proportional to alteration in blood flow and resistance, which can change in response to changes in portal blood flow. In cirrhosis, there is initially an increase in intrahepatic resistance, partly modifiable, and then an increase in splanchnic blood flow, which maintains or further increases portal pressure, giving rise to a hyperdynamic circulatory state with increased cardiac and decreased splanchnic arteriolar tone, both of which further increase portal inflow. Studies in animal models indicate that a number of humoral mediators are involved, including glucagon, prostaglandins, nitric oxide (NO), and endothelium-derived relaxing factor. Changes in intravascular volume also play an important part in the pathophysiology of the hyperdynamic circulation, as do alterations in adrenergic tone in the splanchnic system. These observations have led to new experimental and clinical studies suggesting possible pharmacological treatments for portal hypertension,[5,6] focused on increased intrahepatic vascular resistance as a target, especially through the nitric oxide pathway.

An understanding of portal hypertension in children requires knowledge of the anatomy of the portal system and its development (Figure 15.2). Portal capillaries originate in the mesentery of the intestine and spleen and in the hepatic sinusoids. Capillaries of the superior mesenteric and splenic veins supply the portal vein with nutrient-rich and hormone-rich blood supply. At the hilum of the liver the portal vein divides into two major trunks supplying the right and left lobes of the liver, and these trunks undergo a series of divisions supplying segments of the liver terminating in small branches which pierce the limiting plate of the portal tract and enter the sinusoids through short channels. In fetal life, the ductus venosus connects the umbilical vein and the inferior vena cava, and the umbilical vein joins the left branch of the portal vein. These may persist or remain patent in some situations postnatally. Absence or disconnection of

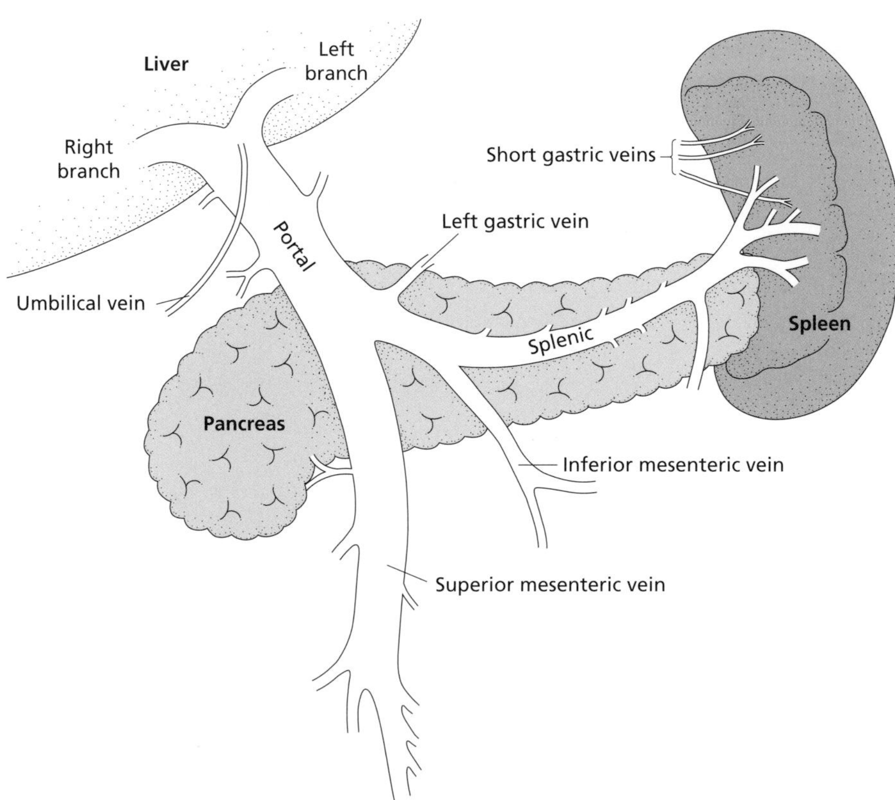

Figure 15.2 The anatomy of the portal venous system. (Reproduced with permission from Sherlock S, Dooley J, *Diseases of the Liver and Biliary System,* 10th ed., Oxford: Blackwell Science, 1998.)

the inferior vena cava, and/or interruption to the azygos system such as occurs in some cases of biliary atresia, may cause special concern.

The partly oxygenated portal venous blood supplements the oxygenated hepatic arterial blood flow to give the liver unique protection against hypoxia. Blood flow from both the hepatic artery and the portal vein is well regulated, allowing the liver to withstand thrombosis of either one of these major vessels.

Portal hypertension due to chronic liver disease may arise due to a prehepatic or an intrahepatic block, where the block may be presinusoidal, sinusoidal, or postsinusoidal. The major pathological effect of portal hypertension is the development of collaterals carrying blood from the portal venous system to the systemic circulation in the upper part of the stomach, the esophagus, the rectum, and in the falciform ligament. These may also drain into the inferior vena cava via the umbilical vein remnant or the left renal vein (Figure 15.3).

Causes of chronic liver disease

In children, a wide range of causes of hepatocellular injury may result in cirrhosis (Table 15.1). These include cholestatic diseases (e.g., biliary secretory disorders or obstruction), as well as infections, toxins, metabolic, vascular, and nutritional disorders. The pattern of progression to cirrhosis in pediatric liver diseases is highly variable. In some conditions, such as neonatal extrahepatic biliary atresia, the development of hepatic fibrosis is extraordinarily rapid, with cirrhosis occurring by 8–16 weeks of age and liver failure by as early as 24 weeks of age. Other disorders, such as cystic fibrosis (CF)-associated

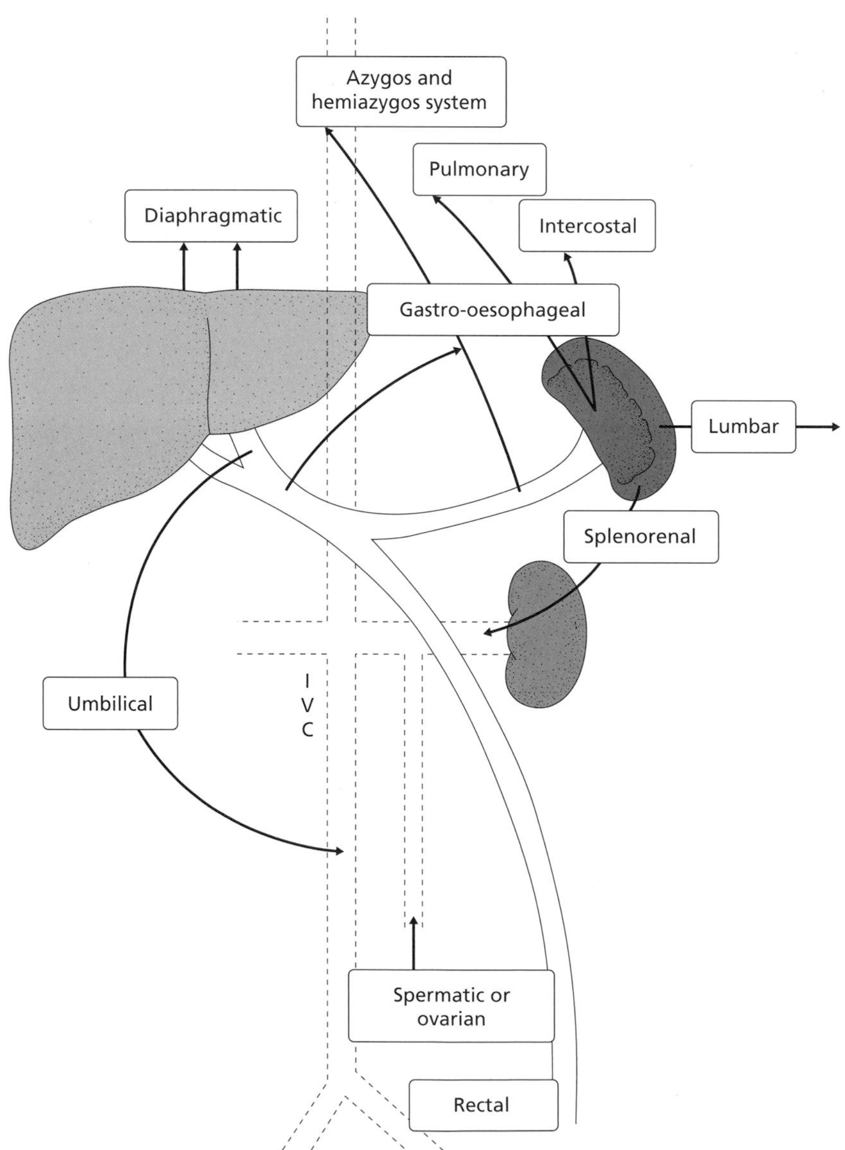

Figure 15.3 Sites of collateral circulation in portal hypertension. (Reproduced with permission from Sherlock S, Dooley J, *Diseases of the Liver and Biliary System*, 10th ed., Oxford: Blackwell Science, 1998.)

Table 15.1 Causes of chronic liver disease in children.

Biliary
Extrahepatic biliary atresia
Choledochal cyst, tumors, stones
Alagille's syndrome, biliary hypoplasia
Familial intrahepatic cholestasis, drugs
Sclerosing cholangitis
Graft-versus-host-disease
Histiocytosis X
Hepatic
Neonatal hepatitis
Hepatitis B ± delta
Hepatitis C
Autoimmune hepatitis
Drugs/toxins
Genetic/metabolic
Carbohydrate defects
Galactosemia, fructosemia, glycogen storage III and IV
Amino acid defects
Tyrosinemia, urea cycle disorders
Metal storage defects
Neonatal hemochromatosis, Wilson's disease
Lipid storage diseases
Gaucher disease, Niemann–Pick type C
Fatty acid β-oxidation defects
Peroxisomal disorders
Zellweger syndrome
Mitochondrial disorders
Respiratory chain defects
Cystic fibrosis
Fibropolycystic disorders*
Vascular
Hepatic vein thrombosis
Budd–Chiari syndrome
Veno-occlusive disease
Cardiac

*Do not cause cirrhosis.

focal biliary cirrhosis, can be compatible with normal liver function for many years, presenting with signs of portal hypertension only in the second decade of life. The importance of genetic influences on outcomes and progression of chronic liver diseases has also been a topic of scientific interest, with specific reference to genetic modifiers in the variance of occurrence and progression of hepatic fibrosis.[3] Despite this wide variation in occurrence and severity, it appears that the cellular mechanisms and factors responsible for the development of liver fibrosis in these two widely differing diseases, and indeed in most chronic liver diseases, are remarkably similar. Activation of hepatic stellate cells and associated increased production of type I collagen have been documented in both biliary atresia[7] and in the focal biliary cirrhosis associated with CF.[8] TGF-β1 is produced in biliary atresia by both injured hepatocytes and bile duct epithelial cells; in cystic fibrosis liver disease, it is expressed predominantly in bile duct epithelium.

Diagnosis of chronic liver disease

Diagnosis is essentially a stepwise process, involving a range of clinical, laboratory, radiological imaging, and pathological investigations:

1 Confirming the presence and type of liver disease
2 Determining the etiology
3 Assessing the extent of complications
4 Determining the prognosis and outcome with regard to liver transplantation.

Chronic liver disease may be either active or inactive, depending on the presence of biochemical or histological evidence of hepatocellular necrosis, apoptosis, and inflammation; and either compensated or decompensated, depending on the presence or absence of clinical or laboratory features of liver failure. In general, morphological and histological classifications are often unhelpful in clinical settings, although certain features may help in determining the cause of the cirrhosis—such as biliary disease, hepatic venous outflow obstruction, and features specific for particular inherited or infective conditions. Grouping disorders that progress to cirrhosis by etiology is helpful because of the framework this provides for diagnosis, prognosis, treatment, and genetic counseling. Ultimately, the presence or absence of liver failure provides the basis for the transition from supportive therapy to considerations of liver transplantation when the condition of end-stage liver disease has been reached (see the section "Overview of Management of Chronic Liver Disease," below).

Clinical presentation

In compensated liver disease, there may be no symptoms or signs. The first indication of liver disease may be an incidental finding of hepatosplenomegaly, splenomegaly alone, or increased serum transaminases. Commonly in cirrhosis, the liver is small and impalpable, but it can be enlarged, hard, or nodular with in some patients a small right lobe or splenomegaly. Cutaneous features such as spider angiomas, prominent periumbilical veins, and palmar erythema may provide a clue to the presence of liver disease (Figure 15.4). Spider angiomas may occur in healthy children under the age of 5 years and are thus not pathognomonic of liver diseases in children, but the appearance of new spider angiomas or more than five or six suggests liver disease. They are frequently observed in the vascular drainage of the superior vena cava, and feature a central arteriole from which radiate numerous fine vessels, ranging from 2 to 5 mm in diameter. The presence of prominent veins radiating from the umbilicus

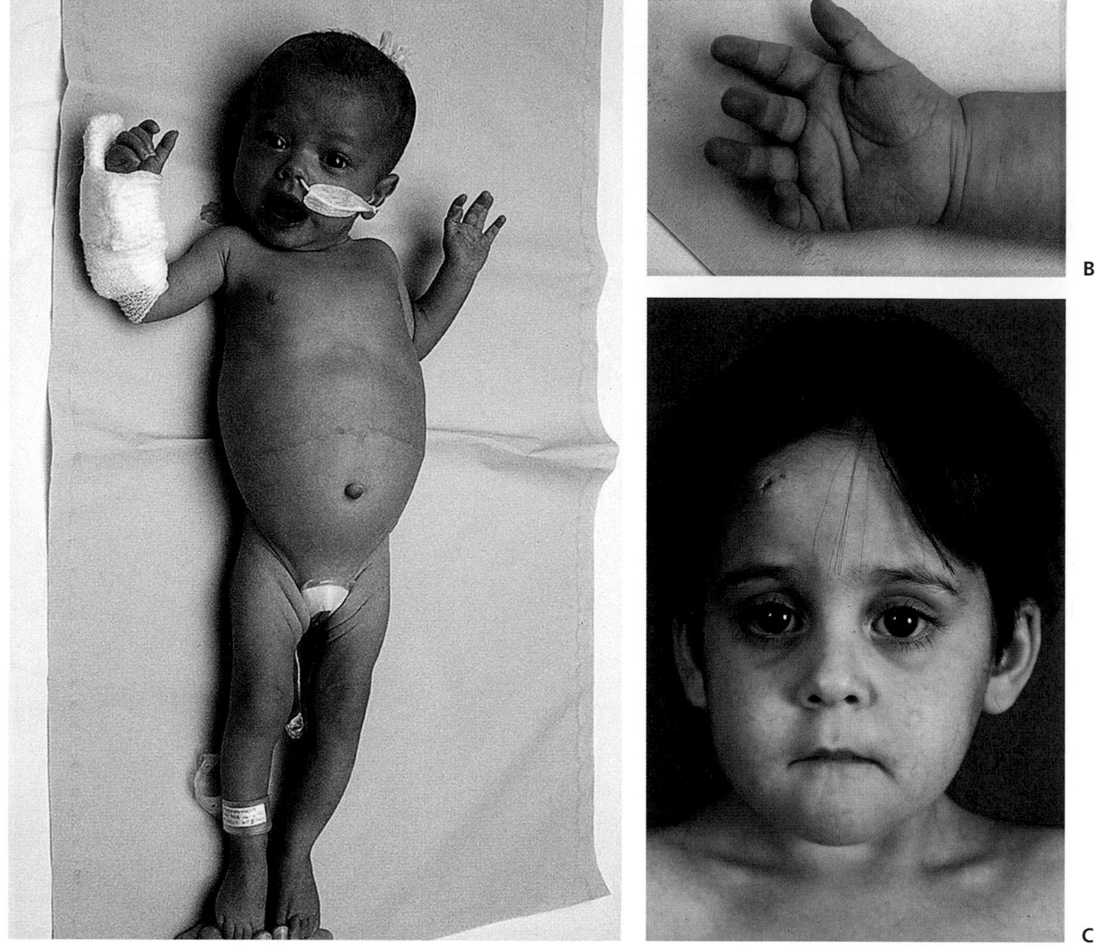

Figure 15.4 Clinical features of biliary cirrhosis in infancy. Jaundice is severe, with wasting, ascites, prominent abdominal veins, clubbing, and hepatosplenomegaly. **A** The abdominal scar is from failed portoenterostomy for biliary atresia. **B** Both plantar and palmar erythema develop early. **C** In older children, facial telangiectasia and spider nevi may be evident.

is an indication of portal hypertension. Other cutaneous features include: easy bruising; fine telangiectasia on the face and upper back (Figure 15.4); white spots, most often on buttocks and arms, which when examined with a lens show the beginnings of spider angiomas; and clubbing of the fingers. On intranasal examination, prominent telangiectasia of the Little area (Kiesselbach area) is common, associated with recurrent epistaxis. In Wilson's disease, specific features include hemolytic anemia, subtle signs of encephalopathy such as personality changes, loss of memory, or school failure, and Kayser–Fleischer rings, sought by an experienced examiner using a slit lamp.

Children with cholestatic liver disease (Table 15.1) will have predominant signs or symptoms of persisting jaundice and/or pruritus, acholic stools, and dark urine. The liver is usually enlarged, and xanthelasma, malnutrition, and deficiency of fat-soluble vitamins (particularly vitamins D and K) may be prominent features. Clubbing is more likely to occur in biliary cirrhosis, and malnutrition and decompensation occur earlier in this form of liver disease.

Decompensated liver disease is characterized by clinical and laboratory findings of liver synthetic failure, and the occurrence of complications of portal hypertension (Table 15.2). As well as the features mentioned above, the major features include malnutrition, ascites, peripheral edema, coagulopathy, and gastrointestinal bleeding. Signs of hepatic

Table 15.2 Complications of cirrhosis in children.

Malnutrition and growth failure
Portal hypertension and variceal bleeding
Hypersplenism
Ascites
Encephalopathy
Coagulopathy
Hepatopulmonary syndrome
Hepatorenal syndrome
Bacterial infections, spontaneous bacterial peritonitis
Hepatocellular carcinoma

encephalopathy are subtle in children. Except for those with biliary cirrhosis, jaundice is a late feature in cirrhosis and indicates very advanced disease. Malnutrition with reduced lean tissue and fat stores as well as poor linear growth is a well-recognized and important feature of chronic liver disease in children.[9–11] Spontaneous bruising caused by impaired hepatic production of clotting factors and thrombocytopenia due to hypersplenism are signs of advanced disease. Cirrhosis with decompensation may also be associated with changes in the systemic and pulmonary circulations, with arteriolar vasodilation, increased blood volume, a hyperdynamic circulatory state, and cyanosis due to intrapulmonary shunting. Renal failure is a late but serious event. Laboratory investigations may reveal elevated alkaline phosphatase, bilirubin, hepatic transaminases, creatinine, and ammonia, but in particular there is abnormal liver synthetic function, reflected by such findings as hypoalbuminemia and prolonged prothrombin time.

Investigations (Table 15.3)

In all forms of suspected liver disease, confirmation will ultimately rest with the interpretation of liver biopsy findings, which may confirm the presence, type, and degree of activity of cirrhosis, and contribute to a diagnosis of the cause of the liver disease. However, a full range of laboratory and imaging investigations should be performed prior to performing a liver biopsy, focusing on determining both the etiology and the severity of the liver disease prior to further confirmation with a liver biopsy. Such investigations may be diagnostic of the underlying cause and may allow appropriate handling of the liver biopsy specimen with respect to specific histological and biochemical analysis, particularly for metabolic disorders. Table 15.3 lists the diagnostic tests that should be considered for children with suspected cirrhosis or chronic liver disease. Cirrhosis may be suggested by ultrasound, where there is abnormal homogeneity of the liver architecture, and an irregular liver edge. The occurrence of esophageal varices should be sought by endoscopy.

Table 15.3 Investigation of chronic liver disease in children.

General
Bilirubin
Aminotransferases
γ-glutamyltransferase
Alkaline phosphatase
Albumin
Cholesterol
Urea and creatinine
Ammonia
α-Fetoprotein
Full blood count
Prothrombin time
PELD or PHD score
Chest radiography
Hepatobiliary and renal ultrasound
Upper gastrointestinal endoscopy
Electrocardiography
Electroencephalography
Liver biopsy
Specific (for diagnosis)
Biliary
Blood and liver tissue culture
Operative cholangiogram
ERCP/MRCP
Hepatobiliary scan
Colonoscopy
Hepatic
Viral serology (TORCH, hepatitis B, C, EBV)
ESR
Autoimmune antibodies, immunoglobulins
Liver copper or iron deposition
General/metabolic
Urinary sugars, amino acids, organic acids, porphyrins, fatty acid degeneration products
Blood sugar (fasting), lactate, pyruvate, urate
Serum amino acids, copper, ceruloplasmin, α_1-antitrypsin, iron ferritin, porphyrins, bile acids
Serum acylcarnitine profile, CPK
Sweat test, CF mutation studies
Protease inhibitor phenotype
Muscle biopsy, liver fibroblasts for specific enzymes
Vascular
Doppler images of hepatic venous blood flow
Digital subtraction angiography
Inferior venacavography
Antithrombin III, protein C, protein S

CF, cystic fibrosis; CPK, creatine phosphokinase; EBV, Epstein–Barr virus; ERCP, endoscopic retrograde cholangiopancreatography; ESR, erythrocyte sedimentation rate; MRCP, magnetic resonance cholangiopancreatography; TORCH, toxoplasmosis, other (congenital syphilis and viruses), rubella, cytomegalovirus, and herpes simplex virus; PELD, Pediatric End-Stage Liver Disease (score); PHD, Pediatric Hepatic Dependency (score).

Liver pathology

Classification of liver pathology in chronic liver diseases is based on morphology, histology, etiology, and degree of activity. Fibrosis is not synonymous with cirrhosis. Marked fibrosis without nodules occurs typically in congenital hepatic fibrosis and granulomatous liver disease, but fibrosis occurs without nodules in the evolution of cirrhosis. Percutaneous needle liver biopsy interpretation difficulties may arise because of small samples and fragmentation of the specimen, or if the specimen is taken from a macronodule, which may look almost normal except for hyperplasia of the hepatocytes or a relative excess of hepatic vein branches.

The morphological classification divides cirrhosis into micronodular, macronodular, and mixed types. Micronodular cirrhosis is characterized by fibrous septa separating small

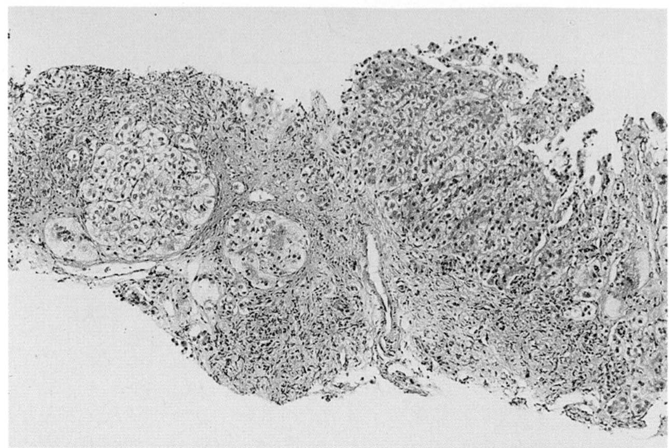

Figure 15.5 Liver histology of biliary cirrhosis, with portal inflammation and fibrosis linking the portal tracts, leading to nodule formation.

(< 3 mm) regeneration nodules of almost uniform size, present throughout the liver. This is most commonly seen in children in the early stages of extrahepatic biliary atresia (Figure 15.5). Macronodular cirrhosis is characterized by nodules up to 5 cm in diameter, separated by irregular septa of varying widths. Regenerative nodules larger than 2 cm in diameter are evidence that the cirrhotic process has persisted for a number of years. This pattern is usually seen in α_1-antitrypsin deficiency, chronic active hepatitis, and Wilson's disease. Many cases, however, have a mixed pattern, and it is known that micronodular cirrhosis can mature into macro-nodular or mixed cirrhosis.

The histological classification is generally more helpful in defining etiology and in management. Cirrhosis is defined as postnecrotic, biliary (periportal), or hepatic venous outflow (cardiac) cirrhosis. Postnecrotic cirrhosis (Table 15.1) is the result of liver cell damage and is most commonly seen in chronic hepatitis due to viral factors, autoimmune factors, or drugs, and is a common sequela of neonatal hepatitis. Features include piecemeal necrosis, bridging fibrosis, collapse of the hepatic lobules, and regeneration, with the development of macronodular cirrhosis. In biliary cirrhosis from cholestatic disorders (Figure 15.5), fibrosis develops from within the portal tracts, extending out into the parenchyma and linking adjacent portal tracts, with little change in the hepatic parenchyma and preservation of the lobular architecture. In neonatal biliary disease, bile duct proliferation is a feature of extrahepatic biliary atresia, and bile duct paucity or hypoplasia is a feature of intrahepatic cholestatic syndromes. Obstruction to hepatic venous outflow due to cardiac lesions with increased right atrial pressure or hepatic vein occlusive disorders leads to centrilobular hemorrhagic necrosis, with fibrosis extending from central veins to portal tracts. In chronic cases, cirrhosis eventually develops, and the initial distinguishing features may be obliterated.

Specific histological patterns occur in Wilson's disease (copper pigment deposition), α_1-antitrypsin deficiency (intracellular periodic acid–Schiff-positive, diastase-resistant inclusions) and storage disorders.

Diagnostic dilemmas

The process of cirrhosis in chronic liver disease may be superimposed on the primary cause and eventually obscure the nature of the original insult. Many forms of liver disease have specific histology patterns early in the disease, but as the disease progresses, patterns merge, leaving morphological and histological classifications unhelpful. In many cases—particularly in cholestatic syndromes causing jaundice, pruritus, dark urine, and pale stools—the cause of the liver damage will be evident on the basis of the history, examination, and imaging techniques.

A high index of suspicion is necessary to diagnose potentially treatable disorders:

- Genetic disorders such as Wilson's disease, galactosemia, hereditary fructosemia, and tyrosinemia type I
- Acquired disorders, such as hepatitis B, hepatitis C, and autoimmune chronic liver disease
- Surgically correctable disorders such as choledochal cysts and biliary stenosis, usually diagnosed by imaging studies or laparotomy.

It is important to differentiate between cirrhosis and presinusoidal causes of portal hypertension such as congenital hepatic fibrosis and extrahepatic portal hypertension. In the latter conditions, there are no signs of chronic liver disease. In congenital hepatic fibrosis, the liver is enlarged and hard, splenomegaly is prominent, and transaminases and synthetic tests are usually normal. Histologically, there are prominent abnormal bile ducts in wide bands of fibrous tissue, but no nodules. Renal cysts on ultrasound or a suggestive family history may provide a clue to this diagnosis (see Chapter 10). In extrahepatic portal hypertension due to portal vein malformation or obstruction, the liver is small, histologically normal, and transaminases are normal. There may be mild derangement of coagulation parameters secondary to an underlying coagulation disorder (e.g., protein C or S deficiency). Ultrasound will demonstrate a portal vein cavernoma or absence of blood flow in the portal system, which may be confirmed on angiography or splenoportography (see Chapters 2, 3, and 19).

Overview of management of chronic liver disease

The primary aims in the management of children with any form of chronic liver disease are:

- To minimize or prevent progressive liver damage by treating the cause, if possible.
- To predict the outcome in order to deliver definitive therapy by liver transplantation.
- To anticipate, prevent, or control the complications.

Specific therapies

With the exception of a few specific therapies aimed at the causes of chronic liver disease—such as chelation therapy in Wilson's disease, diet and nitisinone for tyrosinemia type I,[12,13] phlebotomy for hemochromatosis, the use of antiviral agents in hepatitis B and C, weight management for nonalcoholic steatohepatitis (NASH), and immunotherapy for autoimmune hepatitis—treatment of the cause of most chronic liver diseases is not possible. Nevertheless, resolution of hepatic fibrosis has been observed in many of the above conditions,[2,13] and thus therapies targeting the fibrogenic response to mediate progression of chronic liver disease and its complications are being actively researched experimentally and hold some promise. These include inhibition of hepatic stellate cell activation—e.g., antioxidants, peroxisome proliferator-activated receptor-γ (PPAR-γ) agonists, antifibrogenic agents (e.g., TGF-β antagonists, inhibitors of the endothelin receptor, curcumin, or the renin–angiotensin system)—and agents that regulate the degradation of scar tissue.[14] Nevertheless, no adequate antifibrotic therapy is currently available and in regular clinical use. Ursodeoxycholic acid has been shown to improve liver function and biochemical tests in some pediatric liver disorders, such as cystic fibrosis, but the effects of this agent as an antifibrotic remain largely unproven. Thus, for most patients with cirrhosis and its associated clinical complications, supportive management of the complications and ultimately liver transplantation is the only curative approach.

Predicting outcome

With the advent of liver transplantation as a definitive therapy for many causes of chronic liver disease, a redefinition of the diagnosis of end-stage liver disease is necessary with a view to the predicted outcome, full and frank discussion of treatment options, and timely intervention if the transplant option is to be realized. This allows time for optimizing supportive therapy, evaluating suitability for transplantation, and maximizing the prospects for finding a suitable donor. In addition, complications such as malnutrition, gastrointestinal hemorrhage, encephalopathy, ascites, and infection can be anticipated and prevented whenever possible.

Unfortunately, most available liver function tests have poor predictive value until liver decompensation has taken place, and the occurrence of specific complications such as gastrointestinal hemorrhage or encephalopathy is unpredictable. For all causes of end-stage disease, age, bilirubin, international normalized ratio (INR), growth failure, and albumin were significant for poor outcome in an analysis of data by the Studies of Pediatric Liver Transplantation (SPLIT) Consortium. This Pediatric End-Stage Liver Disease (PELD) score is used as the standard for organ sharing in the United States.[15] A similar but more extensive scoring system for disease severity in children with mild to severe liver disease, the Pediatric Hepatology Dependency (PHD) score, comprises 10 parameters (aspartate transaminase, prothrombin time, albumin, bilirubin, ascites, nutritional support, organ dysfunction, blood product support, sepsis, and intravenous access) and correlates with the PELD score for patients requiring transplantation, but is also a measure of dependency and disease severity in other groups of patients with liver disease.[16] In older studies,[10,11] malnutrition was found to be an important independent risk factor, possibly because major nutritional deficits in energy, protein, lipids, vitamins, and minerals may independently compromise outcome and further compromise liver function per se. Quantitative dynamic liver function tests such as monoethylglycinexylidide (MEGX) formation from lignocaine, and caffeine clearance, have also been evaluated as prognostic indicators of residual functional capacity of the liver, but are no longer used.[17,18] In general, expert clinical evaluation using a range of modalities included in the PELD and/or PHD scores (Table 15.4) is necessary for determining the prognosis and predicting the need for transplantation.

In addition, knowledge of the natural history of particular disease states is of value. In biliary atresia, survival of the native liver after Kasai portoenterostomy is dependent on age, the degree of fibrosis at the time of the procedure,[19] surgical

Table 15.4 Measures for prognostic factors in children with chronic liver disease.

Independent predictors
Bilirubin > 300 μmol/L
Prolonged prothrombin time unresponsive to intravenous vitamin K
Partial thromboplastin time > 20 s
Malnutrition (weight, SD score < 1.5)
Low plasma cholesterol
Ascites
Pediatric End-Stage Liver Disease (PELD): a score for transplant waiting list mortality with an algorithm of five parameters:
Age
Bilirubin
International normalized ratio (INR)
Growth failure
Albumin
Pediatric Hepatology Dependency (PHD): a score for dependency and severity of chronic liver disease with an algorithm of 10 parameters:
Aspartate transaminase
Prothrombin time
Albumin
Bilirubin
Ascites
Nutritional support
Organ dysfunction
Blood product support
Sepsis
Intravenous access

subtype, and the surgical skill according to caseload for the procedure.[20] Failure to clear jaundice following portoenterostomy is a clear prognostic indicator and an indication for early referral for transplantation (see Chapters 5,20). In α_1-antitrypsin deficiency—the most common metabolic disease leading to liver transplantation in children—only 10–15% of the protease-inhibitor type ZZ (PI ZZ) population develops liver disease, with 5–10% of these patients requiring liver transplantation in childhood. The duration of jaundice, severity of histological features, and biochemical abnormalities may predict the outcome in this condition. In tyrosinemia type I, unless controlled by diet and nitisinone, progressive hepatocellular damage is associated with a high incidence of hepatocellular carcinoma by 5 years of age, and ≥ 60% of those presenting by 2 months of age and 25% of those with onset between 2 months and 6 months of age die by 12–15 months of age.[21]

Complications of chronic liver disease

(Table 15.2)

Complications of chronic liver disease are primarily due to impaired hepatic function, which causes nutritional and metabolic disturbances; impaired protein synthesis and coagulopathy; portal hypertension, which causes ascites; variceal hemorrhage, hepatorenal and hepatopulmonary syndromes; and/or cholestasis, which contributes to malabsorption and pruritus. Several of these mechanisms contribute to ascites and encephalopathy. There may also be impaired immunity, with resulting bacterial infection. Hepatocellular carcinoma can complicate any cause of chronic liver disease, particularly tyrosinemia type I and chronic hepatitis B (see Chapter 20).

Malnutrition and nutritional support

A wide range of nutrient deficits occur in chronic liver disease in children (Table 15.5). The liver has a central role in regulating fuel and metabolism, nutrient homeostasis, and absorption of a number of nutrients. Anorexia or an inadequate nutrient intake contribute to malnutrition in chronic liver disease, particularly in infants, who are more vulnerable to the debilitating effects of malnutrition because of their higher energy and growth requirements.[22] Moreover, nutrition plays a crucial role in neurodevelopment, learning, immunity, energy level, and surgical outcomes. Protein–calorie malnutrition, poor growth, vitamin deficiencies, and bone disease influence both short-term and long-term survival, even after liver transplantation. Malnutrition itself may further derange liver function, as the liver requires energy for a number of synthetic, storage, and detoxification functions. Thus, nutritional management is a fundamental part of the management of an infant or child with liver disease.

Malnutrition in pediatric liver disease is a modifiable risk factor.[23] In adults with cirrhosis, enteral nutritional supplements improve nutritional status and liver function, reduce the rate of complications, and prolong survival.[24] In children with biliary atresia, malnutrition is associated with poor outcome after Kasai portoenterostomy; is a major factor associated with transplant waiting list mortality; and is a predictor of post-transplantation morbidity and mortality.[25] Intensive nutritional support can improve nutritional status, as shown in at least one controlled trial[26] and a number of open label studies. The key to optimal nutritional management is a multidisciplinary approach to nutritional surveillance and intervention, including a pediatric dietitian, nurse coordinator, feeding psychologist, and clinician.

Pathophysiology of malnutrition in liver disease

The pathophysiology of malnutrition is complex and multifactorial and includes protein energy malnutrition, deranged carbohydrate metabolism, fat malabsorption, and impaired protein and lipid synthesis.

The body composition of malnourished children with chronic liver disease is similar to that seen in protein-energy malnutrition, and these children are hypermetabolic and thus require high energy intakes.[27] Nutrient intakes may be inadequate because of anorexia and malabsorption or nutritional deprivation because of recurrent variceal bleeding or surgery. Protein intake may be insufficient for somatic growth in children because of dietary manipulation for treatment of encephalopathy and management of ascites. Protein synthesis of albumin, transferrin, and clotting factors is impaired in chronic liver disease. An abnormal serum amino acid profile, with elevated plasma aromatic amino acids (AAA) and depletion of and increased requirement for branched-chain amino acids (BCAAs)[28–30] has major implications. BCAAs comprise 40–50% of the minimum daily requirement for essential amino acids in humans, playing an important regulatory role in protein synthesis, and thus growth and positive nitrogen balance.

Carbohydrate metabolic defects include carbohydrate intolerance, peripheral insulin resistance, hyperinsulinemia, and reduced hepatic glycogen stores.

In cholestatic children, reduced delivery of bile salts to the small intestine and exocrine pancreatic dysfunction result in malabsorption of energy, fat, and fat-soluble vitamins, particularly long chain fats and essential fatty acids. Medium-chain fats are well absorbed, as they do not require bile salts for absorption.

Lipid synthesis is also reduced, including very-low-density lipoproteins and cholesterol. Hypocholesterolemia has been considered to be an adverse factor in predicting the outcome of liver transplantation.

A disturbed growth hormone (GH)–insulin-like growth factor (IGF-1) axis may also contribute to wasting and growth failure in children with liver disease, by virtue of IGF-1 deficiency and GH resistance.[28]

Table 15.5 Nutritional deficits and their management in pediatric liver disease.

Deficit	Evaluation	Management
Energy	Energy balance Intake Absorption Expenditure Nutritional status Anthropometry Body cell mass (TBK) DEXA	Energy supplements to achieve 120–130% RDI Nocturnal enteral nutrition
Protein	Plasma albumin BCAA/AAA ratio Protein stores Muscle mass TBN	Provide 3–4 g/kg/d protein BCAA-enriched protein Albumin infusion (if albumin < 25 g/L)
Fat	Skinfolds Body composition EFA deficiency Plasma lipid profile	Optimize fat absorption (MCT/LCT feeds) Provide saturated fats high in EFA
Fat-soluble vitamins	Plasma 25-OH-D Skeletal radiography (rickets) DEXA Prothrombin time Plasma vitamin E and A	Maximize light exposure Vitamin D-1-α (50 ng/kg) Vitamin K (2.5–5.0 mg/day) Vitamin E (50–400 IU/day) (as TPGS) Vitamin A (5000–10 000 IU/day)
Water-soluble vitamins	Specific levels Blood count	Supplement as requested
Minerals	Specific levels Cardiac evaluation	Supplement as requested

AAA, aromatic amino acids; BCAA, branched-chain amino acids; DEXA, dual-energy X-ray absorptiometry; EFA, essential fatty acids; LCT, long-chain fatty acids; MCT, medium-chain fatty acids; RDI, recommended daily intake; TBK, total body potassium; TBN, total body nitrogen; TPGS, tocopherol polyethyleneglycol-1000 succinate.

Vitamin deficiencies are common and important problems.[29–32] Vitamin K is a necessary cofactor for the conversion of inactive precursors of prothrombin and factors VII, IX, and X into their active forms. In cholestasis, vitamin K malabsorption is the primary cause of a prolonged prothrombin time. In parenchymal liver disease, the synthesis of liver-dependent clotting factors is reduced. Elevated levels of PIVKA-II (a protein induced in the absence of vitamin K) can occur in children with a normal prothrombin time, indicating that these more sensitive markers of vitamin K status should be used in children with chronic liver disease. If vitamin K deficiency is a result of malabsorption, parenteral vitamin K normalizes the prothrombin time, but in advanced liver disease, vitamin K only partially corrects the prolonged prothrombin time, suggesting poor hepatic synthetic function.

Vitamin E deficiency is common, particularly in infants with cholestatic liver diseases, resulting in a distinctive, progressive, but preventable neurological disorder associated with peripheral neuropathy, ophthalmoplegia, and ataxia.

Bone disease results from vitamin D and calcium malabsorption, secondary hyperparathyroidism, and overall protein deficiency.[33,34] Patients with cholestasis who have little or no exposure to sunlight depend primarily on dietary vitamin D to maintain body stores and are particularly likely to develop rickets (defective mineralization) and osteopenia (reduced formation of matrix), with low serum 25-hydroxyvitamin D levels and spontaneous fractures. Total 25-(OH)D and osteocalcin levels are low, suggesting that decreased bone formation, rather than increased bone resorption, is the main determinant of the bone disease.

Vitamin A deficiency is uncommon, but abnormalities of the regulation of the metabolism of retinol-binding proteins and biochemical vitamin A deficiency occur, particularly in infants with biliary atresia. Biochemical deficiencies of water-soluble vitamins, including thiamine and pyridoxine, may occur, and cases of nutritional cardiomyopathy and peripheral neuropathy have been reported.

Of the trace elements, iron, zinc and selenium deficiencies have been reported in children with end-stage liver disease and may be associated with growth failure and poor protein synthesis.

Nutritional assessment

Conventional techniques of assessment such as body weight and weight adjusted for height may not be accurate in patients with liver disease, because of fluid retention manifest by ascites and edema masking the underlying loss of bulk in crucial body compartments. Thus, assessment of malnutrition is best performed using several parameters—particularly those less affected by fluid retention, such as triceps skin folds and arm muscle measurements,[35] biochemical tests for vitamin and micronutrient deficiency, and serial evaluation of growth parameters. The gold standard methods for measuring body composition—such as metabolically active cell mass by total body potassium[11]—are expensive and limited to research methodology.

Nutritional management (Table 15.5)

The goals of nutritional support are to provide adequate calories and nitrogen for protein synthesis, restore and prevent plasma amino acid imbalance, prevent vitamin and trace element deficiency, and achieve normal growth and activity. The clinical evaluation and approach to management for specific nutritional deficits is given in Table 15.5.

Recommended intakes and route of administration. Daily intakes of ≥ 130% of the recommended allowances for age and sex are necessary to compensate for increased energy expenditure, increased requirements, and malabsorption. Protein restriction, derived from experience of encephalopathy in adults, is not applicable to small children. Enteral supplements (by nasogastric feeding if required) are indicated if the child cannot sustain reasonable growth and nutrition via a normal diet. Nocturnal nutritional supplements are a useful means of providing sufficient protein/energy for growth in young children with chronic liver disease,[26] partly because of poor oral intake and partly because there is evidence associating fasting with catabolism. Parenteral nutrition is sometimes required for feed intolerance or gastrointestinal bleeding.

Defined formulas. There are now specialized defined formulas for nutritional supplementation in liver disease (see Chapter 24). The carbohydrate and fat composition (a mix of medium-chain triglycerides and long-chain triglycerides) can provide sufficient absorbed energy, but the protein sources of standard formulas have some disadvantages with regard to abnormalities of protein and BCAA metabolism. There is evidence in controlled trials that diets that have a normal protein intake but are relatively rich in BCAA confer nutritional advantages in children and adults with liver disease.[26,36,37] The use of these with normal to high protein intakes (2–3 g/kg/day) does not invoke hepatic encephalopathy. Complete "hepatic" formulas rich in BCAA-containing medium-chain triglycerides and high in carbohydrate, as well as vitamin and mineral supplements, are available (Generaid Plus; Scientific Hospitals Supplies Ltd., Liverpool, United Kingdom). For older children, the use of oral supplements rich in BCAA is recommended (Generaid, SHS Ltd.; Nutrihep, Nestle Clinical Nutrition, Deerfield, Illinois, USA; Aminoleban, Otsuka Pharmaceuticals, Tokyo, Japan).

Vitamins and minerals. Specific vitamin and mineral therapy should also be considered, including both water-soluble and fat-soluble vitamins and specific trace elements (Table 15.5). If steatorrhea or fat malabsorption is marked, parenteral vitamin K (weekly), and vitamin D (monthly) may be necessary. The latter must be controlled by regular clinical assessment, radiographs of the wrist, and measurement of serum phosphate, calcium, and alkaline phosphatase. Treatment with intravenous bisphosphonates may be necessary.

Fat-soluble vitamin preparations in water-miscible form are best in cholestasis. Vitamin E deficiency can usually be prevented with vitamin E in water-miscible form (D-α-tocopherol polyethyleneglycol-1000 succinate, 25 IU/kg/day; most children require 600–3000 IU/day of water-soluble vitamin A, but as vitamin A toxicity can produce cerebral side effects and hepatotoxicity, the dose should be monitored in patients who do not have significant cholestasis. It is important to recognize that certain specific therapies for liver disease—such as cholestyramine, used for controlling pruritus; penicillamine, used in Wilson's disease; and diuretics, used for ascites—may cause deficiency of trace elements.

Water and electrolytes. Fluid and electrolyte homeostasis is an important part of the nutritional management of children with chronic liver disease. Diminished effective circulating blood volume may explain many of the secondary findings of salt and water retention related to portal hypertension, and reduced oncotic pressure due to hypoalbuminemia. Normally, the diminished circulatory blood volume triggers compensatory hormonal and renal responses to conserve water and sodium. Measures to stabilize and restore effective circulating blood volume help maintain the optimal volume of fluid and sodium balance. This can be achieved by maintaining serum albumin levels by infusions of albumin on a regular basis once significant hypoalbuminemia ensues (< 25 g/L), the avoidance of excessive diuretic therapy, and the use of paracentesis with albumin replacement. These measures help prevent dilutional hyponatremia and water overload, which may compromise growth and cause other alterations in nutrient metabolism.

Ascites and edema

Extravascular fluid accumulation—manifest as peripheral edema, in the peritoneal cavity as ascites, or in the pleural cavity as pleural effusion—is a common complication of cirrhosis and a sign of advanced liver disease. Ascites poses an increased risk for infections, particularly spontaneous bacterial peritonitis, as well as renal failure and mortality. The development of ascites is a predictor of the need for liver transplantation. Clinical signs include pitting and facial edema, abdominal distension, and/or the development of hernias. Renal and circulatory dysfunction, manifest as dilutional hyponatremia, low arterial blood pressure, serum creatinine > 1.2 mg/dL (120 IU/L), and intense sodium retention (urine sodium less than 10 mEq/day) may occur.

In the majority of patients, judicious use of diuretics and maintenance of plasma oncotic pressure will control ascites. Some patients either do not respond to diuretic therapy or have diuretic-induced complications that prevent the use of high doses of these drugs. Patients with gross or refractory ascites resulting in breathing difficulties, abdominal pain, or limitation of movement may require paracentesis, which has risks of inducing hypovolemia (see below). Diagnostic paracentesis is indicated for the diagnosis of unexplained fevers, spontaneous bacterial peritonitis (protein concentration < 20 g/L, leukocytosis), and in the diagnosis of Budd–Chiari syndrome, where an acute onset of ascites is associated with protein concentrations > 20 g/L.

Pathophysiology

The two important determinants of extravascular fluid accumulation are portal venous pressure and plasma oncotic pressure, both of which interact in chronic liver disease. Portal hypertension, hypoalbuminemia, and increased sodium and water retention all contribute to result in fluid redistribution between the intravascular and extravascular spaces. This process may develop insidiously or be precipitated by events such as malnutrition, gastrointestinal bleeding, or infection.

Several theories as to the formation of ascites exist.[38] According to the "arterial vasodilation hypothesis," sodium retention is the consequence of a homeostatic response in which there is underfilling of the arterial circulation secondary to arterial vasodilation in the splanchnic vascular bed. This underfilling is sensed by arterial and cardiopulmonary receptors and activates antinatriuretic factors, resulting in hypervolemia. The retained fluid initially compensates for the disturbance in the arterial circulation and suppresses the activation of sodium-retaining mechanisms. However, as the vasodilation in the splanchnic circulation causes more marked arterial underfilling, the retained fluid does not adequately fill the intravascular compartment, mainly because fluid is leaking continuously into the peritoneal cavity. The sodium-retaining mechanisms then become permanently activated. The development of arteriovenous connections implies the presence of vasoactive hormones.

A somewhat similar "underfilling hypothesis" suggests that there is increased sinusoidal pressure, leading to a cascade of events resulting in fluid retention from elevated portal venous pressure, increased splanchnic volume, decreased systemic vascular resistance, and decreased effective plasma volume. The decreased plasma volume results in increased activity of plasma renin and aldosterone, resulting in renal retention of sodium and water, leading to the accumulation of ascites. These two related hypotheses are supported by the fact that expansion of the plasma volume by methods such as albumin infusion may reverse ascites, decrease levels of renin and aldosterone, and result in a diuresis.

An "overflow hypothesis" speculates that inappropriate renal sodium and water retention is the primary abnormality triggered by the hepatorenal reflex. Some animal studies support this hypothesis, but the fact that the renin–angiotensin–aldosterone system is activated in decompensated cirrhosis argues against it. These various mechanisms may not necessarily be mutually exclusive. Early "overflow" secondary to renal sodium retention may be an initiating factor, but later diminished effective plasma volume with its accompanying hormonal changes may predominate, leading to peripheral arterial vasodilation and a further increase in sodium and water retention.

Whichever mechanism predominates, there is a decreased plasma volume, activation of antinatriuretic factors and the renin–aldosterone system, and sodium retention, all of which are relevant to rational treatment, such as to maintain plasma oncotic pressure and to use aldosterone antagonists. The development of new drugs that inhibit the tubular effect of antidiuretic hormone and increase renal water excretion without affecting urine solute excretion, such as vasopressin receptor antagonists,[39] is of particular interest in treatment.

Treatment

Mild/moderate ascites. Mild ascites causing minimal discomfort or difficulties with mobility or breathing requires no specific treatment in most cases. For moderate ascites, diuretics (drugs that increase sodium excretion by reducing the tubular reabsorption of sodium) are effective in most circumstances. Sequential albumin infusion and "chaser" diuretic therapy can be useful for moderate to severe ascites. Nutritional support, with maintenance of adequate protein homeostasis, is a key factor in the management of ascites in children (Table 15.6). Fluid and salt restriction are usually prescribed in adults, but in children these may have deleterious effects

Table 15.6 Treatment of ascites.

Nutritional support
Avoid excessive sodium intake (< 1–2 mmol/kg)
Spironolactone:
< 3 years 12.5 mg q.i.d.
4–7 years 25 mg q.i.d.
8–11 years 37.5 mg q.i.d.
11 years + 50 mg q.i.d.
± Chlorothiazide + vitamin K supplement
Albumin infusion (if serum albumin < 25 g/L) 2 g/kg or 10 mL/kg + frusemide 2 mg/kg
Paracentesis + albumin infusion for refractory symptomatic ascites

on plasma volume in the short term and nutrition in the medium term.

The initial diuretic of choice is the aldosterone antagonist spironolactone, which requires a flexible dosage regimen, often using doses that are higher than in other disorders that cause fluid retention in children. This takes 2–4 days to take effect, using initial dosages as shown in Table 15.6. The response to diuretic therapy should be evaluated by measuring body weight, urine volume, serum electrolytes, blood urea nitrogen, and sodium excretion. The initial goal of treatment is a negative fluid balance of ≥ 10 mL/kg/day. Higher negative balances risk plasma volume depletion and decline in renal function, which may be preempted by albumin infusion. The response to spironolactone is so reliable that the patient's plasma volume status should be investigated if no significant diuresis is achieved within 2–4 days. Side effects include hyponatremia and hyperkalemia, which are indications for reducing/discontinuing spironolactone. Loop diuretics may be added if there is only a partial response to spironolactone and no reduction in plasma volume. Furosemide (1–2 mg/kg) is most commonly used, particularly with albumin infusion, but chronic use is accompanied by excessive losses of urinary potassium and chloride, which can exacerbate hepatic encephalopathy and plasma volume depletion. Routine replacement of potassium is recommended. Because of the higher toxicity of loop diuretics, thiazide diuretics such as chlorothiazide are preferable for chronic use, often resulting in a satisfactory diuresis at a dosage initially of 2–3 mg/kg/day in association with spironolactone.

Refractory tense ascites. The combination of frequent albumin infusions and large-volume paracenteses is the preferred intervention, based on controlled trials in adults demonstrating relative safety and efficacy.[40] Complete removal of ascites in one tap with intravenous albumin (1 g per 100 mL tapped) is an effective measure in controlling tense ascites. Post-paracentesis circulatory dysfunction and, associated with hyponatremia, renal impairment can be prevented with the further administration of plasma expanders. In cases in which portal hypertension and variceal bleeding are also an issue, a transjugular intrahepatic portosystemic stent shunt (TIPSS) temporarily decreases portal pressure, decompresses the liver, and reduces sinusoidal and splanchnic pressure. This procedure is increasingly being used in pediatric liver centers when a bridging procedure before transplantation is required.[41] Liver transplantation is the only treatment that improves long-term survival.

Variceal bleeding

Variceal hemorrhage is a life-threatening complication of chronic liver disease and develops secondary to cirrhosis and portal hypertension (see also Chapter 19). Management is directed towards emergency therapy and/or prophylaxis against rebleeding. Direct treatment of variceal hemorrhage, or in some selected cases a shunt procedure, are the major approaches, except where liver decompensation coexists, where the ultimate treatment of choice is liver transplantation. Only the submucosal collaterals, such as in the esophagus and stomach and rarely in other parts of the intestine, are associated with gastrointestinal bleeding (Figure 15.6). Collaterals in other parts of the intestine occur at sites of surgery in the gastrointestinal tract, particularly stomas and anastomotic sites. Portal hypertensive gastropathy, which is suggested by dilated mucosal veins and capillaries and mucosal congestion in the stomach, develops particularly in patients who have had variceal obliteration. Most of the data concerning the management of variceal hemorrhage have come from large controlled trials in adults, and the pediatric literature is generally descriptive or anecdotal.

Acute gastrointestinal bleeding in a patient with chronic liver disease requires emergency treatment (Figure 15.7).

Initial management (Figure 15.6)

In all cases of hematemesis, admission to the nearest hospital with blood transfusion facilities is advised because initial melena or a sentinel bleed may precede extensive hematemesis and shock, which require rapid blood transfusion to prevent death. For significant blood loss, initial fluid management in the form of crystalloids followed by red blood cell transfusion is important. In all cases, coagulopathy should be corrected with parenteral vitamin K administration (2–10 mg/kg), fresh frozen plasma (10 mL/kg), or if there is severe thrombocytopenia (platelets $< 70 \times 10^9$), platelet infusion. As soon as the patient is hemodynamically stable, has a blood transfusion available, and a secure intravenous infusion line, referral to a tertiary unit with experience in endoscopy and the management of variceal hemorrhage in children is recommended. Nasogastric intubation is an essential part of management, allowing the documentation of ongoing bleeding and the removal of blood that might precipitate encephalopathy. Unless the bleeding

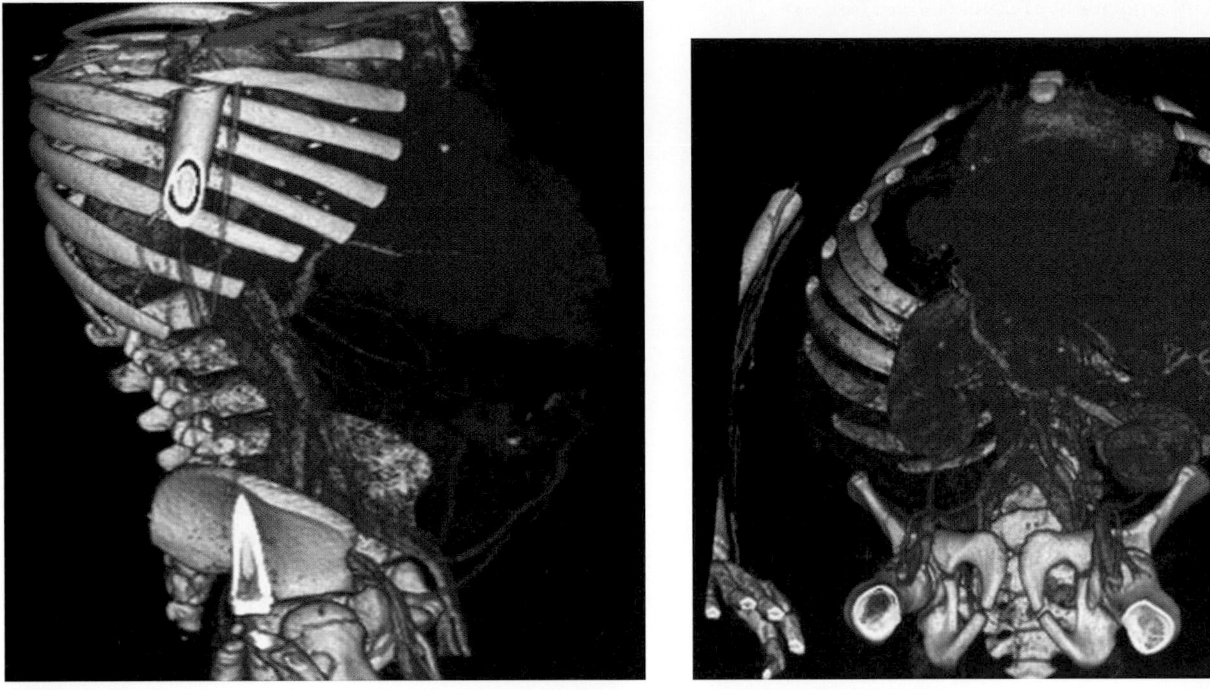

Figure 15.6 Computed-tomographic angiography is a good way of demonstrating varices. This three-dimensional reconstruction shows rectal (**A**) and splenic (**B**) varices.

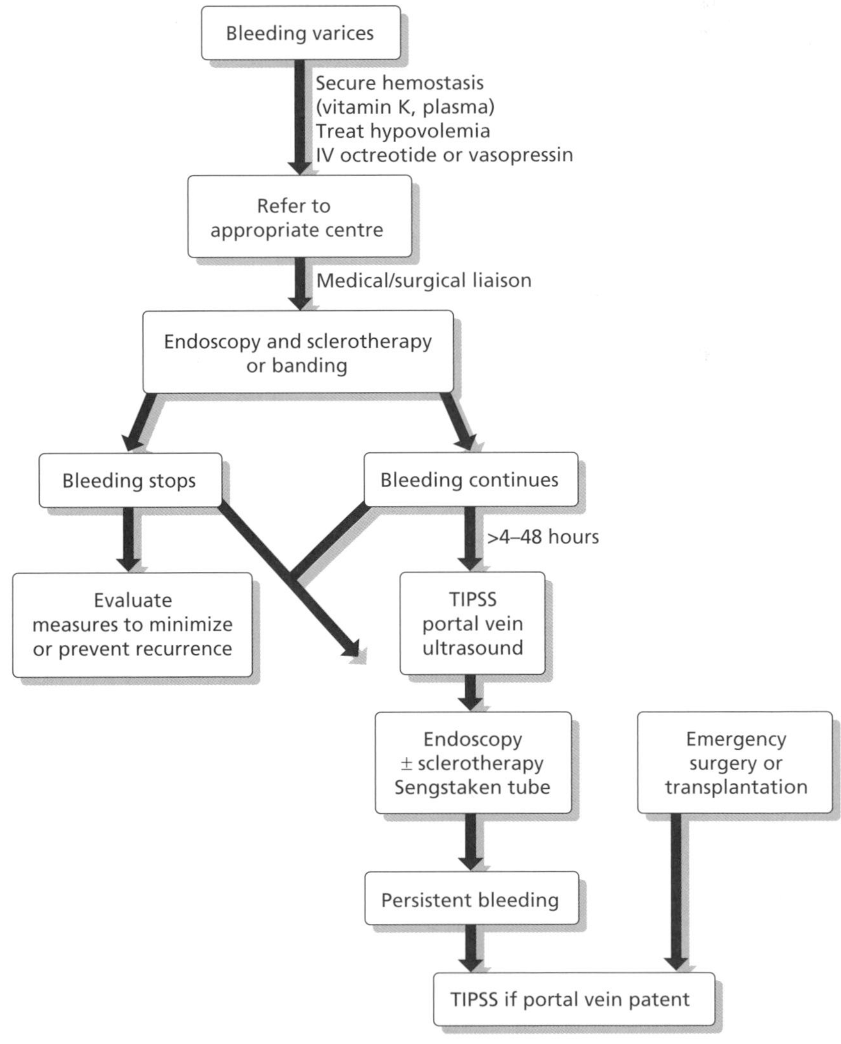

Figure 15.7 Algorithm for the management of bleeding varices. TIPSS, transjugular intrahepatic portosystemic stent shunt.

spontaneously remits, significant bleeding with hypotension impairs hepatic perfusion, causes deterioration of liver function, and precipitates ascites and encephalopathy. Vital signs such as tachycardia and hypotension and a reduction in splenomegaly can be helpful in assessing ongoing blood loss. Prior beta-blocker therapy may mask significant hypotension. Hepatic encephalopathy must be anticipated, and lactulose (0.3–0.4 mL/kg three times/day) should be given.

Pharmacological and endoscopic treatment

A meta-analysis of multiple controlled adult studies clearly shows that endoscopic treatment plus pharmacological treatment is currently the best measure for achieving initial control of significant acute variceal bleeding.[42] Pharmacological therapy is directed towards reducing hepatic vascular resistance (Table 15.7). Somatostatin or its longer-acting analogue octreotide (maximum dose 1 μg/kg/h i.v., or 2–4 μg/kg/dose subcutaneously 8-hourly) have fewer side effects and are the drugs of choice, although there has not been a systematic evaluation in children. The other major splanchnic vasoconstrictors are vasopressin (0.3 U/kg bolus over 20 min, then continuous infusion of 0.3 U/kg/h, usually for 24 h or until the bleeding has ceased) or its inactive precursor terlipressin (Glypressin; 0.01 mg/kg bolus 4–6-hourly or 0.05 mg/kg infusion over 6 h for 24–48 h). Side effects include skin pallor, abdominal colic, and chest pain. An adjunctive vasodilator, such as nitroglycerine in the form of a 10-mg patch, may reduce these effects. As soon as the patient is hemodynamically stable, an experienced endoscopist should document the cause of the hemorrhage. A significant percentage of patients with known varices have bleeding from other sources, including duodenal and gastric ulceration.

Table 15.7 Pharmacotherapy in portal hypertension.

Short-acting splanchnic vasoactive agents
Growth hormone–inhibiting factors
Somatostatin
Octreotide (1 mg/kg/h i.v. infusion or 2–4 mg/kg/dose/8 h s.c.)
Vasoconstrictors
Vasopressin (0.3 units/kg/h infusion for 24 h)
Glypressin (0.01 mg/kg bolus 4–6-hourly or 0.05 mg/kg infusion over 6 h for 24–48 h)
Long-acting splanchnic vasoactive agents
β-Adrenergic receptor blockers
Propranolol (1–5 mg/kg/day in three divided doses)
Atenolol (1 mg/kg/day in two doses)
α-Adrenergic receptor blockers
Clonidine* (10–20 mg/kg/day in three doses)
5-HT receptor antagonists
Ritanserin
Nitrovasodilators
Nitroglycerin* (5–10 mg patches)
Isosorbide-5-nitrate
Diuretics
Spironolactone (1.5–3.0 mg/kg/day in three doses)

*Reported adjunctive effect with propranolol.
5-HT, 5-hydroxytrypramine.

Endoscopic treatment with sclerotherapy or band ligation is often necessary for ongoing hemorrhage. Both techniques are well-described in children.[43,44] In adults, sclerotherapy and ligation have equal efficacy in controlling bleeding, reducing rebleeding, and ablating varices, but there are fewer adverse effects with banding.[45] However, in pediatric patients, the two procedures can be complementary, because in small infants, entrapment of part of the esophageal wall with perforation or bleeding can occur with banding, and sclerotherapy is more appropriate for smaller veins. Banding involves the application of a multiple banding device (the "Six-Shooter") to entrapped varices. Risks include entrapment of mucosa or esophageal wall in smaller children, resulting in ulceration, ischemia, and perforation. Sclerotherapy involves injection of sclerosants such as ethanolamine or sodium tetradecyl sulfate paravariceally or intravariceally in volumes of 0.5–1.0 mL just above the gastroesophageal junction. It is associated with bacteremia, and broad-spectrum antibiotics should be prescribed (amoxicillin, cefuroxime, and metronidazole). Complications include esophageal ulceration, stricture, and pain. Mucosal protecting agents such as sucralfate (1–4 g 6-hourly) may minimize the risk of ulceration and/or stricture formation. Serious complications are rare, but include perforation, thrombotic phenomena, respiratory complications, and rarely pericardial problems.

In rare cases, if the above measures fail to control bleeding, temporary cessation of bleeding can be achieved using balloon tamponade of esophageal and gastric varices with a pediatric Sengstaken–Blakemore tube or a Linton tube. These devices are best inserted under anesthesia at endoscopy. The Sengstaken–Blakemore tube consists of a rubber tube with two balloons, which is passed into the stomach where the first balloon is inflated and withdrawn against the gastroesophageal junction. The second balloon may be inflated in the esophagus at a pressure of 20–30 mmHg but is rarely required, as the pressure on the gastroesophageal junction is usually sufficient to control the bleeding. A Linton tube is a single-balloon device with a pear-shaped single balloon, which is inflated in the stomach and then pulled up against the gastroesophageal junction. Balloon tamponade may be useful temporarily to control bleeding to allow for resuscitation and prevent exsanguination, but should not be used for longer than 24 or 48 h because of the risk of ischemia/ulceration of the esophagus. There is a high incidence of rebleeding when the tubes are removed.

Emergency surgical approaches and emergency portosystemic shunts

Emergency creation of portosystemic shunts or other surgical therapy is usually a last resort for persisting exsanguinating acute variceal hemorrhage, often in patients with gastric variceal bleeding. Other techniques to be considered include transjugular intrahepatic portosystemic shunt (TIPSS), surgical shunts, esophageal transection, and esophagogastric devascularization with splenectomy. TIPSS is an interventional radiological technique and has been used effectively in critically ill adults and children to control intractable bleeding prior to liver transplantation (Figure 15.8). The procedure decreases portal pressure acutely, although up to 60% of emergency TIPSS occlude within 3–12 months, so that it is a bridging procedure only. Pediatric application is limited by size constraints, but in experienced hands it is effective in selected children over the age of 2–5 years and is preferable to major shunt surgery for hepatic causes of portal hypertension.

A

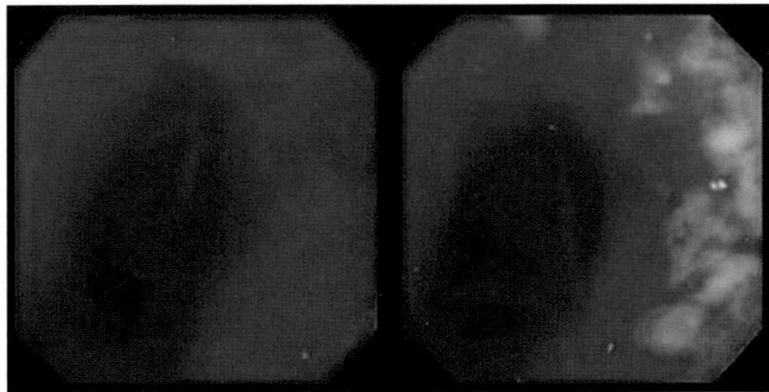

B

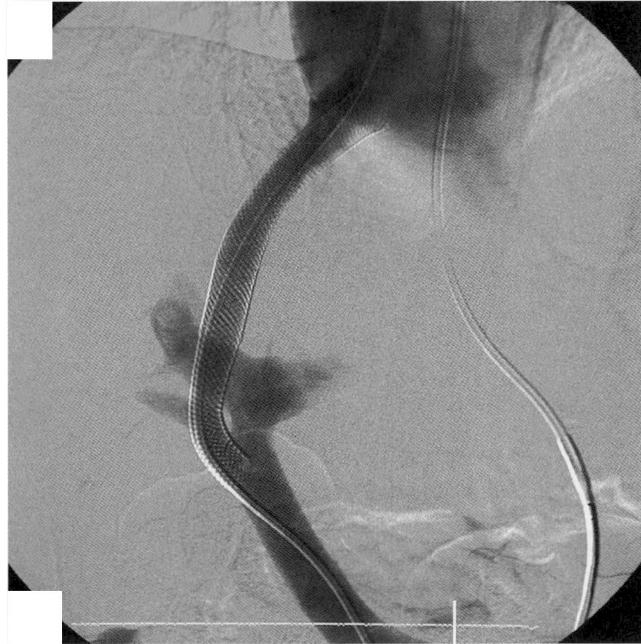

Figure 15.8 Intractable variceal bleeding or ascites may respond to the insertion of a transjugular intrahepatic portosystemic shunt (TIPSS). This venogram (**A**) demonstrates the shunt that has been created by placing a stent between the right hepatic and right portal veins, establishing good flow between the portal vein and the hepatic vein and reducing the portal vein pressure (**B**).

Primary prophylaxis of variceal bleeding

Primary prophylaxis is controversial in recognized cases of portal hypertension with varices. However, it is reasonable to prepare for the possibility by ensuring that the child's caregivers understand the importance of seeking early medical advice by attending the nearest hospital for blood cross-matching and appropriate referral to a tertiary unit. Long-acting vasoactive drugs that reduce splanchnic pressures may be useful in these circumstances (Table 15.7). Beta-blockers, such as propranolol and the more selective atenolol, reduce hepatic arterial and portal vein blood flow and have been studied with respect to reduction in portal pressures to < 12 mmHg, thereby reducing the risk of an initial bleed in adults.[46] A small uncontrolled clinical trial in children suggested a benefit for both primary and secondary prophylaxis.[47] Primary prophylactic sclerotherapy reduced the risk of bleeding, but led to an increase in portal gastropathy in another controlled trial in children.[48]

Prevention of recurrent gastrointestinal bleeding

Direct obliteration of the varices is the treatment of choice for bleeding from esophageal varices. Randomized controlled trials in adults have shown a reduction in the frequency of bleeding and improved survival, and although no randomized controlled trials have been performed in children, several large studies of sclerotherapy and/or banding in children with portal hypertension indicate that this procedure is safe and reduces the chance of rebleeding.[43,44,48] Neither technique reduces portal pressure, and both may cause some interference with the vascular hemodynamics. In some cases, hypersplenism and portal gastropathy become worse temporarily.

Several vasoactive drugs have also now been documented in multiple controlled trials in adults to reduce the risk of rebleeding by reducing portal and systemic pressures.[45] A combination of a nonselective beta-blocker and certain nitrates (e.g., isosorbide 5-mononitrate) are the drugs of choice, with the aim being to achieve a 25% reduction in resting heart rate (Table 15.7). Adverse effects of beta-blockers include reactive airway disease and heart block. Losartan, an angiotensin II (A-II) type 1 receptor blocker, may have a pronounced portal pressure-reducing effect, possibly greater than that of propranolol, but studies have not been conducted in children.[49]

Surgical management of portal hypertension is a major consideration when there is a significant risk of mortality from bleeding and failure of direct variceal obliteration. Such patients should ideally should be evaluated and treated in a transplant center, where the range of surgical options can be assessed. *Surgical portosystemic shunts* may reduce the risk of gastrointestinal bleeding, but they reduce hepatic perfusion and carry a risk of hepatic decompensation and hepatic encephalopathy, and they preclude liver transplantation or make it more difficult. Moreover, randomized controlled trials in adult patients have not shown any significant improvement in survival with portosystemic shunts in patients with intrahepatic causes of portal hypertension. If a shunt operation is contemplated in critically ill patients, then the use of a TIPSS as a bridging procedure is probably the procedure of choice. The surgical procedure of choice for uncontrolled portal hypertension due to intrahepatic disease is liver transplantation.

In non-shunt, non-transplant candidates, an esophageal disconnection/devascularization procedure (Sugiura) may be lifesaving, with the added advantage of a low risk of encephalopathy. Special consideration should be given to shunt surgery in some patients with cystic fibrosis–associated liver disease, when there is a slow evolution of hepatic dysfunction; in patients with congenital hepatic fibrosis, a presinusoidal cause of portal hypertension that is not associated with liver synthetic dysfunction; and in patients with portal vein thrombosis. In these cases, the choice of the type of shunt is determined by the vascular anatomy, the size of the veins, the risk of thrombosis and failure, and the risk of encephalopathy. *"Selective" shunts* such as distal splenorenal or distal splenoadrenal are preferred, except in portal thrombosis, where the Rex shunt, an internal jugular vein graft mesenterico–left portal vein bypass, has the major theoretical advantage of restoring portal flow to the liver, reducing the risk of encephalopathy (see Chapter 19).

Hepatic encephalopathy

Hepatic encephalopathy is a major neuropsychiatric complication of chronic liver disease. It tends to develop slowly in cirrhotic patients, starting with altered sleep patterns and eventually progressing through asterixis to stupor and coma. Precipitating factors include an oral protein load, gastrointestinal bleeding, anesthesia, and the use of sedatives. It is common following shunts for portal hypertension. Hepatic encephalopathy is difficult to recognize in children, particularly in infants. Early symptoms of encephalopathy are subtle and include neurodevelopmental delay, school problems, lethargy, or sleep reversal. Intellectual impairment and personality change may occur in older children, while clouding of consciousness, progressing to stupor and coma, is a late sign. Clinical signs such as ataxia, tremor, and dysdiadochokinesia are difficult to determine in small children.

Pathophysiology

Hepatic encephalopathy appears to be related to four major events: portosystemic shunting; hepatocellular dysfunction; interaction of nitrogen metabolites from the intestine with the central nervous system; and altered neurotransmitter function.[50] Further alterations in brain function can be induced by hypoglycemia (common with fasting in young children) or respiratory alkalosis, leading to a decrease in cerebral perfusion and hypoxemia due to hemodynamic changes. Aggravating factors include gastrointestinal hemorrhage, hypovolemia, hypokalemia, sedatives, anesthetics, sepsis, and high protein intake, which increase the endogenous nitrogen load, thus precipitating overt encephalopathy. Hepatic encephalopathy is rare when liver function is able to remove nitrogenous intestinal metabolites, although portosystemic shunting alone can result in encephalopathy if the patient is given a high-protein diet. Serum ammonia levels do not directly correlate with cerebral state and are not the cause of the encephalopathy. Neuropathologically, there is astrocytic (rather than neuronal) alteration. Magnetic resonance imaging reveals bilateral signal hyperintensity, particularly in globus pallidus, and magnetic resonance spectroscopy shows an increase in the glutamine resonance in the brain, reflecting increased brain ammonia removal. Although the exact molecular mechanisms are not known, excitatory/inhibitory neurotransmitter imbalance leading to dysfunction of the glutamate–nitric oxide system is thought to play a major role. NO is a gaseous, highly reactive, freely diffusible molecule with a short half-life. Increased expression of the neuronal isoform of NO synthase and the uptake of L-arginine (the obligate precursor of NO) has been demonstrated. Hyperammonemia results in increased NO, which may lead to impairment of learning and memory. Other metabolic factors include short-chain fatty acids such as butyrate, valerate, and octanoate, which are increased in the plasma and cerebrospinal fluid and may act synergistically with ammonia. There is also accumulation of inhibitory neurotransmitters in the brain. Neurotransmitters mediate the postsynaptic action of neurones. Inhibitory neurotransmitters may be false (not ordinarily present in the brain) or true (such as the amino acid γ-aminobutyric acid) (GABA), which is produced in the brain by the decarboxylation of glutamic acid. γ-Aminobutyric acid (GABA) has an important role in central nervous system inhibition, and GABA-like activity has been found in portal blood in both animal models and patients with chronic liver failure after gastrointestinal hemorrhage. In experimental models, GABA may produce coma. The GABA receptor is activated not only by GABA but by benzodiazepines. The reversal of encephalopathy in some patients after the administration of a benzodiazepine antagonist supports this hypothesis, although the effect is not entirely consistent. Alterations in neurotransmitter function may also occur as a result of disturbances of amino acid metabolism, particularly the deficiency of branched-chain amino acids and excess of aromatic amino acids.

Diagnosis

Diagnosis of hepatic encephalopathy in children involves a high index of suspicion and careful clinical assessment. While there are agreed criteria with neuropsychiatric tests in adults, these are not applicable to children, and there is no specific laboratory test for encephalopathy. Changes on electroencephalography (EEG) may provide objective evidence of cerebral dysfunction, but the changes are nonspecific and do not correlate with the severity of encephalopathy. Slow waves are prominent on EEG at stage II to III encephalopathy, but may occur in normal children. In chronic encephalopathy, the degree of encephalopathy varies with protein intake, which is an important clue to early diagnosis.

Treatment

This is directed at identifying and treating any precipitating factors, the avoidance of fasting, sedatives, and reducing the nitrogen load from the intestine. While standard therapy in adults for chronic hepatic encephalopathy includes protein restriction,[46] this may result in growth failure and nutritional depletion in children, which may further aggravate glucose and amino acid disturbances. Thus, restriction of dietary and/or intravenous protein to 1–2 g/kg should be used only in acute or very symptomatic encephalopathy, and protein may be reintroduced as the encephalopathy subsides. A reduction in intestinal protein load and bacterial flora in the gastrointestinal tract can be achieved in the short term by enemas, particularly if an acute episode of encephalopathy is precipitated by gastrointestinal hemorrhage, and in the long term by use of broad-spectrum antibiotics and/or lactulose. Antibiotics reduce the amount of bacterial urease available by directly suppressing ammonia-forming bacteria. In children, neomycin is no longer used, as its long-term use has resulted in deafness. Vancomycin hydrochloride has been successfully used in resistant cases.

Lactulose, a nonabsorbable synthetic disaccharide, is the mainstay of treatment for hepatic encephalopathy and should be first-line therapy, since in theory its mode of action may be counteracted by antibiotics. In the colon, the unabsorbed lactulose is metabolized by bacteria, producing lactic acid, causing a drop in pH in the colon and a reduction in ammonia reabsorption.[46] The recommended dose is 0.3–0.4 mL/kg three times a day, sufficient to acidify the stools (pH < 6.0), without significant diarrhea. BCAA-enriched nutritional supplements may be a useful adjunctive therapy for hepatic encephalopathy by reducing muscle protein breakdown and normalizing plasma amino acid profiles, although double-blind randomized studies of BCAAs for chronic encephalopathy in adults have shown conflicting results. Benzodiazepine antagonists might ameliorate some symptoms of hepatic encephalopathy. In addition, sodium benzoate, useful in treating episodic hyperammonemia in urea-cycle disorders, may have application in hepatic encephalopathy unresponsive to lactulose.

Coagulopathy

The liver plays an important role in the maintenance of hemostasis by a complex balance between the production of coagulation proteins, inhibitors of coagulation and removal of fibrin degradation products and coagulation factors. Thus, coagulation disorders are common in chronic liver disease (Table 15.8) due to a combination of vitamin K malabsorption and deficiency, reduced synthesis of coagulation factors and inhibitors of coagulation, thrombocytopenia secondary to hypersplenism, or intravascular coagulopathy. These disturbances are particularly important in the prognostic assessment and in the genesis and management of gastrointestinal bleeding, and may lead to serious complications such as intracerebral bleeding and intravascular coagulopathy.

Table 15.8 Coagulation disturbances and altered hemostasis in chronic liver disease.

Vitamin K malabsorption/deficiency
Vitamin K–dependent coagulation protein deficiencies (factors II, VII, IX, X)
Hypofibrinogenemia and dysfibrinogenemia
Thrombocytopenia
Consumption coagulopathy

Pathophysiology

There are abnormalities of primary hemostasis (interaction between platelets and vessel wall), coagulation (thrombin generation), and fibrinolysis in patients with chronic liver disease, but there is a poor correlation between the risk of bleeding and the peripheral indices of hemostasis.[51] It is possible that the delicate balance between prothrombotic and antithrombotic factors synthesized by the liver might be different in patients with chronic liver disease, so that they might be less prone to bleed unless there are additional factors such as infections. Normal hemostasis is affected by reduced numbers of circulating platelets and platelet function, but platelet counts > 20 000 rarely cause problems.

Once there is liver failure, there is a reduced capacity to clear activated hemostatic proteins and protein inhibitor complexes from the circulation. During liver transplantation, hemorrhage may occur due to the preexisting hypocoagulable state, the collateral circulation caused by portal hypertension, and the increased fibrinolysis that occurs during the operation.

Management

This is directed at prevention or correction of vitamin K deficiency by regular administration of vitamin K. All patients should have oral vitamin K supplements (Table 15.8). Parenteral vitamin K (2–10 mg i.v. daily for 3 days or 5–10 mg per week i.m.) should be given to cholestatic patients with a prolonged prothrombin time. Infusions of fresh frozen plasma (5–10 mL/kg), cryoglobulin, and/or platelet transfusions are effective for transient correction, and should be reserved for invasive procedures such as liver biopsy and for bleeding episodes. However, in children awaiting liver transplantation, the regular use of fresh frozen plasma and platelets, if the prothrombin time is > 40 s prolonged or the

Table 15.9 Pulmonary complications of chronic liver disease.

Intrapulmonary shunts and hypoxemia
Pulmonary hypertension
Pleural effusions
Pneumonia
Restrictive or obstructive airways disease

platelet count is < 20 000, may reduce the risk of hemorrhage. When there is persistent severe coagulation disturbance or persisting bleeding, a reduction in the prothrombin time and bleeding time can be achieved by using desmopressin, which increases levels of factors VIII and IX, or by using specific factor products or recombinant factor VI.[52]

Pulmonary complications of chronic liver disease

Chronic liver disease and cirrhosis have a number of potential pulmonary complications (Table 15.9). In particular, pulmonary vascular abnormalities have been increasingly recognized as important clinical entities that influence survival and liver transplant candidacy in affected patients.

Hepatopulmonary syndrome

The hepatopulmonary syndrome is defined as a triad of liver dysfunction, intrapulmonary arteriovenous shunts, and variable arterial hypoxemia in the presence of hepatic dysfunction or portal hypertension.[53] There is a widened alveolar–arterial oxygen gradient ($AaPo_2$) on room air (> 15 mmHg), with or without hypoxemia, resulting from intrapulmonary vasodilation. This is relatively common in childhood liver disease. Oxygen saturations of < 90% and cyanosis appear to be unrelated to the severity of liver damage, but are associated with the occurrence of clubbing.

Pathophysiology

The defining feature of the hepatopulmonary syndrome is microvascular dilation within the pulmonary arterial circulation.[53] These changes may result from decreased precapillary arteriolar tone alone, or may involve additional mechanisms such as angiogenesis, remodeling, and vasculogenesis. The recognition in experimental models that a unique sequence of molecular alterations leads to endothelin-1 and tumor necrosis factor-α (TNF-α) modulation of pulmonary microvascular tone may lead to the development of novel and effective medical therapies. This vasodilation appears to result from excessive vascular production of vasodilators, particularly nitric oxide, based on the observation that exhaled NO levels are increased in patients with hepatopulmonary syndrome and normalize after liver transplantation. There are intrapulmonary shunts (often seen on chest radiographs), arteriovenous shunts, ventilation–perfusion defects, and portopulmonary venous anastomoses. The degree of cyanosis may be proportionally greater than the hypoxemia. In infants, hypoxemia can be aggravated by poor respiratory effort related to ascites or hepatomegaly. Such patients have dyspnea at rest, particularly when upright, often relieved by lying down.

Diagnosis

Simple transcutaneous techniques of oxygen monitoring can be of diagnostic value.[54] Contrast echocardiography and standard cardiopulmonary testing confirm the diagnosis. Transthoracic microbubble contrast echocardiography is the preferred test. This is performed by injecting agitated saline intravenously during echocardiography, producing microbubbles that are visualized by sonography. This bolus opacifies the right ventricle within seconds and, in the absence of right-to-left shunting, bubbles are absorbed in the lungs. If intrapulmonary shunting characteristic of hepatopulmonary syndrome is present, the left ventricle opacifies at least three heart beats after the right (delayed shunting). This study also ensures that there is no underlying cardiac defect. Ventilation–perfusion scans can demonstrate the presence of extrapulmonary isotope in the cerebral blood and other organs; lung function tests are usually normal.

Management

While no specific treatment for this syndrome has been found, the hypoxemia is improved by oxygen administration, attention to nutrition support, and control of ascites. The hepatopulmonary syndrome may seriously limit tolerance to anesthesia. During or after transplantation, worsening hypoxemia may be improved by using inhaled NO. Some improvement in oxygenation has been observed after transjugular intrahepatic portosystemic shunt procedures. Liver transplantation is the only established effective therapy and will reverse the systemic and pulmonary vascular changes, although recovery may be slow. Hepatopulmonary shunting may recur if there is portal vein obstruction after transplantation, or portopulmonary shunting may develop.[55]

Pulmonary hypertension

This may occur in cirrhosis as a result of failure of degradation of vasoactive substances in the splanchnic circulation associated with portopulmonary venous anastomoses and paraesophageal portosystemic collaterals within the pulmonary venous system. The presenting feature is cyanosis, but early signs include right ventricular hypertrophy or accentuation of the pulmonary vessels on chest radiography.

Pleural effusions and pneumonia

These are common in end-stage liver disease. Pleural effusions have a similar etiology to ascites (see above) and, in association with an increased risk of bacterial infection, increase the risk of pneumonia. The occurrence of fever, cough, or dyspnea indicates a need for appropriate investigations and management.

Obstructive and restrictive pulmonary abnormalities

A variety of these have been detected in patients with chronic liver disease, particularly in α_1-antitrypsin deficiency and in liver disease associated with cystic fibrosis, in which the etiology of these pulmonary complications is due to the primary disease.

Hepatorenal syndrome

This syndrome is a functional progressive renal failure of unknown cause occurring in patients with severe liver disease. It is a serious complication of cirrhosis and carries a poor prognosis. It may be either slowly or rapidly progressive (types I and II , respectively).

Pathophysiology

While the pathogenesis is not fully understood, reduced renal cortical blood flow is central to it.[56] There is also increased splanchnic blood pooling from portal hypertension, further decreasing renal blood flow, possibly related to up-regulated endothelial NO synthase. Renal vasoconstriction may also contribute due to increased production of thromboxane, a potent vasoconstrictor, and a decrease in prostaglandin 2, a dilatory metabolite. A high incidence of glomerulosclerosis and membranoproliferative glomerulonephritis has been documented in children with end-stage liver disease at the time of liver transplantation,[57] probably secondary to chronic reduction in renal cortical blood flow. Efforts to increase glomerular filtration and renal blood flow form the basis of current approaches to supportive medical therapy.

Clinical features and diagnosis

Acute renal failure in children with liver disease may be due to primary renal disease, prerenal failure, or hepatorenal syndrome. It is possible to differentiate them by urinary indices, such as urinary sodium concentrations (< 20 mmol/L in prerenal) and the ratio of urinary to plasma creatinine (> 40 in prerenal). Functional renal failure (the hepatorenal syndrome) presents in two forms. In type 1, the onset is acute, precipitated by gastrointestinal hemorrhage, aggressive diuresis, or an associated deterioration of liver function. It is associated with oliguria, uremia, hyperkalemia, hyponatremia, and a low urinary sodium concentration (< 10 mmol/L). Initial serum creatinine levels double in less than 2 weeks. These features are difficult to distinguish from prerenal failure, which responds to an acute volume expansion, or acute tubular necrosis, in which tubular casts and high urinary sodium (> 30 mmol/L) are found. Plasma volume expansion does not improve renal function in hepatorenal syndrome. Type 2 is characterized by a slower development of oliguric renal failure with a marked reduction in glomerular filtration rate and hyponatremia, again with a low urinary sodium concentration. Serial measurements of urinary sodium concentration and urinary osmolarity help distinguish the condition of acute tubular necrosis, in which the urinary sodium concentration may rise and urine osmolarity is usually equal to plasma osmolarity. These measurements are unreliable if the patient is receiving diuretics, particularly furosemide.

Management

Renal failure has a mortality rate of ≥ 90% in the setting of severe liver disease, but is effectively reversed by liver transplantation. Acute renal failure should initially be managed with volume expansion as a diagnostic therapy, as mentioned above. Following this, temporary reversal of the hepatorenal syndrome can be achieved with combinations of splanchnic vasoconstrictors (octreotide, 3–5 μg/kg/day), or vasopressin analogues (terlipressin, 0.04 mg/kg/day), colloid volume expansion with regular albumin infusions (1–2 g/kg/day), insertion of transjugular intrahepatic portovenous shunts, and improved forms of dialysis.[58] Liver transplantation is tolerated in patients with hepatorenal syndrome, although the preexisting glomerular abnormalities and the post-transplantation nephrotoxic effects of calcineurin inhibitors may partly explain the high rates of renal dysfunction after transplantation.

Bacterial infections

Bacterial infections are common in chronic liver disease, and may precipitate other complications, such as encephalopathy, ascites, and hepatorenal syndrome. Urinary and respiratory tract infections are frequent, and bacteremia commonly results from invasive investigations. Spontaneous bacterial peritonitis is a common serious complication of ascites and should always be excluded in all children with sepsis. Immune deficits associated with chronic liver disease include abnormalities of complement and opsonization, impaired function of Kupffer cells, neutropenia, and alterations in mucosal barriers, particularly the gastrointestinal tract. Portal hypertension makes patients susceptible to frequent bacteremia, perhaps by inducing bacterial translocation of the gut. The specific risk factors for infection are low serum albumin, gastrointestinal bleeding, intensive care unit admission for any cause, and therapeutic endoscopy. Certain infectious agents are more virulent and more common in patients with liver disease. These include *Klebsiella, Escherichia coli, Vibrio, Campylobacter, Yersinia, Plesiomonas, Enterococcus, Aeromonas, Capnocytophaga*, and *Listeria* species, as well as organisms from other species. Preventative measures such as pneumococcal and *Haemophilus influenzae* vaccination, prophylactic antibiotics for invasive procedures, and nutritional support may reduce the risk of specific infection.

Spontaneous bacterial peritonitis

This is a potentially fatal complication of ascites in children. The condition should always be suspected in a patient with ascites and concurrent fever, abdominal pain, or neutrophilia. Common signs in pediatric patients include abdominal distension, vomiting, and diarrhea. Examination may reveal abdominal tenderness with rebound and decreased or absent bowel sounds. Occasionally, spontaneous bacterial peritonitis may be relatively asymptomatic except for fever. The diagnosis is established by abdominal paracentesis, which reveals cloudy fluid with a neutrophil leukocyte count of > 250/mm and a low protein concentration < 20 g/L. Characteristically, spontaneous bacterial peritonitis in children is caused by a single species—often enteric bacteria such as *Klebsiella* spp., *E. coli,* and enterococcus, although *Streptococcus pneumoniae* predominates.[59,60] The presence of multiple species suggests the possibility of bowel perforation and secondary peritonitis. While the final choice of antibiotics is dictated best by the bacteriology, early institution of therapy with a third-generation cephalosporin, such as ceftriaxone or cefotaxime, is recommended. Prophylaxis against this disorder has not been subjected to definitive trials,[61] but clinical experience suggests that it can be achieved by using prophylactic antibiotics during invasive procedures, immunization (as above), and in recurrent cases a prophylactic oral antibiotic such as co-trimoxazole, ciprofloxacin, or norfloxacin.

Pruritus

Pruritus is a debilitating complication of cholestasis that may be a symptom of many chronic pediatric liver diseases, notably Alagille's syndrome, progressive familial intrahepatic cholestasis, and some cases of biliary atresia. Disfiguring xanthomas secondary to hypercholesterolemia may accompany severe pruritus. To date, the pathophysiological link between cholestasis and pruritus is not fully understood. There is an association between pruritus and serum bile acids. Temporary relief may be possible with bile salt reduction following biliary diversion[62] or using the Molecular Adsorbents Recirculating System (MARS), which is an alternative form of hemodialysis that uses a specific filter to remove toxic products, but not albumin.[63]

There is some evidence to suggest a central mechanism for pruritus involving endogenous opioids and serotonin metabolism.[64,65]

Management

Severe pruritus can have a serious impact on patients' quality of life—e.g., sleep disturbances and unremitting distress in infants. The severity is difficult to measure in children, but a five-tier scoring system has been suggested to compare the outcomes of various therapies:[62]

- Grade 1, no pruritus
- Grade 2, mild scratching when distracted
- Grade 3, active scratching without abrasion
- Grade 4, active scratching with abrasions
- Grade 5, cutaneous mutilation with bleeding/scarring

Children with marked pruritus require careful skin care and hygiene and efforts to minimize scratching such as cooling the skin, emollients, avoiding excess sweating, and wearing cotton gloves while sleeping. There are several therapeutic options with different pathophysiological rationales for medical therapy of pruritus: hydrophilic bile acids (e.g., ursodeoxycholic acid), anion exchanger (cholestyramine), histamine H_1-antagonists (e.g., clemastine), hepatic enzyme–inducing drugs (phenobarbital, rifampicin), cannabinoid receptor agonist (dronabinol), serotonin reuptake inhibitors (e.g., sertraline) and, finally, opioid antagonists (e.g., naltrexone). These are variably effective, the most effective being the consistent administration of cholestyramine (difficult to administer because of taste) and/or rifampin.[64] One adult controlled trial found that sertraline appeared to be an effective, well-tolerated treatment for pruritus due to chronic liver disease. Some patients have contraindications or do not respond to all these drugs. Severe intractable pruritus and disfiguring xanthomas may be a relative indication for liver transplantation in patients with progressive chronic liver disease. In patients without progressive liver disease, such as some patients with Alagille's syndrome, other treatment options such as partial biliary diversion or Molecular Adsorbents Recirculating System (MARS)[62,63] have been of benefit.

Molecular Adsorbents Recirculating System

MARS is an alternative form of hemodialysis that uses a specific filter to remove toxic products, but not albumin. It has a role in the management of both acute liver failure and acute-on-chronic liver failure in adults, and there are anecdotal reports of its efficacy in children. It reduces plasma bilirubin, bile salt concentration, normalizes coagulation, and improves encephalopathy in the short term, but it may have a role to play in creating a bridge to transplantation.[66]

Hepatocellular carcinoma

Hepatocellular carcinoma may occur in the setting of chronic liver disease in cirrhosis in childhood. Frequent associations include chronic hepatitis B, in which children with neonatally acquired hepatitis B have developed hepatocellular carcinoma by age of 7 or 8 years;[67] tyrosinemia type I, with an occurrence rate of 37% in patients surviving beyond 2 years of age, although the early use of nitisinone (NTBC) may reduce this risk.[13] Patients may present with abdominal pain and/or abdominal mass, or an increase in α fetoprotein, but hepatocellular carcinoma may be found incidentally at liver transplantation. If hepatocellular carcinoma is associated with chronic liver disease, liver transplantation is the treatment of choice.

Future directions in the management of chronic liver disease complications

The traditional view of the prevention and treatment of the major complications of liver disease, as delineated above, is being challenged by newer concepts of management arising out of improved knowledge of the basic mechanisms of liver injury and developments in cell and molecular biology. Examples include: therapy aimed at slowing/preventing progressive liver injury due to cholestasis, such as antioxidants and ursodeoxycholic acid; measures aimed at preventing fibrogenesis, thus slowing the progression of liver fibrosis and cirrhosis; the experimental use of antifibrotic agents reversing fibrosis; hepatocyte transplantation, in which both animal models and human studies show that hepatocytes survive, function, and participate in regeneration when transplanted into liver or spleen, improving hepatic and enzyme function. In addition, clinical studies have suggested a possible role for gene therapy protocols bridging to transplantation, while future therapy with gene therapy remains elusive.

Case study

The patient was a 4.5-year-old girl with biliary atresia who presented with vomiting, fresh blood and clots, hypovolemic shock, and hemoglobin 4 g/dL. Her body weight was 12.8 kg.

She had been diagnosed with biliary atresia at the age of 6 weeks, by operative cholangiography. She underwent a successful hepatoportoenterostomy and had been free of jaundice since. She had been growing well (75th centile for weight and height). However, at follow-up examinations at the ages of 1, 2, and 4 years, she was found to have persistent hepatosplenomegaly and elevated hepatic transaminases. At the age of 4 years, she developed hypersplenism, with low numbers of erythrocytes, white cells, and platelets, but had normal liver synthetic function (albumin and prothrombin time).

Her only other significant history of illness was a 5-day admission to hospital for dehydration due to gastroenteritis, requiring intravenous fluids, at the age of 2.5 years.

On examination, she was tachycardic (160 beats/min) and hypotensive (80/30), with weak pulses and prolonged capillary refill. She had marked abdominal distension, with hepatosplenomegaly and ascites. She was mildly jaundiced. The respiratory and central nervous system examinations were normal. She had fine telangiectasia on her face, several spider nevi on her back, and obvious abdominal wall veins. She had bruises on her shins.

Initial emergency management. Secure the largest intravenous infusion line possible; obtain blood for cross-matching for transfusion of blood and blood products; hemoglobin and platelet count, international normalized ratio (INR), albumin. Initial fluid management should be crystalloids, such as stable plasma protein solution 20 mL/kg, followed by red blood cell transfusion until hemodynamically stable. Administer vitamin K 10 mg i.m. or i.v. Any coagulopathy should be corrected fresh frozen plasma, and/or platelet infusion. Administer octreotide (maximum dose 1 μg/kg/h i.v., or 2–4 μg/kg/dose subcutaneously 8-hourly for 24 h or until the bleeding has ceased). Nasogastric intubation is an essential part of management, allowing the documentation of ongoing bleeding and the removal of blood, which might precipitate encephalopathy. When hemodynamically stable, endoscopy is indicated for diagnosis and therapy.

The endoscopic findings in the esophagus are shown in Figure 15.9A. There were grade 3–4 varices with cherry red spots, a clot over the surface of one vein just above the gastroesophageal junction, and old blood in the stomach.

Most appropriate approach to controlling/preventing further variceal bleeding. In adults, comparative trials of sclerotherapy and ligation indicate equal efficacy in controlling bleeding, reducing rebleeding, and ablating varices, but fewer adverse effects with banding. The two procedures can be complementary in this age group, and access to both procedures is warranted. Ligation may be technically difficult for smaller varices, particularly in small infants, where entrapment of part of the esophageal wall with perforation or bleeding can occur. In these circumstances, sclerotherapy may be more appropriate, using injection of sclerosant (ethanolamine, or tetradecyl sulfate) either paravariceally or intravariceally, in volumes of 0.5–1.0 mL just above the gastroesophageal junction. Care should be taken to avoid injecting too high above the cardia, as this can increase bleeding from a distal varix. Broad-spectrum antibiotics should be prescribed (amoxicillin, metronidazole). Complications, which should be uncommon in experienced centers, include esophageal ulceration, stricture and pain.

Follow-up. There was no further gastrointestinal bleeding. After recovery between days 2 and 14, her ongoing clinical problems were persisting ascites and peripheral edema.

Laboratory investigations on day 5 were as follows: Hb 9 g/dL, white blood count (WBC) 2400, platelets 75 000, albumin 1.8 g/dL, prothrombin time 17 s, total bilirubin 3.4 mg/dL.

Computed tomography showed an echogenic, nonhomogeneous liver, portal vein thrombosis, extensive paraesophageal and gastric varices, and marked mesenteric edema and ascites, probably secondary to vascular congestion (Figure 15.10).

Appropriate medical therapy for ascites, hypersplenism, portal hypertension, and the risk of further gastrointestinal bleeding. Sequential i.v. albumin infusion (1 g/kg/day for 3 days) and furosemide 2 mg/kg (i.v. or oral), as well as oral spironolactone, which requires a flexible dosage regimen and takes 2–4 days to take effect using an initial dosage of 1 mg/kg q.i.d. The response to diuretic therapy should be evaluated by measuring body weight, urine volume, serum electrolytes and blood urea nitrogen, and sodium excretion. The initial goal of treatment is a negative fluid balance of ≥ 10 mL/kg/day. Higher negative balances risk plasma volume depletion and a decline in renal function. This can be preempted by further albumin infusion. The response to spironolactone is so reliable that the plasma volume status of the patient should be investigated if no significant diuresis is achieved within 2–4 days. Side effects include hyponatremia and hyperkalemia, which are indications for reducing/discontinuing spironolactone.

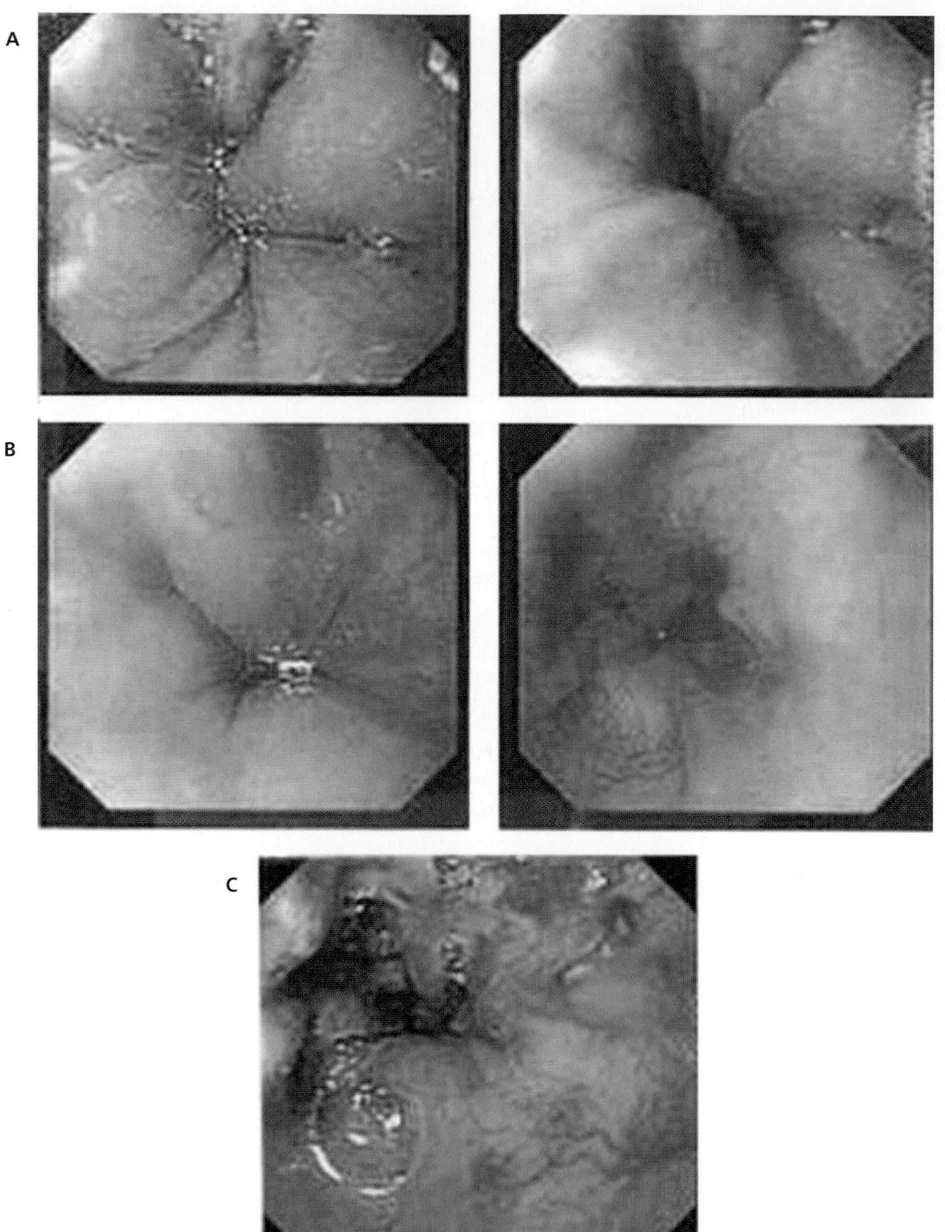

Figure 15.9 Grade 3 esophageal varices, with cherry-red spot (suggesting an immediate risk of bleeding) and recent clot.

There is no specific therapy for the hypersplenism.

Further direct obliteration of the varices should reduce the risk of recurrent bleeding from esophageal varices in the medium term. This does not reduce portal pressure and may cause some interference with the vascular hemodynamics, with worsening of the hypersplenism and portal gastropathy. Several vasoactive drugs have also now been documented in multiple controlled trials in adults to reduce the risk of rebleeding by reducing portal and systemic pressures. A combination of a nonselective beta-blocker (propranolol 1–5 mg/kg/day in three divided doses) and a nitrate (e.g., isosorbide 5-mononitrate) are the drugs of choice, with the aim being to achieve a 20% reduction in the resting heart rate. Adverse effects of beta-blockers include reactive airway disease and heart block. Nutritional supplements with a high-energy diet and multivitamin supplements, including fat soluble vitamins, should be prescribed, along with weekly intramuscular or intravascular vitamin K 5 mg.

Further progress. Three and six weeks later, she underwent a further endoscopy (Figure 15.9B, C). Six weeks after presentation, she was moderately jaundiced, with mild persisting ascites (body weight 12.4 kg). The following laboratory investigations were obtained:

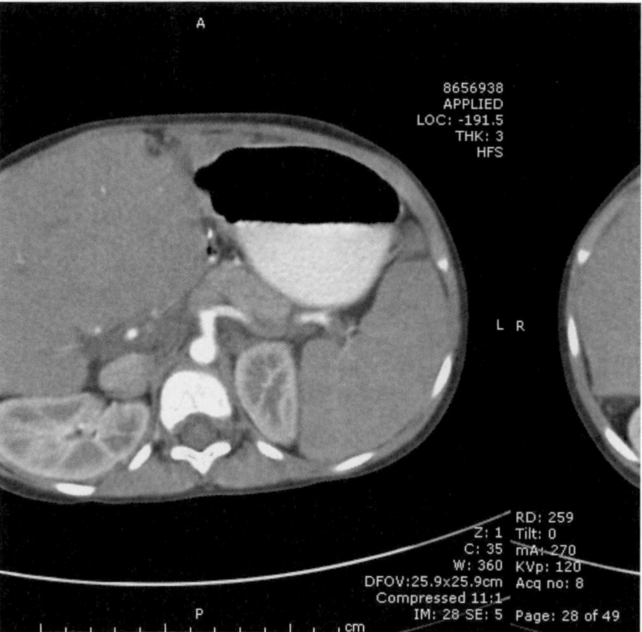

Figure 15.10 Abdominal computed tomogram with contrast, showing partial cavernous transformation of a thrombosed portal vein. From the confluence of the splenic and mesenteric vein, almost no contrast is seen coursing from the expected location of the portal vein. Other images, not shown, showed that the majority of blood was coursing along a very dilated tortuous coronary vein, which could be traced to the gastroesophageal junction, where there were several large varices. The liver is cirrhotic.

- Hb 8.4 g/dL, WBC 3200, platelets 50 000
- Total bilirubin 5 g/dL, conjugated 3.3 g/dL, aminotransferase (AST) 190 IU, alanine aminotransferase (ALT) 240 IU, γ-glutamyltransferase (GGT) 125 IU, serum alkaline phosphatase (SAP) 560 IU
- Serum albumin 2.2 g/dL
- Prothrombin time 19 s
- Partial thromboplastin time 28 s
- INR 2.0

Surgical options for improving portal hypertension. The patient was not a candidate for transjugular intrahepatic portosystemic stent shunt (TIPSS) shunting due to her portal vein thrombosis, and she was not a candidate for surgical shunting due to her underlying liver disease. Splenectomy was not indicated. Given the background of biliary atresia with features of cirrhosis with ongoing hepatic decompensation, as well as the occurrence of extrahepatic portal hypertension with a risk of variceal bleeding and refractory ascites, consideration for liver transplantation is the only viable long-term option. For all causes of end-stage disease, age, bilirubin, and international normalized ratio growth failure and albumin were significant for poor outcome in an analysis of data from the Studies of Pediatric Liver Transplantation (SPLIT) Consortium.

The Pediatric End-Stage Liver Disease (PELD) score is used as the standard for organ-sharing in the United States. A similar but more extensive scoring system for disease severity in children with mild to severe liver disease, the Pediatric Hepatology Dependency (PHD) score comprises 10 parameters (aspartate aminotransferase, prothrombin time, albumin, bilirubin, ascites, nutritional support, organ dysfunction, blood product support, sepsis and intravenous access) and has been found to be in agreement with the PELD score for patients requiring transplantation, but is a measure of dependency and disease severity in more heterogeneous groups of patients with liver disease.

Using these prognostic/severity scores, the patient's PELD score was 24 and her PHD score was 17. Both the PELD score and the PHD score indicate a high risk for death or transplantation within 6 months.

References

1 Sokol RJ, Devereaux M, Dahl R, Gumpricht E. "Let there be bile"—understanding hepatic injury in cholestasis. *J Pediatr Gastroenterol Nutr* 2006;**43**(Suppl 1):S4–9.

2 Kisseleva T, Brenner DA. Hepatic stellate cells and the reversal of fibrosis. *J Gastroenterol Hepatol* 2006;**21**(Suppl 3):S84–7.

3 Bataller R, Brenner DA. Hepatic stellate cells as a target for the treatment of liver fibrosis. *Semin Liver Dis* 2001;**21**:437–51.

4 Guicciardi ME, Gores GJ. Cholestatic hepatocellular injury: what do we know and how should we proceed. *J Hepatol* 2005;**42**: 297–300.

5 Boyer TD. Pharmacologic treatment of portal hypertension: past, present, and future. *Hepatology* 2001;**34**(4 Pt 1):834–9.

6 Rodriguez-Vilarrupla A, Fernandez M, Bosch J, Garcia-Pagan JC. Current concepts on the pathophysiology of portal hypertension. *Ann Hepatol* 2007;**6**:28–36.

7 Ramm GA, Nair VG, Bridle KR, Shepherd RW, Crawford DH. Contribution of hepatic parenchymal and nonparenchymal cells to hepatic fibrogenesis in biliary atresia. *Am J Pathol* 1998;**153**: 527–35.

8 Lewindon PJ, Pereira TN, Hoskins AC, *et al.* The role of hepatic stellate cells and transforming growth factor-beta(1) in cystic fibrosis liver disease. *Am J Pathol* 2002;**160**:1705–15.

9 Kaufman SS, Murray ND, Wood RP, Shaw BW Jr, Vanderhoof JA. Nutritional support for the infant with extrahepatic biliary atresia. *J Pediatr* 1987;**110**:679–86.

10 Shepherd RW, Chin SE, Cleghorn GJ, *et al.* Malnutrition in children with chronic liver disease accepted for liver transplantation: clinical profile and effect on outcome. *J Paediatr Child Health* 1991;**27**:295–9.

11 Chin SE, Shepherd RW, Thomas BJ, *et al.* The nature of malnutrition in children with end-stage liver disease awaiting orthotopic liver transplantation. *Am J Clin Nutr* 1992;**56**:164–8.

12 Holme E, Lindstedt S. Tyrosinaemia type I and NTBC (2-(2-nitro-4-trifluoromethylbenzoyl)-1,3-cyclohexanedione). *J Inherit Metab Dis* 1998;**21**:507–17.

13 Crone J, Moslinger D, Bodamer OA, *et al.* Reversibility of cirrhotic regenerative liver nodules upon NTBC treatment in a child with tyrosinaemia type I. *Acta Paediatr* 2003;**92**:625–8.

14 Wynn TA. Common and unique mechanisms regulate fibrosis in various fibroproliferative diseases. *J Clin Invest* 2007;**117**:524–9.

15 McDiarmid SV, Merion RM, Dykstra DM, Harper AM. Selection of pediatric candidates under the PELD system. *Liver Transpl* 2004;**10**(10 Suppl 2):S23–30.

16 Cowley AD, Cummins C, Beath SV, *et al.* Paediatric hepatology dependency score (PHD score): an audit tool. *J Pediatr Gastroenterol Nutr* 2007;**44**:108–15.

17 Burdelski M, Schutz E, Nolte-Buchholtz S, Armstrong VW, Oellerich M. Prognostic value of the monoethylglycinexylidide test in pediatric liver transplant candidates. *Ther Drug Monit* 1996;**18**:378–82.

18 el-Yazigi A, Shabib S, al-Rawithi S, Yusuf A, Legayada ES, al-Humidan A. Salivary clearance and urinary metabolic pattern of caffeine in healthy children and in pediatric patients with hepatocellular diseases. *J Clin Pharmacol* 1999;**39**:366–72.

19 Weerasooriya VS, White FV, Shepherd RW. Hepatic fibrosis and survival in biliary atresia. *J Pediatr* 2004;**144**:123–5.

20 McKiernan PJ, Baker AJ, Kelly DA. The frequency and outcome of biliary atresia in the UK and Ireland. *Lancet* 2000;**355**:25–9.

21 Grompe M. The pathophysiology and treatment of hereditary tyrosinemia type 1. *Semin Liver Dis* 2001;**21**:563–71.

22 Shepherd RW. Pre- and postoperative nutritional care in liver transplantation in children. *J Gastroenterol Hepatol* 1996;**11**:S7–10.

23 Plauth M, Cabre E, Riggio O, *et al.* ESPEN guidelines on enteral nutrition: liver disease. *Clin Nutr* 2006;**25**:285–94.

24 Utterson EC, Shepherd RW, Sokol RJ, *et al.* Biliary atresia: clinical profiles, risk factors, and outcomes of 755 patients listed for liver transplantation. *J Pediatr* 2005;**147**:180–5.

25 Chin SE, Shepherd RW, Thomas BJ, *et al.* Nutritional support in children with end-stage liver disease: a randomized crossover trial of a branched-chain amino acid supplement. *Am J Clin Nutr* 1992;**56**:158–63.

26 Greer R, Lehnert M, Lewindon P, Cleghorn GJ, Shepherd RW. Body composition and components of energy expenditure in children with end-stage liver disease. *J Pediatr Gastroenterol Nutr* 2003;**36**:358–63.

27 Mager DR, Wykes LJ, Roberts EA, Ball RO, Pencharz PB. Mild-to-moderate chronic cholestatic liver disease increases leucine oxidation in children. *J Nutr* 2006;**136**:965–70.

28 Mager DR, Wykes LJ, Roberts EA, Ball RO, Pencharz PB. Branched-chain amino acid needs in children with mild-to-moderate chronic cholestatic liver disease. *J Nutr* 2006;**136**:133–9.

29 Greer RM, Quirk P, Cleghorn GJ, Shepherd RW. Growth hormone resistance and somatomedins in children with end-stage liver disease awaiting transplantation. *J Pediatr Gastroenterol Nutr* 1998;**27**:148–54.

30 Mager DR, McGee PL, Furuya KN, Roberts EA. Prevalence of vitamin K deficiency in children with mild to moderate chronic liver disease. *J Pediatr Gastroenterol Nutr* 2006;**42**:71–6.

31 Sokol RJ. Fat-soluble vitamins and their importance in patients with cholestatic liver diseases. *Gastroenterol Clin North Am* 1994; **23**:673–705.

32 Sokol RJ, Balistreri WF, Hoofnagle JH, Jones EA. Vitamin E deficiency in adults with chronic liver disease. *Am J Clin Nutr* 1985;**41**:66–72.

33 Sokol RJ, Heubi JE, Balistreri WF. Vitamin E deficiency in cholestatic liver disease. *J Pediatr* 1983;**103**:663–4.

34 Crawford BA, Labio ED, Strasser SI, McCaughan GW. Vitamin D replacement for cirrhosis-related bone disease. *Nat Clin Pract Gastroenterol Hepatol* 2006;**3**:689–99.

35 Klein GL, Soriano H, Shulman RJ, Levy M, Jones G, Langman CB. Hepatic osteodystrophy in chronic cholestasis: evidence for a multifactorial etiology. *Pediatr Transplant* 2002;**6**:136–40.

36 Sokol RJ, Stall C. Anthropometric evaluation of children with chronic liver disease. *Am J Clin Nutr* 1990;**52**:203–8.

37 Charlton M. Branched-chain amino acid enriched supplements as therapy for liver disease. *J Nutr* 2006;**136**(1 Suppl):295–8S.

38 van Erpecum KJ. Ascites and spontaneous bacterial peritonitis in patients with liver cirrhosis. *Scand J Gastroenterol Suppl* 2006; (**243**):79–84.

39 Decaux G. V2-antagonists for the treatment of hyponatraemia. *Nephrol Dial Transplant* 2007;**22**:1853–5.

40 McGibbon A, Chen GI, Peltekian KM, van Zanten SV. An evidence-based manual for abdominal paracentesis. *Dig Dis Sci* 2007;**52**:3307–15.

41 Heyman MB, LaBerge JM. Role of transjugular intrahepatic portosystemic shunt in the treatment of portal hypertension in pediatric patients. *J Pediatr Gastroenterol Nutr* 1999;**29**:240–9.

42 Banares R, Albillos A, Rincon D, *et al.* Endoscopic treatment versus endoscopic plus pharmacologic treatment for acute variceal bleeding: a meta-analysis. *Hepatology* 2002;**35**:609–15.

43 McKiernan PJ, Beath SV, Davison SM. A prospective study of endoscopic esophageal variceal ligation using a multiband ligator. *J Pediatr Gastroenterol Nutr* 2002;**34**:207–11.

44 Goenka AS, Dasilva MS, Cleghorn GJ, Patrick MK, Shepherd RW. Therapeutic upper gastrointestinal endoscopy in children: an audit of 443 procedures and literature review. *J Gastroenterol Hepatol* 1993;**8**:44–51.

45 Stiegmann GV, Goff JS, Michaletz-Onody PA, *et al.* Endoscopic sclerotherapy as compared with endoscopic ligation for bleeding esophageal varices. *N Engl J Med* 1992;**326**:1527–32.

46 Lebrec D. Drug therapy for portal hypertension. *Gut* 2001;**49**: 441–2.

47 Shashidhar H, Langhans N, Grand RJ. Propranolol in prevention of portal hypertensive hemorrhage in children: a pilot study. *J Pediatr Gastroenterol Nutr* 1999;**29**:12–7.

48 Goncalves ME, Cardoso SR, Maksoud JG. Prophylactic sclerotherapy in children with esophageal varices: long-term results of a controlled prospective randomized trial. *J Pediatr Surg* 2000; **35**:401–5.

49 Castano G, Viudez P, Riccitelli M, Sookoian S. A randomized study of losartan vs propranolol: Effects on hepatic and systemic hemodynamics in cirrhotic patients. *Ann Hepatol* 2003;**2**:36–40.

50 Bass NM. Review article: the current pharmacological therapies for hepatic encephalopathy. *Aliment Pharmacol Ther* 2007;**25** (Suppl 1):23–31.

51 Tripodi A, Mannucci PM. J Abnormalities of hemostasis in chronic liver disease: reappraisal of their clinical significance and need for clinical and laboratory research. *J Hepatol* 2007;**46**: 727–33.

52 Ramsey G. Treating coagulopathy in liver disease with plasma transfusions or recombinant factor VIIa: an evidence-based review. *Best Pract Res Clin Haematol* 2006;**19**:113–26.

53 Palma DT, Fallon MB. The hepatopulmonary syndrome. *J Hepatol* 2006;**45**:617–25.

54 Santamaria F, Sarnelli P, Celentano L, *et al.* Noninvasive investigation of hepatopulmonary syndrome in children and adolescents with chronic cholestasis. *Pediatr Pulmonol* 2002;**33**: 374–9.

55 Shah T, Isaac J, Adams D, Kelly D; Liver Units. Development of hepatopulmonary syndrome and portopulmonary hypertension in a paediatric liver transplant patient. *Pediatr Transplant* 2005; **9**:127–31.

56 Salerno F, Gerbes A, Gines P, Wong F, Arroyo V. Diagnosis, prevention and treatment of the hepatorenal syndrome in cirrhosis. *Gut* 2007;**56**:1310–8.

57 Chin SE, Axelsen RA, Crawford DH, *et al.* Glomerular abnormalities in children undergoing orthotopic liver transplantation. *Pediatr Nephrol* 1992;**6**:407–11.

58 Moreau R, Lebrec D. The use of vasoconstrictors in patients with cirrhosis: type 1 HRS and beyond. *Hepatology* 2006;**43**:385–94.

59 Vieira SM, Matte U, Kieling CO, *et al.* Infected and noninfected ascites in pediatric patients. *J Pediatr Gastroenterol Nutr* 2005;**40**: 289–94.

60 Larcher VF, Manolaki N, Vegnente A, Vergani D, Mowat AP. Spontaneous bacterial peritonitis in children with chronic liver disease: clinical features and etiologic factors. *J Pediatr* 1985;**106**: 907–12.

61 Soares-Weiser K, Brezis M, Leibovici L. Antibiotics for spontaneous bacterial peritonitis in cirrhotics. *Cochrane Database Syst Rev* 2001;(**3**):CD002232.

62 Emerick KM, Whitington PF. Partial external biliary diversion for intractable pruritus and xanthomas in Alagille's syndrome. *Hepatology* 2002;**35**:1501–6.

63 Montero JL, Pozo JC, Barrera P, *et al.* Treatment of refractory cholestatic pruritus with molecular adsorbent recirculating system (MARS). *Transplant Proc* 2006;**38**(8):2511–3.

64 Bergasa NV. Pruritus in chronic liver disease: mechanisms and treatment. *Curr Gastroenterol Rep* 2004;**6**:10–6.

65 Ng VL, Balistreri WF. Treatment options for chronic cholestasis in infancy and childhood. *Curr Treat Options Gastroenterol* 2005;**8**: 419–30.

66 Debray D, Yousef N, Durand P. New management options for end-stage chronic liver disease and acute liver failure: potential for pediatric patients. *Paediatr Drugs* 2006;**8**:1–13.

67 Hsu HC, Wu MZ, Chang MH, Su IJ, Chen DS. Childhood hepatocellular carcinoma developed exclusively in hepatitis B surface antigen carriers in three decades in Taiwan: a report of 51 cases strongly associated with rapid development of liver cirrhosis. *J Hepatol* 1987;**5**:260–7.

9 The Liver and Other Organs

16 The Liver in Systemic Illness

Susan V. Beath

The liver inevitably plays a major role in systemic illness. It is the largest organ in the body and takes up to 25% of cardiac output. The presence of a double vascular input from the celiac axis and portal vein exposes the liver to high concentrations of inflammatory mediators, hormones, nutrients, food antigens, drugs, and intestinal microorganisms.

The hepatic veins drain into the inferior vena cava or directly into the right atrium, which means that cardiac dysfunction rapidly leads to hepatic congestion. In addition, the liver is composed of many different cell types—e.g., hepatocytes, endothelial cells, Kupffer cells, biliary epithelial cells, stellate cells, and immune regulatory cells. These cells produce an enormous range of bioactive molecules, including glucose, inflammatory mediators, chemoattractant molecules for cytotoxic CD8 and regulatory T cells, growth factors, hormones, bilirubin, coagulation factors, albumin, and products of drug metabolism. For example, Kupffer cells may cause hepatocyte necrosis by producing harmful soluble mediators, as well as acting as antigen-presenting cells during viral infections of the liver.[1] There is a great potential for extrahepatic disease to influence liver function and for impaired liver function to influence the course of systemic disease.

Cardiac disease and the liver

The pathophysiology of early hepatic dysfunction in heart disease is related to hypoxia, congestion, and low cardiac output.[2] There are recognized risk factors for hepatic ischemia, which include: a history including a Fontan operation, the use of vasopressors, need for intra-aortic balloon counterpropulsion, prolonged aortic clamping times, and diabetes mellitus.[3,4] Dextrocardia and pulmonary stenosis may also be associated with liver disease. Long-term complications of surgery for congenital heart disease may include hepatic fibrosis and portal hypertension, which is often subclinical but is associated with a protein-losing enteropathy or esophageal varices and hemorrhage in severe cases; 35% (34/97) patients listed for heart transplantation had a protein-losing enteropathy, which resolved after successful heart transplantation.[5]

Hypoxia

This type of injury is frequently seen after coronary bypass surgery, especially if the bypass operation has taken longer than 2 h. The evidence that the injury is primarily hypoxic is based on liver histology, in which changes in zone 3 (around the central vein, which is furthest away from arterial blood) are characteristic. A dramatic rise in transaminases, which may be > 10 000 IU/L, occurs 24–48 h after the cardiac surgery. Cholestasis after bypass surgery may occur if the bypass time exceeds 2 h, as demonstrated by a study in which 18.5% of adults who underwent heart valve surgery under bypass developed cholestasis.[6]

Coagulopathy is rare, although clotting may be prolonged because of heparin/warfarin treatment. The liver function tests usually return to normal within weeks, unless hypoxia or a low cardiac output state persist. Biliary sludge, which may lead to obstructive jaundice, is a recognized complication of major cardiac surgery, especially if the child has required a major blood transfusion and is not permitted enteral feeding for more than a few days.[6] The differential diagnosis includes drug toxicity—e.g., both amiodarone and verapamil may cause a cholestatic hepatitis[7]—systemic sepsis, viral hepatitis, congenital risk factors such as α_1-antitrypsin deficiency, Alagille's syndrome, hypopituitarism, and biliary obstruction.

Hepatic congestion

The liver becomes congested when there is an increase in right atrial or ventricular pressure, as in pulmonary atresia, constrictive pericarditis, tetralogy of Fallot, and after the Fontan procedure carried out on univentricular hearts. Sinusoidal engorgement usually causes modest elevations of transaminases, while alkaline phosphatase and bilirubin are typically normal, although there may be a rise in unconjugated hyperbilirubinemia. The clinical features are those of hepatic vein outflow obstruction and include: hepatomegaly, which may be tender; unconjugated hyperbilirubinemia; transaminases 80–200 IU/L; and sinusoidal dilation around

Diseases of the Liver and Biliary System in Children, 3rd edition. Edited by Deirdre Kelly. © 2008 Blackwell Publishing, ISBN: 978-1-4051-6334-7.

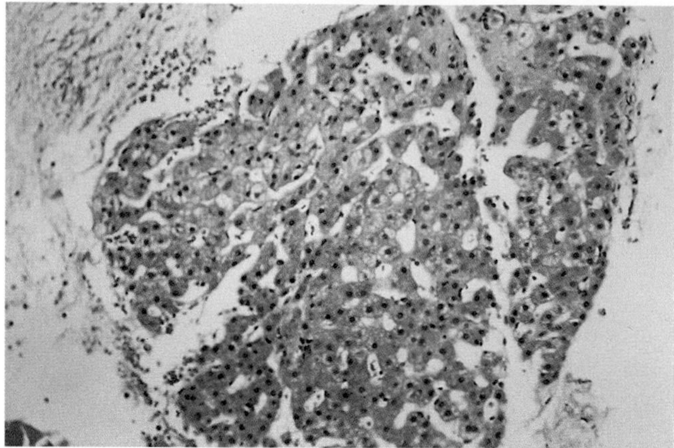

Figure 16.1 Sinusoidal dilation secondary to raised hepatic pressure from constrictive pericarditis due to tuberculosis. The patient improved following pericardectomy and isoniazid treatment.

the central vein on histology. Later, the clinical picture includes: hypoalbuminemia exacerbated by protein-losing enteropathy, ascites, cirrhosis, and portal hypertension. If constrictive pericarditis is the underlying cause of hepatic congestion, the diagnosis may be missed, as cardiac signs and symptoms are minimal. Cardiac catheterization may be required to confirm the diagnosis. In a study of 83 patients with a variety of cardiac disorders, there was a correlation between raised aminotransferases and raised hepatic venous pressures (mean wedge pressure 18 mmHg and free 15 mmHg), which was also related to the presence of centrilobular necrosis and inflammation.[8] The differential diagnosis includes Budd–Chiari syndrome, veno-occlusive disease, and tuberculous pericarditis (Figure 16.1)

Low cardiac output

States secondary to hypoplastic left heart or cardiomyopathy reduce blood flow within the liver parenchyma, producing chronic hypoxia. There may be a compensatory increase in portal vein blood flow to balance the reduction in hepatic arterial flow, so hepatic dysfunction may be minimal unless multiorgan failure has developed due to the low output state.[2] Jaundice and elevated transaminases (100–10 000 IU/L) are usual and tend to be worse with prolonged low-output states. As in acute hypoxic injury, biliary sludge may develop, causing biliary obstruction and an increase in cholestasis (Figure 16.2).[9] Fetal arrhythmias such as supraventricular tachycardia and atrial flutter are associated with a neonatal cholestasis if they persist for more than 2 weeks, but this is reversible upon resolution of the arrhythmia. Babies with arteriovenous block, however, can develop severe cholestasis associated with liver failure and death.[10] The differential diagnosis includes drugs such as amiodarone, viral hepatitis, and in neonates congenital liver disease (e.g., biliary atresia, α_1-antitrypsin deficiency; see Chapters 4 and 5).

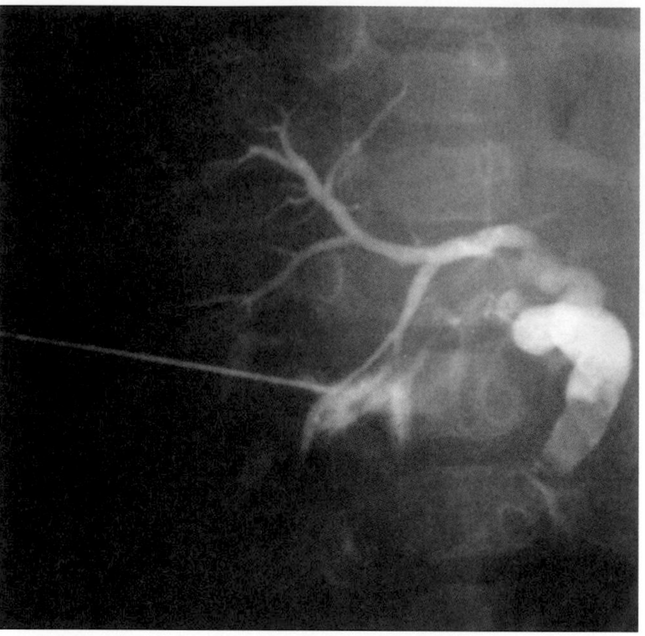

Figure 16.2 Percutaneous transhepatic cholangiogram, demonstrating obstructed biliary tree due to biliary sludge following cardiac surgery.

Cardiac–hepatic syndromes (Table 16.1)

Biliary atresia

In approximately 10% of patients, biliary atresia is associated with congenital heart disease, which may include atrial septal defect, ventricular septal defect, aortic stenosis, pulmonary stenosis, and dextrocardia with or without situs inversus. If severe, the cardiac lesion should be corrected before liver transplantation (Chapter 21).

Alagille's syndrome

Alagille's syndrome is classically associated with cardiac disease (Chapter 4). This multisystem, autosomal-dominantly inherited disease consists of a characteristic triangular-shaped face, failure to thrive, cholestasis often accompanied by severe pruritus, hypoplasia of the intrahepatic bile ducts, butterfly vertebrae, and posterior embryotoxon. The cardiac disease usually consists of peripheral pulmonary stenosis or atresia, but other congenital defects such as Fallot tetralogy may occur (Table 16.1). The clinical phenotype is variable, and 10% of patients have cardiac symptoms only.[11] The diagnosis is usually obvious clinically, but is confirmed by electrocardiography (ECG), which may show right ventricular overload, or by echocardiography. Cardiac catheterization will document pulmonary artery pressures and indicate whether balloon dilation or surgery is required or feasible. Surgery may be necessary before liver transplantation. It is not clear whether the defect regresses after liver transplantation.

Chronic hepatitis

In patients with a severe chronic hepatitis (defined by liver

Table 16.1 Features of cardiac–hepatic syndromes.

Condition	Hepatic features	Cardiac features
Biliary atresia	Cholestasis and cirrhosis	Dextrocardia, ASD, VSD
Alagille's syndrome	Cholestasis, pruritus	Peripheral pulmonary stenosis
Hyperaldosteronism	Edema Fulminant or subacute liver failure	Volume-overloaded ventricles Bounding pulses
Portopulmonary hypertension	Extrahepatic portal hypertension, dyspnea, hypoxemia; liver function tests may be normal, cirrhosis not always present	Right ventricular heart failure Cor pulmonale
Hepatopulmonary syndrome	Cirrhosis and hypoxemia	Marked shunting within the pulmonary capillary Abnormal perfusion scan of pulmonary and systemic circulations
Mitochondrial cytopathy, tyrosinemia type I	High lactate, coagulopathy	Hypertrophic cardiomyopathy

ASD, atrial septal defect; VSD, ventricular septal defect.

biopsy fibrosis score), an association with impaired right ventricular diastolic function was found. This could be monitored by tissue Doppler echocardiography, in which the early diastolic velocity of the tricuspid valve annulus, the isovolumic relaxation time, and peak early myocardial tissue velocity were all found to be most abnormal in patients with the most severe hepatitis, although clinically the patients had no cardiac symptoms.[12]

Cardiomyopathy

Cardiomyopathy may be associated with inherited metabolic disease. Hypertrophic cardiomyopathy may develop as a result of the abnormal tyrosine metabolism in tyrosinemia type I.[13] It is not usually clinically significant and regresses with nitisinone therapy or liver transplantation (Chapters 5, 13, and 21). Cyclosporine and the immune suppressant tacrolimus have been reported to cause dose-dependent hypertrophic cardiomyopathy.[14]

Mitochondrial disease may present with either fulminant liver failure in the neonatal period or progressive neurological deterioration and hypertrophic cardiomyopathy.[15] The diagnosis may be confirmed by ECG, echocardiography, or cardiac biopsy, or may be suspected biochemically on the basis of an elevated plasma lactate and an inability to metabolize a glucose load (Chapters 5 and 13).

Cardiomyopathy may also develop as a consequence of cirrhosis, in which one of the mediators appears to be a natriuretic peptide. A study of 36 adult patients with and without ascites demonstrated a relationship between higher levels of brain natriuretic peptide in the group with ascites and also with thickness of the interventricular septum. All 36 patients with cirrhosis had detectable changes in cardiac function, as assessed by transthoracic two-dimensional echocardiography and radionuclide angiography, in comparison with age-matched volunteers; the changes included increased mean ejection fraction, prolonged deceleration times, left atrial enlargement, and interventricular septal thickening.[16] Another feature of cirrhosis-induced cardiomyopathy is a prolongation of the QT interval.[17]

Chronic fluid retention

Portal hypertension leads to subclinical sodium retention, causing an increase in circulating blood volume and all body fluid compartments (Chapter 15). Initially, this process suppresses the renin–angiotensin–aldosterone system, but as liver disease progresses, the system becomes activated, resulting in further fluid retention. Failure to clear vasodilating molecules such as nitric oxide and hyperaldosteronism in chronic liver disease lead to an increase in cardiac output, and a high-output state with bounding peripheral pulses is apparent.[18]

Systemic hypertension is common after liver transplantation secondary to immunosuppression with steroids, cyclosporine, or tacrolimus, and may also be associated with left ventricular hypertrophy.

Investigation

Various tests are recommended in order to determine the extent and severity of hepatic dysfunction and to screen for coexisting liver disease (Table 16.2) (see also Chapter 2).

Table 16.2 Investigations of liver function in children with cardiac disorders.

Liver function tests	Aspartate transaminase γ-Glutamyltransferase Coagulation tests
Blood culture and viral serology	Hepatitis A, B, and C Adenovirus, coxsackievirus titers
Screen for congenital disease	α_1-Antitrypsin level and phenotype Urinary amino acids and organic acids
Screen for biliary obstruction	Hepatic ultrasound Biliary scintigraphy (e.g., TEBIDA scan)
Liver biopsy ± muscle biopsy if diagnostic uncertainty remains	

TEBIDA, technetium trimethyl 1-bromoiminodiacetic acid.

Table 16.3 Management of cholestasis secondary to cardiac disease.

Fat-soluble vitamins Vitamin A: Arcavit A (5000–25 000 IU/day) Vitamin D: alfacalcidol (50 ng/kg/day) Vitamin E: α-tocopherol (50–500 IU/day) Vitamin K: phytomenadione (1–10 mg/day)
Ursodeoxycholic acid (20–50 mg/kg/day)
Calorie supplements Medium-chain triglyceride: Liquigen (Scientific Hospital Supplies)
Specialized feed containing medium-chain triglyceride Pepti-Junior (Nutricia) Pregestimil (Mead Johnson Nutritionals)

Management

Hepatic dysfunction secondary to heart disease requires supportive management only, since effective treatment of the underlying cardiac lesion leads to improvement of liver function (Table 16.3). As the formation of biliary sludge is a risk with complex cardiac surgery and major blood transfusion, parenteral nutrition is best avoided or combined with enteral feeding to stimulate bile flow. Ursodeoxycholic acid (20–50 mg/kg/day) may be a useful choleretic in children with impaired biliary drainage, as it stimulates bile flow and reduces the formation of insoluble cholesterol and phospholipid aggregates. The development of the inspissated bile syndrome may be resistant to ursodeoxycholic acid, and surgical or radiological intervention with biliary lavage may be necessary (Chapter 19). If cholestasis is prolonged, fat-soluble vitamins, calorie supplements, and medium-chain triglycerides should be prescribed (Chapter 4; Table 16.3). The prognosis depends on the underlying cardiac condition and is good unless a low cardiac output state persists and multiorgan failure develops.

Patent ductus venosus

The physiological effect of a persistent patent ductus venosus is to cause a variable percentage of the cardiac output to bypass the liver. Studies in neonates have shown a correlation between the severity of the shunt (i.e., the flow volume through the patent ductus) and elevated plasma ammonia, serum bilirubin concentrations, and hepaplastin percentage.[19] In the majority of neonates, the ductus venosus closes spontaneously within weeks of birth, but important liver functions such as detoxification and the regulation of coagulation factors and bilirubin metabolism are impaired by a patent ductus in premature neonates as well as those born at term and may explain why neonates are at increased risk of complications of intravenous nutrition when supplied in the first few weeks of life.

Gastrointestinal disease

The gastrointestinal tract is intimately related to the liver anatomically and physiologically. The presence of food in the stomach and duodenum triggers a cascade of hormones responsible for digestion, absorption, and metabolic processing of nutrients. For example, emptying of the gallbladder can be induced by cholecystokinin, which is released from neuroendocrine cells in the duodenum in response to fat or amino acids present in the duodenum.

Impaired enterohepatic circulation of bile

Lack of stimulation to bile flow caused by enteral starvation after major surgery is considered to be the reason for the development of biliary sludge and stones postoperatively.[20] Impaired reabsorption of bile salts in the terminal ileum depletes the bile acid pool, altering the composition of bile and making it more lithogenic. Crohn disease, cystic fibrosis, or surgical resection of the terminal ileum may be associated with impaired bile acid circulation and gallstone formation. Clinical features of terminal ileal disease include: steatorrhea, watery diarrhea secondary to bile salt colitis, intermittent abdominal pain, obstructive jaundice secondary to inspissated bile, gallstones, fat-soluble vitamin deficiency, and anemia secondary to vitamin B_{12} deficiency.

Management

The management of liver disease in children with terminal ileal disease is difficult, as the condition is usually chronic. Metronidazole (20 mg/kg/day), which selectively decontaminates the intestinal tract and reduces deconjugation of bile salts by bacteria, may be useful in reducing abnormalities in liver function tests in patients with Crohn disease.[21]

Cystic fibrosis

This is associated with bile salt malabsorption, and up to 25% of adolescents have evidence of biliary cirrhosis. Risk factors for liver disease appear to be a history of meconium ileus, male gender, and early onset of abnormal liver function in the first decade of life.[22] The liver function tests typically demonstrate transient increases in alkaline phosphatase, γ-glutamyltransferase (GGT), and transaminases. The plasma bilirubin is usually normal unless a gallstone obstructs the common bile duct. The extent of liver disease may be underestimated by liver function tests and abdominal ultrasound, but biliary radioisotope excretion scans may show focal delayed excretion, and liver histology shows portal tract pathology rather than parenchymal changes. Ursodeoxycholic acid has an important role in stimulating bile flow and making the composition of the bile less lithogenic, which appears to protect against further deterioration in liver function in cystic fibrosis (Chapter 12).[23]

Shwachman–Diamond syndrome

Also known as Shwachman disease, this is a rare autosomal-recessive condition that may present as one of the myelodysplastic syndromes.[24] It often presents in the first year of life with growth failure secondary to malabsorption caused by exocrine pancreatic dysfunction. There may be multisystem involvement, particularly of the bone marrow (cyclical neutropenia), in which abnormal clones from the myeloid cell lines may be detected, skeleton (metaphyseal dyschondroplasia of the femoral and humoral head), and liver. Hepatomegaly and moderately elevated hepatic transaminases (80–300 IU/L) were present in over 50% of patients at the time of presentation, although there was some resolution with time.[25] Histology is nonspecific, with macrovesicular fatty change. Some genetic markers have been reported on chromosome 7 in association with acute myelogenous leukemia, and most patients have mutations in the *SBDS* gene, which is expressed in leukocytes. Although the function of the gene is unknown, the *SBDS* gene product is not detected in patients with Shwachman–Diamond syndrome, suggesting that a loss of function underlies the pathophysiology of this genetically heterogeneous disorder.[26]

Celiac disease

Patients with celiac disease frequently have elevated transaminases, and in a large population study carried out in Sweden, this appeared to be associated with an increased chance of developing a variety of liver diseases, including acute hepatitis, primary sclerosing cholangitis, fatty liver, liver fibrosis, and cirrhosis.[27] The risk of liver disease was independent of diabetes mellitus. It was also noted that patients who had previously been diagnosed with liver disease had a 4–6-fold increased risk of developing celiac disease subsequently. In an Italian study of 255 patients with autoimmune cholestasis, 3.5% had celiac disease,[28] and it appears that celiac disease is a risk factor in nonresponse to hepatitis B vaccination.[29]

Inflammatory bowel disease

All forms of inflammatory bowel disease (Crohn disease, ulcerative colitis, and indeterminate colitis) are associated with chronic hepatitis and/or autoimmune sclerosing cholangitis (ASC).[30,31] The pathogenesis of hepatic involvement is not understood, but it is probably related to immune mechanisms such as exposure to cytokines produced in the lamina propria of the intestine and transferred via the portal vein to the liver; the production of autoantibodies; and a reduction in suppressor T cells. The bowel disease usually precedes the liver disease, although chronic active hepatitis and ASC may occur in isolation (see Chapter 8).

Hepatomegaly, with or without jaundice or stigmata of chronic liver disease such as telangiectasia and splenomegaly, is the commonest clinical feature. In ASC, jaundice and abdominal pain are more common. Biochemical liver function tests demonstrate elevated transaminases (100–500 IU/L) and elevated alkaline phosphatase and GGT if cholangitis is present (Chapter 8). Table 16.4 outlines the recommended hepatic investigations and differential diagnosis for inflammatory bowel disease. With the increasing use of anti-tumor necrosis factor (anti-TNF) therapy to treat fistulas, it is

Table 16.4 Differential diagnosis of liver disease and inflammatory bowel disease.

Diagnosis	Investigations
Drug toxicity (e.g., azathioprine, infliximab)	Full drug history, blood levels, liver biopsy
Viral hepatitis	Serology (hepatitis A, B, and C, EBV, CMV, adenovirus, human herpesvirus 6, parvovirus, coxsackie)
Abnormal enteropathic circulation of bile salts	Stool color, trial of ursodeoxycholic acid Small-bowel contrast study to assess terminal ileum Hepatic ultrasound
Autoimmune disease	Autoantibodies (SMA, ANA, ANCA) Immunoglobulins Complement levels Endoscopic cholangiogram MRI cholangiogram Liver biopsy

ANA, antinuclear autoantibodies; ANCA, antinuclear cytoplasmic antibodies; CMV, cytomegalovirus; EBV, Epstein–Barr virus; MRI, magnetic resonance imaging; SMA, smooth muscle autoantibodies.

important to be aware of the handful of case reports describing acute liver failure in association with anti-TNF-α antibody; in one unusual case, infliximab appeared to trigger subfulminant hepatitis B in a patient carrying HB_s antigen.[32]

Management

Inflammatory bowel disease is a chronic condition with considerable morbidity, which is potentially fatal and should be supervised in a regional center by a multidisciplinary team. Remission of both bowel and liver disease can be induced with prednisolone and maintained with azathioprine. Immunosuppression is reduced slowly over months and years while liver function tests and the full blood count are monitored carefully. The course of the liver disease is variable, as the disease may have many relapses and remissions,[33] and it is not necessarily associated with the severity of the bowel disease.

The prognosis is also variable, but children who present before the onset of liver failure have a 5-year survival of over 90%.[30] Liver transplantation may be necessary in a small number of children with aggressive disease or who present late with subacute liver failure. Inflammatory bowel disease may deteriorate or present for the first time after liver transplantation.

Intestinal failure

Intestinal failure and dependence on parenteral nutrition (PN) have significant effects on hepatic function, especially during the first few weeks of life, when the detoxifying capacity of the liver is reduced for physiological reasons.[19] The reduced mucosal integrity of the abnormal gut, the increased risk of sepsis, and the absence of a normal enterohepatic circulation all contribute to portal and pericellular fibrosis, which are characteristic of PN-induced liver disease (see Chapters 4 and 22). Children should be referred before life-threatening complications develop (Table 16.5).[34–39] In children referred for intestinal transplant assessment, hepatomegaly is common and splenomegaly almost invariable (see Chapter 22). Elevations of biliary enzymes, alkaline phosphatase, and GGT occur early, and jaundice is a late sign.[20,40] The differential diagnosis includes gallstones, sepsis, and viral hepatitis. Manganese levels should be measured, as manganese has been associated with PN-related liver disease and toxic concentrations causing a Parkinsonian syndrome may develop in cholestatic infants, as manganese depends on biliary excretion.[41]

Management

Children with chronic intestinal failure should be evaluated in a specialist center.[42] Intestinal adaptation should be encouraged medically, and reconstructive surgery to the intestinal tract should be carried out in appropriate cases. Episodes of sepsis need to be treated aggressively, and the children should be managed at home whenever possible.[43] Treatment with ursodeoxycholic acid and selective decontamination of the gut with metronidazole also have a role. Since the use of lipid emulsions in preterm infants was not associated with beneficial effects on growth in the first antenatal month, it has been suggested that starting lipid infusions should be delayed for some weeks, and reduction or temporary cessation of intravenous lipid during episodes of sepsis or deterioration in liver function, especially bilirubin concentrations, is now recommended.[44,45] The prognosis is universally poor once bilirubin is consistently > 100 μmol/L, and small-bowel transplantation should be considered.[46–48]

Autoimmune liver and joint disease

As the liver is rich in major histocompatibility complex (MHC) antigen-presenting cells, there is considerable potential for recognition by effector T cells and macrophages, with subsequent inflammation. Whilst primary autoimmune liver disease in children has been well defined (see Chapter 8),[30,31,33] there are many overlap syndromes[49] in which liver dysfunction is part of a systemic illness—for example, juvenile chronic arthritis (JCA) and systemic lupus erythematosus (SLE).

JCA, which affects one in 1000 children before the age of 16, rarely presents with systemic features, and hepatic involvement is even more uncommon. In SLE, hepatic disease may be associated with other multiorgan involvement, including fibrosing alveolitis, pericarditis, and autoimmune gut disease.

Clinical features include elevated transaminases, cholestasis, pruritus, and—rarely—acute liver failure.[50] Immunoglobulin subclasses may be raised nonspecifically in any active autoimmune condition, including JCA and SLE. Complement

Table 16.5 Complications in children maintained on parenteral nutrition.

Complication	Incidence	References
Liver disease (abnormal liver function tests)	50%	Protheroe and Beath 1997,[34] Kelly 1998[35]
Pulmonary thromboembolism	35–50%	Dollery *et al.* 1994,[36] Pollard *et al.* 1995[37]
Restricted venous access	15%	Ricour *et al.* 1990,[38] Rodrigues *et al.* 2006[39]

levels may also be raised, but C4 deficiency is associated with autoimmune chronic active hepatitis. Specific autoantibodies such as liver–kidney microsomal antibodies (LKM) are typically found in autoimmune hepatitis type 2, but may develop in an overlap syndrome with arthritis. Liver histology is often not diagnostic, demonstrating nonspecific portal inflammatory changes that are common in many chronic inflammatory diseases affecting the liver. Demonstration of extensive necrosis or fibrosis may contribute prognostic information.

The differential diagnosis of liver dysfunction with joint disease should include: sepsis, especially if the child is on steroids; autoimmune hepatitis type 1 or 2; drug toxicity (see below); and viral hepatitis.

Management

The management of liver disease in systemic JCA or other severe autoimmune conditions is first to treat the underlying condition, which may include nonsteroidal anti-inflammatory drugs or steroids; and secondly, azathioprine to induce and maintain remission. Methotrexate and cyclophosphamide should be avoided if possible because of potential hepatic toxicity. The prognosis is unclear and is related to the course of the joint disease.

The anti-inflammatory drugs used to manage JCA and SLE, especially azathioprine and methotrexate, may also cause hepatic dysfunction, which varies from a low-grade transaminitis of little clinical significance to more severe hepatic dysfunction with cholestasis, pruritus, and impaired synthetic function. Liver histology typically shows fatty change and portal fibrosis in more severe cases.[51] The hepatic lesions subside within days or weeks when the offending drug is withdrawn, although fulminant liver failure has been described.[32]

Obesity

Obesity is associated with fatty liver, which may cause abnormalities of liver function. A review of 310 obese Japanese schoolchildren in whom other forms of liver disease had been excluded found that 24% had an alanine aminotransferase (ALT) level at least 30 IU/L above the upper limit of normal and that most of them (83%) also had an abnormal abdominal ultrasound suggesting fatty infiltration.[52] A review of 742 children aged 2–19 years who had an autopsy carried out between 1993 and 2003 in California showed that fatty liver (defined as 5% or more hepatocytes containing macrovesicular fat) was present in 13%, with the highest rate in obese children (38%).[53] The pathogenesis of fatty liver in obesity is unknown, but it may be due to hyperinsulinemia or insulin resistance. In another Japanese study of 228 obese children, fatty liver, as measured by the serum level of glutamic–pyruvic transaminase (alanine aminotransferase), correlated more closely with high levels of immunoreactive insulin than with skinfold thickness or other anthropometric variables.[54] There may be an important relationship between fatty liver and the more serious entity nonalcoholic steatohepatitis (NASH; see Chapter 11). The natural history of the two conditions is being evaluated currently,[55] and a large multicenter trial of vitamin E and metformin is currently underway.[56]

Endocrine disorders

Diabetes mellitus

Diabetes mellitus causes profound metabolic instability and wide variations in plasma glucose and lipids, even with good insulin control. Hepatic manifestations in diabetes mellitus include hepatomegaly due to excess glycogen and fat stores. This may occur acutely in diabetic ketosis, or chronically if diabetic control is suboptimal. Abdominal pain may occur and is associated with rapid enlargement of the liver and stretching of the liver capsule.[57] Gallstones are another complication of diabetes, which may lead to abdominal pain and abnormal liver function. Hepatic transaminases may be raised, typically up to 80–150 IU/L.[58] Mauriac syndrome, which is now rare, is when poor diabetic control is associated with hepatomegaly due to fatty liver, growth retardation, a moon-shaped face, fat deposition on shoulders and abdomen, and chronic hepatitis.[59] Cirrhosis may develop as a result of severe steatosis and pericentral hepatic fibrosis, but these changes occur gradually and are not likely to present in childhood.[60]

Alström syndrome

This recessively inherited condition is characterized by congenital retinal dystrophy and blindness, hearing impairment, obesity, insulin resistance, and type 2 diabetes mellitus. In a review of 182 patients, a dilated cardiomyopathy and hypertriglyceridemia were the most life-threatening conditions, but hyperinsulinism and type 2 diabetes mellitus had developed by 16 years of age in 82%. The associated obesity explains the presence of fatty liver and fibrosis and also fibrotic infiltrations in multiple other organs, including kidney, heart, lung, pancreas, bladder, and gonads.[61]

Hypopituitarism

Hypopituitarism is a rare disorder in which partial or total failure to produce adrenocorticotropic hormone (ACTH), thyroid-stimulating hormone, growth hormone, and gonadotropins is present. It may present within weeks of birth with neonatal hepatitis, causing elevated transaminases and conjugated hyperbilirubinemia (Chapter 4). Hypoglycemia, failure to thrive, and micropenis are characteristic features which should raise clinical suspicion[62,63] (see Figure 4.7, p. 70). Septo-optic dysplasia may be present, in which case infants may present with roving eye movements and poor vision. Treatment with hydrocortisone and thyroxine is associated with improvement in liver function and growth. Although growth hormone levels are low, it is usually possible to maintain a normal growth velocity by ensuring a good calorie intake until the child is 2 years old. After the age of 2, linear growth is more dependent on growth hormone, which is therefore given by subcutaneous injection. The prognosis for septo-optic dysplasia depends on the severity of the initial lesion and is not related to hormone replacement.

Hypothyroidism

Hypothyroidism leads to a mild unconjugated hyperbilirubinemia, although neonatal hepatitis may develop (Chapter 4).

Hypoparathyroidism

Chronic active hepatitis is associated with type I polyglandular syndrome, in which hypoparathyroidism, adrenal insufficiency, and mucocutaneous candidiasis may occur. This syndrome is rare, and in any single individual only two or three features are present. Onset is usually in infancy or childhood, and the condition may be autosomal-recessive. Patients with this syndrome should be screened for abnormalities of liver function, as chronic hepatitis may remain clinically silent until the onset of liver failure, which is the major cause of mortality.[64]

Turner syndrome

Turner syndrome is characterized by XO genotype and short stature. Modern management involves multidisciplinary working in which growth hormone is given to maximize final adult height and estrogen to achieve feminization. In a clinic of 214 patients, 8.9% had elevated liver enzymes and this tended to be associated with hormonal therapies and was self-limiting, although the long-term effects on liver function and the risk of subsequent intrahepatic cholestasis are not known.[65]

Renal disease

Alagille's syndrome

Alagille's syndrome (Chapter 4) may be associated with renal abnormalities, including renal tubular dysfunction, glomerular nephritis, or cystic changes.[66] Occasionally, the renal disease may predominate, but the hepatic and cardiac manifestations are usually more significant clinically.[11]

Infantile polycystic disease

Infantile polycystic disease is an autosomal-recessive condition that may be associated with congenital hepatic fibrosis. The clinical phenotype is variable, and hepatomegaly usually develops before the age of 10 years. Earlier onset of symptomatic hepatosplenomegaly is associated with a poorer prognosis (Chapter 10). Polycystic kidney disease may also occur in association with Caroli disease (see Figure 6.3, p. 139). Combined liver and kidney transplantation may be necessary in patients with severe symptoms related to recurrent cholangitis and renal failure.

Hepatitis B

The development of glomerulonephritis secondary to chronic hepatitis B has long been recognized and is more common in the developing world (Chapter 6). Treatment is with oral antiviral drugs such as lamivudine and/or adefovir, which reduce viral load and can improve renal function, including remission of proteinuria.[67]

Cirrhosis and renal dysfunction

A variety of glomerular disorders, including increased numbers of sclerotic glomeruli and mesangial proliferation, have been reported in a morphometric study of 17 adult patients with cirrhosis and normal renal biochemistry who were compared with normal control individuals. This may explain the rapidity of onset and severity of hepatorenal syndrome in patients with end-stage liver disease.[68] Similar findings have been observed in children with α_1-antitrypsin deficiency.[69]

Hepatorenal syndrome

Hepatorenal syndrome occurs in fulminant and chronic liver disease. Portal hypertension in association with severe hepatic decompensation results in inappropriate activation of the renin–angiotensin–aldosterone system, the sympathetic nervous system, and arginine vasopressin, all of which contribute to sodium and water retention and the development of ascites. The redistribution of fluid between compartments may reduce renal blood flow, setting in motion several intrarenal events such as increased renal sympathetic activity and vasoconstricting prostaglandins, which precipitate hepatorenal syndrome.[70] Acute tubular necrosis and functional renal failure are accompanied by severe oliguria, and inappropriately low sodium excretion may occur. Hepatorenal syndrome has recently been classified into two types based on the clinical course—a distinction that is important in the context of evaluating new treatment.

Type 1 hepatorenal syndrome is the severe acute-onset form, in which there is nearly 100% mortality unless a timely liver transplant is carried out. *N*-acetylcysteine (150 mg/kg over 2 h followed by 100 mg/kg daily for 5 days) may be useful in type 1 hepatorenal syndrome. Renal function improved from 25 mL/min to a mean of 43 mL/min in 12 adult patients treated with *N*-acetylcysteine, without an improvement in hepatic parameters or other interventions such as hemofiltration.[71] More recently, the role of vasoconstrictors (midodrine and norepinephrine) and vasopressor analogs (ornipressin and terlipressin) has been found to improve renal function significantly in liver transplant candidates with type 1 hepatorenal syndrome and even to reverse hepatorenal syndrome in some studies.[72] The role of volume expansion in managing type 1 hepatorenal syndrome remains unproven.

The type 2 hepatorenal syndrome is less severe, more insidious, and appears responsive to transjugular intrahepatic portosystemic stent shunting (TIPSS).[73] Management of both types includes careful fluid balance, including the use of splanchnic vasoconstrictors and colloid volume expansion, renal dialysis, or hemofiltration in order to maintain perfusion of vital organs (Chapters 7 and 14). Recovery from hepatorenal syndrome usually occurs when portal hypertension is reduced either by TIPSS, or successful liver transplant, or spontaneous recovery of liver function.[74]

Respiratory disease

Respiratory dysfunction does not usually affect liver function, possibly because the liver has a double vascular blood flow and tolerates modest hypoxia (arterial oxygen saturations > 85%).

α_1-Antitrypsin deficiency

Deficiency of α_1-antitrypsin, which is an important cause of neonatal jaundice, may present in adolescence when respiratory symptoms related to pulmonary emphysema coincide with hepatitis and hepatic fibrosis/cirrhosis. The diagnosis is made by detecting low levels of α_1-antitrypsin in plasma and establishing the phenotype (PI ZZ) (see Chapter 4). The clinical phenotype is extremely variable,[75] with some individuals having mild symptoms related to reduced functional residual capacity and hyperinflation,[76] while around 10% develop liver disease and 5% of them will need a liver transplant before the age of 5 years. Prolonged neonatal jaundice (cholestasis persisting more than 6 weeks) appears to be a risk factor for a poorer prognosis.[77]

Hepatopulmonary syndrome (HPS)

Cyanosis secondary to arteriovenous shunting may develop in infants and older children with any form of chronic liver disease. The pathophysiology is not well understood, but may be a consequence of increased circulation of the vasodilatory effects of TNF-α and pulmonary endothelial nitric oxide production, which occurs in cirrhosis.[78] Severe intrapulmonary shunting results and may be an indication for liver transplantation even in children with compensated cirrhosis (Chapters 15 and 21).[79] The chronic hypoxia leads to increased erythropoietin production and an increased red cell mass, which persists for some time even after successful liver transplantation. A useful screening test for patients with chronic liver disease is pulse oximetry, performed in the supine position and repeated in the upright position; a supine oximetry measurement of less than 92% that decreases by more than 4% when the patient is sitting upright is indicative of HPS.[80] The diagnosis is confirmed by excluding a cardiac cause and establishing that there is intrapulmonary arteriovenous shunting on perfusion scans of pulmonary and systemic circulation (see Table 16.2). Angiography is rarely indicated. It is important to differentiate arteriovenous shunting secondary to liver disease from poor respiratory function due to other causes (e.g., cystic fibrosis or pulmonary hypertension; see below), as HPS is reversible after liver transplantation.[81] Another reversible cause of HPS is obstructed hepatic vein outflow, whether caused by stricture or by a coagulation defect, as in Budd–Chiari syndrome. It is important to diagnose Budd–Chiari syndrome early—that is, before the development of ascites—as the lesion may be treated without invasive surgery and the outcome is improved.[82]

Portopulmonary hypertension (PPH)

PPH also occurs in cirrhosis and may be detected during evaluation for liver transplantation; dyspnea, hypoxemia, and right ventricular hypertrophy (in contrast to bilateral ventricular hypertrophy, often seen in children with fluid retention secondary to chronic liver failure) are key signs.[83] The diagnosis is confirmed by contrast-enhanced echocardiography and pulmonary angiography. As in HPS, the pathophysiology is related to failure of the liver to remove vasoactive substances, specifically vasoconstrictors, which results in elevated pressures in the pulmonary arterioles and cor pulmonale (see Table 16.1). Whereas the severity of HPS appears to parallel the severity of liver failure, PPH does not, and may occur in patients with extrahepatic portal hypertension and relatively normal liver function. The two conditions do not coexist, but have been reported to occur sequentially after liver transplantation when the grafted liver became cirrhotic secondary to chronic rejection.[84] Unfortunately, unlike HPS, PPH is not reversed by liver transplantation, and such patients may need to be considered for combined lung and liver transplantation.[85]

Hematological disease

Sickle cell disease

Sickle cell disease is a chronic hemolytic anemia, secondary to a defect in the β polypeptide chain of hemoglobin A, which leads to production of hemoglobin S (HbS). HbS forms insoluble polymers, particularly in conditions of low oxygen saturation. The HbS polymers damage the red cell membrane, which shortens the life of the red cell. HbS increases the viscosity of the blood, and capillary obstruction and sequestration become more likely, which may trigger further HbS polymerization and provoke a "sickling crisis."

The hepatic sinusoids are a common site for sequestration of red blood cells in sickle cell anemia, because of sluggish blood flow and relatively low oxygen saturation in zone 3 around the central vein.

Clinical features

The clinical features vary depending on the phenotype:

- Hemolytic anemia with unconjugated hyperbilirubinemia.
- Splenomegaly develops between 6 months and 5 years, reducing with age and repeated infarction; 10% of children have persistent splenomegaly.
- Hepatomegaly due to sickling, hemosiderosis, or congestive failure.
- Enlargement of both liver and spleen during sickle cell crises.
- Progressive liver disease due to anoxic necrosis and hepatic infarction.
- Pigment gallstones and cholecystitis.
- Viral hepatitis.

The phenotype varies considerably in severity. In a series of 510 adult patients, only 26 had hepatic symptoms (gallstones, hepatomegaly, abnormal liver function tests). Biliary tract lesions were uncommon (Table 16.6).

Although low-grade hemolysis is almost invariable, hepatic lesions are a result of recurrent ischemia and vascular occlusion secondary to sinusoidal sickling during systemic viral infections,[86] rather than biliary lithiasis. Patients with a severe phenotype who have multiple sequestration crises and require repeated blood transfusions may develop iron overload and viral hepatitis.[87]

Diagnosis and management

Biochemical liver function tests may demonstrate a rise in transaminases, alkaline phosphatase, and conjugated bilirubin, particularly during a sickle cell crisis. Gallstones and/or cholecystitis will be obvious on ultrasonography. Liver biopsy is only required if there is difficulty in diagnosis, or for prognostic reasons. Histology may show evidence of vascular lesions, including sinusoidal dilation, perisinusoidal fibrosis, and ischemic necrosis.[88] Portal fibrosis and cirrhosis are particularly associated with iron overload.

There may be difficulty in differentiating abdominal pain due to sickle cell sequestration from cholelithiasis, as in both situations there may be right-sided abdominal pain and tenderness. If biliary symptoms persist in the presence of gallstones, cholecystectomy is recommended (Chapter 19), ensuring that perioperative hypoxia is prevented.

Table 16.6 Lesions of the liver in sickle cell disease.[88]

Pathology	n	%
Sinusoidal dilation	23	89
Perisinusoidal fibrosis	19	73
Ischemic necrosis	5	19
Chronic persistent hepatitis	11	42
Cirrhosis	2	8
Gallbladder stones	20	77
Common bile duct stone	1	4

Bone-marrow transplantation is available for patients who are likely to die in childhood,[89] although it is advisable to evaluate the extent and severity of liver disease first.

Thalassemia

Thalassemia is caused by deficient production of either α or β globin chains and results in a greatly reduced red cell life span (days rather than weeks). Unlike sickle cell disease, sequestration crises do not occur. The main problems in thalassemia are related to the effects of chronic anemia (fatigue, hyperplasia of sites of red cell production such as liver and skull, infections, impaired growth, and absent sexual maturation), hemolysis, and iron overload. Patients with β-thalassemia usually die unless transfused within the first year of life, but if the hemoglobin is maintained above 10.5 g/dL by monthly transfusions given with an iron-chelating agent, desferrioxamine, survival into adult life is possible.

Liver disease in thalassemia

Liver disease is usually secondary to:

- Hemosiderosis, which develops despite iron chelation treatment and may progress to fibrosis and cirrhosis (Figure 16.3).

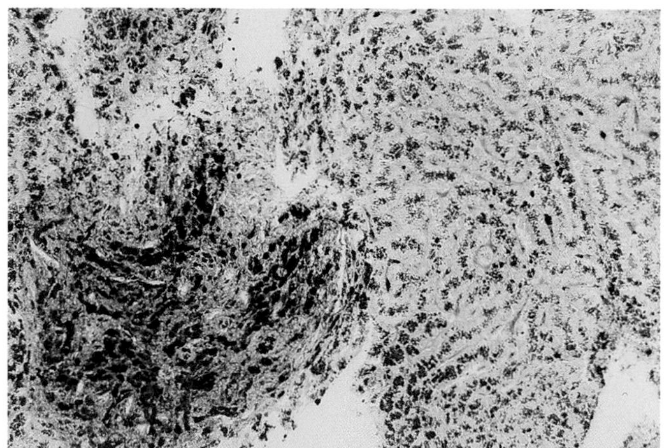

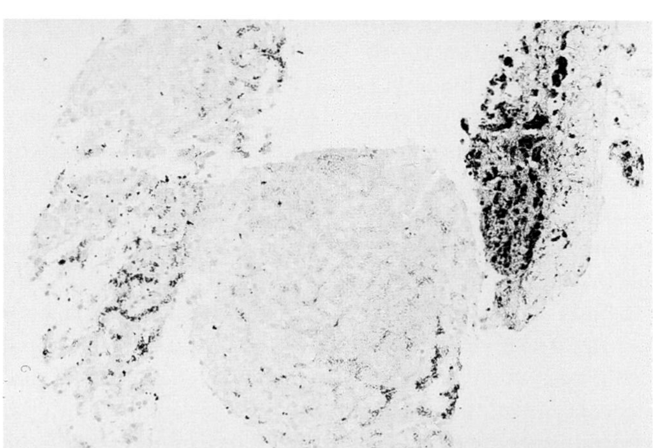

Figure 16.3 Thalassemia. There is marked hemosiderosis involving both hepatocytes and Kupffer cells (**A**), which has almost disappeared 3 years after bone-marrow transplantation (**B**).

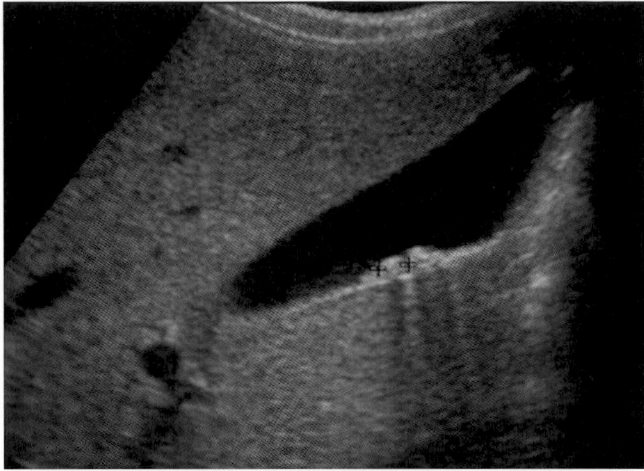

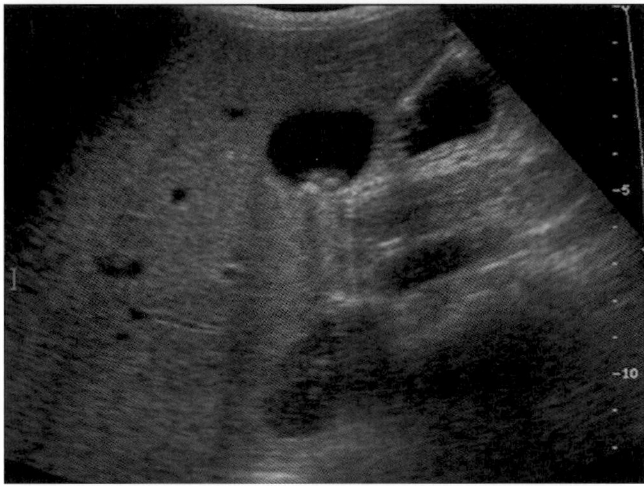

Figure 16.4 Children with thalassemia and severe hemolysis develop gallstones and biliary obstruction. Ultrasonography demonstrates gallstones (**A**) and stones in the common bile duct (**B**).

- Viral hepatitis, which may be secondary to hepatitis B, C or non-A–G (acquired from blood transfusion); patients are also at increased risk of human immunodeficiency virus (HIV) (Chapter 7)
- Gallstones are also common, although usually asymptomatic unless impacted in the common bile duct (Figure 16.4).

The development of extensive iron overload can be predicted in patients with high transfusion requirements (> 100 transfusions). These patients should be evaluated for bone-marrow transplantation before they develop cirrhosis and other major complications of iron overload.[90] Treatment of chronic viral hepatitis C, particularly genotypes 2 and 3, with combination therapy with pegylated interferon and ribavirin is now successful and can be undertaken in children with thalassemia, although the risk of hemolysis with ribavirin is increased and it is necessary to reduce the dose (Chapter 6).

Hemophilia A

Liver disease in classical hemophilia is related to viral hepatitis from infected blood products or factor VIII concentrate. Screening of blood products and prophylactic immunization have greatly reduced the risk of hepatitis B, but many children were infected with hepatitis C and HIV prior to adequate screening in the 1980s. These children are at risk of chronic hepatitis, cirrhosis, and hepatocellular carcinoma (Chapter 6), which may be more aggressive in this group of children (see Figure 6.5, p. 147).[91] Treatment with interferon alpha and ribavirin is effective in approximately 45% of children, depending on genotype (Chapter 6). Liver transplantation is indicated for liver failure, and will also cure the hemophilia.

HIV infection commonly produces abnormal liver function, caused by opportunistic infections, lymphoproliferative disease, or neoplasia related to acquired immune deficiency syndrome (AIDS).[92] The availability of combinations of retroviral drugs in recent years has changed the prognosis of HIV dramatically. The effects of HIV infection can be modified by treatment with three classes of retroviral drugs (nucleoside analogs, nonnucleoside analogs, and protease inhibitors), which reduce the viremia, and restore the CD4 : CD8 ratio. According to the Canadian hemophiliac registry, such combinations of antiviral drugs prolong life for many years, with a median survival of 15 years.[93] However, while the proportion of deaths due to AIDS has reduced, the proportion of deaths due to liver disease has increased in this group, which may be related to the hepatotoxicity of nonnucleoside analog reverse transcriptase inhibitors such as nevirapine, efavirenz, and delavirdine, which are increasingly being used to treat HIV infection.[94] See also the section on acquired immunodeficiency (HIV infection) below.

Hemolytic anemia

Immune-related

Rhesus incompatibility directed against fetal erythrocytes causes brisk hemolysis, which leads to anemia, unconjugated hyperbilirubinemia, and kernicterus if bilirubin levels are not controlled with phototherapy and exchange transfusion if necessary. Rhesus and ABO blood group incompatibility are self-limiting, but a more severe form is described in which Coombs-positive autoantibodies are directed against hepatocytes as well as red cells. Coombs-positive autoimmune hepatitis produces a clinical picture of progressive neonatal hepatitis, which often causes death from sepsis and/or liver failure within the first year of life. Steroids may slow the progression of the disease, and a case report in an infant describes resolution of hemolysis and hepatitis after treatment with an antibody to B lymphocytes (anti-CD20, also known as rituximab), although prolonged hypogammaglobulinemia ensued.[95] Liver transplantation has been attempted, but the disease may recur in the graft.

Red cell fragility

Hereditary spherocytosis commonly presents in the neonatal

period as an episode of unconjugated hyperbilirubinemia, or during intercurrent sepsis because hypoglycemia and acidosis increase red cell fragility. Infection with parvovirus B19 is associated with an aplastic crisis.[96] Hepatic disease consists of cholelithiasis secondary to pigment stones and occasionally cholecystitis. Splenectomy is indicated in children older than 5 years, as this restores the red cell life span to around 100 days, normalizes the plasma hemoglobin, and reduces the risk of obstructive jaundice caused by bile pigment stones.

Aplastic anemia

Aplastic anemia may be a presenting symptom of fulminant liver failure or may develop after successful liver transplantation. The common factor may be a virus (e.g., parvovirus, Epstein–Barr virus), but often the cause is unknown. It is important to consider the possibility of a viral etiology causing simultaneous bone-marrow and liver failure, as many drugs used therapeutically after liver transplantation will exacerbate the bone-marrow disease (e.g., tacrolimus, co-trimoxazole). Some patients have received successful bone-marrow transplantation after successful liver transplantation when the aplastic anemia has been refractory and continuing viral infection has been excluded.[96]

Hemophagocytic lymphohistiocytosis (erythrocytosis)

Hemophagocytic lymphohistiocytosis is primarily a hematological disease in which macrophages, including hepatic Kupffer cells, become excessively activated and phagocytose neighboring cells such as erythrocytes and leukocytes and secrete large quantities of inflammatory cytokines. The disorder may be sporadic, associated with viruses—for example, parvovirus 19, echovirus, or Epstein–Barr virus (EBV). More frequently, however, hemophagocytic lymphohistiocytosis is familial (FHL), and recently it has become possible to define subtypes according to specific genetic mutation defects, which are usually inherited in an autosomal-recessive fashion, although some show X-linked inheritance.[97]

The clinical picture includes hepatosplenomegaly and jaundice, which may resemble neonatal hepatitis, although fulminant liver failure with coagulopathy is more common and may be difficult to distinguish from septicemia. The diagnosis is made by demonstrating erythrophagocytosis in liver or bone marrow (see Figure 5.10, p. 116). In the familial (inherited) type of hemophagocytic lymphohistiocytosis, atypical lymphocytes or histiocytes may be found in the cerebrospinal fluid, which also contains excess protein.

Management consists of support for acute liver failure (Chapters 5 and 7) and cytotoxic therapy. Remission can be achieved with etoposide, methylprednisolone, and methotrexate in at least one-third of cases, but the mortality may be as high as 75% in some groups, which has prompted the use of allogeneic bone-marrow transplantation or stem cell transplantation in high-risk patients (less than 2 years old, familial pattern).[98] Liver transplantation is not indicated.

After bone marrow transplantation

Bone marrow transplantation (BMT) is indicated for many disorders, ranging from acute leukemia to immunodeficiency. Some of the patients may have liver disease with their original disease, while others may have been treated with hepatotoxic drugs as part of their treatment or conditioning pre-BMT. It is not surprising, therefore, that abnormal liver function develops in approximately 30% of patients undergoing BMT.[99] There are many potential causes, including infection, non-A–G hepatitis, graft-versus-host-disease (GVHD), veno-occlusive disease (VOD), and drug toxicity, especially 6-thioguanine.[100,101]

Graft-versus-host-disease

GVHD is a systemic disorder involving skin, gut, lung, eye, pancreas, and liver, typically occurring 7–50 days after BMT (and occasionally after liver or small-bowel transplantation). The acute form presents with a desquamating skin rash and diarrhea, and the liver is involved in 40% of cases, manifested by mild jaundice and hepatomegaly. The immune damage in the liver is directed towards the small bile ducts. The biliary epithelium becomes irregular, with nuclear pleomorphism and vacuolated cytoplasm. There may also be endotheliitis and mild portal tract inflammation, with bile duct loss and cholestasis; the parenchyma is relatively spared (Figure 16.5).

Chronic GVHD is defined as continuing poorly controlled acute GVHD after 100 days. Eighty percent of patients are cholestatic and have complete loss of all bile ducts. Histology of the liver shows bile duct loss, bridging fibrosis, and occasionally cirrhosis (Table 16.7).[88,102] The differential diagnosis of both acute and chronic GVHD includes:

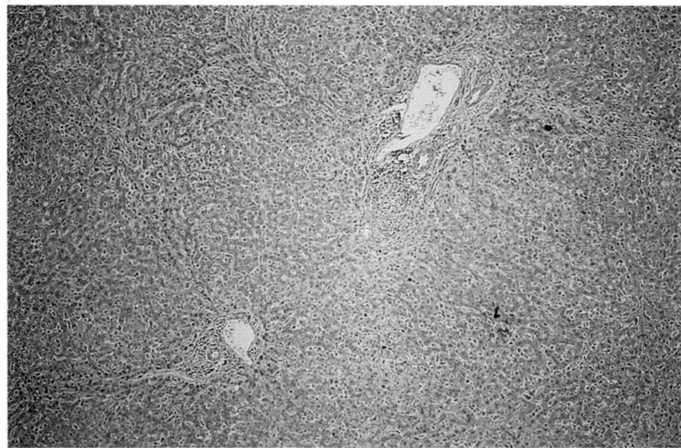

Figure 16.5 Graft-versus-host disease is most common after bone-marrow transplantation. It may affect the skin, intestine, and liver. Liver histology demonstrates loss of bile ducts, which may be irreversible.

Table 16.7 Clinical features of graft-versus-host-disease (GVHD) and veno-occlusive disease (VOD).

	Acute GVHD	Chronic GVHD	VOD
Onset	7–50 days	> 100 days	1–30 days
Clinical	Skin rash Diarrhea	Skin rash Pale stools	Tender hepatomegaly Ascites, elevated jugular venous pressure
Biochemistry	Bilirubin > 50 μmol/L	Bilirubin > 200 μmol/L Raised alkaline phosphatase	Bilirubin > 35 μmol/L Raised alkaline phosphatase
Histology	Vanishing bile ducts	Bile ducts absent	Narrow or occluded vessels

- Viral hepatitis—cytomegalovirus (CMV), EBV, hepatitis A, B, C, other
- Drug toxicity (including parenteral nutrition)
- Biliary obstruction from biliary sludge (occurs in 20% of BMT recipients[99])
- Hepatobiliary infection
- Veno-occlusive disease

Investigations should include: viral serology; abdominal ultrasound to detect sludge, biliary dilation, and portal vein flow; blood, bone marrow, and hepatic culture; and skin, gut, and liver biopsy. The diagnosis is made on the clinical features and the characteristic changes in skin, jejunum, rectal, or liver biopsies, although the liver biopsy may be almost normal in the early stages.

Management. The management of GVHD, irrespective of organ involvement, is to increase immunosuppression with high-dose corticosteroids, cyclosporine (trough levels 200–400 ng/mL monovalent assay) and tacrolimus (trough levels 8–15 ng/L). In addition, azathioprine, antithymocyte globulin, and thalidomide may be useful if the patient has a history of GVHD. Rituximab, an anti-CD20 chimeric monoclonal antibody, has recently been shown to be effective in the treatment of chronic GVHD.[101] Ursodeoxycholic acid is frequently used to encourage enterohepatic recirculation of bile acids and to treat pruritus.[103] The prognosis is related to the control of GVHD and the success of the bone-marrow graft. In rare circumstances, progression to cirrhosis and liver failure may occur. Liver transplantation may be considered if disease in other organs is minimal and the bone-marrow graft has been successful.

Veno-occlusive disease

VOD is a serious complication of BMT that occurs in 20–30% of patients and presents within 30 days of BMT. The clinical features mimic the Budd–Chiari syndrome and include:

- Jaundice (bilirubin > 35 μmol/L)
- Tender hepatomegaly
- Elevated jugular venous pressure
- Ascites or unexpected weight gain.[104,105]

Patients with a history of pretransplant viral hepatitis, radiotherapy, or busulfan conditioning are more likely to develop VOD. In a retrospective, multivariate analysis, the use of ciprofloxacin and vancomycin prophylaxis, 6-thioguanine intensification regimens, methotrexate treatment for GVHD, and abnormal transaminases and alkaline phosphatase pre-BMT were also associated with an increased risk of VOD.[100,106]

The diagnosis is based on clinical criteria:

- Exclusion of other causes of hepatic dysfunction post-BMT (Table 16.7).
- Abdominal ultrasound of the portal vein flow to identify retrograde flow and or an increase in hepatic resistance.
- Liver biopsy, if coagulation permits. Liver histology demonstrates narrowing or occlusion of the terminal hepatic venules, sinusoidal congestion, and necrosis of hepatocytes, with a mild inflammatory infiltrate in the centrilobular zone. Fibrosis and cirrhosis may develop (Figure 16.6).

The management is supportive, including management of cholestasis and diuretics for ascites. Without specific treatment, the prognosis is poor for such patients, especially if they have previously received busulfan conditioning. Historically,

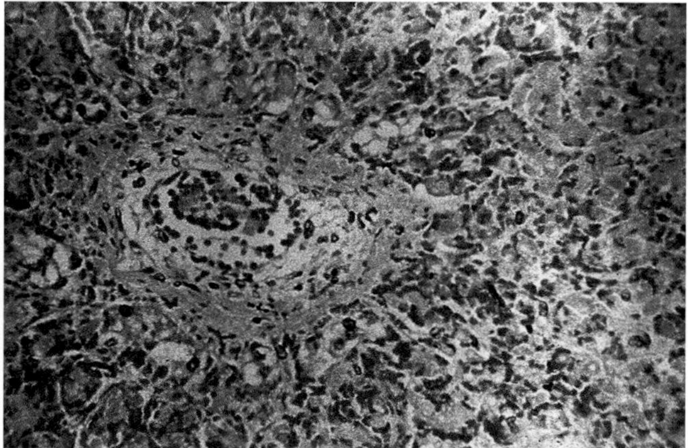

Figure 16.6 Veno-occlusive disease occurs in 26% of patients after bone-marrow transplantation. Liver histology shows occlusion of the terminal venules, sinusoidal congestion, and necrosis of hepatocytes. Fibrosis and cirrhosis may develop.

VOD-induced liver failure had a mortality of 50%. However, the new thrombolytic defibrotide, combined with antithrombin III, achieved complete remission in 13 of 14 patients.[107] The lack of serious toxicity with defibrotide, which is a polydeoxyribonucleotide, is attributed to its lack of systemic anticoagulant effects at the same time as having a local thrombolytic and antithrombotic action. Defibrotide has also been used to treat VOD after liver transplantation.[108] A novel approach described recently in six children who developed VOD refractory to defibrotide after stem cell transplantation involved the use of a protein C concentrate, which normalized prothrombin and partial thromboplastin time and was associated with a reduction in levels of plasminogen activator inhibitor and resolution of clinical and radiological signs of VOD in all the patients.[109]

Hepatobiliary infections

Hepatobiliary infections, especially candidiasis and CMV, are well-recognized features after BMT. Risk factors for fungal infection include neutropenia, recent treatment with myelosuppressive agents, use of broad-spectrum antibiotics, and immunosuppression. Patients present with fever, hepatic dysfunction, and rarely tender hepatomegaly. Investigations should include: C-reactive protein, fungal and bacterial culture of blood, and bone-marrow or liver biopsy, although fungi are notoriously difficult to culture when present in low numbers (Figure 16.7). Abdominal computed tomography scanning and ultrasound may show characteristic multiple, low-attenuation or hypoechoic areas that may represent fungal infection. In the context of immunosuppression and fever unresponsive to broad-spectrum antibiotics, fungal infection is probable and should be treated with liposomal amphotericin (1–3 mg/kg/day) and/or flucytosine (100–200 mg/kg/day) in severe infections.

CMV infection may occur either as a primary infection or a reactivation causing hepatitis or other systemic disease such as CMV enteritis or pneumonitis. Treatment is with intravenous ganciclovir and hyperimmune gammaglobulin. EBV infection may occur, but does not usually cause significant hepatic disease. If high levels of immune suppression are maintained for > 6 months, there is a risk of B-cell lymphoproliferative disease developing.[110]

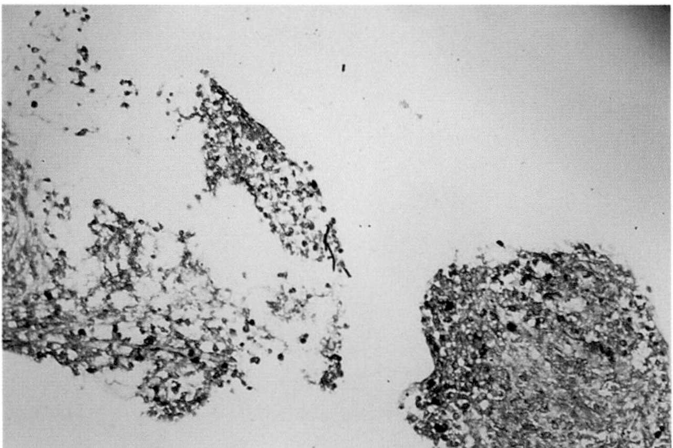

Figure 16.7 Liver biopsy demonstrating hepatic candidiasis in an immune-suppressed patient after liver transplantation (Grocott stain, original magnification × 20).

Malignancy

Infiltration by tumor

Primary tumors such as hepatoblastomas or hepatocellular carcinoma may cause clinically obvious abdominal distension and may be associated with chronic hepatitis B infection or tyrosinemia type I (Chapter 20).

Abnormal liver function tests (elevated alkaline phosphatase and transaminases) are found in up to 30% of patients with Hodgkin disease and may represent increased Kupffer cell activity in the portal tracts.

Tumors such as rhabdomyosarcoma may infiltrate the liver, causing thrombosis of the portal vein or obstruction of the biliary tree. Other tumors, such as peritoneal mesothelioma, may simulate end-stage liver failure and present with jaundice, coagulopathy, wasting, and gross ascites.[111]

Acute leukemia may present with hepatosplenomegaly and elevated transaminases (100–400 IU/L) due to infiltration by malignant clones of lymphocytes. Histology will demonstrate leukemic infiltration of the portal tract, which usually reverses following therapy.

Langerhans histiocytosis

Langerhans histiocytosis, which is characterized by the abnormal clonal proliferation of macrophage-derived cells anywhere in the reticuloendothelial system, has a wide range of presentations and rates of progression. Children presenting with hepatic involvement usually come to notice because of nonspecific concerns relating to appetite, growth, abdominal pain, and an enlarged liver. Liver aminotransferases are elevated, but the serum bilirubin may be normal. Diagnosis can be difficult if signs in other organ systems are minimal, and the first liver biopsy may fail to yield a diagnostic lesion. In a cohort of 220 patients seen between 1987 and 2001, multisystem involvement including lung, liver, and blood was present in one-third (n = 83). Treatment depends on the clinical presentation, but usually involves vinblastine and steroids. The prognosis for patients with liver involvement was relatively poor, with a 5-year survival of 23% in comparison with those with pulmonary disease alone or no multisystem disease, whose 5-year survival was 83% and 94%, repsectively.[112]

Cytotoxic therapy

Cytotoxic treatment for malignancy inevitably affects the liver, which is one of the most metabolically active tissues in the body, but these effects are rarely apparent clinically because of the capacity for hepatic regeneration. Thus, hepatic damage due to chemotherapy is more likely in children who are debilitated by chronic disease or receiving prolonged therapy.[51] The clinical features are variable and related to the drug involved—for example, actinomycin, which is frequently used in the management of Wilms tumor, may be associated with an intense hepatitis sufficient to induce subacute hepatic failure, as in the case of a 10-year-old boy who had an additional risk factor of being a carrier for α_1-antitrypsin deficiency.[113] Radiotherapy of the liver is another risk factor for actinomycin toxicity, especially in small children.[114] Actinomycin has also been reported as a rare cause of VOD in a series of six children, three of whom died,[115] and as a cause of hepatic fibrosis and cirrhosis (see Figure 9.8, p. 211).

Methotrexate hepatotoxicity is usually dose-related, and liver biopsy may show steatosis and portal tract fibrosis in children who have received prolonged courses, and in rare cases fulminant liver failure has ensued. 6-Mercaptopurine (6-MCP), used in maintenance treatment of acute lymphocytic leukemia, is also hepatotoxic and is associated with hepatic necrosis and cholestasis. Fatalities have been reported.[116] Patients receiving 6-MCP should have regular liver function tests, as hepatic damage is reversible if treatment is stopped promptly.

6-Thioguanine is also used to treat leukemia and is mainly used for intensification courses. Although it appears to reduce central nervous system relapse in comparison with 6-mercaptopurine, 6-thioguanine exposure was associated with veno-occlusive disease, and during the long-term follow-up, 13% of the patients (10/75) were referred for evaluation of symptoms suggestive of portal hypertension (thrombocytopenia and splenomegaly) and two presented with gastrointestinal bleeding.[100] This worryingly high incidence has led to the institution of an endoscopy screening program for all children who receive 6-thioguanine as maintenance treatment for acute lymphocytic leukemia.

Doxorubicin is more often associated with cardiomyopathy, but may cause a chemical hepatitis.[117] In patients with preexisting abnormalities of liver function, the dose should be reduced (50% of the normal dose if the bilirubin is > 20 μmol/L; 25% of normal dose if bilirubin > 50 μmol/L).

Azathioprine is no longer commonly used in regimens for treating cancers, but it remains a cytotoxic agent widely used in the management of inflammatory conditions such as ulcerative colitis, arthritis, and following solid-organ transplantation. Rare but serious adverse effects have been reported, including VOD and the development of a hepatocellular carcinoma.[118] The mechanism may be via the metabolite of azathioprine, 6-mercaptopurine, which is a dose-dependent hepatotoxin.

Impaired immune system

Children treated for malignancy are immunocompromised, which increases the incidence of bacterial, viral, and fungal infections that may affect the liver, resulting in liver dysfunction, especially cholestasis. Clinically, fungal infections are insidious in onset, evolving over many days and weeks, usually in the context of neutropenia, serum C-reactive protein > 50 mg/L, malnutrition, broad-spectrum antibiotics, and a high swinging fever (temperature typically 39–40 °C).[119,120] Visceral candidiasis has been reported in which *Candida* species invaded the liver, biliary tract, and portal vein, producing cholestasis and gross hepatosplenomegaly.[121] The positive identification of fungi is very difficult,[122] except in overwhelming infections, and treatment with amphotericin (1–3 mg/kg/day) and/or flucytosine (100–200 mg/kg/day) is therefore often empirical, based on risk factors and clinical suspicion.[123] In systemic candidiasis, prolonged treatment may be required (Figure 16.7).

Immunodeficiency

Children with inherited immunodeficiency syndromes may have associated liver dysfunction because of recurrent bacterial, viral, or opportunistic infection (Figure 16.8). In a review of 147 children with primary immune deficiency who developed abnormal liver function tests, 21 were subsequently found to have sclerosing cholangitis on the basis of radiological and histological criteria.[124] The mechanism of damage is almost always from infecting organisms carried in the intestinal tract, which ascend via the biliary tree and cause a sclerosing cholangitis. The differential diagnosis of sclerosing cholangitis includes primary immune deficiency as well as HIV, autoimmune pancreatitis, portal biliopathy, eosinophilic cholangitis, intra-arterial chemotherapy, and intraductal stone disease.[125] A case report of interleukin-2 receptor-α deficiency provides an example of a different mechanism, in which a congenital immune deficiency state induced a condition mimicking primary biliary cirrhosis by the age of 5 years in a male child of consanguineous parents and was cured by allogenic stem cell transplantation.[126]

CD40 ligand deficiency

This X-linked inherited immunodeficiency is associated with chronic hepatitis, cirrhosis, and opportunistic infections of the biliary tree. Recurrent ascending cholangitis, often due to atypical organisms such as cryptosporidia, eventually causes a sclerosing cholangiopathy that leads to liver failure (Figure 16.9). It may be age-related, as the incidence of liver disease increases with age: by the age of 20 years, 75% of survivors with CD40 ligand deficiency have liver disease,[127] which recurs following liver transplantation. The role of BMT prior to the development of advanced liver disease has been evaluated in eight boys, four of whom survived.[128] A better outcome was associated with younger age at transplant, normal liver histology, and absence of lung damage.[129]

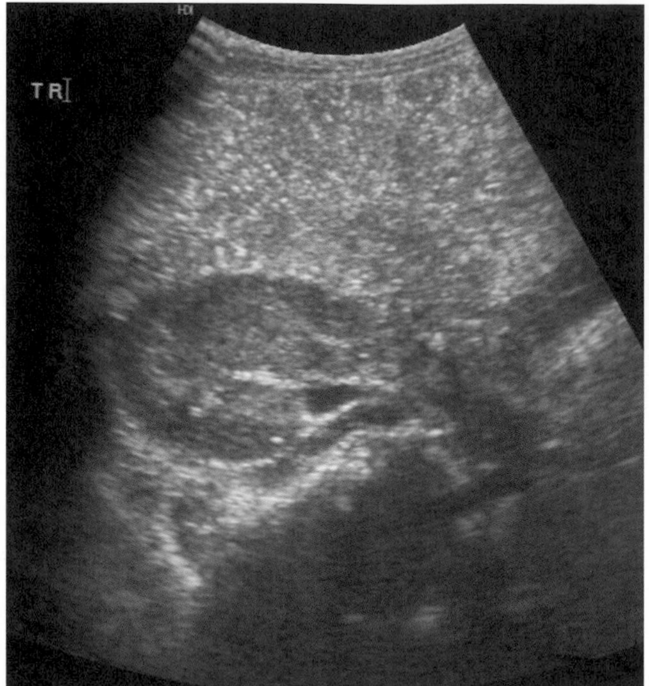

A

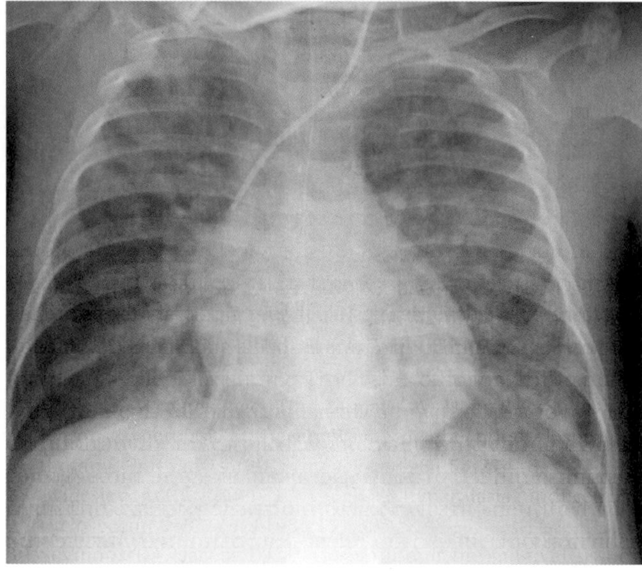

B

Figure 16.8 This infant with severe combined immunodeficiency (SCID) presented with acute liver failure due to fatal *Pneumocystis carinii* infection of the liver with numerous abscesses (**A**) and interstitial lung disease (**B**).

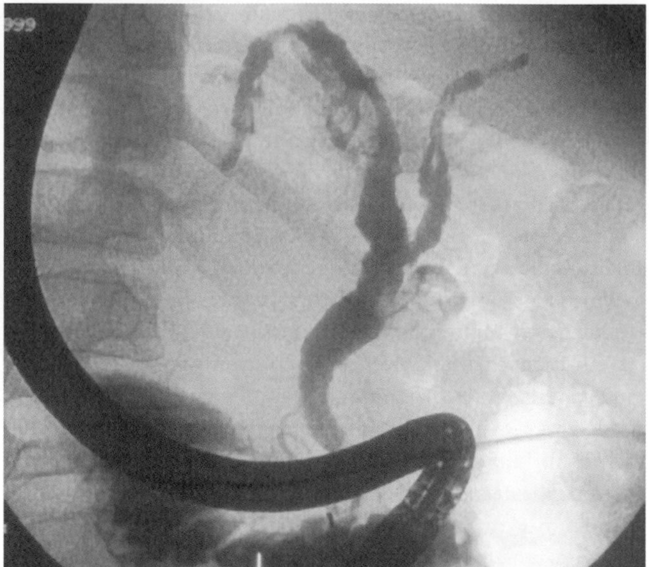

A

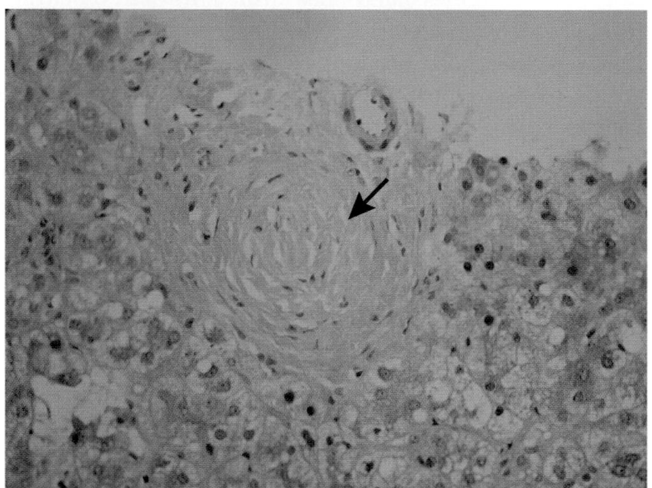

B

Figure 16.9 CD40 ligand deficiency is a rare X-linked immunodeficiency syndrome that is treatable by bone-marrow transplantation. **A** Sclerosing cholangitis secondary to cryptosporidia infection in the liver may develop and is shown in this endoscopic retrograde cholangiopancreatogram, which demonstrates the characteristic dilation and beading of bile ducts. **B** This boy developed liver failure after bone-marrow transplantation, due to graft-versus-host disease and cryptosporidial cholangitis with loss of bile ducts (Masson Trichrome, original magnification × 400).

Acquired immunodeficiency (HIV infection)

Mothers who are HIV-positive have a one in four risk of infecting their babies. Of the reported 26% of babies who acquire HIV from their mothers, approximately 90% of the infants have hepatomegaly and abnormal liver function tests,[92] usually as a consequence of opportunistic infection. These babies are also at risk of hepatitis B and C. Other potential causes of hepatic disease include *Mycobacterium avium-intracellulare*, CMV, lymphomas, and Kaposi sarcoma, all of which may develop in children with HIV. Recurrent or chronic infection of the biliary tree with cryptosporidiosis or other organisms may produce a clinical picture resembling sclerosing cholangitis.[92] Myocarditis and congestive cardiac failure can occur in HIV-infected patients and produce secondary changes in the liver (abnormal liver function tests and fibrosis of the central vein).[130] Perinatal transfer of HIV may be reduced to 8% by administering oral zidovudine antenatally or intravenously during labor to the mother and oral zidovudine to the baby until 6 weeks old.[131]

The long-term medical outlook for children with HIV has improved considerably in countries that can afford the cost of triple treatment with nucleoside analogs, nonnucleoside analogs, and protease inhibitors.[93,132] Another advance in antiviral treatments is the nucleoside reverse transcriptase inhibitor tenofovir, which unlike nucleoside reverse transcriptase inhibitors such as nevirapine is converted to the pharmacologically active metabolite after only two phosphorylation steps and is capable of producing synergistic effects against HIV when combined with other antiretroviral agents.[133] Although toxicity studies in children are awaited, tenofovir appears to be less hepatotoxic than nonnucleoside analog reverse transcriptase inhibitors[94] and is reported to suppress hepatitis B viral replication in patients co-infected with HIV and also to improve synthetic parameters of liver function such as prothrombin time and albumin.[134]

Chronic granulomatous disorders

Granulomas are collections of specialized immune cells such as Kupffer cells, macrophages, or neutrophils, which—in response to infection, toxic injury (drugs and alcohol), or abnormal regulation of the immune system—fuse to form large epithelioid cells with multiple nuclei. Granulomas may appear anywhere in the body, although particular diseases have characteristic patterns (Table 16.8). Numerically the most important causes of granuloma in the liver are tuberculosis, sarcoid, schistosomiasis, and intrinsic liver disease (Figure 16.10).[135] Hepatic granulomas are often clinically silent, but established disease may present as a chronic intrahepatic cholestatic syndrome, portal hypertension, and Budd–Chiari. Even in patients with no respiratory symptoms, exclusion of tuberculosis is extremely important.

The further management of patients with granuloma depends on the final diagnosis, which will become apparent through a systemic evaluation of intestine, chest, joints, eyes, and skin, and will usually require input from other specialists such as a rheumatologist, ophthalmologist, immunologist, and gastroenterologist. Appropriate investigation includes: serology for hepatitis viruses, HIV, chest radiograph, Mantoux test, lung function tests, drug history, liver function testing including organ-specific and non–organ-specific autoantibodies, immunoglobulin subclasses, full blood count and film, erythrocyte sedimentation rate, angiotensin-converting enzyme level, microscopic assessment of stool for ova of schistosomiasis, abdominal ultrasound, gastroduodenoscopy to assess portal hypertension, colonoscopy to evaluate inflammatory bowel disease, and liver biopsy.

Sarcoidosis

Granulomatous disease secondary to sarcoidosis is an uncommon but important cause of liver dysfunction. In adults, respiratory symptoms are prominent, but extrapulmonary sites—especially joints, eyes, and liver—are more usual in children.[136] There is often a long delay between the onset of symptoms such as malaise, weight loss, stiffness, and muscle pain and the diagnosis. Hepatic sarcoidosis can mimic juvenile chronic arthritis,[137] and the international registry of sarcoid arthritis has recorded data in 53 children over 5 years in which 10 had noncaseating granuloma of the liver, 38 had persistent arthritis, and 44 had an inflamed uveal tract, including one child who was blind.[138] Diagnosis depends on excluding other causes of granulomas, although the presence

Table 16.8 Granulomatous conditions affecting the liver: common sites and characteristics.

	Primary site	Associated sites	Special features
Tuberculosis	Lung, lymph node	Intestine, liver	Caseating granulomas secondary to infection with *Mycobacterium tuberculosis*
Sarcoidosis	Lung, ocular, joints	Liver, spleen, bone, heart	Extrapulmonary disease more common in pediatric age 40% have elevated angiotensin-converting enzyme, etiology unknown
Schistosomiasis	Veins of the colon	Portal veins infested by *Schistosoma mansoni*	Ova from adult worms evoke delayed-type hypersensitivity portal hypertension, so-called "pipe stem" fibrosis
Crohn's disease	Intestinal tract	Liver, skin, oral mucosa	May be part of overlap syndrome including chronic active hepatitis, juvenile chronic arthritis
Wegener granulomatosis	Naso-oral cavity	Liver, skin, intestine, heart, kidney	Fibrinoid necrosis of medium-sized arteries, especially of midline structures, resulting in ulcerating granulomas
Chronic granulomatosis disease	Lung, neutrophil dysfunction	Intestine (diarrhea), skin, nodes, liver	X-linked disorder of neutrophil hydrogen peroxide dismutase, *Aspergillus* pneumonia

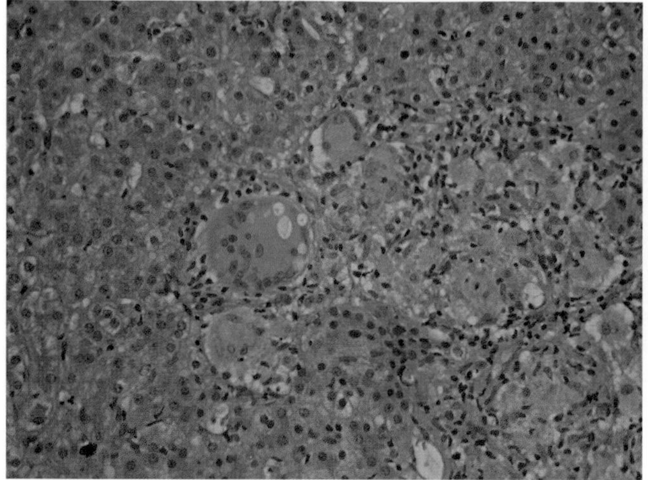
A

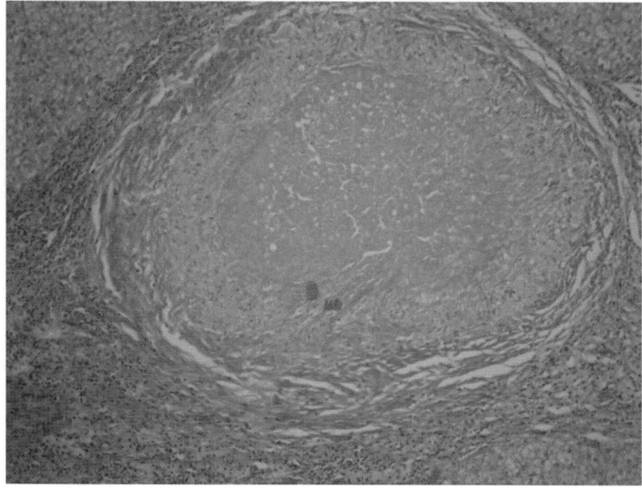
B

Figure 16.10 Granulomas in the liver may be due to many different causes. The lesions range from small aggregates of macrophage-like cells, as in this child with sarcoid (**A**), to caseating granulomas as in this case of tuberculosis (**B**).

of elevated angiotensin enzyme is helpful sometimes (in the patients reported to the international sarcoid arthritis registry, only 14 of 37 patients had a high level of angiotensin-converting enzyme). Mediastinoscopy has a high diagnostic yield if less invasive tests have been inconclusive.[139] Treatment depends on the site and effect of granulomas, but the most usual approach is oral prednisolone (1–2 mg/kg/day). Methotrexate has been used to treat pulmonary disease with some success in adults; however, some hepatic toxicity can be expected, and caution is therefore advised in using this agent in children with hepatic sarcoidosis.[140]

Chronic granulomatous disease

This disorder is an uncommon primary immunodeficiency disease with an estimated incidence of about one in 200 000 births. It is inherited in an X-linked recessive fashion, although autosomal-recessive modes of inheritance are described. Chronic suppurative infections are the most common manifestation, with up to 27% of patients developing liver abscess and staphylococcus being the most usual causative organism.[141] An unusual hepatic manifestation of chronic granulomatous disease is ascites, which has been reported as a consequence of primary bacterial peritonitis, and also separately as a result of portal hypertension secondary to chronic hepatic granulomatosis.[142] The hepatic pathology has been described in a review of male patients aged 5–41 years[143] in which foamy macrophages containing a fine granular golden brown pigment were seen in all seven cases, predominantly in the portal tract areas. Granulomas and associated giant cells were seen in four cases, and when cultured grew *Staphylococcus aureus*. Abscesses are frequently resistant to simple medical treatment with antibiotics, and a multidisciplinary approach is necessary in which precise imaging and percutaneous drainage are often successful. Interferon gamma, which has been used prophylactically, may also be useful in acute infective episodes.[144]

Multisystem pathology

Sepsis

Liver dysfunction commonly develops secondary to severe sepsis.[145] The infection may involve the liver directly, as in hepatitis B, herpes simplex virus, Kawasaki disease, Gram-negative septicemia, and candidiasis,[146] or indirectly as part of the toxic shock and hypoperfusion caused by the inflammatory response—for example, in meningococcal septicemia.

Jaundice and hepatomegaly are early signs, with non-specific elevation in transaminases. Coagulopathy may develop either as part of the liver failure or due to disseminated intravascular coagulation. Ultrasound scanning of the abdomen is helpful in identifying abscesses, fluid collections, or an obstructed biliary tree secondary to biliary sludge or gallstones. The commonest ultrasonic finding in septicemia is an "echo-bright" liver due to hyperplasia of the reticuloendothelial system or fatty change, which may be confirmed histologically.

In Kawasaki disease, acute hydrops of the gallbladder may be detected on ultrasound in addition to hepatomegaly, abnormal liver function tests, and elevated serum total bile acids. Aspiration of the gallbladder may be required in order to prevent perforation (see Figure 19.8B, p. 446).

In shocked patients with hypoperfusion, ischemic necrosis with high transaminases (> 500 IU/L) coagulopathy may develop, which is reversible if supportive treatment for septic shock is commenced promptly.

The differential diagnosis includes:

- An inborn error of metabolism that has become apparent because of septicemia.[147] Biochemical markers for inborn errors of metabolism include a high plasma lactate, increased free fatty acids, especially short-chain species (C6, C8, C10) and relatively low ketone production, suggesting a disorder of β-oxidation (Chapters 5 and 13).[148]

• Drug ingestion. Acetaminophen, rifampicin, azathioprine, Augmentin (potassium clavulanate), solvent abuse, cocaine, and heroin have been associated with liver failure and septicemia.[149,150]

The diagnosis is based on establishing the source of infection and excluding other causes of liver disease. Management is directed towards treating the sepsis and providing support for the liver failure (Chapter 7). The prognosis depends on the etiology of the sepsis. Liver transplantation is only indicated if sepsis is confined to the liver and will not recur after transplantation (e.g., echovirus).

Malnutrition

Malnutrition has profound effects on the functioning of all organs, including the liver.[151] Drug and toxicant clearance is reduced[152] and myocardial and respiratory function are significantly impaired in malnourished intensive-care patients.[153,154] Hepatic and plasma concentrations of glutathione and associated antioxidant systems are reduced in protein energy malnutrition.[155,156] The liver has a large population of Kupffer cells and therefore has a major role in the immune system, which is depressed in malnutrition. In particular, cell-mediated responsiveness and peripheral T-cell counts are reduced, rendering malnourished patients with acute or chronic liver disease especially susceptible to fungal and enteric infections.[122,157] Malnutrition also appears to be a risk factor in major surgical procedures, with an increased operative morbidity and mortality after liver transplantation.[158,159] The consequences of malnutrition are profound, so it is important to institute appropriate nutritional support as soon as possible (see also Table 16.3).[160,161]

Investigations

Abnormal liver function requires systematic investigation. In the setting of systemic disease, evaluation should include:

• A careful history, noting details of drug exposure, blood product transfusion, and family history (see Table 16.2)

• Previous evidence of chronic liver disease—e.g., palmar erythema, hypoxemia, splenomegaly, or obstructive jaundice (e.g., pale stools and dark urine)

• Blood culture, urinalysis, chest radiography

• Total and unconjugated bilirubin, hepatic transaminases, alkaline phosphatase (low in Wilson's disease, high in biliary diseases and some metabolic diseases—e.g., tyrosinemia), albumin

• Prothrombin time, activated partial thromboplastin time, fibrinogen, and D-dimers

• Viral serology (hepatitis A, B, C; EBV; CMV; adenovirus; echovirus; parvovirus; and, if sclerosing cholangitis is suggested by first-line tests, HIV testing)

• α_1-Antitrypsin level, ferritin (for neonatal hemochromatosis)

• Urinalysis for reducing substances, organic acids, and amino acids to screen for inborn errors of metabolism

• An ultrasound of the abdomen, noting the size and echogenicity of the liver, abnormalities of the biliary tree and gallbladder, patency and size of hepatic vessels, portal vein flow, spleen size, and the presence of ascites

• Liver biopsy may be justified if diagnostic and prognostic uncertainty remains.

References

1 Kolios G, Valatas V, Kouroumalis E. Role of Kupffer cells in the pathogenesis of liver disease. *World J Gastroenterol* 2006;**12**: 7413–20.

2 Mathie RT. Hepatic blood flow during cardiopulmonary bypass. *Crit Care Med* 1993;21:572–576.

3 Byhahn C, Strouhal U, Martens S, Mierdl S, Kessler P, Westphal K. Incidence of gastrointestinal complications in cardiopulmonary bypass patients. *World J Surg* 2001;**25**:1140–4.

4 Raman JS, Kochi K, Morimatsu H, Buxton B, Bellomo R. Severe ischemic early liver injury after cardiac surgery. *Ann Thorac Surg* 2002;**74**:1601–6.

5 Bernstein D, Naftel D, Chin C, *et al.* Outcome of listing for cardiac transplantation for failed Fontan: a multi-institutional study. *Circulation* 2006;**114**:273–80.

6 Michalopoulos A, Alivizatos P, Geroulanos S. Hepatic dysfunction following cardiac surgery: determinants and consequences. *Hepatogastroenterology* 1997;**4**:779–83.

7 Morse RM, Valenzuela GA, Greenwald TP, Eulie PJ, Wesley RC, McCallum RW. Amiodarone-induced liver toxicity. *Ann Intern Med* 1988;**109**:838–40.

8 Myers RP, Cerini R, Sayegh R, *et al.* Cardiac hepatopathy: clinical, hemodynamic, and histologic characteristics and correlations. *Hepatology* 2003:**37**:393–400.

9 Lee SP, Hayashi A, Young SK. Biliary sludge: curiosity or culprit? *Hepatology* 1994;**20**:523–5.

10 Sant'Anna AM, Fouron JC, Alvarez F. Neonatal cholestasis associated with fetal arrhythmia. *J Pediatr* 2005;**146**:277–80.

11 Alagille's D, Estrada A, Hadchouel M, Gautier M, Odievre M, Dommergues JP. Syndromic paucity of intralobular bile ducts (Alagille's syndrome or arteriohepatic dysplasia): review of 80 cases. *J Pediatrics* 1987;**110**:195–200.

12 Polat TB, Urganci N, Yalcin Y, *et al.* Evaluation of cardiac function by tissue Doppler imaging in children with chronic hepatitis. *J Pediatr Gastroenterol Nutr* 2006;**43**:222–7.

13 Kvittingen EA. Tyrosinaemia type 1—an update. *J Inherit Metab Dis* 1991;**14**:554–62.

14 Atkison P, Joubert G, Barron A, *et al.* Hypertrophic cardiomyopathy associated with tacrolimus in paediatric transplant patients. *Lancet* 1995;**345**:894–6.

15 Poulton J, Brown GK. Investigation of mitochondrial disease. *Arch Dis Childhood* 1995;**73**:94–6.

16 Wong F, Siu S, Liu P, Blendis LM. Brain natriuretic peptide: is it a predictor of cardiomyopathy in cirrhosis? *Clin Sci* 2001;**10**: 621–8.

17 Al Hamoudi W, Lee SS. Cirrhotic cardiomyopathy. *Ann Hepatol* 2006;**5**:132–9.

18 Blendis L, Wong F. The hyperdynamic circulation in cirrhosis: an overview. *Pharmacol Ther* 2001;**89**:221–31.

19 Murayama K, Nagasaka H, Tate K, *et al.* Significant correlations between the flow volume of patent ductus venosus and early neonatal liver function: possible involvement of patent ductus venosus in postnatal liver function. *Arch Dis Child Fetal Neonatal Ed* 2006:**91**:F175–9.

20 Hofman AF. Defective biliary secretion during total parenteral nutrition: probable mechanisms and possible solutions. *J Pediatr Gastroenterol Nutr* 1995;**20**:376–90.

21 Capron JP, Gineston JL, Herve MA, Braillon A. Metronidazole in prevention of cholestasis associated with total parenteral nutrition. *Lancet* 1983;**i**:446–7.

22 Colombo C, Battezzati PM, Crosignani A, *et al.* Liver disease in cystic fibrosis: a prospective study on incidence, risk factors and outcome. *Hepatology* 2002;**35**:1374–82.

23 Balistreri WF. Bile acid therapy in pediatric hepatobiliary disease: the role of ursodeoxycholic acid. *J Pediatr Gastroenterol Nutr* 1997;**2**:573–89.

24 Sokolic RA, Ferguson W, Mark HF. Discordant detection of monosomy 7 by GTG-banding and FISH in a patient with Shwachman–Diamond syndrome without evidence of myelodysplastic syndrome or acute myelogenous leukemia. *Cancer Genet Cytogenet* 1999;**115**:106–13.

25 Mack DR, Forstner GG, Wilschanski M, Freedman MH, Durie PR. Shwachman syndrome: exocrine pancreatic dysfunction and variable phenotypic expression. *Gastroenterology* 1996;**111**: 1593–602.

26 Woloszynek JR, Rothbaum RJ, Rawls AS, *et al.* Mutations of the *SBDS* gene are present in most patients with Shwachman–Diamond syndrome. *Blood* 2004;**104**:3588–90.

27 Ludvigsson JF, Elfström P, Broome U, Ekbom A, Montgomery SM. Celiac disease and risk of liver disease: a general population-based study. *Clin Gastroenterol Hepatol* 2007;**5**:63–9.

28 Volta U, Rodrigo L, Granito A, *et al.* Celiac disease in autoimmune cholestatic liver disorders. *Am J Gastroenterol* 2002;**97**: 2609–13.

29 Park SD, Markowitz J, Pettei M, *et al.* Failure to respond to hepatitis B vaccine in children with celiac disease. *J Pediatr Gastroenterol Nutr* 2007;**44**:431–5.

30 Mieli-Vergani G, Vergani D. Autoimmune hepatitis. *Arch Dis Child* 1996;**74**:2–5.

31 Gregorio GV, Portmann B, Reid F, *et al.* Autoimmune hepatitis in childhood: a 20-year experience. *Hepatology* 1997;**25**: 541–7.

32 Millonig G, Kern M, Ludwiczek O, Nachbaur K, Vogel W. Subfulminant hepatitis B after infliximab in Crohn's disease: need for HBV screening? *World J Gastroenterol* 2006;**12**:974–6.

33 Maggiore G, Alvarez F, Bernard O. Autoimmune chronic hepatitis. In: Buts JP, Sokal EM, eds. *Management of Digestive and Liver Disorders in Infants and Children.* Amsterdam: Elsevier, 1993: 567–75.

34 Protheroe SM, Beath SV. Nutritional support in liver disease. In: Ryan SW, ed. *Baillière's Clinical Paediatrics—Nutritional Support*, vol. 5. London: Saunders, 1997: 215–31.

35 Kelly DA. Liver complications of pediatric parenteral nutrition-epidemiology. *Nutrition* 1998;**14**:153–7.

36 Dollery CM, Sullivan ID, Bauraind O, Bull C, Milla PJ. Thrombosis and embolism in long term central venous access for parenteral nutrition. *Lancet* 1994;**344**:1043–5.

37 Pollard A, Sreeram N, Wright JG, Beath SV, Booth IW, Kelly DA. ECG and echocardiographic diagnosis of pulmonary thromboembolism associated with central venous lines. *Arch Dis Child* 1995;**73**:147–50.

38 Ricour C, Gorski AM, Goulet O. Home parenteral nutrition in children: 8 years of experience with 112 patients. *Clin Nutr* 1990;**9**:65–71.

39 Rodrigues AF, van Mourik IDM, Sharif K, *et al.* Management of end stage central venous access in children referred for possible small bowel transplantation. *J Pediatr Gastroenterol Nutr* 2006;**42**:427–33.

40 Black DD, Suttle EA, Whitington PF. The effect of short term total parenteral nutrition on hepatic function in the neonate: a prospective randomized study demonstrating alteration of hepatic canalicular function. *J Pediatrics* 1981;**99**: 445–8.

41 Fell JME, Reynolds AP, Meadows N, *et al.* Manganese toxicity in children receiving long term parenteral nutrition. *Lancet* 1996;**347**:1218–21.

42 Sudan D, DiBaise J, Torres C, *et al.* A multidisciplinary approach to the treatment of intestinal failure. *J Gastrointest Surg* 2005; **9**:165–76.

43 Stringer MD, Puntis JWL. Short bowel syndrome. *Arch Dis Child* 1995;**73**:170–3.

44 Koletzko B, Goulet O, Hunt J, *et al.* Guidelines on paediatric parenteral nutrition of the European Society of Paediatric Gastroenterology, Hepatology and Nutrition (ESPGHAN) and the European Society for Clinical Nutrition and Metabolism (ESPEN), supported by the European Society of Paediatric Research (ESPR). *J Pediatr Gastroenterol Nutr* 2005;**41**(Suppl 2):S1–87.

45 Krohn K, Koletzko B. Parenteral lipid emulsions in paediatrics. *Curr Opin Nutr Metab Care* 2006;**9**:319–23.

46 Beath SV, Booth IW, Murphy MS, *et al.* Nutritional care and candidates for small-bowel transplantation. *Arch Dis Child* 1995;**73**:348–50.

47 Beath SV, Needham SJ, Kelly DA, *et al.* Clinical features and prognosis of children assessed for isolated small bowel or combined small bowel and liver transplantation. *J Pediatr Surg* 1997;**32**:459–61.

48 Kaufman SS, Atkinson JB, Bianchi A, *et al.* Indications for pediatric intestinal transplantation. *Pediatr Transplant* 2001;**5**: 80–7.

49 Gohlke F, Lohse AW, Dienes HP, *et al.* Evidence for overlap syndrome of autoimmune hepatitis and primary sclerosing cholangitis. *J Hepatology* 1996;**24**:699–705.

50 Pearson RD, Swenson I, Schenk EA, Klish WJ, Brown MR. Fatal multisystem disease with immune enteropathy heralded by juvenile rheumatoid arthritis. *J Pediatr Gastroenterol Nutr* 1989;**8**:259–65.

51 Tang H, Neuberger J. Methotrexate in gastroenterology—dangerous villain or simply misunderstood? *Aliment Pharmacol Ther* 1996;**10**:851–8.

52 Tazawa Y, Noguchi H, Nishinomiya F, Takada G. Serum alanine aminotransferase activity in obese children. *Acta Paediatr* 1997;**86**:238–41.

53 Schwimmer JB, Deutsch R, Kahen T, Lavine JE, Stanley C, Behling C. Prevalence of fatty liver in children and adolescents. *Pediatrics* 2006;**118**:1388–93.

54 Kawasaki T, Hashimoto N, Kikuchi T, Takahashi H, Uchiyama M. The relationship between fatty liver and hyperinsulinemia in obese Japanese children. *J Pediatr Gastroenterol Nutr* 1997; **24**:317–21.

55 Rashid M, Roberts EA. Nonalcoholic steatohepatitis in children. *J Pediatr Gastroenterol Nutr* 2000;**30**:48–53.

56 Patton HM, Sirlin C, Behling C, Middleton M, Schwimmer JB, Lavine JE. Pediatric nonalcoholic fatty liver disease: a critical appraisal of current data and implications for future research. *J Pediatr Gastroenterol Nutr* 2006;**43**:413–27.

57 Lecomte M, Gottrand F, Stukens C, Lecomte-Houcke M. Acute steatosis in an 8 year old boy with insulin-dependent diabetes mellitus. *J Pediatr Gastroenterol Nutr* 1997;**25**:98–100.

58 Falchuk KR, Conlin D. The intestinal and liver complications of diabetes mellitus. *Adv Intern Med* 1997;**38**:269–86.

59 Lorenz G, Bärenwald G. Histological and electron-microscopic liver changes in diabetic children. *Acta Hepatogastroenterol (Stuttg)* 1979;**26**:435–8.

60 Nagore N, Scheur P. Pathology of diabetes mellitus. *J Pathol* 1988;**156**:155–60.

61 Marshall JD, Bronson RT, Collin GB, *et al.* New Alström syndrome phenotypes based on the evaluation of 182 cases. *Arch Intern Med* 2005;**165**:675–83.

62 Kaufman FR, Costin G, Thomas DW, Sinatra FR, Roe TF, Neustein HB. Neonatal cholestasis and hypopituitarism. *Arch Dis Child* 1984;**59**:787–9.

63 Spray CH, Mckiernan P, Waldron KE, Shaw N, Kirk J, Kelly DA. Investigation and outcome of neonatal hepatitis in infants with hypopituitarism. *Acta Paediatr* 2000;**89**:951–4.

64 Michele TM, Fleckenstein J, Sgrignoli AR, Thuluvath PJ. Chronic active hepatitis in the type I polyglandular autoimmune syndrome. *Postgrad Med J* 1994;**70**:128–31.

65 Wasniewska M, Bergamaschi R, Matarazzo P, *et al.* Increased liver enzymes and hormonal therapies in girls and adolescents with Turner syndrome. *J Endocrinol Invest* 2005;**28**:720–6.

66 Martin SR, Garel L, Alvarez F. Alagille's syndrome associated with cystic renal disease. *Arch Dis Child* 1996;**74**:232–5.

67 Fabrizi F, Dixit V, Martin P. Meta-analysis: anti-viral therapy of hepatitis B virus-associated glomerulonephritis. *Aliment Pharmacol Ther* 2006;**24**:781–8.

68 Wagrowska-Danilewicz M, Danilewicz M, Sikorska B. Glomerular and interstitial renal findings in patients with liver cirrhosis and normal renal function. The histomorphometric study. *Gen Diagn Pathol* 1996;**14**:353–7.

69 Noble-Jamieson G, Mowat AP, Thiru S, Barnes N. Severe hypertension after liver transplantation in children with alpha-1-antitrypsin deficiency. *Arch Dis Child* 1990;**65**;1217–9.

70 Davison AM. Hepatorenal failure. *Nephrol Dial Transplant* 1996;**11**(Suppl 8):24–31.

71 Holt S, Goodier D, Marley R, *et al.* Improvement in renal function in hepatorenal syndrome with *N*-acetylcysteine. *Lancet* 1999;**353**:294–5.

72 Schmidt LE, Ring-Larsen H. Vasoconstrictor therapy for hepatorenal syndrome in liver cirrhosis. *Curr Pharm Des* 2006; **12**:4637–47.

73 Wong F, Blendis L. New challenge of hepatorenal syndrome: prevention and treatment. *Hepatology* 2001;**34**:1242–51.

74 Moore, K. The hepatorenal syndrome. *Clin Sci* 1997;**92**:433–43.

75 Schwarzenberg SJ, Sharp HL. Pathogenesis of α_1-antitrypsin deficiency-associated liver disease. *J Pediatr Gastroenterol Nutr* 1990;**10**:5–12.

76 Greenough A, Pool JB, Ball C, Mieli-Vergani G, Mowat AP. Functional residual capacity related to hepatitic disease. *Arch Dis Child* 1988;**63**:850–82.

77 Francavilla R, Castellaneta SP, Hadzic N, *et al.* Prognosis of alpha-1-antitrypsin deficiency related liver disease in the era of pediatric liver transplantation. *J Hepatol* 2000;**32**:986–92.

78 Zhang J, Ling Y, Tang L, *et al.* Pentoxifylline attenuation of experimental hepatopulmonary syndrome. *J Appl Physiol* 2007;**102**:949–55.

79 Lange PA, Stoller JK. The hepatopulmonary syndrome. *Ann Intern Med* 1995;**122**:521–9.

80 Deibert P, Allgaier HP, Loesch S, *et al.* Hepatopulmonary syndrome in patients with chronic liver disease: role of pulse oximetry. *BMC Gastroenterol* 2006;**6**:15.

81 Abrams GA, Jaffe CC, Hoffer PB, Binder HJ, Fallon MB. Diagnostic utility of contrast echocardiography and lung perfusion scan in patients with hepatopulmonary syndrome. *Gastroenterology* 1995;**109**:1283–8.

82 Cauchi JA, Oliff S, Baumann U, *et al.* The Budd–Chiari syndrome in children: the spectrum of management. *J Pediatr Surg* 2006;**41**:1919–23.

83 Milani A, Basso M, Fiorini A, Pardeo M, Romano C. [Hepatopulmonary syndrome and porto-pulmonary hypertension. Nosologic features and etiopathogenic considerations; in Italian.] *Recenti Prog Med* 2001;**92**:158–63.

84 Shah T, Isaac J, Adams D, Kelly D. Development of hepatopulmonary syndrome and portopulmonary hypertension in a paediatric transplant patient. *Pediatr Transplant* 2005;**9**:127–31.

85 Herve P, Le Pavec J, Sztrymf B, Decante B, Savale L, Sitbon O. Pulmonary vascular abnormalities in cirrhosis. *Best Pract Res Clin Gastroenterol* 2007;**21**:141–59.

86 Koduri PR, Patel AR, Pinar H. Acute sequestration caused by parvovirus B19 infection in a patient with sickle cell anemia. *Am J Hematol* 1994;**47**:250–1.

87 Hatton CS, Bunch C, Weatherall DJ. Hepatic sequestration in sickle cell anaemia. *Br Med J (Clin Res Ed)* 1985;**290**:744–5.

88 Charlotte F, Bachir D, Nenert M, *et al.* Vascular lesions of the liver in sickle cell disease. A clinicopathological study in 26 living patients. *Arch Pathol Lab Med* 1995;**119**:46–52.

89 Walters MC, Patience M, Leisenring W, *et al.* Bone marrow transplantation for sickle cell disease. *N Engl J Med* 1996:**335**: 369–76.

90 Lucarelli G, Clift RA, Gamimberti M, *et al.* Marrow transplantation for patients with thalassemia: results in class 3 patients. *Blood* 1996;**87**:2082–8.

91 Tong MJ, el-Farra N, Reikes AR, Co RL. Clinical outcomes after transfusion-associated hepatitis C. *N Engl J Med* 1995;**332**: 1463–6.

92 Lefkowitch JH. Pathology of AIDS-related liver disease. *Dig Dis* 1994;**12**:321–30.

93 Arnold DM, Julian JA, Walker IR. Mortality rates and causes of death among all HIV-positive individuals with haemophilia in Canada over 21 years of follow-up. *Blood* 2006;**108**:460–4.

94 Kontorinis N, Dieterich DT. Toxicity of non-nucleoside analogue reverse transcriptase inhibitors. *Semin Liver Dis* 2003; **23**:173–82.

95 Gorelik M, Debski R, Frangoul H. Autoimmune hemolytic anemia with giant cell hepatitis: case report with review of the literature. *J Pediatr Hematol Oncol* 2004;**26**:837–9.

96 Perkins JL, Neglia JP, Ramsay NK, Davies SM. Successful bone marrow transplantation for severe aplastic anemia following orthotopic liver transplantation: long-term follow-up and outcome. *Bone Marrow Transplant* 2001;**28**:523–6.

97 Ueda I, Ishii E, Morimoto A, Ohga S, Sako M, Imashuku S. Correlation between phenotypic heterogeneity and gene mutational characteristics in familial hemophagocytic lymphohistiocytosis (FHL). *Pediatr Blood Cancer* 2006;**46**:484–8.

98 Hirst WJ, Layton DM, Singh S, *et al.* Haemophagocytic lymphohistiocytosis: experience at two UK centres. *Br J Haematol* 1994;**88**:731–9.

99 Barker CC, Anderson RA, Sauave RS, Butzner JD. GI complications after pediatric patients post-BMT. *Bone Marrow Transplant* 2005;**31**:51–8.

100 Ravikumara M, Hill FG, Wilson's DG, *et al.* 6-Thioguanine-related chronic hepatotoxicity and variceal haemorrhage in children treated for acute lymphoblastic leukaemia—a dual centre experience. *J Pediatr Gastroenterol Nutr* 2006;**42**:535–8.

101 Knapp AB, Crawford JM, Rappeport JM, Gollan JM. Cirrhosis as a consequence of graft versus host disease. *Gastroenterology* 1987;**67**:513–9.

102 Zaja F, Bacigalupo A, Patriarca F, *et al.* Treatment of refractory chronic GVHD with rituximab: a GITMO study. *Bone Marrow Transplant* 2007;**40**:273–7.

103 Farthing MJG, Clark ML, Sloane JP, Powles RL, McElwain TJ. Liver disease after bone marrow transplantation. *Gut* 1982;**23**: 465–74.

104 Fried RH, Murakami CS, Fisher LD, Willson RA, Sullivan KM, McDonald GB. Ursodeoxycholic acid treatment of refractory chronic graft-versus-host disease of the liver. *Ann Intern Med* 1992;**116**:624–9.

105 Reiss U, Cowan M, McMillan A, Horn B. Hepatic venoocclusive disease in blood and bone marrow transplantation in children and young adults: incidence, risk factor, and outcome in a cohort of 241 patients. *J Pediatr Hematol Oncol* 2002;**24**:746–50.

106 McDonald GB, Sharma P, Mathews DE, Shulman HM, Thomas E. Veno-occlusive disease of the liver after bone marrow transplantation: diagnosis, incidence, and pre-disposing factors. *Hepatology* 1984;**4**:116–22.

107 Styler MJ, Crilley P, Biggs J, *et al.* Hepatic dysfunction following busulfan and cyclophosphamide myeloablation: a retrospective, multicentre analysis. *Bone Marrow Transplant* 1996;**18**: 171–6.

108 Haussman U, Fischer J, Eber S, Scherer F, Seger R, Gungor T. Hepatic veno-occlusive disease in pediatric stem cell transplantation: impact of pre-emptive anti-thrombin III replacement and combined antithrombin III/defibrotide therapy. *Haematologica* 2006:**91**:795–800.

109 Mor E, Pappo O, Bar-Nathan N, *et al.* Defibrotide for the treatment of veno-occlusive disease after liver transplantation. *Transplantation* 2001;72:1237–1240.

110 Eber SW, Gungor T, Veldman A, *et al.* Favorable response of pediatric stem cell recipients to human protein C concentrate substitution for veno-occlusive disease. *Pediatr Transplant* 2007;**11**:49–57.

111 Forman SJ, Sullivan JL, Wright C. Epstein–Barr virus related malignant B cell lymphoplasmacytic lymphomas following allogenic bone marrow transplantation for aplastic anemia. *Transplantation* 1987;**44**:244–8.

112 Harrison RF, Bowker CM, Beath SV, Young JA. Cytological appearances of malignant peritoneal mesothelioma in a child: a case report. *Cytopathology* 1996;**7**:145–9.

113 Braier J, Latella A, Balancini B, *et al.* Outcome in children with pulmonary Langerhans cell histiocytosis. *Pediatr Blood Cancer* 2004;**43**:765–9.

114 Ruchelli ED, Horn M, Taylor SR. Severe chemotherapy-related hepatic toxicity associated with MZ protease inhibitor phenotype. *Am J Pediatr Hematol Oncol* 1990;**12**:351–4.

115 Ludwig R, Weirich A, Abel U, Hofmann W, Graf N, Tournade MF. Hepatotoxicity in patients treated according to the nephroblastoma trial and study SIOP-9/GPOH. *Med Pediatr Oncol* 1999;**33**:462–9.

116 D'Antiga L, Baker A, Pritchard J, Pryor D, Mieli-Vergani G. Veno-occlusive disease with multi-organ involvement following actinomycin-D. *Eur J Cancer* 2001;**37**:1141–8.

117 Laidlaw ST, Reilly JT, Suvarna SK. Fatal hepatotoxicity associated with 6-mercaptopurine therapy. *Postgrad Med J* 1995;**71**:639.

118 Coker RJ, James ND, Stewart JS. Hepatic toxicity of liposomal encapsulated doxorubicin. *Lancet* 1993;**341**:756.

119 Russman S, Zimmerman A, Krahenbuhl S, Kern B, Reichen J. Veno-occlusive, nodular regenerative hyperplasia and hepatocellular carcinoma after azathioprine treatment in a patient with ulcerative colitis. *Eur J Gastroenterol Hepatol* 2000;**13**: 287–90.

120 Stone HH, Kolb LD, Currie CA, Geheber CE, Cuzzell JZ. *Candida* sepsis: pathogenesis and principles of treatment. *Ann Surg* 1974;**179**:697–711.

121 Anttila VJ, Ruutu P, Bondestam S, *et al.* Hepatosplenic yeast infection in patients with acute leukemia: a diagnostic problem. *Clin Infect Dis* 1994;**18**:979–81.

122 Hacking CN, Goodrick MJ, Chisholm M. Hepatobiliary candidiasis in chronic lymphatic leukaemia. *BMJ* 1989;**299**:1568.

123 Rolando N, Harvey F, Brahm J. Fungal infection, a common unrecognised complication of acute liver failure. *J Hepatol* 1991;**12**:1–9.

124 de Repentigny L, Reiss E. Current trends in immunodiagnosis of candidiasis and aspergillosis. *Rev Infect Dis* 1984;**6**:301–12.

125 Rodrigues F, Davies EG, Harrison P, *et al.* Liver disease in children with primary immune deficiencies. *J Pediatr* 2004;**145**: 333–9.

126 Abdalian R, Heathcote EJ. Sclerosing cholangitis: a focus on secondary causes. *Hepatology* 2006;**44**:1063–74.

127 Aoki CA, Roifman CM, Lian ZX, *et al.* IL-2 receptor alpha deficiency and features of primary biliary cirrhosis. *J Autoimmun* 2006;**27**:50–3.

128 Hayward AR, Levy J, Facchetti F, *et al.* Cholangiopathy and tumors of the pancreas, liver, and biliary tree in boys with x-linked immunodeficiency with hyper-IgM. *J Immunol* 1997; **158**:977–83.

129 Khawaja K, Gennery AR, Flood TJ, Abinun M, Cant AJ. Bone marrow transplantation for CD40 ligand deficiency: a single center experience. *Arch Dis Child* 2001;**84**:508–11.

130 Gennery AR, Khawaja K, Veys P, *et al.* Treatment of CD40 ligand deficiency by hematopoietic stem cell transplantation: a survey of the European experience, 1993–2002. *Blood* 2004; **103**:1152–7.

131 Hardman TC, Purdon SD. The cardiological complications associated with HIV infection and acquired immune deficiency syndrome (AIDS). *Br J Cardiol* 2002;**9**:593–9.

132 Connor EM, Sperling RS, Gelber R, *et al.* Reduction of maternal–infant transmission of human immunodeficiency virus type 1 with zidovudine treatment. *N Engl J Med* 1994;**331**:1173–80.

133 Palella FJ, Delaney KM, Moorman AC, *et al.* Declining morbidity and mortality among patients with advanced HIV infection. *N Engl J Med* 1998;**338**:853–60.

134 Fung HB, Stone EA, Piacenti FJ. Tenofovir disoproxil fumarate: a nucleotide reverse transcriptase inhibitor for the treatment of HIV infection. *Clin Ther* 2002;**24**:1515–48.

135 Matthews GV, Cooper DA, Dore GJ. Improvements in parameters of end-stage liver disease in patients with HIV/HBV cirrhosis treated with tenofovir. *Antivir Ther* 2007;**12**:119–22.

136 James DG, Sherlock S. Sarcoidosis of the liver. *Sarcoidosis* 1994;**11**:2–6.

137 Rizzato G. Extrapulmonary presentation of sarcoidosis. *Curr Opin Pulm Med* 2001;**7**:295–7.

138 Sarigol SS, Hay MH, Wyllie R. Sarcoidosis in preschool children with hepatic involvement mimicking juvenile rheumatoid arthritis. *J Pediatr Gastroenterol Nutr* 1999;**28**:510–2.

139 Lindsley CB, Petty RE. Overview and report on international registry of sarcoid arthritis in childhood. *Curr Rheumatol Rep* 2000;**2**:343–8.

140 Yanardag H, Caner M, Kaynak K, Uygun S, Demirci S, Karayei T. Clinical value of mediastinoscopy in the diagnosis of sarcoidosis: an analysis of 68 cases. *Thorac Cardiovasc Surg* 2006;**54**: 198–201.

141 Lower EE, Baughman RP. Prolonged use of methotrexate for sarcoidosis. *Arch Intern Med* 1995;**155**:846–51.

142 Winkelstein JA, Marino MC, Johnston RBJ, *et al.* Chronic granulomatous disease. Report on a national registry of 368 patients. *Medicine* 2000;**79**:155–69.

143 Castro M, Balducci L, Ciuffetti C, Lucidi V, Torre A, Bella S. [Ascites as an unusual manifestation of chronic granulomatous disease in childhood; in Italian.] *Pediatr Med Chir* 1992;**14**: 317–9.

144 Nakhleh RE, Glock M, Snover DC. Hepatic pathology of chronic granulomatous disease of childhood. *Arch Pathol Lab Med* 1992;**116**:71–5.

145 Hague RA, Eastham EJ, Lee RE, Cant AJ. Resolution of hepatic abscess after interferon gamma in chronic granulomatous disease. *Arch Dis Child* 1993;**69**:443–5.

146 Gimson AE. Hepatic dysfunction during bacterial sepsis. *Intensive Care Med* 1987;**13**:162–6.

147 Kimura A, Inoue O, Kato H. Serum concentrations of total bile acids in patients with acute Kawasaki syndrome. *Arch Ped Adolesc Med* 1996;**150**:289–92.

148 Waggoner DD, Buist NRM, Donnell GN. Long-term prognosis in galactosaemia: results of a survey of 350 cases. *J Inherit Metab Dis* 1990;**13**:802–18.

149 Morris AAM, Leonard JV. Early recognition of metabolic decompensation. *Arch Dis Child* 1997;**76**:555–6.

150 Marks V, Chapple PAL. Hepatic dysfunction in heroin and cocaine users. *Br J Addict* 1967;**62**:189–95.

151 Meadows R, Verghese A. Medical complications of glue sniffing. *South Med J* 1996;**89**:455–62.

152 Alleyne GAO, Halliday D, Waterlow JC. Chemical composition of organs of children who died of malnutrition. *Br J Nutr* 1969;**23**:783–90.

153 Bidlack WR, Hamilton Smith C. The effect of nutritional factors on hepatic drug and toxicant metabolism. *J Am Diet Assoc* 1984;**84**:892–8.

154 Meakins JL, Christou NV, Shizgal HM, MacLean LD. Therapeutic approaches to anergy in surgical patients. Surgery and levamisole. *Ann Surg* 1979;**190**:286–96.

155 Sheldon GF, Petersen SR. Malnutrition and cardiopulmonary function: relation to oxygen transport. *JPEN J Parenter Enteral Nutr* 1980;**4**:376–83.

156 Shi EC, Fisher R, McEvoy M, Vantol R, Rose M, Ham JM. Factors influencing hepatic glutathione concentrations: a study in surgical patients. *Clin Sci* 1982;**62**:279–83.

157 Becker K, Leichsenring M, Gana L, Bremer HJ, Schirmer RH. Glutathione and association antioxidant systems in protein energy malnutrition: results of a study in Nigeria. *Free Radic Biol Med* 1995;**18**:257–63.

158 Gross RL, Newberne PM. Role of nutrition in immunologic function. *Physiol Rev* 1980;**60**:188–302.

159 Shaw BW, Wood RP, Gordon RD, *et al.* Influence of selected patient variables and operative blood loss on 6 month survival following liver transplantation. *Semin Liver Dis* 1985;**5**:385–93.

160 Beath S, Brook G, Kelly D, McMaster P, Mayer D, Buckels J. Improving outcome of liver transplantation in babies less than 1 year. *Transplant Proc* 1994;**26**:180–2.

161 Beath SV, Kelly DA, Booth IW. Nutritional support in liver disease. *Arch Dis Child* 1993;**69**:545–9.

17 Skin Disorders in Liver Disease

Indra D.M. van Mourik and Michelle Thomson

Pediatric skin disorders account for 10–15% of family practitioner consultations. Their prevalence in children with liver disease is unknown, but may be even higher. The enormous variety of skin diseases poses a considerable diagnostic challenge to the nondermatologist, and appropriate treatment may be delayed.[1]

In the context of pediatric hepatology, skin disorders can be separated into three groups:

- Common incidental skin conditions such as acne, warts, eczema, drug rashes and infections due to common bacteria, viruses or fungi
- Dermatological manifestations of an underlying systemic disorder such as xanthelasma, associated with cholestasis or spider nevi in chronic liver disease
- Skin disorders following liver transplantation, including:
  - —Side effects of immunosuppressant drugs
  - —Direct results of immunosuppression, including bacterial, viral, fungal, and protozoal infections
  - —Graft-versus-host disease
  - —Cutaneous malignancies

This chapter first deals with the structure and function of normal skin as a basis for understanding skin pathophysiology, dermatological manifestations of liver disease in general, and skin conditions in the immunocompromised host.

Structure and function of normal skin

Skin structure

The skin is divided into three layers: the epidermis, dermis, and subcutaneous layer.[2]

Epidermis

The epidermis is a multilayered structure that renews itself continuously by cell division in the basal layer. It consists of:

- Keratinocytes, which move peripherally from the basal layer, giving rise to successive layers of cells that lose their nuclei and eventually die as they reach the surface
- Melanocytes, melanin-producing dendritic cells
- Langerhans cells, important antigen-presenting cells bearing major histocompatibility (MHC) class II antigens
- Merkel cells, involved in sensation and mainly seen on digital pads, lips and in the oral cavity

The epidermal appendages are apocrine sweat glands, hair, sebaceous glands, nails, and teeth.

Dermis

The dermis forms the bulk of the skin and contains connective-tissue fibers (mainly collagen, with some elastin and reticulin) lying beneath the epidermis, giving the skin its ability to stretch and mold. Blood vessels, nerves, lymphatics, and muscles, as well as cells such as leukocytes, histiocytes, fibroblasts, and mast cells are found in this layer.

Subcutaneous layer

The subcutaneous layer mainly contains fat, sweat glands, and blood vessels.

Skin function

The skin is a vital part of the body with numerous functions, including:

- Physical barrier to antigens or bacteria (intact stratum corneum, lipids in sebaceous glands, suppressant effect of normal skin flora on pathogens, presence of granulocytes, macrophages and killer T cells)
- Prevention of excessive absorption or loss of water and regulation of internal temperature (sweat glands)
- Pigmentation, preventing injury from ultraviolet light
- Vitamin D synthesis by sunlight in the epidermis
- Sensation of pain, touch, and temperature
- Involvement in immunological reactions (Langerhans cells, secretory IgA, T cells and B cells)

Dermatological manifestations of liver disease

Jaundice

Jaundice (icterus), a yellow discoloration of the skin and mucous membranes, is the most obvious sign of liver disease

Diseases of the Liver and Biliary System in Children, 3rd edition. Edited by Deirdre Kelly. © 2008 Blackwell Publishing, ISBN: 978-1-4051-6334-7.

and is best seen in the conjunctivae. It is detectable when the serum level of bilirubin exceeds 2 mg/dL (34 µmol/L), although in neonates it may not be detected unless the level exceeds 5 mg/dL (85 µmol/L). The differential diagnosis and management are discussed elsewhere in this book (Chapter 4).

Palmar erythema

Palmar erythema, or "liver palms," is a nonspecific red discoloration of the palms and fingertips of the hand indicative of a hyperdynamic circulation, which is associated with chronic liver disease and cirrhosis.

Spider nevi

Spider nevi, or spider angiomas, are telangiectases consisting of a central arteriole with superficially radiating small vessels, resembling spiders' legs, and are mainly observed in the superior vena cava distribution area (i.e., above the nipple line) (Figure 17.1). Characteristically, the whole lesion will blanch when pressure is applied to the center of the spider, and during episodes of severe or prolonged hypotension they may disappear. They can be successfully treated with laser therapy.[3]

Although spider nevi do occur in healthy people, especially at puberty, the presence of more than five is suggestive of chronic liver disease. An increase in number or size of spider nevi may suggest progressive liver damage (cirrhosis), but also occurs in pregnancy or in girls taking the contraceptive pill.

White nails (Terry nails)

White nails are a common feature of chronic liver disease (cirrhosis) in adults, but are less frequently seen in children.

Pruritus

Pruritus is a distressing symptom of cholestasis or inborn errors of bile acid metabolism. Symptoms range from mild to severe intractable pruritus, which interferes with the patient's daily activity and sleep. Intractable pruritus may be an indication for liver transplantation.

The exact mechanism of pruritus is uncertain. Cholestasis leads to an accumulation in plasma of substances which are normally excreted into bile (e.g., bilirubin, cholesterol, and bile acids). High levels of bile acids may damage hepatocyte membranes, triggering the release of pruritogenic substances, which interact with nerve endings in the skin.[4,5]

The skin in patients with generalized pruritus is often very dry and varies from a normal appearance, through mild flakiness with a few scratch marks, to severe excoriation with scars and nodules.

Treatment of pruritus is empirical and unsatisfactory. Good skin care is essential. As dryness of the skin is a prominent feature, avoidance of soap and liberal use of emollients are strongly recommended. Alternative treatments such as evening primrose oil and aromatherapy, and a wide range of drugs and therapies including ursodeoxycholic acid, phenobarbitone, rifampicin, cholestyramine, histamine antagonists, ondansetron, plasmapheresis, and phototherapy (Chapter 4) are used with variable success. Partial external diversion of bile has been attempted in patients with pruritus unresponsive to medical treatment, again with highly variable success rates.[6]

More recent studies have implicated increased opioid neurotransmission/neuromodulation in the central nervous system as a contributor to pruritus in cholestasis, suggesting that oral opiate antagonists—for example, naloxone—may provide long-term relief from pruritus.[7] Although the exact mechanism of opiate involvement is still unknown, the beneficial effects of opiate antagonists have been shown in different randomized, blinded, placebo-controlled trials.[8–10] Finally, subjective amelioration of pruritus following intravenous administration of ondansetron to cholestatic patients may suggest that altered serotonergic neurotransmission may also contribute to this form of pruritus.[7]

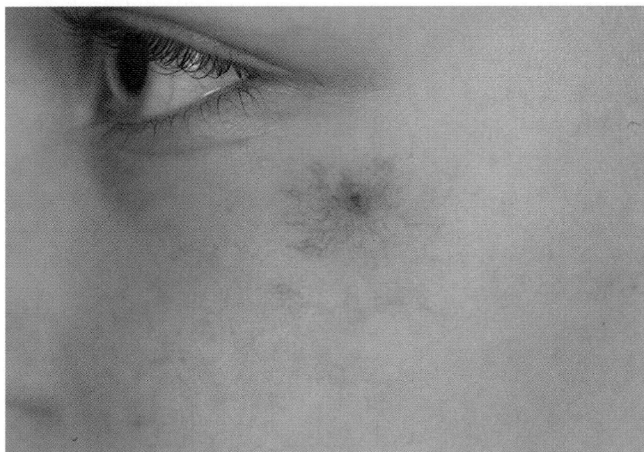

Figure 17.1 Spider nevus on a young girl's cheek, which is suggestive of chronic liver disease. Spider nevi are also found in pregnancy, at puberty, and in girls taking the contraceptive pill, although usually in fewer numbers.

Xanthelasma

Orange-yellow lipid deposits of cholesterol in the skin are known as xanthelasmas. They are seen in children with elevated plasma cholesterol due to chronic cholestasis secondary to intrahepatic biliary hypoplasia such as Alagille's syndrome.[11] They rarely present before the age of 16 months. The commonest sites are areas of mild trauma, the elbows, knees, and at flexures. Xanthelasmas regress with management of hypercholesterolemia and following liver transplantation.

Purpura

Purpura is extravasation of red cells in the skin, which presents with red patches that do not blanch on pressure. Purpura in liver disease usually reflects thrombocytopenia secondary to hypersplenism and portal hypertension, or skin fragility due to steroids.

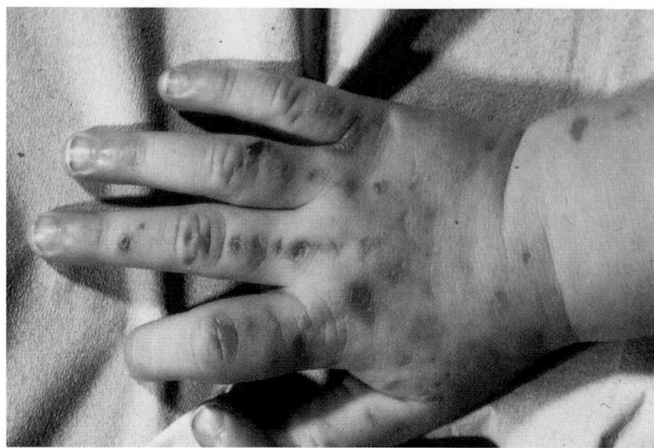

Figure 17.2 Photosensitive porphyria-like skin lesions in a child with Alagille's syndrome. She had elevated urinary porphyrins, which were thought to be secondary to liver dysfunction.

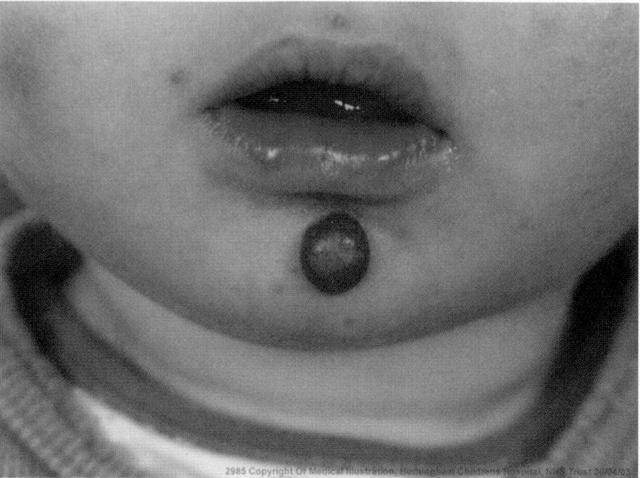

Figure 17.3 Hemangioma on a child's chin. Hemangiomas may be single or multiple. They may be a sign of other hemangiomas elsewhere—e.g., the liver.

Photosensitivity

Photosensitivity with abnormal liver function may be due to porphyria cutanea tarda. Early cutaneous features are blister formation and erosions on the backs of the hands, the forearms, and the face following exposure to sunlight. The areas heal with scarring and milia formation. Later, there may be hyperpigmentation, hypertrichosis, and pseudosclerodermatous thickening of the skin.

Similar photosensitive blistering eruptions, associated with elevated plasma and urinary porphyrins (raised coproporphyrin isomer I and III fraction), have been described in children with Alagille's syndrome (Figure 17.2). It is unclear whether the elevated porphyrins are secondary to liver dysfunction or associated with the deletion of chromosome 20 in this condition. The lack of similar lesions in other hepatic disorders associated with comparable porphyrin abnormalities does suggest that other factors may be involved in the pathogenesis of these cutaneous lesions.[12]

Carotenemia

This yellow/orange discoloration of the skin, in particular of the palms, soles, and feet, may occur in otherwise healthy children due to excess dietary β-carotene. Its importance is that it may be mistaken for jaundice. In some children, it may be associated with low serum retinol-binding protein (RBP4) levels, resulting in slow uptake and release of vitamin A by the liver and subsequent inhibition of conversion of carotene to vitamin A. The resulting hypercarotenemia and low vitamin A levels do not respond to vitamin A supplementation.[13]

Hemangioma

Rarely, infants are born with multiple angiomas of the skin and internal organs. The skin lesions look like small strawberry nevi, which are present at birth or arise shortly afterwards and, although they may appear anywhere on the body, have a predilection for the head, neck, and napkin area (Figure 17.3). The lesions contain both capillary and "cavernous" vascular elements, rapidly increase in size to often dome-shaped, red/purple extrusions, and may bleed if traumatized. Although the skin lesions would normally undergo spontaneous resolution with time, the associated hepatic and intestinal angiomas may lead to severe complications and, depending on the extent of disease and organs affected, often have a poor prognosis (see Chapters 10 and 19).

Gianotti–Crosti syndrome

Gianotti–Crosti syndrome, or papular acrodermatitis of childhood, is a nonspecific viral exanthema that may accompany hepatitis B infection. There are erythematous, nonitchy papules on the face and extremities. Other clinical findings are generalized lymphadenopathy, and in children with hepatitis there is hepatomegaly and biochemical and histological evidence of acute or chronic hepatitis.

Lichen planus and hepatitis C infection

Lichen planus is an idiopathic inflammatory disease of the skin and mucous membranes. The pathogenesis is not fully understood, but several reports have suggested a relationship between oral lichen planus and chronic liver disease, especially hepatitis C virus (HCV) infection. In several case–control studies, the prevalence of HCV was higher in patients with lichen planus than in controls, although such an association may not be significant in some geographical areas.[14,15] However, in view of the possible association, screening patients with oral lichen planus for antibodies to HCV is recommended.

Neonatal lupus erythematosus

Neonatal lupus erythematosus (NLE) is an autoimmune disease characterized by congenital heart block, thrombocytopenia, hepatobiliary disease, and/or transient skin lesions of subacute cutaneous lupus. In contrast to adult lupus, the lesions have a predilection for the face, especially the periorbital region.[16] The skin lesions typically resolve without scarring, although dyspigmentation may persist for many months and some may have residual telangiectasias. Children with skin signs of neonatal lupus should be evaluated for cardiac, hepatobiliary,[17] and hematologic[18] manifestations.

Skin manifestations of malnutrition

Infants with chronic liver disease are particularly at risk of malnutrition (see Chapters 4, 15, and 16).[19] Deficiencies in calories, protein, essential fatty acids, minerals, and trace elements (particularly zinc and selenium) may eventually lead to skin abnormalities.

Dietary protein deficiency (kwashiorkor) may result in nonspecific skin changes, ranging from pigmentary changes (hyperpigmentation or hypopigmentation) to flexural erosions, desquamation, and dry, depigmented, and pluckable hair. In children with reduced calorie intake (marasmus), the skin may appear dry and wrinkled. Similar changes can be found as a result of longstanding essential fatty acid deficiency, but the main feature is a dry, flaky skin (ichthyosis) with hyperpigmentation (Figure 17.4).

Zinc deficiency occasionally complicates liver disease and may lead to exudative eczematous lesions around the orifices and on the hands and feet, similar to those found in acrodermatitis enteropathica, an inborn error of zinc metabolism. Selenium deficiency may lead to loss of hair pigment.

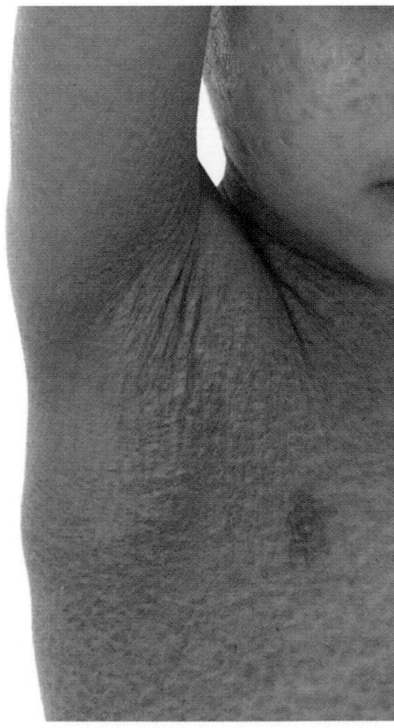

Figure 17.4 Dry, flaky skin (ichthyosis), often seen in long-standing essential fatty acid deficiency, which is secondary to fat malabsorption in liver disease.

All of these conditions are reversible with appropriate dietary supplementation.

Dermatological complications of liver transplantation

The skin in the immunocompromised host

Environmental conditions and skin microorganisms, which have little significance in the normal host, may have quite devastating effects in the immunocompromised patient. Protection by an intact well-functioning skin is essential, but may be compromised by various factors uniquely associated with the immunosuppression. In the first place, the integrity of the skin may be breached by the use of long-term central lines, intravenous devices, and invasive diagnostic procedures, allowing easy invasion of pathogens. Second, immunosuppressant drugs such as corticosteroids cause atrophy of the skin, thus compromising the first-line barrier, while other immunosuppressant drugs (cyclosporine, tacrolimus, etc.) lead to granulocytopenia, neutropenia, and neutrophil defects, or alteration of T-cell and B-cell function, thereby reducing the second-line defences against pathogens. Finally, longstanding antimicrobial therapy may alter the normal skin flora (e.g., staphylococci, coryneforms, and some Gram-negative bacilli such as *Acinetobacter* spp.), allowing colonization with potential pathogens. Once colonized, the immunocompromised host is at continuous risk of acquiring infection with these organisms.[20]

Cutaneous side effects of immunosuppressive drugs

Hypertrichosis (hirsutism)

Cyclosporine therapy causes a reversible, dose-dependent increase in the growth of body hair, more frequently seen in younger transplant patients (Figure 17.5).[21] Vellus hair (thin, short hair without pigment, which takes over from lanugo hair in hair follicles after birth) converts to terminal hair, which is longer, coarser, and darker, and existing terminal hair becomes thicker. The mechanism of this follicular stimulation is unknown. It may be exacerbated by the use of systemic steroids.[22,23] Laser hair removal is effective, but repeated treatment is required in order to maintain improvement.[24]

Retrospective studies in adult renal transplant recipients receiving cyclosporine found that 40–60% had hirsutism, with a slightly higher incidence in dark-skinned patients, suggesting predisposing genetic factors.[25,26] The incidence of hypertrichosis in children receiving cyclosporine after liver transplantation is approximately 30%, and the impact of its cosmetic effect, particularly in teenagers, is substantial.[27]

Gingival hyperplasia

Gingival hyperplasia is a recognized side effect of cyclosporine and of the antihypertensive drug nifedipine, which is frequently used after liver transplantation (Chapter 21).

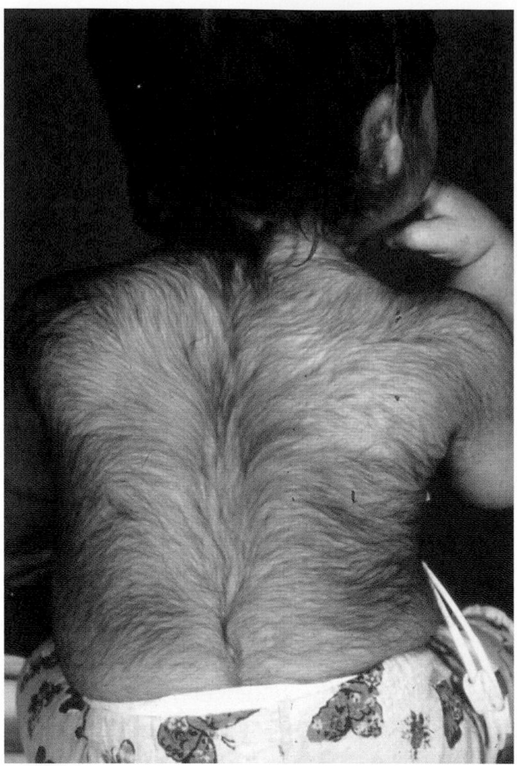

Figure 17.5 Immunosuppression with cyclosporine commonly causes excessive hirsutism, which resolves on reduction of the drug.

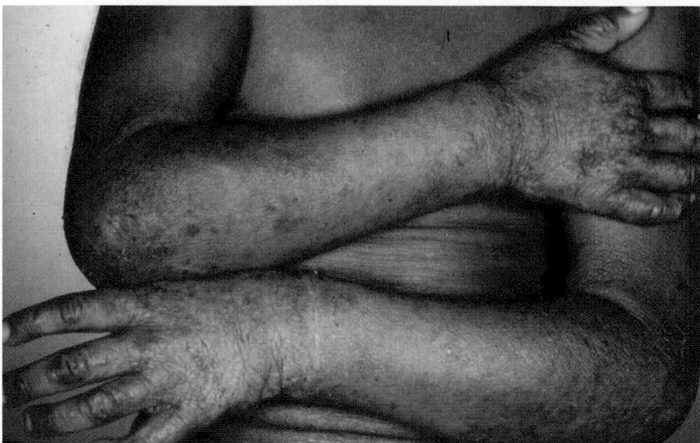

Figure 17.6 Red, scaly skin with exaggerated skin markings (lichenification) are a sign of chronic eczema. It is difficult to treat in children who also have pruritus due to cholestasis. Eczema may also become exacerbated after transplantation, particularly with cyclosporine treatment.

Eczema

Atopic dermatitis, or eczema, is a common skin disorder in infancy and childhood, affecting 5–7% of children before the age of 5 years. It may be particularly troublesome in children with liver disease before or after transplantation.

In infants and younger children, the main affected areas are the face and extensor surfaces of the extremities, while in older children and adults, the flexural areas are predominantly involved. Chronic eczema (Figure 17.6) appears red, scaly, and lichenified (thickened, with exaggerated skin markings), while acute exacerbations are characterized by edema, oozing, crusting, and excoriation. The main symptom is pruritus, which may be not only difficult to manage, but also difficult to differentiate from pruritus due to cholestasis in children with both conditions.

Immunocompromised children with atopic dermatitis have an increased risk of secondary bacterial infection of the eczematous lesions, leading to crusting and weeping.

Occasionally, eczema appears for the first time or becomes more severe in children after transplantation who are receiving cyclosporine. This is paradoxical, because cyclosporine is used to treat eczema, and may indicate a role for infection in the pathogenesis of eczema. There is no clear relationship with cyclosporine dose, but the eczema may improve when immunosuppression is reduced.

First-line treatment of eczema involves soap substitutes, bath oils, and emollient creams (e.g., aqueous cream and combinations of white soft paraffin and liquid paraffin) to moisturize the skin and reduce pruritus secondary to xeroderma (dry skin). More inflamed areas should be treated with topical steroids, which are available in increasing strengths from hydrocortisone 0.5–1%, to Eumovate (clobetasone butyrate 0.05%) or Betnovate (betamethasone 0.1%). In superimposed bacterial or fungal infection, an ointment combining a steroid and antibacterial or anticandidal agent is necessary, such as Canesten HC, Terra-Cortril, or Vioform HC. A body suit made of tubular bandages is comforting at night. Sometimes a double layer of bandages, with the inner layer wet ("wet wraps"), is helpful for extreme pruritus. Ichthammol-impregnated bandages are useful for lichenified eczema on the limbs.

In more resistant cases of chronic eczema, long-term use of topical and systemic corticosteroids is limited because of numerous side effects. In recent years, other, immunomodulatory forms of treatment have been explored, including topical tacrolimus ointment. Large multicenter studies have recently shown that its long-term use in both adults and children with severe atopic eczema is both efficacious and safe.[28–30]

Acne vulgaris

Acne vulgaris affects most adolescents during puberty, when changes in the hair follicle and sebaceous glands are stimulated by hormones. Drug-induced acne rarely occurs before puberty, in the "unprimed" prepubertal follicles. Adolescents and adults treated with high-dose corticosteroids for autoimmune hepatitis or after transplantation may develop acne for the first time, or experience an exacerbation of preexisting acne.[31]

Steroid-induced acne is reversible, and generally appears 2–3 weeks after initiation of high-dose prednisolone therapy. It may be mild or severe, extending beyond the usual

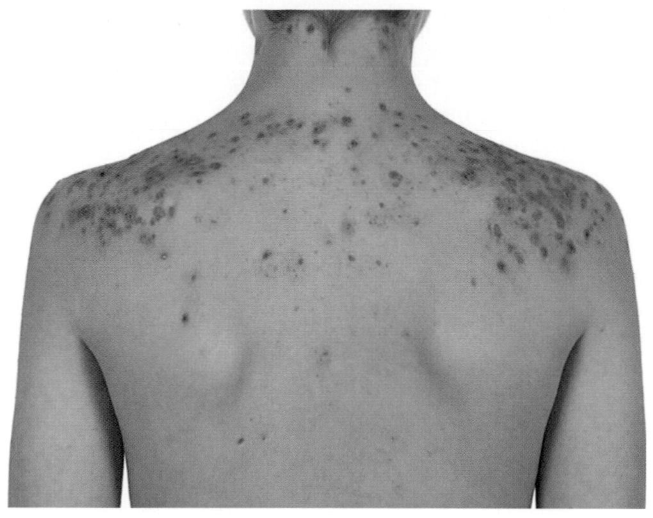

Figure 17.7 Treatment with steroids after transplantation or for autoimmune hepatitis can lead to sever acne with extensive atrophic scarring.

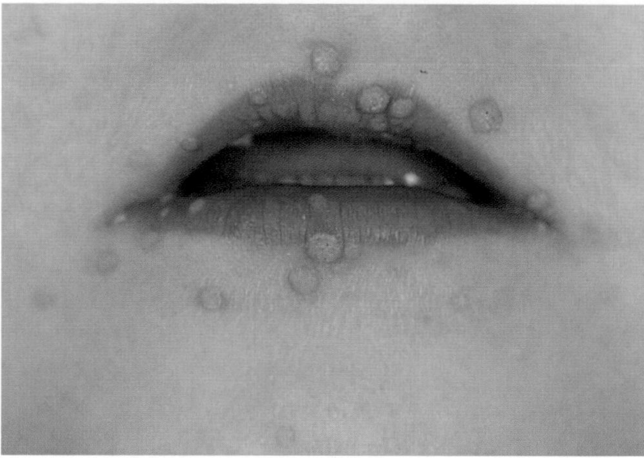

Figure 17.8 Warts are common in post-transplantation patients because of immunosuppression. This child receiving cyclosporine therapy had warts on the hands that spread to the face. Warts can be treated conservatively with keratolytic paints or destructively using cryotherapy.

distribution sites to the arms, the whole central back, and down to the buttocks. Acne vulgaris is characterized by comedones, papules and pustules, nodules and cysts, and finally scar formation (Figure 17.7). In steroid-induced acne, pustules predominate, and the eruption is often strikingly monomorphic. Cyclosporine may also provoke acne as part of its effect on the hair follicle.

Mild forms of acne should be treated with topical preparations such as benzoyl peroxide or retinoic acid, alone or in combination with topical antibiotics (tetracyclines, erythromycin, or clindamycin). In moderate cases, treatment should include a combination of topical preparations with systemic oxytetracycline or erythromycin.[32] Minocycline, an oral preparation of tetracycline, should be avoided, as it can cause a lupus-like hepatitis. The more potent anti-acne drugs, cyproterone acetate and isotretinoin, are potentially hepatotoxic and therefore contraindicated.

Other steroid-induced skin manifestations

Striae, facial erythema, atrophic and friable skin, purpura, and telangiectasia are all well-recognized cutaneous side effects of prolonged high-dose steroid use. Apart from erythema, these changes are irreversible.

Cutaneous lesions in immunocompromised hosts

Viral infections

Cutaneous viral infections in healthy individuals are common, benign, and self-limiting, but they may be devastating in immunocompromised hosts, so early diagnosis and treatment are vital. The most important cutaneous virus infections in the context of liver transplantation are human papillomaviruses (HPV), molluscum contagiosum, herpes simplex virus (HSV), varicella-zoster virus (VZV), and cytomegalovirus (CMV).

Human papillomavirus. Viral warts (verrucae) are one of the commonest cutaneous manifestations of long-term immunosuppressive therapy and may be so numerous as to be disfiguring (Figure 17.8).[26] The warts may reflect primary infection or reactivation of previously acquired latent virus. Studies in adult renal transplant recipients have shown a link between HPV and cutaneous malignancies, although other factors such as ultraviolet exposure and the type of immunosuppressive drug also play a role.

Common warts, palmar and plantar warts. Warts and verrucas (plantar warts). Warts can be treated conservatively with keratolytic paints or destructively by cryotherapy. In immunosuppressed children, cryotherapy is often ineffective, as well as painful. If the child requires a general anesthetic for another reason, the warts may be curetted or frozen at the same time, but unfortunately they may recur. Repeated treatment may be required until immunosuppression can be reduced. If the warts are asymptomatic, treatment may not be indicated. There is some evidence that topical imiquimod 5% cream may benefit immunosuppressed adults with recalcitrant warts, but studies in children with transplants have not been performed.[33]

Plane warts. These are tiny, flat, flesh-colored warts, usually occurring on the back of hands and on the face. They usually resolve spontaneously, and treatment is not indicated.

Condyloma acuminatum. These are genital warts, located on the penis, vulva, or perianal area, which usually present as small, cauliflower-like lesions. They are common in childhood, particularly in children undergoing immunosuppression. They are best treated with podophyllin paint under general anesthetic if there are numerous warts.

Molluscum contagiosum. Molluscum contagiosum is caused by a poxvirus. The umbilicated, white or whitish-yellow papules occur anywhere on the body and may be very extensive in immunosuppressed patients, responding to reduction in immunosuppressive therapy. There is no specific treatment, as they eventually resolve spontaneously. If symptomatic, cryotherapy or individual enucleation with a needle is possible.

Herpes simplex virus. Primary herpes simplex infection due to HSV type 1 presents in immunocompetent children as a cold sore with mild to moderate stomatitis. Immunocompromised patients suffer primary HSV-1 infection as severe herpetic gingivostomatitis with extensive blisters and erosions on buccal mucosa and lips. Conjunctivitis and keratitis may also occur (Figure 17.9).

As the virus persists in sensory ganglia, the patient remains at risk of recurrent herpes infection, which usually presents as cold sores on the lips, with occasional spread to the esophagus.

The diagnosis is based on the clinical features and positive electron microscopy of cultured fluid from vesicles. Serology is helpful only in primary HSV infection.

Cutaneous HSV infection in immunosuppressed patients should always be treated systemically (acyclovir), with reduction of immunosuppression in more extensive infections.

Varicella-zoster virus. The presentation of varicella (chickenpox) in immunosuppressed patients resembles that in healthy children, with fever, malaise, and a characteristic skin rash, but the disease may be more severe and lead to serious complications such as hemorrhagic varicella, postinfectious encephalomyelitis, and pneumonia. The virus remains dormant in dorsal root ganglia and may reactivate, leading to herpes zoster (shingles). In immunosuppressed hosts, reactivation is more likely and may lead to recurrent varicella and/or disseminated disease with visceral involvement, which may be fatal. Treatment of both forms of varicella includes a reduction in immunosuppressive therapy, intravenous acyclovir, and zoster immunoglobulin (ZIg).

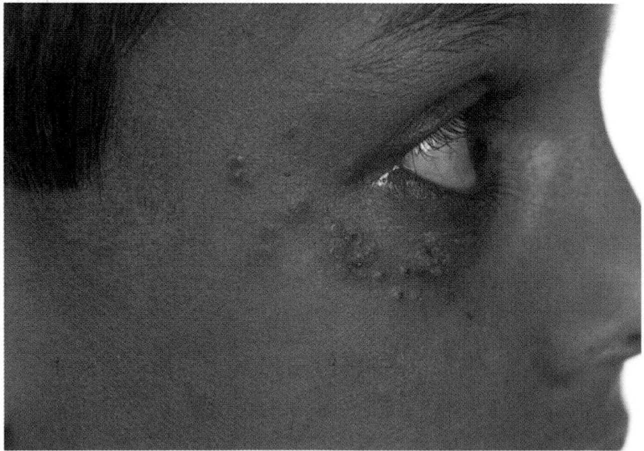

Figure 17.9 Herpes simplex infection around the eye is characterized by monomorphic vesicles and erosions. Treatment is with acyclovir and reduction in immunosuppression, if relevant.

Cytomegalovirus. CMV infection in immunocompromised hosts rarely presents with cutaneous manifestations, but as a febrile illness with arthralgia and myalgia or disseminated disease with visceral involvement. A few patients with primary or reinfection with CMV have presented with erythema multiforme with the typical "target lesions" or blisters.

Fungal infections of the skin

Fungal infections are common in immunocompromised patients, some reviews reporting an incidence as high as 70–85%. They include (i) infections that commonly affect normal individuals but in immunocompromised hosts present in a more severe and extensive form; and (ii) "opportunistic" fungal infections with organisms unlikely to invade a normal host.[34,35]

This chapter covers only the superficial mycoses involving the outermost layers of the skin, the nails, the hair, and mucous membranes. The main pathogens in this group are the dermatophytes and yeasts.[36,37]

Dermatophytoses. Infections with dermatophytes, or ringworm fungi, are confined to the superficial stratum corneum, nails, and hair and are usually acquired from contact with keratin debris carrying fungal spores. There are three genera of dermatophytes: *Trichophyton*, *Microsporum*, and *Epidermophyton*, of which more than 40 species are recognized world-wide. Some are anthropophilic (i.e., transmitted from person to person), while others are zoophilic (i.e., passed from animals to humans).

Diagnosis is confirmed by microscopic detection of fungal hyphae in skin scrapings, nail clippings or plucked hair or a positive culture. Treatment includes topical broad-spectrum antifungal agents such as miconazole (Daktarin) or clotrimazole (Canesten) in cases of very limited infection, or oral griseofulvin where the fungal infection is more extensive. More potent systemic antifungals include itraconazole and terbinafine, but these are not licensed in children at present and are potentially hepatotoxic. For drug doses, see Table 17.1.

Tinea pedis (athlete's foot). This presents as scaling, itchy skin between the toes, often spreading to the entire sole. A foul odor may be present. Vesicles may occur, particularly during warm weather, rupturing to leave a ring-like ragged border. It is a relatively uncommon condition in immunocompetent prepubertal children, where the diagnosis of contact dermatitis is more likely. However, the incidence is increasing in immunosuppressed children in this age group.

Table 17.1 Drug dosages in dermatological conditions.

Drug	Dosage	Frequency (route)
Antibacterial		
Carbenicillin	25–100 mg/kg/dose (max. 5 g)	4–6 h (i.m./i.v.)
Co-trimoxazole	2.5 mg/kg/dose	12 h (i.v./oral)
Erythromycin	10–25 mg/kg/dose	6–8 h (oral)
Flucloxacillin	25–50 mg/kg/dose (max. 2 g)	4–6 h (i.v.)
	10 mg/kg/dose (max. 250 mg)	6 h (oral)
Gentamicin	7.5 mg/kg/dose	Single (i.v./i.m.)
Oxytetracycline	250–500 mg/dose (NOT/kg)	6 h (oral)
Penicillin		
Benzylpenicillin (penicillin G)	30–60 mg/kg/dose (max. 3 g)	4–6 h (i.v.)
Phenoxymethylpenicillin (penicillin V)	7.5–15 mg/kg/dose (max. 500 mg)	6 h (oral)
Ticarcillin	50 mg/kg/dose (max. 3 g)	4–6 h (i.v.)
Vancomycin	15 mg/kg/dose (max. 500 mg)	Single (i.v. over 2 h)
Antifungal		
Amphotericin (liposomal)	1 mg/kg	Daily (i.v. over 1 h)
	Then increase over 2–4 days to 2–3 mg/kg	Daily (i.v.)
Fluconazole	4 (or 8) mg/kg (max. 200 mg)	Stat. (oral/i.v.)
	Then 2 (or 4–8) mg/kg (max. 100 mg)	Daily (oral/i.v.)
Flucytosine	400–1200 mg/m^2/dose (max. 2 g)	6 h (oral./i.v.)
Griseofulvin	10–20 mg/kg (max. 1 g)	Daily (oral)
Ketoconazole	3–5 mg/kg/dose (max. 400 mg)	12–24 h (oral)
Miconazole	7.5–15 mg/kg/dose (max. 1.2 g)	8 h (i.v. over 1 h)
Antiviral		
Acyclovir	250–500 mg/m^2/dose	8 h (i.v. over 1 h)
Ganciclovir	2.5–5 mg/kg/dose	8–12 h (i.v. over 1 h)

The condition may resolve without treatment, but often recurs.

Tinea corporis. Dermatophyte infection of the trunk, legs, arms, or face produces annular scaly, itchy lesions with an inflammatory edge and central clearing (Figure 17.10). It may have spread from another site (e.g., tinea cruris) or from an external source, animal or human.

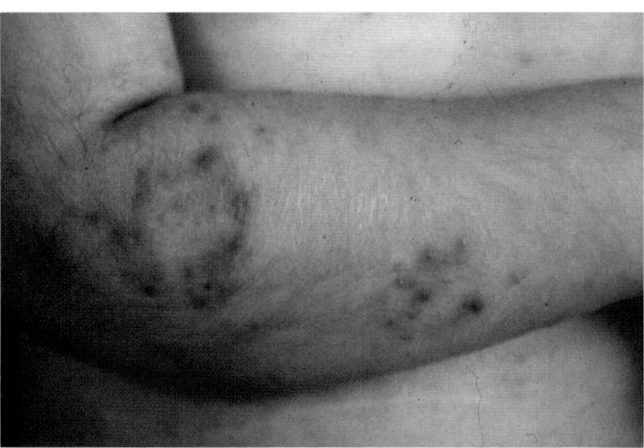

Figure 17.10 Tinea corporis (ringworm) is common in children, but may be more severe in immunosuppressed children after liver transplantation. The annular lesion with an inflammatory edge and central clearing should be noted.

Tinea capitis. Dermatophyte infection of the scalp and hair produces varying degrees of scaling, patchy hair loss, and areas of suppuration (kerion) (Figure 17.11). The few hairs in the affected areas are usually broken just above the surface of the scalp, and in some cases the fungi can be detected by their yellow-green fluorescent appearance under the Wood light (long-wave ultraviolet light). This infection always requires systemic treatment for at least 6 weeks.

Tinea unguium. Onychomycosis due to dermatophyte infection more often affects toenails than fingernails, and is frequently associated with tinea pedis. It usually starts as yellow-white, irregular distal nail dystrophy, which spreads slowly proximally, eventually producing a thickened, friable, opaque, yellow nail (Figure 17.12). If treatment is required, it must be systemic.

Tinea cruris. Uncommon in children and usually occurring in young adult males, tinea cruris is a symmetrical, red, itchy

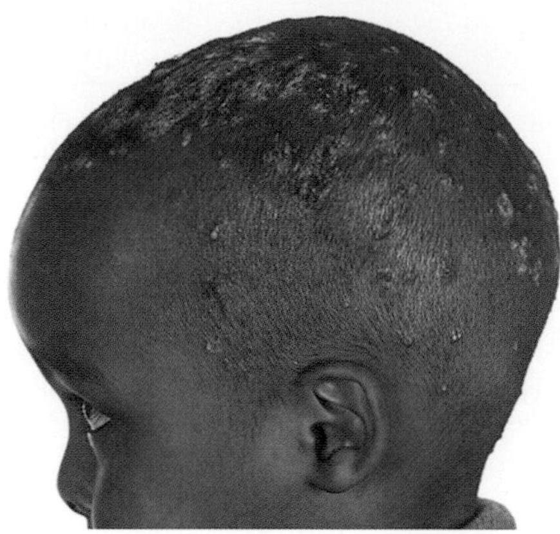

Figure 17.11 Tinea capitis is a dermatophytic infection of the head, with scaling, patchy hair loss, and areas of suppuration (kerion). It requires systemic therapy.

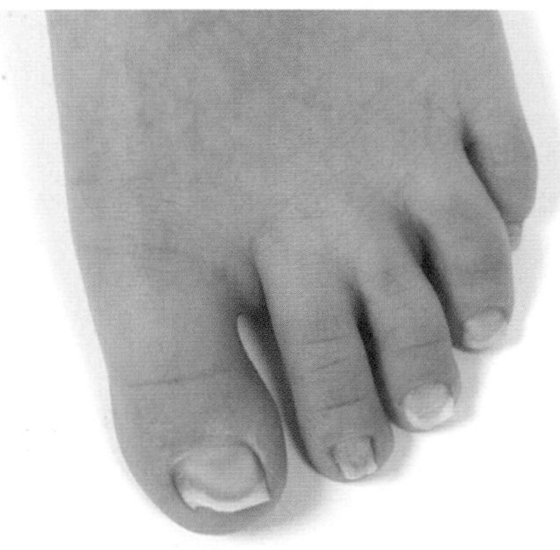

Figure 17.12 Tinea unguium is frequently associated with tinea pedis. The lateral and distal discoloration of the large toenail and a thickened, dystrophic second toenail should be noted.

eruption with a scaly edge and central clearing, which spreads from the groin and pubic region to the inner thighs.

Superficial yeast infections

Pityriasis (tinea) versicolor. This common condition is characterized by light-brown scaly patches on the trunk, neck, shoulders, and upper arms. In immunosuppressed patients, the rash may extend to the scalp, face, abdomen, groin, and legs. The causative organism, *Malassezia furfur*, is a normal skin commensal. The diagnosis is clinical and includes demonstration of a greenish, golden-yellow, or pink fluorescence under the Wood light. Treatment with topical agents such as selenium sulfide, miconazole, clotrimazole, or econazole is usually effective, although the infection may relapse in places where the topical agents have not been applied properly.

Candidiasis. Candida albicans is a normal commensal of the human digestive tract and can be isolated from the mouth and intestinal tract in 30–50% of the normal population and from the genital tract in up to 20% of normal women. Infection of skin and mucous membranes (candidiasis) is usually derived from the patient's own reservoir. Topical and systemic steroid treatment, immunosuppression, and long-term use of broad-spectrum antibiotics predispose to candidiasis.

Adequate treatment of superficial candidiasis is usually achieved with topical antifungal preparations such as nystatin, clotrimazole, amphotericin, or miconazole. In more widespread infections, systemic antidermatophytes such as ketoconazole, miconazole and fluconazole (Table 17.1) are indicated. Griseofulvin is ineffective against *Candida* spp. Liposomal amphotericin is the drug of choice for severe or intractable candidiasis. Flucytosine, a synthetic antifungal drug, is only active against yeasts, but has been demonstrated to have a synergistic effect with amphotericin.

Oral candidiasis. This is characterized by white, curd-like plaques inside the mouth, which can be scraped off, leaving inflamed and friable mucosa. In severe cases, the disease may spread to the oropharynx and esophagus. Localized lesions should clear within 2 weeks of the start of topical treatment with nystatin oral suspension, amphotericin, or miconazole gel (Daktarin). In extensive infections, systemic treatment is indicated.

Chronic paronychia. This is a chronic inflammatory process affecting the proximal nail fold and nail matrix, caused by bacteria or *C. albicans*. Simple measures such as keeping the fingers dry and avoiding finger-sucking and nail-biting will help. Treatment should be with topical or, if this is unsuccessful, with oral preparations.

Cutaneous candidiasis. Cutaneous candidiasis occurs in moist areas, such as body flexures (intertrigo) and skin that has been occluded with bandages or adhesive tape. Lesions start as vesicles or pustules, which may coalesce and erupt, leaving an erythematous area surrounded by an irregular, scaling margin. The clinical diagnosis of candidiasis is confirmed by microscopic demonstration of *C. albicans* in scrapings of the lesions or by culture from swabs. Topical treatment is usually adequate, but systemic therapy is indicated for widespread infection.

Pityrosporum folliculitis. In this acneiform condition, which is seen frequently in immunosuppressed children, small follicular papules and pustules are present on the trunk, in the absence of other features of acne. It responds well to treatment with antifungal agents such as miconazole.

Other opportunistic fungal infections

Cutaneous aspergillosis. Aspergillosis is a common fungal infection in immunocompromised hosts. The primary cutaneous form of aspergillosis, however, is uncommon and in most cases develops at entry sites of intravenous catheters or where splints were strapped to the skin. The lesions are erythematous or violaceous, edematous, indurated plaques that evolve into necrotic ulcers covered with a black eschar. They may be painful and pruritic, in contrast to ecthyma gangrenosum, which looks identical and evolves in quite a similar way. The diagnosis is confirmed by demonstrating dermal hyphae in a skin biopsy. Cultures of biopsied lesions may yield *Aspergillus flavus*, *A. fumigatus*, *A. niger* or, less commonly, *A. terreus*. Blood cultures are rarely positive.

Secondary cutaneous aspergillosis may follow hematogenous spread of invasive aspergillosis in immunocompromised hosts, and presents as cutaneous maculopapular lesions, which eventually become pustular and evolve into ulcers covered with a black eschar. Diagnosis is again made by microscopy and culture of a skin biopsy, and blood cultures are more likely to be positive.

Serological tests for the presence of *Aspergillus* antibodies (precipitin test to detect precipitating antibodies) or *Aspergillus* antigens (latex particle agglutination test for *Aspergillus* galactomannan, a cell wall glycoprotein) in immunocompromised hosts are not very helpful in establishing the diagnosis and are frequently false-negative, due to a delayed or absent immune response.

Treatment includes removal of any foreign body such as intravenous lines and catheters, local wound care, and intravenous antifungal treatment with liposomal amphotericin B (Table 17.1).

Cutaneous cryptococcosis. This uncommon condition in immunocompromised patients may present as primary cutaneous cryptococcosis or the more common secondary cutaneous disease, which occurs in 10–15% of patients with disseminated disease.

There may be single or multiple nodules, vesicles, ulcers or abscesses, predominantly located on the head, trunk or limbs, or small maculopapular lesions resembling molluscum contagiosum. The diagnosis is confirmed by demonstrating the organism, *Cryptococcus neoformans*, in aspirates from blister fluid and in cultured fluid, ulcer drainage, or skin biopsy specimens. In most patients with disseminated disease, latex agglutination tests for the presence of cryptococcal antigen in body fluids will be positive, although serology is usually negative. All patients with cutaneous cryptococcosis should be investigated for disseminated infection. Treatment with systemic antifungal preparations such as amphotericin B, with or without flucytosine, should be commenced as soon as possible.

Cutaneous histoplasmosis. This very rare infection with *Histoplasma capsulatum* is usually self-limiting in the general population, but in immunocompromised hosts it frequently progresses to disseminated disease. Cutaneous involvement is rare and presents as papules, plaques, and ulcers, which may progress to purpuric lesions and abscesses. Occasionally, aggressive erysipelas or cellulitis-like eruptions develop. The diagnosis is confirmed by demonstrating the organism in skin biopsies, as culture growth is too slow to establish an early diagnosis. Serological precipitin and agglutination assays are unreliable and often negative in immunocompromised patients. Treatment should consist of amphotericin B, often given in combination with flucytosine for its additive and synergistic effect.

Unusual fungal skin infections

Cutaneous trichosporonosis. In its mild form, infection with *Trichosporon beigelii* causes a superficial hair infection, which presents as firmly attached, irregular, soft, light-brown nodules along the midshafts of the hairs (white piedra). It particularly affects young adults and is found worldwide, although it is most common in tropical and subtropical regions. The diagnosis is confirmed by microscopic detection of the hyphae on the hairs, as well as culturing of the organism. The simplest treatment option is to shave or clip the hair in the affected area, followed by topical application of clotrimazole or miconazole cream.

Secondary cutaneous trichosporonosis usually presents as multiple, erythematous, maculopapular lesions, which may develop into necrotic ulcers. Histopathological examination of skin biopsies reveals the organism, and the diagnosis can be confirmed by positive blood cultures. Serological tests are often false-negative. Intravenous amphotericin B is an effective treatment, provided the patient is not neutropenic.

Others. Cutaneous infections in the immunocompromised host may also be caused by an array of unusual fungi which, in the past, were often considered as contaminants and whose classification creates great confusion. Examples are certain yeasts, such as *Geotrichum candidum*, *Rhodotorula*, *Saccharomyces* and *Torulopsis* species, dermatophytic fungi such as *Alternaria*, *Curvularia*, and *Drechslera*, and hyaline molds such as *Fusarium*, *Penicillium*, and *Paecilomyces*. Skin lesions vary enormously, but many begin as a pigmented papule or vesicle, which subsequently progresses to necrosis. A positive culture is essential for the correct diagnosis, as on histological examination of skin biopsies it is often impossible to differentiate between the various types of fungal organisms. Amphotericin B is the drug of choice, with imidazoles for amphotericin-resistant cases.[38]

Bacterial skin lesions

Gram-negative infections. Gram-negative bacilli such as *Escherichia coli*, *Klebsiella pneumoniae*, and *Pseudomonas aeruginosa* are responsible for most serious skin infections in immunocompromised patients. Skin manifestations include cellulitis, subepidermal bullae, subcutaneous abscesses, and rarely toxic epidermal necrolysis (TEN).

Ecthyma gangrenosum, usually due to *P. aeruginosa*, is commonest in severely neutropenic patients. It begins as a painless, round, erythematous macule, which may have a small vesicle on its surface. Later it becomes indurated and bullous or pustular, and subsequently the skin sloughs and forms a gangrenous ulcer with a gray-black eschar surrounded by an erythematous halo. It is commonest in intertriginous regions, but may also appear on the extremities, face, or trunk. It may be associated with a high temperature, tachycardia, tachypnea, and hypotension. The diagnosis is confirmed by positive cultures from a skin biopsy specimen or blood cultures. Treatment is aggressive with high doses of intravenous carboxypenicillins, such as carbenicillin or ticarcillin, in combination with an aminoglycoside (Table 17.1). Persistent neutropenia during treatment and multiple skin lesions are poor prognostic features.[39]

Gram-positive infections. Skin infections by Gram-positive bacteria do not differ in character from those in immunocompetent patients, but may be more severe and are more often associated with systemic involvement.

Streptococcal infections. Streptococcal infection of the skin and subcutaneous tissue presents as cellulitis, an erythematous, hot, swollen area, often on the leg. There may be blisters and even skin necrosis with malaise, high fever and rigors. Treatment consists of intravenous penicillin, although in some cases surgical debridement of severely necrotic areas may be necessary.

Staphylococcal infections. These can take various forms, as outlined below.

- Folliculitis. This is an infection of the superficial part of a hair follicle with *Staphylococcus aureus*, leading to a small pustule on an erythematous base, centered on the follicle. In mild forms, treatment consists of topical preparations (e.g., benzoyl peroxide, alone or in combination with topical antibiotics similar to those used in the treatment of acne). In severe cases, systemic antibiotics such as flucloxacillin or erythromycin may be required (Table 17.1).
- Furunculosis ("boils"). This is characterized by painful, inflammatory nodules due to deep infection of hair follicles by *S. aureus* (Figure 17.13). Over a period of time, the lesion becomes fluctuant and once the central necrotic core has been discharged, the boil resolves. In immunosuppressed patients, treatment is with intravenous flucloxacillin.
- Impetigo. This is a superficial skin infection caused by *S. aureus*, alone or in combination with hemolytic streptococci. There is an initial small blister or pustule, which rapidly increases in size, ruptures and leaves a raw, exuding surface, which then dries and forms the typical golden-yellow crust. Impetigo may appear anywhere on the body, even in immunocompetent patients, and in immunosuppressed patients should be treated with systemic flucloxacillin or erythromycin.

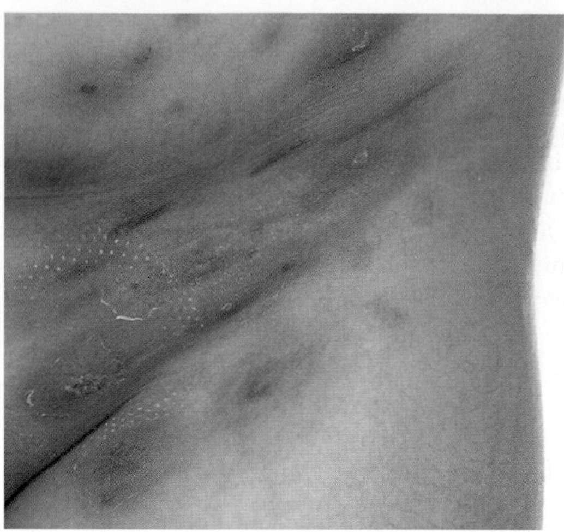

Figure 17.13 Staphylococcal infection leads to furunculosis (boils). Systemic treatment is required in immunosuppressed patients, as the condition can lead to disfiguring scars.

- Staphylococcal scalded skin syndrome (SSSS). This is generally thought of as a disease of healthy infants and children, but when seen in adults it predominantly occurs in immunosuppressed individuals. It is caused by the production of a toxin by some staphylococcal phage types, which splits the dermis, causing the superficial epidermis to peel off and leaving a skin resembling severe scalding. In immunocompromised patients, it is often associated with severe sepsis, with positive blood cultures for *S. aureus*, and treatment should include a course of intravenous antibiotics (flucloxacillin).

Corynebacterial infections. Coryneforms, or diphtheroids, are normal skin commensals which cause minor problems in healthy individuals (e.g., erythrasma). Cutaneous infections in immunocompromised patients occur in severely neutropenic patients previously treated with broad-spectrum antibiotics. They mainly present as cellulitis or subcutaneous abscess at the site of a puncture wound or intravenous catheter. A few cases have been reported in which corynebacteria infection presented as an erythematous maculopapular rash, initially on the trunk, followed by diffuse spread and a more pustular appearance. Clinical diagnosis requires confirmation from blood and skin biopsy cultures. Treatment is difficult, as the organism is resistant to most antibiotics except vancomycin.

Mycobacterial infections. Both *Mycobacterium tuberculosis* and atypical mycobacteria may cause cutaneous disease. Primary skin infections, usually caused by the atypical mycobacteria *M. marinum, M. chelonae, M. kansasii,* and *M. haemophilium,* occur in normal and immunosuppressed hosts. The commonest presentation is a pigmented, granulomatous nodule with an erythematous halo on an extremity, although a wide variety of lesions, such as cellulitis or panniculitis, may occur.

Systemic symptoms are not usually present, although in immunocompromised hosts the infection may disseminate to multiple cutaneous sites or ulcerate, leading to superinfection.

Skin manifestations of disseminated *M. tuberculosis* infection in immunocompromised hosts include recurrent episodes of skin and soft-tissue abscesses of the extremities with symptom-free intervals in between and often minimal systemic symptoms. The diagnosis is confirmed by histological identification of acid-fast bacilli and positive cultures. Treatment should be with appropriate antituberculous chemotherapy.

Nocardial infections. Nocardia spp. infection, especially with *N. asteroides*, is strongly associated with immunosuppression and may be focal or disseminated. Skin manifestations include pustules, cellulitis, or ulcers, and are usually secondary to disease in the lungs. The diagnosis is often difficult, as *Nocardia* is not easily detected in cultures or histological sections. Treatment consists of adequate surgical drainage, if required, in combination with co-trimoxazole.

Cutaneous malignancies

Susceptibility to skin cancer after transplantation is multifactorial. Predisposing risk factors include older age at the time of transplant, lighter skin type, solar keratosis, greater sunlight exposure, higher rejection rate in the first year after transplant, and level of immunosuppression.[40,41] More recent research, mainly in renal transplant recipients, has indicated that genetic variation in the enzymes involved in free radical metabolism in the skin might also be associated with the development of skin cancer.[42]

Cutaneous lymphomas occur with increased incidence in transplant recipients.[43] They are predominantly of B-cell origin and in many cases are associated with Epstein–Barr virus infection.[44] Cutaneous T-cell lymphomas have been rarely described in this group, and their etiology is ill-understood. Reduced immune surveillance, chronic antigenic stimulation caused by transplant grafts, and the direct oncogenic effect of immunosuppressive drugs have all been suggested as mechanisms.[45] It is likely that immunosuppressive treatment (cyclosporine, tacrolimus) causes an imbalance in the T-cell regulatory systems, resulting in an expanded T-cell subpopulation. In both conditions, the early skin changes are nonspecific (Figure 17.14), but the later stages are characterized by exfoliative generalized erythroderma and lymphadenopathy. The definitive diagnosis is made by skin biopsy.

Nonmelanoma skin cancer (NMSC) is increasingly recognized as a complication of long-term immunosuppression in solid-organ transplant recipients.[46] Studies in adult renal transplant recipients have shown an annual incidence rate of 6.5%, increasing to 10.5% at more than 10 years after transplantation.[47] Major contributing factors are exposure to ultraviolet radiation (i.e., high levels of sun exposure), drug-induced immunosuppression, and HPV infection. The occurrence of skin cancer in transplanted children is an extremely rare event during childhood, and in a study of pediatric transplant recipients in the United Kingdom, a number of pigmented lesions were identified, but no skin cancer was found (Figure 17.15).[48,49] Although still rare in childhood, these lesions occur at a younger age and lead to a higher morbidity and mortality than in immunocompetent individuals.

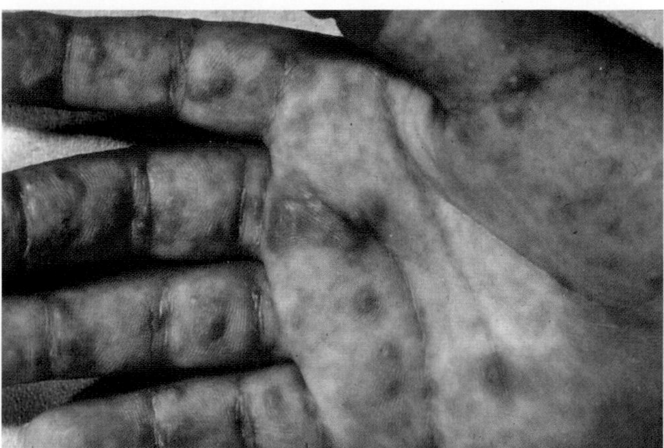

Figure 17.14 This papular skin rash was secondary to T-cell infiltration of the skin, which resolved on reduction of immunosuppression.

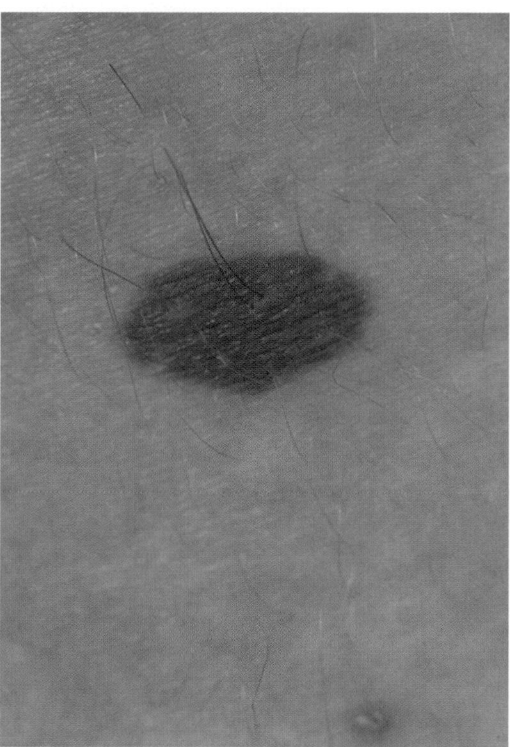

Figure 17.15 This pigmented lesion is a congenital nevus, which is benign. Transplant recipients are more likely to develop skin cancer and melanoma because of long-term immunosuppression, and thus pigmented lesions need to be scrutinized.

Dysplastic skin lesions in adult transplant recipients include actinic or solar keratosis, Bowen disease, squamous cell carcinoma and, less commonly, basal cell carcinoma and malignant melanoma, all of which are uncommon in children. Warts, following infection with HPV, are common in both groups and rarely become malignant (warty dysplasia), particularly on sun-exposed skin areas.[50,51]

Early detection and treatment of skin malignancies is necessary to avoid metastatic spread. Management strategies should focus on regular full-skin check and nodular examination, aggressive treatment of established malignancies (including reduction in immunosuppression), and prophylactic measures to reduce the risk of additional photodamage and malignant transformation.[52]

Preventative measures include minimizing immunosuppression and avoiding excessive sun exposure, and this advice should be routinely provided to parents and children undergoing transplantation. Children should be advised to use adequate sun block and wear protective clothing.

As it may be difficult to differentiate between benign and dysplastic lesions, any skin lesion that suddenly appears, changes color or size, becomes itchy or painful, or starts bleeding, oozing or crusting, should be seen by a dermatologist and a skin biopsy performed to confirm the diagnosis and commence appropriate treatment.

Graft-versus-host disease

Acute graft-versus-host disease (GVHD) remains a major cause of morbidity and mortality following bone-marrow transplantation, affecting the liver, skin, and gut (Chapter 16). It is very rare following liver transplantation.[53]

Cutaneous acute GVHD presents between 7 days and 7 weeks after transplantation, with a maculopapular rash, which may look like measles, accompanied by palmar and plantar erythema and sometimes edema (Figure 17.16). The rash may be pruritic or feel like sunburn. The lesions coalesce and spread to the trunk, face, and extremities. Sometimes the rash becomes bullous and progresses to toxic epidermal necrolysis.

The diagnosis can be confirmed by skin biopsy, which shows dermoepidermal clefts, necrosis of keratinocytes surrounded by lymphocytes ("satellite cell necrosis"), vacuolization of basal epidermal cells, and edema.

Cutaneous lesions in chronic GVHD are itchy, flat-topped, red-purple shiny papules resembling lichen planus. Later, the skin may thicken and look like scleroderma, with hyperpigmentation and hypopigmentation.

Nonspecific skin rashes

Rashes in immunosuppressed patients vary enormously in their presentation and represent a wide variety of underlying diagnoses.[54] Histopathological interpretation is difficult without an informed dermatological differential diagnosis. In some cases, the diagnosis may become more obvious at a later stage, and careful documentation, including medical illustration and review by a dermatologist, are therefore essential.

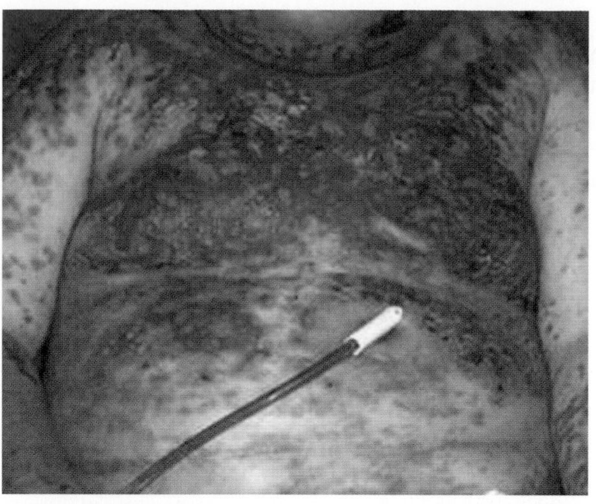

A

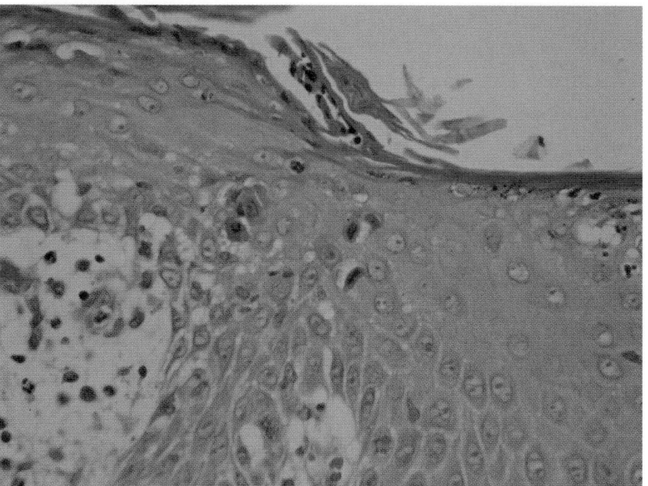

B

Figure 17.16 Cutaneous graft-versus-host disease (GVHD) presents with a maculopapular rash, which may be pruritic. **A** The lesions coalesce and spread to the trunk, face, and extremities. **B** A skin biopsy, which showed inflammatory changes and apoptotic keratinocytes centrally on hematoxylin–eosin stains, typical of severe GVHD. (Original magnification: 400×).

Liver disease induced by treatment of dermatological conditions

A number of frequently used treatments for common skin conditions may potentially induce liver dysfunction.

Chinese herbal medicine for atopic eczema

Chinese herbal mixtures have been used to treat atopic eczema for many years. Their efficacy has attracted public attention, and clinical trials in children and adults have shown marked benefit, although other reporters have not been able to replicate these results.[55–57] Hepatotoxicity, ranging from mild to acute liver failure, has been a problem with some Chinese herbal remedies, although the results are heterogeneous.[58]

Methotrexate treatment of psoriasis

Methotrexate is a first-line systemic therapy for psoriasis, as it is highly efficacious for severe disease. However, chronic administration of methotrexate is associated with a risk of hepatic damage and hepatic fibrosis. Liver function tests (LFTs) are indicated before and during methotrexate therapy. If there are persistent elevations (two to three times normal) in LFTs, methotrexate should be discontinued until they normalize; if elevations persist for more than 2 months, a liver biopsy is indicated.[59] A new method, measurement of serum aminoterminal propeptide of type III procollagen (PIIINP), might reduce the need for routine liver biopsy, as it is a marker of fibrosis.[60]

Approach to diagnosis of dermatological lesions

A practical approach to the diagnosis of skin disorders in immunosuppressed children after transplantation is outlined in Figure 17.17. A dermatological history is essential, including the patient's own history and family history, as well as a detailed review of systemic and topical therapy. As previous treatment can be just as important in determining the cause of a rash. This, in combination with a careful documentation of the site and/or distribution of lesions and a description of the characteristics of individual lesions, may in many cases offer sufficient information for a correct diagnosis to be made.

Further investigations and/or referral to a dermatologist are indicated if the patient is systemically unwell, if the diagnosis is not clear, or if there is suspicion of skin malignancy.[61]

Techniques

Skin scrapings for mycology

The scaly edge of the lesion should be carefully scraped with a scalpel blade onto black paper and sent to the microbiology laboratory for microscopic examination and mycological culture.

Nail clippings

Nail clippings should be taken as proximally as possible, to optimize the chances of identifying fungus on microscopy or culture.

Scalp lesions

Scalp lesions should be examined under ultraviolet light (Wood light) to detect fluorescence, although some ringworm species do not fluoresce. Plucked hairs from the edge of a lesion can be sent for microscopic examination and culture.

Skin cultures

Pus or vesicle fluid can be swabbed directly. Samples for bacteriological examination should be sent either dry or in a transport medium, while virological samples should be sent in a special viral transport medium. In the case of blisters, the base should be scraped for electron-microscopic examination.

Skin biopsies

A punch or incisional biopsy should be performed, preferably under local anesthesia. A fresh lesion should be selected for biopsy, as older lesions may show secondary changes, which make histological interpretation more difficult.[62]

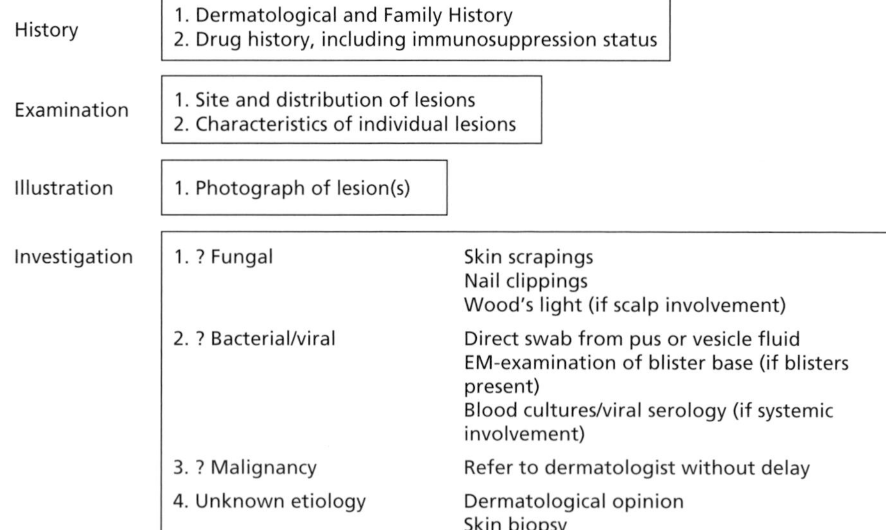

Figure 17.17 A practical approach to the diagnosis of skin lesions.

It should be established beforehand from the laboratory what transport medium is required. Formaldehyde is routine for light microscopy, but is unsuitable for fat-containing lesions—for example, xanthomas. Glutaraldehyde is usual for electron microscopy. If there is any doubt, and for skin to be cultured for microorganisms, the specimen should be placed on a saline-soaked gauze swab and conveyed directly to the laboratory.

Case study

Patient RW was diagnosed with gastroschisis and, following initial repair, developed associated gastrointestinal dysmotility, requiring long-term parenteral nutrition. Because of a lack of venous access due to multiple venous thromboses, he successfully underwent isolated small-bowel transplantation. Four months after transplantation, he developed a generalized erythematous, maculopapular rash, sparing his face and confluent on his palms and soles, with no vesicles or mucosal involvement (Figure 17.16A). A clinical suspicion of graft-versus-host disease (GVHD) was confirmed on skin biopsy, which showed inflammatory changes and apoptotic keratinocytes centrally on hematoxylin–eosin stains, typical of severe GVHD (Figure 17.16B). Immunosuppression was stepped up by giving high doses of intravenous corticosteroid treatment, which was slowly tapered over the next few weeks and subsequently changed to oral prednisolone when the rash gradually improved.

Comment. GVHD is unusual following isolated liver transplantation, but more common after isolated bowel or combined liver and bowel transplantation. It may present simply with skin manifestations or with diarrhea. It usually responds to an increase in immunosuppression, unless there is preexisting immunodeficiency (see also Chapter 22).

References

1 Morelli JG, Weston WL. Skin. In: Hathaway WE, Hay WW, Groothuis JR, Paisley JW, eds. *Current Paediatric Diagnosis and Treatment.* London: Prentice Hall International, 1993: 372–91.

2 Graham-Brown R, Burns T, eds. *Lecture Notes on Dermatology.* Oxford: Blackwell Scientific, 1990.

3 Scheepers JH, Quaba AA. Treatment of nevi aranei with the pulsed tunable dye laser at 585 nm. *J Pediatr Surg* 1995;**30**:101–4.

4 Gregorio GV, Ball CS, Mowat AP, Mieli-Vergani G. Effect of rifampicin in the treatment of pruritus in hepatic cholestasis. *Arch Dis Child* 1993;**69**:141–3.

5 Jones EA, Bergasa NV. Why do cholestatic patients itch? *Gut* 1996;**38**:644–5.

6 Connolly CS, Kantor GR, Menduke H. Hepatobiliary pruritus: what are effective treatments? *J Am Acad Dermatol* 1995;**33**:801–5.

7 Jones EA, Bergasa NV. Evolving concepts of the pathogenesis and treatment of pruritus of cholestasis. *Can J Gastroenterol* 2000;**14**: 33–40.

8 Bergasa NV, Alling DW, Talbot TL, *et al.* Relief from the intractable pruritus of chronic cholestasis associated with oral nalmefene therapy. *Hepatology* 1991;**14**:154A.

9 Bergasa NV, Alling DW, Talbot TL, *et al.* Nalmefene therapy is associated with the relief of pruritus of cholestasis: results of a double-blind randomised placebo-controlled trial. *Hepatology* 1993;**18**:177A.

10 Kjellberg F, Tramer MR. Pharmacological control of opioid-induced pruritus: a quantitative systematic review of randomized trials. *Eur J Anaesthesiol* 2001;**18**:346–57.

11 Garcia MA, Ramonet M, Ciocca M, *et al.* Alagille's syndrome: cutaneous manifestations in 38 children. *Pediatr Dermatol* 2005;**22**:11–4.

12 Poh-Fitzpatrick MB, Zaider E, Sciales C, *et al.* Cutaneous photosensitivity and coproporphyrin abnormalities in the Alagille's syndrome. *Gastroenterology* 1990;**99**:831–5.

13 Attard-Moltano S, Evans N, Sherwood RA. Carotinaemia with low vitamin A levels and retinol-binding protein. *J Inherit Metab Dis* 1992;**15**:929–30.

14 Lodi G, Giuliana M, Majorana A, *et al.* Lichen planus and hepatitis C virus: a multicentre study of patients with oral lesions and a systematic review. *Br J Dermatol* 2004;**151**:1172–81.

15 Laeijendecker R, Van Joost TH, Tank B, Neumann HA. Oral lichen planus and hepatitis C virus infection. *Arch Dermatol* 2005;**141**:906–7.

16 Weston WL, Morelli JG, Lee LA. The clinical spectrum of anti-Ro positive cutaneous neonatal lupus erythematosus. *J Am Acad Dermatol* 1999;**40**:675–81.

17 Lee LA, Sokol RJ, Buyon JP. Hepatobiliary disease in neonatal lupus: prevalence and clinical characteristics in cases enrolled in a national registry. *Paediatrics* 2002;**109**: E11.

18 Watson R, Kang JE, May M, *et al.* Thrombocytopenia in the neonatal lupus syndrome. *Arch Dermatol* 1988;**124**:560–3.

19 Beath SV, Booth IW, Kelly DA. Nutritional support in liver disease. *Arch Dis Child* 1993;**69**:545–9.

20 Fritsch P, Schuler G, Hintner H, eds. *Current Problems in Dermatology: Immunodeficiency and Skin.* Basle: Karger, 1989.

21 Euvrard S, Kanitakis J, Cochat P, Cambazard F, Claudy A. Skin diseases in children with organ transplants. *J Am Acad Dermatol* 2001;**44**:932–9.

22 Tosi A, Misciali C, Piraccini BM, Peluso AM, Bardazzi F. Drug-induced hair loss and hair growth: incidence, management and avoidance. *Drug Saf* 1994;**10**:310–7.

23 Yamamoto S, Kato R. Hair growth-stimulating effects of cyclosporin A and FK506, potent immunosuppressants. *J Dermatol Sci* 1994;**7**(Suppl):S47–54.

24 Morley S, Gault D. Hair removal using the long-pulsed ruby laser in children. *J Clin Laser Med Surg* 2000;**18**:277–80.

25 Bencini PL, Montagnino G, Sala F, De Vecchi A, Crosti C, Tarantino A. Cutaneous lesions in 67 cyclosporin-treated renal transplant recipients. *Dermatologica* 1986;**172**:24–30.

26 Chugh KS, Sharma SC, Singh V, Sakhuja V, Jha V, Gupta KL. Spectrum of dermatological lesions in renal allograft recipients in a tropical environment. *Dermatology* 1994;**188**:108–12.

27 Van Mourik IDM, Nagle A, Kelly DA. Conversion from Sandimmune to Neoral in stable paediatric liver transplant recipients. *Hepatology* 1997;**26**:432.

28 Assmann T, Homey B, Ruzaicka T. Topical tacrolimus for the treatment of inflammatory skin diseases. *Expert Opin Pharmacother* 2001;**2**:1167–75.

29 Reitamo S, Wollenberg A, Schopf E, *et al.* Safety and efficacy of 1 year of tacrolimus ointment monotherapy in adults with atopic dermatitis. The European Tacrolimus Ointment Group. *Arch Dermatol* 2000;**136**:999–1006.

30 Schachner LA, Lamerson C, Sheehan MP, *et al.* Tacrolimus ointment 0.03% is safe and effective for the treatment of mild to moderate atopic dermatitis in pediatric patients: results from a randomized, double-blind, vehicle-controlled study. *Pediatrics* 2005;**116**:e334–42.

31 Munro CS. Acne. *J R Coll Physicians Lond* 1997;**31**:360–3.

32 Prudy S, de Berker D. Acne. *BMJ* 2006;**333**:949–53.

33 Harwood CA, Perrett CM, Brown VL, *et al.* Imiquimod cream 5% for recalcitrant cutaneous warts in immunosuppressed individuals. *Br J Dermatol* 2005;**152**:122–9.

34 Denning DW. *Pocket Reference to Opportunistic Fungal Infections.* London: Science Press, 1994.

35 Philpot C. Mycological examination of skin. In: Marks R, Dykes P, Motley R, eds. *Clinical Signs and Procedures in Dermatology.* London: Dunitz, 1993: 158–72.

36 Richardson MD, Warnock DW, eds. *Fungal Infection: Diagnosis and Management.* Oxford: Blackwell Scientific, 1993.

37 Gulec AT, Demirbilek M, Seckin D, *et al.* Superficial fungal infections in 102 renal transplant recipients: a case–control study. *J Am Acad Dermatol* 2003;**49**:187–92.

38 Vartivarian SE, Anaissie EJ, Bodey GP. Emerging fungal pathogens in immunocompromised patients: classification, diagnosis and management. *Clin Infect Dis* 1993;**17**(Suppl 2):S487–491.

39 Kuhls TL, Leach CT. Infections in pediatric liver transplant recipients. In: Patrick CC, ed. *Infections in Immunocompromised Infants and Children.* New York: Churchill Livingstone, 1992: 231–50.

40 Haagsma EB, Hagens VE, Schaapveld M, *et al.* Increased cancer risk after liver transplantation: a population based study. *J Hepatol* 2001;**34**:84–91.

41 Mithoefer AB, Supran S, Freeman RB. Risk factors associated with the development of skin cancer after liver transplantation. *Liver Transplantation* 2002;**8**:939–44.

42 Marshall SE, Bordea C, Haldar NA, *et al.* Glutathione *S*-transferase polymorphisms and skin cancer after renal transplantation. *Kidney Int* 2000;**58**:2186–93.

43 Pascual J, Torrelo A, Teruel JL, Bellas C, Marcen R, Ortuno J. Cutaneous T cell lymphomas after renal transplantation. *Transplantation* 1992;**53**:1143–5.

44 McGregor JM, Yu CC, Lu QL, Cotter FE, Levison DA, MacDonald DM. Posttransplant cutaneous lymphoma. *J Am Acad Dermatol* 1993;**29**:549–54.

45 Ward HA, Russo GG, McBurney E, Millikan LE, Boh EE. Posttransplant primary cutaneous T-cell lymphoma. *J Am Acad Dermatol* 2001;**44**:675–80.

46 Penn I, Brunson ME. Cancers after cyclosporine therapy. *Transplant Proc* 1988;**20**(3 Suppl 3):885–92.

47 Ramsay HM, Fryer AA, Reece S, Smith AG, Harden PN. Clinical risk factors associated with nonmelanoma skin cancer in renal transplant recipients. *Am J Kidney Disease* 2000;**36**:168–76.

48 Euvrard S, Kanitakis J, Cochat P, Claudy A. Skin cancers following pediatric organ transplantation. *Dermatol Surg* 2004;**30**: 616–21.

49 Thomson MA, Suggett NR, Nightingale PG, *et al.* Skin surveillance of a UK paediatric transplant population. *Br J Dermatol* 2007; **156**:45–50.

50 Blohme I, Larko O. Skin lesions in renal transplant patients after 10 years of immunosuppressive therapy. *Acta Derm Venereol* 1990;**70**:491–4.

51 Blohme I, Larko O. Premalignant and malignant skin lesions in renal transplant patients. *Transplantation* 1994;**37**:165–7.

52 Otley CC, Pittelkow MR. Skin cancer in liver transplant recipients. *Liver Transpl* 2000;**6**:253–62.

53 Vogelsang GB, Hess AD, Santos GW. Acute graft-versus-host disease: clinical characteristics in the cyclosporin era. *Medicine* 1988;**67**:163–74.

54 Chren MM, Lazarus HM, Bickers DR, Landefeld S. Rashes in immunocompromised cancer patients. *Arch Dermatol* 1993;**129**: 175–81.

55 Sheehan MP, Atherton DJ. One-year follow up of children treated with Chinese medicinal herbs for atopic eczema. *Br J Dermatol* 1994;**130**:488–93.

56 Sheehan MP, Rustin MH, Atherton DJ, *et al.* Efficacy of traditional Chinese herbal therapy in adult atopic dermatitis. *Lancet* 1992;**340**:13–7.

57 Fung AY, Look PC, Chong LY, *et al.* A controlled trial of traditional Chinese herbal medicine in Chinese patients with recalcitrant atopic dermatitis. *Int J Dermatol* 1999;**38**:387–92.

58 Zhang W, Leonard T, Bath-Hextall F, *et al.* Chinese herbal medicine for atopic eczema. *Cochrane Database Syst Rev* 2005;(**2**): CD002291.

59 British Association of Dermatologists. Psoriasis Guideline 2006 (available at: http://www.bad.org.uk/healthcare/guidelines/psoriasis_guideline_(Final_update)_280906.pdf).

60 Chalmers RJ, Kirby B, Smith A, *et al.* Replacement of routine liver biopsy by procollagen III aminopeptide for monitoring patients with psoriasis receiving long-term methotrexate: a multicentre audit and health economic analysis. *Br J Dermatol* 2005;**152**: 444–50.

61 Allen U, Smith CR, Prober CG. The value of skin biopsies in febrile, neutropenic, immunocompromised children. *Am J Dis Child* 1986;**140**:459–61.

62 Parham DM, Wilson's RT, Callihan TR. Skin biopsies. In: Patrick CC, ed. *Infections in Immunocompromised Infants and Children.* New York: Churchill Livingstone, 1992: 787–804.

18 Dental Care of Children with Liver Disease

Marie-Therese Hosey and Victoria Clark

Children with liver disease and liver transplantation require specialist dental care. Even simple dental treatment requires careful management, because of the children's inadequate drug and protein metabolism and tendency toward prolonged bleeding. Children with liver disease and liver grafts are more likely to have hypoplastic defects of the enamel of their teeth, delayed eruption of the primary dentition, intrinsic green staining of both primary and permanent teeth and the oral soft tissues, and an increased susceptibility to dental caries or cyclosporine-induced gingival overgrowth.[1–6] In this chapter, a brief discourse on the relevant areas of dental development and disease will be presented and then the oral implications of liver disease and liver transplantation will be examined and guidelines suggested.

Formation and composition of enamel and dentine

Mature enamel is a crystalline material, in the form of hydroxyapatite, that is 96% by weight mineral and as such is the hardest calcified tissue in the human body. Enamel is laid down in an incremental fashion from the tip of the cusp to the cervical margin, and it is possible to see a microscopic neonatal line marking the border between the enamel matrix that is formed before birth and that formed after.[7] Hard tissue formation in the crowns of primary incisor teeth starts between the 13th and 16th weeks of intrauterine life and continues until enamel calcification is completed 3 months after birth.[8]

Dental disease

There has been little change in the proportion of children with actively decayed primary teeth over the last 10 years. The incidence of dental disease is higher in Northern Ireland and Scotland, in ethnic minority groups, and in children from low-income and single-parent families. It has been identified that children who are medically compromised may be more susceptible to poor oral health and subsequent caries development. There is therefore an opportunity for nondental health professionals to promote caries prevention in this group of patients by encouraging attendance at the dentist and maintaining good oral health. Of recent interest is the possible beneficial effect of sonic toothbrushes in children with gingival overgrowth.[9–13] The frequent administration of liquid medicines sweetened with sucrose has significantly contributed to an increased incidence of dental caries in children with chronic medical disorders. Unfortunately, there is also evidence to suggest that medically compromised children have a much higher proportion of untreated carious lesions than the average child, brush their teeth less often, and seldom use fluoride supplements.[14] In addition, children who have had invasive dental or medical procedures are more likely to be afraid of dental treatment and either avoid attending the dentist altogether or cooperate poorly.

Dental caries

Children with liver disease have been reported to have "generalized dental discomfort," "chronic marginal gingivitis and advanced carious destruction," and "absent oral hygiene."[1] Seow *et al.* reported a high prevalence of untreated dental caries (Figure 18.1) and also noted that the teeth had enlarged pulp chambers.[2] The latter finding is a morphological feature that might make pulpal exposure and subsequent loss of vitality of the carious tooth more likely. Children with liver disease therefore not only appear to have a predilection for tooth decay, but may also be more likely to lose their teeth as a result. Although the pediatric dentist is skilled in the management of anxious children, behavioral management techniques require care, patience, and time. For many children with liver disease, the time available for completion of the dental treatment is limited by the overriding urgency of transplant surgery. Dental treatment under general anesthesia is therefore often the only option, although this does little to foster a future positive attitude toward dental care. To avoid this, these children are best referred before problems arise to a specialist pediatric dentist, who can then

Diseases of the Liver and Biliary System in Children, 3rd edition. Edited by Deirdre Kelly. ISBN: 978-1-4051-6334-7.

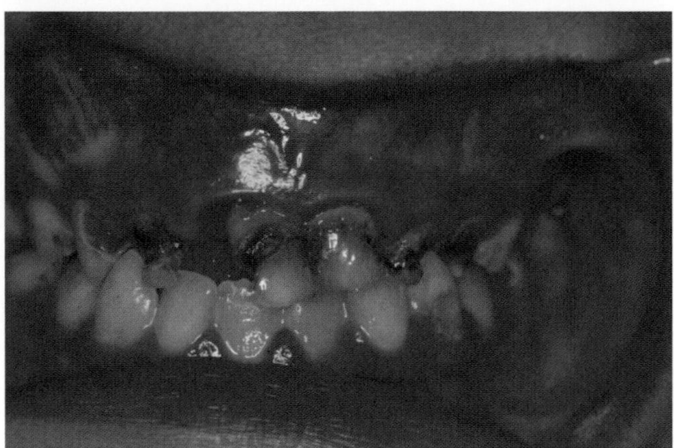

Figure 18.1 Anterior view of a 6-year-old child with rampant dental caries of the primary dentition.

institute preventative and acclimatization therapies in good time.

It has been recommended that high-speed suction should be used for children with liver disease during operative dental procedures, to guard against ingestion of blood,[15–17] and that the dose of amide local anesthetic solutions (lignocaine) used during operative dental procedures should be reduced. These children might also require antihemolytic agents to aid hemostasis following dental surgery or tooth extraction. General anesthesia is best provided by an anesthetist suitably experienced in managing children with compromised liver function, in a hospital facility. Dental treatment under general anesthetic should be combined with other medical procedures whenever possible—for example, a liver biopsy or endoscopy—to reduce the number of anesthetics received and antibiotic prophylaxis required.

Periodontal disease

Diseases of the periodontal tissues begin in childhood. Dental plaque initiates an inflammatory reaction, modulated by the immune response, microbial species, and genetic predisposition. Periodontal disease progresses from gingivitis to gradual loss of the attachment of the tooth to the surrounding connective tissues and bone, causing tooth mobility, bleeding, pocketing, and eventual abscess and tooth loss.

Prevention of dental disease

Many children with liver disease require nutritional supplementation, and such supplements often contain high proportions of nonmilk extrinsic sugars that are highly cariogenic. It is important that the parents are not confused by contradictory messages about diet; this requires a degree of pragmatism by the dental team and places a greater burden upon them to deliver stringent preventive care together with the restorative treatment that will doubtless ensue. It is helpful if the dietician and physician can, where possible, limit the frequency of the dietary supplements to mealtimes and prescribe sugar-free medications in order to reduce the incidence of dental caries.

Teeth should be brushed twice daily with a 1000-ppm fluoride toothpaste, which is then spat out rather than rinsed out with water, to reduce caries. The use of fluoride—either professionally applied or prescribed as supplements or rinses—is also recommended for these high-risk children. Chlorhexidine delivered as a gel, varnish, or rinse reduces the bacterial load, and possibly also the risk of bacteremia,[6,18] as well as preventing caries and periodontal disease. All susceptible fissures should be sealed using fissure sealants, and the use of xylitol chewing gum should be considered.[13,18]

Intrinsic dental pigmentation

Dental discoloration can arise from extrinsic sources such as chromogenic bacteria, food pigment, dye, and tobacco. Intrinsic discoloration is found in many conditions, including: fluorosis, tetracycline ingestion, lepromatous leprosy, and hemolytic diseases of the newborn and congenital erythropoietic porphyria. The earliest reports of intrinsic green-pigmented primary teeth were published over 50 years ago in children with hyperbilirubinemia caused by rhesus incompatibility.

Intrinsically pigmented green primary and permanent teeth, alveolar bone, and oral mucosa have been widely reported in children with liver disease.[1,2,4,5,19,20–24] It is thought that this pigment is deposited in the enamel organ during tooth formation as biliverdin, the oxidation product of the bilirubin molecule, in those areas of dentine and enamel that were undergoing calcification during the period when the child was jaundiced.[4] Indeed, Seow *et al.* in 1991 reported that the green pigment extended into the roots of the affected primary teeth, but stopped at the stage of root development that corresponded to the time when the child received a liver graft.[2]

However, owing to the very high mineral content of enamel and dentine, biochemical and histological examination is difficult and there are no radiographic or histological abnormalities associated with the pigmentation.[3,23] As yet, the exact nature of the pigment is unknown, but it is conceivable that it might not be equally distributed in both enamel and dentine.[3,19]

The deposition of intrinsic stain may occur during hard tissue formation postnatally or in utero,[1–4,19–22] but recent clinical evidence strongly suggests that the pigment is deposited after birth, as primary molar teeth are more deeply stained than the primary incisors since a greater proportion of the primary molar crown is formed after birth (Figure 18.2).[5,19]

A

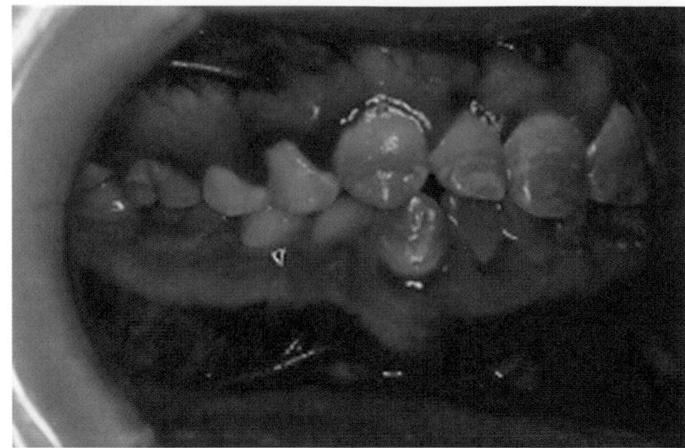

B

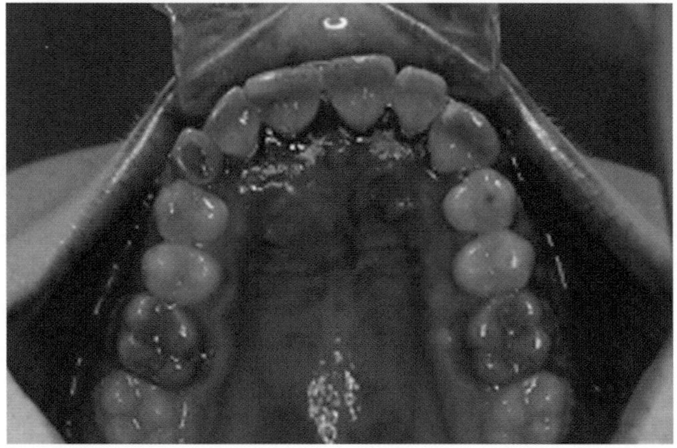

Figure 18.2 A Buccal view of the permanent dentition. **B** Maxillary view of the permanent dentition. This is the dentition of a 16-year-old girl with partial green intrinsic staining. Pigments were deposited during the formation of the incisors and first permanent molars at the time of birth. Subsequently developing premolar teeth are unaffected after transplantation.

Treatment of discolored teeth

There is a variety of treatment choices for improving the aesthetics of discolored permanent anterior teeth. In many cases, there is a hierarchy of treatment options and these should be pursued in a logical, stepwise order. Vital bleaching is one of the simplest techniques, involving the external application of either hydrogen peroxide or carbamide peroxide gel. The application can either be applied by a dentist in the dental setting or by the use of custom-fitted trays by the patient at home. The results have been shown to be variable, and are both untried in green stained teeth and unlikely to improve the appearance when dentine is stained.[25] More advanced techniques involve the use of adhesive dental materials. These materials are now widely used to restore the aesthetics of a child's discolored permanent incisor teeth. Composite restorations (white fillings) and porcelain veneers can easily be applied to the labial surface of the incisor teeth to camouflage unsightly intrinsic discoloration. There are many color-modifying adhesive materials which, used singly or in combination, can restore a child's smile throughout the formative years. These techniques are nondestructive of tooth tissue and the technique does not require local anesthesia. These veneers extend into the space between the teeth and underneath the gingival margin; it is therefore imperative that the child should have scrupulous oral hygiene, otherwise there will be increased plaque retention, leading to caries and periodontal disease. In adulthood, porcelain crowns may be the treatment of choice to mask the discoloration fully, but these cannot be provided sooner than the third decade of life, since not only is the immature dental pulp too large, risking exposure during crown preparation, but also the gingival contour shrinks back during adolescence, leaving unsightly crown margins visible if the definitive restoration is provided too early.

Enamel hypoplasia in children with liver disease

The mineralized enamel contains a history of the child's early life. Enamel does not remodel, and so disturbances during development remain in the tooth as a permanent record.[26] Enamel hypoplasia is a quantitative defect of enamel, visually and morphologically identified as involving the surface of the enamel and associated with a reduced thickness. The defective enamel may have shallow or deep pits or wide or narrow grooves, arranged horizontally in a linear fashion or generally distributed around all or part of the enamel surface. Enamel defects can be hereditary or acquired and can be associated with numerous systemic disorders. The presence of enamel defects in permanent teeth has been reported to be between 30% and 49%.[26]

Enamel hypoplasia is much less common in primary teeth than their permanent successors. It has been attributed to various factors such as fever, local infection, nutritional deficiency, prolonged hypocalcemia, and steroid therapy. Trauma to the mineralizing primary teeth caused by pressure of the laryngoscope on the alveolar ridge during intubation has also been suggested as an etiological factor.[27]

Enamel hypoplastic defects may be more prevalent in children with liver disease. Seow *et al.* found enamel hypoplasia in each of the nine children in their study and reported that these defects ranged from minor breaks in the enamel to large areas in which the enamel was missing altogether.[2] However, in a more recent study, Hosey *et al.* found hypoplastic defects in only six of their 55 pediatric liver-graft recipients, despite the fact that many of the children lived in a fluoridated area; however, this might be attributable to the high proportion of children with dentition in the sample.[5] These hypoplastic primary teeth are more susceptible to caries, necessitating stringent preventive therapy.[2,5]

Dental treatment of hypoplastic teeth

Hypoplastic first permanent molars are more susceptible to caries, and so dental management focuses on caries prevention by limiting sugar frequency and providing motivation toward good oral hygiene and the use of topical fluorides and fissure sealants. Although these teeth are sometimes extracted as part of an elective orthodontic treatment plan,[28] this is not always the treatment of choice and many have to be restored so that masticatory function and pleasing aesthetics are maintained. Unaesthetic hypoplastic permanent incisor teeth can be restored using the same adhesive techniques as previously described.

Table 18.1 Birmingham Children's Hospital prophylactic antibiotic regimen.

Oral antibiotics should be commenced prior to dental procedure and be continued for a total of 48 h, as follows:
• One dose prior to treatment and continued for 48 h of:
—Child 1 mo–1 y: Augmentin 0.25 mL/kg of 125/31 suspension t.d.s.
—Child 1–6 y: Augmentin 5 mL of 125/31 suspension t.d.s.
—Child 6–12 y: Augmentin 5 mL of 250/62 suspension t.d.s.
Child 12–18 y: Augmentin 250/125—1 tablet t.d.s.

Augmentin: proprietary preparation of amoxicillin sodium (or amoxicillin trihydrate) and potassium clavulanate.

Guidelines for the dental management of children with liver disease

The following are suggested guidelines for the dental management of children with liver disease.

• Parents need active encouragement to ensure that their child receives lifelong dental care. Parents can become so overwhelmed by the medical treatment that they simply forget that continued dental care is vital to the health of the child. Early involvement of the dental team helps overcome this problem and enables parents and children to benefit fully from preventive care and acclimatization therapy.

• Children with liver disease are at risk of dental caries. They need early referral to a specialist pediatric dental service for coordination of their preventive therapy. Shared dental care may be appropriate with the primary dental care provider and the specialist pediatric dental service, to reduce the burden of care for these children. Preventive management will include dietary control, fluoride supplements, fissure sealants, and oral hygiene instruction.

• Invasive dental treatment such as extractions needs to be carried out by a specialist in pediatric dentistry in consultation with a physician, to ensure that the appropriate medical precautions are taken—e.g., antihemolytic agents, broad-spectrum antibiotics. If it is carried out in association with another invasive procedure such as liver biopsy, intravenous antibiotics (amoxicillin, metronidazole, and cefotaxime) should be given for 24–48 h.

• Children who require treatment under general anesthesia need to be treated in a hospital environment where there are medical facilities and trained medical staff available. Where possible, medical and dental therapies should be combined under the same general anesthetic—e.g., extractions and liver biopsy.

• High-speed suction during operative dental procedures should be used to guard against ingestion of blood.

• The dose of amide local anesthetic solutions (lignocaine) should be reduced.

• When nutritional support is required, it is helpful if the dietician and physician can, where possible, limit the frequency of the dietary supplements to mealtimes and prescribe sugar-free medications. Since this is rarely possible, it is vital that these children are referred early to a pediatric dentist so that rigorous preventive therapy can be provided.

• Parents should be made aware of the likelihood of the occurrence of intrinsic green discoloration and enamel hypoplasia, but should be reassured that there are techniques available that can alleviate compromised dental aesthetics, appropriate to the age and dental development of the child.

Care of transplant recipients

Delayed eruption in pediatric liver transplantation

Delayed eruption of the primary dentition has been reported in 29–40% of pediatric liver-graft recipients.[2,5] The prevalence has been found to be as high as 48% in malnourished children (Figure 18.3) shows delayed emergence of upper primary incisors in a 22-month-old liver-graft recipient. There is little variation in primary tooth eruption times

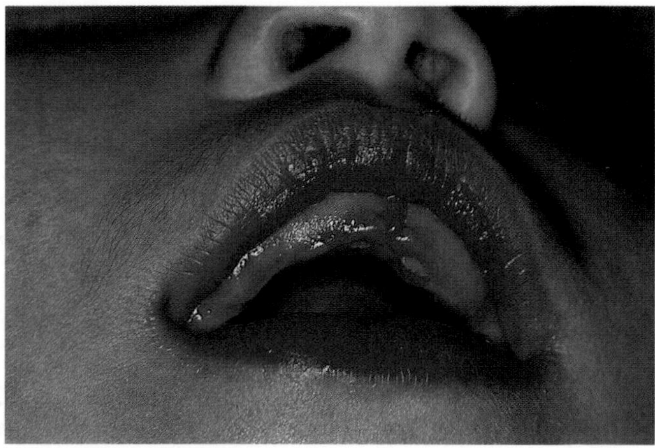

Figure 18.3 Delayed emergence of upper primary incisors in a 22-month-old child after liver transplantation. The upper central incisors are partially erupted, but there is no sign of the lateral incisors. This may be related to gingival overgrowth.

between different populations or between sexes. Delayed eruption of the primary dentition is found in children with chromosomal abnormalities, such as Down syndrome, and in hypothyroidism and hypopituitarism, but there are also local causes such as ectopic crypt position, supernumerary teeth and lack of space.

Tooth eruption ultimately depends upon the imbalance of forces acting on the tooth and the forces resisting its movement.[29] In this way, the resilience, texture, or thickness of the overlying oral mucosa may counteract the forces of eruption and impede the emergence of the tooth.[30] The timing of primary tooth emergence is related to general somatic growth, nutritional status, prematurity, and birth weight.[31,32] Moreover, studies of severely malnourished children in Peru have shown that these children not only suffer from delayed eruption, but are also more susceptible to dental caries.[33,34] Although children with delayed eruption of the primary dentition catch up on the population norms after the second year of life, once the nutritional difficulties have been resolved,[35] malnourished children after liver transplantation still fail to catch up on their dental eruption, despite nutritional support.

Corticosteroid therapy and delayed eruption

Corticosteroid therapy is known to slow the rate of statural growth and skeletal maturation in children,[36] and possibly also to cause delayed eruption of the permanent dentition. There have been no direct reports of delayed eruption in the primary dentition attributable to steroid therapy, but it is possible that this is due to the hitherto small number of infant transplant recipients.

Cyclosporine and delayed eruption of the primary dentition

Cyclosporine causes gingival overgrowth, and as such it might also be implicated in the delayed eruption of both primary and permanent teeth, although there is little research evidence to support this theory.

Management of delayed eruption

Palliative treatment such as the use of teething rings, sugar-free hard and fibrous foods on which to gnaw, teething gels, and systemic analgesia are recommended to the parents of children with delayed primary tooth eruption. Forewarning parents—especially parents of children who have been severely malnourished—of the likelihood of delayed eruption also helps allay parental anxiety.

Correcting the underlying medical condition—for example, discontinuing corticosteroid medication and providing nutritional support—is often sufficient to facilitate eruption of previously delayed teeth. Surgical intervention may be necessary in some cases, but fortunately most of the delayed primary teeth appear to erupt eventually. Indeed, adopting a wait-and see approach might avoid unnecessary and traumatic surgical therapy.

Cyclosporine-induced gingival overgrowth in transplant recipients

The supporting tissues of the teeth consist of the marginal and attached gingiva, the periodontal ligament, cementum covering the dentine on the root, and the alveolar bone.

Periodontal diseases are a group of acute and chronic infections that affect these tissues. Such conditions often begin during childhood as inflammation of the gum margin, with redness, swelling, and bleeding on brushing. Chronic gingivitis increases steadily between the ages of 5 and 9 years and is closely associated with the amount of plaque, debris, and calculus.[10]

The severity of the gingivitis is increased when oral hygiene is impaired, but it can be reversed with effective plaque control. Gingival overgrowth deepens the pocket between the gingival tissues and the teeth and therefore increases plaque retention. The hyperplastic gingival tissue caused by cyclosporine often has marked inflammatory changes and consequently bleeds readily. Liver-graft recipients are predisposed to diseases of the periodontal tissues. Gingival overgrowth is the only known oral side effect of cyclosporine therapy and was first reported in the early 1980s.[37,38] The reported prevalence of cyclosporine-induced gingival overgrowth in transplant recipients is between 8% and 100%.[5,39–41] This variation in the prevalence of gingival overgrowth could be attributed to differences in individual sensitivity, either between different HLA-B37 phenotypes or between different fibroblast populations.[37,42–44] Indeed, elevation of genes responsible for the turnover of extracellular matrix (ECM) within fibroblasts may be implicated (Figure 18.4).[45]

Pediatric liver-graft recipients

The prevalence of cyclosporine-induced gingival overgrowth in the pediatric liver transplant population has been found to be between 51% and 100% (Table 18.2).[2–5,15,41]

Pathogenesis of gingival overgrowth

Cyclosporine-induced gingival overgrowth is firm and pink, with focal lobulations and a stippled surface consisting primarily of a highly vascularized connective tissue with an overlying irregular, multilayered, parakeratinized epithelium of variable thickness. The predominant feature is a proliferation of collagen fibers in the corium, which are lightly distributed, in a foamy basophilic ground substance. There is a marked plasma cell, macrophage, and T-cell infiltrate, and modification of the appearance of gingival fibroblasts.

Gingival overgrowth may be caused by cyclosporine creating an imbalance between tissue formation and degradation, thereby inducing connective-tissue accumulation or inhibition of matrix breakdown and associated with various other mediators of inflammation, growth, and soft-tissue modeling. Contemporary research has therefore largely focused on the mechanisms of gingival overgrowth at a subcellular level.[37,39,46–55]

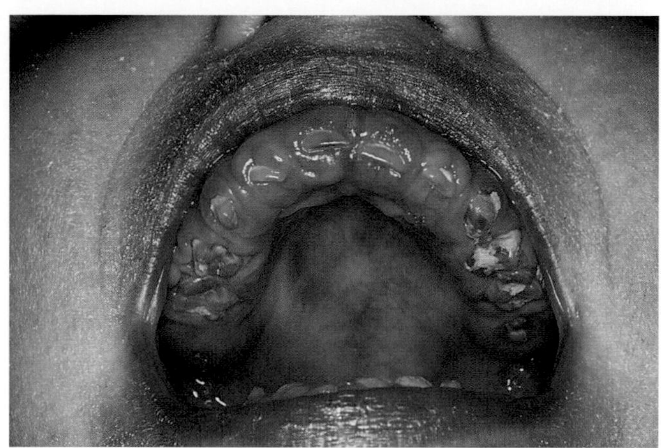
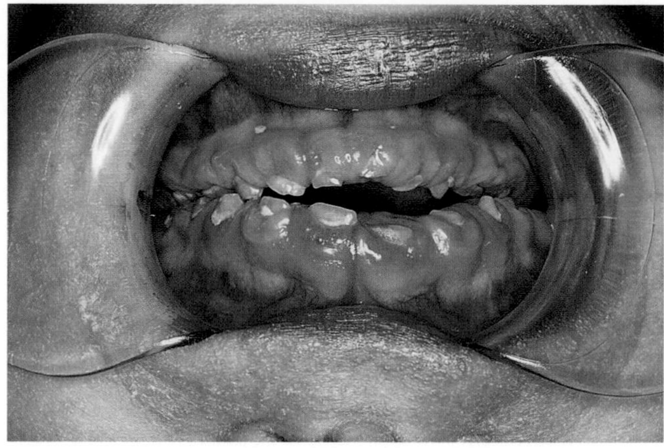

Figure 18.4 Severe gingival overgrowth after liver transplantation in a child receiving both cyclosporine and nifedipine. **A** Note the poor oral hygiene and calculus deposits. **B** The teeth are dysplastic and have severe intrinsic green pigmentation from prolonged jaundice.

Table 18.2 The prevalence of gingival overgrowth in previous studies of liver-graft recipients.

First author (ref.)	Date	Patients (n)	Mean age Months (range)	Medical diagnosis	Gingival overgrowth (%)	Other comments
Svirsky[15]	1989	1	37	OLT	100	
Ross[41]	1989	21	100 (24–192)	OLT	Not reported	Increased plaque index in patients, but no correlation between trough cyclosporine, therapy duration, or comitant nifedipine medication
Seow[2]	1991	7	39 (1–34)	OLT	86	Gingival overgrowth worsened with therapy duration
Funakoshi[3]	1992	5	53	OLT	100	No relation between gingival overgrowth and dose or therapy duration
Zaia[4]	1993	1	84	OLT	100	
Hosey[5]	1995	55	56 (8–194)	OLT	51	No relation between trough cyclosporine level and the severity of gingival overgrowth or between concomitant nifedipine therapy and presence of gingival overgrowth. Significant inverse relation between cyclosporine duration and overgrowth severity

Gingival overgrowth and cyclosporine dosage

Although the relationships between both cyclosporine dosage and serum trough level and gingival overgrowth have been extensively investigated, the results are controversial. Animal[56] and in vitro[57] studies have confirmed a relationship, but although some clinical studies have supported these findings,[58,59] others have not.[5,40,41,60–62] It has been suggested that there is a "threshold dose" below which the biological effect of the drug or one of its metabolites on the gingival tissues is dispelled.[37,39,42]

Age and cyclosporine-induced gingival overgrowth

The risk of cyclosporine-induced gingival overgrowth is greatest in adolescents,[60] which may be due to the added effect of growth hormone on the fibroblastic response, or the effect of estrogen and progesterone on gingival tissues or periodontal vasculature. The effect of the duration of cyclosporine therapy on gingival overgrowth in humans has not been established,[56] although in young children this might be the most critical factor.[62] There is resolution of the gingival response once the drug has been discontinued.[42]

The influence of plaque on cyclosporine-induced gingival overgrowth

The severity of cyclosporine-induced gingival overgrowth is related to gingival irritants, such as dental plaque, calculus, imperfections in dental restorations, orthodontic appliances, and the effects of mouth breathing.[37,38,60–66] Transplant recipients have been reported to have a significantly increased level of plaque, which might explain why gingival overgrowth is more prominent in areas where dental plaque has accumulated.[41,60,61,64]

There is a correlation between poor oral hygiene and the presence of gingival overgrowth. The mild chronic irritation caused by dental plaque may promote the hyperplastic effect of cyclosporine on the gingiva and act as a reservoir for the drug.[60,63] However, not all studies have demonstrated that dental plaque is a significant etiological factor.[58,67] Indeed, Tyldesley and Rotter reported that even frequent oral hygiene procedures were insufficient to eliminate gingival overgrowth.[38] Nevertheless, Ross *et al.*, in a controlled study, found that levels of both plaque and gingivitis were increased in liver-graft recipients.[41] Clearly, large multicenter studies are required in order to clarify the relationship between dental plaque and gingival overgrowth.

Neoral cyclosporine preparation

The Neoral preparation of cyclosporine improves the bioavailability of cyclosporine after liver grafting, but the increased exposure to cyclosporine might increase drug-related adverse effects.

Concomitant nifedipine medication and gingival overgrowth

Nifedipine not only causes gingival overgrowth,[68,69] but also acts synergistically with cyclosporine on the gingival tissues (Figure 18.4).[40,65,70] This may be due to similarities in the mechanism of action of the two drugs at the cellular level.[71]

Management of gingival overgrowth

Children with liver grafts need to be taught to acquire and then retain excellent oral hygiene skills. The health of their periodontal tissues needs to be monitored throughout their lives, and they need constant encouragement to keep up the best possible standard of oral cleanliness. Poor oral hygiene and periodontal disease predispose to transient bacteremia, and excellent oral hygiene—possibly augmented with a chlorhexidine oral rinse—is therefore beneficial. For antibacterial medication, metronidazole and azithromycin have been shown to effectively reduce the amount of gingival overgrowth.[72] For a few, surgical excision of the overgrown tissue (gingivectomy) or gingival recontouring (gingivoplasty) may be required to improve aesthetics and to reduce plaque retention by allowing adequate access for effective plaque removal. Alternatively, a change of immunosuppression to tacrolimus or mycophenolate mofetil (see Chapter 21) may be beneficial. Gingival overgrowth has been reported in patients taking tacrolimus,[73] but this growth is less than in patients taking cyclosporine.

Transferring patients from cyclosporine to tacrolimus normally resolves the gingival overgrowth, but this does not always happen and persistent overgrowth can occur.[73] Azathioprine has been shown to lower gingival overgrowth; this may be by exerting a protective effect directly through its anti-inflammatory properties or by reducing the cyclosporine dosage required.[66,73]

Prophylactic antibiotic therapy

Bacteremia of dental origin follows even the simplest dental procedure, but especially all minor oral surgical procedures in children; with multiple tooth extractions causing the greatest proportion of positive blood cultures. For invasive procedures such as subgingival scaling, dental extractions, and surgery that involves the gingival tissues, antibiotic prophylaxis is usually recommended.[18]

There is at present controversy as to the necessity for antibiotic cover following solid organ transplant. The American Academy of Pediatric Dentistry recommends prophylactic antibiotic therapy for organ transplant and immunocompromised patients, since they may be at risk from bacteremia produced by invasive dental procedures. They advise a course of amoxicillin 50 mg/kg (maximum 2 g) orally 1 h before the dental procedure. Clindamycin 20 mg/kg (maximum 600 mg) orally 1 h before the dental procedure is recommended for children who are allergic to penicillin.[74] The protocol devised at Birmingham Children's Hospital for all children after liver transplantation recommends the same prophylaxis as for children with significant cardiac conditions (Tables 18.1, 18.2).[75]

Guidelines for the dental management of pediatric liver-graft recipients

The dental management of pediatric recipients of liver transplants should be based on the following guidelines.

Before liver transplantation

- Good oral hygiene is probably the most important factor in reducing the risk of significant infection in susceptible individuals. Intensive oral hygiene therapy, preventive care, and careful parental counseling are of paramount importance if good oral health is to be maintained. This is best achieved when liver transplantation is first contemplated, since dental care is then seen by the family as being an integral part of the child's treatment.
- It is important that each child who is likely to be scheduled for liver grafting has a full dental examination, so that potential sources of infection can be treated and preventive therapy commenced. Where possible, active treatment should be completed before transplantation; this includes the removal of any teeth that are of dubious prognosis, since these may become a nidus of infection in the immunocompromised child.

• Children who already attend their local general dental practice regularly should be advised to continue, in order to "normalize" their lives as much as possible. Nevertheless, oral care still needs to be coordinated by a specialist pediatric dentist who is not only skilled in the management of medically compromised children but is also capable of coordinating the various medical and dental specialties into a framework for the better oral care of the child.

After liver transplantation

• Following liver transplantation, patients require routine dental check-ups, frequent topical fluoride application, and reinforcement of preventive advice. Tooth brushing can be complemented with chlorhexidine oral rinse or gel, and the use of a sonic toothbrush might be suggested. Fluoride supplementation should be considered, especially if the child lives in a nonfluoridated area, to reduce the risk of tooth decay.

• Parents should be made aware that delayed eruption of the primary dentition sometimes occurs, and palliative treatment—for example, the use of teething rings—should be recommended. The development of the dentition should be monitored, but parents can be reassured that these teeth generally do erupt eventually and often without recourse to surgical intervention.

• Gingival overgrowth in liver-graft recipients is most common and severe in adolescents. Good oral hygiene is vital to reduce the risk of periodontal disease. A sonic toothbrush may be helpful in this cohort. Although gingivectomy and gingivoplasty are rarely required in younger children, these procedures may be necessary in adolescents.

• Antibiotic prophylaxis should be given to all children in the first year after transplantation during high immunosuppression and continued in those children who have significant cardiac condition.[76] It should be given for invasive dental procedures involving gingival bleeding, including scaling surgery and dental extractions, since such patients may be at risk from bacteremia produced by invasive dental therapy. Oral amoxicillin (50 mg/kg in a single dose 1 h prior to the procedure) will eliminate most odontogenic bacteria. Erythromycin and clindamycin are recommended for children who are allergic to penicillin (Table 18.1).

• Regular surveillance of the head and neck region should be performed.

References

1 Shapiro BM, Gallagher FE, Needleman HL. Dental management of the patient with biliary atresia. *Oral Surg Oral Med Oral Pathol* 1975;**40**:742–7.

2 Seow WK, Shepherd RW, Ong TH. Oral changes associated with end-stage liver disease and liver transplantation: implications for dental management. *ASDC J Dent Child* 1991;**58**:474–80.

3 Funakoshi Y, Ohishita C, Moritani Y, Hieda T. Dental findings of patients who underwent liver transplantation. *J Clin Pediatr Dent* 1992;**16**:259–62.

4 Zaia AA, Graner E, De Almeida OP, Scully C. Oral changes associated with biliary atresia and liver transplantation. *J Pediatr Dent* 1993;**18**:39–42.

5 Hosey MT, Gordon G, Kelly DA, Shaw L. Oral findings in children with liver transplants. *Int J Paediatr Dent* 1995;**5**:29–34.

6 Sheehy EC, Roberts GJ, Beighton D, O'Brien G. Oral health in children undergoing liver transplantation. *Int J Paediatr Dent* 2000;**10**:109–19.

7 Bath-Balogh M, Fehrenbach MJ. *Dental Embryology, Histology and Anatomy.* Philadelphia: Saunders, 1997.

8 Lunt RC, Law DB. A review of the chronology of eruption of deciduous teeth. *J Am Dent Assoc* 1974;**89**:872–9.

9 Attwood D, Blinkhorn AS, MacMillan AS. A three-year follow-up study of the dental health of 12- and 15-year-old school children in Glasgow. *Community Dent Health* 1990;**7**:143–8.

10 O'Brian M. *Children's Dental Health in the United Kingdom.* London: Office of Population Census & Surveys, UK, 1993.

11 Scottish Intercollegiate Guideline Network (SIGN) 63. *Prevention of Dental Caries in Children of High Caries Risk.* Edinburgh: SIGN Executive, Royal College of Physicians, 2006.

12 Smith JM, Hwong CS, Salamonik EB, *et al.* Sonic tooth brushing reduces gingival overgrowth in renal transplant recipients. *Pediatr Nephrol* 2006;**21**:1753–9.

13 Scottish Intercollegiate Guideline Network (SIGN) 47. *Prevention of Dental Caries in Children of High Caries Risk.* Edinburgh: SIGN Executive, Royal College of Physicians, 2000.

14 Franco E, Saunders CP, Roberts GJ. Dental disease, caries related microflora and salivary IgA of children with severe congenital cardiac disease: an epidemiological and oral microbial survey. *Pediatr Dent* 1996;**18**:228–35.

15 Svirsky JA. Dental management of patients after liver transplantation. *Oral Surg Oral Med Oral Pathol* 1989;**67**:541–6.

16 Little JW. Dental treatment of the liver transplant patient. *Oral Surg Oral Med Oral Pathol* 1992;**73**:419–26.

17 Glassman P, Wong C, Gish R. A review of liver transplantation for the dentist and guidelines for dental management. *Special Care Dentistry* 1993;**13**:74–80.

18 Sheehy EC, Heaton N, Smith P, Roberts GJ. Dental management of children undergoing liver transplantation. *Pediatr Dent* 1999;**21**:272–80.

19 Marsland EA, Gerrard JW. Intrinsic staining of teeth following icterus gravis. *Br Dent J* 1953;**12**:305–10.

20 Herbert FL, Delcambre TJ. Unusual case of green teeth resulting from neonatal hyperbilirubinemia. *ASDC J Dent Child* 1987;**54**:54–6.

21 Genot MT, Golan HP, Porter PJ, Kass EH. Effect of administration of tetracycline in pregnancy on the primary dentition of the offspring. *J Oral Med* 1970;**25**:75–9.

22 Van Cleynenbreugel D, Demars-Fremault C. [Analysis of deciduous tooth discoloration, before and after liver transplantation; in French.] *Actual Odontostomatol (Paris)* 1990;**172**:545–8.

23 Majewski RF, Hess J, Kabani S, Ramanathan G. Dental findings in a patient with biliary atresia. *J Clin Pediatr Dent* 1993;**18**:33–7.

24 Morisaki I, Abe K, Tong LS, Kato K, Sobue S. Dental findings of children with biliary atresia: report of seven cases. *ASDC J Dent Child* 1990;**57**:220–3.

25 Wray A, Welbury R. *Treatment of Intrinsic Discoloration in Permanent Anterior Teeth in Children and Adolescents*, rev. ed. 2004. London: Royal College of Surgeons of England (available at: http://www.rcseng.ac.uk/fds/clinical_guidelines/documents/discolor.pdf).

26 Fearne JM, Elloi TJC, Wong FS, Davis GR, Boyde A, Jones SJ. Deciduous enamel defects in low birth-weight children: correlated X-ray microtomographic and backscattered electron imaging study of hypoplasia and hypomineralisation. *Anat Embryol* 1994;**189**:375–81.

27 Noren JG, Ranggard L, Klingberg G, Persson C, Nilsson K. Intubation and mineralization disturbances in the enamel of primary teeth. *Acta Odontol Scand* 1993;**51**:271–5.

28 Mackie IC, Blinkhorn AS, Davies PHJ. The extraction of first permanent molars during the mixed dentition period—a guide to treatment planning. *J Paediatr Dent* 1989;**5**:85–92.

29 Kardos TB. The mechanism of tooth eruption. *Br Dent J* 1996; **181**:91–5.

30 Di Biase DD. Mucous membrane and delayed eruption. *Dent Pract Dent Rec* 1971;**21**:241–9.

31 Infante PF, Owen GM. Relation of chronology of deciduous tooth emergence to height, weight and head circumference in children. *Arch Oral Biol* 1973;**18**:1411–7.

32 Fadavi S, Punwani IC, Adeni S, Vidyasagar D. Eruption pattern in the primary dentition of premature low-birth-weight children. *ASDC J Dent Child* 1992;**59**:120–2.

33 Alvarez JO, Eguren JC, Caceda J, Navia JM. The effect of nutritional status on the age distribution of dental caries in the primary teeth. *J Dent Res* 1990;**69**:1564–6.

34 Alvarez JO, Caceda J, Woolley TW, *et al.* The longitudinal study of dental caries in the primary teeth of children who suffered from infant malnutrition. *J Dental Res* 1993;**72**:1573–6.

35 Delgado H, Habicht JP, Harborough C. Nutritional status and the timing of deciduous tooth eruption. *Am J Clin Nutr* 1975;**28**: 216–24.

36 Blodgett FM, Burgin L, Iezzoni D, Gribetz D, Talbot NB. Effects of prolonged cortisone therapy on the statural growth, skeletal maturation and metabolic status of children. *N Engl J Med* 1956;**254**:636–41.

37 Wysocki GP, Gretzinger HA, Laupacis A, Ulan RA, Stiller CR. Fibrous hyperplasia of the gingiva: a side effect of cyclosporin A therapy. *Oral Surg Oral Med Oral Pathol* 1983;**55**:274–8.

38 Tyldesley WR, Rotter E. Gingival hyperplasia induced by cyclosporin-A. *Br Dent J* 1984;**157**:305–9.

39 Seymour RA, Jacobs DJ. Cyclosporin and the gingival tissues. *J Clin Periodontol* 1992;**19**:1–11.

40 Thomason JM, Seymour RA, Rice N. The prevalence and severity of cyclosporin and nifedipine-induced gingival overgrowth. *J Clin Periodontol* 1993;**20**:37–40.

41 Ross PJ, Nazif M, Zullo T, Zitelli B, Guevara P. Effects of Cyclosporin A on gingival status following liver transplantation. *ASDC J Dent Child* 1989;**56**:56–9.

42 Hassell TM, Stanek EJ. Evidence that healthy human gingiva contains functionally heterogeneous fibroblast subpopulations. *Arch Oral Biol* 1983;**28**:617–25.

43 Daly CG. Resolution of cyclosporin A (CsA)-induced gingival enlargement following reduction in CsA dosage. *J Clin Periodontol* 1992;**19**:143–5.

44 Thomason JM, Seymour RA, Ellis JS, *et al.* Determinants of gingival overgrowth severity in organ transplant patients. An examination of the role of HLA phenotype. *J Clin Periodontol* 1996;**23**:628–34.

45 Dannewitz B, Edrich C, Tomakidi P, *et al.* Elevated gene expression of MMP-1, MMP10, and TIMP-1 reveal changes of molecules involved in turn-over of extracellular matrix in cyclosporine-induced gingival overgrowth. *Cell Tissue Res* 2006;**325**:513–22.

46 Yamasaki A, Rose GG, Pinero GJ, Mahan CJ. Ultrastructure of fibroblasts in cyclosporin A-induced gingival hyperplasia. *J Oral Pathol* 1987;**16**:129–34.

47 Barber MT, Savage NW, Seymour GJ. The effect of cyclosporin and lipopolysaccharide on fibroblasts: implications for cyclosporin-induced gingival overgrowth. *J Periodontol* 1992;**63**:397–404.

48 Romanos GE, Schroter-Kermani C, Hinz N, Bernimoulin JP. Distribution of fibronectin in healthy, inflamed and drug-induced gingival hyperplasia. *J Oral Pathol Med* 1992;**21**:256–60.

49 Schincaglia GP, Forniti F, Cavallini R, Piva R, Calura G, del Senno L. Cyclosporin-A increases type I procollagen production and mRNA level in human gingival fibroblasts in vitro. *J Oral Pathol Med* 1992;**21**:181–5.

50 Williamson MS, Miller BK, Plemons J, Rees T, Iacopino AM. Cyclosporine A upregulates interleukin-6 gene expression in human gingiva: possible mechanism for gingival overgrowth. *J Periodontol* 1994;**65**:895–903.

51 Seymour RA, Thomason JM, Ellis JS. The pathogenesis of drug-induced gingival overgrowth. *J Clin Periodontol* 1996;**23**:165–75.

52 Thomason JM, Sloan P, Seymour RA. Immunolocalization of collagenase (MMP-1) and stromelysin (MMP-3) in the gingival tissues of organ transplant patients medicated with cyclosporin. *J Clin Periodontol* 1998;**25**:554–60.

53 Thomas DW, Newcombe RG, Osborne GR. Risk factors in the development of cyclosporine-induced gingival overgrowth. *Transplantation* 2000;**69**:522–6.

54 Das SJ, Parkar MH, Olsen I. Upregulation of keratinocyte growth factor in cyclosporin A-induced gingival overgrowth. *J Periodontol* 2001;**72**:745–52.

55 Wright HJ, Chapple IL, Matthews JB. TGF-beta isoforms and TGF-beta receptors in drug-induced and hereditary gingival overgrowth. *J Oral Pathol Med* 2001;**30**:281–9.

56 Fu E, Nieh S, Chang HL, Wang SL. Dose-dependent gingival overgrowth induced by cyclosporin in rats. *J Periodontol* 1995; **66**:594–8.

57 Coley C, Jarvis K, Hassell T. Effect of cyclosporine A on human gingival fibroblasts in vitro [abstract]. *J Dent Res* 1986;**65**:353.

58 Seymour RA, Smith DG, Rogers SR. The comparative effects of azathioprine and cyclosporin on some gingival health parameters of renal transplant patients. *J Clin Periodontol* 1987;**14**:610–3.

59 Somacarrera ML, Hernández G, Acero J, Moskow BS. Factors related to the incidence and severity of cyclosporin-induced gingival overgrowth in transplant patients. A longitudinal study. *J Periodontol* 1994;**65**:671–5.

60 Daley TD, Wysocki G, Day C. Clinical and pharmacologic correlations in cyclosporine-induced gingival hyperplasia. *Oral Surg Oral Med Oral Pathol* 1986;**62**:417–21.

61 Karpinia KA, Matt M, Fennell RS 3rd, Hefti AF. Factors affecting cyclosporine-induced gingival overgrowth in pediatric renal transplant recipients. *Pediatr Dent* 1996;**18**:450–5.

62 Seymour RA, Smith DG. The effect of a plaque control programme on the incidence and severity of cyclosporin-induced gingival changes. *J Clin Periodontol* 1991;**18**:107–10.

63 Pernu HE, Pernu LM, Huttunen KR, Nieminen PA, Knuttila MLE. Gingival overgrowth among renal transplant recipients related to immunosuppressive medication and possible local background factors. *J Periodontol* 1992;**63**:548–53.
64 Bartold PM. Cyclosporine and gingival overgrowth. *J Oral Pathol* 1987;**16**:463–8.
65 McGaw T, Lam S, Coates J. Cyclosporin-induced gingival overgrowth: correlation with dental plaque scores, gingivitis scores, and cyclosporin levels in serum and saliva. *Oral Surg Oral Med Oral Pathol* 1987;**64**:293–7.
66 Wilson's RF, Morel A, Smith D, *et al.* Contribution of individual drugs to gingival overgrowth in adult and juvenile renal transplant patients treated with multiple therapy. *J Clin Periodontol* 1998;**25**:457–64.
67 Margiotta V, Pizzo I, Pizzo G, Barbaro A. Cyclosporin- and nifedipine-induced gingival overgrowth in renal transplant patients: correlations with periodontal and pharmacological parameters, and HLA-antigens. *J Oral Pathol Med* 1996;**25**:128–34.
68 Singer DL, Zebrowski EJ. Nifedipine: effects in vitro on gingival fibroblasts. *J Dent Res* 1988;**67**:332.
69 Salo T, Oikarinen KS, Oikarinen AI. Effect of phenytoin and nifedipine on collagen gene expression in human gingival fibroblasts. *J Oral Pathol Med* 1990;**19**;404–7.
70 Slavin J, Taylor J. Cyclosporin, nifedipine, and gingival hyperplasia. *Lancet* 1987;**ii**:739.
71 Nishikawa S, Tada H, Hamasaki A, *et al.* Nifedipine-induced gingival hyperplasia: a clinical and in vitro study. *J Periodontol* 1991;**62**:30–5.
72 Chand DH, Quattrocchi J, Poe SA, Terezhalmy GT, Strife CF, Cunningham RJ. Trial of metronidazole vs. azithromycin for treatment of cyclosporine-induced gingival overgrowth. *Pediatr Transplant* 2004;**8**:60–4.
73 Ellis JS, Seymour RA, Taylor JJ, Thomason JM. Prevalence of gingival overgrowth in transplant patients immunosuppressed with tacrolimus. *J Clin Periodontol* 2004;**31**:126–31.
74 American Academy of Pediatric Dentistry Clinical Affairs Committee; American Academy of Pediatric Dentistry Council on Clinical Affairs. Guideline on antibiotic prophylaxis for dental patients at risk for infection. [American Academy of Pediatric Dentistry reference manual 2007–2008.] *Pediatr Dent* 2007–2008; **29**(7 Suppl):202–4 (available at: http://www.aapd.org/media/Policies_Guidelines/G_AntibioticProphylaxis.pdf).
75 Gould FK, Elliot TSJ, Foweraker J, *et al.* Guidelines for the prevention of endocarditis: report of the Working Party of the British Society for Antimicrobial Chemotherapy. *J Antimicrob Chemother* 2006;**57**:1035–42.
76 Graham C, Baumann U. *Antibiotic Prophylaxis in Liver and Small Bowel Transplant.* Birmingham, England: Birmingham Children's Hospital, 2006.

10 Surgical Management of Liver Disease

19 Surgical Disorders of the Liver and Bile Ducts and Portal Hypertension

Alastair J.W. Millar

The bile ducts

Biliary atresia, choledochal cysts, spontaneous perforation of the bile duct, and inspissated bile syndrome are the most common "surgical" causes of jaundice in infants. Biliary atresia is the most common abnormality presenting in the neonatal period. Early diagnosis is essential, as delay in treatment may result in irreversible liver damage.

Biliary atresia

Congenital atresia of the bile ducts is a unique pathological entity that has no analogy with any disease process in the bile ducts of older patients. It is characterized as a destructive inflammatory process of unknown etiology which affects a variable length of the biliary tract. Untreated infants develop biliary cirrhosis and die of liver failure within the first 2 years of life. The first clear report of the natural history of the condition was published by the Edinburgh pediatrician, John Thomson in 1891,[1] but it was not until 1928 that Ladd[2] described surgical correction of a small number of cases of the so-called "correctable" type of atresia, in which the atretic segment is limited to the common bile duct, whilst the proximal biliary tree within the liver is patent. Ladd performed anastomotic procedures in six of the 11 cases he explored.[3]

A majority of affected infants, however, have a surgically "uncorrectable" type of biliary atresia, in which the atresia extends into the proximal bile ducts. All of these children died within a year or two of their disease until a novel method of treatment was introduced from Japan in the late 1950s.[4] Kasai reported the identification of microscopic biliary channels within the proximal atretic tissue in the porta hepatis and showed that exposure of these channels by radical resection of the biliary tract could result in effective drainage of bile. Although this work was initially greeted with a considerable degree of scepticism outside of Japan, successful results were eventually achieved in centers throughout the world, and the Kasai portoenterostomy is now accepted as the standard operation for the condition.

Incidence

Biliary atresia is a rare disease with a frequency of approximately one in 10 000–16 000 live births. The incidence is similar in many countries, as shown by recent studies in France and the United Kingdom, with a slightly increased frequency seen in the Far East.[5–7] There is a slight female preponderance in most large series, but only rarely is there any significant family history of liver or biliary disease. Thirteen instances of familial biliary atresia have been documented.[8,9]

Etiology

The true etiology of biliary atresia is unknown, although embryological, infective, hormonal, and anatomical hypotheses have been suggested.

Embryological and genetic abnormality. Approximately 10% of children with biliary atresia have associated extrahepatic abnormalities, which include polysplenia, situs inversus, interrupted inferior vena cava, and cardiac defects. These associations, have been termed the "biliary atresia splenic malformation (BASM) syndrome" (Table 19.1).[10] The critical period of early development for all the affected components of this syndrome (biliary, inferior vena cava, portal vein, splenic) is from 25 to 40 days of gestation, and hence an embryopathic insult at this early stage of development would help to explain the coincident anomalies. Also described was a possible relationship between BASM and antenatal events in the mother, the most common of which was maternal diabetes, a condition that is known to cause fetal malformations such as transposition of the great vessels.

The embryological development of the biliary tree and liver is complex. There are histological and immunohistochemical similarities between the developing hepatobiliary system at 11–13 weeks' gestation and the appearance of established biliary atresia. Bile is produced by hepatocytes from 12 weeks' gestation and coincident with this there are remodeling, selection, and deletion of fetal bile ducts originating from the ductal plate membrane to form the definitive

Diseases of the Liver and Biliary System in Children, 3rd edition. Edited by Deirdre Kelly. © 2008 Blackwell Publishing, ISBN: 978-1-4051-6334-7.

Table 19.1 Abnormalities associated with the biliary atresia splenic malformation (BASM) syndrome.[10]

Anomaly	Frequency	Comment
Preduodenal portal vein	75%	
Polysplenia	90%	
Situs inversus	50%	Usually with normal position of heart
Malrotation	50%	
Interruption of inferior vena cava	30%	Venous drainage by azygos veins
Cardiac anomalies	30%	May be mode of presentation
Intrapulmonary shunting	5%	Increasingly apparent in long-term survivors
Double spleen/splenunculi	2–5%	
Asplenia	2–5%	
Pancreatic anomalies	2–5%	E.g., annular pancreas
Immotile cilia syndrome	1%	Bronchiectasis, sinusitis

pattern of proximal intrahepatic bile ducts. It has been suggested that biliary atresia without syndromic features may represent an arrested development of these biliary radicals.[11]

A small number of cases of biliary atresia have been detected antenatally on maternal ultrasound scans from 17 weeks.[12–14] Cases have been identified on fetal ultrasound scans showing evidence of "subhepatic cysts." γ-glutamyltransferase (GGT) is an enzyme of fetal liver origin that can be found in amniotic fluid from the second trimester onward and relates to in utero bile production and fetal defecation.[15] A large study of amniotic fluid sampling showed that patients born with biliary atresia had minimal levels of amniotic fluid GGT dating back to 18 weeks' gestation.[16]

There have been reports of isolated cases of biliary atresia associated with trisomy.[17–19] The frequency of twinning in biliary atresia is no greater than that expected in a normal population, with most being discordant for the disease.[20,21]

Infective factors. Isolated cases of biliary atresia have followed infection with rubella and the Epstein–Barr virus.[22,23] Much of the interest in infection has focused on experimental work with the hepatotropic RNA viruses, reovirus and rotavirus. Liver disease and hyperbilirubinemia could be induced in 21-day-old weanling mice after inoculation with reo-3 virus.[24] Similar experiments with rotavirus have reproduced some of the histological and anatomical features of biliary atresia—although not usually the typical extrahepatic appearance and sequelae.[25–27] In one model, there was strain-specific targeting of biliary epithelium.[28] The mechanism of injury is thought to be due to a specific T cell–mediated immune response with an interferon gamma–rich proinflammatory "footprint" present at the time of diagnosis. In mice with genetic loss of interferon gamma (IFN-γ), the inflammatory and fibrosing obstruction of extrahepatic bile ducts did not occur.[29]

Although some clinical studies have suggested that there is a high incidence of positive serology against reovirus type 3 in infants with biliary atresia, others have disputed this.[30–32] Viral-like particles have only been identified from a single case of biliary atresia, and further studies using sophisticated techniques such as polymerase chain reaction (PCR) have proved negative.[33,34]

Seasonal variation and a winter predilection for biliary atresia have been identified in some cohort studies and provide some evidence for a possible viral etiology.[35,36] However, larger, less well-controlled studies have failed to confirm this observation.[37]

Anatomical factors. A common pancreaticobiliary channel has been demonstrated in 60% of cases of biliary atresia and in over 80% of children with congenital choledochal cysts.[38,39] Endoscopic retrograde cholangiography (ERCP) findings in 28 infants with biliary atresia were compared with seven infants with neonatal hepatitis syndrome. The mean length of the pancreaticobiliary channels in the former was 5.1 mm, compared with 1.3 mm in the latter, suggesting a possible role for the malformation in etiology.

Animal observations. Biliary atresia has been described in lambs and calves in New South Wales, Australia.[40] A common factor in this, and in previous outbreaks of the disease, was the restriction of grazing to particular areas of land when the maternal animals were in the early stages of pregnancy. The authors suggested that perhaps a plant toxin might be involved in the etiology of the biliary atresia, although they failed to identify a specific substance during their investigation.

Pathogenesis

Biliary atresia is a cholangiopathic panductular disease, which in most infants is present at birth. Progression of the condition results in cholestasis, hepatic fibrosis, and cirrhosis. Bile duct plugging, ductular proliferation, portal edema, a small-cell infiltrate, and variable giant-cell formation characterize the histological appearances of the liver.[41] A pronounced inflammatory reaction, particularly at the porta hepatis, with a dense small-cell infiltrate, is not uncommon.[42] This feature appears to be related to the child's age, as older infants may show a diminution in the inflammatory change.[43] An aberrant expression of cellular mediators of inflammation, such as intercellular adhesion molecules (ICAM) and vascular adhesion molecules (VCAM), has been detected in cases of biliary atresia but not in other cases of neonatal cholestasis. On the other hand, in one study of the inflammatory infiltrate and its relationship with clinical outcome, the immunohistochemical patterns of immune-mediated inflammation in biliary atresia differed significantly from those observed in infants with non–biliary atresia cholestatic jaundice.[44] The authors did note that an improved prognosis in biliary atresia was associated with a reduction in the expression of the macrophage marker CD68 in the liver and biliary remnants, and a reduction in ICAM expression on infiltrating cells within bile duct tissue. Experimentally induced biliary atresia using rotavirus in neonatal mice showed overexpression of interferon gamma by neonatal hepatic T cells, with tropism of primed $CD8^+$ for extrahepatic bile ducts and their epithelial lining and loss of $CD8^+$ cells, remarkably suppressed duct injury, prevented luminal obstruction, and restored bile flow.[45] In the human, the predominant inflammatory infiltrates are $CD4^+$ lymphocytes and macrophages. Levels of adhesion molecules and cytokines increase progressively in the first 6 months after portoenterostomy. Persistently high levels have been associated with clinical indicators for early transplantation.[46] This work has particular relevance in the use of immunosuppressive medication—steroids in particular—after the Kasai operation and fits in with information from molecular genetic microarray research suggesting that there is increased expression of immune-regulatory genes in biliary atresia.[47]

The inflammatory process affects the intrahepatic ducts in all cases of biliary atresia, and intrahepatic ducts do not show dilation on ultrasonography or cholangiography. Radiologically, they have the appearance of a "cloud" radiating from the porta hepatis (Figure 19.1). This appearance does not change in the long term, even in those who have had a good response to portoenterostomy and satisfactory bile drainage.

The lumen of the extrahepatic duct is obliterated by inflammatory tissue at a variable level, and this macroscopic appearance forms the basis for the commonest pathological classification. There are three main types of obliteration (Figure 19.2), of which type 3 (obliteration at the level of the porta hepatis) is the commonest, occurring in 85–90% of cases. Obstruction at the level of the common hepatic duct (type 2) or common bile duct (type 1) is much less common, but carries a better prognosis. In about 5% of cases, cysts can occur proximal or distal to the obliterated duct. However, the cyst wall in such cases is invariably thickened and communicates poorly with intrahepatic ducts, and this appearance should not be confused with true choledochal cystic dilation.

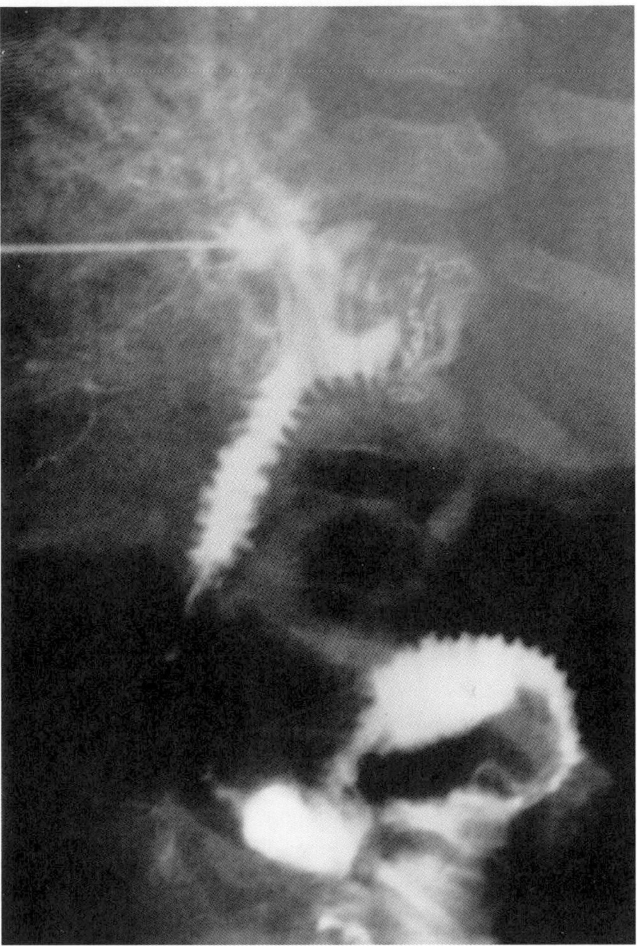

Figure 19.1 A percutaneous cholangiogram in a child who had previously undergone a Kasai portoenterostomy. There is free-flow of contrast into the Roux loop. The bile ducts are very abnormal and show the typical cloud-like appearance of biliary atresia.

Role of screening

There has been interest in a screening program for biliary atresia because of the delay that may occur before these infants reach specialist centers.[48] Tandem mass spectrometry to measure conjugated bile acids in dried blood spots obtained from newborn infants has proved disappointing.[49] Although screening for conjugated bilirubin in liquid blood was both sensitive and specific for the diagnosis of biliary atresia, it has not proved possible to transfer this technique to dry blood spots. In a pilot study to screen the stool color of infants for the early diagnosis of biliary atresia in Taiwan, an infant stool color card was used to screen 78 184 infants, and 26 of 29 infants with biliary atresia were picked up by stool color card testing before 60 days of age.[50] This had good sensitivity

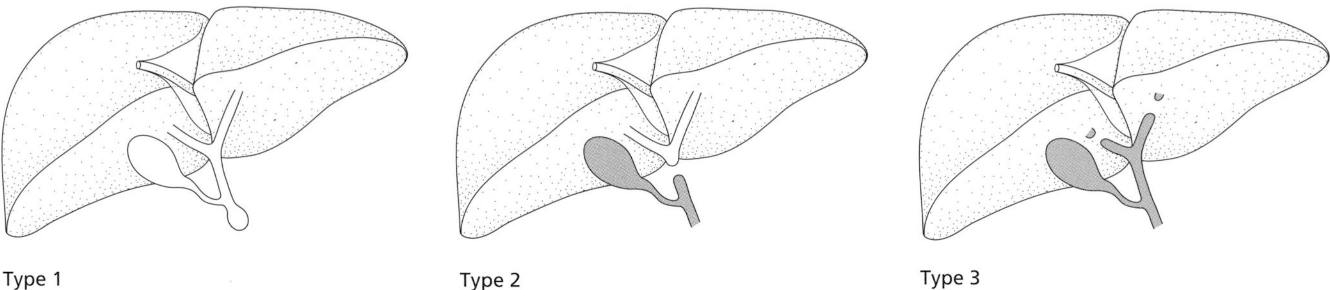

Figure 19.2 Classification of biliary atresia (based on the Japanese Association of Pediatric Surgeons classification). Type 1: atresia affecting the common bile duct, often associated with proximal biliary cyst. Type 2: atresia affecting the common hepatic duct. Type 3: obliteration and atresia affecting the whole of the extrahepatic biliary tree.

(89.7%) and specificity (99.9%), but a poor positive predictive value (28.6%). It is imperative that primary-care practitioners should be alerted to the simple observation of pale stools and that pediatricians investigate and exclude biliary atresia in all infants who have persistent conjugated jaundice after 14 days of age.[51,52]

Clinical features and diagnosis (see also Figures 4.4, 4.5, 4.7)

Infants with biliary atresia present with:

- Conjugated hyperbilirubinemia
- Dark urine and pale, acholic stools

These signs are present from birth, although birth weight and gestation are usually normal. At first, the infants feed and thrive appropriately. Lack of fat-soluble vitamin K absorption may eventually result in a coagulopathy, particularly if the child is receiving oral vitamin K supplements or is breastfed, and a number of the infants present with abnormal bleeding, which may be intracranial. On examination, the liver is enlarged, and in older infants there may be ascites and splenomegaly. In all cases, liver function tests are abnormal, with raised serum bilirubin > 100 μm/L (conjugated > 80%) and a rise in alkaline phosphatase and GGT, suggesting duct obstruction; however, neither is specific for biliary atresia.

An accurate diagnosis of biliary atresia is established preoperatively in approximately 95% of cases by excluding medical causes of conjugated hyperbilirubinemia (particularly α_1-antitrypsin deficiency) and identifying the characteristic histological appearances of a percutaneous liver biopsy (see Chapter 4). The following investigations may be particularly helpful:

- Hepatobiliary ultrasound will exclude other surgical causes of jaundice, such as choledochal cyst and obstructed extrahepatic ducts due to inspissated bile. An absent gallbladder or one with an irregular outline is suggestive of biliary atresia in a fasting infant.[53] In some cases, a well-defined triangular area of high reflectivity corresponding to fibrotic ductal remnants at the porta hepatis may be seen on ultrasound (the "triangular cord" sign).[54]
- Radionuclide hepatobiliary imaging using iminodiacetic acid (IDA) derivatives fails to show bile excretion into the bowel within 24 h in cases of biliary atresia and discriminates between this condition and most causes of the neonatal hepatitis syndrome.[55] Phenobarbitone pretreatment (5 mg/kg/day for 3–5 days) improves the accuracy.
- Magnetic resonance cholangiography (MRC) may be used to visualize the bile ducts and gallbladder of nonbiliary atresia infants with cholestatic jaundice and therefore exclude biliary atresia. This method had a diagnostic accuracy of 98%, a sensitivity of 100%, and a specificity of 96% in one series of 23 patients.[56]
- If the diagnosis remains unclear even after liver biopsy, then consideration should be given to ERCP if available. This is technically possible in about 90% of infants, and biliary atresia can be confidently excluded if the whole of the biliary tree is imaged, although false-positive results may follow from technical failures in cannulation.[57] Normal bile ducts were successfully demonstrated in 43 of 50 ERCPs, and six of the seven cases in which visualization of the bile ducts failed proved to be cases of biliary atresia at subsequent laparotomy.
- An alternative to ERCP is provided by laparoscopy and operative cholangiography.
- The role of endoscopic ultrasound in the diagnosis of biliary atresia has not yet been evaluated (Chapter 2).

Surgery (Figure 19.3)

The operation for biliary atresia initially proposed by Kasai in 1959 has changed little since its first description, although numerous modifications have been proposed.[58] There is now substantial consensus over most aspects of the actual operation, but there is less in areas involving the role of postoperative drainage and the use of steroids, prophylactic antibiotics, and the treatment of cholangitis.[59]

The biliary tree is approached via a right-sided transverse incision, which can be extended across the midline.[60] If the diagnosis has not been established preoperatively, then an operative cholangiogram is obtained via a catheter in the gallbladder. If there is bile in a normal-looking gallbladder,

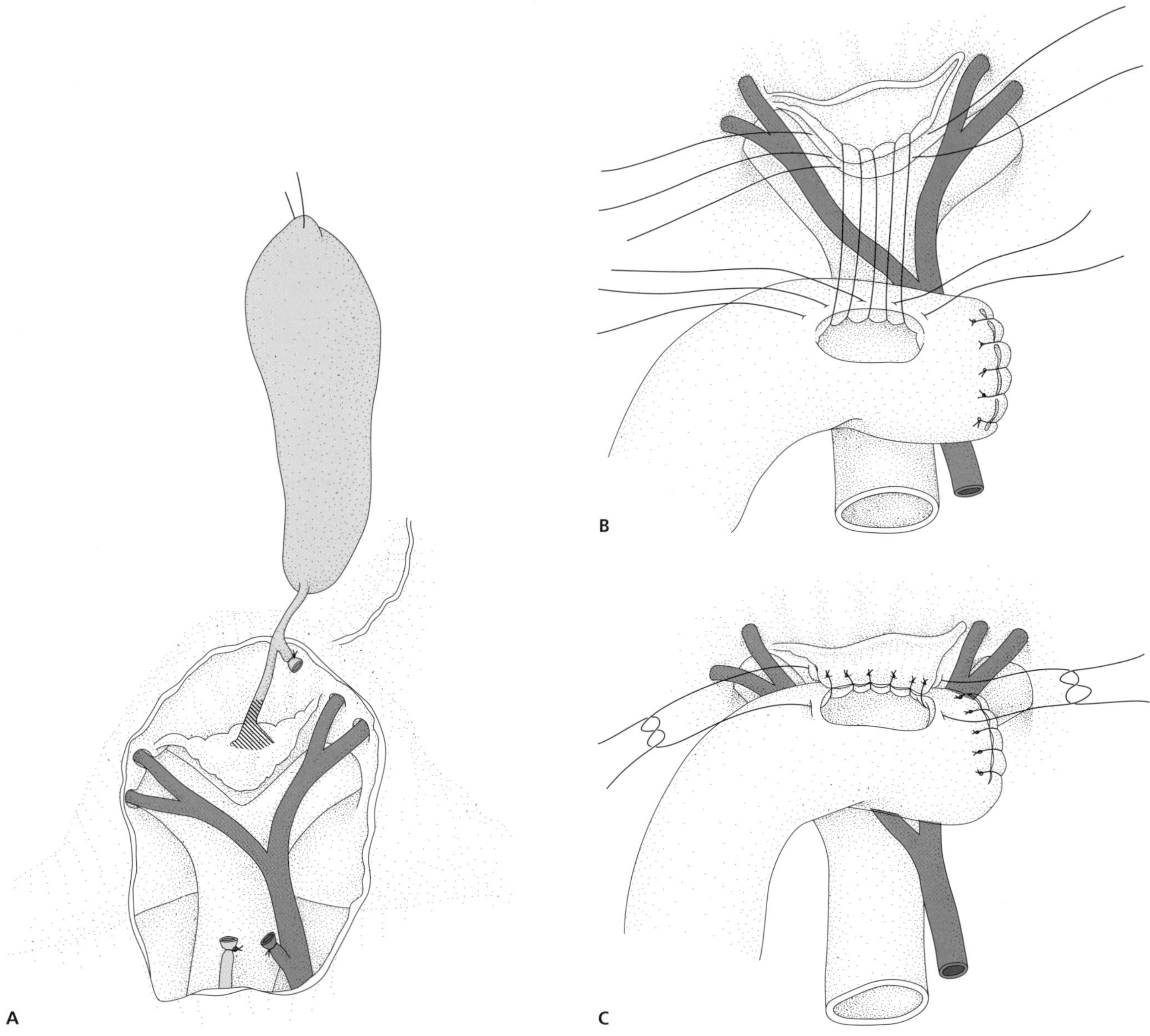

Figure 19.3 Three stages in the portoenterostomy operation for biliary atresia (Kasai operation). **A** The gallbladder and remnants of the bile ducts are mobilized completely into the porta hepatis. **B** All residual bile duct tissue is excised, and a Roux loop of jejunum is prepared for anastomosis to the cut surface in the porta hepatis. **C** The Roux loop is anastomosed to the porta hepatis.

the diagnosis of biliary atresia is excluded. It must be emphasized that only complete visualization of the whole of the biliary tree will exclude biliary atresia at this stage. The hepatic suspensory ligaments may be divided and the liver rotated to expose its inferior surface in the incision. This maneuver provides maximal exposure of the porta hepatis. The gallbladder remnant is dissected, and the obliterated biliary tract is divided distally and elevated to separate it from the underlying portal vein and adjacent hepatic artery. It is then dissected free and transected high at the level of the porta hepatis without entering liver parenchyma. A complete resection of the extrahepatic biliary tree is advisable in all types of biliary atresia, except for the uncommon case in which there is a significant remnant of patent bile duct in the porta hepatis. Biliary continuity is restored using a Roux loop, which is anastomosed to the transected tissue in the porta hepatis as a portoenterostomy (Figure 19.1).

In some cases of biliary atresia, operative cholangiography may show a patent lower common bile duct in continuity with the gallbladder, the atretic process being restricted to the common hepatic and hepatic ducts. Reconstruction of the biliary tract using the gallbladder (portocholecystostomy) after resection of the remnants of the bile ducts has been suggested as an effective method of preventing postoperative cholangitis. Unfortunately, postoperative complications are not uncommon with this technique.

Currently, a revision or re-do portoenterostomy is not recommended in the United Kingdom, as it is associated with only a small chance of success. It also increases the technical difficulty of any subsequent liver transplantation.

Infants tolerate portoenterostomy very well, and early postoperative complications are unusual. As with many other pediatric operations, minimally invasive techniques are being investigated. Early evidence is that the outcomes appear to be equivalent to those with the open technique, with low morbidity.[61–63]

Postoperative care and long-term complications after portoenterostomy

Intravenous antibiotics are given in the immediate postoperative period, and are replaced by 1 month of oral antibiotic prophylaxis after the return of bowel activity. Choleretics (cholestyramine, ursodeoxycholic acid, and phenobarbitone) and vitamins A, D, E, and K are prescribed for at least 1 year. Steroids have been recommended in the belief that they might reduce scar tissue formation and provide improvement in bile flow after portoenterostomy. No controlled trials have been published to confirm or deny the efficacy of steroids, although there is some observational evidence to support their use.[64–67] There is wide variation in the dosage, time for starting treatment, and duration, and prospective trials are in progress to define the best practice (Table 19.2).[68]

Complications of the portoenterostomy operation include:

- Ascending bacterial cholangitis
- Cirrhosis and portal hypertension
- Metabolic and nutritional consequences of cholestasis
- Intrahepatic cyst formation
- Hepatopulmonary syndrome and pulmonary hypertension
- Malignant changes in the liver (rare)

Ascending bacterial cholangitis. This serious complication occurs most commonly in the first year following portoenterostomy. Episodes of infection have been recorded in approximately 40–50% of the infants in most series and occur in those who have achieved at least some degree of bile flow.[69] The condition is characterized by worsening jaundice, fever, and acholic stools. The diagnosis is confirmed by blood culture or by percutaneous liver biopsy. A wide range of organisms may be identified, including *Escherichia coli* and *Proteus* and *Klebsiella* species, but it is important to treat suspected cases early and empirically with broad-spectrum antibiotics such as ceftazidime, amoxicillin, ciprofloxacin, and gentamicin or piperacillin before the detailed results of investigation are available.

Table 19.2 Protocol for management of biliary atresia after portoenterostomy.

Preoperative management (commencing 24–48 h before surgery)	
Medication	
Neomycin	12.5 mg/kg/dose t.d.s. oral
Metronidazole	7.5 mg/kg/dose t.d.s. oral
Lactulose	5 mL b.i.d. oral
Blood tests	
Full blood count, liver function tests, clotting screen, group and cross-match	
Operation	
Operative cholangiogram if bile in gallbladder	
Portoenterostomy	
Postoperative management	
Pain relief:	
Epidural for first 36–48 h, followed by acetaminophen	
Intravenous fluids:	
Oral feeding with return of bowel activity	
Steroids (optional 2-week course—value not yet proven)	
E.g., day 1, methylprednisolone i.v. 20 mg, decreasing 2.5 mg daily to 5 mg/day, then prednisolone 5 mg daily, orally for 1 week	
Antibiotics: i.v. for 5 days	
Gentamicin i.v.	2.5 mg/kg/dose t.d.s. (levels needed)
Amoxicillin i.v.	25 mg/kg/dose t.d.s.
Antibiotic prophylaxis (started on postoperative day 6)	
Cephalexin	12.5 mg/kg/dose b.i.d. for 1 month
Or ciprofloxacin	5–10 mg/kg/dose b.i.d.(oral) with extended prophylaxis daily dose
Longer-term oral medication	
Ranitidine	1 mg/kg/dose t.d.s.
Phenobarbitone	5 mg/kg/dose nocte
UDCA	10 mg/kg/dose b.i.d.
Vitamin A	5000 IU/day
Vitamin D	50 ng/kg/day (alfacalcidol)
Vitamin E	50 mg/day
Vitamin K	1–2 mg/day
Management of postoperative cholangitis	
Septic screen	
Liver biopsy for culture	
Intravenous antibiotics:	
Ceftazidime	30 mg/kg t.d.s. for 10 days
Amoxicillin	20 mg/kg t.d.s. for 10 days
Or ciprofloxacin	4–7 mg/kg/dose 12 h i.v. for 10 days
If temperature does not settle after 5 days or returns on discontinuation of antibiotics, do ascitic tap and liver biopsy for bacteriological culture and further therapy based on the culture and sensitivity.	
Second-line treatment is:	
Meropenem	10–20 mg/kg/dose 8 h
Vancomycin	15 mg/kg loading dose then 10 mg/kg/dose with levels after the fourth dose

UDCA, ursodeoxycholic acid.

A number of modifications have been made to Kasai's original portoenterostomy operation to try to reduce the incidence of cholangitis. These have included diversion stomas and the formation of antireflux valves in the Roux loop.[70] However, despite the theoretical benefits of such modifications, in practice they confer little additional benefit, and equally good results are obtained with the use of a long Roux loop.[71]

Cholangitis may occur some years after a portoenterostomy procedure in a child with otherwise good liver function. It is important in such a case to exclude a partial obstruction of the Roux loop, perhaps secondary to an adhesion or twist causing partial obstruction, as this can be relieved by surgery. Percutaneous transhepatic cholangiography (PTC) and radionuclide hepatic imaging are essential diagnostic measures for identifying the site of the obstruction in these cases. Prolonged antibiotic prophylaxis is necessary, particularly if there is no obstruction of the Roux loop. If cholangitis recurs frequently despite these measures, with deteriorating liver function, then liver transplantation should be considered.

Portal hypertension. Hepatic fibrosis is always present at the time of portoenterostomy and is reflected in an increase in portal venous pressure.[72,73] Approximately 60% of children who survive to 2 years will have endoscopic evidence of esophageal varices, although only about half of these will ever bleed.[74] The severity of the varices in older children is not related to the original degree of liver fibrosis or to the number of episodes of cholangitis.[69,74] As the average age at first bleed is about 3 years, some centers recommend endoscopic assessment of the upper gastrointestinal tract from 2 years of age.[37,75] Bleeding was found to be more common in those who were persistently jaundiced and in those who had suffered recurrent attacks of cholangitis.

The initial treatment of bleeding varices is supportive, with restoration of blood volume plus correction of coagulopathy and thrombocytopenia. Endoscopic sclerotherapy or variceal banding, with or without a Sengstaken tube, may be required for the control of severe bleeding.[76,77] Transjugular intrahepatic portosystemic shunt (TIPSS) has been used for infants with bleeding esophageal varices but is technically difficult, mainly due to periportal fibrosis and small portal veins. The frequency of repeat interventions is also higher in comparison with adults[78] (see also Chapter 15). The development and rupture of a splenic artery aneurysm is a rare but potentially fatal complication of long-standing portal hypertension in girls. Screening with an annual ultrasound scan is advised, and arteriographic embolization is indicated if an aneurysm is identified.[79]

Metabolic and nutritional consequences of post-Kasai cholestasis. Persisting cholestasis and diminished bile flow may cause malabsorption of fat and fat-soluble vitamins.[80] This may manifest as vitamin K–dependent coagulopathy. Intestinal absorption of calcium may be impaired and hydroxylation of vitamin D reduced as a consequence of hepatic fibrosis or cirrhosis, and it is therefore not surprising that changes in bone mass and clinical evidence of osteomalacia and rickets may occur. Osteoporosis and low levels of serum 25-hydroxyvitamin D were found in 16 of 20 jaundiced and three of 22 nonjaundiced patients with biliary atresia in one series. The role of vitamin E malabsorption in children who have undergone portoenterostomy is unclear, although neurological signs such as abnormal eye movements have been reported in cases of long-term vitamin E deficiency associated with cholestatic syndromes. Usually, vitamin deficiencies can be avoided by adequate oral supplementation. In severe cholestasis, parenteral supplements may be necessary. Malabsorption of long-chain triglycerides and fatty acids occurs in cholestatic patients, and replacing formula feeds with medium-chain triglyceride–enriched feeds often improves weight gain and steatorrhea. However, an adequate intake of essential fatty acids must be maintained. Copper and zinc metabolism may be abnormal in children after portoenterostomy, and high serum copper and low serum zinc levels have been reported in long-term survivors both with and without cholestasis[81,82] (see also Chapter 15).

Intrahepatic cyst formation. Biliary cystic changes may occur in the livers of long-term survivors and may be associated with recurrent attacks of cholangitis. The morphological appearances of the cysts have been classified into:[72]

- Discrete cysts not communicating with the enterostomy—type A
- Discrete cysts communicating with the enterostomy—type B
- Diffuse cystic dilations of the bile ducts—type C

Thirty-nine patients (25%) in a series of 154 who had undergone portoenterostomies between 1992 and 2000 developed jaundice and had intrahepatic cystic changes.[83] Single cysts were present in 23 patients and multiple cysts in 16. Jaundice and cholangitis were presenting signs in 13 and 15 patients in the respective groups. Interestingly, the cysts in seven patients decreased in size during courses of prolonged antibiotic treatment.

Single large cysts may be drained either percutaneously or via a cystoenterostomy operation, but repeated cholangitis in children with cystic change is an indication for liver transplantation.

Hepatopulmonary syndrome and pulmonary hypertension. As in other types of chronic liver disease, hypoxia with cyanosis on standing (platypnea) and exertion, dyspnea, and finger clubbing may be presenting features of diffuse intrapulmonary shunting and vascular dilation in long-term survivors of portoenterostomy. The mechanism responsible for these abnormalities is not known, although they appear to be more common in children with BASM.[84] Routine monitoring of peripheral oxygen saturation is essential to detect this syndrome early. The diagnosis is confirmed using arterial blood gas estimations with and without inspired oxygen. Ventilation–perfusion radionuclide lung scans are used to quantify the degree of shunting. This severe complication is resistant to conventional therapy, and liver transplantation is the only treatment.

Pulmonary hypertension can also develop in biliary atresia patients and may be caused by vasoactive substances such as endothelin and prostaglandin F_2, which are either not metabolized in the liver or are secreted by endothelial cells.[85] Assessments of pulmonary function and pulmonary hemodynamics should be part of the long-term follow-up in these children.

Malignant changes in the liver. Malignant changes (both cholangiocarcinoma and hepatocellular carcinoma) in cirrhotic livers of postportoenterostomy children have been reported.[86,87]

Results of portoenterostomy

The results of portoenterostomy have improved remarkably since 1974, when the median survival times were less than 1 year. After 1975, the survival, aided by earlier diagnosis and improved surgical technique, increased to a median of 18 years, and this has now been achieved in up to 60% of patients.[88]

A number of variables have been studied in an attempt to predict the effectiveness of the portoenterostomy procedure; some have been derived from perioperative data—e.g., age at surgery, macroscopic appearance of the bile ducts,[89] microscopic analysis of the resected specimen, and histopathology of the liver. The extent of histological abnormality (degree of fibrosis) at the time of surgery may indicate a poorer prognosis, but this has not been a consistent finding. The degree of portal hypertension at the time of the Kasai operation has been shown to correlate with a shorter time to transplantation, thus reflecting liver pathophysiology in a more functional way.[90]

The surgeon's experience has also been implicated as an important prognostic factor, although this has been disputed.[6,91] Perhaps more importantly, improved outcomes have been demonstrated with larger caseloads and more experience in specialized centers, as well as better communication between major centers and more peripheral units.[5,6,48,89,92]

The age at which surgery is carried out is the single most widely quoted prognostic variable, although some observers have shown little relationship in the majority of infants who are < 10 weeks of age.[93] However, uncorrected atresia of the bile ducts does result in progressive intrahepatic disease, and a clear detrimental effect of age on survival has been demonstrated in infants who are older than 100 days at the time of the portoenterostomy operation.[8]

In summary, the postoperative volume of bile flow is probably related to the size of bile ductules at the porta hepatis (> 100 μm), whilst the long-term quality of survival in those with adequate bile flow depends on the severity of secondary liver damage at the time of surgery and the incidence and severity of postoperative cholangitis.[43,94]

Approximately 70–80% of infants will show evidence of bile flow after surgery, which will be adequate to ensure survival to 5 years of age in more than 60%.[43,48] Furthermore, series in Japan, France, the United States, and Britain have suggested that about 30–40% of the children may survive to 10 years of age with their native liver intact, although approximately 40% have abnormal liver function tests, and in one French series 63 of 212 patients (23%) operated on between 1968 and 1983 were alive with their native liver 20 years after surgery, although all but two had signs of cirrhosis.[8,43,67,82,93–95]

Quality of life

Ohi has summarized the clinical status of 80 patients who survived for more than 10 years with their native liver.[96] Although over 70% were clinically well, one or more complications were recorded in 29% of the patients, who had a variety of symptoms and signs of liver dysfunction, including: 23 (29%) with increased fatigue, 10 (12.5%) with pruritus, four (5%) with abdominal pain, three (4%) with hepatopulmonary syndrome, three (4%) with jaundice, and two (2.5%) with recurrent pyrexia.

An assessment of the occupations of 82 patients showed that 44 were at school or college and 34 in work, and that four described themselves as housewives; six had married and four women had children. Valayer analyzed 25 patients over 15 years of age and did not find any specific problems related to puberty or sexual development, which was normal in all cases.[84,97]

Detailed quality-of-life assessments of a cohort of 25 Japanese patients were compared with an age-matched cohort of 21 from the United Kingdom.[88] The results showed that there were no significant differences between the assessments of the Japanese and British patients with regard to physical and social functioning, bodily pain, or emotional status, although there were marginal differences in indices of general health and vitality. Importantly, the study showed the similarity of results that can be achieved after portoenterostomy in different centers in the world. Only about 15% of infants operated on for biliary atresia will have a truly normal long-term existence, and even then late (adult) deterioration of liver function has been observed.[98]

Transplantation (see Chapter 21)

Biliary atresia is the commonest indication for liver transplantation during childhood.[99] Transplantation was initially used for survivors of the Kasai operation with life-threatening complications (e.g., variceal bleeding and chronic liver failure). However, with increasing experience in transplantation, early liver replacement has been undertaken in infants who have failed to respond to portoenterostomy.[100]

Some authors have suggested that transplantation should be performed as a primary procedure during infancy as an alternative to the portoenterostomy operation, but this ignores the potential for long-term survival in a significant proportion of children.[97] Kasai portoenterostomy should remain the first operation of choice and primary transplantation should be reserved for patients with advanced liver disease who present with hepatosplenomegaly, low albumin levels, growth failure, and severe complications of portal hypertension. The outcome for the complementary treatments of portoenterostomy and transplantation is now a long-term survival rate of over 85%, with expected catch-up growth and normal development.[101–103]

Choledochal cysts

Choledochal cysts are rare congenital localized dilations of the bile ducts. They are more common in *Asian* ethnic groups and their incidence is estimated to be about one in 100 000 live births in Western countries. More than two-thirds of cases are diagnosed in children under 10 years of age, and girls outnumber boys by about 3 : 1.

Anatomy and classification

The classification of choledochal cysts is based on that proposed by Todani *et al.* (Figure 19.4).[104] Type I cysts may be either cystic or fusiform and account for more than 70% of cases in most series. Next in frequency are type IVa cysts—i.e., multiple cystic dilations of the extrahepatic and intrahepatic ducts. Type II (diverticulum), type III (choledochocele), type IVb (multiple extrahepatic cysts), and type V (multiple in Caroli's disease, or single intrahepatic duct cysts) are very

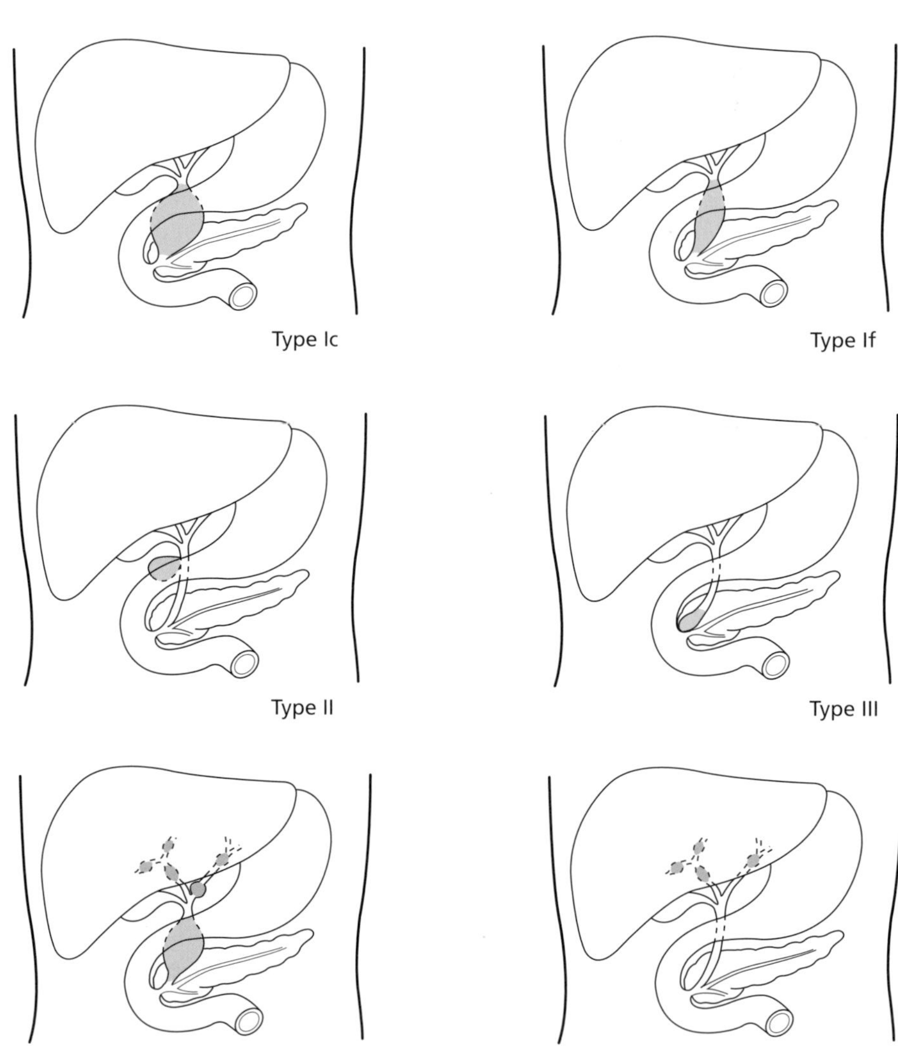

Figure 19.4 Classification of choledochal cysts. Type I dilations may be cystic (Ic) or fusiform (If) and typically associated with pancreaticobiliary malunion. Other types are: II (diverticulum), III (choledochocele), IVa (multiple cystic dilations of the extrahepatic and intrahepatic ducts), IVb (multiple extrahepatic cysts), and V (single or multiple intrahepatic duct cysts).

rare. Pancreaticobiliary malunion (see below) without cystic biliary dilation has been termed a *forme fruste* choledochal cyst, but it should be treated in a similar way to a fusiform choledochal cyst.

Pancreaticobiliary malunion

Choledochal cysts are frequently associated with an abnormal junction between the terminal common bile duct and the pancreatic duct, in which the ducts unite well outside the duodenal wall and are therefore not surrounded by the normal sphincter mechanism.[105] This abnormal long common channel, which often exceeds 5–10 mm in length, encourages reflux of pancreatic juice into the biliary tree, and high concentrations of pancreatic enzymes are then found in the bile. This may predispose to the development of bile duct and gallbladder cancer in adults.[105,106] Less frequently, bile refluxes into the pancreatic duct, precipitating pancreatitis. Pancreaticobiliary malunion is common in type I and IVa choledochal cysts, but is rarely seen with other varieties.

Pathology

In type Ic cysts, the choledochal dilation typically starts just above the duodenum and ends abruptly just below the bifurcation of the common hepatic duct. The gallbladder is often normal in size but may be enlarged, with a tortuous and dilated cystic duct. The wall of a choledochal cyst is thickened and composed of fibrous tissue, with occasional elastic and smooth-muscle fibers. The epithelial lining may be ulcerated, particularly in older children. In adults, epithelial metaplasia and dysplasia occur.[107] Hepatic histology varies from normal to mild periportal fibrosis through to biliary cirrhosis. Hilar duct strictures may be found with type IVa cysts.[108] Other biliary abnormalities are uncommon.[109] Portal hypertension may develop secondary to portal vein compression, or from hepatic fibrosis or cirrhosis. Malformations outside the biliary tree are rare.[110,111]

Etiology and pathogenesis

There are two principal theories. The first suggests that a choledochal cyst arises because of an acquired weakness of the wall of the bile duct secondary to reflux of pancreatic juice.[111–113] However, pancreaticobiliary malunion is not found in all patients with a choledochal cyst, and it may occur in others without duct dilation. The second theory proposes that obstruction of the distal common bile duct is the key event.[111] A stenosis is often seen just below a type I cyst, but whether this is congenital or acquired is unclear. Genetic factors appear to be likely, in view of the female preponderance and geographical distribution of the condition. However, familial choledochal cysts have rarely been reported, and twin studies have not identified any clear genetic predisposition.[114]

Clinical presentation

Choledochal cysts can present at any age, but most are diagnosed before 10 years.[110] Specific age groups present in different ways:

- Prenatal diagnosis. Choledochal cysts can be detected by ultrasound scan as early as 15 weeks' gestation.[13,110] Most are type I cystic lesions. Postnatally, affected infants who are otherwise well should be treated with early surgery (< 3 months), particularly if they are jaundiced. Some will have a cystic variant of biliary atresia, but progressive enlargement of the cyst during gestation and subsequent demonstration of dilated intrahepatic bile ducts favor true choledochal pathology.[115] Liver fibrosis may develop rapidly and is reversible by early surgery.[116] Early treatment also reduces the risks of cholangitis, progressive jaundice, and cyst perforation. The results of surgical treatment at this age are generally excellent.[12,117]
- Infants typically present with obstructive jaundice. Vomiting, fever, failure to thrive, and an abdominal mass may be noted. Even with pancreaticobiliary malunion, hyperamylasemia is not found, because the amylase concentration in pancreatic juice is low until about 1 year of age.[118,119] However, biliary concentrations of pancreatic lipase, elastase, and trypsin are significantly elevated in infants with a common channel.[119,120]
- Older children often present with abdominal pain. Of 72 children in the King's College Hospital series, 50 (69%) presented with jaundice, which was associated with abdominal pain in half and a palpable mass in seven.[110] In infants the jaundice is frequently persistent, but in older children it is often intermittent. In this same series, 13 children (18%) presented with recurrent abdominal pain alone, and plasma and/or biliary amylase values were elevated in all. The classic triad of jaundice, pain, and a right hypochondrial mass was present in only four (6%).

Diagnostic delay is common, highlighting the need for adequate investigation of jaundice, pancreatitis, or a dilated common bile duct.[110] A choledochal cyst should always be included in the differential diagnosis of jaundice and pancreatitis. On ultrasonography, the common bile duct diameter measures up to 3.5 mm in healthy children and up to 2 mm in infants.[121] A persistently dilated bile duct needs to be investigated further. Children with recurrent severe abdominal pain should have a plasma amylase level measured. The hyperamylasemia associated with pancreaticobiliary malunion can be accompanied by acute pancreatitis, but some children have only "biochemical" pancreatitis.[119,120] In these cases, hyperamylasemia may result from either diffusion of pancreatic amylase through the denuded epithelium of the cyst, or from cholangiovenous reflux of amylase-rich fluid induced by high choledochal pressure.

Complications

Choledochal cysts are prone to complications, which may be the presenting feature. These include:

• Cholangitis—presents with progressive jaundice, abdominal pain, fever, and often rigors. The causative organism is usually a Gram-negative organism.
• Rupture—typically occurs spontaneously in children under 4 years of age.[110,122] Intraperitoneal rupture causes biliary peritonitis, whereas retroperitoneal rupture is less dramatic. Clinical features include abdominal pain and distension, vomiting, fever, mild jaundice, and biliary ascites. Definitive surgery may be possible at the time of diagnosis, but temporary T-tube drainage of the choledochal cyst and delayed surgery once the inflammation has subsided and after the anatomy has been clarified is a safe alternative.
• Pancreatic disease—pancreaticobiliary malunion may be associated with recurrent acute pancreatitis, chronic pancreatitis, pancreatic duct protein plugs, and calculi.
• Gallstones—there was an 8% incidence in one Japanese series.
• Portal hypertension—may be secondary to portal vein compression, hepatic fibrosis, or cirrhosis.
• Malignant changes—this is a well-recognized complication, mainly affecting adults, although older children are also at risk.[123,124] A 12-year-old girl with a type IVa cyst and a long common channel complicated by carcinoma has been reported.[125] The age-related cancer risk has been estimated to be 0.7% in the first decade, 7% in the second decade, and 14% after 20 years of age.[126] Pancreaticobiliary ductal malunion is an important predisposing factor. The risk of malignancy is greatest in patients who have been treated with internal drainage of a choledochal cyst (cystoenterostomy).[127] Even after cyst excision, malignancy may affect incompletely excised extrahepatic ducts or dilated intrahepatic ducts, indicating the need for lifelong surveillance.[128] Malignant change carries a poor prognosis.

Investigations

Biochemical liver function tests may be normal or show evidence of obstructive jaundice. Hyperamylasemia may be detected during episodes of abdominal pain. Clotting abnormalities should be excluded in jaundiced patients.

Ultrasonography is the initial investigation of choice. The size, contour, and position of the cyst, the proximal bile ducts, vascular anatomy, and hepatic echotexture can all be accurately assessed together with signs of any complications. ERCP provides excellent visualization of the cyst, ductal anatomy, and pancreaticobiliary junction. PTC is an alternative. Both investigations are invasive and associated with a small risk of complications such as iatrogenic pancreatitis or biliary sepsis, and both are best performed under general anesthesia in children. ERCP should be avoided during an episode of acute pancreatitis. Magnetic resonance cholangiopancreatography (MRCP) is noninvasive and does not require the use of contrast agents or irradiation (Figure 19.5).[129] Bile and pancreatic secretions have a high signal intensity on T2-weighted images. However, definition of the pancreatic duct and common channel may be suboptimal, especially in infants, and calculi may be overlooked.[130] Ongoing developments may overcome these problems.[131]

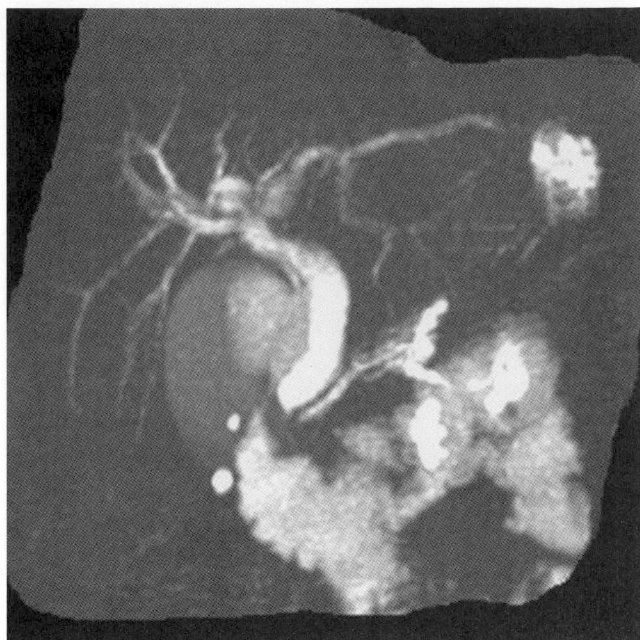

Figure 19.5 Magnetic resonance cholangiopancreatography of a 4-year-old girl who presented with pancreatitis. It shows a fusiform choledochal cyst and pancreaticobiliary malunion, with the pancreatic duct joining the distal bile duct at some distance from the ampulla. Total excision of the cyst, with a Roux-en-Y hepaticojejunostomy to the confluence of the hepatic ducts, is indicated. Distally, the pancreatic duct junction with the bile duct has to be protected. The conjunction can be identified with the assistance of intraoperative choledochoscopy.

Hepatobiliary scintigraphy may be useful in selected cases—e.g., in the jaundiced infant in whom a cystic variant of biliary atresia is suspected, or in some cases of cyst rupture. Radioisotope scanning is also useful for assessing biliary drainage after surgery. Computed tomography (CT) is helpful in evaluating pancreatitis. Laparoscopy and angiography are rarely necessary. In many patients, a detailed ultrasound scan supplemented by intraoperative cholangiography provides sufficient anatomical information, but ERCP or MRCP offer more definitive preoperative imaging[131] (Figure 19.5; see also Figures 4.8 and 4.9).

Surgical management

Radical cyst excision and hepaticoenterostomy is the optimum treatment for the more common types of choledochal cyst.[109,132] In experienced centers, the procedure can be performed safely at all ages with minimal morbidity. Simple anastomosis of the cyst to a loop of bowel (cystoenterostomy) should rarely, if ever, be undertaken, because of the inevitable long term morbidity (cholangitis, cholelithiasis,

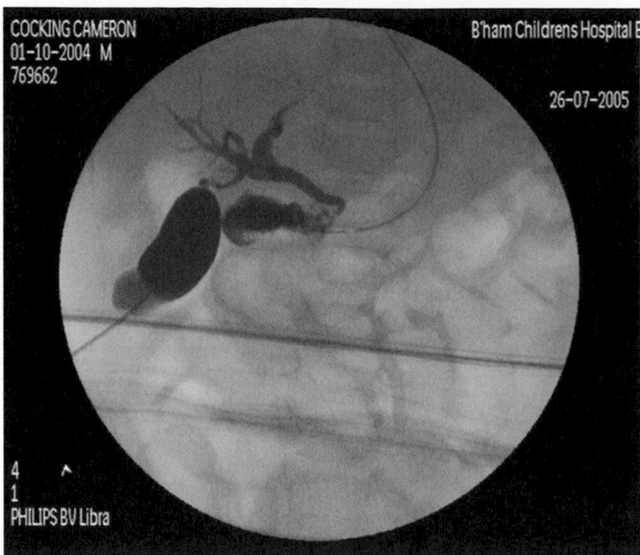

Figure 19.6 Operative cholangiogram via the gallbladder in a 1-year-old boy presenting with cholangitis. He had undergone duodenoduodenostomy for duodenal atresia in the first week of life. This shows dilated bile ducts and the cystic duct entering the right hepatic duct. Surgery included cholecystectomy and hepaticojejunostomy, with resection of the fusiform choledochal cyst. This case emphasizes the not infrequently associated biliary abnormalities seen in patients with foregut atresia.

pancreatitis, anastomotic stricture, biliary cirrhosis, and malignancy).[119,133]

Intravenous vitamin K is given to correct any coagulopathy, and prophylactic intravenous broad-spectrum antibiotics are given at the start of surgery. If the anatomy of the choledochal cyst has not been defined in detail preoperatively, operative cholangiography is carried out (Figure 19.6). A sample of bile is aspirated from the cyst for culture and measurement of pancreatic enzyme concentrations. The extrahepatic cyst is completely excised, oversewing the distal common bile duct just above its junction with the pancreatic duct. The exact distal anatomy can be clearly identified with perioperative endoscopy. The common hepatic duct is divided at the level of the bifurcation, the left hepatic duct opened, and a wide hilar bilioenteric anastomosis is constructed with a Roux loop of jejunum.[134,135] Hepaticojejunostomy is preferable to hepaticoduodenostomy, as the incidence of long-term complications is significantly increased with a duodenal anastomosis.[136] Any dilated proximal intrahepatic ducts and a dilated common channel should be inspected and cleared of debris. A liver biopsy is performed.

Preliminary T-tube drainage of a choledochal cyst is occasionally required for patients with cyst rupture or uncontrolled cholangitis. Cyst excision can then be performed when the patient is fit. Occasionally, portal hypertension or dense inflammation make radical excision hazardous, and intramural resection of the inner layer of the posterior wall of the cyst avoids damaging the portal vessels.[137] Patients with advanced biliary cirrhosis should be considered for liver transplantation.

In fusiform choledochal dilations, endoscopic sphincterotomy or transduodenal sphincteroplasty have been reported to provide short-term relief of symptoms, but this approach fails to address the long-term hazards of pancreaticobiliary malunion. Types II and III cysts have been successfully managed by more conservative approaches.[138,139] Localized, symptomatic type V cysts can be treated by hepatic resection, but more diffuse disease complicated by recurrent cholangitis and stone formation may require liver transplantation (see Caroli's disease, Chapter 10).

Results and complications

Radical cyst excision and hepaticoenterostomy achieve consistently good results.[110,132,140] Regression of hepatic fibrosis and early biliary cirrhosis has been recorded after surgery.[141] Early postoperative complications such as anastomotic leakage, bleeding, acute pancreatitis, and intestinal obstruction are rare. Long-term complications may be evident clinically or from routine biochemical liver function tests and ultrasound scan. An anastomotic stricture may develop up to 10 or more years postoperatively; there was a median of 14 years and a 9% complication rate in another Japanese series of 200 children followed for a mean of 11 years. Revision surgery was necessary for cholangitis due to anastomotic or ductal strictures, common channel calculi, and adhesive bowel obstruction. Biliary complications were more likely with type IVa cysts, or after anastomosis to the common hepatic duct. Reoperation was not required after hilar hepaticoenterostomy for type I choledochal cysts. There were no instances of malignancy. Anastomotic strictures were very rare in children undergoing surgery before 5 years of age.

Late postoperative cholangitis should be investigated using a combination of ultrasound, MRC, biliary scintigraphy, and/or PTC (with antibiotic prophylaxis). Although interventional radiological techniques may be able to remove stones and dilate strictures, surgery is usually required to revise a bilioenteric anastomotic stricture. Pancreatitis may develop years after cyst excision in patients with a common channel containing protein plugs or calculi, but this is rare after appropriate primary surgery. Endoscopic sphincterotomy may be valuable in such cases. Malignancy has been reported after choledochal cyst excision (see above), but adequate primary surgery should minimize this risk.[142,143]

Spontaneous perforation of the bile duct

Spontaneous perforation of the bile duct was first described in 1932 by Dijkstra, and since then over 70 cases have been reported in the literature.[144–147] The perforation occurs at the junction of the cystic and common hepatic ducts and is usually described as "punched-out." There is usually no obvious cause, although transient biliary obstruction, perhaps due to inspissated bile and a sudden increase in biliary pressure, seems likely in some cases. A developmental weakness of the bile duct has been suggested, but embryological studies of the development of the biliary tract have not identified any possible cause for this.[148,149]

Presentation and diagnosis

Clinical presentation is from 2 to 24 weeks of age, with abdominal distension accompanied by jaundice and acholic stools. Differential diagnoses include perforation associated with choledochal cysts, trauma, and *Ascaris* infestation of the bile duct.[147,150]

The infants usually have unremarkable birth histories and development until a rapid onset of generalized peritonitis, or an insidious onset of obstructive jaundice, pale stools, and dark urine. Three types of presentation have been described as acute peritonitis, localized peritonitis, and bile duct stenosis.[151] Of the three, localized peritonitis is the commonest type of presentation, manifesting as abdominal distension, intermittent vomiting, failure to thrive, and ascites. The vomiting may be severe enough to suggest an erroneous diagnosis of gastric outlet obstruction.[152] Often the infant is not pyrexial. Bile in the peritoneal cavity presents with greenish staining of hydroceles, hernial sacs, and the umbilicus.

Bile leakage in the porta hepatis results in severe inflammatory change, which can rarely cause a secondary stenosis of the lower portion of the common bile duct.[43]

Abdominal ultrasound may show a complex mass around the bile duct and duodenum, free intraperitoneal fluid, and in some cases dilated intrahepatic ducts. Biochemical liver function tests are abnormal, with a mild, conjugated hyperbilirubinemia and raised alkaline phosphatase and GGT levels. Biliary radionuclide imaging may show isotope within the peritoneal cavity, or a PTC will demonstrate a leak (Figure 19.7).

Treatment

The treatment is surgical in all cases. A laparotomy and cholangiogram performed with a catheter placed in the gallbladder, which may be thick-walled from the surrounding inflammation, will confirm the site of perforation and indicate whether there is any distal common bile duct obstruction from inspissated bile or stricture formation. Lilly *et al.* suggested a conservative surgical approach using peritoneal drainage alone.[153] However, except in patients with very small perforations and no evidence of distal bile duct obstruction, a more interventional method is preferable, as deaths have occurred from persistent bile leaks when peritoneal drainage has been used as the sole technique. A small T-tube can be placed in the common bile duct to provide a controlled biliary fistula and to allow recovery from the biliary peritonitis. This is left in situ for 2 weeks and then removed if repeat T-tube cholangiography shows no evidence of distal obstruction. In late-presenting cases, it may be necessary to resect a secondary bile duct atresia and reestablish biliary drainage via a hepaticojejunostomy.[154]

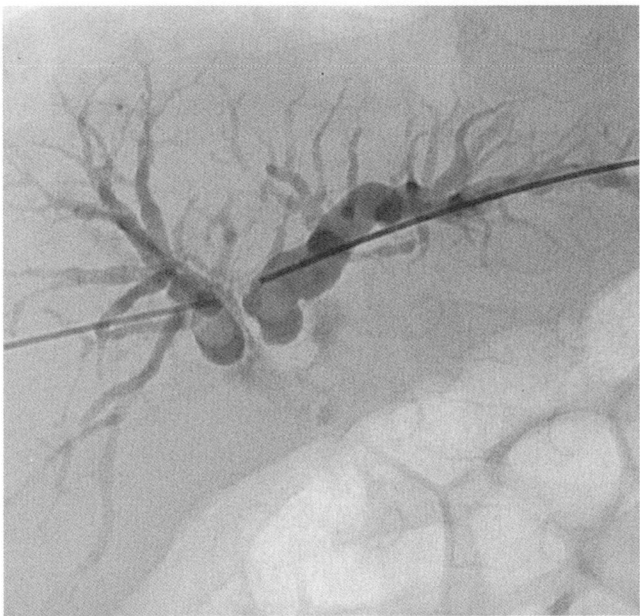

Figure 19.7 Percutaneous transhepatic cholangiogram (PTC) in a 6-week-old infant with jaundice from biliary obstruction secondary to spontaneous bile duct perforation. The dilated right and left hepatic ducts have been punctured at PTC with 22-gauge Chiba needles and contrast has been injected. Strictures involving the confluence of the right and left ducts are shown, with rounded filling defects in both main ducts due to biliary sludge. No contrast is seen in the extrahepatic bile duct and duodenum. The findings were confirmed at laparotomy, and a hepaticojejunostomy was carried out.

Inspissated bile syndrome

Bile duct obstruction caused by plugs of thickened bile was first described by Ladd in 1935.[3] The incidence increased during the 1950s and 1960s, perhaps because of the prevalence of untreated rhesus disease of the newborn associated with prolonged hemolysis and precipitation of bilirubin within the common bile duct (see also Chapter 16).

Infants with short bowel syndrome may have a history of episodes of dehydration, parenteral nutrition, prematurity, or diuretic therapy.[155] A prospective ultrasound study of neonates receiving parenteral nutrition visualized biliary sludge in 44% and discrete gallstones in 5% of cases.[156] Occasionally there are cholangiographic anomalies, such as an abnormal entry of the common bile duct into the duodenum or a hepatocystic duct anomaly, which may explain why some infants seem predisposed to develop inspissated bile syndrome. Although intraluminal obstruction is caused by inspissated bile, the two older patients in a series of nine cases had obstruction caused by distinct gallstones (at 4 and 6 months).[157]

Diagnosis and treatment

The differential diagnosis of inspissated bile syndrome in the neonatal period includes biliary atresia, but the diagnosis is usually obvious on abdominal ultrasonography, which may reveal dilated intrahepatic and extrahepatic bile ducts secondary to impacted inspissated bile in the distal common bile duct. Radionuclide scans will confirm biliary obstruction but are not diagnostic. The definitive investigation is PTC or laparoscopic cholangiography. Occasionally, this can be therapeutic, as flushing the biliary tree via a small catheter may clear the obstruction.[157] In some cases, irrigation can be similarly achieved with ERCP. If this fails, a laparotomy is indicated to decompress the biliary tree. The common bile duct is opened, the inspissated material washed out, and free distal drainage is reestablished (confirmed by cholangiography).

The use of choleretic agents (e.g., ursodeoxycholic acid 20 mg/kg/d) and biliary motility drugs (e.g., cholecystokinin) has recently been introduced to help avoid the need for surgery, as there is evidence that the lack of gallbladder activity during prolonged parenteral nutrition may potentiate the development of inspissated bile.

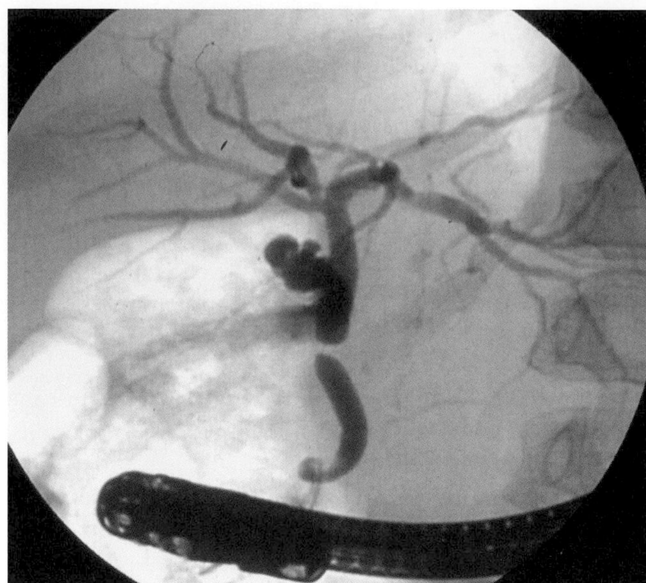

Figure 19.8 Endoscopic retrograde cholangiopancreatography in a 4-year-old girl who presented with intermittent jaundice. Treatment includes placement of an endoscopic stent or surgical removal of the isolated biliary stricture.

Benign bile duct strictures

Strictures of the extrahepatic bile ducts in children may result from trauma, surgery, radiotherapy for malignant disease, and spontaneous perforation.[158] Another type of idiopathic benign stricture has been described in seven children (six girls and one boy); these cases were not associated with any obvious etiological factor and were designated by the authors as "idiopathic."[155,159] They were characterized by a specific combination of histological features, which included fibrosis and chronic inflammation of the wall of the bile duct, loss of epithelium, and epithelial hyperplasia and regenerative changes. At least three of these four features were present in each case.

These isolated strictures (Figure 19.8) differ from the multiple strictures observed in sclerosing cholangitis, a condition in which the epithelium remains intact. In addition, long-term follow-up of the children with idiopathic lesions did not reveal any recurrence after resection or the development of any other disease. A similar condition has been described in adults, and hepaticojejunostomy is the treatment of choice in all age groups.[160]

Bile duct tumors

Painless obstructive jaundice is the presenting feature of these very rare lesions, which may be misdiagnosed as choledochal cysts or cholelithiasis. The diagnosis depends on accurate imaging of the biliary tract using a combination of ultrasonography, CT, MRCP, and ERCP. Malignant tumors occur more frequently than benign lesions (Table 19.3).[161–173]

Malignant

Rhabdomyosarcoma is the commonest primary tumor of the bile duct in children, and it should always be considered in the differential diagnosis of obstructive jaundice.[174] Approximately 100 cases have been reported to date. The median age at presentation is 3.4 years, and there is no gender predominance. Clinical signs include obstructive jaundice, fever, weight loss, and abdominal distension. Scanning of the biliary tract shows an extrahepatic mass, with solid material within dilated intrahepatic and extrahepatic bile ducts. PTC is useful in defining the extent of the tumor within the bile ducts. Local or distant spread is present in 30–40% of cases at the time of presentation.[175]

Macroscopically, the tumors are polypoid, with grape-like projections filling the lumen of the bile duct. Histological examination shows typical features of embryonal rhabdomyosarcoma with botryoid features. The cells are of mesenchymal origin and have a myxomatous appearance, with eosinophilic cytoplasm. The botryoid polyps are hypocellular and edematous. The tumor infiltrates beneath the bile duct epithelium and into the liver parenchyma, and it may also infiltrate surrounding structures such as the pancreas, stomach, and inferior vena cava and may even cause obstruction to the portal vein from external compression.

Until recently, the survival of these patients was dismal, with an average life expectancy of 6 months. However, an aggressive approach to treatment using a combination of chemotherapy, surgery, and radiotherapy has improved the outlook, with an estimated overall 5-year survival rate of 66% in a series of 25 children treated since 1972. The survival rate for the children who did not have metastatic disease at the time of presentation was 78%.[175]

Table 19.3 Specific conditions associated with childhood cholelithiasis.

Condition	Etiological factors	Reference
Cystic fibrosis	Abnormalities of biliary lipid and mucin composition. Common bile duct stenosis	Anagnostopoulos *et al.* 1993[161]
Down syndrome	Prenatal factors may be important, since calculi have been detected soon after birth	Toscano *et al.* 2001,[162] Sakopoulos *et al.* 2002[163]
Cardiac/liver transplantation	Multifactorial (hemolysis, cyclosporine-induced changes in bile and lipid metabolism, gallbladder stasis, furosemide therapy)	Sakopoulos *et al.* 2002[163]
Childhood cancer	Multifactorial (ileal conduit, parenteral nutrition, abdominal surgery, repeated blood transfusions, and abdominal radiotherapy)	Mahmoud *et al.* 1991[164]
Bone-marrow transplantation	Blood transfusions/chemotherapy	Safford *et al.* 2001[165]
Spinal surgery/injury	Immobilization, disturbed calcium hemostasis, blood transfusion	Teele *et al.* 1987[166]
Hepatobiliary trauma	Hemobilia	Reif *et al.* 1991[167]
Selective IgA deficiency	Gallbladder sepsis. Decreased bile acid pool due to intestinal losses	Danon *et al.* 1983[168]
Dystrophia myotonica	Impaired gallbladder emptying	Schwindt *et al.* 1969[169]
Chronic intestinal pseudo-obstruction	Impaired gallbladder motility	Shimotake *et al.* 1993[170]
Cholestatic/cirrhotic liver disease	Alagille's syndrome, PFIC, Gilbert syndrome and Wilson's disease	Lykavieris *et al.* 2001[171]
Congenital anomalies	Fibrosis around the distal common bile duct after surgical repair	Tchirkow *et al.* 1980,[172] Mali *et al.* 2007[173]

Carcinoma may arise in the biliary tracts of patients with untreated choledochal cysts. It has also been reported in residual extrahepatic and intrahepatic bile ducts after successful cyst excision.[142,176] The youngest case of carcinoma in a patient with no predisposing cause was a girl who was 17 years of age.[177] Surgical resection is required, if possible.

Liposarcoma. One case of this tumor has been reported in a child aged 2 years and 4 months, who had presented with jaundice and fever. The diagnosis was confirmed at postmortem.[178]

Benign

Inflammatory pseudotumor. The etiology of inflammatory pseudotumors of the bile duct is not known, although it has been suggested that they may arise in response to a local chemical or infective irritant. The macroscopic appearance of a resected lesion is of an encapsulated mass of yellow-brown tissue surrounding a compressed bile duct. Histological features consist of a mass of collagenous tissue with a mixed inflammatory cell infiltrate. Surgical resection and reconstruction of the biliary tract with a Roux loop of jejunum is curative.

Papilloma. Papillomas of the bile duct have been reported twice in children.[179] Surgical excision is essential, as they may develop areas of dysplasia and carcinoma.

Granular-cell tumor. There have been four reports of granular-cell tumors in children under 15 years of age.[180] These lesions are thought to arise from Schwann cells, and they are positive for S100 protein immunoreactivity, which is a neural marker.[181] The clinical presentation is with a stricture of the bile duct, and histology shows cells containing granular eosinophilic cytoplasm. Infiltration of surrounding structures may complicate surgical resection.

Cholelithiasis

Epidemiology

Estimates of the prevalence of gallstones in children vary depending on geographic area and age—0.5% of neonates in Germany, 0.13–0.2% of infants and children in Italy, and less than 0.13% of children in Japan.[162,182–184] Most studies of cholelithiasis in childhood show a bimodal distribution, with a small peak in infancy and a steadily rising incidence from early adolescence onward. In early childhood, boys and girls are similarly affected, but a clear female predisposition emerges during adolescence. Studies in Western children have shown a consistent increase in both the prevalence of gallstones and the incidence of cholecystectomy for cholelithiasis during the last three decades.[185–190] This may reflect improved detection due to the widespread use of diagnostic ultrasonography, and/or a genuine increase in the incidence of cholelithiasis.

Pathogenesis

There are four major types of gallstone: mixed cholesterol, pure cholesterol, and black or brown pigment stones. Mixed cholesterol stones are the commonest variety in adults, but are also found in obese adolescent girls. They develop from cholesterol supersaturation of bile in the presence of bile stasis; noncholesterol components include calcium salts and proteins. All four stone types can occur in children, but black pigment stones are relatively common and are seen in hemolytic disorders and in association with total parenteral nutrition.[191] Black pigment stones are formed from supersaturation of bile with calcium bilirubinate. Brown pigment stones are associated with biliary stasis and infection, and form more often in the bile ducts than the gallbladder. Rarely, calculi are composed of pure calcium carbonate.[192,193]

Biliary sludge is composed of mucin, calcium bilirubinate, and cholesterol crystals and appears echogenic on ultrasound but does not cast an acoustic shadow. Gallbladder sludge is typically found in association with total parenteral nutrition/fasting, pregnancy, sickle-cell disease, treatment with ceftriaxone or octreotide, and after bone-marrow transplantation. The natural history of biliary sludge is variable; it may disappear spontaneously or progress to gallstone formation. Persistent sludge may cause biliary tract complications.

Many etiological factors have been associated with cholelithiasis in children (Table 19.3). The dominant ones are biliary stasis, excess bilirubin load, and lithogenic bile.[194]

Hemolytic disorders

These include sickle-cell disease, hereditary spherocytosis, and thalassemia major. In each, the incidence of gallstones increases with age. The prevalence of pigment stones in sickle-cell anemia is approximately 10–15% in children under 10 years of age, but up to 40% in those aged 10–18 years.[195,196] About 10–20% of children with hereditary spherocytosis have evidence of cholelithiasis.[197] In thalassemia, gallstones are rare before 5 years of age but thereafter between 4 and 14% of children are affected.[198] Pigment stones may also complicate hemolytic uremic syndrome, ABO or rhesus incompatibility, and cardiac valve replacement. In the newborn, an excessive bilirubin load combined with an immature bilirubin excretion mechanism has been linked to pigment stone formation.

Ileal resection/disease

Ileal resection or disease is an unequivocal risk factor for cholelithiasis.[199] Symptomatic gallstones occur in 10–20% of children with short bowel syndrome.[200] Children with Crohn's disease affecting the terminal ileum are similarly at risk. The most likely mechanism is a disturbance of the normal enterohepatic circulation of bile salts causing a relative bile salt deficiency, which leads to incomplete solubilization of unconjugated bilirubin and calcium bilirubinate stones.

Total parenteral nutrition

The association between total parenteral nutrition (TPN) and biliary sludge/cholelithiasis is well established. Fasting and TPN promote biliary stasis by impairing both the enterohepatic circulation of bile acids and cholecystokinin-induced gallbladder contraction.[201] Premature infants are particularly susceptible to this complication. In a prospective sonographic study of 41 infants receiving TPN, gallbladder sludge was detected in 18 (44%) after a mean period of 10 days.[202] In 12 infants, the sludge cleared within 1 week of enteral feeding, but two of the remaining patients went on to develop asymptomatic gallstones.

Other risk factors

Adolescents with cholelithiasis typically have an adult pattern of risk factors—i.e., female gender, obesity, and sometimes teenage pregnancy.[167] Estrogens increase cholesterol excretion, whilst progesterone reduces bile acid excretion and slows gallbladder emptying.[194] Rapid weight loss is a risk factor in adults. Biliary obstruction and stasis from choledochal cysts and biliary strictures are known to promote gallstone formation. Numerous specific disorders have been associated with an increased incidence of gallstones in children (Table 19.3).

Clinical features

These are age-dependent.

• Infancy. In recent years, the number of reports of infants with gallstones has increased significantly. Gallstones have even been detected in the fetus.[203] Premature infants are more at risk, probably because of impaired gallbladder contractility, repeated blood transfusions, furosemide therapy, phototherapy, decreased bile acid output, and systemic or biliary infection.[204–206] Gallstones are frequently asymptomatic in infants, but they can cause nonspecific symptoms such as poor feeding and vomiting or give rise to acute cholecystitis, obstructive jaundice, or biliary perforation.[155,206]

• Childhood. Hemolytic disorders, ileal resection, and total parenteral nutrition are among the conditions predisposing to cholelithiasis in this age group.[187] Symptomatic children usually complain of abdominal pain in the right upper quadrant or epigastrium, associated with nausea and vomiting. Occasionally, the presentation is with obstructive jaundice or pancreatitis.

• Adolescence. More often, the patients are girls who are overweight and have a positive family history, but cholelithiasis due to other causes may also present in this age group.[187] There does not appear to be an association with the oral contraceptive pill.[207] Fatty food intolerance, biliary colic, and acute or chronic cholecystitis are reported in most patients with symptomatic stones.

Diagnosis

A clinical suspicion of cholelithiasis is readily confirmed by an ultrasound scan in a fasting patient. Gallstones are solitary or multiple, mobile, and typically cast an acoustic shadow; stones as small as 1.5 mm can be detected by ultrasound. Gallbladder wall thickness and common bile duct dilation can also be assessed. The sensitivity and specificity of ultrasound exceeds 95% for gallbladder cholelithiasis, but only 50–75% of common bile duct stones are detected. Between 20% and 50% of stones in children are radiopaque.

Radioisotope scanning with technetium Tc 99 m diisopropyl iminodiacetic acid (DISIDA) is highly sensitive and specific in the diagnosis of acute cholecystitis. Nonvisualization of the gallbladder in an otherwise patent biliary system suggests acute cholecystitis. MRC is being increasingly used to investigate complicated gallstone disease. With common bile duct stones, endoscopic retrograde cholangiography offers the additional advantage of therapeutic intervention.

Management

Nonsurgical. Infants with spontaneously resolving cholelithiasis have been reported by several authors.[155,190,206] Early surgery should therefore be avoided in the asymptomatic infant with gallbladder calculi. Clinical and ultrasound monitoring is appropriate, provided the infant has no other evidence of biliary tract disease. In infants remaining dependent on TPN, cholecystokinin or ursodeoxycholic acid may be helpful in clearing biliary sludge.[208]

In older children, the management of asymptomatic gallbladder calculi of nonhemolytic origin is controversial, as the natural history of the condition is poorly defined. Many children remain asymptomatic for at least a few years.[209] However, the likelihood of spontaneous resolution of cholelithiasis in older children is low (particularly if stones are calcified), and the child is at risk of gallstone complications for life.

Dissolution therapy for gallstones in children is of doubtful benefit. Despite prolonged treatment, low dissolution rates and high recurrence rates have been observed in adults with cholesterol stones. Calcified and pigment stones and patients with a nonfunctioning gallbladder are not amenable to treatment. Ursodeoxycholic acid is ineffective in children with radiolucent calculi complicating cystic fibrosis.[210]

Extracorporeal shock-wave lithotripsy of gallstones has rarely been reported in children, although successful treatment of a child with a single obstructing 7-mm stone in the distal common bile duct has been reported.[211]

Surgical. Symptomatic or complicated gallstone disease usually requires surgery. Cholecystectomy, either laparoscopic or through a small incision, is the standard treatment for gallbladder stones.[212] In the hemolytic disorders, asymptomatic calculi deserve special consideration. In hereditary spherocytosis, cholecystectomy is indicated for children with asymptomatic calculi who are undergoing splenectomy for hematological reasons.[197] Prophylactic cholecystectomy at the time of splenectomy is not indicated in those who do not have gallstones.[213] In sickle-cell anemia opinion is divided. Reasons for favoring elective cholecystectomy for asymptomatic stones include the increasing risk of complications with age, the higher morbidity of emergency surgery, and the difficulty of distinguishing cholecystitis from a sickle-cell abdominal crisis.[214,215] Perioperative complications are minimized by preoperative blood transfusion to correct anemia and reduce the proportion of hemoglobin S, together with avoidance of acidosis, hypovolemia, and hypothermia. Laparoscopic cholecystectomy is advantageous in these patients, and may obviate the need for preoperative blood transfusion in some cases.

Choledocholithiasis. Common bile duct stones are relatively uncommon, but children with sickle-cell disease and infants have a higher incidence.[189,206,216,217] Obstructive jaundice, cholangitis, and/or acute pancreatitis may occur. MRC may be helpful in diagnosis, but endoscopic retrograde cholangiography (ERC) also offers the opportunity for intervention.

There are several approaches to managing choledocholithiasis. ERC and sphincterotomy with stone retrieval can be undertaken before or after laparoscopic cholecystectomy, even in small infants.[218] Early ERC is recommended for common duct stones causing obstructive jaundice or cholangitis. Gallstone pancreatitis is less straightforward, since the stone usually passes spontaneously, after which laparoscopic cholecystectomy can be undertaken.[212] Surgical approaches to choledocholithiasis include cholecystotomy and irrigation in small infants or, in older children, choledochotomy and stone removal or transduodenal sphincteroplasty.[219] Some centers have used percutaneous retrieval techniques. In infants with a common bile duct stone, a short period of observation is often worthwhile if the infant is well, since spontaneous passage has been described, although with increasing laparoscopic expertise a primary laparoscopic exploration of the common bile duct has been advocated, with endoscopic sphincterotomy being used only for those with residual obstruction.[155,220]

Biliary dyskinesia

Biliary dyskinesia is defined as symptomatic biliary colic without cholelithiasis, with pain typically precipitated by fatty meals, and is becoming increasingly recognized as a cause of abdominal pain in children.[221–223] The diagnosis is suggested if there is an ejection fraction of < 35% as assessed either by cholecystokinin-stimulated hepatobiliary isotope scan, ultrasonography after a fatty meal, or computed tomography after a Lipomul challenge. In some centers in the United States, biliary dyskinesia has become the most frequent indication for cholecystectomy.[224] However—on a cautionary note—in one study of 55 patients with biliary dyskinesia (< 35% ejection fraction on hepatobiliary iminodiacetic acid scanning), 35 underwent cholecystectomy and 20 did not receive surgery. After a 2-year follow-up period, a similar

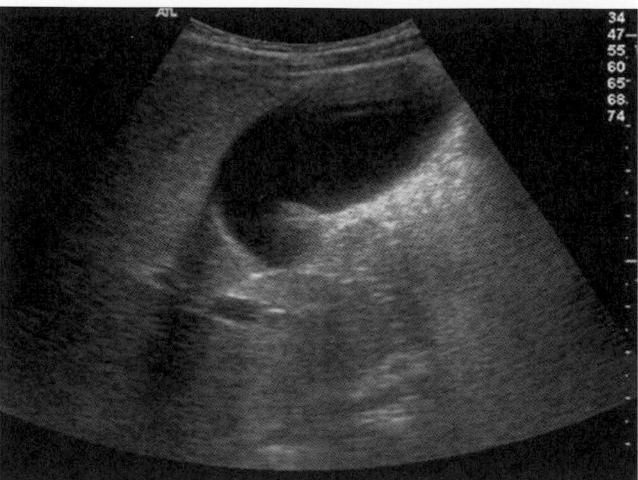

Figure 19.9 Acalculus cholcystitis is part of Kawasaki syndrome, in which the gall bladder is much distended. With resolution of the inflammatory process, the gallbladder settles spontaneously.

number in both groups showed improvement. Of all the patient characteristics evaluated, only weight loss was found to be significant for determining positive patient outcomes.[225]

Acalculous cholecystitis

Severe acute distension of the gallbladder in the absence of any other biliary tract disease is rare. If infection, ischemia, or chemical irritation supervenes, acute acalculous cholecystitis may occur. In Western countries, acute acalculous cholecystitis may develop after shock, trauma, cardiac surgery, burns, systemic sepsis, *Salmonella* infection, and parenteral nutrition.[226] In the tropics, *Salmonella typhi* infection and ascariasis should be considered, although no etiological factors are identifiable in some cases.[227] Acalculous cholecystitis has also been described in Kawasaki disease (Figure 19.9).

Clinical features include abdominal pain, vomiting, fever, localized tenderness and, in half of the cases, a palpable right upper quadrant mass. Laboratory investigations reveal leukocytosis, raised acute-phase reactants, hyperbilirubinemia, and mild hyperamylasemia. The differential diagnosis includes appendicitis, but this is readily distinguished by ultrasound, which shows a markedly distended gallbladder with a thickened edematous wall.

Initial management is conservative with antibiotics, intravenous fluids, and bowel rest. Cholecystectomy or cholecystostomy is indicated if there is progressive clinical deterioration, a persistent tender mass, and/or increasing gallbladder distension on ultrasound.

Congenital vascular abnormalities

The portal venous system develops from paired vitelline and umbilical veins, which drain the yolk sac and placenta, respectively. These veins intercommunicate around the embryonic duodenum and supply the developing hepatic sinusoids. There is also a constant venous anastomosis between the left portal vein and the hepatic veins, known as the ductus venosus, which allows placental blood from the left umbilical vein to bypass the hepatic sinusoids and empty directly into the right heart. Selective atrophy of these embryonic veins leaves the final arrangement as a single post-duodenal portal vein and an umbilical vein, which eventually atrophies to become the ligamentum teres, but which retains its connection with the left branch of the portal vein.[228]

Minor changes in the embryology of the portal venous system can result in major anatomical abnormalities of the portal vein, which include:

- A preduodenal position
- Cavernous transformation
- Duplication
- Congenital portosystemic communications

The formation of the inferior vena cava (IVC) is also a very complex process and is the end result of the coalescence of several venous channels. Anatomical abnormalities—for example, absence of the IVC—may be associated with abnormalities of the portal venous system.

Congenital portocaval shunts

These manifest as abnormal communications between the portal and systemic venous systems. They include extrahepatic congenital portocaval shunts, which have been classified into type 1, when portal venous blood is completely diverted from the liver into the vena cava; and type 2, when there is only partial portal blood flow into the cava.[229]

At an early stage in the normal development of the portal venous system, blood flows from the left umbilical vein into the ductus venosus, which acts as a bypass to the retrohepatic portion of the IVC. This arrangement allows the shunting of oxygenated placental blood directly into the heart via the IVC. Approximately 40–50% of umbilical blood traverses the ductus venosus, the remainder flowing through the liver sinusoids.[230] Closure of the ductus venosus and total flow of portal blood through the liver sinusoids are a consequence of the cessation of flow in the umbilical vein on the first day of life; the process is completed within 15–20 days of birth.

A congenital portocaval shunt and absence of the portal venous supply to the liver was first described by John Abernethy in 1793 in a 13-year-old girl with multiple malformations.[231] Since then, at least 12 type 1 cases have been described.[228,229,232] Type 1 cases occur commonly in girls and are usually associated with other anomalies (e.g., polysplenia, biliary atresia, cardiac anomalies, and liver tumors). The shunt itself is compatible with normal liver function, although in later life it may predispose to hepatic encephalopathy and liver tumors.[233]

Type 2 portocaval (side-to-side) shunts are less common.[229] Initial reports suggested that they presented in adult life with encephalopathy; however, the widespread use of abdominal ultrasound has led to their increased recognition at all ages, and an association with the development of hepatopulmonary syndrome has been noted.[234–239]

A familial incidence of type 2 shunts was reported in three brothers, two of whom presented at 3 and 5 years of age with encephalopathy. Symptoms and biochemical abnormalities were reversed successfully in two of the children, who underwent surgical shunt closure.[240] Cases presenting in infancy may be jaundiced.

The treatment of these shunts requires precise imaging and intraoperative measurement of portal vein pressures. Type 1 shunts are not treatable by conventional means, although transplantation has been performed for the associated liver anomaly. Type 2 shunts should be closed to prevent later encephalopathy, although it is important to ensure that the liver can tolerate the increase in portal venous flow without excessive rises in portal pressure.[241] Embolization with interventional radiology has also been reported both in humans and in dogs, where the anomaly is seen much more frequently.[233,242]

Hepatoportal arteriovenous communications

Abnormal communications between the hepatic arterial system and the portal venous system have been described within the liver. Such fistulas may be isolated congenital abnormalities and may present with severe portal hypertension, gastrointestinal bleeding, and failure to thrive (Figure 19.10). Occasionally, they may form part of a vascular syndrome such as Osler–Weber–Rendu syndrome (hereditary hemorrhagic telangiectasia).[243] Fistulas can also arise after blunt liver trauma or penetrating injury, including liver biopsy and surgery.[244]

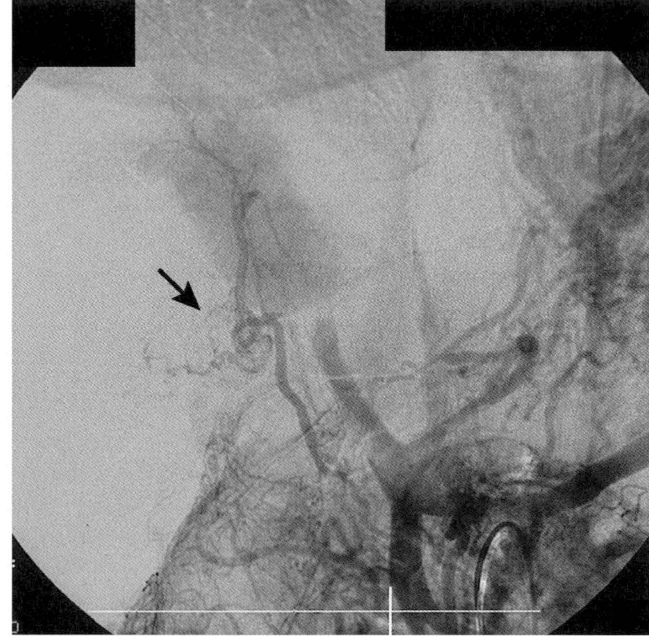

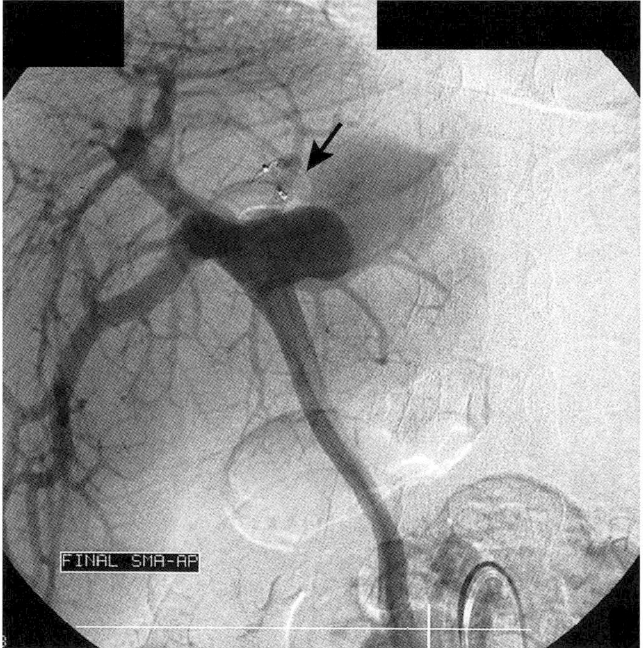

Figure 19.10 **A** The catheter aortogram shows an enlarged hepatic artery draining through a congenital arterioportal fistula into a left portal vein varix. **B** The superior mesenteric arterioportogram demonstrates that there is no main portal vein flow into the liver, due to reversal of portal flow via the fistula. There are a few portal vein collaterals draining portal blood into the caudate lobe, but most of the flow is through portosystemic collaterals in the upper abdomen. **C** After embolization of the fistula (seen as two small metallic rings), there is normal portal vein flow into the liver, with no collaterals. Doppler ultrasonography 24 h after embolization demonstrated thrombosis of the left portal vein varix.

Presentation during infancy with failure to thrive, splenomegaly, gastrointestinal upset with watery diarrhea, and bleeding has been described.[245] Ultrasound and Doppler flow studies of the portal vein proved crucial to the correct diagnosis and characteristically showed pulsatile portal venous flow with reversal during diastole. The diagnosis is confirmed by mesenteric arteriography, which shows the site and degree of the aberrant communication.

Fistulas confined to one segment of the liver are amenable to treatment with hepatic resection or embolization using a large (Amplatzer) device.[246] Multiple or bilobar fistulas can be controlled with multiple trials of superselective transarterial embolization or operative hepatic arterial ligation.[247] However, excessive embolization may cause significant ischemia of the liver and gut and should be undertaken only by experts. Collateral vessels may develop, with a recurrence of symptoms, which may be severe enough to warrant liver transplantation.[248]

Portal hypertension

Portal hypertension can be caused by a wide variety of conditions, each with a different natural history. It frequently presents with bleeding from esophageal varices, which is the commonest cause of serious gastrointestinal hemorrhage in children. Precise diagnosis, a sound understanding of the therapeutic options, and a multidisciplinary approach are essential for successful management.

Definition and pathophysiology

The portal vein carries blood to the liver from the gastrointestinal tract and spleen, contributing two-thirds of the liver's blood supply. The right and left portal veins undergo several divisions to supply each of the liver segments. Terminal portal tract branches supply the hepatic sinusoids.

Portal venous pressure is the product of:

- Blood flow—increased in cirrhosis due to splanchnic vasodilation.
- Vascular resistance—within the liver, this includes both fixed components (fibrosis and architectural distortion) and dynamic components (sinusoidal vascular tone).

A rise in portal pressure leads to splenomegaly and the development of portosystemic collaterals at various sites: the distal esophagus and gastric cardia (esophageal and gastric varices); the anal canal (anorectal varices); the falciform ligament (umbilical varices); and varices in the abdominal wall and retroperitoneum. The junction between mucosal and submucosal varices in the lower 2–5 cm of the esophagus is the usual site of rupture leading to variceal bleeding.[249] Portal hypertension is defined by an increased hepatic venous pressure gradient (> 5 mmHg), which is the difference between wedge hepatic venous pressure (an indicator of portal venous pressure) and free hepatic venous pressure. A gradient of more than 12 mmHg is necessary for the development of esophageal varices.[250] Although the relationship is not linear, the risk of variceal bleeding is increased in larger varices and in those with a higher internal pressure and wall tension.[251] In established cirrhosis, the risk of variceal bleeding is related to the severity of the liver disease.

Classification, etiology, and clinical features

Portal hypertension (PHT) in children may be due to:

- Primary venous obstruction at a prehepatic level (e.g., portal vein obstruction), intrahepatic level (e.g., hepatoportal sclerosis), or posthepatic level (e.g., Budd–Chiari syndrome). Rarely, an arterioportal venous fistula causes portal hypertension in an unobstructed system.
- Intrinsic liver disease (e.g., cirrhosis, fibrosis, nodular hyperplasia).

Chronic liver disease is the commonest overall cause of portal hypertension, but portal vein occlusion (PVO) is the most frequent cause of extrahepatic portal hypertension. Occasionally, the picture is mixed, as in cirrhosis complicated by portal vein thrombosis. Presentation is typically with acute gastrointestinal hemorrhage (hematemesis and/or melena) and/or splenomegaly, or as part of the manifestation of chronic liver disease. Varices, ascites, and bleeding in patients with cirrhosis identify four clinical stages, of increasing severity:

- Stage 1: no varices, no ascites
- Stage 2: varices, no ascites
- Stage 3: ascites, with or without varices
- Stage 4; bleeding, with or without ascites[94]

Children with PVO typically present with variceal bleeding at a younger mean age (5 years) than those with cirrhosis (8 years), but the onset of hemorrhage can occur at any age.[37] The risk of bleeding in PVO may decrease with advancing age, concomitant with the spontaneous development of portosystemic collaterals.[252] A small proportion of children with PVO have small varices, which do not bleed.[253]

An upper respiratory tract infection and, historically, aspirin therapy may be a precipitant. Anecdotal reports suggest that air transport is an additional trigger. Splenomegaly may be associated with evidence of hypersplenism. However, unlike cirrhotic patients, humoral immunity is preserved in those with PVO. Ascites usually denotes the presence of chronic liver disease, but may occur transiently after a major variceal bleed in those with extrahepatic portal hypertension. Encephalopathy may complicate an episode of bleeding in cirrhotic patients, but is rarely detectable in children with PVO.

Portal hypertension may cause mucosal edema in the small intestine, leading to malabsorption, protein loss, and failure to thrive. Growth failure is common in cirrhosis and can also be found in children with PVO.[254,255] In established PHT, dilated cutaneous collateral veins carry blood away from the umbilicus toward the tributaries of the vena cava (caput medusae). In long-standing disease, varices around the common bile duct may cause bile duct dilation and rarely obstructive jaundice. Rarely, pulmonary hypertension may coexist with portal hypertension, more often in children with cirrhosis than those with PVO.[256,257]

Prehepatic

Portal vein occlusion. PVO accounts for approximately 30% of all children with bleeding esophageal varices.[258,259] Many etiological factors have been implicated (Table 19.4).[260]

Umbilical vein catheterization in the newborn, with or without infusion of irritant solutions, and umbilical sepsis are recognized precipitants in up to 30% of patients.[252] However, small prospective studies indicate that this is a rare complication of umbilical catheters.[261] Thrombophilic disorders may predispose to portal vein thrombosis, but the results of investigations have to be interpreted cautiously. Circulating levels of natural anticoagulant proteins (protein C, protein S, and antithrombin III) are commonly decreased as a result of PVO.[262,263] Currently, the minority of patients with PVO with a true inherited thrombophilia can usually only be established by investigation of family members.

The pattern of portomesenteric venous obstruction may provide a clue to etiology.[264] In myeloproliferative disorders and severe thrombophilia, extensive thrombosis involving portal, mesenteric, splenic, hepatic, and deep veins may be present. Intra-abdominal sepsis (local inflammation and/or portal pyemia) and trauma may cause PVO, with or without involvement of the superior mesenteric vein. Rarely, isolated splenic vein obstruction is found and may be associated with pancreatitis.[265]

Table 19.4 Causes of portal vein occlusion.[260]

General factors
Developmental malformations
Septicemia
Thrombophilia
Myeloproliferative disorders
Paroxysmal nocturnal hemoglobinuria
Protein C deficiency
Protein S deficiency
Antithrombin III deficiency
Factor V Leiden mutation
Antiphospholipid antibodies (includes lupus anticoagulant and anticardiolipin)
Factor II (prothrombin) gene mutation (G20210A)
Homocystinemia
Local factors
Umbilical sepsis, catheterization, infusion of irritant solutions
Intra-abdominal sepsis and portal pyemia
Abdominal trauma (including surgical)
Structural lesions—e.g., portal vein web
Cholangitis/choledochal cyst
Pancreatitis
Malignant disease/lymphadenopathy
Splenectomy

In the majority of children with isolated PVO, the etiology is unknown. The portal vein is typically replaced by multiple venous collaterals, the so-called portal vein cavernoma. Associated anomalies are uncommon, but include congenital heart disease, anomalous IVC, choledochal cyst, intestinal malrotation, duodenal atresia, and craniofacial dysostosis.[264,266]

Intrahepatic

The intrahepatic causes of portal hypertension are diverse. Some conditions predominantly affect the venous circulation through the liver (e.g., hepatoportal sclerosis, schistosomiasis, and veno-occlusive disease), but the majority are intrinsic diseases of the liver (e.g., cirrhosis, fibrosis, nodular hyperplasia).

Hepatoportal sclerosis. In a small proportion of children with portal hypertension, the portal vein is patent but there is presinusoidal venous obstruction from subendothelial thickening of intrahepatic portal venous radicles.[267,268] There are striking similarities to idiopathic portal hypertension in Japan and noncirrhotic portal fibrosis in India.[269] Biochemical liver function is normal. Initially, liver histology is relatively normal, but portal tract fibrosis subsequently develops. Angiography confirms intrahepatic portal vein obstruction. The etiology of this condition is unknown. Most cases are not progressive and respond well to treatment of symptomatic esophageal varices.

Veno-occlusive disease. In this form of hepatic venous obstruction, there is a toxic injury to the sinusoidal endothelium, leading to occlusion of centrilobular veins and hepatic venules, sinusoidal congestion, and hepatocyte necrosis. In the West Indies, South Africa, India, and the Middle East, the condition is associated with ingestion of toxins (pyrrolizidine alkaloids) found in food or herbal teas.[270] In Western countries, veno-occlusive disease is seen after irradiation and/or cytotoxic drug–induced injury to the liver.[271,272] A high incidence has been recorded in bone-marrow transplant recipients.

The clinical features are similar to those in Budd–Chiari syndrome, with a rapid onset of painful hepatomegaly and ascites. If the child survives the acute stage, cirrhosis and portal hypertension may develop. After bone-marrow transplantation, the onset is usually manifest by jaundice, abdominal pain, ascites, and weight gain within 1 month of grafting, but one-third of patients are asymptomatic[273] (Chapter 16). Treatment is largely supportive and includes the administration of diuretics and *N*-acetylcysteine. Thrombolytic therapy is of limited benefit, but defibrotide, a drug with antithrombotic and thrombolytic properties, has shown promise in uncontrolled studies.[274] Low-dose heparin and ursodeoxycholic acid may have prophylactic roles.[272,275]

Cirrhosis and congenital hepatic fibrosis (see Chapters 10 and 15). Biliary atresia is the commonest cause of portal hypertension in this category, but there are many other conditions, including cystic fibrosis, autoimmune hepatitis, α_1-antitrypsin deficiency, and congenital hepatic fibrosis.

Posthepatic

Budd–Chiari syndrome. This is due to hepatic venous thrombosis, typically secondary to an underlying myeloproliferative disorder or thrombophilic state and rarely membranous obstruction to the inferior vena cava at the cavoatrial junction.[276–278] Most patients are young adults, and the condition is rarely seen in children.[279] In adolescent girls, the oral contraceptive pill may precipitate onset. Similar clinical features develop after hepatic vein occlusion from trauma, malignancy, or surgery and with retrohepatic IVC obstruction.

The clinical features include hepatomegaly, intractable ascites, symptoms and signs of portal hypertension, and progressive cachexia. Jaundice is variable. The caudate lobe is frequently spared because of its independent venous drainage directly into the IVC. Caudate lobe hypertrophy may compress the cava, causing lower limb edema (Figure 19.11). The onset may be acute (when symptoms of abdominal pain, distension, and diarrhea may be severe), but is more often chronic.

Chronic constrictive pericarditis may cause liver damage similar to that seen in chronic Budd–Chiari syndrome. Echocardiography should help confirm the diagnosis. Treatment, which may include pericardectomy, leads to progressive resolution of the hepatic changes.

Investigation

Hematology

A full blood count may show anemia, leukopenia, and/or thrombocytopenia from hypersplenism. The prothrombin time is commonly prolonged in patients with intrinsic liver disease or Budd–Chiari syndrome. In PVO, the prothrombin time is often slightly prolonged in association with a reduced factor VII concentration. The presence of reduced procoagulant and anticoagulant protein concentrations in PVO is probably due to reduced portal blood flow and/or portosystemic shunting.[263] In patients with Budd–Chiari syndrome, an underlying myeloproliferative disorder or thrombophilic state should be excluded by bone-marrow aspirate, and estimation of protein C, protein S, factor V Leiden, and lupus anticoagulant.

Biochemical liver function tests

In PVO, plasma albumin may be reduced following a variceal bleed, but biochemical liver function is essentially normal. Intrahepatic diseases usually cause abnormal liver function, but routine biochemistry can be normal in well-compensated cirrhosis. In Budd–Chiari syndrome, both liver and renal function may be disturbed.

Abdominal ultrasound scan

This confirms nonspecific features of portal hypertension such as large collateral veins and splenomegaly. The hepatic echotexture may indicate the presence of chronic liver disease. Color Doppler flow studies provide information on the direction and velocity of flow in the portal vein, hepatic veins, and vena cava.

Gastrointestinal endoscopy

Endoscopy can be used to evaluate gastroesophageal and anorectal varices and mucosal features of portal hypertension at all ages. Esophageal varices are graded according to severity. Large varices may show "red signs" of recent or impending variceal hemorrhage; these stigmata include "cherry-red spots" and "varices on varices" (see Figure 15.9). Endoscopic ultrasound assessment of submucosal and paraesophageal varices is a distinct advance, with diagnostic accuracy (see Chapter 2). Portal gastropathy is characterized by mucosal hyperemia and dilated submucosal veins.

CT and magnetic resonance imaging

Both modalities are useful in evaluating focal liver lesions associated with portal hypertension and in Budd–Chiari syndrome. In the latter, the findings depend on the duration and degree of venous obstruction; in chronic cases, there is splenomegaly and ascites and the liver parenchyma shows patchy contrast enhancement and caudate lobe hypertrophy. In PVO, a variable degree of liver atrophy may be seen.

Angiography

Magnetic resonance angiography is increasingly being used as a noninvasive alternative to conventional angiography. It confirms the diagnosis of PVO and assesses the patency and caliber of veins throughout the portomesenteric system. Angiography is particularly important when considering portosystemic shunt surgery, including meso-Rex surgery, and when assessing patients with a thrombosed or abnormal portal vein before liver transplantation. Conventional angiography can be performed by several routes, but the commonest is by indirect portography. Direct splenoportography after percutaneous needle puncture of the spleen also makes it possible to measure splenic pulp pressure (an index of portal hypertension), which may be of value in assessing anastomotic portal vein strictures after transplantation. Percutaneous transhepatic portography is occasionally used. Hepatic venography shows a typical "spiderweb" pattern of venous collaterals around hepatic vein thrombosis in Budd–Chiari syndrome. Inferior vena cavography or magnetic resonance venography may be necessary to determine the patency of the IVC or the intrahepatic portal and Rex veins.

Percutaneous liver biopsy

If there are no contraindications, a biopsy is usually

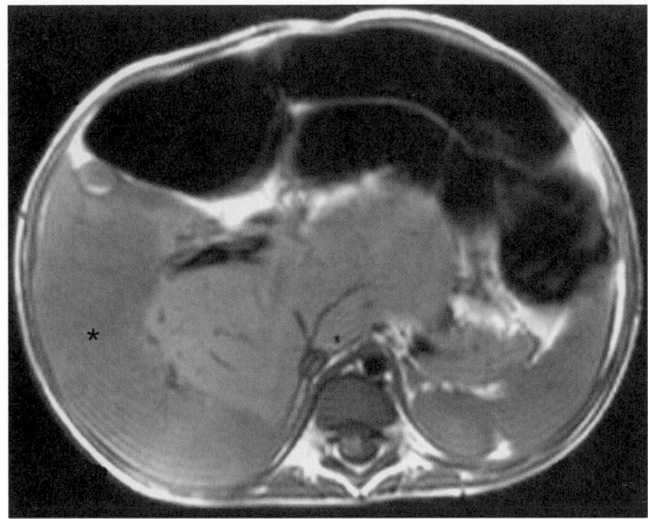

A

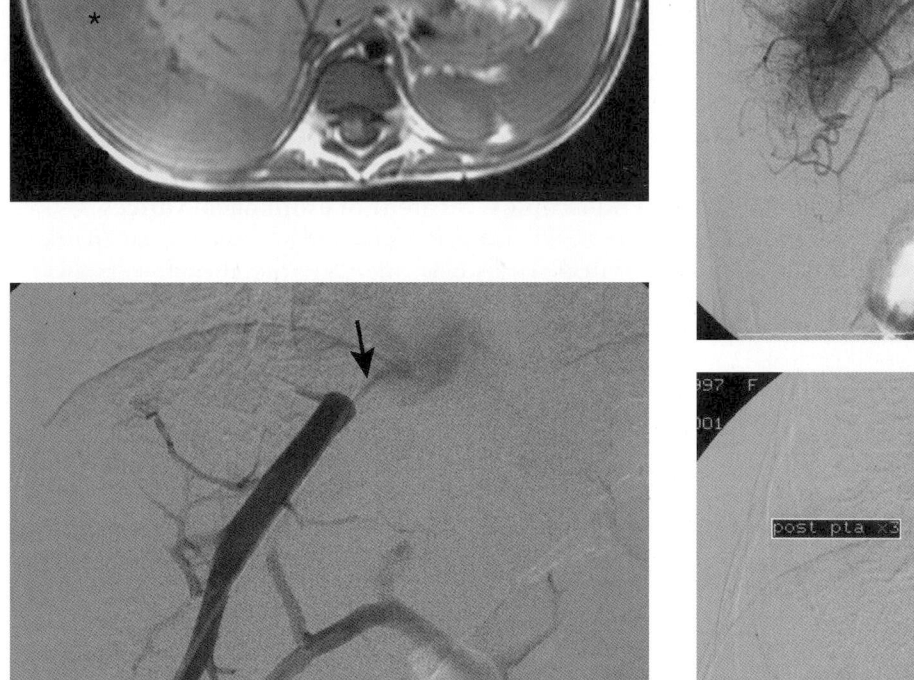

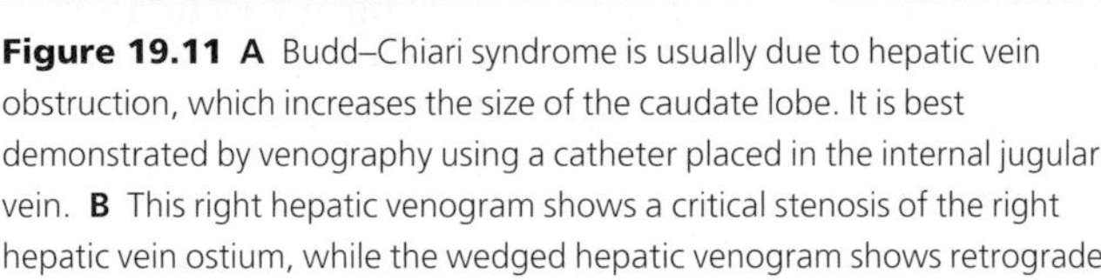

B

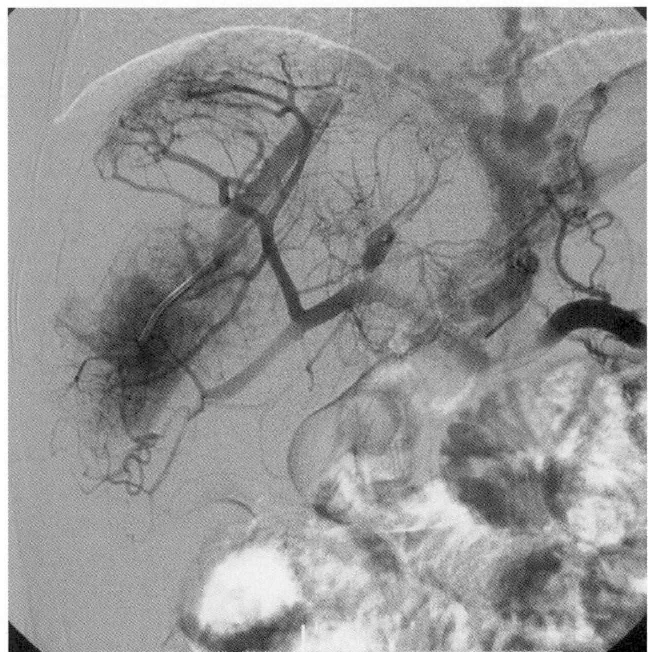

C

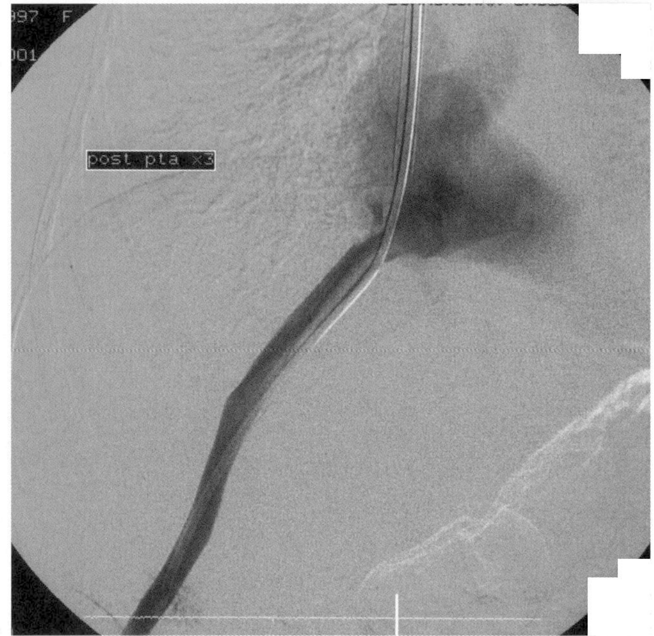

D

Figure 19.11 A Budd–Chiari syndrome is usually due to hepatic vein obstruction, which increases the size of the caudate lobe. It is best demonstrated by venography using a catheter placed in the internal jugular vein. **B** This right hepatic venogram shows a critical stenosis of the right hepatic vein ostium, while the wedged hepatic venogram shows retrograde filling of the portal vein and filling of varices in the upper abdomen as a result of the portal hypertension (**C**). **D** After balloon angioplasty and dilation, the right hepatic vein stenosis has been abolished, with improved blood flow, a reduction in the pressure gradient, and resolution of the portal hypertension.

undertaken to diagnose any underlying liver disease. In extrahepatic PVO, the liver architecture is normal, but mild periportal fibrosis may be seen. In hepatic vein obstruction, liver biopsy typically shows marked venous congestion around central venules, with hepatocyte necrosis; in chronic cases, there is progression to hepatic fibrosis and cirrhosis.

Management

If portal vein thrombosis develops acutely and is diagnosed promptly, anticoagulant or thrombolytic treatment may restore normal patency.[280,281]

In established portal hypertension, treatment includes the emergency management of active bleeding and the prevention of recurrent bleeding after a first episode (secondary prophylaxis). Primary prophylaxis should be considered in patients who have never bled. In children with good liver function and bleeding varices (e.g., PVO or congenital hepatic fibrosis), treatment is focused on portal hypertension, whereas in cirrhotic patients management is heavily influenced by the severity of their liver disease.

Emergency management of variceal bleeding

(Table 19.5; see also Chapter 15, Figure 15.7 and Table 15.7) Bleeding from esophageal varices is life-threatening and requires hospital admission. The mortality is closely related to the severity of any underlying liver disease.

Somatostatin reduces splanchnic blood flow and portal pressure with minimal short-term side effects, but its plasma half-life is less than 3 min. Octreotide, a long-acting analog of somatostatin, has a plasma half-life of more than 1 h and has largely superseded vasopressin and terlipressin treatment, which have side effects due to systemic vasoconstriction. Most, but not all, studies in adults have shown that octreotide is effective in controlling acute variceal bleeding, particularly when used in combination with endoscopic therapy.[282]

Balloon tamponade is rarely required to control active variceal bleeding. A Sengstaken-type tube can be inserted by an experienced clinician after the airway has been secured by endotracheal intubation. Only the gastric balloon need be inflated, and correct positioning has to be verified by radiography. Moderate traction is applied by taping the tube to the side of the face; excessive traction may cause mucosal ulceration or catastrophic balloon displacement. The balloon is deflated after 12–24 h at the time of endoscopy. Balloon deflation may be followed by severe bleeding, especially with gastric fundic varices.

Table 19.5 A guide to the emergency management of bleeding esophageal varices.

Resuscitation

- Airway (must be secure)
- Breathing (give oxygen if shocked)
- Circulation: insert two intravenous cannulae (22 G or larger) and commence intravenous fluids (5% dextrose if well perfused, colloid if poorly perfused)

Investigation

- Full blood count, clotting, urea, creatinine, electrolytes, liver function tests
- Blood cultures and cross-match (at least two units of packed red cells)
- Monitor and maintain blood glucose
- Accurate monitoring of (a) fluid balance and (b) cardiorespiratory status
- Watch for encephalopathy

Treatment

- Nil by mouth
- Ranitidine 1 mg/kg i.v. t.d.s. and oral sucralfate
- Intravenous antibiotics if evidence of sepsis
- Ensure that an appropriate-sized pediatric Sengstaken tube is available
- Transfuse packed red cells slowly aiming, for Hb approximately 10 g/dL (avoid overtransfusion)
- Give vitamin K 1–10 mg slowly i.v.
- Correct coagulopathy with fresh frozen plasma and platelets
- Octreotide infusion: bolus dose of 1 μg/kg i.v. (maximum 50 μg) over 5 min followed by infusion at 1–3 μg/kg/h (maximum 50 μg/h) via dedicated line. Continue infusion until 24 h after bleeding ceases and wean off slowly over 24 h
- Consider prophylaxis against encephalopathy if poor liver function
- Urgent upper gastrointestinal endoscopy within 24 h to confirm source of bleeding and to treat varices by banding or sclerotherapy

Endoscopic treatment of esophageal varices

Injection sclerotherapy. Introduced by Crafoord and Frenckner in 1939, endoscopic injection sclerotherapy (EIS) was a standard technique for inducing variceal thrombosis for many years, but has largely been superseded by esophageal banding.[281,283] EIS is applicable to all age groups and is best performed with the patient under general anesthesia with an endotracheal tube in place. It is now only used in small infants, in whom it is not possible to pass the endoscope with the banding equipment. A variety of injection techniques and sclerosants have been used, with 5% ethanolamine oleate being most widely used.[284] Between 1 and 3 mL of sclerosant are injected into each of the major variceal columns just above the gastroesophageal junction).[285] Para-variceal injection or a combination of the two is equally efficacious.

Varices should be initially injected every 1–2 weeks and then at monthly intervals until sclerosis is complete. Patients are given oral sucralfate for 48 h and ranitidine for 2 weeks after each injection session to reduce complications due to ulceration.[286] An endoscopic review is carried out after 6 months and then annually, but only large recurrent varices require treatment.

Tissue adhesives such as cyanoacrylate have been used as an alternative sclerosant in adults. This liquid preparation transforms into a solid after injection into a varix, thereby achieving hemostasis. It may be advantageous in treating gastric varices and endoscopically accessible ectopic varices. The possibility of postinjection venous embolization of cyanoacrylate is a potential concern in children, although gastric varices may be best addressed by direct suture or portosystemic shunt surgery.[287,288]

Efficacy, safety and late sequelae. EIS is a highly effective treatment for esophageal varices and can control bleeding in most cases.[258] Five to six injection sessions may be required. Long-term efficacy in children with PVO has been documented at a mean follow-up of 9 years after complete sclerosis.[289] Gastric variceal bleeding can be managed by injection of thrombin,

TIPPS, or portosystemic shunt surgery. EIS alone was effective in more than 80% of cases.[290]

Complications. Transient retrosternal discomfort and fever are common after EIS and usually resolve within 48 h.[291] Antibiotic prophylaxis is given to patients who are at risk of bacterial endocarditis, those with cirrhosis and ascites, and those who are immunosuppressed. Major complications of sclerotherapy include esophageal stricturing (which responds to dilation), recurrent esophageal varices, and interim bleeding.[258] Some children experience intermittent dysphagia and heartburn secondary to esophageal dysmotility and gastroesophageal reflux.[292] Dissemination of the injected sclerosant causing distant complications has been rarely reported. The potential long-term risk of neoplasia is a concern, but there are very few reports of this potential association and systematic studies have failed to support a link.[293,294]

Variceal ligation (banding). In this technique, the varix is aspirated into a transparent cylinder fitted onto the end of a flexible endoscope, and an elastic band is released by a tripwire passing through the biopsy channel. Introduced by Stiegmann *et al.* in 1989, endoscopic variceal ligation (EVL) causes strangulation of the varix, which then thromboses and sloughs.[295] Treatment begins with ligation of the most distal varix in the esophagus just above the cardia. Up to four bands can be applied to the varices at each session; the treatment is repeated after 1–2 weeks and then monthly until the varices have been obliterated. Multiple-band devices allow the application of several bands with a single pass of the endoscope.[77]

In adults, EVL is regarded as the method of choice for treating active variceal bleeding and for preventing rebleeding from esophageal varices. Whilst EVL and EIS are similarly effective, EVL offers more rapid eradication with fewer treatment sessions and lower complication rates. Esophageal ulcers caused by banding are more superficial and resolve more quickly than those induced by sclerotherapy, and the incidence of esophageal stricture and systemic complications is lower.[296,297]

Several small studies have confirmed the safety and efficacy of EVL in children.[77,298,299] Variceal eradication is achieved after a median of two to four sessions. Reported complications have included interim bleeding, esophageal perforation, and recurrent varices. Currently, technical difficulties render the technique more hazardous in small children (< 10 kg) and if there is brisk bleeding. Variceal banding has also been used successfully to prevent a first bleed in children with portal hypertension and enlarging varices. In one prospective study, 28 of 37 children with portal hypertension and varices had eradication of varices with a mean of two band ligation sessions.[300] EVL and EIS are not mutually exclusive, and a combination of the two can be particularly useful in some children.[301]

Ectopic varices

The development of varices at sites other than the esophagus or stomach (ectopic varices) poses a small risk of bleeding in the long term. This risk is greatest in PVO.[302,303] Ectopic varices are more common in the duodenum, at sites of previous intestinal anastomoses, and around stomas. Bleeding from ectopic varices should prompt investigation by endoscopy, possibly capsule endoscopy, and angiography. Recurrence is common after local resection, and portosystemic shunting or liver transplantation, depending on the underlying pathology, are often required to control persistent bleeding. In contrast, significant bleeding from anorectal varices and hemorrhoids, which are found in up to one-third of children with portal hypertension, is uncommon and can often be controlled by local measures such as injection sclerotherapy or banding.[303]

Gastric varices

Many gastric varices are fundic and directly contiguous with lower esophageal varices. Most are present at the initial endoscopy and are eradicated during the treatment of esophageal varices. However, 5–10% of patients develop significant gastric varices after treatment of esophageal varices using EIS. Bleeding from gastric varices may respond to EIS, but this is much less likely if the gastric varices are isolated and not contiguous with esophageal varices.[288,304] Alternative sclerosants, such as bovine thrombin and cyanoacrylate, have been used successfully in adults but have not been evaluated in children.[305] Banding of gastric varices is associated with a high rebleeding rate. If sclerotherapy is ineffective or inappropriate, then a TIPSS or surgical shunting or local devascularization procedure should be considered in patients with satisfactory liver function.[288,306]

Surgery for portal hypertension

Surgical shunts. Shunt surgery and endoscopic therapy are complementary procedures in the management of portal hypertension.[307]

Indications for surgery are:

- Uncontrolled bleeding from esophageal varices (not responding to at least two sessions of banding or sclerotherapy) in children with PVO or those with chronic liver disease and reasonable liver function
- Bleeding gastric or ectopic varices that cannot be controlled endoscopically
- Massive splenomegaly causing severe hypersplenism or abdominal pain
- Lack of access to expert endoscopy

However, a case can be made for mesoportal bypass surgery as prophylactic therapy in children with extrahepatic PVO and cavernoma, because of the added benefit of not only relieving PHT but also redirecting portal venous blood into the liver.[307]

In a small proportion of children, venous anatomy or occlusion may preclude shunt surgery.[308–310] Many types of

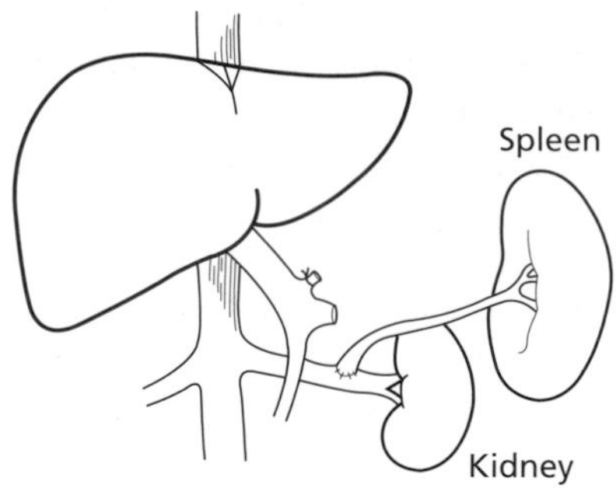

1. A Distal splenorenal (Warren)

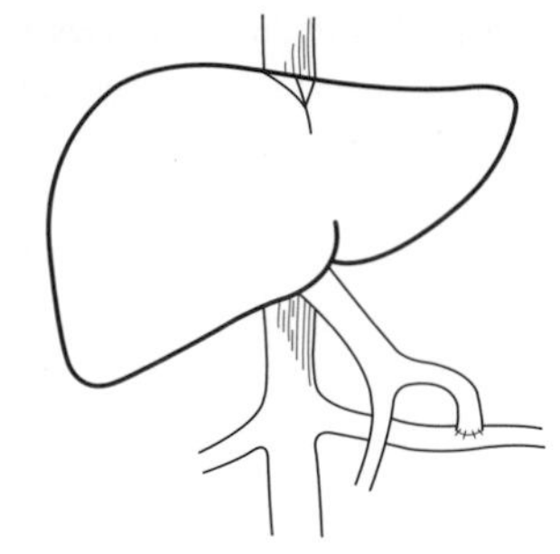

B Proximal splenorenal

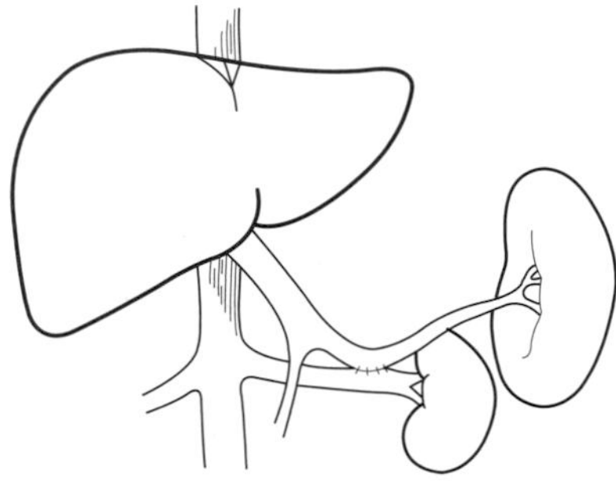

C Side-to-side splenorenal

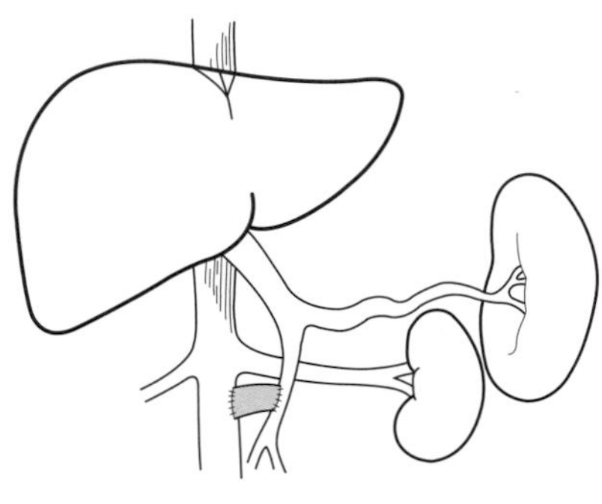

D Mesocaval

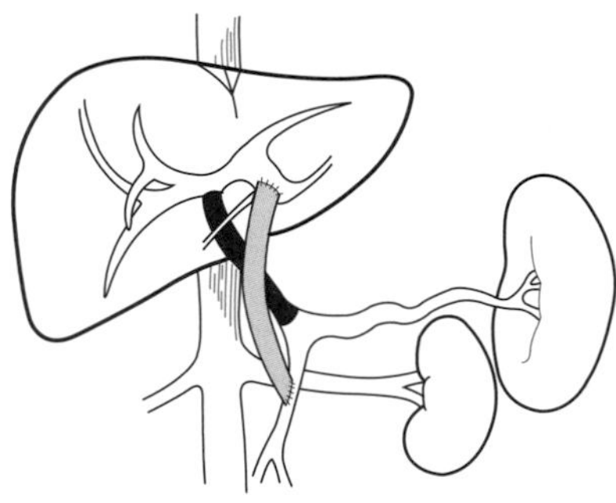

2. Mesoportal (Rex)

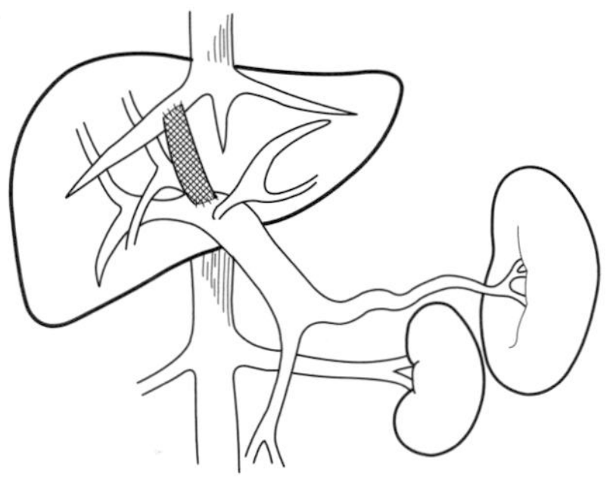
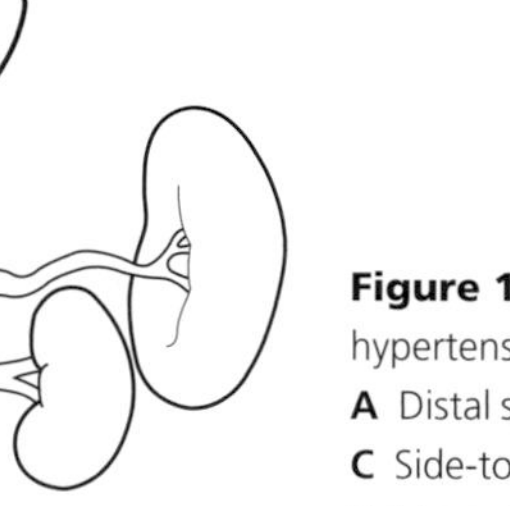

3. TIPSS

Figure 19.12 Shunt procedures for portal hypertension. 1. Portosystemic shunts. **A** Distal splenorenal. **B** Proximal splenorenal. **C** Side-to-side splenorenal. **D** Mesocaval. 2. Mesenterico–left portal (Rex) shunt. 3. Transjugular intrahepatic portosystemic stent shunt (TIPSS).

portosystemic shunt have been described, but mesocaval and splenorenal shunts have been used most often in children (Figure 19.12). The distal splenorenal (Warren) shunt is considered to be a selective shunt, in that it achieves gastrosplenic variceal decompression whilst maintaining portal perfusion.[311] The results of the mesocaval interposition shunt using a segment of autologous jugular vein have been generally good. Growth velocity frequently improves after successful portosystemic shunting.[312]

Shunt thrombosis is a major complication and frequently manifests as recurrent variceal bleeding. It is more likely in children under 5 years.[313] Shunt patency can be assessed directly by a variety of imaging modalities, including color Doppler ultrasound imaging of the shunt, magnetic resonance angiography, and conventional angiography, or indirectly by ultrasound examination of flow patterns in the portomesenteric and systemic veins. This is confirmed by an improvement in hypersplenism as evidenced by an increase in platelet counts, a reduction in splenomegaly, and regression of esophageal varices observed endoscopically.

Encephalopathy is a well-recognized complication of portosystemic shunt surgery in cirrhotic patients. Detailed long-term studies have demonstrated that the risk is extremely small in those with PVO.[309,313] Alagille's *et al.* investigated a cohort of patients with PVO up to 24 years after portosystemic shunt surgery using a battery of clinical, psychometric, and encephalographic tests and found no instance of encephalopathy.[314] In contrast, improvement in some areas of cognitive function has been documented after restoration of normal portal blood flow into the liver by means of the Rex shunt, which lends credence to the premise that there are some subtle neurological consequences to diversion of portal blood away from the liver.[315]

Rarely, progressive pulmonary hypertension may develop in children with PVO after portosystemic shunt surgery.[316] This may be a consequence of vasoactive substances bypassing the liver.

The introduction of the mesenterico–left portal (Rex) shunt has significantly broadened the indications for shunt surgery in PVO.[310] In this shunt, a vein graft is interposed between the superior mesenteric vein and the (intrahepatic) left portal vein, which is located in the Rex recessus adjacent to the falciform ligament (Figure 19.12). The portal vein occlusion is bypassed, hepatic portal blood flow is restored, and portal hypertension is corrected. The operation requires the presence of an adequate caliber, a patent intrahepatic left portal vein, and patent splenic and mesenteric veins; this must be established preoperatively by magnetic resonance angiography, ultrasound, and/or retrograde hepatic venography. This shunt is a valuable option for selected children with PVO, since it restores normal physiology. However, it is not feasible in all cases. Shunt failure is a potential problem, but medium-term follow-up studies indicate that excellent results can be achieved with autologous vein grafts (Figure 19.13).[317]

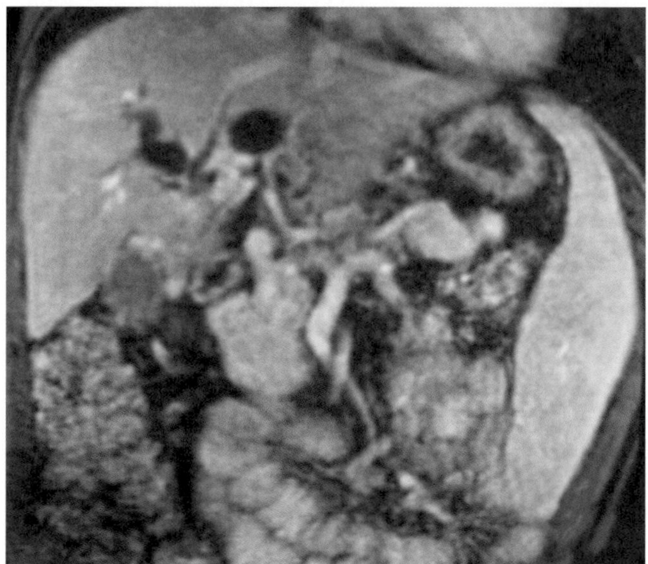

A

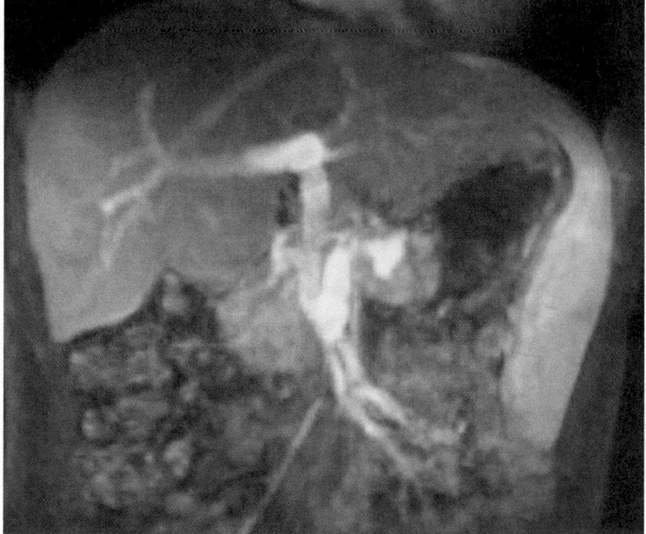

B

Figure 19.13 CT scan with contrast of a patient with portal cavernoma **A** prior to MesoRex shunt showing dilated bile ducts, portal cavernoma, a small liver and large spleen. **B** CT scan taken 2 years later shows a patent shunt with good flow into the liver, a liver of increased size, resolution of the biliopathy and cavernoma and a smaller spleen indicating normalization of splanchnic venous flow into the liver and its beneficial effects.

Nonshunt surgery. Other surgical techniques for controlling variceal bleeding have been disappointing in the long term because of a high rate of rebleeding. Splenectomy alone, suture ligation of varices, and esophagogastric transection have generally only yielded short-term success, except in gastric variceal bleeding from isolated splenic vein thrombosis, when splenectomy may be curative. Radical devascularization procedures have been more successful, but these often include splenectomy, which renders the child susceptible to life-threatening infection.[318] Splenectomy is rarely indicated for massive splenomegaly causing severe hypersplenism or abdominal pain, but shunt surgery should also be considered in such cases. Splenic embolization is an alternative, but its effects may be temporary and the procedure is not without morbidity.[319] In cystic fibrosis–related portal hypertension, some authors have recommended partial splenectomy for hypersplenism, but this is not generally recommended.[320,321]

Liver transplantation. Liver transplantation is the treatment of choice for most children with variceal bleeding complicating end-stage chronic liver disease. Endoscopic treatment of esophageal varices provides effective control of hemorrhage in children with biliary atresia awaiting transplantation.[75] However, sclerotherapy is best avoided immediately before transplantation.[322] In children with variceal bleeding from cystic fibrosis liver disease, endoscopic therapy and/or surgical portosystemic shunting are potential options if liver and lung function are well preserved, but others are best managed by transplantation.[323]

Previous portosystemic shunting does not compromise survival after liver transplantation, although operative morbidity is less likely in those who have had a distal splenorenal or mesocaval shunt, both of which avoid surgery around the porta hepatis.[324]

Surgery for Budd–Chiari syndrome. Rarely, posthepatic portal hypertension has a radiologically or surgically treatable cause, such as a caval web. Many children with hepatic vein thrombosis are successfully managed by medical therapy directed at controlling ascites and preventing progressive venous thrombosis. Portal decompression is necessary for variceal bleeding, deteriorating liver function associated with zonal necrosis on liver biopsy, and intractable ascites. Portosystemic shunting converts the portal vein into a venous outflow tract. Occasionally, more complex shunts are needed in those with IVC obstruction.[75] These procedures are potentially hazardous, and TIPSS is a less invasive alternative (Figure 19.12).[279] Liver transplantation is indicated for fulminant liver failure or cirrhosis, but recurrence of Budd–Chiari syndrome in the graft is a risk, and patients with thrombophilia usually require long-term anticoagulation.[325]

Primary prophylaxis of variceal bleeding

Beta-blockers. Propranolol reduces portal pressure by causing splanchnic vasoconstriction and reducing cardiac output. Randomized controlled trials have shown it to be effective in preventing the first variceal bleed and rebleeding in adults with cirrhosis.[305,326] Uncontrolled studies in children suggest a possible benefit with few side effects, but there are no controlled data.[327] If there are no contraindications to β-blockade (e.g., asthma), primary prophylaxis may be worthwhile in children with PVO or cirrhosis and large varices. Therapy should aim to reduce the resting pulse rate by 25%.

Endoscopic therapy. Prophylactic use of injection sclerotherapy or banding is controversial. A small proportion of patients with PVO never bleed. The single prospective, randomized controlled trial in children (predominantly with intrahepatic disease) showed no survival advantage for prophylactic sclerotherapy of esophageal varices and suggested that treatment might promote bleeding from portal gastropathy or gastric varices, which are less amenable to endoscopic treatment.[328] Trials of prophylactic sclerotherapy in adults with cirrhosis have yielded conflicting results, whilst those with banding have shown a benefit in comparison with no active treatment.[305,329] However, a definite advantage for banding over β-blocker therapy has not been established, and a randomized trial is in progress in the United Kingdom. At present, primary endoscopic prophylaxis cannot be recommended except in situations in which a child may be returning to an environment where treatment is limited.

Transjugular intrahepatic portosystemic stent shunt

This procedure involves the percutaneous insertion of a guidewire via the jugular vein into a hepatic vein. Under radiological guidance, a needle is then advanced over the wire from the hepatic vein into the right or left portal vein. A balloon catheter is used to dilate this intrahepatic tract, and an expandable metal stent is deployed between the hepatic and portal veins (Figure 19.12).

The indications for TIPSS in children include refractory acute variceal bleeding and recurrent variceal bleeding in those awaiting liver transplantation (serving as a bridge to transplantation).[330] Selected patients with Budd–Chiari syndrome or intractable ascites may also benefit. Portal vein occlusion and uncorrected coagulopathy are contraindications.

In adults, the technique is effective and associated with low procedural complication rates, but major risks include stent occlusion and hepatic encephalopathy.[331] The incidence of stent occlusion increases with time. Prophylactic stent dilation may help maintain long-term patency. These and other complications, as well as the technical demands of the procedure, have limited its role in children. Nevertheless, TIPSS has been successfully performed in children as young as 3 years and as small as 13 kg.[330] Long-term patency rates in children are not yet known.

Liver trauma

The liver is the most commonly injured solid abdominal organ.[332,333] Damage may result from blunt, penetrating, or iatrogenic trauma, and mortality rates are related to the type of insult. Additional injuries to the head, thorax, and limbs are not uncommon in cases of blunt hepatic trauma, which is associated with a considerable amount of force. Road-traffic crashes account for the majority of blunt liver injuries in children, followed by recreational accidents and damage secondary to child abuse. Diagnostic procedures such as needle biopsy may occasionally result in significant hemorrhage from the liver parenchyma. Penetrating trauma is unusual in children, and accounted for only 4% of 328 injuries in one large series.[334] Children with a "blush" seen on abdominal CT with contrast have higher transfusion requirements and a greater risk of mortality, and this would be an indication for possible immediate arterial embolization or laparotomy.[335] It is noteworthy that more than half of the penetrating injuries reported in North American series are the result of gunshot wounds (Table 19.6, 19.7)[334,336,337]

Mortality rates are greater after blunt than after penetrating trauma. There is little protection from flexible ribs, and a protuberant abdomen and major disruption of the organ may occur without any associated rib fractures. The right lobe is injured four times more frequently than the left lobe, the posterior segments being the most vulnerable. Historically, it was estimated that up to 40% of young children with major liver injuries died before, or soon after, reaching hospital.[336]

The risk to the liver of seat-belt compression during rapid deceleration of motor vehicles has been reported in recent years. The mechanism of injury includes compression of the thorax and abdomen, hyperflexion of the trunk, and shearing of the peritoneal attachments of the liver. The children may present in the emergency department with evidence of intraperitoneal hemorrhage and a "seat-belt sign" of bruising across the chest and abdomen. The severity of the injury is related to the impact speed of the vehicle, and this type of

Table 19.6 Causes of liver injury in 328 children admitted to a North American regional pediatric trauma center (San Diego, California) over a period of 13 years and 311 children admitted to a similar trauma center in Cape Town, South Africa—emphasizing the different patterns of injury seen in developing countries.[334,336]

Cause	Percentage of all injuries	
	San Diego	Cape Town
Pedestrians struck by vehicles	39	75
Vehicle passengers	34	12
Falls or blows to abdomen	13	8
Bicycle injuries	5	0.1
Child abuse	5	5
Penetrating injuries	4	Not recorded

Table 19.7 Nineteen complications (13.6%) encountered during the conservative management of 140 children with liver trauma.[337]

Bile leak	5
Ruptured hematoma	3
Hemobilia	2
Pneumonia	2
Abscess	1
Septicemia	1
Surgical intervention	5 (bile duct injury, infected hematoma, avulsed renal pedicle)

injury can occur with all types of restraint such as lap belts, lap-and-shoulder belts, and even child car seats.[338] It should be emphasized, however, that all these restraints minimize the frequency of head injuries. A review of 42 injured children aged between 2 months and 15 years who had been restrained automobile passengers showed that 26 (62%) had sustained significant intra-abdominal injuries even though they were wearing seat belts; 19 (45%) had visible belt-related bruising of the abdominal wall, and visceral injuries included the spleen, bowel, kidney, stomach, and pancreas; five had sustained liver injuries.[338]

Recreational injuries are an important cause of trauma in children, particularly bicycle handlebars.[339] It has been observed that although subcutaneous bruising is a poor indicator of underlying organ damage, the small cross-sectional area of the handlebar results in a powerful impact to a small area of the abdominal wall, which is enough to cause organ rupture.

Parenchymal liver damage is well recognized as a possible sequel of child abuse. There may be no obvious external signs of trauma on the abdominal wall, and the clinical history is commonly unclear or misleading. There is a high mortality rate associated with this type of injury, and in the past many of the victims died before they reached hospital.[340] In a review of 8000 cases of pediatric trauma in which 22 cases were due to child abuse, the mortality in this group, which included six cases of liver trauma, was 45%.[341]

Subcapsular hepatic hematomas may present in the newborn period and were identified in 118 (15%) of 783 neonatal autopsies by French and Waldstein.[342] The etiology is probably a combination of abdominothoracic compression during delivery and decreased clotting function. In 31 cases, the lesions were > 3 cm in diameter, and in one baby there was intraperitoneal hemorrhage from rupture of the liver capsule. The hematomas are recognized 2–5 days after birth from the association of hepatic enlargement and anemia. Occasionally, an affected infant may become shocked, and the intraperitoneal blood may cause discoloration of the periumbilical region and/or the scrotum. The diagnosis is confirmed with ultrasound and CT scanning.[343] If surgery is required, after correction of any clotting abnormality with vitamin K, fresh frozen plasma and cryoprecipitate perihepatic packing is the preferred treatment, with removal of the packs after 48 h.

Presentation and investigation

Trauma to the liver may be suspected with clinical evidence of signs of bruising, bicycle handlebar marks, or seat-belt marks over the upper abdomen or right chest wall. Peritonism and/or shock may be present with severe injuries (Table 19.7). It is important to suspect intra-abdominal or thoracic injury in this clinical setting.

Signs of child abuse such as multiple bruises, poor nutrition, and unexplained fractures should prompt investigation for liver injury.[341]

Investigations:

- Plain radiography is of limited value except for detecting foreign bodies such as bullets after penetrating trauma.
- Ultrasonography is quick, portable, and does not expose the child to ionizing radiation, but it is operator-dependent and may be technically difficult in the recently injured child. It can accurately detect free intraperitoneal fluid. However, solid organ injuries may be overlooked in as many as one-third of patients.[344] Ultrasound is most useful in the subsequent monitoring of children with blunt liver injury managed nonoperatively. Other investigations include CT, peritoneal lavage, radionuclide scanning, and angiography. Only a minority of very unstable patients cannot undergo at least one of these tests. Appropriate tests are essential, as the initial clinical evaluation of a child with abdominal trauma may be incorrect in approximately 25% of cases.[345]
- An abdominal CT scan is the investigation of choice after major blunt abdominal trauma in the hemodynamically stable child.[346] Although there is debate about the value of oral contrast at the time of CT, intravenous contrast is invaluable.[347] CT allows the visualization of parenchymal tears (Figure 19.14), disruption of major blood vessels, and an assessment of the volume of any free intraperitoneal blood. Evidence of a "blush" of contrast confirms active bleeding

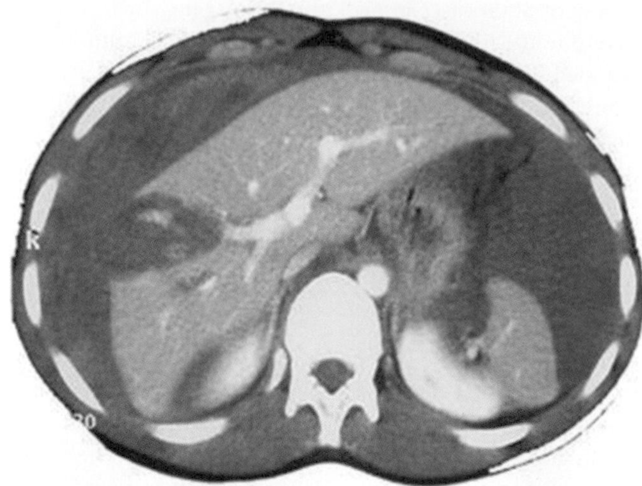

A

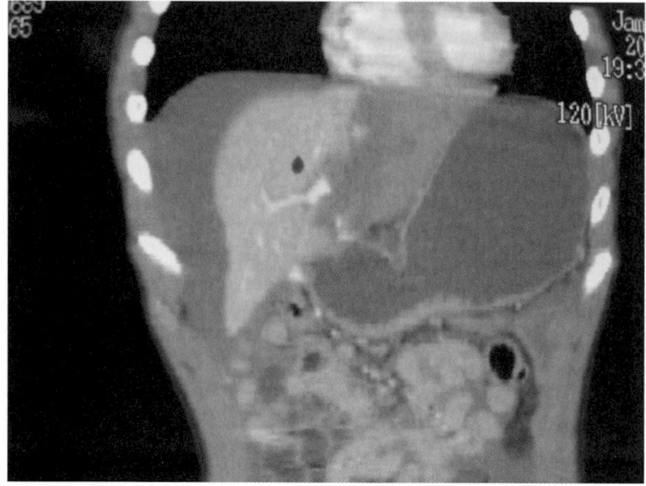

B

Figure 19.14 A An axial computed tomogram (CT) in the portal venous phase with contrast enhancement, in a child following blunt abdominal trauma. The deep fracture in the right lobe, with a "blush" of contrast indicating ongoing bleeding, should be noted. There is a large amount of blood in the peritoneal cavity. Surgical intervention is indicated. **B** Coronal CT of a child after blunt abdominal trauma, showing hypoperfusion of the left liver, a "blush" of contrast indicating ongoing hemorrhage, and a large amount of fluid (blood) surrounding the liver. The stomach is also dilated. Urgent laparotomy and resection of the almost completely avulsed left lateral segment was required in this case.

and should prompt urgent intervention. Nonperfused liver segments may also be detected.[348] As well as providing an assessment of liver damage, CT may allow the identification of injuries to other organs, including the diaphragm. It also assists in the detection of late complications such as bile leaks and abscess formation.

• Diagnostic peritoneal lavage is potentially misleading in children, because the presence of intraperitoneal blood is not by itself an indication for laparotomy.[346] However, in centers without ready access to CT scanning, it remains a sensitive method of detecting free blood in the abdomen and may be helpful in selected cases of blunt abdominal injury.

• Laparoscopy may have a role in the assessment of liver injury, but it requires a general anesthetic and its accuracy is limited. It should not be used to supplant well-validated, noninvasive imaging techniques.[349]

• Liver scintiscanning is particularly valuable in the diagnosis and management of biliary tract injuries after blunt abdominal trauma.[350]

• Angiography is useful for the assessment of complex hepatic trauma, but its most valuable role lies in the management of severe bleeding and the complication of hemobilia with arterial embolization.

Liver injury may be accompanied by a rapid rise in blood transaminase levels.[351]

Management (Figure 19.15)

In recent years, it has become clear that the majority of liver injuries in children can be managed either nonoperatively or with the aid of relatively simple surgical procedures.[332,333,352,353] In contrast, the relatively small number of children with severe parenchymal disruption require a high degree of radiological and surgical expertise, and the mortality rates in these children may be greater than 30%. The results of treatment are related to the cause of trauma; mortality rates recorded in one series were 25% for shotgun injuries, 19% for blunt trauma, and 1% for stab wounds.[333]

Nonoperative treatment

Nonoperative treatment of blunt liver injury is now the accepted management strategy, provided hemodynamic stability is maintained after initial resuscitation. Careful observation, frequent monitoring, and precise fluid management are essential. Additional requirements are nasogastric decompression, antibiotics, bed rest, transfusion, and ready access to an operating room. Children with evidence of continuing intra-abdominal bleeding require urgent laparotomy, as do those with bowel perforation or deep penetrating trauma. Recent guidelines suggest that a transfusion requirement of $\geq$ 25 mL/kg in the first 2 h after injury has a predictive accuracy of 88% and 95% for operative intervention and for major hepatic disruption.[334] Using this strategy, 87% of 328 patients were managed conservatively, with a mortality rate of 17%. Associated severe injuries and sepsis caused most of the deaths, and only three were related to the liver trauma. A further review of 140 cases of nonoperative management revealed a 14% complication rate, which included hematoma rupture, infection, bile leaks, and three deaths (2.1%; Table 19.7).[337]

After major liver injuries, observation usually continues in hospital for 7–10 days. Evidence-based guidelines suggest that children with uncomplicated isolated liver injuries can be discharged home sooner (after 5 days), but activity should be restricted for 3–6 weeks and contact sports avoided for 2–3 months.[354] Usually, the damaged parenchyma and surrounding hematoma are absorbed to form localized collections

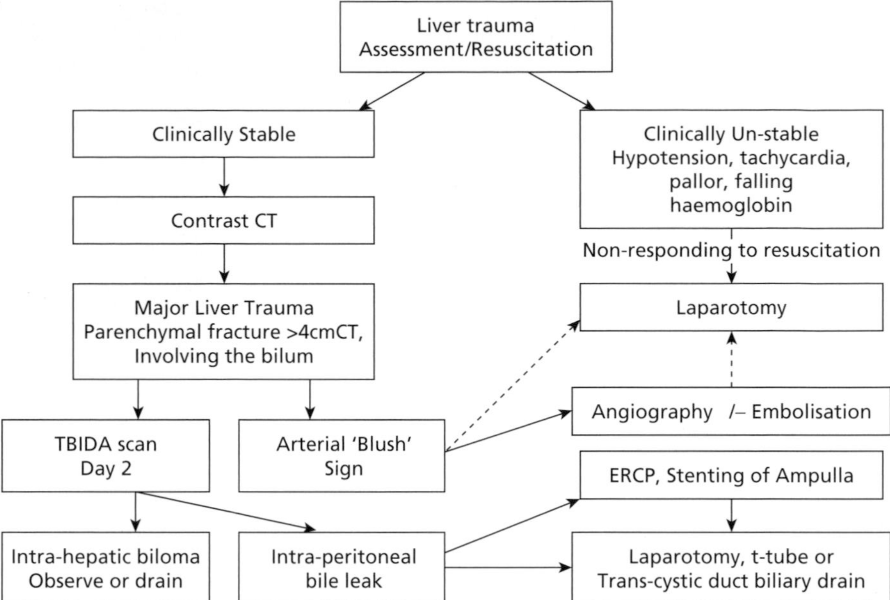

Figure 19.15 An algorithm for the management of liver trauma, incorporating conservative and surgical treatment. The hemodynamically unstable child who becomes stable after volume replacement can undergo computed tomography scanning.

of fluid within weeks, and these resolve over the following 3–4 months.

Surgical treatment

Although nonoperative management is successful in the majority of children with blunt liver trauma, a small number require urgent surgical intervention for persistent bleeding. The need for emergency surgical intervention is related more to the volume of intraperitoneal blood loss than to the extent of parenchymal disruption observed on a CT examination.[355,356] In isolated blunt liver trauma, surgery should be seriously considered once volume replacement exceeds 40 mL/kg.

Prompt arrest of major bleeding is critical to prevent prolonged hypotension, an abdominal compartment syndrome with renal failure, and the secondary complications of coagulopathy, acidosis and hypothermia, all of which exacerbate hemorrhage. Intraoperative use of a cell saver, rapid infusers, and blood warmers is helpful.

Rapid exposure of the abdominal cavity is achieved by a midline incision (or a broad transverse incision in a small child). Confirmation of the nature of the liver injury is followed by compression of the hepatic artery and portal vein in the porta hepatis (the Pringle maneuver), together with local packing to reduce bleeding from the torn parenchyma. This is followed by a rapid search for major injuries to other organs in the abdomen. Continued severe bleeding after the Pringle maneuver suggests the possibility of a tear in the IVC or hepatic veins (retrohepatic or suprahepatic). Improved access to the liver can be obtained by subcostal extensions of the midline incision or vertical extension of a transverse incision. Thoracotomy incisions are not necessary unless there is evidence of a major intrathoracic injury.

Surgical resection of a severely damaged liver requires wide exposure but is rarely required now that the efficacy of intraoperative perihepatic packing has been proven. A key paper suggesting the value of this technique was published in 1981, reporting the survival of nine of 10 patients who had been treated with packing after other methods of obtaining vascular control had failed.[357] Increasing application of the technique has established the value of emergency packing in arresting hemorrhage, reducing operating time, and reducing the incidence of complications from prolonged hypotension. Packing can be highly efficacious if used appropriately. Injuries to the bile ducts in severe liver trauma are frequently encountered and should be delineated by intraoperative cholangiography. Bile leakage often manifests as biliary ascites with increasing abdominal distension and raised serum bilirubin during early convalescence in patients who are managed nonoperatively. The diagnosis can be confirmed by radioisotope scanning.[350] Most patients can be managed with a combination of external drainage and reduction in the intraluminal pressure in the bile ducts by either endoscopic biliary stenting, placement of a T-tube in the bile duct, or a transcystic duct drain after cholecystectomy. Complete disruption of the right or left hepatic ducts would require a Roux-en-Y hepaticojejunostomy. Long-term outcomes are excellent.

Interventional radiology

Arterial embolization is widely used for the control of arterial bleeding in many organs, and selective hepatic arterial occlusion has been used both as an adjunct to conservative management or as a preliminary maneuver to reduce hemorrhage before surgical exploration of the liver.[358] Pseudoaneurysms and arteriovenous fistulas—both rare complications of liver trauma—can frequently be managed using embolization techniques.[359] Bile leaks are typically managed by percutaneous drainage, with or without ERCP, and temporary internal stenting of the bile ducts.[360]

In summary, most cases of blunt liver trauma in children can be successfully managed nonoperatively. The challenge is the early selection of patients who will require surgery for ongoing bleeding. In the small proportion of patients who require surgical intervention, perihepatic packing should be the procedure of choice, with removal of the packs after 24–48 h at a second laparotomy. Hepatic resection is now reserved for the occasional patient in whom bleeding is not controlled by packing. Interventional radiology plays a significant role in some patients. Radioisotope studies are useful for detecting bile duct injuries.

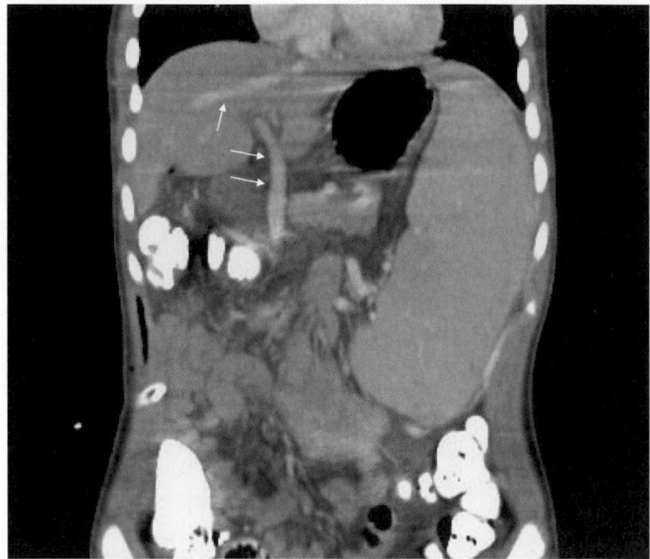

Figure 19.16 Coronal plane CT scan with contrast done on the first post operative day after meso-rex shunt, as an ultrasound scan could not clearly identify flow in the shunt. Note the small liver after prolonged portal vein thrombosis and marked splenomegaly (22 cm). The shunt is shown to be patent with good flow into the liver (arrows) measuring 10cm in length and 11 mm in diameter. Also noted are varices in the splenic hilum.

Case study

A 12-year-old well-grown boy was referred from a regional center with a history of hematemesis. His hemoglobin at presentation was 5 g/dL and he had received 400 mL of packed cells. He was commenced on octreotide intravenous infusion and ranitidine and was transferred to the liver unit. Five years previously, he had been investigated for splenomegaly, and a diagnosis of portal vein thrombosis had been made on the basis of abdominal ultrasonography and CT scan (Figure 19.16). No predisposing cause had been identified; specifically, perinatal sepsis, umbilical vein catheterization, and a thrombophilic diathesis were excluded. The α_1-antitrypsin phenotype was PI MZ. A liver biopsy had shown no significant fibrosis.

He appeared clinically well and stable. He was above the 50th percentile for height and weight. There were no signs of chronic liver disease. Abdominal examination revealed splenomegaly 10 cm below the left costal margin, and the liver was impalpable. A complete blood count showed a hemoglobin level of 11.1 g/dL (after transfusion), hypersplenism with a white blood count of 2.1×10^9/L, neutrophils 1.1, and platelets 32×10^9/L. The prothrombin time was 15 s, fibrinogen was 1.4 mg%, and the partial thromboplastin time was 37 s. Liver function tests were normal. Upper gastrointestinal endoscopy showed grade 3 esophageal varices and red color changes, but no gastric varices or gastropathy. The duodenum was normal. He had four bands placed on varices in the lower esophagus. Ultrasound scanning identified a shrunken liver with a normal echotexture and echogenic sludge in the gallbladder, with multiple stones. No normal portal vein was identified. There was some antegrade portal flow to the liver in a number of tortuous veins at the porta hepatis. A 19-cm splenomegaly was recorded.

He underwent several banding procedures until all of the varices had been obliterated. During this period (6 months), he developed marked portal hypertensive gastropathy, observed at endoscopy, and progressive hypersplenism, with the splenomegaly increasing in size to 22 cm. He had one further bleed after inadvertent use of a nonsteroidal anti-inflammatory agent.

He was referred for consideration for a mesoportal bypass. Retrograde hepatic angiography failed to show a convincing Rex vein, but there was cross-filling, right to left, of portal veins in the umbilical fissure. A decision was made to carry out surgery with the aim of attempting a mesoportal bypass, but if this was not possible, then a distal splenorenal shunt.

At laparotomy, there was evidence of marked portal hypertension, with multiple large tortuous portal veins present, particularly around the gallbladder. The gallbladder was thick-walled and filled with stones. The liver was small but had a normal appearance. There was no obvious Rex vein, but there was a single vein in the inferior part of the umbilical fissure just large enough for a shunt to be attempted and with branches to left and right. The superior mesenteric vein was also partially thrombosed. A 10-cm length of left internal jugular vein was procured from the neck, and the graft was sutured to the vein at the Rex recessus and distally to a patent area of the superior mesenteric vein.

The postoperative course was uneventful. Lack of clarity on a surveillance ultrasound prompted a CT with contrast on the first postoperative day (Figure 19.16), which showed a patent shunt and good hepatopetal flow. One year after the shunt, the patient was well, with no further bleeding. The shunt was still patent, with increased flow (velocity on ultrasound of 37 cm/s) without flow in the cavernoma. The spleen size declined to 19 cm on ultrasound and the hypersplenism was resolving, with a current complete blood count showing hemoglobin 13.2 g/dL, white blood cell count 4.1, and platelets 65 × 10^9/L. He continued to receive warfarin anticoagulation, with a prothrombin time of 21 s. Liver function was normal, and serum albumin had improved from 40 g/L to 47 g/L. A follow-up endoscopy 9 months after the operation showed a normal appearance at the gastroesophageal junction, with no visible varices or evidence of portal gastropathy. Endoscopic ultrasound showed no evidence of submucosal varices. The family reported that he seemed brighter and more energetic than before the shunt procedure. He had undergone a growth spurt of 6 cm in height.

Comments. This young man had a portal vein thrombosis of unknown cause and developed a cavernoma (with tortuous collateral vessels around the portal vein). The first-line treatment is variceal ablation with band ligation, but his portal hypertension progressed, with portal gastropathy and varices around the gallbladder. Occasionally, these may lead to biliary obstruction. He had an effective mesoportal bypass procedure for portal vein thrombosis and cavernoma, despite reduced Rex vein patency. He characteristically had a growth spurt after shunt surgery, which is thought to be due to reinstating portal blood flow to the liver. Although he was asymptomatic for 5 years after the initial presentation, earlier referral for surgical intervention might have been advantageous, as Rex vein patency may decline with age.

Acknowledgments

The author would like to acknowledge the contribution made to this chapter in the first and second editions of this book (1999, 2004), by Professor Edward Howard and Mr Mark Davenport of King's College Hospital, London, and Professor Mark Stringer of St. James's Hospital, Leeds, United Kingdom.

References

1 Thomson J. On congenital obliteration of the bile ducts. *Edinb Med J* 1891;**37**:523–31.

2 Ladd WE. Congenital atresia and stenosis of the bile ducts. *J Am Med Assoc* 1928;**91**:1082–5.

3 Ladd WE. Congenital obstruction of the bile ducts. *Ann Surg* 1935;**102**:742–51.

4 Kasai MS. A new operation for "non-correctable" biliary atresia with hepatic portoenterostomy. *Shujyutsu* 1959;**13**:733–9.

5 Chardot C, Carton M, Spire-Bendelac N, Le Pommelet C, Golmard JL, Auvert B. Epidemiology of biliary atresia in France: a national study 1986–96. *J Hepatol* 1999;**31**:1006–13.

6 McKiernan PJ, Baker AJ, Kelly DA. The frequency and outcome of biliary atresia in the UK and Ireland. *Lancet* 2000;**355**: 25–9.

7 Nio M, Ohi R, Miyano T, *et al.* Five- and 10-year survival rates after surgery for biliary atresia: a report from the Japanese Biliary Atresia Registry. *J Pediatr Surg* 2003;**38**:997–1000.

8 Davenport M, Kerkar N, Mieli-Vergani G, Mowat AP, Howard ER. Biliary atresia: the King's College Hospital experience (1974–1995). *J Pediatr Surg* 1997;**32**:479–85.

9 Cunningham ML, Sybert VP. Idiopathic extrahepatic biliary atresia: recurrence in sibs in two families. *Am J Med Genet* 1988; **31**:421–6.

10 Davenport M, Savage M, Mowat AP, Howard ER. Biliary atresia splenic malformation syndrome: an etiologic and prognostic subgroup. *Surgery* 1993;**113**:662–8.

11 Tan CE, Driver M, Howard ER, Moscoso GJ. Extrahepatic biliary atresia: a first-trimester event? Clues from light microscopy and immunohistochemistry. *Pediatr Surg* 1994;**29**:808–14.

12 Redkar R, Davenport M, Howard ER. Antenatal diagnosis of congenital anomalies of the biliary tract. *J Pediatr Surg* 1998;**33**: 700–4.

13 Mackenzie TC, Howell LJ, Flake AW, Adzick NS. The management of prenatally diagnosed choledochal cysts. *J Pediatr Surg* 2001;**36**:1241–3.

14 Iwai N, Deguchi E, Sasaki Y, Idoguchi K, Yanagihara J. Antenatal diagnosis of biliary atresia (noncorrectable cyst type): a case report. *Eur J Pediatr Surg* 1999;**9**:340–2.

15 MacGillivray TE, Adzick NS. Biliary atresia begins before birth. *Pediatr Surg Int* 1994;**9**:116–7.

16 Muller F, Oury JF, Dumez Y, Boué J, Boué A. Microvillar enzyme assays in amniotic fluid and fetal tissues at different stages of development. *Prenat Diagn* 1988;**8**:189–98.

17 Danks DM. Prolonged neonatal obstructive jaundice: a survey of modern concepts. *Clin Pediatr (Phila)* 1965;**4**:499–510.

18 Alpert LI, Strauss L, Hirschhorn K. Neonatal hepatitis and biliary atresia associated with trisomy 17–18 syndrome. *N Engl J Med* 1969;**280**:16–20.

19 Strauss L, Valderrama E, Alpert L. Biliary tract anomalies: the relationship of biliary atresia to neonatal hepatitis. *Birth Defects* 1972;**8**:135–45.

20 Schweizer P, Kerremans J. Discordant findings in extrahepatic bile duct atresia in 6 sets of twins. *Z Kinderchir* 1988;**43**:72–5.

21 Silveira TR, Salzano FM, Howard ER, Mowat AP. Extrahepatic biliary atresia and twinning. *Braz J Med Biol Res* 1991;**24**:67–71.

22 Strauss L, Bernstein J. Neonatal hepatitis in congenital rubella. A histopathological study. *Arch Pathol* 1968;**86**:317–27.

23 Weaver LT, Nelson R, Bell TM. The association of extrahepatic bile duct atresia and neonatal Epstein–Barr virus infection. *Acta Paediatr Scand* 1984;**73**:155–7.

24 Phillips PA, Keast D, Papadimitriou JM, Walters MN, Stanley NF. Chronic obstructive jaundice induced by Reovirus type 3 in weanling mice. *Pathology* 1969;**1**:193–203.

25 Parashar K, Tarlow MJ, McCrae MA. Experimental reovirus type 3-induced murine biliary tract disease. *J Pediatr Surg* 1992; **27**:843–7.

26 Riepenhoff-Talty M, Schaekel K, Clark HF, *et al.* Group A rotaviruses produce extrahepatic biliary obstruction in orally inoculated newborn mice. *Pediatr Res* 1993;**33**:394–9.

27 Chan RY, Tan CE, Czech-Schmidt G, Petersen C. Computerized three-dimensional study of a rotavirus model of biliary atresia: comparison with human biliary atresia. *Pediatr Surg Int* 2005;**21**:615–20.

28 Allen SR, Jafri M, Donnelly B, *et al.* Effect of rotavirus strain on the murine model of biliary atresia. *J Virol* 2007;**81**:1671–9.

29 Shivakumar P, Campbell KM, Sabla GE, *et al.* Obstruction of extrahepatic bile ducts by lymphocytes is regulated by IFN-gamma in experimental biliary atresia. *J Clin Invest* 2004; **114**:322–9.

30 Morecki R, Glaser JH, Cho S, Balistreri WF, Horwitz MS. Biliary atresia and reovirus type 3 infection. *N Engl J Med* 1984;**310**: 1610.

31 Dussaix E, Hadchouel M, Tardieu M, Alagille's D. Biliary atresia and reovirus type 3 infection. *N Engl J Med* 1984;**310**:658.

32 Brown WR, Sokol RJ, Levin MJ, *et al.* Lack of correlation between infection with reovirus 3 and extrahepatic biliary atresia or neonatal hepatitis. *J Pediatr* 1988;**113**:670–6.

33 Morecki R, Glaser JH, Johnson AB, Kress Y. Detection of reovirus type 3 in the porta hepatis of an infant with extrahepatic biliary atresia: ultrastructural and immunocytochemical study. *Hepatology* 1984;**4**:1137–42.

34 Iwami D, Ohi R, Chiba T, *et al.* Detection of reovirus type 3 in patients with biliary atresia by polymerase chain reaction (PCR). In: Ohi R, ed. *Biliary Atresia: Proceedings of the Fifth International Sendai Symposium on Biliary Atresia, Sendai, Japan, May 27–29, 1991.* Tokyo: Icom Associates, 1991: 7–10.

35 Strickland AD, Shannon K. Studies in the etiology of extrahepatic biliary atresia: time-space clustering. *J Pediatr* 1982; **100**:749–53.

36 Yoon PW, Bresee JS, Olney RS, James LM, Khoury MJ. Epidemiology of biliary atresia: a population-based study. *Pediatrics* 1997;**99**:376–82.

37 Houwen RH, Kerremans II, van Steensel-Moll HA, van Romunde LK, Bijleveld CM, Schweizer P. Time-space distribution of extrahepatic biliary atresia in The Netherlands and West Germany. *Z Kinderchir* 1988;**43**:68–71.

38 Chiba T, Ohi R, Mochizuki I. Cholangiographic study of the pancreaticobiliary ductal junction in biliary atresia. *J Pediatr Surg* 1990;**25**:609–12.

39 Miyano T, Suruga K, Suda K. Abnormal choledocho-pancreatico ductal junction related to the etiology of infantile obstructive jaundice diseases. *J Pediatr Surg* 1979;**14**:16–26.

40 Harper P, Plant JW, Unger DB. Congenital biliary atresia and jaundice in lambs and calves. *Aust Vet J* 1990;**67**:18–22.

41 Haas JE. Bile duct and liver pathology in biliary atresia. *World J Surg* 1978;**2**:561–9.

42 Dillon P, Belchis D, Tracy T, Cilley R, Hafer L, Krummel T. Increased expression of intercellular adhesion molecules in biliary atresia. *Am J Pathol* 1994;**145**:263–7.

43 Davenport M, Howard ER. Macroscopic appearance at portoenterostomy—a prognostic variable in biliary atresia. *J Pediatr Surg* 1996;**31**:1387–90.

44 Davenport M, Gonde C, Redkar R, *et al.* Immunohistochemistry of the liver and biliary tree in extrahepatic biliary atresia. *J Pediatr Surg* 2001;**36**:1017–25.

45 Shivakumar P, Sabla G, Mohanty S, *et al.* Effector role of neonatal hepatic $CD8^+$ lymphocytes in epithelial injury and autoimmunity in experimental biliary atresia. *Gastroenterology* 2007;**133**: 268–77.

46 Narayanaswamy B, Gonde C, Tredger JM, Hussain M, Vergani D, Davenport M. Serial circulating markers of inflammation in biliary atresia—evolution of the post-operative inflammatory process. *Hepatology* 2007;**46**:180–7.

47 Bezerra JA. The next challenge in pediatric cholestasis: deciphering the pathogenesis of biliary atresia. *J Pediatr Gastroenterol Nutr* 2006;**43**(Suppl 1):S23–9.

48 Mieli-Vergani G, Howard ER, Portman B, Mowat AP. Late referral for biliary atresia—missed opportunities for effective surgery. *Lancet* 1989;**i**:421–3.

49 Mushtaq I, Logan S, Morris M, *et al.* Screening of newborn infants for cholestatic hepatobiliary disease with tandem mass spectrometry. *BMJ* 1999;**319**:471–7.

50 Chen SM, Chang MH, Du JC, *et al.* Screening for biliary atresia by infant stool color card in Taiwan. *Pediatrics* 2006;**117**:1147–54.

51 Hussein M, Howard ER, Mieli-Vergani G, Mowat AP. Jaundice at 14 days of age: exclude biliary atresia. *Arch Dis Child* 1991;**66**:1177–9.

52 Mowat AP, Davidson LL, Dick MC. Earlier identification of biliary atresia and hepatobiliary disease: selective screening in the third week of life. *Arch Dis Child* 1995;**72**:90–2.

53 Farrant P, Meire HB, Mieli-Vergani G. Ultrasound features of the gall bladder in infants presenting with conjugated hyperbilirubinaemia. *Br J Radiol* 2000;**73**:1154–8.

54 Park WH, Choi SO, Lee HJ. The ultrasonographic "triangular cord" coupled with gallbladder images in the diagnostic prediction of biliary atresia from infantile intrahepatic cholestasis. *J Pediatr Surg* 1999;**34**:1706–10.

55 Dick MC, Mowat AP. Biliary scintigraphy with DISIDA. A simpler way of showing bile duct patency in suspected biliary atresia. *Arch Dis Child* 1986;**61**:191–2.

56 Avni FE, Segers V, De Maertelaer V, *et al.* The evaluation by magnetic resonance imaging of hepatic periportal fibrosis in infants with neonatal cholestasis: preliminary report. *J Pediatr Surg* 2002;**37**:1128–33.

57 Iinuma Y, Narisawa R, Iwafuchi M, *et al.* The role of endoscopic retrograde cholangiopancreatography in infants with cholestasis. *J Pediatr Surg* 2000;**35**:545–9.

58 Kasai M. Treatment of biliary atresia with special reference to hepatic porto-enterostomy and its modifications. *Prog Pediatr Surg* 1974;**6**:5–52.

59 Davenport M, Ure BM, Petersen C, Kobayashi H. Surgery for biliary atresia—is there a European consensus? *Eur J Pediatr Surg* 2007;**17**:180–3.

60 Howard E. Surgery for biliary atresia. In: Spitz L, Coran GA, eds. *Pediatric Surgery,* 5th ed. London: Chapman and Hall Medical, 1995: 551–61 (Rob and Smith's operative surgery, vol. 3.).

61 Martinez-Ferro M, Esteves E, Laje P. Laparoscopic treatment of biliary atresia and choledochal cyst. *Semin Pediatr Surg* 2005;**14**: 206–15.

62 Dutta S, Woo R, Albanese CT. Minimal access portoenterostomy: advantages and disadvantages of standard laparoscopic and robotic techniques. *J Laparoendosc Adv Surg Tech A* 2007;**17**: 258–64.

63 Aspelund G, Ling SC, Ng V, Kim PC. A role for laparoscopic approach in the treatment of biliary atresia and choledochal cysts. *J Pediatr Surg* 2007;**42**:869–72.

64 Dillon PW, Owings E, Cilley R, Field D, Curnow A, Georgeson K. Immunosuppression as adjuvant therapy for biliary atresia. *J Pediatr Surg* 2001;**36**:80–5.

65 Meyers RL, Book LS, O'Gorman MA, *et al.* High-dose steroids, ursodeoxycholic acid, and chronic intravenous antibiotics improve bile flow after Kasai procedure in infants with biliary atresia. *J Pediatr Surg* 2003;**38**:406–11.

66 Escobar MA, Jay CL, Brooks RM, *et al.* Effect of corticosteroid therapy on outcomes in biliary atresia after Kasai portoenterostomy. *J Pediatr Surg* 2006;**41**:99–103.

67 Kobayashi H, Yamataka A, Koga H, *et al.* Optimum prednisolone usage in patients with biliary atresia postportoenterostomy. *J Pediatr Surg* 2005;**40**:327–30.

68 Muraji T, Nio M, Ohhama Y, *et al.* Postoperative corticosteroid therapy for bile drainage in biliary atresia—a nationwide survey. *J Pediatr Surg* 2004;**39**:1803–5.

69 Ecoffey C, Rothman E, Bernard O, Hadchouel M, Valayer J, Alagille's D. Bacterial cholangitis after surgery for biliary atresia. *J Pediatr*1987;**111**:824–9.

70 Saeki M, Nakano M, Hagane K, Shimizu K. Effectiveness of an intussusceptive antireflux valve to prevent ascending cholangitis after hepatic portojejunostomy in biliary atresia. *J Pediatr Surg* 1991;**26**:800–3.

71 Ohi R. Long-term results of hepatic portoenterostomy. In: Howard ER, ed. *Surgery of Liver Disease in Children.* London: Butterworth-Heinemann, 1991: 60–71.

72 Kasai M, Okamoto A, Ohi R, Yabe K, Matsumura Y. Changes of portal vein pressure and intrahepatic blood vessels after surgery for biliary atresia. *J Pediatr Surg* 1981;**16**:152–9.

73 Ohi R, Mochizuki I, Komatsu K, Kasai M. Portal hypertension after successful hepatic portoenterostomy in biliary atresia. *J Pediatr Surg* 1986;**21**:271–4.

74 Kang N, Davenport M, Driver M, Howard ER. Hepatic histology and the development of esophageal varices in biliary atresia. *J Pediatr Surg* 1993;**28**:63–6.

75 Stringer MD, Howard ER, Mowat AP. Endoscopic sclerotherapy in the management of esophageal varices in 61 children with biliary atresia. *J Pediatr Surg* 1989;**24**:438–42.

76 Hall RJ, Lilly JR, Stiegmann GV. Endoscopic esophageal varix ligation: technique and preliminary results in children. *J Pediatr Surg* 1988;**23**:1222–3.

77 McKiernan PJ, Beath SV, Davison SM. A prospective study of endoscopic esophageal variceal ligation using a multiband ligator. *J Pediatr Gastroenterol Nutr* 2002;**34**:207–11.

78 Huppert PE, Goffette P, Astfalk W, *et al.* Transjugular intrahepatic portosystemic shunts in children with biliary atresia. *Cardiovasc Intervent Radiol* 2002;**25**:484–93.

79 Evans HM, Sharif K, Brown RM, Platt C, Crisp WJ, Kelly DA. Fatal and life threatening rupture of splenic artery aneurysms in children with portal hypertension. *Pediatr Transplant* 2004;**8**: 192–5.

80 Cywes C, Millar AJ. Assessment of the nutritional status of infants and children with biliary atresia. *S Afr Med J* 1990;**77**: 131–5.

81 Endo M, Fuchimoto Y, Ukiyama E, *et al.* Evaluation of postoperative zinc and copper dynamics in infants and children with biliary atresia, with special reference to progression of liver cirrhosis. In: Ohi R, ed. *Biliary Atresia: Proceedings of the Fifth International Sendai Symposium on Biliary Atresia, Sendai, Japan, May 27–29, 1991.* Tokyo: Icom Associates, 1991: 210–4.

82 Suita S, Ikeda K, Doki T, *et al.* Zinc status and its relations to growth retardation in children with biliary atresia. *J Pediatr Surg* 1987;**22**:401–5.

83 Bu LN, Chen HL, Ni YH, *et al.* Multiple intrahepatic biliary cysts in children with biliary atresia. *J Pediatr Surg* 2002;**37**: 1183–7.

84 Valayer J. Conventional treatment of biliary atresia: long-term results. *J Pediatr Surg* 1996;**31**:1546–51.

85 Soh H, Hasegawa T, Sasaki T, *et al.* Pulmonary hypertension associated with postoperative biliary atresia: report of two cases. *J Pediatr Surg* 1999;**34**:1779–81.

86 Kulkarni PB, Beatty E Jr. Cholangiocarcinoma associated with biliary cirrhosis due to congenital biliary atresia. *Am J Dis Child* 1977;**131**:442–4.

87 Brunati A, Feruzi Z, Sokal E, *et al.* Early occurrence of hepatocellular carcinoma in biliary atresia treated by liver transplantation. *Pediatr Transplant* 2007;**11**:117–9.

88 Howard ER, MacLean G, Nio M, Donaldson N, Singer J, Ohi R. Survival patterns in biliary atresia and comparison of quality of life of long-term survivors in Japan and England. *J Pediatr Surg* 2001;**36**:892–7.

89 Davenport M, Saxena R, Howard E. Acquired biliary atresia. *J Pediatr Surg* 1996;**31**:1721–3.

90 Duché M, Fabre M, Kretzschmar B, Serinet MO, Gauthier F, Chardot C. Prognostic value of portal pressure at the time of Kasai operation in patients with biliary atresia. *J Pediatr Gastroenterol Nutr* 2006;**43**:640–5.

91 Lloyd D, Jones M, Dalzell M. Surgery for biliary atresia. *Lancet* 2000;**355**:1099–100.

92 Serinet MO, Broué P, Jacquemin E, *et al.* Management of patients with biliary atresia in France: results of a decentralized policy 1986–2002. *Hepatology* 2006;**44**:75–84.

93 Tagge DU, Tagge EP, Drongowski RA, Oldham KT, Coran AG. A long-term experience with biliary atresia. Reassessment of prognostic factors. *Ann Surg* 1991;**214**:590–8.

94 Shneider BL, Brown MB, Haber B, *et al.* A multicenter study of the outcome of biliary atresia in the United States, 1997 to 2000. *J Pediatr* 2006;**148**:467–74.

95 Lykavieris P, Chardot C, Sokhn M, Gauthier F, Valayer J, Bernard O. Outcome in adulthood of biliary atresia: a study of 63 patients who survived for over 20 years with their native liver. *Hepatology* 2005;**41**:366–71.

96 Ohi R. Biliary atresia: long-term outcomes. In: Howard ER, Stringer MD, Colombani PM, eds. *Surgery of the Liver, Bile Ducts and Pancreas in Children,* 2nd ed. London: Arnold, 2002: 133–47.

97 Hadzić N, Davenport M, Tizzard S, Singer J, Howard ER, Mieli-Vergani G. Long-term survival following Kasai portoenterostomy: is chronic liver disease inevitable? *J Pediatr Gastroenterol Nutr* 2003;**37**:430–3.

98 Hadzic A, Vloka J, Hadzic N, Thys DM, Santos AC. Nerve stimulators used for peripheral nerve blocks vary in their electrical characteristics. *Anesthesiology* 2003;**98**:969–74.

99 Salt A, Noble-Jamieson G, Barnes ND, *et al.* Liver transplantation in 100 children: Cambridge and King's College Hospital series. *BMJ* 1992;**304**:416–21.

100 Beath S, Pearmain G, Kelly D, McMaster P, Mayer A, Buckels J. Liver transplantation in babies and children with extrahepatic biliary atresia. *J Pediatr Surg* 1993;**28**:1044–7.

101 van Mourik ID, Beath SV, Brook GA, *et al.* Long-term nutritional and neurodevelopmental outcome of liver transplantation in infants aged less than 12 months. *J Pediatr Gastroenterol Nutr* 2000;**30**:269–75.

102 Barshes NR, Lee TC, Balkrishnan R, Karpen SJ, Carter BA, Goss JA. Orthotopic liver transplantation for biliary atresia: the U.S. experience. *Liver Transpl* 2005;**11**:1193–200.

103 McKiernan, P, Baker, HJ, Lloyd, C *et al.* The British Paediatric Surveillance Unit study of biliary atresia-outcome at 13 years. *Lancet* 2000;**355**:25–29.

104 Todani T, Watanabe Y, Narusue M, Tabuchi K, Okajima K. Congenital bile duct cysts: Classification, operative procedures, and review of thirty-seven cases including cancer arising from choledochal cyst. *Am J Surg* 1977;**134**:263–9.

105 Iwai N, Yanagihara J, Tokiwa K, Shimotake T, Nakamura K. Congenital choledochal dilatation with emphasis on pathophysiology of the biliary tract. *Ann Surg* 1992;**215**:27–30.

106 Yamauchi S, Koga A, Matsumoto S, Tanaka M, Nakayama F. Anomalous junction of pancreaticobiliary duct without congenital choledochal cyst: a possible risk factor for gallbladder cancer. *Am J Gastroenterol* 1987;**82**:20–4.

107 Komi N, Tamura T, Tsuge S, Miyoshi Y, Udaka H, Takehara H. Relation of patient age to premalignant alterations in choledochal cyst epithelium: histochemical and immunohistochemical studies. *J Pediatr Surg* 1986;**21**:430–3.

108 Todani T, Watanabe Y, Fujii T, Toki A, Uemura S, Koike Y. Congenital choledochal cyst with intrahepatic involvement. *Arch Surg* 1984;**119**:1038–43.

109 Stringer MD. Choledochal cysts. In: Howard ER, Stringer MD, Colombani PM, eds. *Surgery of the Liver, Bile Ducts and Pancreas in Children,* 2nd ed. London: Arnold, 2002: 149–68.

110 Stringer MD, Dhawan A, Davenport M, Mieli-Vergani G, Mowat AP, Howard ER. Choledochal cysts: lessons from a 20 year experience. *Arch Dis Child* 1995;**73**:528–31.

111 Spitz L. Experimental production of cystic dilatation of the common bile duct in neonatal lambs. *J Pediatr Surg* 1977;**12**:39–42.

112 Babbitt DP. [Congenital choledochal cysts: new etiological concept based on anomalous relationships of the common bile duct and pancreatic bulb.] *Ann Radiol (Paris)* 1969;**12**:231–40.

113 Han SJ, Hwang EH, Chung KS, Kim MJ, Kim H. Acquired choledochal cyst from anomalous pancreatobiliary duct union. *J Pediatr Surg* 1997;**32**:1735–8.

114 Lane GJ, Yamataka A, Kobayashi H, Segawa O, Miyano T. Different types of congenital biliary dilatation in dizygotic twins. *Pediatr Surg Int* 1999;**15**:403–4.

115 Kim WS, Kim IO, Yeon KM, Park KW, Seo JK, Kim CJ. Choledochal cyst with or without biliary atresia in neonates and young infants: US differentiation. *Radiology* 1998;**209**:465–9.

116 Lugo-Vicente HL. Prenatally diagnosed choledochal cysts: observation or early surgery? *J Pediatr Surg* 1995;**30**:1288–90.

117 Suita S, Shono K, Kinugasa Y, Kubota M, Matsuo S. Influence of age on the presentation and outcome of choledochal cyst. *J Pediatr Surg* 1999;**34**:1765–8.

118 Davenport M, Stringer MD, Howard ER. Biliary amylase and congenital choledochal dilatation. *J Pediatr Surg* 1995;**30**:474–7.

119 Todani T, Urushihara N, Morotomi Y, *et al.* Characteristics of choledochal cysts in neonates and early infants. *Eur J Pediatr Surg* 1995;**5**:143–5.

120 Urushihara N, Todani T, Watanabe Y, Uemura S, Morotomi Y, Wang ZQ. Does hyperamylasemia in choledochal cyst indicate true pancreatitis? An experimental study. *Eur J Pediatr Surg* 1995;**5**:139–42.

121 Hernanz-Schulman M, Ambrosino MM, Freeman PC, Quinn CB. Common bile duct in children: sonographic dimensions. *Radiology* 1995;**195**:193–5.

122 Ando K, Miyano T, Kohno S, Takamizawa S, Lane G. Spontaneous perforation of choledochal cyst: a study of 13 cases. *Eur J Pediatr Surg* 1998;**8**:23–5.

123 Yamaguchi M. Congenital choledochal cyst. Analysis of 1433 patients in the Japanese literature. *Am J Surg* 1980;**140**:653–7.

124 Bismuth H, Krissat J. Choledochal cystic malignancies. *Ann Oncol* 1999;**10**(Suppl 4):94–8.

125 Iwai N, Deguchi E, Yanagihara J, *et al.* Cancer arising in a choledochal cyst in a 12-year-old girl. *J Pediatr Surg* 1990;**25**: 1261–3.

126 Voyles CR, Smadja C, Shands WC, Blumgart LH. Carcinoma in choledochal cysts. Age-related incidence. *Arch Surg* 1983;**118**: 986–8.

127 Todani T, Watanabe Y, Toki A, Urushihara N. Carcinoma related to choledochal cysts with internal drainage operations. *Surg Gynecol Obstet* 1987;**164**:61–4.

128 Kobayashi S, Asano T, Yamasaki M, Kenmochi T, Nakagohri T, Ochiai T. Risk of bile duct carcinogenesis after excision of extrahepatic bile ducts in pancreaticobiliary maljunction. *Surgery* 1999;**126**:939–44.

129 Matos C, Nicaise N, Devière J, *et al.* Choledochal cysts: comparison of findings at MR cholangiopancreatography and endoscopic retrograde cholangiopancreatography in eight patients. *Radiology* 1998;**209**:443–8.

130 Lam WW, Lam TP, Saing H, Chan FL, Chan KL. MR cholangiography and CT cholangiography of pediatric patients with choledochal cysts. *AJR Am J Roentgenol* 1999;**173**:401–5.

131 Kim SH, Lim JH, Yoon HK, Han BK, Lee SK, Kim YI. Choledochal cyst: comparison of MR and conventional cholangiography. *Clin Radiol* 2000;**55**:378–83.

132 Miyano T, Yamataka A, Kato Y, *et al.* Hepaticoenterostomy after excision of choledochal cyst in children: a 30-year experience with 180 cases. *Pediatr Surg* 1996;**31**:1417–21.

133 Kaneko K, Ando H, Watanabe Y, *et al.* Secondary excision of choledochal cysts after previous cyst-enterostomies. *Hepatogastroenterology* 1999;**46**:2772–5.

134 Todani T, Watanabe Y, Toki A, Urushihara N, Sato Y. Reoperation for congenital choledochal cyst. *Ann Surg* 1988;**207:**142–7.

135 Stringer MD. Wide hilar hepaticojejunostomy: the optimum method of reconstruction after choledochal cyst excision. *Pediatr Surg Int* 2007;**23**:529–32.

136 Shimotakahara A, Yamataka A, Yanai T, *et al.* Roux-en-Y hepaticojejunostomy or hepaticoduodenostomy for biliary reconstruction during the surgical treatment of choledochal cyst: which is better? *Pediatr Surg Int* 2005;**21**:5–7.

137 Lilly JR. Total excision of choledochal cyst. *Surg Gynecol Obstet* 1978;**146**:254–6.

138 O'Neill JA Jr, Templeton JM Jr, Schnaufer L, Bishop HC, Ziegler MM, Ross AJ 3rd. Recent experience with choledochal cyst. *Ann Surg* 1987;**205**:533–40.

139 Dohmoto M, Kamiya T, Hünerbein M, Valdez H, Ibanegaray J, Prado J. Endoscopic treatment of a choledochocele in a 2-year-old child. *Surg Endosc* 1996;**10**:1016–8.

140 Todani T. Choledochal cysts. In: Stringer MD, Oldham KT, Mouriquand PDE, Howard ER, eds. *Pediatric Surgery and Urology Long-Term Outcomes.* Philadelphia: Saunders, 1998: 417–29.

141 Yeong ML, Nicholson GI, Lee SP. Regression of biliary cirrhosis following choledochal cyst drainage. *Gastroenterology* 1982;**82**: 332–5.

142 Yoshikawa K, Yoshida K, Shirai Y, *et al.* A case of carcinoma arising in the intrapancreatic terminal choledochus 12 years after primary excision of a giant choledochal cyst. *Am J Gastroenterol* 1986;**81**:378–84.
143 Yamamoto J, Shimamura Y, Ohtani I, *et al.* Bile duct carcinoma arising from the anastomotic site of hepaticojejunostomy after the excision of congenital biliary dilatation: a case report. *Surgery* 1996;**119**:476–9.
144 Dijkstra CH. Graluistorting in ie buikholte bij een zuigeling. *Maandschr Kindegeneeskd* 1932;**1**:409–14.
145 Fitzgerald RJ, Parbhoo K, Guiney EJ. Spontaneous perforation of bile ducts in neonates. *Surgery* 1978;**83**:303–5.
146 Hammoudi SM, Alauddin A. Idiopathic perforation of the biliary tract in infancy and childhood. *J Pediatr Surg* 1988;**23**:185–7.
147 Davenport M, Heaton ND, Howard ER. Spontaneous perforation of the bile duct in infants. *Br J Surg* 1991;**78**:1068–70.
148 Johnston JH. Spontaneous perforation of the common bile-duct in infancy. *Br J Surg* 1961;**48**:532–3.
149 Tan CE, Moscoso GJ. The developing human biliary system at the porta hepatis level between 29 days and 8 weeks of gestation: a way to understanding biliary atresia. Part 1. *Pathol Int* 1994;**44**:587–99.
150 Witcombe JB. *Ascaris* perforation of the common bile duct demonstrated by intravenous cholangiography. *Pediatr Radiol* 1978;**7**:124–5.
151 Chardot C, Iskandarani F, De Dreuzy O, *et al.* Spontaneous perforation of the biliary tract in infancy: a series of 11 cases. *Eur J Pediatr Surg* 1996;**6**:341–6.
152 Kumar V, Chattopadhyay A, Bhat N, Rao PL. Spontaneous biliary perforation presenting as gastric outlet obstruction. *Indian J Pediatr* 2001;**68**:361–3.
153 Lilly JR, Weintraub WH, Altman RP. Spontaneous perforation of the extrahepatic bile ducts and bile peritonitis in infancy. *Surgery* 1974;**75**:664–73.
154 Spigland N, Greco R, Rosenfeld D. Spontaneous biliary perforation: does external drainage constitute adequate therapy? *J Pediatr Surg* 1996;**31**:782–4.
155 St-Vil D, Yazbeck S, Luks FI, Hancock BJ, Filiatrault D, Youssef S. Cholelithiasis in newborns and infants. *J Pediatr Surg* 1992;**27**:1305–7.
156 Schirmer WJ, Grisoni ER, Gauderer MW. The spectrum of cholelithiasis in the first year of life. *Pediatr Surg* 1989;**24**:1064–7.
157 Heaton ND, Davenport M, Howard ER. Intraluminal biliary obstruction. *Arch Dis Child* 1991;**66**:1395–8.
158 Howard ER. Benign extrahepatic bile duct obstruction and cholestatic syndromes. In: Howard ER, Stringer MD, Colombani PM, eds. *Surgery of the Liver, Bile Ducts and Pancreas in Children*, 2nd ed. London: Arnold, 2002: 175–87.
159 Bowles MJ, Salisbury JR, Howard ER. Localized, benign, non-traumatic strictures of the extrahepatic biliary tree in children. *Surgery* 2001;**130**:55–9.
160 Verbeek PC, van Leeuwen DJ, de Wit LT, *et al.* Benign fibrosing disease at the hepatic confluence mimicking Klatskin tumors. *Surgery* 1992;**112**:866–71.
161 Anagnostopoulos D, Tsagari N, Noussia-Arvanitaki S, Sfougaris D, Valioulis I, Spyridakis I. Gallbladder disease in patients with cystic fibrosis. *Eur J Pediatr Surg* 1993;**3**:348–51.
162 Toscano E, Trivellini V, Andria G. Cholelithiasis in Down's syndrome. *Arch Dis Child* 2001;**85**:242–3.
163 Sakopoulos AG, Gundry S, Razzouk AJ, Andrews HG, Bailey LL. Cholelithiasis in infant and pediatric heart transplant patients. *Pediatr Transplant* 2002;**6**:231–4.
164 Mahmoud H, Schell M, Pui CH. Cholelithiasis after treatment for childhood cancer. *Cancer* 1991;**67**:1439–42.
165 Safford SD, Safford KM, Martin P, Rice H, Kurtzberg J, Skinner MA. Management of cholelithiasis in pediatric patients who undergo bone marrow transplantation. *J Pediatr Surg* 2001;**36**: 86–90.
166 Teele RL, Nussbaum AR, Wyly JB, Allred EN, Emans J. Cholelithiasis after spinal fusion for scoliosis in children. *J Pediatr* 1987;**111**:857–60.
167 Reif S, Sloven DG, Lebenthal E. Gallstones in children. Characterization by age, etiology, and outcome. *Am J Dis Child* 1991;**145**:105–8.
168 Danon YL, Dinari G, Garty BZ, Horodniceanu C, Nitzan M, Grunebaum M. Cholelithiasis in children with immunoglobulin A deficiency: a new gastroenterologic syndrome. *J Pediatr Gastroenterol Nutr* 1983;**2**:663–6.
169 Schwindt WD, Bernhardt LC, Peters HA. Cholelithiasis and associated complications of myotonia dystrophica. *Postgrad Med* 1969;**46**:80–3.
170 Shimotake T, Iwai N, Yanagihara J, Tokiwa K, Fushiki S. Biliary tract complications in patients with hypoganglionosis and chronic idiopathic intestinal pseudoobstruction syndrome. *J Pediatr Surg* 1993;**28**:189–92.
171 Lykavieris P, Hadchouel M, Chardot C, Bernard O. Outcome of liver disease in children with Alagille's syndrome: a study of 163 patients. *Gut* 2001;**49**:431–5.
172 Tchirkow G, Highman LM, Shafer AD. Cholelithiasis and cholecystitis in children after repair of congenital duodenal anomalies. *Arch Surg* 1980;**115**:85–6.
173 Mali V, Wagener S, Sharif K, Millar AJ. Foregut atresias and bile duct anomalies: rare, infrequent or common? *Pediatr Surg Int* 2007;**23**:889–95.
174 EE, Perez-Atayde AR, Schuster SR. Botryoid rhabdomyosarcoma of the biliary tract. *Am J Surg Pathol* 1981;**5**:643–52.
175 Spunt SL, Lobe TE, Pappo AS, *et al.* Aggressive surgery is unwarranted for biliary tract rhabdomyosarcoma. *J Pediatr Surg* 2000;**35**:309–16.
176 Watanabe Y, Toki A, Todani T. Bile duct cancer developed after cyst excision for choledochal cyst. *J Hepatobiliary Pancreat Surg* 1999;**6**:207–12.
177 Czaja MJ, Goldfarb JP, Cho KC, Biempica L, Morehouse HT, Abelow A. Bile duct carcinoma in an adolescent. *Am J Gastroenterol* 1985;**80**:486–9.
178 Soares FA, Landell GA, Peres LC, Oliveira MA, Vicente YA, Tone LG. Liposarcoma of hepatic hilum in childhood: report of a case and review of the literature. *Med Pediatr Oncol* 1989;**17**:239–43.
179 Arif Mateen Khan M, Thomas DM, Howard ER. Pancreatitis in childhood associated with villous adenoma of the ampulla of Vater. *Br J Surg* 1996;**83**:1211.
180 Reynolds EM, Tsivis PA, Long JA. Granular cell tumor of the biliary tree in a pediatric patient. *J Pediatr Surg* 2000;**35**:652–4.
181 Cheslyn-Curtis S, Russell RC, Rode J, Dhillon AP. Granular cell tumour of the common bile duct. *Postgrad Med J* 1986;**62**:961–3.
182 Wendtland-Born A, Wiewrodt B, Bender SW, Weitzel D. [Prevalence of gallstones in the neonatal period; in German.] *Ultraschall Med* 1997;**18**:80–3.

183 Palasciano G, Portincasa P, Vinciguerra V, *et al.* Gallstone prevalence and gallbladder volume in children and adolescents: an epidemiological ultrasonographic survey and relationship to body mass index. *Am J Gastroenterol* 1989;**84**:1378–82.

184 Nomura H, Kashiwagi S, Hayashi J, *et al.* Prevalence of gallstone disease in a general population of Okinawa, Japan. *Am J Epidemiol* 1988;**128**:598–605.

185 Takiff H, Fonkalsrud EW. Gallbladder disease in childhood. *Am J Dis Child* 1984;**138**:565–8.

186 Bailey PV, Connors RH, Tracy TF Jr, Sotelo-Avila C, Lewis JE, Weber TR. Changing spectrum of cholelithiasis and cholecystitis in infants and children. *Am J Surg* 1989;**158**:585–8.

187 Grosfeld JL, Rescorla FJ, Skinner MA, West KW, Scherer LR 3rd. The spectrum of biliary tract disorders in infants and children. Experience with 300 cases. *Arch Surg* 1994;**129**:513–8; discussion 518–20.

188 Waldhausen JH, Benjamin DR. Cholecystectomy is becoming an increasingly common operation in children. *Am J Surg* 1999; **177**:364–7.

189 Kumar R, Nguyen K, Shun A. Gallstones and common bile duct calculi in infancy and childhood. *Aust N Z J Surg* 2000;**70**:188–91.

190 Miltenburg DM, Schaffer R 3rd, Breslin T, Brandt ML. Changing indications for pediatric cholecystectomy. *Pediatrics* 2000;**105**: 1250–3.

191 O'Brien CB, Berman JM, Fleming CR, Malet PF, Soloway RD. Total parenteral nutrition gallstones contain more calcium bilirubinate than sickle cell gallstones [abstract]. *Gastroenterology* 1986;**90**:1752A.

192 Wu SS, Casas AT, Abraham SK, Billmire DF, Smergel EM, de Chadarevian JP. Milk of calcium cholelithiasis in children. *J Pediatr Surg* 2001;**36**:644–7.

193 Sayers C, Wyatt J, Soloway RD, Taylor DR, Stringer MD. Gallbladder mucin production and calcium carbonate gallstones in children. *Pediatr Surg Int* 2007;**23**:219–23.

194 Afdhal NH. Epidemiology, risk factors, and pathogenesis of gallstones. In: Afdhal NH, ed. *Gallbladder and Biliary Tract Diseases.* New York: Dekker, 2000: 127–46.

195 Bond LR, Hatty SR, Horn ME, Dick M, Meire HB, Bellingham AJ. Gall stones in sickle cell disease in the United Kingdom. *Br Med J (Clin Res Ed)* 1987;**295**:234–6.

196 Webb DK, Darby JS, Dunn DT, Terry SI, Serjeant GR. Gall stones in Jamaican children with homozygous sickle cell disease. *Arch Dis Child* 1989;**64**:693–6.

197 Croom RD 3rd, McMillan CW, Orringer EP, Sheldon GF. Hereditary spherocytosis. Recent experience and current concepts of pathophysiology. *Ann Surg* 1986;**203**:34–9.

198 Kalayci AG, Albayrak D, Güneş M, Incesu L, Agaç R. The incidence of gallbladder stones and gallbladder function in beta-thalassemic children. *Acta Radiol* 1999;**40**:440–3.

199 Davies BW, Abel G, Puntis JW, *et al.* Limited ileal resection in infancy: the long-term consequences. *J Pediatr Surg* 1999;**34**: 583–7.

200 Georgeson K, Brown P. Short bowel syndrome. In: Stringer MD, Oldham KT, Mouriquand PDE, Howard ER, eds. *Pediatric Surgery and Urology Long-Term Outcomes.* Philadelphia: Saunders, 1998: 237–42.

201 Jawaheer G, Pierro A, Lloyd DA, Shaw NJ. Gall bladder contractility in neonates: effects of parenteral and enteral feeding. *Arch Dis Child Fetal Neonatal Ed* 1995;**72**:F200–2.

202 Matos C, Avni EF, Van Gansbeke D, Pardou A, Struyven J. Total parenteral nutrition (TPN) and gallbladder diseases in neonates. Sonographic assessment. *J Ultrasound Med* 1987;**6**:243–8.

203 Stringer MD, Lim P, Cave M, Martinez D, Lilford RJ. Fetal gallstones. *J Pediatr Surg* 1996;**31**:1589–91.

204 Lehtonen L, Svedström E, Kero P, Korvenranta H. Gall bladder contractility in preterm infants. *Arch Dis Child* 1993;**68**(1 Spec No):43–5.

205 Halpern Z, Vinograd Z, Laufer H, Gilat T, Moskowitz M, Bujanover Y. Characteristics of gallbladder bile of infants and children. *J Pediatr Gastroenterol Nutr* 1996;**23**:147–50.

206 Debray D, Pariente D, Gauthier F, Myara A, Bernard O. Cholelithiasis in infancy: a study of 40 cases. *J Pediatr* 1993; **122**:385–91.

207 Vessey M, Painter R. Oral contraceptive use and benign gallbladder disease; revisited. *Contraception* 1994;**50**:167–73.

208 Rintala RJ, Lindahl H, Pohjavuori M. Total parenteral nutrition-associated cholestasis in surgical neonates may be reversed by intravenous cholecystokinin: a preliminary report. *J Pediatr Surg* 1995;**30**:827–30.

209 Bruch SW, Ein SH, Rocchi C, Kim PC. The management of nonpigmented gallstones in children. *J Pediatr Surg* 2000;**35**: 729–32.

210 Colombo C, Bertolini E, Assaisso ML, Bettinardi N, Giunta A, Podda M. Failure of ursodeoxycholic acid to dissolve radiolucent gallstones in patients with cystic fibrosis. *Acta Paediatr* 1993;**82**: 562–5.

211 Sokal EM, De Bilderling G, Clapuyt P, Opsomer RJ, Buts JP. Extracorporeal shock-wave lithotripsy for calcified lower choledocholithiasis in an 18-month-old boy. *J Pediatr Gastroenterol Nutr* 1994;**18**:391–4.

212 Holcomb GW 3rd, Morgan WM 3rd, Neblett WW 3rd, Pietsch JB, O'Neill JA Jr, Shyr Y. Laparoscopic cholecystectomy in children: lessons learned from the first 100 patients. *J Pediatr Surg* 1999;**34**:1236–40.

213 Sandler A, Winkel G, Kimura K, Soper R. The role of prophylactic cholecystectomy during splenectomy in children with hereditary spherocytosis. *J Pediatr Surg* 1999;**34**:1077–8.

214 Alexander-Reindorf C, Nwaneri RU, Worrell RG, Ogbonna A, Uzoma C. The significance of gallstones in children with sickle cell anemia. *J Natl Med Assoc* 1990;**82**:645–50.

215 Winter SS, Kinney TR, Ware RE. Gallbladder sludge in children with sickle cell disease. *J Pediatr* 1994;**125**:747–9.

216 Newman KD, Powell DM, Holcomb GW 3rd. The management of choledocholithiasis in children in the era of laparoscopic cholecystectomy. *Pediatr Surg* 1997;**32**:1116–9.

217 Ware R, Filston HC, Schultz WH, Kinney TR. Elective cholecystectomy in children with sickle hemoglobinopathies. Successful outcome using a preoperative transfusion regimen. *Ann Surg* 1988;**208**:17–22.

218 Guelrud M, Mendoza S, Jaen D, Plaz J, Machuca J, Torres P. ERCP and endoscopic sphincterotomy in infants and children with jaundice due to common bile duct stones. *Gastrointest Endosc* 1992;**38**:450–3.

219 Mah D, Wales P, Njere I, Kortan P, Masiakos P, Kim PC. Management of suspected common bile duct stones in children: role of selective intraoperative cholangiogram and endoscopic retrograde cholangiopancreatography. *J Pediatr Surg* 2004;**39**: 808–12.

220 Bonnard A, Seguier-Lipszyc E, Liguory C, *et al.* Laparoscopic approach as primary treatment of common bile duct stones in children. *Pediatr Surg* 2005;**40**:1459–63.

221 Hadigan C, Fishman SJ, Connolly LP, Treves ST, Nurko S. Stimulation with fatty meal (Lipomul) to assess gallbladder emptying in children with chronic acalculous cholecystitis. *J Pediatr Gastroenterol Nutr* 2003;**37**:178–82.

222 Dumont RC, Caniano DA. Hypokinetic gallbladder disease: a cause of chronic abdominal pain in children and adolescents. *J Pediatr Surg* 1999;**34**:858–61; discussion 861–2.

223 Campbell BT, Narasimhan NP, Golladay ES, Hirschl RB. Biliary dyskinesia: a potentially unrecognized cause of abdominal pain in children. *Pediatr Surg Int* 2004;**20**:579–81.

224 Vegunta RK, Raso M, Pollock J, *et al.* Biliary dyskinesia: the most common indication for cholecystectomy in children. *Surgery* 2005;**138**:726–31; discussion 731–3.

225 Scott Nelson R, Kolts R, Park R, Heikenen J. A comparison of cholecystectomy and observation in children with biliary dyskinesia. *J Pediatr Surg* 2006;**41**:1894–8.

226 Tsakayannis DE, Kozakewich HP, Lillehei CW. Acalculous cholecystitis in children. *J Pediatr Surg* 1996;**31**:127–30; discussion 130–1.

227 Ameh EA. Cholecystitis in children in Zaria, Nigeria. *Ann Trop Paediatr* 1999;**19**:205–9.

228 Joyce AD, Howard ER. Rare congenital anomaly of the portal vein. *Br J Surg* 1988;**75**:1038–9.

229 Howard ER, Davenport M. Congenital extrahepatic portocaval shunts—the Abernethy malformation. *J Pediatr Surg* 1997;**32**: 494–7.

230 Meyer WW, Lind J. The ductus venosus and the mechanism of its closure. *Arch Dis Child* 1966;**41**:597–605.

231 Abernethy J. Account of two instances of uncommon formation in the viscera of the human body. *Philos Trans R Soc London* 1793;**83**:59–66.

232 Howard ER. Etiology of portal hypertension and congenital anomalies of the portal venous system. In: Howard ER, Stringer MD, Colombani PM, eds. *Surgery of the Liver, Bile Ducts and Pancreas in Children,* 2nd ed. London: Arnold, 2002: 287–95.

233 Ishii Y, Inagaki Y, Hirai K, Aoki T. Hepatic encephalopathy caused by congenital extrahepatic portosystemic venous shunt. *J Hepatobiliary Pancreat Surg* 2000;**7**:524–8.

234 Raskin NH, Bredesen D, Ehrenfeld WK, Kerlan RK. Periodic confusion caused by congenital extrahepatic portacaval shunt. *Neurology* 1984;**34**:666–9.

235 Barsky MF, Rankin RN, Wall WJ, Ghent CN, Garcia B. Patent ductus venosus: problems in assessment and management. *Can J Surg* 1989;**32**:271–5.

236 Laverdiere JT, Laor T, Benacerraf B. Congenital absence of the portal vein: case report and MR demonstration. *Pediatr Radiol* 1995;**25**:52–3.

237 Manning N, Impey L, Lindsell D, Lakhoo K. Prenatally diagnosed portocaval shunt and postnatal outcome: a case report. *Prenat Diagn* 2004;**24**:537–40.

238 Cheung KM, Lee CY, Wong CT, Chan AK. Congenital absence of portal vein presenting as hepatopulmonary syndrome. *J Paediatr Child Health* 2005;**41**:72–5.

239 Tercier S, Delarue A, Rouault F, Roman C, Bréaud J, Petit P. Congenital portocaval fistula associated with hepatopulmonary syndrome: ligation vs liver transplantation. *Pediatr Surg* 2006; **41**:e1–3.

240 Uchino T, Endo F, Ikeda S, Shiraki K, Sera Y, Matsuda I. Three brothers with progressive hepatic dysfunction and severe hepatic steatosis due to a patent ductus venosus. *Gastroenterology* 1996;**110**:1964–8.

241 Howard ER. Encephalopathy without cirrhosis: hunt the shunt. *Gut* 1999;**45**:329–30.

242 Léveillé R, Pibarot P, Soulez G, Wisner ER. Transvenous coil embolization of an extrahepatic portosystemic shunt in a dog: a naturally occurring model of portosystemic malformations in humans. *Pediatr Radiol* 2000;**30**:607–9.

243 Zentler-Munro PL, Howard ER, Karani J, Williams R. Variceal haemorrhage in hereditary haemorrhagic telangiectasia. *Gut* 1989;**30**:1293–7.

244 Davenport M, Redkar R, Howard ER, Karani J. Arterioportal hypertension: a rare complication of partial hepatectomy. *Pediatr Surg Int* 1999;**15**:543–5.

245 Heaton ND, Davenport M, Karani J, Mowat AP, Howard ER. Congenital hepatoportal arteriovenous fistula. *Surgery* 1995; **117**:170–4.

246 Kumar N, de Goyet J de V, Sharif K, McKiernan P, John P. Congenital, solitary, large, intrahepatic arterioportal fistula in a child: management and review of the literature. *Pediatr Radiol* 2003;**33**:20–3.

247 Norton SP, Jacobson K, Moroz SP, *et al.* The congenital intrahepatic arterioportal fistula syndrome: elucidation and proposed classification. *J Pediatr Gastroenterol Nutr* 2006;**43**:248–55.

248 Stringer MD, McClean P, Arthur RJ, Lintott D. Congenital hepatoportal arteriovenous fistula. *Surgery* 1996;**119**:235–6.

249 Arakawa M, Masuzaki T, Okuda K. Pathomorphology of esophageal and gastric varices. *Semin Liver Dis* 2002;**22**:73–82.

250 Garcia-Tsao G, Groszmann RJ, Fisher RL, Conn HO, Atterbury CE, Glickman M. Portal pressure, presence of gastroesophageal varices and variceal bleeding. *Hepatology* 1985;**5**:419–24.

251 Lebrec D. Ectopic varices in patients with portal hypertension. *Arch Surg* 1980;**115**:890.

252 Webb LJ, Sherlock S. The aetiology, presentation and natural history of extra-hepatic portal venous obstruction. *Q J Med* 1979;**48**:627–39.

253 Lykavieris P, Gauthier F, Hadchouel P, Duche M, Bernard O. Risk of gastrointestinal bleeding during adolescence and early adulthood in children with portal vein obstruction. *J Pediatr* 2000;**136**:805–8.

254 Sarin SK, Bansal A, Sasan S, Nigam A. Portal-vein obstruction in children leads to growth retardation. *Hepatology* 1992;**15**:229–33.

255 Mehrotra RN, Bhatia V, Dabadghao P, Yachha SK. Extrahepatic portal vein obstruction in children: anthropometry, growth hormone, and insulin-like growth factor I. *J Pediatr Gastroenterol Nutr* 1997;**25**:520–3.

256 Silver MM, Bohn D, Shawn DH, Shuckett B, Eich G, Rabinovitch M. Association of pulmonary hypertension with congenital portal hypertension in a child. *J Pediatr* 1992;**120**:321–9.

257 Schuijtvlot ET, Bax NM, Houwen RH, Hruda J. Unexpected lethal pulmonary hypertension in a 5-year-old girl successfully treated for biliary atresia. *J Pediatr Surg* 1995;**30**:589–90.

258 Howard ER, Stringer MD, Mowat AP. Assessment of injection sclerotherapy in the management of 152 children with oesophageal varices. *Br J Surg* 1988;**75**:404–8.

259 Maksoud JG, Gonçalves ME, Porta G, Miura I, Velhote MC. The endoscopic and surgical management of portal hypertension in children: analysis of 123 cases. *J Pediatr Surg* 1991;**26**: 178–81.

260 Stringer MD. Pathogenesis and management of esophageal and gastric varices. In: Howard ER, Stringer MD, Colombani PM, eds. *Surgery of the Liver, Bile Ducts and Pancreas in Children*, 2nd ed. London: Arnold, 2002: 297–314.

261 Yadav S, Dutta AK, Sarin SK. Do umbilical vein catheterization and sepsis lead to portal vein thrombosis? A prospective, clinical, and sonographic evaluation. *J Pediatr Gastroenterol Nutr* 1993;**17**:392–6.

262 Dubuisson C, Boyer-Neumann C, Wolf M, Meyer D, Bernard O. Protein C, protein S and antithrombin III in children with portal vein obstruction. *J Hepatol* 1997;**27**:132–5.

263 Fisher NC, Wilde JT, Roper J, Elias E. Deficiency of natural anticoagulant proteins C, S, and antithrombin in portal vein thrombosis: a secondary phenomenon? *Gut* 2000;**46**:534–9.

264 Stringer MD, Heaton ND, Karani J, Olliff S, Howard ER. Patterns of portal vein occlusion and their aetiological significance. *Br J Surg* 1994;**81**:1328–31.

265 Lenthall R, Kane PA, Heaton ND, Karani JB. Segmental portal hypertension due to splenic vein obstruction: imaging findings and diagnostic pitfalls in four cases. *Clin Radiol* 1999;**54**: 540–4.

266 Odièvre M, Pigé G, Alagille's D. Congenital abnormalities associated with extrahepatic portal hypertension. *Arch Dis Child* 1977;**52**:383–5.

267 Mikkelsen WP, Edmondson HA, Peters RL, Redeker AG, Reynolds TB. Extra- and intrahepatic portal hypertension without cirrhosis (hepatoportal sclerosis). Ann Surg 1965;**162**:602–20.

268 Carson JA, Tunell WP, Barnes P, Altshuler G. Hepatoportal sclerosis in childhood: a mimic of extrahepatic portal vein obstruction. *J Pediatr Surg* 1981;**16**:291–6.

269 Okudaira M, Ohbu M, Okuda K. Idiopathic portal hypertension and its pathology. *Semin Liver Dis* 2002;**22**:59–72.

270 Steenkamp V, Stewart MJ, Zuckerman M. Clinical and analytical aspects of pyrrolizidine poisoning caused by South African traditional medicines. *Ther Drug Monit* 2000;**22**:302–6.

271 Kullendorff CM, Békássy AN. Hepatic veno-occlusive disease in Wilms' tumor. *Eur J Pediatr Surg* 1996;**6**:338–40.

272 DeLeve LD, Shulman HM, McDonald GB. Toxic injury to hepatic sinusoids: sinusoidal obstruction syndrome (veno-occlusive disease). *Semin Liver Dis* 2002;**22**:27–42.

273 Shulman HM, Hinterberger W. Hepatic veno-occlusive disease—liver toxicity syndrome after bone marrow transplantation. *Bone Marrow Transplant* 1992;**10**:197–214.

274 Chopra R, Eaton JD, Grassi A, *et al.* Defibrotide for the treatment of hepatic veno-occlusive disease: results of the European compassionate-use study. *Br J Haematol* 2000;**111**:1122–9.

275 Attal M, Huguet F, Rubie H, *et al.* Prevention of hepatic veno-occlusive disease after bone marrow transplantation by continuous infusion of low-dose heparin: a prospective, randomized trial. *Blood* 1992;**79**:2834–40.

276 Valla DC. Hepatic vein thrombosis (Budd–Chiari syndrome). *Semin Liver Dis* 2002;**22**:5–14.

277 Odell JA, Rode H, Millar AJ, Hoffman HD. Surgical repair in children with the Budd–Chiari syndrome. *J Thorac Cardiovasc Surg* 1995;**110**:916–23.

278 Cauchi JA, Oliff S, Baumann U, *et al.* The Budd–Chiari syndrome in children: the spectrum of management. *J Pediatr Surg* 2006;**41**:1919–23.

279 Gentil-Kocher S, Bernard O, Brunelle F, *et al.* Budd–Chiari syndrome in children: report of 22 cases. *J Pediatr* 1988;**113**: 30–8.

280 Rehan VK, Cronin CM, Bowman JM. Neonatal portal vein thrombosis successfully treated by regional streptokinase infusion. *Eur J Pediatr* 1994;**153**:456–9.

281 Parker MJ, Joubert GI, Levin SD. Portal vein thrombosis causing neonatal cerebral infarction. *Arch Dis Child Fetal Neonatal Ed* 2002;**87**:F125–7.

282 Abraldes JG, Bosch J. Somatostatin and analogues in portal hypertension. *Hepatology* 2002;**35**:1305–12.

283 Crafoord C, Frenckner P. New surgical treatment of varicose veins of the oesophagus. *Acta Otolaryngol* 1939;**27**:422–9.

284 Stringer MD. Portal hypertension: injection sclerotherapy of esophageal varices. In: Stringer MD, Oldham KT, Mouriquand PDE, Howard ER, eds. *Pediatric Surgery and Urology Long-Term Outcomes*. Philadelphia: Saunders, 1998: 430–8.

285 Stringer MD. Pathogenesis and management of esophageal and gastric varices. In: Howard ER, Stringer MD, Colombani PM, eds. *Surgery of the Liver, Bile Ducts and Pancreas in Children*, 2nd ed. London: Arnold, 2002: 297–314.

286 Kumar A, Mehta SR, Joshi V, Kasthuri AS, Narayanan VA. Ranitidine for the prevention of complications following endoscopic sclerotherapy for esophageal varices. *J Assoc Physicians India* 1993;**41**:584, 589.

287 Roesch W, Rexroth G. Pulmonary, cerebral and coronary emboli during bucrylate injection of bleeding fundic varices. *Endoscopy* 1998;**30**:S89–90.

288 Millar AJ, Brown RA, Hill ID, Rode H, Cywes S. The fundal pile: bleeding gastric varices. *J Pediatr Surg* 1991;**26**:707–9.

289 Stringer MD, Howard ER. Longterm outcome after injection sclerotherapy for oesophageal varices in children with extrahepatic portal hypertension. *Gut* 1994;**35**:257–9.

290 Paquet KJ, Lazar A. Current therapeutic strategy in bleeding esophageal varices in babies and children and long-term results of endoscopic paravariceal sclerotherapy over twenty years. *Eur J Pediatr Surg* 1994;**4**:165–72.

291 Sauerbruch T, Holl J, Ruckdeschel G, Förstl J, Weinzierl M. Bacteriaemia associated with endoscopic sclerotherapy of oesophageal varices. *Endoscopy* 1985;**17**:170–2.

292 Greenholz SK, Hall RJ, Sondheimer JM, Lilly JR, Hernandez-Cano AM. Manometric and pH consequences of esophageal endosclerosis in children. *J Pediatr Surg* 1988;**23**:38–41.

293 Kokudo N, Sanjo K, Umekita N, Harihara Y, Tada Y, Idezuki Y. Squamous cell carcinoma after endoscopic injection sclerotherapy for esophageal varices. *Am J Gastroenterol* 1990;**85**:861–4.

294 Dina R, Cassisa A, Baroncini D, D'Imperio N. Role of esophageal brushing cytology in monitoring patients treated with sclerotherapy for esophageal varices. *Acta Cytol* 1992;**36**:477–9.

295 Stiegmann GV, Goff JS, Sun JH, Davis D, Bozdech J. Endoscopic variceal ligation: an alternative to sclerotherapy. *Gastrointest Endosc* 1989;**35**:431–4.

296 Young MF, Sanowski RA, Rasche R. Comparison and characterization of ulcerations induced by endoscopic ligation of esophageal varices versus endoscopic sclerotherapy. *Gastrointest Endosc* 1993;**39**:119–22.

297 Helmy A, Hayes PC. Review article: current endoscopic therapeutic options in the management of variceal bleeding. *Aliment Pharmacol Ther* 2001;**15**:575–94.
298 Fox VL, Carr-Locke DL, Connors PJ, Leichtner AM. Endoscopic ligation of esophageal varices in children. *J Pediatr Gastroenterol Nutr* 1995;**20**:202–8.
299 Price MR, Sartorelli KH, Karrer FM, Narkewicz MR, Sokol RJ, Lilly JR. Management of esophageal varices in children by endoscopic variceal ligation. *J Pediatr Surg* 1996;**31**:1056–9.
300 Celińska-Cedro D, Teisseyre M, Woynarowski M, Socha P, Socha J, Ryzko J. Endoscopic ligation of esophageal varices for prophylaxis of first bleeding in children and adolescents with portal hypertension: preliminary results of a prospective study. *J Pediatr Surg* 2003;**38**:1008–11.
301 Poddar U, Thapa BR, Singh K. Band ligation plus sclerotherapy versus sclerotherapy alone in children with extrahepatic portal venous obstruction. *J Clin Gastroenterol* 2005;**39**:626–9.
302 Lebrec D, Benhamou JP. Ectopic varices in portal hypertension. *Clin Gastroenterol* 1985;**14**:105–21.
303 Heaton ND, Davenport M, Howard ER. Incidence of haemorrhoids and anorectal varices in children with portal hypertension. *Br J Surg* 1993;**80**:616–8.
304 Sarin SK. Long-term follow-up of gastric variceal sclerotherapy: an eleven-year experience. *Gastrointest Endosc* 1997;**46**:8–14.
305 Binmoeller KF, Borsatto R. Variceal bleeding and portal hypertension. *Endoscopy* 2000;**32**:189–99.
306 Heaton ND, Howard ER. Complications and limitations of injection sclerotherapy in portal hypertension. *Gut* 1993;**34**:7–10.
307 Superina R, Shneider B, Emre S, Sarin S, de Ville de Goyet J. Surgical guidelines for the management of extra-hepatic portal vein obstruction. *Pediatr Transplant* 2006;**10**:908–13.
308 Bismuth H, Franco D, Alagille's D. Portal diversion for portal hypertension in children. The first ninety patients. *Ann Surg* 1980;**192**:18–24.
309 Prasad AS, Gupta S, Kohli V, Pande GK, Sahni P, Nundy S. Proximal splenorenal shunts for extrahepatic portal venous obstruction in children. *Ann Surg* 1994;**219**:193–6.
310 de Ville de Goyet J, Alberti D, Clapuyt P, *et al.* Direct bypassing of extrahepatic portal venous obstruction in children: a new technique for combined hepatic portal revascularization and treatment of extrahepatic portal hypertension. *J Pediatr Surg* 1998;**33**:597–601.
311 Warren WD, Salam AA, Hutson D, Zeppa R. Selective distal splenorenal shunt. Technique and results of operation. *Arch Surg* 1974;**108**:306–14.
312 Kato T, Romero R, Koutouby R, *et al.* Portosystemic shunting in children during the era of endoscopic therapy: improved postoperative growth parameters. *J Pediatr Gastroenterol Nutr* 2000;**30**:419–25.
313 Valayer J, Branchereau S. Portal hypertension: portosystemic shunts. In: Stringer MD, Oldham KT, Mouriquand PDE, Howard ER, eds. *Pediatric Surgery and Urology Long-Term Outcomes.* Philadelphia: Saunders, 1998: 439–46.
314 Alagille's D, Carlier JC, Chiva M, Ziadé R, Ziadé M, Moy F. Long-term neuropsychological outcome in children undergoing portal-systemic shunts for portal vein obstruction without liver disease. *J Pediatr Gastroenterol Nutr* 1986;**5**:861–6.
315 Mack CL, Zelko FA, Lokar J, *et al.* Surgically restoring portal blood flow to the liver in children with primary extrahepatic portal vein thrombosis improves fluid neurocognitive ability. *Pediatrics* 2006;**117**:e405–12.
316 Levine OR, Harris RC, Blanc WA, Mellins RB. Progressive pulmonary hypertension in children with portal hypertension. *J Pediatr* 1973;**83**:964–72.
317 Bambini DA, Superina R, Almond PS, Whitington PF, Alonso E. Experience with the Rex shunt (mesenterico–left portal bypass) in children with extrahepatic portal hypertension. *J Pediatr Surg* 2000;**35**:13–8; discussion 18–9.
318 Uchiyama M, Iwafuchi M, Ohsawa Y, *et al.* Long-term results after nonshunt operations for esophageal varices in children. *J Pediatr Surg* 1994;**29**:1429–33.
319 Brandt CT, Rothbarth LJ, Kumpe D, Karrer FM, Lilly JR. Splenic embolization in children: long-term efficacy. *J Pediatr Surg* 1989;**24**:642–4; discussion 644–5.
320 Thalhammer GH, Eber E, Uranüs S, Pfeifer J, Zach MS. Partial splenectomy in cystic fibrosis patients with hypersplenism. *Arch Dis Child* 2003;**88**:143–6.
321 Kelly DA, de Ville de Goyet J. Commentary [on ref. 320]. *Arch Dis Child* 2003;**88**:145–6.
322 Vickers CR, O'Connor HJ, Quintero GA, Aerts RJ, Elias E, Neuberger JM. Delayed perforation of the esophagus after variceal sclerotherapy and hepatic transplantation. *Gastrointest Endosc* 1989;**35**:459–61.
323 Stringer MD, Price JF, Mowat AP, Howard ER. Liver cirrhosis in cystic fibrosis. *Arch Dis Child* 1993;**69**:407.
324 Mazzaferro V, Todo S, Tzakis AG, Stieber AC, Makowka L, Starzl TE. Liver transplantation in patients with previous portasystemic shunt. *Am J Surg* 1990;**160**:111–6.
325 Srinivasan P, Rela M, Prachalias A, *et al.* Liver transplantation for Budd–Chiari syndrome. *Transplantation* 2002;**73**:973–7.
326 Hayes PC, Davis JM, Lewis JA, Bouchier IA. Meta-analysis of value of propranolol in prevention of variceal haemorrhage. *Lancet* 1990;**336**:153–6.
327 Shashidhar H, Langhans N, Grand RJ. Propranolol in prevention of portal hypertensive hemorrhage in children: a pilot study. *Pediatr Gastroenterol Nutr* 1999;**29**:12–7.
328 Gonçalves ME, Cardoso SR, Maksoud JG. Prophylactic sclerotherapy in children with esophageal varices: long-term results of a controlled prospective randomized trial. *J Pediatr Surg* 2000;**35**:401–5.
329 Lay CS, Tsai YT, Teg CY, *et al.* Endoscopic variceal ligation in prophylaxis of first variceal bleeding in cirrhotic patients with high-risk esophageal varices. *Hepatology* 1997;**25**:1346–50.
330 Heyman MB, LaBerge JM. Role of transjugular intrahepatic portosystemic shunt in the treatment of portal hypertension in pediatric patients. *J Pediatr Gastroenterol Nutr* 1999;**29**:240–9.
331 Jalan R, Lui HF, Redhead DN, Hayes PC. TIPSS 10 years on. *Gut* 2000;**46**:578–81.
332 Cywes S, Bass DH, Rode H, Millar AJ. Blunt liver trauma in children. *Injury* 1991;**22**:310–4.
333 Stone HH, Ansley JD. Management of liver trauma in children. *Pediatr Surg* 1977;**12**:3–10.
334 Gross M, Lynch F, Canty T Sr, Peterson B, Spear R. Management of pediatric liver injuries: a 13-year experience at a pediatric trauma center. *J Pediatr Surg* 1999;**34**:811–6; discussion 816–7.
335 Eubanks JW 3rd, Meier DE, Hicks BA, Joglar J, Guzzetta PC. Significance of "blush" on computed tomography scan in children with liver injury. *J Pediatr Surg* 2003;**38**:363–6; discussion 363–6.

336 Debakey ME, Howard JM, Mikesky WE. Injuries of the liver in 300 consecutive patients. *Surg Gynecol Obstet* 1956;**103**:323–37.
337 MacGillivray DC, Valentine RJ. Nonoperative management of blunt pediatric liver injury—late complications: case report. *J Trauma* 1989;**29**:251–4.
338 Tso EL, Beaver BL, Haller JA Jr. Abdominal injuries in restrained pediatric passengers. *J Pediatr Surg* 1993;**28**:915–9.
339 Clarnette TD, Beasley SW. Handlebar injuries in children: patterns and prevention. *Aust N Z J Surg* 1997;**67**:338–9.
340 Gornall P, Ahmed S, Jolleys A, Cohen SJ. Intra-abdominal injuries in the battered baby syndrome. *Arch Dis Child* 1972;**47**:211–4.
341 Cooper A, Barlow B, Niemirska M, Gandhi R. Fifteen years' experience with penetrating trauma to the head and neck in children. *J Pediatr Surg* 1987;**22**:24–7.
342 French CE, Waldstein G. Subcapsular hemorrhage of the liver in the newborn. *Pediatrics* 1982;**69**:204–8.
343 Iino S, Sawada T, Kusunoki T. Case report. Computed tomography in neonatal subcapsular hemorrhage of the liver. *J Comput Assist Tomogr* 1981;**5**:416–7.
344 Coley BD, Mutabagani KH, Martin LC, *et al.* Focused abdominal sonography for trauma (FAST) in children with blunt abdominal trauma. *J Trauma* 2000;**48**:902–6.
345 Meyer AA, Crass RA. Abdominal trauma. *Surg Clin North Am* 1982;**62**:105–11.
346 Mackway-Jones K, Molyneux E, Phillips B, Wieteska S. *Advanced Paediatric Life Support: the Practical Approach*, 3rd ed. London: BMJ, 2001.
347 Shankar KR, Lloyd DA, Kitteringham L, Carty HM. Oral contrast with computed tomography in the evaluation of blunt abdominal trauma in children. *Br J Surg* 1999;**86**:1073–7.
348 Vock P, Kehrer B, Tschaeppeler H. Blunt liver trauma in children: the role of computed tomography in diagnosis and treatment. *J Pediatr Surg* 1986;**21**:413–8.
349 Elliott DC, Rodriguez A, Moncure M, *et al.* The accuracy of diagnostic laparoscopy in trauma patients: a prospective, controlled study. *Int Surg* 1998;**83**:294–8.
350 Sharif K, Pimpalwar AP, John P, Johnson K, Donnell S, De Ville De Goyet J. Benefits of early diagnosis and preemptive treatment of biliary tract complications after major blunt liver trauma in children. *J Pediatr Surg* 2002;**37**:1287–92.
351 Hennes HM, Smith DS, Schneider K, Hegenbarth MA, Duma MA, Jona JZ. Elevated liver transaminase levels in children with blunt abdominal trauma: a predictor of liver injury. *Pediatrics* 1990;**86**:87–90.
352 Landau A, van As AB, Numanoglu A, Millar AJ, Rode H. Liver injuries in children: the role of selective non-operative management. *Injury* 2006;**37**:66–71.
353 Richie JP, Fonkalsrud EW. Subcapsular hematoma of the liver. Nonoperative management. *Arch Surg* 1972;**104**:781–4.
354 Stylianos S. Evidence-based guidelines for resource utilization in children with isolated spleen or liver injury. The APSA Trauma Committee. *J Pediatr Surg* 2000;**35**:164–7; discussion 167–9.
355 Moulton SL, Lynch FP, Hoyt DB, *et al.* Operative intervention for pediatric liver injuries: avoiding delay in treatment. *J Pediatr Surg* 1992;**27**:958–62; discussion 963.
356 Ruess L, Sivit CJ, Eichelberger MR, Taylor GA, Bond SJ. Blunt hepatic and splenic trauma in children: correlation of a CT injury severity scale with clinical outcome. *Pediatr Radiol* 1995; **25**:321–5.
357 Feliciano DV, Mattox KL, Jordan GL Jr. Intra-abdominal packing for control of hepatic hemorrhage: a reappraisal. *J Trauma* 1981;**21**:285–90.
358 Pain JA, Heaton ND, Karani JB, Howard ER. Selective arterial embolisation for hepatic trauma. *Ann R Coll Surg Engl* 1991;**73**: 189–93.
359 Görich J, Rilinger N, Brado M, *et al.* Non-operative management of arterial liver hemorrhages. *Eur Radiol* 1999;**9**:85–8.
360 Castagnetti M, Houben C, Patel S, *et al.* Minimally invasive management of bile leaks after blunt liver trauma in children. *J Pediatr Surg* 2006;**41**:1539–44.

20 Primary Hepatic Tumors

Bruce Morland and Jean de Ville de Goyet

Liver tumors are relatively rare in childhood, but may be associated with a range of diagnostic, genetic, therapeutic, and surgical problems sufficient to tax even the most experienced clinician. This chapter outlines the epidemiology, etiology, pathology, initial workup, and management of liver tumors, concentrating on the commoner malignant tumors, hepatoblastoma, and hepatocellular carcinoma. Advice on the diagnosis and management of some of the benign tumors seen in children is included, with general guidelines on the selection of patients for surgery or liver transplantation.

Epidemiology

Table 20.1 indicates the nature and frequency of hepatic tumors seen in children.[1] The incidence of hepatic tumors in childhood is consistently quoted from many series as being in the region of 0.5–2.5 per million population.[2] Data collected from the West Midlands Regional Children's Tumor Registry[3] in the United Kingdom has reported the incidence to be 1.2 per million person-years. The incidence of hepatoblastoma (the commonest malignant tumor) was 0.77, and for hepatocellular carcinoma (HCC) it was 0.09—somewhat lower than other published series.

Table 20.1 The incidence of hepatic tumors in childhood (adapted from Weinberg and Finegold 1986).[1]

Type of tumor	n	%
Malignant		
Hepatoblastoma	532	43
Hepatocellular carcinoma	284	23
Sarcoma	79	6
Benign		
Hemangioma/hemangioendothelioma	166	13
Mesenchymal hamartoma	75	6
Adenoma	22	2
Focal nodular hyperplasia	22	2
Other	57	5

Thus, on average in the United Kingdom, approximately 10–15 children with hepatoblastoma and one or two children with hepatocellular carcinoma are diagnosed each year. There is a male preponderance of 1.8 : 1 for all malignant tumors, consistent with other series.

Hepatoblastoma presents in a younger age group, being an uncommon diagnosis over the age of 4 years. Hepatocellular carcinoma has its peak onset in early adolescence, although the range is wide. The older age at onset for hepatocellular carcinoma may well reflect its close association with other underlying disease processes.

These data have been recently confirmed in an overview conducted by the Automated Childhood Cancer Information system.[4] At a population level, there has been a dramatic increase in survival in countries in which a modern health system has been implemented, although the increased survival is lower for hepatocarcinomas in comparison with hepatoblastomas.

Etiology

Many etiological factors have been linked with the development of malignant hepatic tumors in childhood (Table 20.2). Broadly speaking, genetic influences are particularly important in the development of hepatoblastoma, whereas environmental factors and coexisting liver disease are strongly associated with hepatocellular carcinoma.

The link between hepatoblastoma and congenital overgrowth abnormalities—including Beckwith–Wiedemann syndrome, Simpson–Golabi–Behmel syndrome, and hemihypertrophy—has been well described.[5–8] Molecular interest has focused on the short arm of chromosome 11, and common genetic links with other embryonal tumors such as Wilms tumor and rhabdomyosarcoma. The WAGR (Wilms tumor, aniridia, genital anomalies, and mental retardation) locus at 11p13,[9] and a second Wilms tumor locus at 11p15.5,[10] have been the stimuli for much of the research efforts. Loss of heterozygosity

Diseases of the Liver and Biliary System in Children, 3rd edition. Edited by Deirdre Kelly. © 2008 Blackwell Publishing, ISBN: 978-1-4051-6334-7.

Table 20.2 Conditions associated with hepatoblastoma and hepatocellular carcinoma.

Hepatoblastoma	Hepatocellular carcinoma
Beckwith–Wiedemann syndrome	Hepatitis B
Hemihypertrophy	Hepatitis C
Familial adenomatous polyposis	Hereditary tyrosinemia
	α_1-Antitrypsin deficiency
Gardner syndrome	Cirrhosis secondary to biliary atresia
Glycogen storage disease type I	Glycogen storage disease type I
Trisomy 18	Neurofibromatosis
Fetal alcohol syndrome	
Prematurity and low birthweight	Familial adenomatous polyposis
Maternal exposure to:	Drug/toxin exposure:
Oral contraceptives	Androgens
Gonadotropins	Oral contraceptives
Metals	Methotrexate
Petroleum products	Aflatoxins
Paints and pigments	
Paternal exposure to:	Fanconi anemia
Metals	
Meckel diverticulum	

for a recessive allele at 11p15.5 in two patients with hepatoblastoma, mapping to an area in the region of insulin-like growth factor-2 (IGF-2), has been demonstrated.[11] The loss of heterozygosity for 11p15.5 in a patient with Beckwith–Wiedemann syndrome and hepatoblastoma has also been reported.[12] The same locus has been linked with the development of rhabdomyosarcoma.[13] The likely mechanism for tumorigenesis is the loss of a tumor-suppressor gene from this region. Other investigators have been able to demonstrate that in addition to loss of heterozygosity, loss of genomic imprinting can result in hepatoblastoma.[14,15] There appears therefore to be compelling evidence to suggest a common genetic link between the pathogenesis of hepatoblastoma, rhabdomyosarcoma, and some cases of Wilms tumor, 11p15.5, and the Beckwith–Wiedemann syndrome. However, the position is far from clear and still requires further investigation. The facts that loss of heterozygosity can occur at several separate 11p loci and that IGF-2 is not implicated in all tumors are examples of why confusion still reigns.[16]

Other genes have now been implicated in the development of some cases of hepatoblastoma, particularly in cases associated with adenomatous polyposis coli (APC, also known as familial adenomatous polyposis) and Gardner syndrome, now mapped to chromosome 5q.[12,13,17,18] The adenomatous polyposis coli gene (*APC*) exerts its tumor-suppressor effects through the Wnt signaling pathway. In a normally functioning pathway, *APC* promotes destruction of β-catenin by binding to it. With loss of function of *APC* by mutation, β-catenin protein accumulates in the cell, acting as a promoter for a number of downstream oncogenic promoters. Mutations of these phosphorylation sites on exon 3 of the *APC* gene have been associated with other types of cancer, and in recent years, a high incidence (up to 80%) of such mutations has been observed in hepatoblastomas.[19–21] It has been suggested that as many as 5–10% of cases of hepatoblastoma may be associated with familial adenomatous polyposis (FAP).[13,22,23] There are important health implications for survivors of childhood hepatoblastoma with a family history of FAP. These children may have up to a 50% incidence of adenomatous polyps in later life, and it is important that they should receive appropriate screening. This raises the question of screening for hepatoblastoma infants of parents with a known history of FAP and colorectal screening for family members of children who develop hepatoblastoma for FAP.[23,24] With the availability of *APC* germline mutation analysis, many now advocate mutation screening in all patients diagnosed with hepatoblastoma.[25]

Other commonly observed genetic abnormalities seen in hepatoblastoma are trisomies of chromosomes 20, 2, and 8,[26] but due to the relative rarity of these tumors, the frequency of genetic abnormalities has been difficult to determine. With newer, more sensitive techniques such as fluorescence in-situ hybridization (FISH), it appears that such genetic abnormalities may occur in up to 50% of patients with hepatoblastoma.[27]

There is a strong link with hepatocellular carcinoma and hepatitis B virus (HBV) infection. The incidence of HCC in chronic HBV carriers is approximately 100 times greater than in the HBV-negative population,[28] and HCC is more common in areas that have high rates of endemic HBV infection. Chen *et al.*[29] reported 100% positivity for HBV infection in Taiwan, and Chan *et al.*[30] described 64% positivity in Hong Kong among children with HCC—both areas with very high endemic levels of HBV infection. Although integration of the HBV genome into the HCC genome can be demonstrated at a molecular level,[31] this event in itself is not necessarily oncogenic, and a second, as yet unidentified, promoter is probably necessary for the development of tumor. It has been postulated that environmental influences may be the reason why the incidence of HCC varies geographically and that it may not simply be a reflection of the prevalence of endemic HBV infection.[32] Promoters could also be genetic variations specific to a population, modifying cellular growth characteristics that in turn would encourage neoplasm formation independently of a direct genetic HCC-type aberration.[33] Evidence from the hemophiliac population[34] suggests that patients infected with hepatitis C virus also have an increased cumulative risk of developing liver cancer and that this risk may be significantly increased when there is coinfection with human immunodeficiency virus-1 (HIV-1).

The relationship between the development of HCC and cirrhosis is unclear. Cirrhosis of any origin and dysplastic regenerating nodules have long been considered to be the likely precursors of HCC because of their frequent association with HCC occurrence, but other genetic mechanisms may be involved. Wong *et al.*[33] identified an 8q copy number gain in a group of 12 noncirrhotic HCCs arising in a homogeneous population. From the cytogenetics, it appears that some HCC genetic alterations may be specific to etiological factors (particularly HBV infection); it has recently been suggested that progressive familial intrahepatic cholestasis (PFIC), associated with the mutation ABCB11—causing deficiency of the bile salt export pump (BSEP), a membrane canalicular bile acid transporter—represents a specific and previously unrecognized risk for HCC in young children.[35] Recently, α_1-antitrypsin deficiency was added to this list, again with a slightly different mechanism for carcinogenesis, in which liver injury would result not from the classical concept of a "gain of toxic function" mechanism, but from abnormal and chronic regenerative signaling from the sick cells to younger, less sick hepatocytes. Chronic regeneration in the presence of tissue injury leads to adenomas and ultimately to carcinomas.[36] It is suggested that the latter mechanism may explain hepatocarcinogenesis in other chronic liver diseases—e.g., genetic disorders, viral hepatitis, or nonalcoholic steatohepatitis.[36] This hypothesis could be evaluated using multicenter analysis for rare disease, such as glycogen storage disease type III, in which a specific risk for HCC has recently been reported.[37]

In general, although the histological features of HCC in children are similar to those seen in adults, there is underlying cirrhosis in only about one-third of pediatric cases.[38,39] This is in contrast to adult HCC, in which 70–90% of tumors are associated with cirrhosis. In cases associated with tyrosinemia type I, cirrhosis is an invariable finding.[40] In cases associated with biliary atresia,[5,41] the development of HCC is not universally associated with cirrhosis, and in cases of cholestasis that may not be associated with cirrhosis (e.g., arteriohepatic dysplasia), there appears to be no predisposition to malignant transformation. Thus, whilst the development of cirrhosis clearly has a part to play in oncogenesis, the exact relationship remains unclear. The finding of giant-cell hepatitis was at one stage thought to be the premalignant transformation important in the development of HCC, since this is commonly associated with a variety of hepatic pathologies (α_1-antitrypsin deficiency, familial cholestasis, etc.). However, the lack of data supporting the onset of HCC in idiopathic giant-cell hepatitis sheds doubt on the exact mechanisms underlying malignant transformation.

From the genetic point of view, dedifferentiation leading to HCC is characterized by increasing chromosomal instability and insertional mutagenesis, leading to an accumulation of structural chromosomal aberrations with losses and gains of defined chromosomal regions. Gains of regions 1q and 8q and losses of 8p are very frequently found using high-resolution microarray comparative genomic hybridization,[42] with frequent mutations in the *CTNNB1* (encoding β-catenin), *TP53*, *AXIN1*, *CTF1*, *PIK3CA*, and *KRAS* genes.[43] In accordance with the latter findings and the clinical characteristics of HCC, a predictor of bad biological behavior and a specific set of identifier genes have been identified that make it possible to categorize HCC into six subgroups. This classification has potential therapeutic implications, since 50% of the tumors were related to Wnt or Akt pathway activation, which may in turn be targeted by specific inhibiting therapies.[43]

Pathology

Malignant tumors

Hepatoblastoma

Historically, a number of classification systems have been used to define the pathological features of hepatoblastoma. Following the formation of the Childhood Epithelial Liver Tumors—International Criteria (CELTIC) group in 1990, international agreement has been sought on a number of issues, including histopathological classification of hepatocellular tumors, staging of tumors, and definitions of response.[44]

The pathology working party of the CELTIC group has agreed on the classification of hepatoblastoma into four groups, based on the work of Weinberg and Finegold.[1] These are: fetal; embryonal; macrotrabecular; and small-cell undifferentiated (Figure 20.1).

- Fetal. The pure epithelial tumors contain fetal cells, embryonal cells, or admixtures of the two. Fetal cells are characterized by being smaller than normal hepatocytes, with a low nucleocytoplasmic ratio and small nucleoli. Mitotic figures are usually uncommon and the cells form into canaliculi, which may contain bile. Some areas may contain abundant intracytoplasmic glycogen, producing a lobulated appearance alongside the acidophilic cytoplasm of other areas of tumor cells.

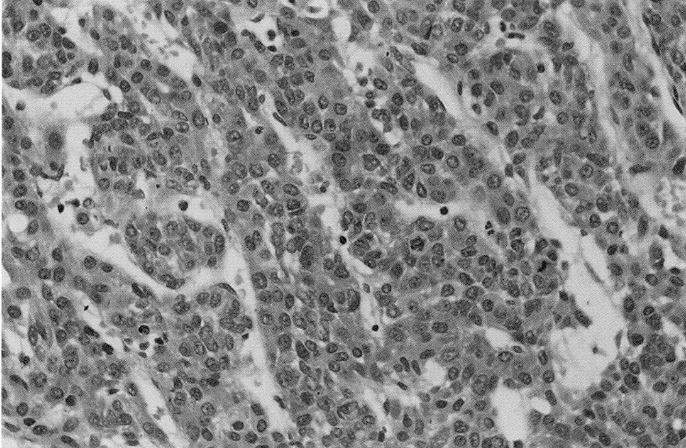

Figure 20.1 The histological diagnosis of hepatic tumors includes invasion of normal liver tissue by malignant cells, which are smaller than normal hepatocytes, with a low nuclear cytoplasmic ratio and small nucleoli. The cells may be fetal, embryonal, macrotrabecular, or small-cell undifferentiated (hematoxylin and eosin, original magnification × 82).

• Embryonal cells are smaller and less well-differentiated and have higher mitotic activity, scanty cytoplasm, and little glycogen. The cells frequently form tubular structures and may resemble the early ducts of the embryonal liver. In many tumors, a neoplastic mesenchymal component may accompany the epithelial cells. This usually takes the form of small, immature spindle cells, but fibrous or osteoid stroma mimicking osteosarcoma can sometimes be seen. Tumors consisting entirely of malignant sarcomatous elements should be classified as hepatic sarcomas (see below).
• Macrotrabecular tumors commonly contain characteristic fetal cells separated by a macrotrabecular network, which may be indistinguishable from hepatocellular carcinoma.
• Undifferentiated tumors are characterized by small cells with scanty cytoplasm. These cells can be similar in appearance to other "small blue cell" tumors of childhood such as neuroblastoma, rhabdomyosarcoma, and lymphoma. Morphological features suggesting differentiation (e.g., muscle fibers in rhabdomyosarcoma) and immunohistochemical techniques can help distinguish between these tumors and undifferentiated hepatoblastoma.

It appears that histology may be an important independent prognostic factor and that patients with exclusively fetal pathology have improved survival.[45,46] Treatment strategies for such patients are therefore focusing on minimal chemotherapy, in the hope that some of the long-term side effects of treatment can be avoided. On the other hand, an unfavorable outcome may be associated with small-cell undifferentiated histology,[47] variant hepatoblastoma with "cholangioblastic features" (personal observation),[48] or a variant type of hepatoblastoma, described recently as "transitional liver cell tumor"[49,50] (see below).

A study of the cytokeratin expression profile of hepatoblastomas suggests that hepatoblastomas recapitulate liver development and probably result from malignant transformation of precursor cells, as a consequence of blockage of normal development (the blockage arresting a clone of cells in a primitive phenotype that is able to proliferate with variable degrees of differentiation). Interestingly, the latter profile shows a correlation between immunoexpression and differentiation, suggesting that hepatoblastomas follow the stages of normal development.[51]

Hepatocellular carcinoma

Macroscopically, these tumors are usually multifocal and invasive, commonly involving both lobes and frequently associated with vascular invasion, extrahepatic extension, or both at the time of diagnosis. Areas of hemorrhage and necrosis are common, and the lesions themselves vary in consistency from soft to firm. This significantly reduces the resectability rate. Czauderna *et al.*[52] report only a 36% complete tumor resection rate in a series of 39 children recorded by the International Society of Pediatric Oncology over a 4-year time period.

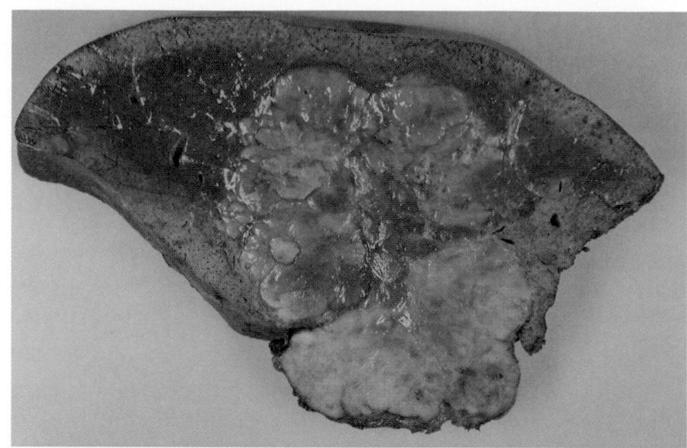

A

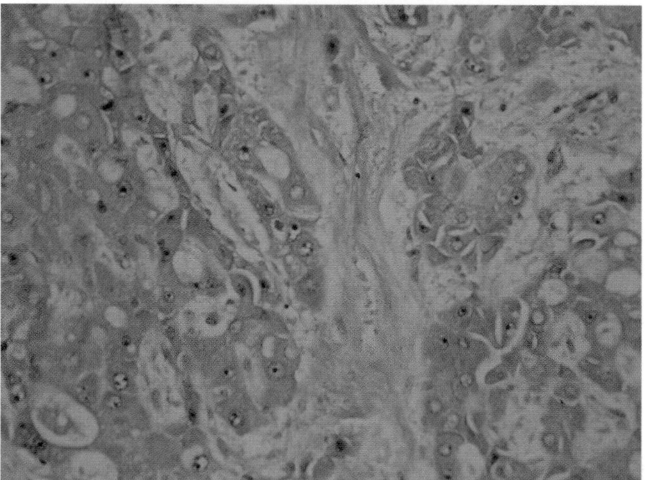

B

Figure 20.2 Fibrolamellar carcinoma usually develops in older children. It is a slow-growing tumor and may resemble focal nodular hyperplasia. **A** The cut surface demonstrates the extent of the tumor. **B** Microscopically, there are large, densely eosinophilic tumor cells separated by cellular fibrous lamellae.

The microscopic features distinguishing hepatocellular carcinoma from hepatoblastoma are the presence of tumor cells larger than normal hepatocytes, broad cellular trabeculae, considerable nuclear pleomorphism, nucleolar predominance, frequent tumor giant cells, and absence of hemopoiesis.[1,53]

The fibrolamellar variant of HCC is probably a separate clinical entity. It arises in older children and young adults, almost invariably in the absence of underlying cirrhosis. The prognosis with these tumors is more favorable than with the normal variant of HCC. Histologically, the tumor cells are plump, with deeply eosinophilic cytoplasm and a marked fibrous stroma separating epithelial cells into trabeculae (Figure 20.2).[54]

Transitional liver cell tumor

Prokurat *et al.*[49] coined the term "transitional liver cell tumor." This appears to be a histologically distinct group of tumors that develop in children who are older than those traditionally presenting with hepatoblastoma. The histology of these tumors does not show the classical features of either hepatoblastoma or hepatocellular carcinoma, but often a mixture of the two. The tumors have also been analyzed and newly classified by Zimmermann.[50] The disease appears to have an aggressive clinical course, and of the seven patients described by Prokurat *et al.*, only one remained alive and disease-free at the time of the report. The authors also reported overexpression of β-catenin in these tumors, which may also explain their aggressive behavior.[49,55]

Other malignant tumors

Sarcoma. The commonest malignant tumor in childhood apart from hepatoblastoma and HCC is undifferentiated (embryonal) sarcoma, sometimes referred to as malignant mesenchymoma.[56] The lesions are usually large and single and may resemble benign mesenchymal hamartomatous lesions. The presence of extensive hemorrhage and necrosis usually indicates the malignant nature of these tumors. Although macroscopically the tumor may appear to be well demarcated from adjacent normal liver, there is usually extensive microscopic invasion. Microscopically, the cells are spindle-shaped, with elongated and irregular nuclei and an underlying myxoid stroma. Lack of rhabdomyoblastic differentiation may help distinguish this type of lesion from rhabdomyosarcoma, but it may be difficult to differentiate from other mesenchymal malignancies such as liposarcoma and chondrosarcoma. Sarcomas may be challenging for the pathologist, and immunohistochemical and ultrastructural studies may be helpful. Although there is an overlap of patterns of immunohistological stains and ultrastructural features, it is possible to distinguish between undifferentiated embryonal sarcoma and biliary rhabdomyosarcoma.[57] The latter diagnosis may be important, since the surgical anatomy of these two tumors differs (either predominantly intraparenchymatous, or more central and involving the portal tracts and bile ducts, respectively)—and this in turn has an impact on the potential radicality of resection. Additional investigations for more detailed diagnosis include flow cytometry and cytogenetics (Figure 20.3).[57]

The exact relationship between undifferentiated sarcoma of the liver and benign mesenchymal hamartoma remains unclear. Anecdotal reports mention "malignant transformation" of mesenchymal hamartoma or associated diseases.[58–61] The exact position remains unclear, but the presence of common histological features at the periphery of malignant lesions,[62] the presence of aneuploidy,[63] and the recent finding that similar cytogenetic alterations may be found in both tumor types[64–67] hints at this possible relationship, with recurrent observations of balanced translocations involving a common breakpoint, 19q13.4.[68–71] A possible histogenetic link (with a common origin of benign and malignant tumors from undifferentiated mesenchymal cells) has also been postulated.[1,62,71,72]

Rare tumors. Rhabdomyosarcoma of both the biliary tree and liver parenchyma,[73,74] primary rhabdoid tumor of the liver,[75] primary non-Hodgkin lymphoma of the liver,[76] hepatic liposarcoma,[77] and germ-cell tumors of the liver[78] have all been described in children, but are extremely rare findings.

Benign tumors

Vascular tumors

The commonest benign tumors of the liver are vascular in origin. The lesions may be solitary or multiple. Histologically, they can be divided into two groups: hemangioma and hemangioendothelioma.[79–81]

Hemangioendotheliomas are divided into infantile or type I lesions, and epithelioid or type II lesions.

Cavernous hemangiomas have no malignant potential and may be entirely asymptomatic; they are sometimes found routinely at autopsy in adults as well as in children. The lesions usually consist of large, thin-walled channels lined with flat endothelium. Areas of calcification, thrombosis, and fibrosis are commonly seen (Chapter 10).

Infantile hemangioendothelioma (type I) is seen mostly in neonates and infants and can grow rapidly, with various related clinical symptoms (hepatomegaly, congestive heart failure, Kasabach–Merritt syndrome, failure to thrive, jaundice, or spontaneous rupture). It consists of channels of varying

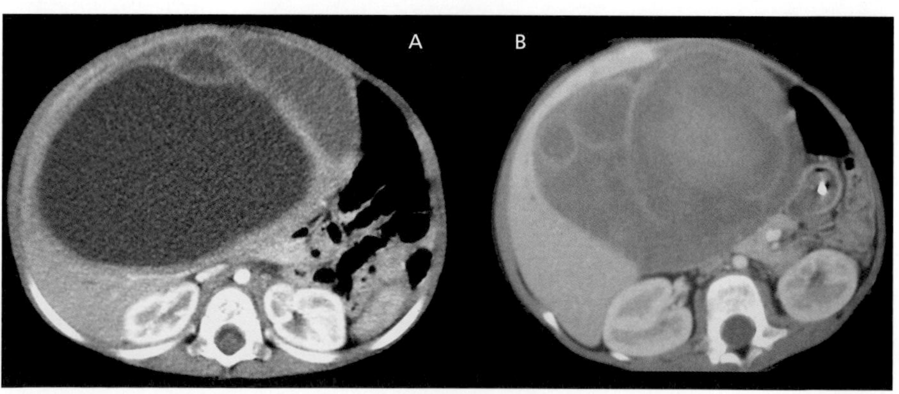

Figure 20.3 Cystic tumors: mesenchymal hamartoma (**A**) and sarcoma (**B**). Both tumor types are usually single, but they are large and multicystic. Although sarcomas are more typically diagnosed in older children, the age range for both tumor types overlap and sarcomas may resemble benign mesenchymal hamartomatous lesions (both on ultrasonography and CT/MRI). The presence of extensive hemorrhage and necrosis usually indicates a malignant nature and should prompt a biopsy.

size lined with often plump endothelial cells. Epithelioid hemangioendothelioma (type II) lesions appear to be more aggressive, demonstrating variability in endothelial cell size and shape and with ill-formed vascular spaces, although mitoses are infrequent. There is a degree of overlap between types I and II; both may show areas of fibrosis and calcification, but type II lesions are positive for factor VIII-related antigen. The latter finding is helpful in diagnosing type II tumors, which are rare in children but appear as low-grade malignancies in the adult population and may have even more aggressive behavior in children (personal observations). The lack of vascular invasion and absence of mitotic activity usually makes it relatively easy to differentiate between malignant angiosarcoma and hemangioendothelioma (Figures 20.4, 20.5).

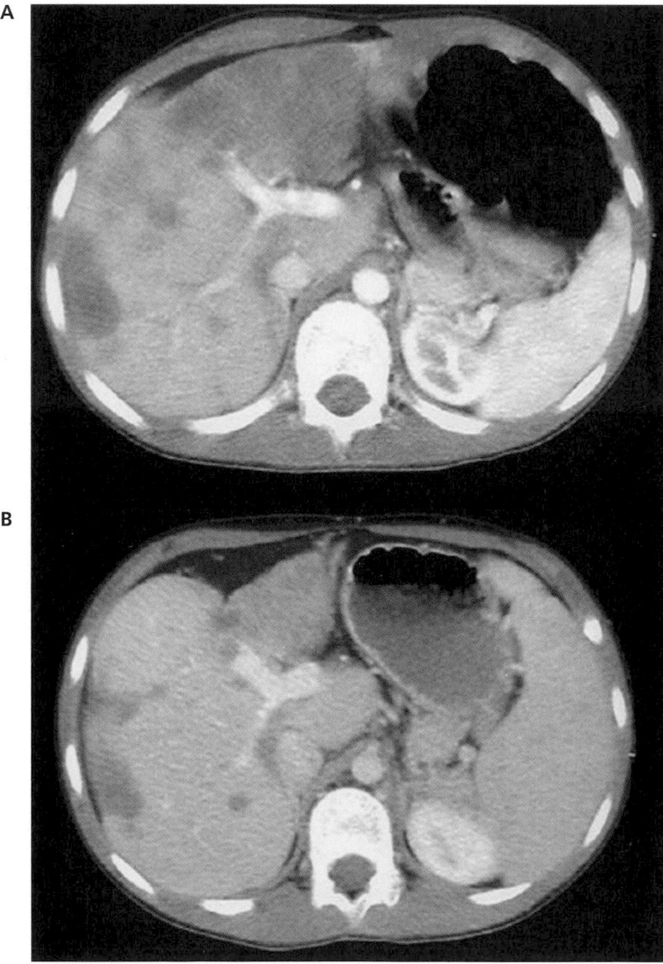

Figure 20.4 Hepatic epithelioid hemangioendothelioma in a 10-year-old child. Computed-tomographic appearance before **A** and after **B** chemotherapy (with carboplatin and etoposide), showing a response to the chemotherapy, which was associated with resolution of clinical symptoms. (Reproduced with permission from Sharif *et al.*, *British Journal of Cancer* 2004.[92])

Mesenchymal hamartoma

These lesions are usually found in children under the age of 2 years and commonly present with abdominal distension. The lesions, often very large in size, are not encapsulated and bulge into the adjacent parenchyma. Both solid and cystic areas are seen, and there is a lack of hemorrhage and necrosis. Histologically, there is an irregular, bland mesenchyme, with variable vascularization. Biliary structures, often cystic, can be identified, although there are no portal tracts present. The gelatinous stroma contains serous or viscous fluid, and pseudolymphatic spaces can be identified. The lesions have been considered not to have any malignant potential[82] (Chapter 10), but recent observations suggest a possible relation with sarcomas (see above).

Focal nodular hyperplasia

These rare benign tumors of childhood may be single or multiple. They are not encapsulated and are usually within the substance of the liver, although some have been reported to be pedunculated. The typical appearance is one of stellate fibrosis, with the septa containing blood vessels and bile ducts with surrounding inflammatory infiltration. The hepatic parenchyma between the septa may be hyperplastic and may be confused with nodular regenerative hyperplasia (Figure 20.5).[83]

Chromosomal gains or losses are typical of neoplasia and may help differentiate focal nodular hyperplasia from other tumors when the precise diagnosis is not clear. Genome-wide microsatellite analysis comparing focal nodular hyperplasia has shown that gross chromosomal alterations are absent in focal nodular hyperplasia, while various features of chromosomal losses or gains are common in hepatocellular carcinoma.[84,85] This may be a useful tool in establishing a clear diagnosis—a precondition for instituting clinical observation and conservative management of focal nodular hyperplasia nodules.

Adenoma

Hepatic adenoma in children has the same features as in adults. Adenomas can occur at any age from birth and have also been reported in the fetus in utero.[86] Whereas there is a strong correlation between oral contraceptive use and adult-onset hepatic adenoma, there appears to be no link between maternal use of contraceptives and childhood adenoma.[87] Adenomas have been reported in patients receiving anabolic steroids, in glycogen storage disease type I, familial diabetes mellitus, transfusion-related hemosiderosis, and galactosemia. Histologically, the lesions may be partially encapsulated and consist of thick cords of benign hepatocytes that lack portal structures and bile ducts.

Cell-biological evaluation using tissue microarray analysis may help diagnose these tumor types more precisely, since studies suggest that in the dysplasia–carcinoma pathway, changes in ploidy are followed by cellular proliferation and overexpression of p53 and Rb1 proteins (down-regulation of

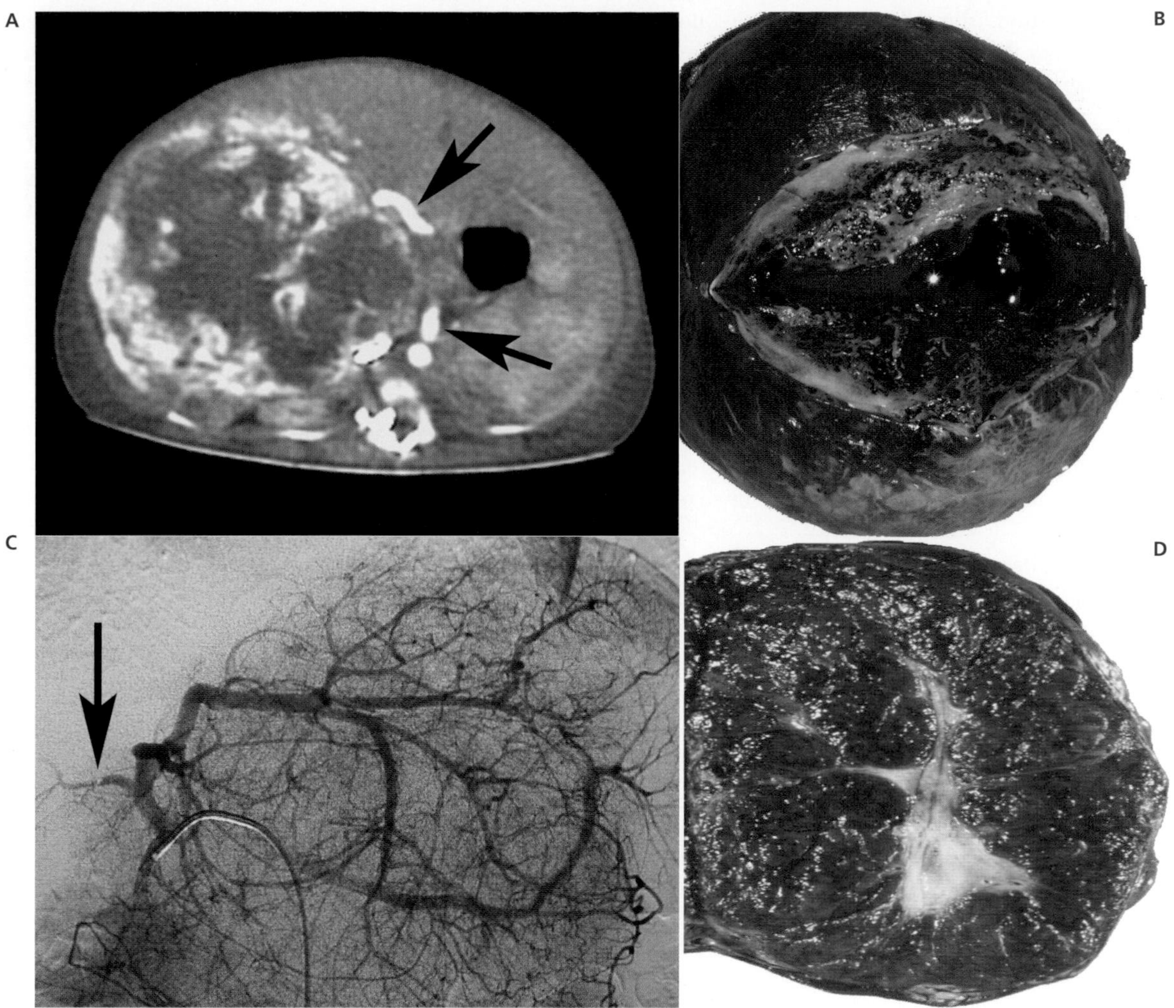

Figure 20.5 Tumors with a high arterial vascular supply. **A** Infantile hemangioendothelioma (appearance on magnetic resonance angiography). The arrows show the large-diameter arterial supply (from the celiac trunk and common hepatic artery). **B** Macroscopic view of the resected mass. **C** Focal nodular hyperplasia (appearance on conventional angiography). The arrow shows a normal right hepatic artery, for comparison with the large left arterial supply. **D** Macroscopic view of a split tumor with the typical central scar.

tumor-suppressor genes).[88] On this basis, adenoma can be distinguished from carcinoma, but not from dysplasia.

Malignant tumors

Clinical features

Hepatoblastoma

Hepatoblastoma is most commonly seen in children under the age of 18 months and is rare after the age of 3 years. There is a male predominance of 3 : 2. The commonest presenting feature is of a palpable abdominal mass with abdominal distension, but other features, including anorexia, weight loss, pain, vomiting, and jaundice have also been reported (Table 20.3).[3,89]

One of the more unusual presenting features of hepatoblastoma is its association with sexual precocity due to the release of human chorionic gonadotropic hormone (β-HCG) by the tumor. Osteoporosis is said to occur in up to 20% of cases and when severe can lead to bone fractures and vertebral compression.[90] The tumor may rupture spontaneously, producing an acute abdomen and hemoperitoneum.

Table 20.3 Signs and symptoms of liver tumors in children.

	Hepatoblastoma (%)	Hepatocellular carcinoma (%)
Abdominal mass	71	58
Weight loss	24	21
Anorexia	22	22
Pain	18	16
Vomiting	13	10
Jaundice	7	10

Physical examination should also focus on possible syndromes that may be associated with hepatoblastoma (Beckwith–Wiedemann, hemihypertrophy, etc.; see Table 20.2). During history-taking, inquiries should be made about familial associations such as hereditary polyposis coli, drug and toxin exposure, etc.

Hepatocellular carcinoma

The clinical features are very similar to those seen with hepatoblastoma (Table 20.3). HCC tends to present at a slightly older age than hepatoblastoma and is very rare in infancy. Jaundice, whilst uncommon, occurs slightly more often in HCC than hepatoblastoma. Sexual precocity and osteoporosis are not features of HCC. A search for signs of underlying liver cirrhosis (splenomegaly due to portal hypertension, spider nevi, etc.) should be sought as a possible clue to underlying etiological factors.

The rare fibrolamellar type of HCC is seen in an older age group (median age 26.4 years)[54] and occurs in noncirrhotic livers. Abdominal mass is the commonest presentation and systemic symptoms are unusual. These tumors have a more favorable prognosis and are less likely to undergo early metastatic spread.

Other malignant tumors

Malignant mesenchymal tumors of the liver represent approximately 10% of the primary malignant tumors of childhood. The commonest of these is undifferentiated (embryonal) sarcoma. Malignant mesenchymal tumors tend to present in a similar fashion, with abdominal pain, mass, and fever. In some cases, the presentation may be relatively acute after the tumor bleeds within the liver, with anemia and abdominal pain caused by the sudden volume increase and liver capsule distension. This mode of presentation is relatively typical of embryonal sarcoma. The latter tumor is often cyst-like, with the tumor mass being very poorly structured and myxoid, mimicking liquid on computed tomography (CT) or ultrasonography. The dislocation of the tumor by the hematoma may make the formal diagnosis difficult, and this typical mode of presentation in small children should help in diagnosing these rare cases (Figure 20.3). α-Fetoprotein (AFP) is normal, there are no abnormalities of the full blood count and liver enzymes, and serum bilirubin is rarely elevated.

Epithelioid hemangioendothelioma is a rare and unique neoplasm, now considered to be a separate entity from hemangioma and angiosarcoma,[91] and has a low-to-intermediate grade of malignancy. It is mostly seen in young adults, but can be observed in teenagers and children, in whom it appears to have more aggressive behavior, with rapid growth and a tendency toward extrahepatic spread (personal observations).[92] Coincidental diagnosis is possible, but most cases are diagnosed late with symptoms related to tumor growth—abdominal pain, Budd–Chiari phenomena, portal hypertension, or liver failure. Since this tumor tends to be multifocal and widespread in the liver at diagnosis,[81,93,94] only a limited number of patients can be considered for surgery, and the role of transplantation in children is not clear (Figure 20.4). New chemotherapy approaches appear to be useful and may help in selecting candidates for transplantation on the basis of the response to chemotherapy, as has already been done successfully for hepatoblastoma cases.[92]

Diagnostic investigations

Laboratory tests

Full blood count. Anemia (usually normocytic, normochromic) is seen in at least 50% of children with hepatoblastoma.[3,95] The platelet count is also often abnormal, with up to one-third of patients demonstrating thrombocytosis (often in excess of 1000×10^9/L),[96] and fewer patients having thrombocytopenia. Thrombocytosis is thought to be related to increased levels of circulating thrombopoietin.[97] Thrombocytosis is less common in HCC patients, but polycythemia is sometimes seen.

Liver function tests. These are commonly normal in hepatoblastoma, but are more frequently abnormal in HCC, presumably due to the greater incidence of underlying cirrhosis or hepatitis.[86,89]

α-Fetoprotein (AFP) is a useful diagnostic and prognostic marker and can be helpful in monitoring disease progress and the response to therapy. From 28 days' gestation onward, the developing fetus produces AFP, reaching maximum levels around 14 weeks. There is a steady decline to term, and the fall continues over the first year of life, when normal adult levels are usually reached. AFP levels may be higher in premature infants. The vast majority of hepatoblastoma patients[3,98–100] and over two-thirds of HCC patients[29] have elevated levels of AFP at presentation. Levels tend to be higher in patients with more bulky disease and metastases and therefore have prognostic significance. A return of AFP levels to normal following treatment indicates remission, while persistently abnormal results should alert the clinician to the possibility of residual tumor or relapse. Malignant yolk sac tumors may rarely present as a primary hepatic tumor. These tumors also secrete AFP, and the presence of elevated serum AFP is therefore not specific for hepatoblastoma/HCC. If β-HCG is elevated at diagnosis, it can be used like AFP to monitor the response of hepatic tumors to therapy.

Other markers. The fibrolamellar variant of HCC is usually associated with normal AFP values, but elevation of vitamin B_{12}-binding proteins, especially transcobalamin I100, makes them useful markers that can also be used to monitor disease response and progression.[101]

Other markers, including elevated urinary cystathionine, elevated serum cholesterol, insulin-like growth factor-2, ferritin, carcinoembryonic antigen, and γ-prothrombin, have all been reported in malignant liver tumors, but are nonspecific and of limited benefit in diagnosis and follow-up.

Imaging

The aim in imaging assessment of any childhood liver tumor is to determine the site and characteristics of the lesion and to establish whether any metastases are present, whilst also giving some indication of the suitability of the lesion for surgical resection.

Abdominal radiography. A plain radiograph of the abdomen will often show a mass effect from the hepatic lesion itself, and in addition the presence of any calcification. This investigation provides very little diagnostic information alone, and since the majority of children will probably have an ultrasound or CT scan as the first-line imaging method, it is not mandatory in all patients.

Ultrasonography. This will often confirm that the lesion originates in the liver and can help distinguish between other common pediatric abdominal tumors that present with a palpable mass (e.g., Wilms tumor and neuroblastoma). The size of the tumor can be defined and measured and information can be obtained on the presence of cystic features, which may be suggestive of a benign lesion. Vascular structures can be identified (hepatic arteries, hepatic veins, portal veins, and inferior vena cava) and Doppler studies performed to confirm flow rates and patency. Ultrasonography may be particularly helpful in differentiating benign hepatic hemangiomas or hemangioendotheliomas, by defining the vascular features of these tumors. However, magnetic resonance imaging (MRI) is now the preferred imaging technique for vascular tumors. Although some authors have reported a reasonable predictive accuracy for the extent and resectability of liver tumors using ultrasound,[102] the additional information gleaned from CT and/or MRI makes these mandatory additional explorations in the investigation of liver tumors.

Computed tomography. CT scanning provides detailed information about the anatomical limits of liver tumors. Intravenous contrast medium should always be used in order to define vascular landmarks and assess the patency of vessels (Figures 20.6, 20.7). Typically, malignant tumors are of low attenuation and demonstrate patchy enhancement with contrast. Vascular lesions may be hard to define without contrast, but show dense peripheral enhancement with gradual filling of the central areas following intravenous contrast. CT scanning will also define the presence of para-aortic lymph-node metastases, although these tend to be uncommon.

Magnetic resonance imaging. This is now increasingly available, allowing comparisons to be made with CT scanning. MRI scanning provides good definition of tumor and surrounding infiltration, allowing accurate assessment of segmental involvement. This has important implications for clinical staging and any proposed surgical interventions. The vascular anatomy can also be demonstrated, and this may avoid the need for hepatic angiography (Figure 20.8).

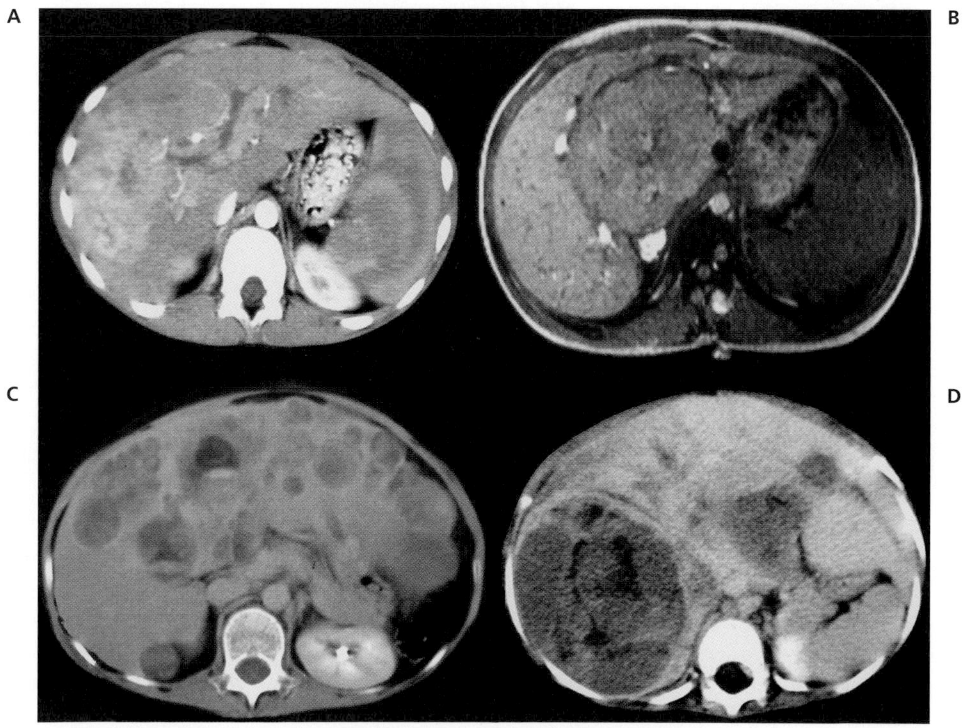

A B C D

Figure 20.6 Computed-tomographic appearances of hepatocarcinoma.
A, B Fibrolamellar hepatocarcinomas.
C, D Classical hepatocarcinomas, originating in normal liver. Hepatocarcinomas are usually multifocal and invasive, commonly involving both lobes at diagnosis. Areas of hemorrhage and necrosis are common in the usual type. Vascular invasion and thrombosis (portal or hepatic veins) are usually associated with rapid progression and a poor short-term prognosis. Fibrolamellar hepatocarcinomas are fibrous, solid tumors, often better delineated, and have remarkably slow growth.

A B C D E F

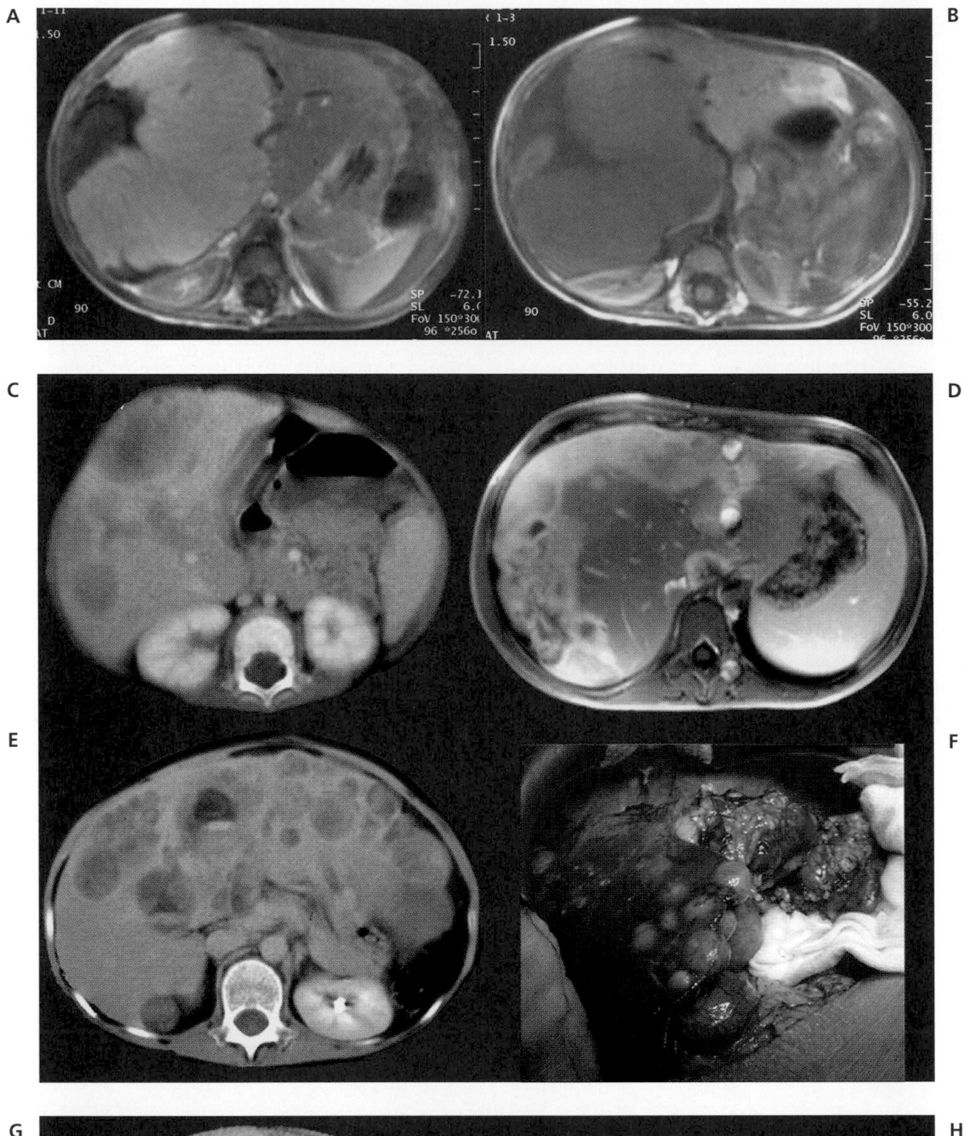

G H

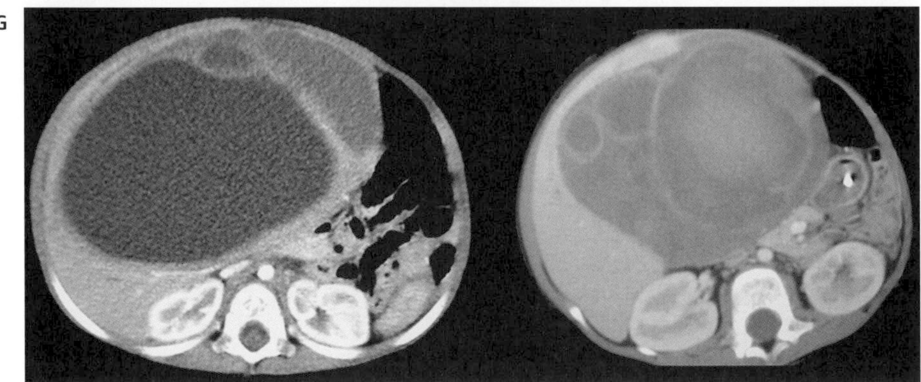

Figure 20.7 Hepatic tumors are best diagnosed by CT scan which demonstrates a large hepatoblastoma before (**A**) and after intravenous contrast (**B**). It may also help to differentiate solid tumors such as hepatoblastoma (**C**) epitheloid haemangioendothelioma (**D**) and hepatocarcinoma (**E**) from cystic tumors such as mesenchymal hamartoma (**G**) and sarcoma (**H**). The cut surface of hepatocarcinoma is shown in **F**.

Hepatic angiography. This may be required before surgery if the vascular anatomy has not been clearly demonstrated on MRI scanning.

Chest radiography. A chest radiograph should be performed to exclude pulmonary metastases. If normal, a CT scan of the chest should be undertaken before the start of therapy, since up to 50% of metastases may not be visible on chest radiography alone.[99]

Positron-emission tomography (PET)—best synchronized with CT or MRI for better anatomical localization of findings—is a

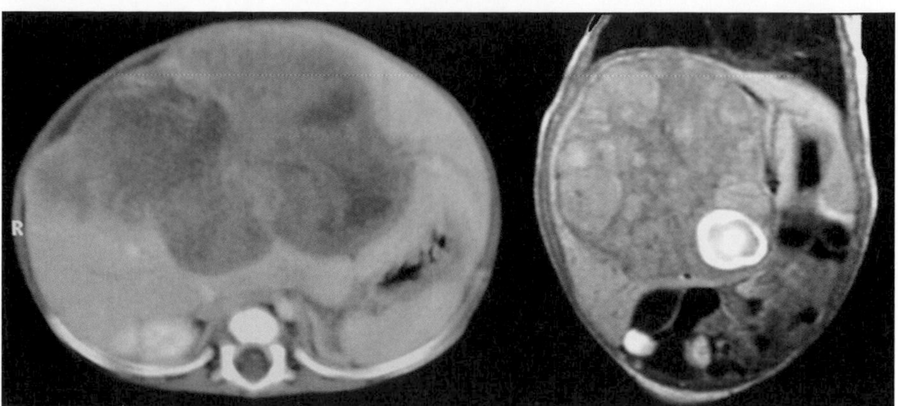

Figure 20.8 Extensive involvement of all segments of the liver with a multifocal hepatoblastoma, as seen on this magnetic resonance image, is an indication for transplantation.

new and interesting tool when available. The scintigram reveals spots of high metabolism and may make it possible to identify extrahepatic sites that may not be detected with other imaging modalities. This method has been very useful for localizing relatively early metastases and recurrences of disease before any mass effect was detectable on routine checks.

Biopsy

Although clinical and laboratory clues can lead to a presumptive diagnosis in the majority of children with liver tumors, caution has to be exercised at all times. For example, although a 2-year-old child with grossly elevated AFP and a liver mass is most likely to have a hepatoblastoma, it is important to exclude other diagnoses, such as malignant germ-cell tumor or hepatocellular carcinoma. This is particularly relevant when chemotherapy is being contemplated prior to definitive surgery. In the majority of cases, therefore, it is mandatory to take an initial biopsy. Due to the multifocal nature of many liver tumors, a "blind" biopsy may not yield samples that contain tumor. It is therefore best to perform a percutaneous biopsy of the liver mass using a Tru-Cut or Menghini needle under CT guidance. In addition, the use of imaging may alert the operator to bleeding from the biopsy site. Fine-needle aspiration may be unsatisfactory, as only minimal amounts of tissue may be obtained, which can be notoriously difficult to interpret with any degree of certainty. Caution must be exercised in attempting biopsies in lesions that are highly vascular, which may be difficult to distinguish clinically from a benign vascular anomaly or a highly vascular malignant tumor. In these circumstances, the safest approach is to undertake an open biopsy through a minilaparotomy in order to be able to visualize the liver and treat any bleeding at the time of surgery. There is a risk of seeding malignant cells along the biopsy track, although the risk is greatest in hepatocellular tumors, which are less responsive to subsequent chemotherapy than hepatoblastomas.

Clinical staging

The International Society of Pediatric Oncology (*Société Internationale d'Oncologie Pédiatrique*, SIOP) has introduced a staging system based on preoperative assessment and the location of the tumor. The original *Pre*treatment *Ext*ent of Disease (PRETEXT) staging system divides patients into four groups, depending on the section or sections (groups of segments) involved and also takes into account vascular involvement of the portal veins and/or inferior vena cava (IVC), extrahepatic extension, and distant metastases.[103] In a recent revision of the PRETEXT system, greater clarity has been provided about the liver sections themselves, including the caudate lobe, which was previously ignored. Much greater detail is also provided for documenting extrahepatic disease (Figure 20.9; Tables 20.4, 20.5).[104] The PRETEXT system has now been evaluated in a large number of children with hepatoblastoma. It demonstrates a slight tendency to overstage patients, but has reliable interobserver reproducibility and, perhaps most importantly, has a superior positive predictive value for survival in comparison with other staging systems.[105]

Treatment

Modern management of malignant hepatic tumors consists of a combination of chemotherapy and surgical resection, with the highest cure rates being associated with complete surgical resection.

Chemotherapy

Hepatoblastoma. The 3-year overall survival rates of children with hepatoblastoma have improved from 25% to around 80% over the past 20 years as a result of progress in the evaluation of chemotherapy regimens.[4,89,106,107] Although surgical resection is essential for long-term cure, the emphasis in each therapeutic modality has changed over time. Evans *et al.*[106] noted that the use of postoperative adjuvant chemotherapy conferred a survival advantage on children

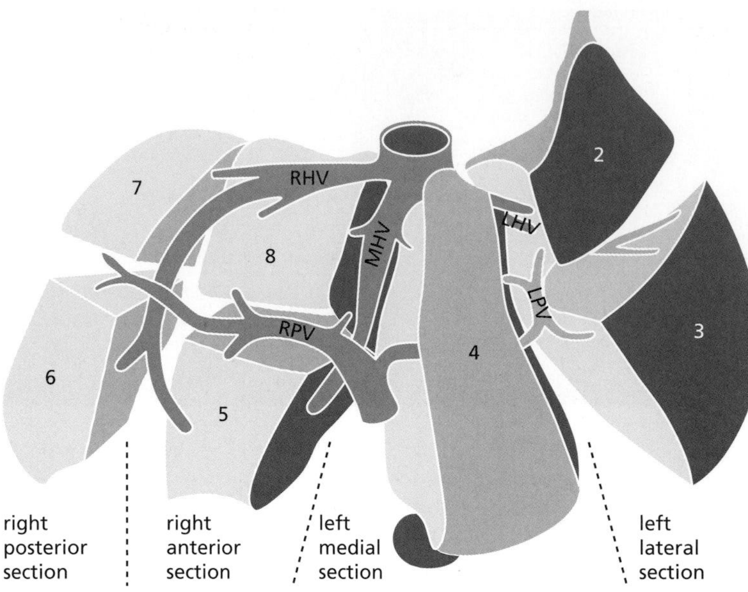

Figure 20.9 Exploded frontal view of the segmental anatomy of the liver. The liver segments are grouped into four sections: segments II and III (left lateral section); segments IVa and IVb (left medial section); segments V and VIII (right anterior section); and segments VI and VII (right posterior section). (Reproduced with permission from Roebuck *et al., Pediatric Radiology* 2007.[104])

Table 20.4 Definitions of *Pre*treatment *Ext*ent of Disease (PRETEXT) numbers.

PRETEXT no.	Definition
I	One section is involved and three adjoining sections are free
II	One or two sections are involved, but two adjoining sections are free
III	Two or three sections are involved, and no two adjoining sections are free
IV	All four sections are involved

Table 20.5 2005 *Pre*treatment *Ext*ent of Disease (PRETEXT) staging system: additional criteria.

Caudate lobe involvement	C	C1	Tumor involving the caudate lobe	All C1 patients are at least PRETEXT II
		C0	All other patients	
Extrahepatic abdominal disease	E	E0	No evidence of tumor spread in the abdomen (except M or N)	Add suffix "a" if ascites is present—e.g., E0a
		E1	Direct extension of tumor into adjacent organs or diaphragm	
		E2	Peritoneal nodules	
Tumor focality	F	F0	Patient with solitary tumor	
		F1	Patient with two or more discrete tumors	
Tumor rupture or intraperitoneal hemorrhage	H	H1	Imaging and clinical findings of intraperitoneal hemorrhage	
		H0	All other patients	
Distant metastases	M	M0	No metastases	
		M1	Any metastases (except E and N)	Add suffix to indicate location
Lymph-node metastases	N	N0	No nodal metastases	
		N1	Abdominal lymph-node metastases only	
		N2	Extra-abdominal lymph-node metastases (with or without abdominal lymph-node metastases)	
Portal vein involvement	P	P0	No involvement of the portal vein or its left or right branches	Add suffix "a" if intravascular tumor is present—e.g., P1a
		P1	Involvement of either the left or right main branch of the portal vein	
		P2	Involvement of the main portal vein	
Involvement of the IVC and/or hepatic veins	V	V0	No involvement of the hepatic veins or IVC	
		V1	Involvement of one hepatic, vein, but not the IVC	Add suffix "a" if intravascular tumor is present—e.g., V3a
		V2	Involvement of two hepatic veins, but not the IVC	
		V3	Involvement of all three hepatic veins and/or the IVC	

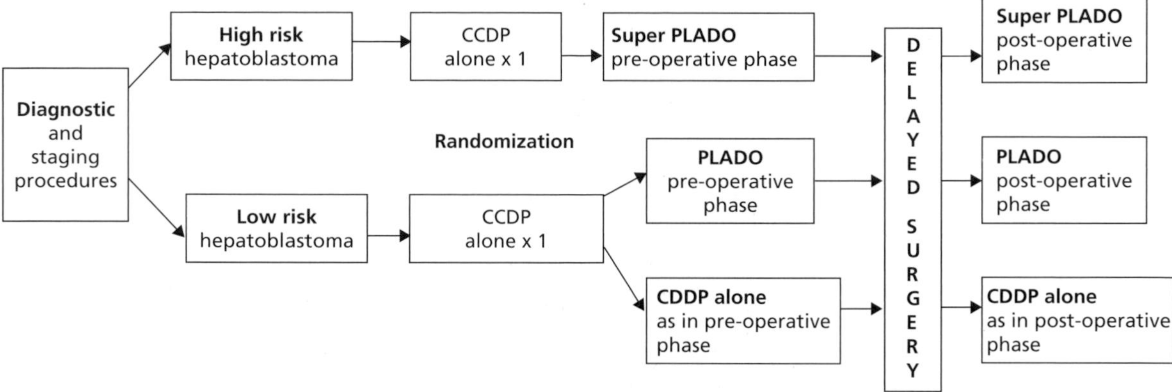

Figure 20.10 Treatment plan for the SIOPEL-3 study chemotherapy regimen: CDDP, cisplatin 80 mg/m^2 every 14 days (four cycles preoperatively, two cycles postoperatively); PLADO, cisplatin 80 mg/m^2, doxorubicin 60 mg/m^2 every 21 days (three cycles + 1 CDDP alone preoperatively, two cycles postoperatively); SuperPLADO, day 1 cisplatin 80 mg/m^2, day 15 carboplatin 500 mg/m^2 and doxorubicin 60 mg/m^2 (every 28 days), four courses CDDP, three courses Carbo/Dox preoperatively, two courses Carbo/Dox, one course CDDP postoperatively.

with completely resected hepatoblastoma and HCC, whereas the preoperative use of similar chemotherapy regimens in unresectable tumors was disappointing. Combinations of cyclophosphamide and vincristine (VCR) with other agents including adriamycin, actinomycin-D, and 5-fluorouracil (5-FU) demonstrated that despite an initial response, only 12% of children were disease-free at 2 years.[53] The introduction of cisplatin in the early 1980s led to a subsequent improvement in the response rate in patients treated either with cisplatin alone or in combination with vincristine/5-fluorouracil and in those who had proved resistant to previous chemotherapy.[108,109] As adriamycin (doxorubicin) had also been shown to be effective as a single agent,[110] chemotherapy regimens containing both cisplatin and doxorubicin (PLADO) were a logical step forward.[111,112] In the first International Society of Pediatric Oncology Liver Trial (SIOPEL-1), PLADO chemotherapy was tested in a multinational setting for the preoperative management of malignant liver tumors. The 5-year event-free and overall survival figures were 66% and 75%, respectively.[113] In a large randomized study by the Children's Cancer Group and Pediatric Oncology Group,[114] PLADO chemotherapy was compared with cisplatin, 5-FU, and VCR. No significant differences in the overall or event-free survival (EFS) were seen between the two chemotherapy schedules, although PLADO consistently outperformed cisplatin/5-FU/VCR (5-year EFS 69% vs. 57%; $P = 0.09$). More toxicity was observed in the PLADO arm, including two cardiac deaths from cumulative doses of 640 mg/m^2 of doxorubicin—dose levels we today would never consider appropriate in these young children.

Building on the good results achieved with a combination of cisplatin and doxorubicin, and an ability to stratify patients into those with good risk and poorer risk, the SIOPEL group planned a pilot study of cisplatin monotherapy in standard risk patients (defined as PRETEXT I–III tumors, without vascular invasion, extrahepatic disease, or metastases) and an intensified chemotherapy approach in high-risk tumors with the addition of carboplatin to PLADO or "SuperPLADO."[115] For the standard risk group, the 3-year overall survival with cisplatin monotherapy was 91%. On the basis of this result, a randomized study (SIOPEL-3) was planned to compare cisplatin against PLADO in this standard risk group. The study closed in 2006, and the results are anticipated soon. For high-risk patients, the SIOPEL-2 study achieved a 3-year event-free survival of 53%, and this arm of treatment was carried over and continued into SIOPEL-3 (Figures 20.10–20.13).

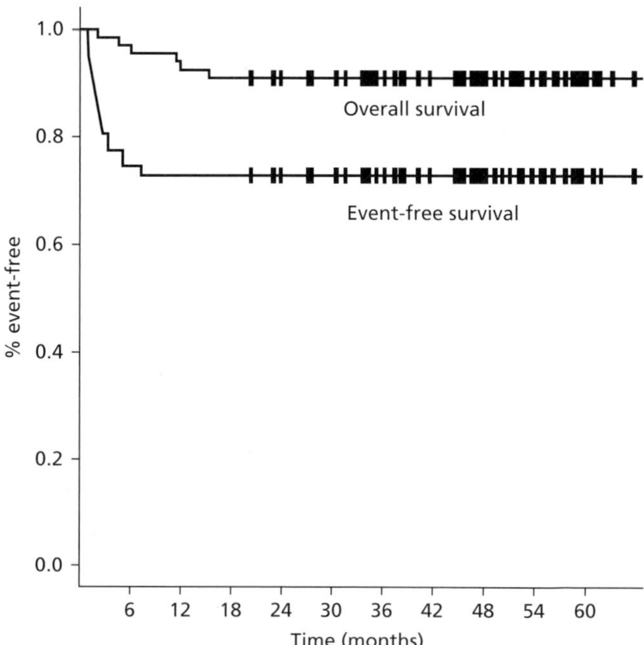

Figure 20.11 Overall survival for patients treated in SIOPEL-2 with "standard-risk" chemotherapy.

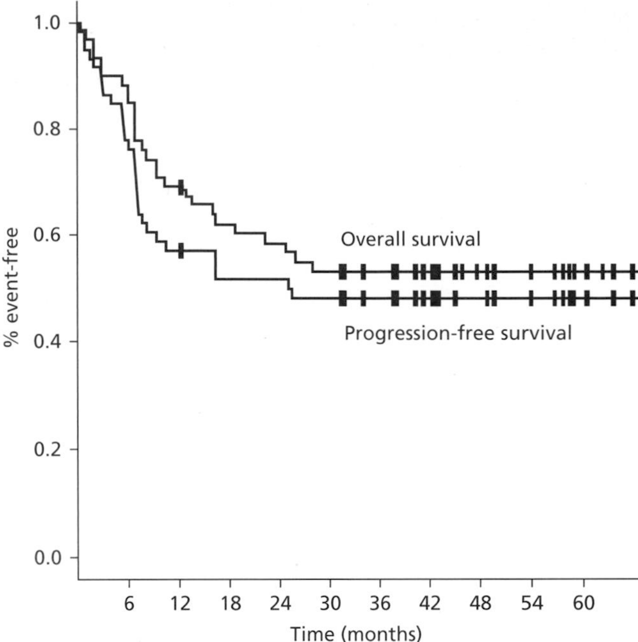

Figure 20.12 Overall and progression-free survival for patients treated in SIOPEL-2 with "high-risk" chemotherapy.

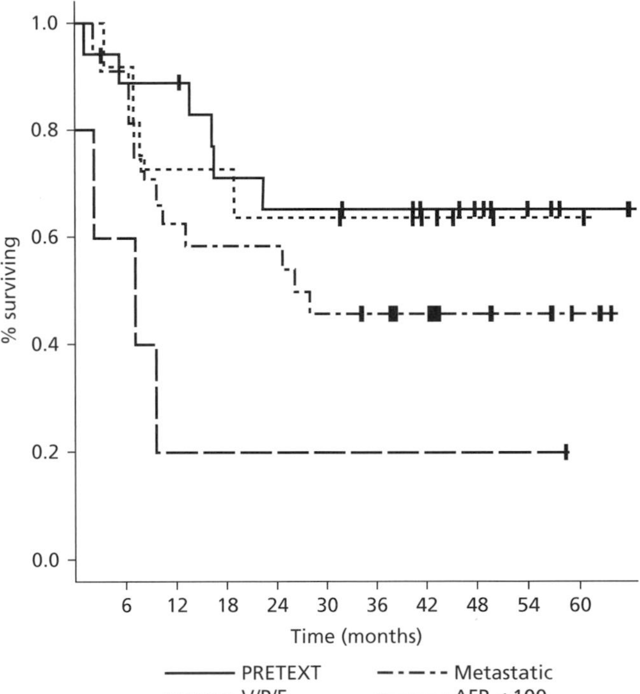

Figure 20.13 Overall survival for high-risk patients treated in SIOPEL-2 in accordance with the PRETEXT IV classification, intra-abdominal extrahepatic disease (V/P/E), presence of metastases, and α-fetoprotein < 10.

The results from the SIOPEL group and those from the Intergroup Liver Tumor Study in the United States strongly suggest that cisplatin is the most effective agent in the management of hepatoblastoma. It was therefore a logical step to try to increase the intensity of platinum treatment in the hope that more patients could be cured. The SIOPEL approach has been to devise a dose-dense regimen of weekly cisplatin at a dosage of 70 mg/m^2 in combination with 3-weekly doxorubicin (60 mg/m^2). This regimen is currently being piloted prospectively in the SIOPEL-4 study. The Intergroup Liver Tumor Study approach was to intensify platinum delivery by alternating carboplatin (700 mg/m^2) and cisplatin (100 mg/m^2) every 2 weeks and randomize against the "standard" arm of cisplatin, 5-FU, VCR (C5V) in high-risk tumors.[116] The results of this randomization showed an inferior outcome for the platinum-intensive arm (1-year event-free survival 37%, vs. 57% for the C5V arm). However, critics have pointed out that substituting cisplatin with carboplatin is not necessarily an intensification of therapy, as there is some evidence that carboplatin is an inferior agent to cisplatin.[117]

SIOPEL-3 recommended the use of "SuperPLADO" in a nonrandomized study for high-risk tumors (PRETEXT IV and metastatic patients). The study has recently closed to recruitment, but early results are encouraging, and this may partly be reflected in the suggestion that there should be more liberal use of liver transplantation in patients with metastatic disease that has cleared with preoperative chemotherapy, in addition to the effectiveness of the chemotherapy alone.

PLADO chemotherapy has a number of problematic side effects, and regular toxicity monitoring throughout treatment is essential. Doxorubicin is cardiotoxic in a cumulative, dose-dependent manner. Prolonged infusion of at least 48 hours' duration may reduce the cardiotoxic effects[118] and improve cytotoxicity by increasing drug exposure to tumor cells.[119] Patients should have echocardiograms before treatment, after alternate cycles of PLADO to a cumulative dose of 300 mg/m^2, and then prior to each cycle of chemotherapy. This is particularly important if the child is subsequently considered for liver transplantation (see below). Current chemotherapy protocols try to restrict the cumulative doses of anthracyclines to 300 mg/m^2.

Cisplatin is both ototoxic and nephrotoxic. Regular monitoring of renal function by radioisotope clearance methods (chromium ethylenediaminetetraacetic acid) and serum electrolytes (e.g., hypomagnesemia) is important. Audiograms are necessary to detect the onset of high-frequency hearing loss, characteristic of cisplatin toxicity, which may produce profound speech and language delay in young children.[120] The aims of the next SIOPEL study (SIOPEL-6) in standard-risk hepatoblastoma will be to administer cisplatin monotherapy with an otoprotectant, in the hope that this disabling side effect of treatment can be avoided in children, the vast majority of whom will be long-term survivors of their disease (Figure 20.14).

The outlook for patients with recurrent disease remains poor. Alternative rescue chemotherapy regimens must be considered, including the use of conventional cytotoxic agents and

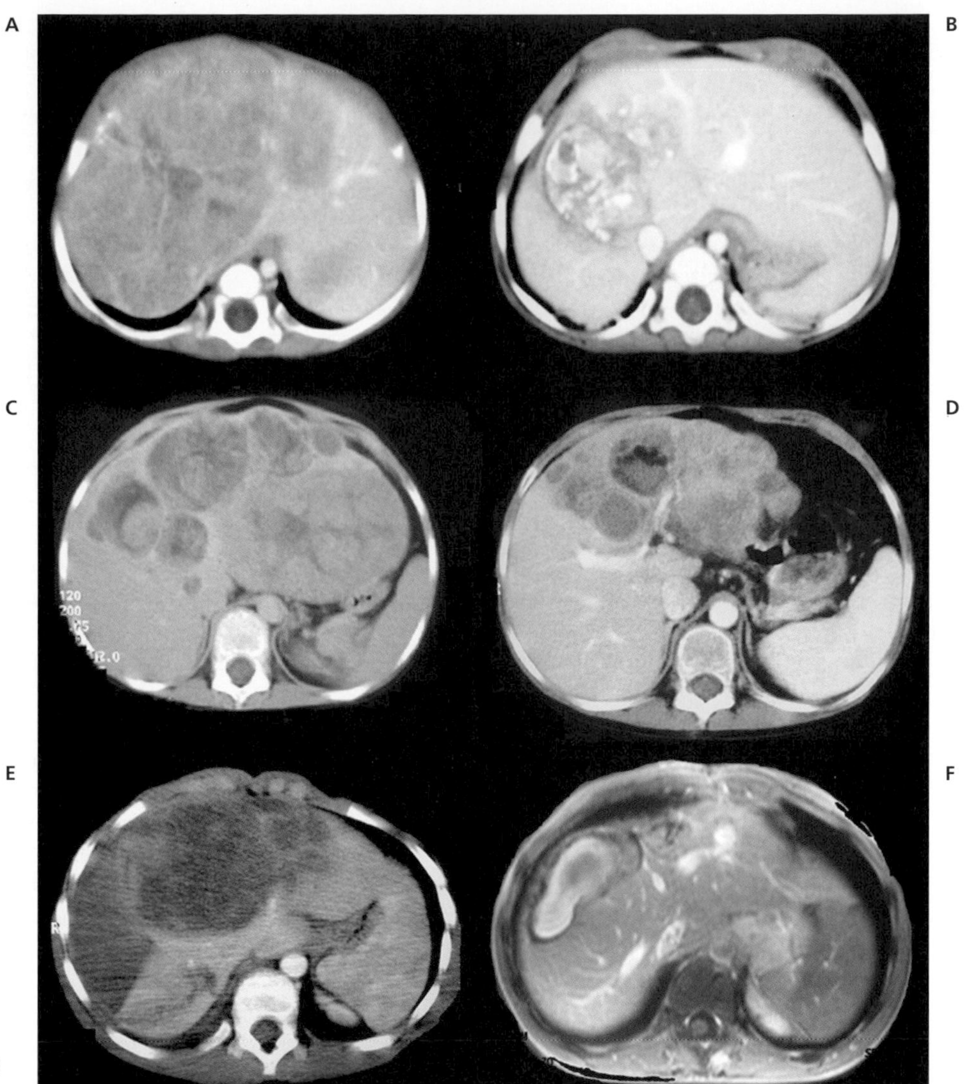

Figure 20.14 The effect of chemotherapy on primary tumor size in various tumor types (A, C, E: before chemotherapy; B, D, F: after chemotherapy. **A, B** Hepatoblastoma. **C, D** Hepatocarcinoma. **E, F** Undifferentiated embryonal sarcoma.

antiangiogenic and targeted drugs. As an example, improving chemotherapy using *MDR1* modulators may be an alternative in the treatment of high-risk, multifocal, or recurrent hepatoblastomas, as suggested by clinical observations and experimentation: increased *MDR1* gene expression and up-regulation of membrane P-glycoprotein have been shown in cells after every course of chemotherapy, and in a mouse model, PSC-833 (valspodar), an *MDR1* inhibitor, significantly improved the shrinkage of tumor after chemotherapy.[121]

Hepatocellular carcinoma. Although traditionally hepatocellular carcinoma has been managed in a similar fashion to hepatoblastoma, the impact of chemotherapy is probably less well defined. There is no doubt that responses to PLADO chemotherapy can be achieved, with response rates in the order of 50%.[111,112] Subsequent complete surgical resection, however, is only possible with a smaller percentage of HCC tumors than with hepatoblastoma. In the SIOPEL experience, response rates of 49% and resection rates of 36% were achieved, but 51% of patients never became operable. Overall survival rates at 5 years were 28%.[39] Experience in the United States is very similar.[122] Patients with localized disease, although this is a rare occurrence (17% in the series), had an encouraging outcome, with 5-year event-free survival estimates of 88%, but for all patients the 5-year survival was only 19%. This probably reflects the surgical nature of the disease, rather than the impact of chemotherapy. In the American study, no difference was observed in randomization between vincristine, 5-FU, and cisplatin versus cisplatin and doxorubicin chemotherapy. Recent reviews of the adult literature highlight the problems with HCC, including a lack of translational research, difficulty in conducting multicenter clinical trials, lack of availability of new agents, adequacy of tools for measuring meaningful clinical benefits, etc.[123,124] In the SIOPEL group, an attempt to conduct at a large international trial of HCC in children and young adults using thalidomide in combination with PLADO as an antiangiogenic drug[125] has floundered, mainly as a result of the complexities of conducting such studies in rare tumors across many sites under the impact of the European Clinical Trial Directive's bureaucracy.

The fibrolamellar variant of HCC is usually a slow-growing tumor, which metastasizes late and can be treated surgically without the need for adjuvant chemotherapy. It was at one time thought that this variant of HCC had a more favorable outcome, but a recent study in the United States suggests that the proportion of patients with advanced disease, the response to chemotherapy, and the outcome do not differ from those in conventional HCC.[126]

Hepatic hemangiomas. The clinical spectrum of these benign tumors is wide, and they may be associated with significant morbidity and mortality; clinical manifestations range from asymptomatic limited lesions to widespread invasion of the liver parenchyma, with neonatal congestive heart failure (massive vascular shunting) or fulminant liver failure–like syndrome and death. There has been little rationale for decision-making in early management and in the choice between corticosteroids and other pharmaceutical agents, surgical hepatic artery ligation or surgical resection, embolization, or liver replacement.[126,127] Moreover, precisely evaluating the effectiveness of these various methods and their contribution to curing the disease is difficult if one takes into account the natural history of spontaneous regression of these hemangiomas.

In order to collect data on a broad basis and improve the understanding of these tumors and their biological and clinical behavior, a registry has been recently opened and a management algorithm has been proposed.[127]

Other tumors. Other malignant tumors of the liver are relatively rare and historically have a poor prognosis. Treatment should be dictated by the histological diagnosis.

Sarcomatous lesions tend nowadays to be managed, like hepatoblastomas, with combined surgical and multiagent chemotherapy regimens, as well as adjuvant radiotherapy treatment. Undifferentiated embryonal sarcoma of the liver, for example, has been considered a very aggressive neoplasm with an unfavorable prognosis, but recent reports suggest that it should no longer regarded as such, since modern chemotherapy regimens can allow significant tumor mass reduction, thereby allowing radical surgery in an increasing number of cases.[128–131]

In the pediatric population, epithelioid hemangioendothelioma is uncommon and typically presents as a nonresectable tumor; it appears to be a more aggressive tumor in comparison with those in adults, and transplantation may not be a suitable management option as in adults. The role of chemotherapy as the first-line or only treatment needs to be rediscussed. It appears from recent reports that ifosfamide-based chemotherapy is not effective.[94,132] However, a regimen combining carboplatin, cisplatin, and adriamycin stabilized the disease in one patient, and carboplatin and etoposide brought about a partial response followed by stabilized disease in another.[94] In addition, Pinet *et al.*[133] have reported a complete response after carboplatin and etoposide in an aggressive form of pleural epithelioid hemangioendothelioma. Overall, using carboplatin and etoposide and further studying their effect on epithelioid hemangioendotheliomas appears worthwhile.

Response to therapy. The response to therapy can be monitored by serial assessment of:

- Imaging findings. Repeat CT scans or ultrasonography will document shrinkage of the hepatic tumor, while chest radiography or chest CT scans will monitor the progress of pulmonary metastases.
- AFP levels in tumors that secrete AFP. Patients with a good response to chemotherapy have a rapid fall in serum AFP levels,[99] whereas a failure to return to normal limits in the absence of radiographically evident disease is highly suspicious for minimal residual disease. An increase in AFP after the initiation of chemotherapy is usually a sensitive marker of relapse or treatment failure.
- Transcobalamin levels in fibrolamellar HCC may be a guide to response.

Eighty-six percent of hepatoblastomas respond to PLADO chemotherapy, while the response rate in hepatocellular carcinomas is only 43%.[112]

Surgery

Selection for surgery. It is clear that complete cure depends on effective resection of the tumor after chemotherapy. Careful assessment of postchemotherapy imaging with CT scans, MRI, or hepatic angiography is essential to establish that the main portal vein is patent and that there will be sufficient liver remaining after resection. In the majority of cases, the tumor will be localized to one half of the liver and compensatory hypertrophy of the contralateral side occurs, so that liver insufficiency after surgery is unusual. Tumors that remain multifocal, central in location, or involve the portal vein after chemotherapy are not resectable, and these patients should be considered for liver replacement unless there is extrahepatic disease that has not responded to chemotherapy.

Surgical resection techniques. Conventional resection techniques are based on the segmental anatomy of the liver.[134] Precise knowledge of the anatomical landmarks and previous surgical experience are the most important factors for obtaining a high rate of complete resection, and concentrating these cases in expert surgical units in which these operations are carried regularly and with a minimum of risk should be recommended.[135–137] In the majority of cases, resection of the hemiliver (left or right) or extended resection of one side plus additional segments from the opposite side is required. Major liver resections can nowadays be performed with minimal perioperative morbidity and mortality. For well-selected patients with conventionally "unresectable" tumors, liver transplantation is emerging as an essential approach.[135] In children, the use of special techniques such as ex-vivo surgery followed by autotransplantation of the liver remnant, or prolonged vascular exclusion with cold perfusion of the liver, are extremely rarely used as the indications are limited and because of the increased technical risks associated with the small size of the vessels.

Surgery is carried out through a wide upper transverse incision. Standard techniques include isolation and suture ligation of the hepatic artery and portal vein branches to the portion of the liver being resected, followed by division of the liver parenchyma along the line of demarcation that has been produced. Most liver surgeons employ special instruments such as an ultrasonic scalpel or a water jet for dividing the liver. These techniques divide the liver parenchyma but leave the vascular and biliary structures intact for subsequent coagulation with diathermy for small structures or suture ligation. The hepatic veins draining the area can be suture-ligated early on in the procedure, but if access is difficult, this step can be delayed until after complete division of the liver. Clamping of the vascular supply (portal vein and hepatic artery) or vascular exclusion (vascular inflow and vena cava) has been suggested in order to reduce blood loss during difficult hepatectomies. While this accelerates the procedure and eventually limits the blood loss, it also causes liver ischemia, thus increasing the risk of postoperative liver dysfunction (especially when the residual liver is small). Most liver surgeons now prefer a meticulous division of the liver, steadily achieving hemostasis and avoiding vascular clamping. While the operating time may be prolonged, this approach is associated with more rapid hepatic recovery and patient discharge. Hemostasis at the cut surface is aided by the use of bipolar diathermy for dividing the liver and of argon diathermy for final hemostasis of the cut surface. Application of a layer of fibrin glue reduces the postoperative risk of leakage of blood or bile (Figure 20.15).

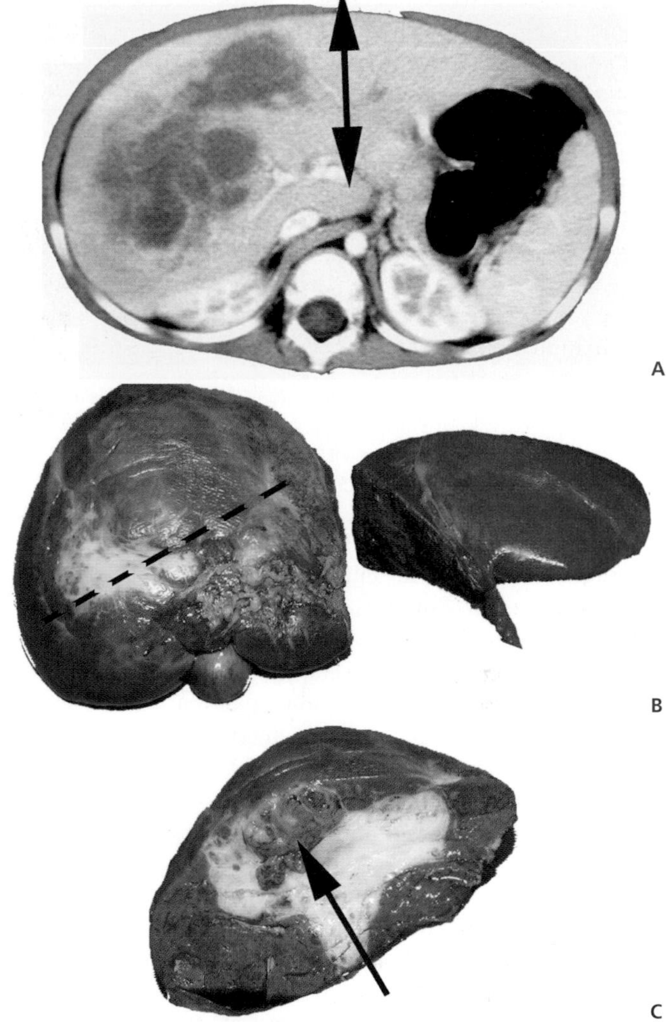

Figure 20.15 Extended right hepatectomy for large hepatoblastoma. **A** Preoperative computed tomography shows the tumor location and extension from the right liver toward the left. The arrow indicates the liver resection line. **B** Intraoperative view showing the resected liver (left side) and the remaining healthy parenchyma (right side). **C** Macroscopic appearance of the tumor at section (resection along the dotted line shown in B). The large white areas represent fibrotic and necrotic transformation of the tumor, but a viable node is still visible (arrow).

Liver transplantation. With excellent results and survival rates, liver transplantation nowadays has a definitive role to play and must be considered for the treatment of patients with unresectable liver tumors. In the context of organ shortage, case selection and correct timing are cornerstones not only for the appropriate use of this surgical option, but also for a successful outcome. Using transplantation as an alternative helps avoid unnecessary attempts to intensify chemotherapy in a vain effort to achieve surgical resectability in difficult cases, along with the related morbidity. Overall, active extrahepatic residues after chemotherapy are formal contraindications, and although a good response of the main tumor site to chemotherapy is not a prerequisite for a good outcome after transplantation, it is an excellent indicator that the biological behavior of the tumor is favorable.[94,138–140] Until now, transplantation has been mostly carried out in patients with hepatoblastoma, with indications including: multifocal tumor (PRETEXT IV at diagnosis); large, solitary tumor (PRETEXT IV, involving all four sectors of the liver); or unifocal, centrally located PRETEXT II and III tumors involving the main hilar structures or all three main hepatic veins, with excellent results when the transplantation is performed as the first operation (see below) (Figure 20.16). Interestingly, macroscopic venous invasion (portal vein, hepatic veins,

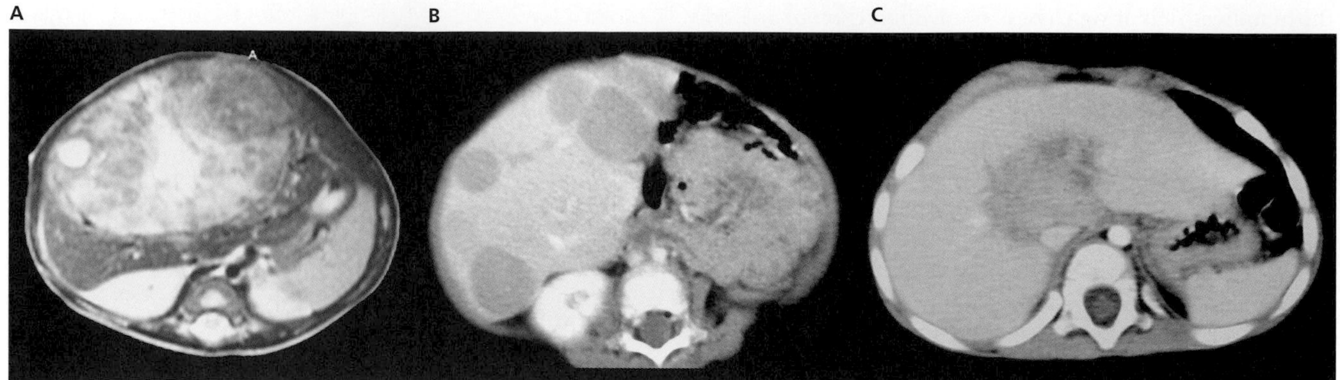

Figure 20.16 Non-resectable hepatoblastomas are an indication for transplantation. Typically, PreTExt IV hepatoblastomas (B) are unresectable and must be considered for transplantation unless there is extrahepatic spread. Selected cases with PreTExt III (B) or PreTExt II (C) tumors may be considered for primary transplantation due to their anatomical position, the difficulty in achieving a radical resection, and/or the risk of secondary liver failure related to insufficient residual liver mass or vascular complications. In the latter cases, heroic attempt at difficult resection should not be encouraged.

vena cava) and previous lung metastases in hepatoblastoma patients are not a contraindication for transplantation if these sites are completely resected during the transplant operation or cleared after chemotherapy or transplantation.[138,140]

Currently, the recommendations regarding the indications in HCC developing in a cirrhotic liver are mainly based on experience gained in adult patients, known as the Milan criteria:[141] no more than three tumors, each no more than 3 cm in size; or a single tumor no more than 5 cm in diameter. In adult patients, survival in the range of 70–80% can be expected in highly selected patients. Recent studies suggest that in an otherwise normal liver, it may be possible to increase the current size cut-off points to 6.5 or 7 cm. In HCC, vascular invasion and lymph-node involvement are contraindications for transplantation.

Epithelioid hemangioendothelioma typically presents as a nonresectable tumor, both in adults and in children; in the pediatric group, the tumor behavior appears to be more aggressive than in adults, with rapid growth and a risk of recurrence. Transplantation may not be a suitable management option, and it is possible that only patients who are responsive to chemotherapy should be considered for transplantation.[94] In selected patients with benign liver tumors, transplantation may be considered when the tumor is associated with local complications (compression, ascites, Budd–Chiari phenomenon), or even life-threatening problems, such as cardiac failure in multifocal neonatal hemangiomas.

Hepatoblastoma. Hepatoblastoma is the most frequently resected tumor. However, the timings for the operation recommended by various international groups differ, and it is interesting to compare the outcomes of two studies—one (SIOPEL-1) an international study (predominantly European) and one in the United States (INT-0098)—both of which were conducted in the early 1990s.[113,114,142] In SIOPEL-1, the vast majority of patients had delayed surgery after preoperative chemotherapy, with only 13 of 154 patients having primary resections. In contrast, 50 of 173 patients in the American study had a primary resection (stage I and II tumors). Once chemotherapy had been given, a complete resection rate of 77% was achieved in SIOPEL-1, in comparison with 62% in INT-0098. Given the importance of surgical resection in liver tumors, this result would seem to favor the SIOPEL strategy, but other issues are disguised. Localized tumors with favorable histology may need minimal chemotherapy, and the INT-0098 study demonstrated a 100% survival rate in this group with primary surgical resection followed by four cycles of doxorubicin (240 mg/m^2 cumulative dose). Treating these patients with preoperative PLADO chemotherapy may therefore be unjustified. The difficulty with diagnosis in infants and neonates is well recognized, with an error rate of 23% in some cases not relying on primary resection.[143]

A concern that unfavorable, chemotherapy-resistant tumors[47] might be missed if reliance is placed on small initial biopsies has also been raised as an argument in favor of primary resection. The debate is still continuing, and recent articles are continuing to promote primary resection as the best practice where feasible.[144] Although some patients present with resectable disease, most patients do not, and all such patients should undergo chemotherapy before surgery. As chemotherapy produces a shrunken and sclerotic tumor mass, the resection line may pass close to this without fear of incomplete resection, as long as the margin itself is clear of tumor.[135,136] This is different from the situation with other malignant tumors, in which a clear margin of at least 1 cm is recommended. Histological examination of hepatoblastomas resected after chemotherapy reveals that much of the residual tumor mass is in fact sterilized disease, with smaller nests of persistent tumor within tumors.

The other option for surgical management of hepatoblastoma is consideration for liver transplantation. In our own series,[138,145,146] we compared the outcome for patients treated with partial hepatectomy or liver transplantation. Patient selection is crucial for transplantation, but in suitably selected candidates it is a viable option for local therapy. The most significant predictor of a good outcome after liver transplantation appears to be the demonstration of chemosensitivity, and we observed a 100% survival rate in this group in comparison with 60% survival in poor responders to chemotherapy, as has been suggested in other series.[147] This is in line with the further observation that the presence of lung metastases at diagnosis is not a contraindication for transplantation if the metastases clear during chemotherapy.

Overall, current results suggest that liver transplantation is a good option in patients with unresectable lesions and no extrahepatic disease at the time of transplant.[138,147,148] Liver transplantation is a poor option for patients with recurrent disease or in whom incomplete excision was achieved previously.[138,149] In a review of the worldwide experience of 147 liver transplantations for hepatoblastoma by Otte *et al.*,[139] the 6-year post-transplant survival was reported to be 82% for patients receiving "primary" transplants and only 30% for patients receiving "rescue" transplants (Figure 20.17).

The issue of liver transplantation is associated with special challenges for the administration of chemotherapy. This is why early identification of patients is essential, so that they can be listed and donor searches initiated. In many cases in the past, donors were not found before planned preoperative chemotherapy had been completed. This then leads to a need to "tread water" whilst a donor is found, with the risk of additional cumulative doses of doxorubicin and the danger of cardiotoxicity. Currently, an active split-liver transplant program allows the allocation of a liver graft around the time of conventional surgery and avoids additional chemotherapy.[138] Another excellent alternative is to procure a left liver graft from a living related donor, allowing planning of this

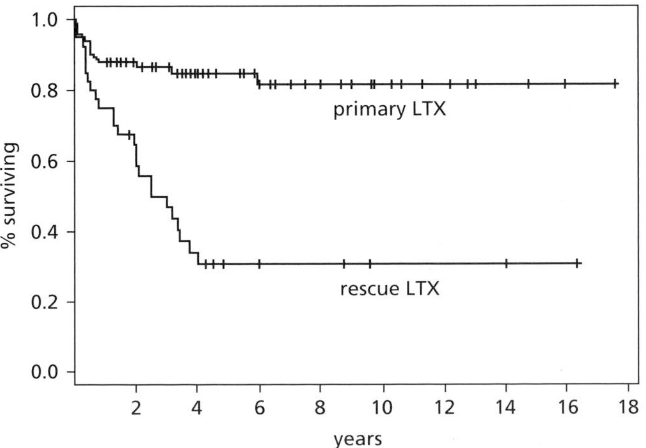

Figure 20.17 Overall survival outcomes after primary and rescue transplantation. (Reproduced with permission from Otte *et al.*, *Pediatric Blood and Cancer* 2004.[139])

elective operation at the right time in accordance with the chemotherapy schedule.[150] In addition, the added problems of cumulative cisplatin exposure can add to concerns about cross-reactivity with critical nephrotoxic drugs administered after transplantation (e.g., cyclosporine).[151] However, in patients in whom early transplantation can be undertaken, the administration of postoperative chemotherapy should be considered. With close scrutiny of serum levels of immunosuppressive drugs during therapy, we have not encountered serious postoperative chemotherapy-related problems.

Hepatocellular carcinoma and other malignant tumors. Resection of hepatocellular carcinoma in children with cirrhotic livers secondary to an underlying metabolic disease is unlikely to achieve a cure, as these tumors are multifocal. Liver transplantation may thus be considered for unresectable HCC, but only for patients who have HCC nodes less than 5 cm in diameter and an absence of vascular invasion (absence of thrombosis). For those who need transplantation, the waiting time to obtain a liver graft may be a limiting factor, allowing the tumor to grow and spread; transplantation should be performed within 3–4 months of diagnosis. Using the option of living-donor transplantation may be a solution for those who are likely to have a longer wait on the list.[152]

Patients with HCC and sarcomas in a noncirrhotic liver should be considered for resection on the basis of the imaging findings, as described above. Techniques as outlined above are used, but it should be emphasized that a clear resection margin of at least 1 cm should be sought in order to maximize cure rates. Epithelioid hemangioendothelioma is also often diffuse or multifocal in the liver at diagnosis and thus unresectable in most cases. Whereas in adults it is reported to be a low-grade malignancy with very slow growth (thus justifying liver transplantation for quality-of-life reasons), its behavior appears to be much more aggressive in children and the role of transplantation may be questioned. Transplantation may be reasonable only for those with slowly growing tumors.

Patients with unresectable HCC and other rarer malignant tumors have received varying treatments, including embolization and hepatic artery ligation, but without any real evidence of benefit. Current research includes chemoembolization using agents injected into the hepatic artery at angiography, and the results with this are awaited.

Radiotherapy

It is difficult to define the role of radiotherapy in the management of hepatoblastoma, since patients have traditionally been managed with combinations of surgery and chemotherapy and have not received radiotherapy in isolation.[153] Current studies do not recommend the use of radiotherapy for either the primary tumor or lung metastases. The use of radiotherapy is presently restricted to palliation of recurrent disease or treatment of residual disease following surgery.

Hepatic artery chemoembolization

Because of the overwhelming importance of rendering tumors resectable, other methods of reducing the bulk of the primary tumor have also been attempted. One such approach is hepatic artery chemoembolization (HACE), which may have a role to play in some cases, although it is not in widespread use. In this technique, intra-arterial chemotherapy is administered in combination with an embolizing compound. The theory behind HACE is that a higher concentration of anticancer drug can be applied directly to the tumor, whilst protecting the normal liver (supplied mainly by portal blood). The embolic effects of the treatment are aimed at prolonging the "dwell time" of the drug within the tumor, reducing the first-pass metabolic effects, and causing direct ischemic damage to the tumor. The use of transarterial chemoembolization in adults with HCC has been well described, and some studies have been able to demonstrate improved survival.[154,155] Experience with HACE in children with hepatoblastoma or HCC is limited, but a number of publications have suggested the procedure is safe, even in very small children, and that the majority of tumors shrink with treatment, often becoming resectable, so that the method can serve as a "bridge" whilst transplantation is awaited. The exact place of such therapy is unclear, but it needs to be considered as part of any combined therapeutic strategy in managing residual bulk tumor.[156–161] As transarterial chemoembolization may be associated with thrombosis of some of the hepatic artery branches, or even of the main (right, left or both) arterial branches, it may interfere with subsequent surgical resection. Transarterial chemoembolization should thus be considered after a multidisciplinary discussion and with the surgical options at the end of the treatment being taken into account.

Benign tumors

Hemangiomas and hemangioendotheliomas

The commonest benign tumors are hemangiomas and infantile hemangioendotheliomas (Table 20.1). The natural history of these lesions is one of gradual progression and enlargement during the first 6 months of life. There may be other cutaneous hemangiomatous lesions that suggest the diagnosis, but most children will present with progressive abdominal distension, and a minority have spontaneous hemorrhage. Cardiac failure is a common presentation in hemangioendothelioma, due to the enormous vascular load of these tumors. Neonates presenting with cardiac failure often have features of congenital heart disease, which may cause a delay in diagnosis. Other presentations include bruising/petechiae from thrombocytopenia (Kasabach–Merritt syndrome)[162] and intravascular consumptive coagulopathy.

The diagnosis is obtained with imaging methods, including ultrasound, CT, or MRI. Biopsy is rarely required and may be dangerous (Chapter 19).

A number of therapeutic options are available. However, since spontaneous resolution may occur, a "watch-and-wait" policy can be adopted in asymptomatic children. If treatment is necessary, it should be tailored to individual cases. Surgical resection, ligation of hepatic arteries, or embolization may be possible with isolated lesions[163] (Chapter 19). These techniques are associated with significant mortality, ranging from 18% to 50%.

Medical treatment options include steroid therapy, radiotherapy, and chemotherapy with cyclophosphamide. Most clinicians tend to adopt an approach involving initial treatment with steroids, progressing to chemotherapy if no response is seen. However, patients who present with spontaneous hemorrhage require immediate surgery, which may involve hepatic artery ligation and/or resection of the lesion. Radiotherapy tends to be reserved for resistant cases, in view of the potential for a second malignancy within the radiation site.[164] Recent interest has focused on the use of interferon alfa 2a therapy in life-threatening hemangiomas, including hepatic lesions.[165] Treatment is undoubtedly effective, appears to be relatively free from significant side effects, and may have better results in terms of mortality than either surgical or other medical approaches.

Epithelioid hemangioendotheliomas (type II) are rare tumors in children. They are more commonly seen in young women and are considered to be low-grade malignancies with very slow growth, associated with prolonged survival without treatment.[81,166,167] However, it appears that they can have more aggressive behavior in children (personal observations). Only a limited number of epithelioid hemangioendotheliomas can be managed by partial resection, since the tumor tends to be widespread within the liver at the time of diagnosis. Because of the slow growth and low metastatic potential of the tumor, liver transplantation has been considered acceptable for adult patients. These tumors can metastasize, but patients with a recurrence following transplantation can have satisfactory and long-term survival.[167] Only a few children with epithelioid hemangioendotheliomas have undergone transplantation and the general outcome has been poor, with rapid recurrence and malignant tumor behavior, followed by death (personal observations).[168] For this reason, the indication for transplantation in children should be considered carefully.

Mesenchymal hamartoma

Mesenchymal hamartoma is a rare tumor, typically seen in children under 2 years of age. The majority of children present with abdominal distension, and the physical examination reveals a large, smooth, nontender mass. The tumors are usually well demarcated, and resection by lobectomy (extended or not) is the treatment of choice.[169]

Adenomas

Adenomas are extremely rare in the pediatric age group,

but can occur at any age. In children, there is an association with glycogen storage disease type I and galactosemia, while in adults and adolescents there is a well-recognized link with oral contraceptive use—in these cases, cessation of the pill may allow resolution. The adenomas are usually diagnosed with ultrasound and confirmed by CT scan or radioisotope imaging using technetium Tc 99m sulfur colloid, as adenomas do not take up the isotope.

Persistent cases in adults require resection because of the risks of malignancy and rupture with intraperitoneal bleeding. Whilst adenomas are not thought to be premalignant in children, they can be difficult to distinguish from a well-differentiated hepatocellular carcinoma, and if there is any doubt resection should be undertaken.

Focal nodular hyperplasia

Focal nodular hyperplasia (FNH) is also rare in the pediatric age group and occurs more commonly in girls than boys. The vast majority of cases are asymptomatic, although some patients present with an abdominal mass or pain. Histologically, the lesions have features of a well-localized area of liver cell hyperplasia around a fibrous central scar, which shows up clearly on CT or MRI scans. Colloid scans are usually positive, as there are sufficient reticuloendothelial cells within the mass to take up the isotope. Surgical resection is only required for symptomatic patients, as there is no risk of malignancy.

Case study

A 2½-year-old girl was referred with a short history over 3 weeks of becoming increasingly unwell with "viral symptoms," associated with an increasingly distended abdomen. Hepatic enlargement was noted by the family practitioner, and a referral to the local hospital was made. A liver mass was detected on ultrasound imaging, and she was referred to the regional pediatric oncology center. The physical examination revealed huge abdominal swelling with a firm liver, palpable to the level of the umbilicus. A full blood count revealed low hemoglobin at 8 g/dL and a slightly raised platelet count at 439×10^9/L. Serum biochemistry showed slightly deranged liver function, with alanine aminotransferase (ALT) 47 IU/L and aspartate aminotransferase (AST) 116 IU/L, but normal bilirubin. Serum lactate dehydrogenase (LDH) was markedly elevated at 2996 IU/L and serum AFP was raised at 39 204 kU/L (rising to > 82 000 kU/L a week later before the start of treatment). MRI of the liver showed an extensive, multifocal tumor involving all sections of the liver (PRETEXT IV), but with no vascular, nodal, or extrahepatic spread. There were no lung metastases on a CT scan of the chest.

Chemotherapy was commenced in accordance with the high-risk arm of the SIOPEL-3 protocol. Cycles of cisplatin (80 mg/m^2) were alternated with carboplatin (500 mg/m^2) and doxorubicin (60 mg/m^2) every 2 weeks. The patient responded well to treatment, with visible shrinkage of the liver mass and a rapid fall in the level of AFP. On reassessment imaging after four cycles of chemotherapy, despite the good response, none of the liver sections was free of tumor, and a decision to list her for transplantation was made. A donor liver became available after the sixth cycle of chemotherapy, at which point the AFP level had nearly normalized to 12 kU/L.

At surgery, however, suspicious areas of extrahepatic disease were identified—a small calcified nodule under the right surface of the liver, a possible lymph node close to the pancreatic head, and a small tumor nodule attached to the lesser curve of the stomach. All three areas were excised, and transplantation was abandoned. Subsequent histology showed that there was no viable tumor in the liver and lymph-node mass and that there were regressive chemotherapy changes, with scanty viable tumor cells in the lesion removed from the lesser curve of the stomach.

A further course of cisplatin chemotherapy was given, with evidence of further tumor regression in the liver and normalization of the AFP to < 10 kU/l. In view of the clinical and pathological response to chemotherapy, a decision was made to relist the patient for transplantation, although it was recognized that this was a high-risk procedure. She underwent liver transplantation soon after, before receiving any further chemotherapy, and made excellent postoperative progress. Three further cycles of chemotherapy were given after transplantation, with a very close eye being kept on renal function and tacrolimus immunosuppression doses. Treatment was completed uneventfully.

Three years after completion of the treatment, the patient is alive and well, with no evidence of tumor recurrence and with a healthy, functioning graft.

References

1 Weinberg AG, Finegold MJ. Primary hepatic tumors in childhood. In: Finegold MJ, ed. *Pathology of Neoplasia in Children and Adolescents—Major Problems in Pathology*. Philadelphia: Saunders, 1986: 333–72.

2 Dimmick JE, Rogers PCJ, Blair G. Hepatic tumors. In: Pochedly C, ed. *Neoplastic Diseases of Childhood*. Chur, Switzerland: Harwood Academic, 1994:973–1010.

3 Mann JR, Kasthuri N, Raafat F, *et al*. Malignant hepatic tumours in children: incidence, clinical features and aetiology. *Paediatr Perinat Epidemiol* 1990;**4**:276–89.

4 Stiller CA, Pritchard J, Steliarova-Foucher E. Liver cancer in European children: incidence and survival 1978–1997. Report for the Automated Childhood Cancer Information System Project. *Eur J Cancer* 2006;**42**:2115–23.

5 Fraumeni JF Jr, Miller RW, Hill JA. Primary carcinoma of the liver in childhood: an epidemiological study. *J Nat Cancer Inst* 1968;**40**:1087–99.

6 Geiser CF, Baez A, Schindler AM, Shih VE. Epithelial hepatoblastoma associated with congenital hemihypertrophy and

cystathioninuria: presentation of a case. *Pediatrics* 1970;**46**:66–73.

7 Sotelo-Avila C, Gonzalez-Crussi F, Fowler JW. Complete and incomplete forms of Beckwith–Wiedemann syndrome: their oncogenic potential. *J Pediatr* 1980;**96**:47–50.

8 Li M, Shuman C, Fei YL, *et al.* GPC3 mutation analysis in a spectrum of patients with overgrowth expands the phenotype of the Simpson–Golabi–Behmel syndrome. *Am J Med Genet* 2001;**102**:161–8.

9 Koufos A, Hansen MF, Lampkin BC. Loss of alleles at loci on human chromosome 11 during genesis of Wilms' tumor. *Nature* 1984;**309**:170–4.

10 Koufos A, Grundy P, Morgan K. Familial Wiedemann–Beckwith syndrome and a second Wilms' tumor locus both map to 11p15.5. *Nature* 1989;**44**:711–9.

11 Koufos A, Hansen MF, Copeland NG, Jenkins NA, Lampkin BC, Cavenee WK. Loss of heterozygosity in three embryonal tumours suggests a common pathogenetic mechanism. *Nature* 1985;**316**:330–4.

12 Little MH, Thomson DB, Hayward DK, Smith PJ. Loss of alleles on the short arm of chromosome 11 in a hepatoblastoma from a child with Beckwith–Wiedemann syndrome. *Hum Genet* 1988; **79**:186–9.

13 Scrable HJ, Witte DP, Lampkin BC, Cavenee WK. Chromosomal localisation of the human rhabdomyosarcoma locus by mitotic recombination mapping. *Nature* 1987;**320**:645–7.

14 Simms LA, Reeve AE, Smith PJ. Genetic mosaicism at the insulin locus in liver associated with childhood hepatoblastoma. *Genes Chromosomes Cancer* 1995;**13**:72–3.

15 Rainier S, Dobry CJ, Feinberg AP. Loss of imprinting in hepatoblastoma. *Cancer Res* 1995;**55**:1836–8.

16 Byrne JA, Simms LA, Little MH, Algar EM, Smith PJ. Three non-overlapping regions of chromosome arm 11p allele loss identified in infantile tumors of the adrenal and liver. *Genes Chromosomes Cancer* 1993;**8**:104–11.

17 Kingston JE, Herbert A, Draper GJ, Mann JR. Association between hepatoblastoma ans polyposis coli. *Arch Dis Child* 1983; **58**:959–62.

18 Oda H, Imai Y, Nakasuru Y, *et al.* Somatic mutations of the *APC* gene in sporadic hepatoblastoma. *Cancer Res* 1996;**56**:3320–3.

19 Jeng YM, Wu MZ, Mao TL, Chang MH, Hsu HC. Somatic mutations of beta-catenin play a crucial role in the tumorigenesis of sporadic hepatoblastoma. *Cancer Lett* 2000;**152**:45–51.

20 Udatsu Y, Kusafuka T, Kuroda S, Miao J, Okada A. High frequency of beta-catenin mutations in hepatoblastoma. *Pediatr Surg Int* 2001;**17**:508–12.

21 Koch A, Denkhaus D, Albrecht S, Leuschner I, Von Schweintz D, Pietsch T. Childhood hepatoblastomas frequently carry a mutated degradation targeting box of the β-catenin gene. *Cancer Res* 1999;**59**:269–73.

22 Phillips M, Dicks-Mireaux C, Kingston J, *et al.* Hepatoblastoma and polyposis coli (familial adenomatous polyposis). *Med Pediatr Oncol* 1989;**17**:441–7.

23 Aretz S, Koch A, Uhlhaas S, *et al.* Should children at risk for familial adenomatous polyposis be screened for hepatoblastoma and children with apparently sporadic hepatoblastoma be screened for *APC* germline mutations? *Pediatr Blood Cancer* 2006;**47**:811–8.

24 Thomas D, Pritchard J, Davidson R, McKiernan P, Grundy RG, de Ville de Goyet J. Familial hepatoblastoma and *APC* gene mutations: renewed call for molecular research. *Eur J Cancer* 2003;**39**:2200–4.

25 Sanders RP, Furman WL. Familial adenomatous polyposis in two brothers with hepatoblastoma: implications for diagnosis and screening. *Pediatr Blood Cancer* 2006;**47**:851–4.

26 Stocker JT. Hepatoblastoma. *Semin Diagn Pathol* 1994;**11**:136–43.

27 Surace C, Leszl A, Perilongo G, Rocchi M, Basso G, Sainati L. Fluorescent in situ hybridization (FISH) reveals frequent and recurrent numerical and structural abnormalities in hepatoblastoma with no informative karyotype. *Med Pediatr Oncol* 2002;**39**:536–9.

28 Hall AJ, Winter PD, Wright R. Mortality of hepatitis B positive blood donors in England and Wales. *Lancet* 1985;**i**:91–3.

29 Chen WJ, Lee JC, Hung WT. Primary malignant tumour of liver in infants and children in Taiwan. *J Pediatr Surg* 1988;**23**:457–61.

30 Chan KL, Fan ST, Tam PK, Chiang AK, Chan GC, Ha SY. Paediatric hepatoblastoma and hepatocellular carcinoma: retrospective study. *Hong Kong Med J* 2002;**8**:13–7.

31 Brechot C, Pourcel C, Louise A, Rain B, Tiollais P. Presence of integrated hepatitis-B virus DNA in cellular DNA of human hepatocellular carcinoma. *Nature* 1980;**286**:533–5.

32 Perilongo G, Pontisso P, Basso G. Can primary cancer of the liver in Western countries be prevented? Pediatric point of view. *Med Pediatr Oncol* 1990;**18**:57–60.

33 Wong N, Lai P, Lee SW, *et al.* Assessment of genetic changes in hepatocellular carcinoma by comparative genomic hybridization analysis. *Am J Pathol* 1999;**154**:37–43.

34 Darby SC, Ewart DW, Giangrande PLF, *et al.* Mortality from liver cancer and liver disease in haemophiliac men and boys in UK given blood products contaminated with hepatitis C. *Lancet* 1997;**350**:1425–31.

35 Knisely AS, Strautnieks SS, Meier Y, *et al.* Hepatocellular carcinoma in ten children under five years of age with bile salt export pump deficiency. *Hepatology* 2006;**44**:478–86.

36 Perlmutter DH. Pathogenesis of chronic liver injury and hepatocellular carcinoma in alpha-1-antitrypsin deficiency. *Pediatr Res* 2006;**60**:233–8.

37 Demo E, Frush D, Gottfried M, *et al.* Glycogen storage disease type III—hepatocellular carcinoma a long-term complication? *J Hepatol* 2007;**46**:492–8.

38 Jones E. Primary carcinoma of the liver with associated cirrhosis in infants and children. Report of a case. *Arch Pathol* 1960; **70**:5–12.

39 Czauderna P. Adult type vs. childhood hepatocellular carcinoma—are they the same or different lesions? Biology, natural history, prognosis, and treatment. *Med Pediatr Oncol* 2002;**39**:519–23.

40 Weinberg AG, Mize CE, Worthen HG. The occurrence of hepatoma in the chronic form of hereditary tyrosinemia. *J Pediatr* 1976;**88**:434–8.

41 Kohno M, Kitatani H, Wada H, *et al.* Hepatocellular carcinoma complicating biliary cirrhosis caused by biliary atresia: report of a case. *J Pediatr Surg* 1995;**30**:1713–6.

42 Steinemann D, Skawran B, Becker T, *et al.* Assessment of differentiation and progression of hepatic tumors using array-based comparative genomic hybridization. *Clin Gastroenterol Hepatol* 2006;**4**:1283–91.

43 Boyault S, Rickman DS, De Reyniès A, *et al.* Transcriptome classification of HCC is related to gene alterations and to new therapeutic targets. *Hepatology* 2007;**45**:42–52.

44 MacKinlay GA, Pritchard J. A common language for childhood liver tumours. *Pediatr Surg Int* 1992;**7**:325–6.

45 Finegold MJ. Tumors of the liver. *Semin Liver Dis* 1994;**14**: 270–81.

46 von Schweinitz D, Wischmeyer P, Leuschner I, *et al.* Clinicopathological criteria with prognostic relevance in hepatoblastoma. *Eur J Cancer* 1994;**30A**:1052–8.

47 Haas JE, Feusner JH, Finegold MJ. Small cell undifferentiated histology hepatoblastoma may be unfavorable. *Cancer* 2001;**92**: 3130–4.

48 Zimmermann A. Hepatoblastoma with cholangioblastic features ("cholangioblastic hepatoblastoma") and other liver tumors with bimodal differentiation in young patients. *Med Pediatr Oncol* 2002;**39**:487–91.

49 Prokurat A, Kluge P, Kościesza A, Perek D, Kappeler A, Zimmermann A. Transitional liver cell tumors (TLCT) in older children and adolescents: a novel group of aggressive hepatic tumors expressing beta-catenin. *Med Pediatr Oncol* 2002;**39**: 510–8.

50 Zimmermann A. The emerging family of hepatoblastoma tumours: from ontogenesis to oncogenesis. *Eur J Cancer* 2005;**41**:1503–14.

51 Cajaiba MM, Neves JI, Casarotti FF, *et al.* Hepatoblastomas and liver development: a study of cytokeratin immunoexpression in twenty-nine hepatoblastomas. *Pediatr Dev Pathol* 2006;**9**:196–202.

52 Czauderna P, Mackinlay G, Perilongo G, *et al.* Hepatocellular carcinoma in children: results of the first prospective study of the International Society of Pediatric Oncology group. *J Clin Oncol* 2002;**20**:2798–804.

53 Haas JE, Muczynski KA, Krailo M, *et al.* Histopathology and prognosis in childhood hepatoblastoma and hepatocarcinoma. *Cancer* 1989;**64**:1082–95.

54 Craig JR, Peters R, Edmondson HA, Omata M. Fibrolamellar carcinoma of the liver: a tumor of adolescents and young adults with distinctive clinicopathologic features. *Cancer* 1980;**46**: 372–9.

55 Yamaoka H, Ohtsu K, Sueda T, Yokoyama T, Hiyama E. Diagnostic and prognostic impact of beta-catenin alterations in pediatric tumors. *Oncol Rep* 2006;**15**:551–6.

56 Stocker JT, Ishak KG. Undifferentiated (embryonal) sarcoma of the liver: report of 31 cases. *Cancer* 1978;**42**:336–48.

57 Nical K, Savel V, Moore J, Teot L, *et al.* Distinguishing undifferentiated embryonal sarcoma of the liver from biliary tract rhabdomyosarcoma: a children's oncology group study. *Pediatr Dev Pathol* 2007;**10**:89–97.

58 Lauwer YG, Grant LD, Donnelly WH, *et al.* Hepatic undifferentiated (embryonal) sarcoma arising in a mesenchymal hamartoma. *Am J Surg Pathol* 1997;**21**:1248–54.

59 Ramanujam TM, Ramesh JC, Goh DW, *et al.* Malignant transformation of mesenchymal hamartoma of the liver, case report and review of literature. *J Pediatr Surg* 1999;**34**:1684–6.

60 de Chadarévian JP, Pawel BR, Faerber EN, Weintraub WH. Undifferentiated (embryonal) sarcoma arising in conjunction with mesenchymal hamartoma of the liver. *Mod Pathol* 1994;**7**:490–3.

61 Begueret H, Trouette, Vielh P, *et al.* Hepatic undifferentiated embryonal sarcoma: malignant evolution of mesenchymal hamartoma? Study of one case with immunohistochemical and flow cytometric emphasis. *J Hepatol* 2001;**34**:178–9.

62 Stocker JT, Ishak KG. Mesenchymal hamartoma of the liver: report of 30 cases and review of the literature. *Pediatr Pathol* 1983;**1**:245–67.

63 Otal TM, Hendricks JB, Pharis P, Donnelly WH. Mesenchymal hamartoma of the liver. *Cancer* 1994;**74**:1237–42.

64 Speleman F, De Telder V, De Potter KR, *et al.* Cytogenic analysis of a mesenchymal hamartoma of the liver. *Cancer Genet Cytogenet* 1989;**40**:29–32.

65 Sawyer JR, Roloson GJ, Bell JM, *et al.* Telometric association in the progression of chromosome aberrations in pediatric solid tumours. *Cancer Genet Cytogenet* 1989;**40**:29–32.

66 Mascarello JT, Krous HF. Second report of translocation involving 19q13.4 in a mesenchymal hamartoma in the liver. *Cancer Genet Cytogenet* 1992;**58**:141–2.

67 Bove KE, Blough RI, Soukup S. Third report of t(19q)(13.4) in mesenchymal hamartoma of liver with comments on link to embryonal sarcoma. *Pedia Develop Pathol* 1998;**1**:438–42.

68 Sharif K, Ramani P, Lochbühler H, Grundy R, de Ville de Goyet J. Recurrent mesenchymal hamartoma associated with 19q translocation. A call for more radical surgical resection. *Eur J Pediatr Surg* 2006;**16**:64–7.

69 Rakheja D, Margraf LR, Tomlinson GE, Schneider NR. Hepatic mesenchymal hamartoma with translocation involving chromosome band 19q13.4: a recurrent abnormality. *Cancer Genet Cytogenet* 2004;**153**:60–3.

70 Rajaram V, Knesevich S, Bove KE, Perry A, Pfeifer JD. DNA sequence of the translocation breakpoints in undifferentiated embryonal sarcoma arising in mesenchymal hamartoma of the liver harbouring the t(11;19)(q11;q13.4) translocation. *Genes Chromosomes Cancer* 2007;**46**:508–13.

71 Talmon GA, Cohen S. Mesenchymal hamartoma of the liver with an interstitial deletion involving chromosome band 19q13.4. *Arch Pathol Lab Med* 2006;**130**:1216–8.

72 Parham DM, Kelly DR, Donnelly DH. Immunohistochemical and ultrastructural spectrum of hepatic sarcomas of childhood: evidence for a common histogenesis. *Mod Pathol* 1991;**4**:648–53.

73 Ruymann FB, Raney RB, Crist WM, Lawrence W, Lindberg RD, Soule EH. Rhabdomyosarcoma of the biliary tree in childhood. *Cancer* 1985;**56**:575–81.

74 Horowitz ME, Etcubanas E, Webber BL, *et al.* Hepatic undifferentiated (embryonal) sarcoma and rhabdomyosarcoma in children. *Cancer* 1987;**59**:396–402.

75 Parham DN, Peiper SC, Robicheaux G, *et al.* Malignant rhabdoid tumor of the liver. *Arch Path Lab Med* 1988;**112**:61–4.

76 Miller S, Wollner N, Meyers PA, Exelby P, Jereb B, Miller DR. Primary hepatic or hepatosplenic non-Hodgkin's lymphoma in children. *Cancer* 1983;**52**:2285–8.

77 Soares FA, Landell GA, Peres LC, Oliveira MA, Vincente YA, Tone LG. Liposarcoma of hepatic hilum in childhood: report of a case and review of the literature. *Med Pediatr Oncol* 1989;**17**: 239–243.

78 Mann JR, Pearson D, Barrett A, Raafat F, Barnes JM, Wallendszus KR. Results of the United Kingdom Children's Cancer Study Group's malignant germ cell tumor studies. *Cancer* 1989;**63**:1657–67.

79 Dehner LP, Ishak KG. Vascular tumors of the liver in infants and children. *Arch Pathol* 1971;**92**:101–11.

80 Weiss SW, Enzinger FM. Epithelioid hemangioendothelioma: a vascular tumour often mistaken for carcinoma. *Cancer* 1982;**50**: 970–81.

81 Ishak KG, Sesterhenn IA, Goodman ZD, Rabin L, Stromeyer FW. Epithelioid hemangioendothelioma of the liver: a clinicopathologic and follow-up study of 32 cases. *Hum Pathol* 1984;**15**:839–52.

82 Srouji MN, Chatten J, Schulman WM, Ziegler MM, Koop CE. Mesenchymal hamartomas of the liver in infants. *Cancer* 1978;**42**:2483–9.

83 Stocker JT, Ishak KG. Focal nodular hyperplasia of the liver: a study of 21 pediatric cases. *Cancer* 1981;**48**:336–45.

84 Nakayama S, Kanbara Y, Nishimura T, *et al.* Genome-wide microsatellite analysis of focal nodular hyperplasia: a strong tool for the differential diagnosis of non-neoplastic liver nodule from hepatocellular carcinoma. *J Hepatobiliary Pancreat Surg* 2006;**13**:416–20.

85 Kellner U, Jacobsen A, Kellner A, Mantke R, Roessner A, Rocken C. Comparative genomic hybridization. Synchronous occurrence of focal nodular hyperplasia and hepatocellular carcinoma in the same liver is not based on common chromosomal alterations. *Am J Clin Pathol* 2003;**119**:265–71.

86 Lack EE, Ornvold K. Focal nodular hyperplasia and hepatic adenoma: a review of eight cases in the pediatric age group. *J Surg Oncol* 1986;**33**:129–33.

87 Dehner LP, Parker ME, Franciosi RA, Drake RM. Focal nodular hyperplasia and adenoma of the liver: a pediatric experience. *Am J Pediatr Med Oncol* 1979;**1**:85–93.

88 Van Dekken H, Verhoef C, Wink J, *et al.* Cell biological evaluation of liver cell carcinoma, dysplasia and adenoma by tissue micro-array analysis. *Acta Histochem* 2005;**107**:161–71.

89 Exelby PR, Filler RM, Grosfeld JL. Liver tumors in children in the particular reference to hepatoblastoma and hepatocellular carcinoma: American Academy of Pediatrics Surgical Section Survey—1974. *J Pediatr Surg* 1975;**10**:329–37.

90 Teng CT, Daeschner CWJ, Singleton EB, *et al.* Liver diseases and osteoporosis in children: I. Clinical observations. *J Pediatr* 1961;**59**:684–702.

91 Awan S, Davenport M, Portmann B, Howard ER. Angiosarcoma of the liver. *J Pediatr Surg* 1996;**31**:1729–32.

92 Sharif K, English M, Ramani P, *et al.* Management of hepatic epithelioid haemangio-endothelioma in children: what option? *Br J Cancer* 2004;**90**:1498–501.

93 Makhlouf HR, Ishak KG, Goodman ZD. Epithelioid hemangioendothelioma of the liver: a clinicopathologic study of 137 cases. *Cancer* 1999;**85**:562–82.

94 Van Beers B, Roche A, Mathieu D, *et al.* Epithelioid hemangioendothelioma of the liver: MR and CT findings. *J Comput Assist Tomogr* 1992;**16**:420–4.

95 Lack EE, Neave C, Vawter GF. Hepatoblastoma—a clinical and pathologic study of 54 cases. *Am J Surg Pathol* 1982;**6**:693–705.

96 Shafford EA, Pritchard J. Extreme thrombocytosis as a diagnostic clue to hepatoblastoma. *Arch Dis Child* 1993;**69**:171.

97 Nickerson HJ, Silberman TL, McDonald TP. Hepatoblastoma, thrombocytosis and increased thrombopoietin. *Cancer* 1980;**45**: 315–7.

98 Pritchard J, da Cunha A, Cornbleet MA, Carter CJ. Alpha fetoprotein monitoring of response to adriamycin in hepatoblastoma. *J Pediatr Surg* 1982;**17**:429–30.

99 Stringer MD, Hennayake S, Howard ER, *et al.* Improved outcome for children with hepatoblastoma. *Br J Surg* 1995;**82**:386–91.

100 Paradinas FJ, Melia WM, Wilkinson ML, *et al.* High serum vitamin B_{12} binding capacity as a marker of the fibrolamellar variant of hepatocellular carcinoma. *BMJ* 1982;**285**:840–2.

101 Wheeler K, Pritchard J, Luck W, Rossiter M. Transcobalamin I as a "marker" for fibrolamellar hepatoma. *Med Pediatr Oncol* 1986;**14**:227–9.

102 de Campo M, de Campo JF. Ultrasound of primary hepatic tumours in childhood. *Pediatr Radiol* 1988;**19**:19–24.

103 Vos A. Primary liver tumours in children. *Eur J Surg Oncol* 1990;**21**:101–5.

104 Roebuck DJ, Aronson D, Clapuyt P, *et al.* 2005 PRETEXT: a revised staging system for primary malignant liver tumours of childhood developed by the SIOPEL group. *Pediatr Radiol* 2007;37:123–32.

105 Aronson DC, Schnater JM, Staalman CR, *et al.* Predictive value of the pretreatment extent of disease system in hepatoblastoma: results from the International Society of Pediatric Oncology Liver Tumor Study Group SIOPEL-1 Study. *J Clin Oncol* 2005; **23**:1245–52.

106 Evans AE, Land VJ, Newton WA, Randolph JR, Sather HN, Tefft M. Combination chemotherapy in the treatment of children with malignant hepatoma. *Cancer* 1982;**50**:821–6.

107 Plaschkes J, Perilongo G, Shafford E, *et al.* SIOP trial report —overall preliminary results of SIOPEL-1 for the treatment of hepatoblastoma (HB) with preoperative chemotherapy—continuous infusion cisplatin and doxorubicin (PLADO) [abstract]. *Med Pediatr Oncol* 1994;**23**:170.

108 Douglass EC, Reynolds M, Finegold M, Cantor AB, Glicksman A. Cisplatin, vincristine, and fluorouracil therapy for hepatoblastoma: a Pediatric Oncology Group Study. *J Clin Oncol* 1993;**11**:96–9.

109 Douglass EC, Green AA, Wrenn E, *et al.* Effective cisplatin (DDP) based chemotherapy in the treatment of hepatoblastoma. *Med Pediatr Oncol* 1985;**13**:187–90.

110 Weinblatt ME, Siegel SE, Siegel MM. Preoperative chemotherapy for unresectable primary hepatic malignancies in children. *Cancer* 1982;**50**:1061–4.

111 Ortega JA, Krailo MD, Haas JE, *et al.* Effective treatment of unresectable or metastatic hepatoblastoma with cisplatin and continuous infusion doxorubicin chemotherapy: a report from the Children's Cancer Study Group. *J Clin Oncol* 1991;**9**:2167–76.

112 Plaschkes J, Perilongo G, Shafford E. Preoperative chemotherapy cisplatin and doxorubicin for the treatment of hepatoblastoma and hepatocellular carcinoma. Brief update of the SIOP liver tumour study (SIOPEL-1) [abstract]. *Med Pediatr Oncol* 1995;**25**:256.

113 Pritchard J, Brown J, Shafford E, *et al.* Cisplatin, doxorubicin, and delayed surgery for childhood hepatoblastoma: a successful approach—results of the first prospective study of the International Society of Pediatric Oncology. *J Clin Oncol* 2000;**18**:3819–28.

114 Ortega JA, Douglass EC, Feusner JH, *et al.* Randomized comparison of cisplatin/vincristine/fluorouracil and cisplatin/continuous infusion doxorubicin for treatment of pediatric hepatoblastoma: a report from the Children's Cancer Group and the Pediatric Oncology Group. *J Clin Oncol* 2000;**18**:2665–75.

115 Perilongo G, Shafford E, Maibach R, *et al.* Risk-adapted treatment for childhood hepatoblastoma: final report of the second study of the International Society of Pediatric Oncology—SIOPEL 2. *Eur J Cancer* 2004;**40**:411–21.

116 Malogolowkin M, Katzenstein H, Krailo M, *et al.* Intensified platinum therapy is an ineffective strategy for improving outcome in pediatric patients with advanced hepatoblastoma. *J Clin Oncol* 2006;**24**:2879–84.

117 Dall'Igna P, Cecchetto G, Dominici C, *et al.* Carboplatin and doxorubicin (CARDOX) for nonmetastatic hepatoblastoma: a discouraging pilot study. *Med Pediatr Oncol* 2001:**36**:332–4.

118 Legha SS, Benjamin RS, Mackay B, *et al.* Reduction of doxorubicin cardiotoxicity by prolonged intravenous infusion. *Ann Intern Med* 1982;**96**:133–9.

119 Rich PS, Occhipinti SJ, Skramstad KS. Schedule optimization of adriamycin in sarcoma 180 in vitro [abstract]. *Proc Am Assoc Cancer Res* 1979;**20**:61.

120 Brock P, Pritchard J, Bellman S, Pinkerton CR. Ototoxicity of high-dose cisplatinum in children. *Med Pediatr Oncol* 1988;**16**:368–9.

121 Warmann S, Hunger M, Teichmann B, Flemming P, Gratz KF, Fuchs J. The role of *MDR1* gene in the development of multidrug resistance in human hepatoblastoma: clinical course and in vivo model. *Cancer* 2002;**95**:1795–801.

122 Katzenstein HM, Krailo MD, Malogolowkin MH, *et al.* Hepatocellular carcinoma in children and adolescents: results from the Pediatric Oncology Group and the Children's Cancer Group Intergroup Study. *J Clin Oncol* 2002;**20**:2789–97.

123 Nowak AK, Chow PKH, Findlay M. Systemic therapy for advanced hepatocellular carcinoma: a review. *Eur J Cancer* 2004;**40**:1474–84.

124 Thomas MB, Zhu AX. Hepatocellular carcinoma: the need for progress. *J Clin Oncol* 2005;**23**:2892–9.

125 Lin AY, Brophy N, Fisher GA, *et al.* Phase II study of thalidomide in patients with unresectable hepatocellular carcinoma. *Cancer* 2004;**103**:119–25.

126 Katzenstein HM, Krailo MD, Malogolowkin MH, *et al.* Fibrolamellar hepatocellular carcinoma in children and adolescents. *Cancer* 2003;**97**:2006–12.

127 Christison-Lagay ER, Burrows PE, Alomari A, *et al.* Hepatic haemangiomas: subtype classification and development of a clinical practice algorithm and registry. *J Pediatr Surg* 2007;**42**:62–8.

128 Kassarjian A, Zurakowski D, Dubois J, Paltiel HJ, Fishman SJ, Burrows PE. Infantile hepatic hemangiomas: clinical and imaging findings and their correlation with therapy. *AJR Am J Roentgenol* 2004;**182**:785–95.

129 Bisogno G, Pilz T, Perilongo G, *et al.* Undifferentiated sarcoma of the liver in childhood. A curable disease. *Cancer* 2002;**94**:252–7.

130 Baron PW, Majlessipour F, Bedros AA, *et al.* Undifferentiated embryonal sarcoma of the liver successfully treated with chemotherapy and liver resection. *J Gastrointest Surg* 2007;**11**:73–5.

131 Weitz J, Klimstra DS, Cymes K, *et al.* Management of primary liver sarcomas. *Cancer* 2006;**109**:1391–6.

132 Dietze O, Davies SE, Williams R, *et al.* Malignant epithelioid haemangioendothelioma of the liver: a clinicopathological and histochemical study of 12 cases. *Histopathology* 1989;**15**:225–37.

133 Pinet C, Magnan A, Garbe L, *et al.* Aggressive form of pleural epithelioid haemangioendothelioma: complete response after chemotherapy. *Eur Respir J* 1999;**14**:237–8.

134 Couinaud C. *Le Foie: études anatomiques et chirurgicales.* Paris: Masson, 1957.

135 Pham TH, Iqbal CW, Grams JM, *et al.* Outcomes of primary liver cancer in children: an appraisal of experience. *J Pediatr Surg* 2007;**42**:834–9.

136 Ang JP, Heath JA, Donath S, Khurana S, Auldist A. Treatment outcomes for hepatoblastomas: an institution's experience over two decades. *Pediatr Surg Int* 2007;**23**:103–9.

137 Lin CC, Chen CL, Cheng YF, Chiu KW, Jawan B, Hsaio CC. Major hepatectomy in children: approaching blood transfusion-free. *World J Surg* 2006;**30**:1115–9.

138 Pimpalwar AP, Sharif K, Ramani P, *et al.* Strategy for hepatoblastoma management: transplant versus nontransplant surgery. *J Pediatr Surg* 2002:**37**:240–5.

139 Otte JB, Pritchard J, Aronson DC, *et al.* Liver transplantation for hepatoblastoma: results from the International Society of Pediatric Oncology (SIOP) Study SIOPEL-1 and review of the World experience. *Pediatr Blood Cancer* 2004;**42**:74–83.

140 Otte JB, de Ville de Goyet J. The contribution of transplantation to the treatment of liver tumors in children. *Semin Pediatr Surg* 2005;**14**:233–8.

141 Mazzaferro V, Regalia E, Doci R. Liver transplantation for the treatment of small hepatocellular carcinomas in patients with cirrhosis. *N Engl J Med* 1996;**334**:693–9.

142 Schnater JM, Aronson DC, Plaschkes J, *et al.* Surgical view of the treatment of patients with hepatoblastoma: results from the first prospective trial of the International Society of Pediatric Oncology Liver Tumor Study Group (SIOPEL-1). *Cancer* 2002;**94**:1111–20.

143 von Schweinitz D, Gluer S, Mildenberger H. Liver tumours in neonates and very young infants: diagnostic pitfalls and therapeutic problems. *Eur J Pediatr Surg* 1995;**5**:72–6.

144 Finegold MJ. Chemotherapy for suspected hepatoblastoma without efforts at surgical resection is bad practice. *Med Pediatr Oncol* 2002;**39**:484–6.

145 Al-Qabandi W, Jenkinson HC, Buckels JA, *et al.* Orthotopic liver transplantation for unresectable hepatoblastoma: a single center's experience. *J Pediatr Surg* 1999;**34**:1261–4.

146 Achilleos OA, Buist LJ, Kelly DA, *et al.* Unresectable hepatic tumors in childhood and the role of liver transplantation. *J Pediatr Surg* 1996;**31**:1563–7.

147 Molmenti EP, Wilkinson K, Molmenti H, *et al.* Treatment of unresectable hepatoblastoma with liver transplantation in the pediatric population. *Am J Transplant* 2002;**2**:535–8.

148 Srinivasan P, McCall J, Pritchard J, *et al.* Orthotopic liver transplantation for unresectable hepatoblastoma. *Transplantation* 2002;**74**:652–5.

149 Otte JB, Aronson D, Vraux H, *et al.* Preoperative chemotherapy, major liver resection and transplantation for primary malignancies in children. *Transplant Proc* 1996;**28**:2392–4.

150 Chardot C, Saint Martin C, Gilles A, *et al.* Living-related liver transplantation and vena cava reconstruction after total hepatectomy including the vena cava for hepatoblastoma. *Transplantation* 2002;**73**:90–2.

151 Arora N, McKiernan PJ, Beath SV, de Ville de Goyet J, Kelly DA. Concomitant basiliximab with low-dose calcineurin inhibitors in children post-liver transplantation. *Pediatr Transplant* 2002;**6**:214–8.

152 Shah SA, Cleary SP, Tan JC, *et al.* An analysis of resection vs transplantation for early hepatocellular carcinoma: defining the optimal therapy at a single institution. *Ann Surg Oncol* 2007;**14**: 2608–14.

153 Habrand JL, Nehme D, Kalifa C, *et al.* Is there a place for radiation therapy in the management of hepatoblastoma and hepatocellular carcinomas in children? *Int J Rad Oncol Biol Phys* 1992;**23**:525–31.

154 Llovet JM, Real MI, Montana X, *et al.* Arterial embolisation or chemoembolisation versus symptomatic treatment in patients with unresectable hepatocellular carcinoma: a randomised controlled trial. *Lancet* 2002;**359**:1734–9.

155 Lo CM, Ngan H, Tso WK, *et al.* Randomized controlled trial of transarterial lipiodol chemoembolization for unresectable hepatocellular carcinoma. *Hepatology* 2002;**35**:1164–71.

156 Oue T, Fukuzawa M, Kusafuka T, Kohmoto Y, Okada A, Imura K. Transcatheter arterial chemoembolization in the treatment of hepatoblastoma. *J Pediatr Surg* 1998;**33**:1771–5.

157 Nakagawa N, Cornelius AS, Kao SC, Nakajima Y, Nakada K. Transcatheter oily chemoembolization for unresectable malignant liver tumors in children. *J Vasc Interv Radiol* 1993;**4**:353–8.

158 Han YM, Park HH, Lee JM, *et al.* Effectiveness of preoperative transarterial chemoembolization in presumed inoperable hepatoblastoma. *J Vasc Interv Radiol* 1999;**10**:1275–80.

159 Arcement CM, Towbin RB, Meza MP, *et al.* Intrahepatic chemoembolization in unresectable paediatric liver malignancies. *Pediatr Radiol* 2000;**30**:779–85.

160 Czauderna P, Zbrzezniak G, Stoba C, *et al.* Preliminary experience with hepatic arterial chemoembolization (HACE) in paediatric liver neoplasms [abstract]. *Med Pediatr Oncol* 2001;**37**:239.

161 Malogolowkin MH, Stanley P, Steele DA, Ortega JA. Feasibility and toxicity of chemoembolization for children with liver tumors. *J Clin Oncol* 2000;**18**:1279–84.

162 Skopec LL, Lakatua DJ. Non-immune fetal hydrops with hepatic hemangioendothelioma and Kasabach–Merritt syndrome. A case report. *Pediatr Pathol* 1989;**9**:87–93.

163 Davenport M, Hansen L, Heaton ND, Howard ER. Hemangioendothelioma of the liver in infants. *J Pediatr Surg* 1995;**30**:44–8.

164 Cornelius AS, Womer RB, Jakacki R. Multiple hemangioendotheliomas of the liver. *Med Pediatr Oncol* 1989;**17**:501–4.

165 Boon LM, Burrows PE, Paltiel HJ, *et al.* Hepatic vascular anomalies in infancy: a twenty-seven-year experience. *J Pediatr* 1996; **129**:346–54.

166 Uchimura K, Nakamuta M, Osoegawa M, *et al.* Hepatic epithelioid hemangioendothelioma. *J Clin Gastroenterol* 2001;**32**:431–4.

167 Läuffer JM, Zimmermann A, Krähenbühl L, Triller J, Baer HU. Epithelioid hemangioendothelioma of the liver. A rare hepatic tumor. *Cancer* 1996;**78**:2318–27.

168 Calder CJ, Raafat F, Buckels JAC, Kelly DA. Orthotopic liver transplantation for type 2 hepatic infantile haemoangioendothelioma. *Histopathology* 1996;**28**:271–3.

169 Lack EE. Mesenchymal hamartoma of the liver. *Am J Pediatr Hematol Oncol* 1986;**8**:91–8.

11 Transplantation

21 Liver Transplantation

Deirdre A. Kelly and David Mayer

The successful development of pediatric liver transplantation has dramatically changed the prognosis for many babies and children dying of end-stage liver failure and is now the accepted therapy for this condition.

The most important elements in improving survival after liver transplantation have been:

- Better preoperative management of hepatic complications and nutritional support
- Innovative surgical techniques to expand the donor pool
- Improvements in postoperative immunosuppression

The consequent improvement in the survival rate has extended the range of indications for liver transplantation in children to include semielective liver replacement and transplantation for metabolic liver disease and unresectable hepatic tumors. Increasing experience has also refined the precise indications for liver transplantation. As the short-term survival has improved, interest has focused on quality of life and long-term survival.

Indications for liver transplantation

Liver transplantation is the standard therapy for acute or chronic liver failure (Table 21.1; Figure 21.1).

Chronic liver disease

Neonatal liver disease

Biliary atresia remains the commonest indication for liver transplantation in children, accounting for 74% of children undergoing transplantation below the age of 2 years.[1,2] Despite the professional emphasis on early diagnosis and management of this condition, in practice many children are still referred too late to benefit from a palliative Kasai portoenterostomy (Chapters 4 and 19). Urgent transplantation is required for those children who have an unsuccessful Kasai portoenterostomy or who develop nutritional or hepatic complications.[3]

Diseases of the Liver and Biliary System in Children, 3rd edition. Edited by Deirdre Kelly. © 2008 Blackwell Publishing, ISBN: 978-1-4051-6334-7.

Table 21.1 Indications for liver transplantation.

Chronic liver failure
Neonatal liver disease
Biliary atresia
Idiopathic neonatal hepatitis
Cholestatic liver disease
Alagille's syndrome
Familial intrahepatic cholestasis (FIC)
Nonsyndromic biliary hypoplasia
Inherited metabolic liver disease
α_1-Antitrypsin deficiency
Cystic fibrosis
Glycogen storage disease type IV
Tyrosinemia type I
Wilson's disease
Chronic hepatitis
Autoimmune
Idiopathic
Postviral (hepatitis B, C, other)
Immunodeficiency
Other
Cryptogenic cirrhosis
Fibropolycystic liver disease ± Caroli syndrome
Acute liver failure
Fulminant hepatitis
Autoimmune
Halothane exposure
Acetaminophen poisoning
Viral hepatitis (A, B, C, E, or non-A–G)
Metabolic liver disease
Fatty acid oxidation defects
Neonatal hemochromatosis
Tyrosinemia type I
Wilson's disease
Inborn errors of metabolism
Crigler–Najjar type I
Familial hypercholesterolemia
Primary oxalosis
Organic acidemia
Urea cycle defects
Liver tumors
Benign tumors
Unresectable malignant tumors

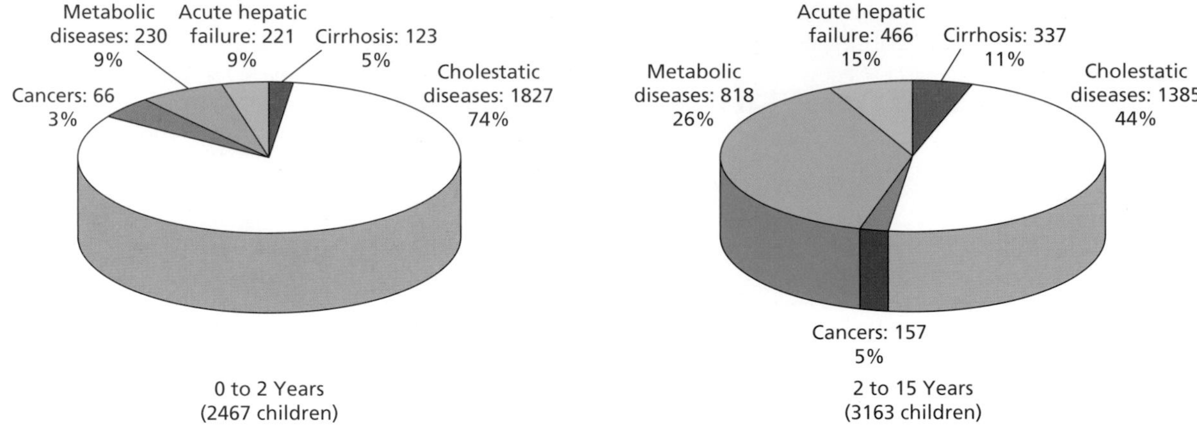

Figure 21.1 Primary indications for liver transplantation in pediatric patients, 1988–2005. (European Liver Transplant Registry.)

Cholestatic liver disease

The outcome of cholestatic liver disease in infancy, such as Alagille's syndrome, nonsyndromic biliary hypoplasia, familial intrahepatic cholestasis, is variable. Liver transplantation is indicated for the development of cirrhosis and portal hypertension, development of malnutrition or growth failure unresponsive to nutritional support, or intractable pruritus that is resistant to maximum medical therapy or biliary diversion.[4]

Inherited metabolic liver disease

α_1-Antitrypsin deficiency is the commonest form of inherited metabolic liver disease presenting in childhood in Europe. Although 50–70% of children may develop persistent liver disease progressing to cirrhosis, only 20–30% require transplantation in childhood.[5,6] The management of tyrosinemia type I has changed dramatically since the introduction of nitisinone (NTBC), which prevents the formation of toxic metabolites and produces rapid clinical improvement. Use of this drug has altered the natural history of the disease and the indications for transplantation.[7–9] Before the introduction of NTBC, liver transplantation was indicated for acute or chronic liver failure, or the development of hepatic dysplasia or hepatocellular carcinoma (HCC). Liver transplantation is now only indicated for those children who have a poor quality of life, do not respond to NTBC, or in whom hepatic malignancy is thought to have developed.[10] Routine monitoring of children with tyrosinemia type I being treated with NTBC includes ultrasound, computed tomography (CT), or magnetic resonance imaging (MRI) to detect the development of nodules and/or early HCC in association with regular α-fetoprotein levels. A persistent or sustained rise in α-fetoprotein may indicate the early development of HCC, which should be confirmed by the detection of hepatic dysplasia on liver biopsy.[11–13]

Wilson's disease is a rare indication for liver transplantation in childhood (Chapter 14), but is indicated for those children who present with advanced liver disease (Wilson's score > 6), fulminant liver failure, or who have progressive hepatic disease despite penicillamine therapy.[14,15]

As the long-term survival improves in children with cystic fibrosis (CF), liver transplantation has become a viable alternative and this is now the commonest indication in adolescents in some centers. Hepatic decompensation is a late feature of CF liver disease, but portal hypertension is common and bleeding from esophageal varices may be a serious recurrent problem. Selection for liver transplantation is indicated only for those children with hepatic decompensation (falling serum albumin, prolonged coagulation unresponsive to vitamin K), severe malnutrition, or complications of portal hypertension unresponsive to medical management—ascites or uncontrolled variceal bleeding.[16,17] Careful assessment of pulmonary function is required, as severe lung disease (< 50% of lung function) may indicate the necessity for a heart, lung, and liver transplant.[18] Thus, early liver transplantation is indicated for children with moderate lung disease prior to the development of significant irreversible lung disease.[19] Preoperative management of respiratory disease is important and should include vigorous physiotherapy, intravenous antibiotics, and DNase. Postoperative antibiotics should be based on known bacterial colonization and antibiotic sensitivity.

The majority of children with glycogen storage disease type I should respond to appropriate medical and nutritional management. Transplantation is indicated only for those children who develop multiple hepatic adenomata or in whom metabolic control has a significant effect on quality of life. Glycogen storage disease types III and IV may progress to cirrhosis, and this may be an indication for transplantation because of hepatic dysfunction.[20,21]

Chronic hepatitis

Autoimmune liver disease types I and II. The majority of children with autoimmune liver disease types I or II respond to immunosuppression with prednisolone or azathioprine (Chapter 8). Liver transplantation is indicated for children who have advanced portal hypertension or do not respond to immunosuppression despite the use of second-line drugs such as cyclosporine, tacrolimus, and mycophenolate mofetil, or those who present with fulminant hepatic failure.[22] Children with autoimmune hepatitis type II are more likely to present in fulminant hepatic failure and have an increased requirement for liver transplantation (Chapter 8).

Most children with chronic hepatitis B or C will be asymptomatic carriers in whom the development of cirrhosis, portal hypertension, and/or HCC may evolve over 20–30 years. Although the main indication for transplantation is the development of chronic liver failure, recurrence with hepatitis B or C post-transplantation is likely in 90% of patients without prophylactic therapy, such as lamivudine, adefovir, hepatitis B immunoglobulin, or post transplant antiviral therapy.[23]

Fibropolycystic liver disease

Fibropolycystic liver disease is a rare indication for liver transplantation in childhood, as liver function usually remains normal for many years in these children, even if they develop severe portal hypertension. Liver replacement is only indicated if hepatic decompensation occurs in association with portal hypertension or hepatic enlargement interferes with quality of life. The disease may be associated with infantile polycystic kidney disease, and both liver and kidney replacement will be required, usually at the time of renal replacement (Chapter 10).

Primary immunodeficiency

As bone-marrow transplantation for primary immunodeficiency has become successful, it is clear that many children with these diseases have associated liver disease. The most common immunodeficiency is CD40 ligand deficiency (hyper-IgM syndrome), in which recurrent cryptosporidial infection of the gut and biliary tree lead to sclerosing cholangitis. In this group of children, it is important to carry out bone-marrow transplantation before the development of significant liver disease or to consider combined liver and bone marrow transplantation, if necessary.[24] More recent developments have identified a range of rare diseases, such as interleukin-12 deficiency, which may be associated with chronic liver disease, although the efficacy of liver transplantation has not been established.

Timing of transplantation for children with chronic liver failure

As many children with cirrhosis and portal hypertension have well-compensated liver function, the timing of liver transplantation may be difficult to predict. Biochemical decompensation can be predicted by studying the lidocaine metabolite monoethylglycinexylidide (MEGX),[25] as serial estimates of MEGX formation and excretion over time may be useful predictors in individual patients. In practice, the need for liver transplantation is indicated by a persistent rise in total bilirubin > 150 μmol/L, prolongation of prothrombin ratio (INR > 1.4), and a fall in serum albumin < 35 g/L.[26] These parameters have been used to develop the Pediatric End-Stage Liver Disease (PELD) score to predict death, and their accuracy has been confirmed in predicting the need for liver transplantation—although in 53% of cases the calculated score was not used to determine allocation, as many centers bypass the system.[27,28]

As protein-energy malnutrition is a known complication of chronic liver disease in the developing child, serial evaluation of nutritional parameters may be an alternative guide to early hepatic decompensation. A progressive reduction of fat stores (triceps skinfold) or protein stores (mid-arm muscle area) despite nutritional support usually predicts hepatic decompensation.[29]

Children with complex hepatic complications, such as chronic hepatic encephalopathy, refractory ascites, intractable pruritus, or recurrent variceal bleeding despite optimum management, require prompt referral for transplantation. Variceal hemorrhage that is not controlled by variceal banding or endoscopic sclerotherapy may be temporarily managed by the insertion of a transjugular intrahepatic portosystemic shunt (Chapters 2, 15, and 19). This technique reduces portal vein pressure and prevents variceal hemorrhage, allowing sufficient time for preoperative nutritional support and the search for an appropriate donor.

A particularly important aspect in the timing of liver transplantation is consideration of psychosocial development. Children with chronic liver disease have a significant reduction of developmental motor skills, which may be reversed following liver transplantation if it is performed early enough.[3,30] Thus, any significant delay in developmental parameters is an indication for referral for liver transplantation.

It is essential that children with chronic liver disease should be referred for transplantation before the complications of their liver disease adversely impair the quality of their lives and before growth and development are retarded.

Acute liver failure

The indications for liver transplantation for acute liver failure vary depending on whether the disease process is due to fulminant hepatitis or secondary to an inborn error of metabolism (Chapters 5, 7, and 13). In general, children with acute liver failure should be referred early to a specialist unit with facilities for transplantation in order to provide time for stabilization and to find an appropriate donor organ.

Fulminant hepatitis

There are four main aims in the management of children with fulminant hepatitis who require transplantation:

- To assess the prognosis for recovery or liver transplantation
- To prevent or treat hepatic complications while awaiting a donor organ/regeneration of native liver
- To provide hepatic support
- To provide psychosocial support and information for parents

The current information on the prognosis for children with fulminant hepatitis is based on previous experience in the pretransplantation era, information from adult studies, and more recently information from pediatric studies.[31,32]

Poor prognostic factors for children with fulminant hepatitis requiring listing for liver transplantation are as follows:

- Non-A–G hepatitis
- Rapid onset of coma, with progression to grade III or IV hepatic coma
- Diminishing liver size
- Falling transaminases
- Increasing bilirubin (> 300 μmol/L)
- Persistent coagulopathy (prothrombin time > 40 s, INR > 4)

Unlike adults, children with fulminant hepatitis may have severe coagulopathy but mild encephalopathy, and therefore both are not required prior to listing for liver transplantation.[33] This has now been accepted by the Liver Advisory Group in the United Kingdom, who have agreed different criteria for listing infants with acute liver failure.[34]

All children with grade III hepatic coma, or those who have persistent coagulopathy (prothrombin time > 40, INR > 4) and have no evidence of irreversible brain damage from cerebral edema or hypoglycemia, should be listed for transplantation. As current medical management for cerebral edema is unsatisfactory and methods of determining irreversible brain damage are unreliable, this may be a difficult decision. Cerebral CT scans may detect gross cerebral edema, hemorrhage, or infarction; they may alter selection for transplantation, but are not usually helpful in the early stages. Monitoring of cerebral edema by measuring intracranial pressure has improved the selection of recipients, but not the overall survival. Assessment of cerebral blood flow is not helpful, as this may be reduced in hepatic failure, but assessment of cerebral perfusion pressure may be more sensitive (Chapter 7).

Electroencephalography (EEG) may demonstrate a reduction in electrical activity and ultimately brain death, although these results must be interpreted cautiously in ventilated patients or those treated with thiopentone, as the EEG tracing is affected by sedation and anesthetic drugs.

Acetaminophen poisoning

Selection of patients with acetaminophen poisoning may be particularly difficult. Children and adolescents have a lower incidence of liver failure with acetaminophen overdose than adults, possibly because of the effect of hepatic maturation and glutathione production.[35] Transplantation is more likely if the overdose was taken with another drug (e.g., LSD, Ecstasy), or with alcohol.[36]

Children should be considered for liver transplantation if there is a persistent coagulopathy (INR > 4), metabolic acidosis (pH < 7.3), elevated creatinine (> 300 mmol/L), or rapid progression to hepatic coma grade III. In some children, cerebral edema may persist despite evidence of hepatic regeneration and recovery and it may influence their postoperative recovery.

Metabolic liver disease

Acute liver failure may be the presenting feature of inherited metabolic liver disease, such as Wilson's disease and tyrosinemia type I (Chapters 5, 13, and 14). The clinical presentation is more likely to be subacute, and liver failure occurs in the presence of underlying cirrhosis. Selection for liver transplantation is on the basis of nonresponse to medication or severe coagulopathy, as jaundice and encephalopathy may not be obvious.[14] Diminishing liver size does not occur, because of the underlying cirrhosis.

Infants with neonatal hemochromatosis who present within days or weeks of birth with severe coagulopathy and encephalopathy may be candidates for liver transplantation if medical management using the "antioxidant cocktail" has failed (Chapters 5, 7).[37]

Inborn errors of metabolism

Certain inborn errors of metabolism are secondary to hepatic enzyme deficiencies (Chapters 5 and 13). Liver transplantation is indicated for these conditions if the hepatic enzyme deficiency leads to:

- Irreversible liver disease/liver failure and/or hepatoma
- Severe extrahepatic disease

Diseases in which the inborn error of metabolism leads to liver failure (tyrosinemia type I, Wilson's disease, or α_1-antitrypsin deficiency; see above) are managed as acute or chronic liver failure.

Severe extrahepatic disease

In these diseases (Table 21.1), the liver functions normally, but the missing hepatic enzyme leads to severe extrahepatic disease—such as kernicterus in Crigler–Najjar type I, coronary artery disease in familial hypercholesterolemia, and systemic oxalosis in primary oxaluria.

Selection for transplantation is difficult. It is important to evaluate the quality of life of the child on medical management and to consider the potential mortality and morbidity of the primary disease in comparison with the risks, complications, and outcome following liver transplantation.

The timing of transplantation in these disorders depends on:

- The rate of progression of the disease
- The quality of life of the affected child
- The development of severe irreversible extrahepatic disease.

Crigler–Najjar type I

The timing of transplantation for this inherited disorder of unconjugated hyperbilirubinemia depends on:

- The quality of the child's life—i.e., how many hours of phototherapy per day are required to control the unconjugated bilirubin levels
- The potential development of irreversible structural brain damage secondary to kernicterus

In general, it is appropriate to transplant these children between the ages of 3 and 5 years in order to reduce disruption to their education. The most appropriate transplant operation for these children is now auxiliary liver transplantation (see below)[38] or hepatocyte transplantation.[39]

Organic acidemia

Children with propionic acidemia or methylmalonic acidemia are at lifelong risk of recurrent metabolic acidosis and long-term brain damage. Liver replacement is considered palliative treatment for these conditions, as the enzyme deficiency affects all body tissue. It should be considered early for children who have a particularly severe phenotype or family history (Chapters 5 and 13). Very careful preoperative management, including preoperative dialysis and perioperative hemofiltration to control acidosis, is essential to ensure good operative control. Until recently, orthotopic liver replacement has been considered necessary to provide adequate enzyme supplementation. It is possible that auxiliary liver transplantation may be sufficient for mildly affected patients.[38]

Familial hypercholesterolemia

Children who are homozygous are prone to premature development of coronary artery disease and thus should be transplanted before coronary artery disease is irreversible. In view of recent progress with gene therapy for this condition, auxiliary liver transplantation or gene therapy may be more appropriate treatment strategies.[40]

Primary oxalosis

Ideally, liver replacement in this condition should be prior to the development of severe irreversible renal failure. As this is often not possible, liver and kidney replacement may be required simultaneously.[41] As deficiency of the enzyme alanine-glyoxylate aminotransferase results in an overproduction of oxalate, these children are not suitable for auxiliary liver transplantation.

Liver tumors

Potential indications for liver tumors include unresectable benign tumors causing hepatic dysfunction, and unresectable malignant tumors (hepatoblastoma or HCC) that are refractory to chemotherapy without evidence of extrahepatic metastases (Chapter 20).

The preoperative evaluation should include a meticulous search for extrahepatic metastases, with CT scanning of chest and abdomen and regular monitoring of serum α-fetoprotein to detect relapse or recurrence outside the liver; and careful assessment of cardiac function, because of the cardiotoxic effects of drugs such as daunorubicin. The timing of transplantation is crucial and it is best planned electively during the course of chemotherapy or at completion.[42] Bone-marrow suppression at the time of transplantation is supported with administration of granulocyte-stimulating factors.

Children with rhabdomyosarcomas are usually unsuitable for transplantation because of the extent of the tumor and the presence of extrahepatic metastases (Chapter 20).

Pretransplant evaluation (Table 21.2)

Evaluation of the patient before transplantation should:

- Assess the severity of the liver disease and the presence or absence of hepatic complications
- Establish the urgency of transplantation
- Assess whether the operation is technically feasible
- Consider any significant contraindications to successful transplantation
- Establish whether the transplant operation is appropriate for the child and family
- Prepare the child and family psychologically

Pretransplant assessment of severity of liver disease

The indications for transplantation should be critically evaluated, the diagnosis should be reviewed, the prognosis should be considered, and alternative medical or surgical therapy should be evaluated. It is essential to evaluate whether liver transplantation will improve the quality of life for both child and family.

Hepatic function

The histological diagnosis should be reviewed and if necessary liver histology should be obtained. The decision to list for transplantation is usually based on serial deterioration in hepatic function, as indicated by:

- Albumin (< 35 g/L)
- Coagulation time (INR > 1.4)
- Rising bilirubin (> 150 μmol/L)

The extent of portal hypertension can be estimated by establishing the size of the portal vein on ultrasound and by visualizing esophageal and gastric varices by gastrointestinal endoscopy, which also establishes the presence of gastritis and/or peptic ulceration.

Renal function

The main abnormalities of renal function in children with either acute or chronic liver failure include renal tubular acidosis, glomerulonephritis, acute tubular necrosis, and hepatorenal syndrome. Careful assessment of renal function is necessary in order to modify the potentially nephrotoxic effects of post-transplantation immunosuppression and to assess the necessity of perioperative renal support. Children

Table 21.2 Pretransplantation assessment.

Nutritional status
Height, weight, triceps skinfold, mid-arm muscle area
Identification of hepatic complications
Ascites, hepatosplenomegaly, varices on endoscopy
Cardiac assessment
ECG, echo, chest radiography (cardiac catheterization, if required)
Respiratory function
Oxygen saturation*, ventilation–perfusion scan*, lung function tests†
Neurological and developmental assessment
EEG, Bayley developmental scales, Stanford–Binet intelligence scales
Renal function
Urea, creatinine, electrolytes
Urinary protein/creatinine ratio
Chromium EDTA (if available)
Dental assessment
Imaging
Ultrasound of liver and spleen for vascular anatomy
Wrist radiography for bone age and rickets
MRI/angiography‡
Serology
Cytomegalovirus
Epstein–Barr virus
Varicella zoster
Herpes simplex
Hepatitis A, B, C
HIV
Measles
Hematology
Full blood count, platelets, blood group

* If cyanosed.
† In cystic fibrosis.
‡ If portal vein anatomy equivocal.
ECG, electrocardiography; EDTA, ethylenediaminetetraacetic acid; EEG, electroencephalography; HIV, human immunodeficiency virus; MRI, magnetic resonance imaging.

with pretransplantation exposure to nephrotoxic drugs (e.g., with cystic fibrosis and hepatoblastoma) are particularly at risk.

Hematology

Full blood count, platelets, coagulation indices, and blood group are obtained. Human leukocyte antigen (HLA) matching is not required.

Serology

It is important to establish immunity to previous infection (Table 21.2). As donor grafts are matched for cytomegalovirus (CMV) status if possible, assessment of previous infection with CMV is important. Children who are negative for Epstein–Barr virus (EBV) are more likely to develop a primary infection after transplantation and have a higher risk of developing post-transplantation lymphoproliferative disease. In some parts of the world (Chapter 23), many donors and recipients will be hepatitis B–positive, and this needs to be taken into consideration. Human immunodeficiency virus (HIV) infection is no longer a contraindication for transplantation.

Imaging

The most important technical information required is the vascular anatomy and patency of the hepatic vessels. Most of the necessary information is obtained by color flow Doppler ultrasound examination of the liver and spleen. MRI or conventional angiography may be required for visualizing abnormal anatomy, such as the hypovascular syndrome, or to determine the extent of portal vein thrombosis.

Evidence of retrograde flow and/or a small portal vein (< 4 mm at the porta hepatis) suggests severe portal hypertension and increases the urgency of liver transplantation.

Children with congenital liver disease, such as biliary atresia, may have an increased incidence of abnormal vasculature. The hypovascular syndrome consists of an absent inferior vena cava, preduodenal or absent portal vein, azygous drainage from the liver, and polysplenia syndrome. It may be associated with situs inversus, dextrocardia, or left atrial isomerism.[43] Angiography is advised to determine the position and size of these abnormal vessels.

Liver transplantation causes important hemodynamic changes during the operative and anhepatic phases. It is essential therefore to have baseline information on cardiac and respiratory function. Most of the information required will be obvious from electrocardiography (ECG), echocardiography, or oxygen saturation.

Cardiac assessment

Particular attention should be paid to children who have congenital cardiac disease—for example, atrial and ventricular septal defects, which are associated with biliary atresia. Peripheral pulmonary stenosis is a known feature of Alagille's syndrome. Cardiomyopathy may develop secondary to tyrosinemia type I and the organic acidemias, or as a result of chemotherapy of malignant tumors. Cardiac catheterization may be necessary to determine whether: (i) cardiac function is adequate to withstand the hemodynamic changes during the operation; (ii) corrective surgery is required preoperatively; or (iii) the cardiac defect is inoperable and liver transplantation is contraindicated.

Respiratory assessment

A minority of children with end-stage liver disease develop intrapulmonary shunts (hepatopulmonary syndrome). This potentially reversible complication of liver disease requires early consideration for liver transplantation. The clinical signs of cyanosis and digital clubbing and reduced oxygen saturation indicate a need for pulmonary function studies, ventilation–perfusion scans, bubble echocardiography, and/or cardiac catheterization.[44,45]

Neurodevelopmental assessment

The aim of liver transplantation is to improve the quality of life after transplantation. Thus, it is necessary to identify any existing neurological or psychological defects that may not be reversible after transplantation. Psychological and developmental assessment of children with clinical liver disease can be carried out using standard tests such as the Griffiths developmental scale (for children under the age of 5 years), Bayley developmental scales, or Stanford–Binet intelligence scales (children of all ages).[46]

Dental assessment

Chronic liver disease has an adverse effect on the growth and development of young children, including their dentition. Clinical problems before transplantation include hypoplasia with staining of the teeth and gingival hyperplasia related to poor hygiene. As gingival hyperplasia may be a significant problem after transplantation, secondary to cyclosporine immunosuppression, it is important to establish good methods of dental hygiene before transplantation[47] (Chapter 18).

Contraindications for transplantation

As surgical skills have improved, there are now fewer contraindications to liver transplantation resulting from technical restrictions. Portal vein thrombosis, age, and size are no longer contraindications for transplantation.[3] However, experience has shown that certain medical conditions are not curable by transplantation. The contraindications for liver transplantation include:

- The presence of severe systemic sepsis, particularly fungal sepsis, at the time of surgery
- Malignant hepatic tumors with extrahepatic spread, because of rapid recurrence
- Severe extrahepatic disease that is not reversible following liver transplantation—e.g., severe cardiopulmonary disease for which corrective surgery is not possible, or severe structural brain damage
- Severe systemic oxalosis with cardiac involvement, as these children develop significant hypotension and do not withstand the hemodynamic disturbances after transplantation
- Mitochondrial cytopathies with multisystem involvement[48]
- Alpers disease and valproate toxicity, because of the progression of neurodegeneration
- Giant-cell hepatitis with autoimmune hemolytic syndrome, because of disease recurrence

Initially, HIV positivity was a contraindication to transplantation, but with current effective treatment regimens, HIV-positive children can now be considered if necessary.[49] Although hepatitis B and C recur after transplantation, postoperative therapy is possible and thus transplantation is acceptable.[23,50]

Children with a higher risk at surgery include those with:

- Previous surgery, because of technical difficulties with adhesions and potential small-bowel perforation
- Portal vein thrombosis, as vein grafts may be required

Preparation for transplantation

Immunization

Live vaccines are usually contraindicated in the immunosuppressed child at least for 12 months after transplantation, and so it is important to ensure that routine immunizations are complete—for example, diphtheria, pertussis, tetanus, and polio; Prevnar or Pneumovax for protection from streptococcal pneumonia; and Hib for protection against *Haemophilus influenzae*. In children older than 6 months, measles, mumps, rubella and varicella vaccination should be offered. Ideally, hepatitis A and B vaccination should be prescribed before transplantation. Recent studies suggest that some live vaccines can be safely given after transplantation.[51]

Management of hepatic complications

The treatment of specific hepatic complications is an important part of preoperative management. Variceal bleeding should be managed as described elsewhere (see Chapters 15 and 19) with esophageal banding or sclerotherapy, vasopressin, or octreotide infusion.

Esophageal banding is preferred to injection sclerotherapy for children on the active liver transplant list, as the inevitable development of postsclerotherapy variceal ulcers may be adversely affected by post-transplantation immunosuppression.[52] In older children with uncontrolled variceal bleeding, the insertion of a transjugular intrahepatic portosystemic stent (TIPSS) shunt has proved an effective management strategy (Chapters 15 and 19).[53,54]

Sepsis—particularly ascending cholangitis and spontaneous bacterial peritonitis—requires effective treatment with appropriate broad-spectrum antibiotics. Cefuroxime (20 mg/kg/dose t.d.s.); amoxicillin (25 mg/kg/dose t.d.s.) and metronidazole (8 mg/kg/dose t.d.s.) are useful first-line drugs until bacterial cultures are positive. In children with acute liver failure, prophylactic antifungal therapy with either fluconazole or liposomal amphotericin is essential. Children should be suspended from the transplant list during episodes of significant sepsis.

Salt and water retention leading to ascites and cardiac failure should be effectively managed with diuretics and salt and water restriction. It is essential to consider intervention with hemodialysis and/or hemofiltration if acute renal failure or hepatorenal failure develop. Hemodialysis is rarely required in chronic liver failure unless there is acute decompensation, but hemodiafiltration may be necessary in acute liver failure to control cerebral edema and/or coagulopathy. Preoperative hemodialysis and perioperative hemofiltration are essential for children undergoing transplantation for organic acidemia. Recent trials in adults have evaluated a modified dialysis method using the Molecular Adsorbents Recirculating System (MARS), which may improve short-term survival in end-stage liver failure. Trials have not yet been conducted in children.[55]

Nutritional support

A number of important advances in the understanding of the pathophysiology of malnutrition in liver disease have led to improved nutritional strategies and improved outcomes after transplantation. The aim of nutritional therapy is to maintain or improve nutritional status and thus improve morbidity and mortality after transplantation. A high-calorie protein feed, 150–200% of the recommended energy intake (EAR), is required (Table 21.3). It may be difficult to provide this high-energy intake with standard feeds, particularly in fluid-restricted children, and a modular feed may therefore be appropriate for young babies. It is usually necessary to provide these feeds by nocturnal nasogastric enteral feeding or continuous feeding. If enteral feeding is not tolerated due to ascites, variceal bleeding, or recurrent hepatic complications, parenteral nutrition in normal amounts is required. Although there may be reluctance to use amino acid and lipid solutions in this situation, the calorific value of these essential nutrients overcomes the potential problems of encephalopathy and lipid catabolism.[29]

Psychological preparation

The most important aspect of the transplant assessment is the psychological counseling and preparation of the child and family. A skilled multidisciplinary team, including a play therapist and psychologist, is essential to the success of this preparation. Parents and appropriate relatives must be fully informed of the necessity for liver transplantation in their child and of the risks, complications, and long-term implications of the operation. Psychological preparation in children older than 2 years is essential and can be successfully achieved through innovative play therapy and toys and books suitable for children (Chapter 24).

Particularly careful counseling is necessary for parents of children who are being considered for liver transplantation because of an inborn error of metabolism. As their children are not dying from liver disease, these parents may find it more difficult to accept the risks and complications of the operation, the potential mortality, and the necessity for long-term immunosuppression. Parents of children who require transplantation for acute liver failure may be too distressed fully to appreciate the significance and implications of liver transplantation and will require ongoing counseling and education postoperatively. Children who survive the liver transplant operation for acute liver failure should have post-operative counseling and play therapy to help them come to terms with their transplant.

On the waiting list

Many families find the waiting time before transplantation very stressful, and continued support from the multidisciplinary team is required. Mortality on the waiting list used to be as high as 25% before the development of reduction hepatectomy, which has dramatically reduced deaths on the waiting list to 5%. Although there are continual problems with donor shortages, particularly for small children, the development of living related liver transplantation and the split-liver graft program has alleviated this problem.[56–58]

Liver transplant surgery

Liver transplantation involves three operations—the donor operation, the back table operation, and the recipient operation. The logistics of coordinating these operations together with transplantation of other organs from the same multi-organ donor are complex, and the surgeon relies heavily on the services of the transplant coordinators. Liver grafts can be

Table 21.3 Nutritional support in infants and children undergoing liver transplantation.*

Nutrient	Preoperative	Postoperative
Carbohydrate	Glucose polymer 15–20 g/kg/day	Glucose polymer 6–8 g/kg/day
Protein	Low-salt protein 3–4 g/kg/day	Whole protein 2.5–3.0 g/kg/day
Fat	50–70% MCT 8 g/kg/day	80–90% LCT 5–6 g/kg/day
Energy intake (EAR)	120–150%	120%

*Best provided as a modular feed in infants and as calorie supplements in older children.
EAR, estimated average requirement; LCT, long-chain triglyceride; MCT, medium-chain triglyceride.

retrieved from heart-beating cadavers, from non–heart-beating donors, or from live donors (see below).

The role of the transplant coordinator

Potential cadaveric organs are notified to the procurement coordinator, who is responsible for establishing their suitability for transplantation, coordinating the multidisciplinary procurement team, and making arrangements at the donor hospital. Other duties include promotion of organ donation, education of health service professionals, and donor family support. The recipient coordinator is responsible for organizing the recipient operation, including travel arrangements for the patient, organization of theaters, anesthesia, blood bank and intensive care, care of the recipient's family during the operation, and postoperative follow-up. The live donor coordinator is responsible for coordinating the live donation assessment process and transplant procedure.

Liver grafts from cadaveric donors

The recipient of a cadaveric graft is selected on the basis of a compatible blood group, size matching, medical urgency, and time on the waiting list. Occasionally, blood group O may be given to blood groups A or B, if medically necessary. When possible, grafts from CMV-positive donors are not given to CMV-negative recipients, but medical urgency may dictate otherwise. In contrast to kidney transplantation, there is no benefit from HLA matching, and hyperacute rejection is exceptionally rare in liver transplantation even in the presence of a positive cytotoxic cross-match.

Most cadaver livers are retrieved from heart-beating donors who satisfy the criteria for brainstem death. However, livers can also be used from donors who have died after a brief period of cardiac arrest (non–heart-beating donors, NHBD) usually after withdrawal of life support on an intensive-care unit. Good results can be obtained using these livers, provided that the donor was previously fit and did not suffer a prolonged period of hypoxia or hypotension, and that the organs were rapidly preserved with cold perfusate shortly after the diagnosis of cardiac death and transplanted expeditiously. These donor livers are, however, associated with a slightly increased risk of primary nonfunction and of developing intrahepatic biliary strictures.

Proper care of the donor is essential to maintain good-quality organs from heart-beating donors. Brainstem death results in loss of central regulatory mechanisms that control the cardiovascular, respiratory, and endocrine systems. Donor resuscitation is directed at optimizing tissue perfusion and oxygenation, maintaining normal blood glucose and body temperature, and controlling sepsis. With the increasing demands for cadaver organs, previous constraints on donor suitability have been relaxed. There is no absolute age limit, although younger donors are preferable for pediatric recipients. Malignancy (except brain tumors) and uncontrolled bacterial sepsis or viral infections such as HIV remain absolute contraindications. Abnormal liver function tests may be misleading, and thus the macroscopic appearance of the liver during organ retrieval is an important factor in selection. A hard fibrotic or frankly cirrhotic liver is clearly unusable, as is a grossly fatty liver. If there is any doubt, histological examination of a frozen section of the liver may be helpful.

The multiorgan donor operation

The liver is retrieved from a cadaver donor as part of an integrated multiorgan operation in which the kidneys, pancreas, heart, lungs, bowel, and other viscera may all be removed simultaneously for transplantation. The heart-beating donor is maintained on a ventilator in the operating theater until the moment of circulatory arrest. Paralyzing agents are given to prevent spinal reflexes, and broad-spectrum antibiotics are given to prevent infection. The organs are removed through a full-length midline incision. The iliac vessels and the superior or inferior mesenteric vein are identified and prepared for cannulation. The liver is inspected with particular care to identify anomalous arterial anatomy. The porta hepatis is dissected, dividing the common bile duct close to the duodenum, and the common hepatic artery is traced to its origin from the aorta. The cardiothoracic organs are then mobilized and heparin is administered to achieve full anticoagulation. At this stage, ventilation is discontinued, the abdominal organs are perfused with ice-cold preservation solution, and the abdomen is packed with ice slush to achieve rapid cooling. Once the cardiothoracic organs have been removed, the liver dissection is completed. The hepatic artery is taken in continuity with a patch of aorta at the origin of the celiac trunk. The portal vein is divided at its confluence with the superior mesenteric and splenic veins, the infrahepatic vena cava is divided just above the origins of the renal veins, and the suprahepatic vena cava is divided at its junction with the right atrium. After removal of the liver, the hepatic artery and portal vein are flushed again with preservation solution and the bile duct is rinsed free of bile. The liver, immersed in cold preservation solution, is hermetically sealed in plastic bags and transported in a freezer box packed with ice. Iliac, splenic, and superior mesenteric vessels are also removed, since they may be required for vascular conduits in the recipient, especially if the liver is split (see below).

The back table operation, liver reduction, and liver splitting

The back table operation is performed at the recipient hospital and is synchronized with the recipient operation. For a whole-liver graft, the back table operation is relatively straightforward; extraneous tissue is cleared from the graft and vascular pedicles are checked for tributaries that require ligation. However, the majority of pediatric liver transplants require a liver reduction operation to be performed in order to generate either a single reduced-size graft or a pair of split-liver grafts.

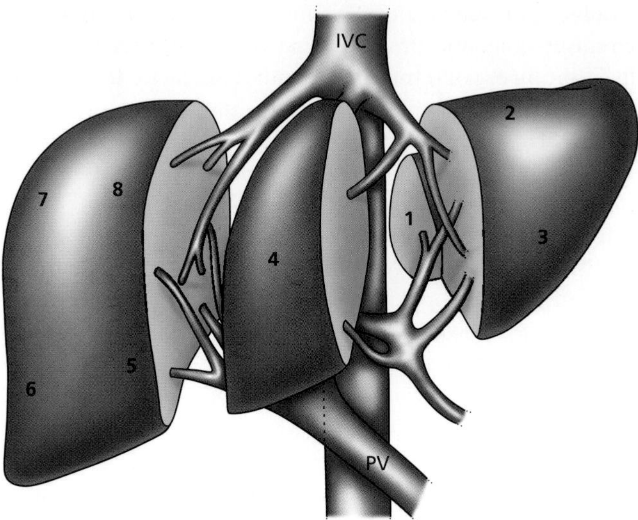

Figure 21.2 Schematic diagram of the liver, showing the eight segments. The left lateral segments, II and III, are most commonly used for reduction hepatectomy and split-liver, living related donor, or auxiliary liver transplantation.

The majority of children needing liver transplantation are aged less than 5 years. In contrast, there are very few small pediatric organ donors. The shortage of suitable size-matched donor livers stimulated the development of innovative techniques to produce small grafts suitable for children on the transplant waiting list.[59] The principles of liver reduction are based on the work of Couinaud, who described the segmental anatomy of the liver[60] on the basis of blood supply and biliary drainage. The liver is composed of eight segments, including the caudate lobe (segment I), three other segments (II–IV) of the anatomical left lobe, and four segments (V–VIII) of the right lobe[61] (Figure 21.2). Depending on the relative size of the donor and the recipient, a graft from a larger donor can usually be tailored to fit into a smaller pediatric recipient. A full right or left lobe graft may be needed for a larger child, whereas a left lateral segmental graft (segments II and III) or occasionally a monosegment[62] is most commonly required for small children and infants.

Liver reduction was first used by Bismuth in Paris and proposed as a potential solution to the severe shortage of small pediatric livers.[63] Although the initial results were poor, the introduction of University of Wisconsin liver preservation solution[64] and technical modifications improved graft survival to match, or even surpass, the results with whole livers in small children and infants.[59,65] In the United States, partial liver grafts now account for 32% of all pediatric grafts and 56% of transplants in recipients aged less than 1 year, with excellent results.[66] In particular, reduced grafts have a lower incidence of hepatic artery thrombosis in comparison with equivalent-sized whole-liver grafts in small children. The technique of liver reduction was modified to allow split-liver grafting, so that a single liver could be used for two recipients.[67]

For split-liver grafts, the liver can be divided along the principal plane to provide full left and right lobes. More commonly, it is divided along the plane of the falciform ligament to provide a left lateral segmental graft (segments II and III) for pediatric transplantation, and an extended right lobe graft (segments IV–VIII) for transplantation into a larger child or adult. We usually preserve the common bile duct, portal vein, and hepatic artery together with the inferior vena cava, with the right graft. The left lateral segmental graft is drained by the left hepatic vein; microvascular techniques are required for the arterial anastomosis to the donor left hepatic artery and a Roux loop of jejunum is required for biliary reconstruction.

Liver reduction/splitting is performed either in situ as part of the donor operation or ex situ on the back table. In-situ liver reduction or splitting has the advantage that the surgery is performed on a well-perfused, functioning liver without the risk of warm ischemia during back table surgery. It also allows meticulous hemostasis at the cut surface. However, in-situ division adds about 2 hours to the operating time at the donor hospital, with the attendant risk of donor instability and, perhaps, compromise to other donor organs. Because of concerns about primary graft dysfunction due to prolonged cold ischemia, ex-situ splitting is usually restricted to livers from stable young donors, whereas in-situ split grafts may have wider applications.[68,69]

The recipient operation

In the early days of liver transplantation, the operation was frequently complicated by extensive bleeding from raw surfaces, particularly in patients with adhesions from previous upper abdominal surgery. Patients with advanced liver disease have portal hypertension, thrombocytopenia, and deranged coagulation. During a long operation in a patient with poor liver function, hypothermia exacerbates the coagulopathy. A better understanding of coagulation disorders, improved monitoring, and more sophisticated hemostatic techniques have greatly reduced transfusion requirements.

Anesthetic monitoring includes serial measurements of blood gases, electrolytes, hemoglobin, and platelet count, together with coagulation indices, including thromboelastography. The thromboelastograph gives a pictorial representation of blood clotting, and its interpretation allows the anesthetist to determine whether there is a defect in clotting factors or platelets, or whether antifibrinolytic drugs such as aprotinin are indicated.

The recipient liver transplant operation is carried out through a bilateral subcostal incision, often with an upper midline extension. The operation can be divided into two phases: total hepatectomy, in which the old liver is dissected and removed; and liver graft implantation.

Total hepatectomy

In the virgin abdomen, hepatectomy is usually straightforward.

However, if there has been previous upper abdominal surgery with bleeding, bile leakage, or local sepsis, then the dissection may be much more difficult (this is commonly the case following a previous Kasai portoenterostomy for biliary atresia). The liver is mobilized by division of adhesions to surrounding structures. The porta hepatis is dissected, and the bile duct (or Kasai portoenterostomy), hepatic artery, and portal vein are divided. The liver is then removed by dividing the hepatic veins, which drain into the inferior vena cava. Alternatively, the old liver can be removed in continuity with the retrohepatic vena cava. The latter technique may be necessary in cases of liver cancer, such as hepatoblastoma, in order to ensure complete excision of the tumor.

Graft implantation

Once the liver graft has been removed from the cold preservation fluid, it starts to warm; the smaller the liver, the more rapid the warming. The vascular anastomoses are therefore carried out expeditiously in order to minimize warm ischemic injury. For a whole graft, the vena cava and portal vein are anastomosed to the equivalent recipient vessels, with care being taken not to constrict the anastomoses when tying the sutures. For a left lateral segment graft, a triangular incision is made on the anterior aspect of the recipient vena cava for anastomosis of the graft left hepatic vein. Following completion of the venous anastomoses, the liver is flushed with a warm rinsing solution to remove cold preservation fluid, and the venous clamps are removed. Following reperfusion of the liver from the portal vein, the arterial anastomosis is carried out. The site depends on the anatomy and relative calibers of the donor and recipient arteries. Most commonly, the donor celiac artery is anastomosed to the bifurcation of the recipient hepatic and gastroduodenal or splenic arteries.

In small children and those with aberrant vessels, we often employ vascular conduits. A hypoplastic portal vein (commonly associated with biliary atresia) can be replaced with a donor iliac vein. Similarly, a donor arterial graft may be needed to act as a conduit from the recipient aorta to the donor hepatic artery.

The final anastomosis is to the graft bile duct. In adults and larger children without previous biliary pathology, the donor and recipient common bile ducts are joined together. Children with biliary atresia and those weighing less than 40 kg require a choledochojejunostomy using a Roux-en-Y loop of recipient jejunum. Biliary complications are more common in small children,[70] partly due to the small caliber of the donor bile duct and partly due to the more tenuous blood supply to the bile duct of a reduced-size liver.

Once the anastomoses have been completed, the operative field is checked for hemostasis and coagulopathy corrected. Bleeding at this stage may originate from raw areas following the hepatectomy, from the surgical suture lines, or from the graft itself. During the first hour after reperfusion there is usually evidence that the liver is working, with spontaneous correction of acidosis and clotting factors, and production of bile. In a proportion of cases (up to 25% of small children), the liver graft may be too large to permit abdominal closure without compromising hepatic venous outflow and also ventilation. In such circumstances, we usually insert a temporary patch of prosthetic material or bio-artificial collagen into the abdominal wall before closing the skin. A large graft will rapidly shrink, and a prosthetic patch can usually be removed after a few days.[71]

Living-donor liver transplantation

The shortage of suitable donors for small children prompted Broelsch and colleagues[72] to adapt the techniques of split cadaveric liver transplantation to obtain partial liver grafts from living donors. There are several potential advantages of living related transplantation. Firstly, it improves the supply of liver grafts for small children who might otherwise die whilst waiting for a suitable cadaveric organ. Secondly, live donation allows optimal timing of the transplant as an elective procedure, and reduces the stress of waiting for a suitable organ. Thirdly, a high-quality graft is obtained from a healthy individual, with minimal preservation time.[73]

Against the benefits to the recipient, however, must be set the potential risks to the donor. Partial hepatectomy, even in a healthy individual, is associated with a small but appreciable degree of morbidity. There have been reports of several donor deaths; the risk of donor mortality is estimated at between 0.1% and 0.5%, depending on whether a smaller left graft or a larger right liver graft is taken.[74] The operation is also associated with significant morbidity, which also relates to the extent of the hepatectomy.[75] Donor complications include bile leaks and hemorrhage from the cut surface, wound pain, infection, and incisional hernia, and a surprisingly high incidence of gastritis and peptic ulceration. Potential donors require careful assessment to ensure that they can provide a graft of suitable size, quality, and blood group to the recipient without excessive risk to the donor. Donation must be altruistic, without coercion by other family members. All donors should have a formal psychological assessment and be counseled about the perioperative risks and possible long-term complications of the procedure. Preoperative investigations include liver function tests, serology, and imaging to assess the size of the intended segmental graft as well as details of its vascular and biliary anatomy. Imaging may indicate abnormal graft parenchyma, in particular fatty change; if there is any doubt, a liver biopsy may be necessary. Imaging is also essential to estimate the size of the potential graft; transplantation from a healthy donor requires a liver graft that weighs at least 0.8% of the recipient's body weight.

For a child, the liver graft from a live donor is usually a left lateral graft (segments II and III), although a full left or right lobe graft may be needed for larger children. Recipients receiving a relatively small graft may develop small-for-size syndrome, characterized by synthetic dysfunction, transaminitis, and prolonged cholestasis.[76] During the left lateral donor operation, the left branches of the hepatic artery, portal vein, and bile duct and the left hepatic vein are identified, and the liver parenchyma is divided along the line of the falciform ligament. The vascular and biliary structures are then divided and the graft is flushed with cold preservation fluid. Implantation is similar to that used for left lateral segmental cadaver grafts (see above). Microsurgical techniques are required for the arterial anastomosis, to reduce the risk of thrombosis. Following the introduction of this technique, excellent results were reported from Japan, where there is a severe shortage of cadaver donors.[77] In the United States, approximately one-third of pediatric liver transplants are now obtained from living donors, and the results compare favorably with those obtained using cadaver grafts.[78] In the United Kingdom, an active policy on split-liver transplantation (donor livers being offered preferentially to centers willing to split them) has largely obviated the need for live donor transplantation in children. Clearly, parents considering live donation must be fully informed of the risks of the procedure and the prospects of finding a cadaver graft before making a decision.

Auxiliary liver transplantation

Auxiliary liver transplantation involves transplantation of a donor liver graft without removal of the entire native liver. Its purpose is to retain the native liver in case of spontaneous recovery, or for future gene therapy. It is of value in metabolic liver diseases in which there is a functionally normal liver but transplantation is indicated for severe extrahepatic disease (e.g., Crigler–Najjar type I). In this situation, only a small amount of normal liver is needed to compensate for the metabolic defect, and it is usually sufficient to replace the left lateral segments (II and III) with an equivalent donor graft. Reports suggest that this is successful in reducing the levels of unconjugated bilirubin in Crigler–Najjar type I.[38] This operation is not indicated for metabolic liver disease such as primary oxalosis, in which the enzyme deficiency contributes to an excess of oxalate production, or in metabolic diseases such as Wilson's disease or tyrosinemia, in which there is a risk of malignancy in the retained liver.

Auxiliary liver transplantation may also be considered for patients with fulminant or subfulminant hepatic failure when there is potential for the original liver to recover.[79] This requires a large auxiliary graft, usually replacing a right or an extended right lobe. Survival rates may be less than with conventional transplantation.[80] It is contraindicated when the liver disease is irreversible (e.g., seronegative hepatitis), but may have a role in reversible toxic injuries such as acetaminophen poisoning. Once the native liver has recovered, immunosuppression is gradually withdrawn and the liver graft atrophies due to chronic rejection.

Postoperative management

Ventilation

Although it is possible to extubate some patients in the operating room, it is generally advisable to stabilize the patient in the intensive-care unit (ICU) to ensure that liver function is satisfactory, with good hepatic artery and portal vein flow on Doppler ultrasound, before discontinuing ventilation. Moreover, large upper abdominal incisions are painful in the early postoperative period, necessitating epidural analgesia, intravenous morphine (according to body weight), or alfentanil (0.5 mg/kg/min), which may depress respiration. Young infants with severe malnutrition due to chronic liver disease or patients in hepatic coma due to fulminant liver failure may spend a prolonged period in the ICU, but the majority of patients return to the ward within 24–48 h postoperatively.

Fluid management

The principles of fluid management are to maintain circulating volume by providing two-thirds of maintenance fluids with crystalloid, while half-replacing wound drain losses with 4.5% albumin as long as urine output is in excess of 1 mL/kg/h and central venous pressure is satisfactory (> 5–6 mmHg). Due to fluid losses, patients are often vasoconstricted and relatively hypovolemic on returning from theaters, especially if there has been preoperative ascites, hypothermia, and the use of intraoperative inotropes. Extra colloid fluid replacement with 4.5% albumin and inotropes, such as dopamine (2–5 mg/kg/min), may be necessary. Hemoglobin should be maintained between 8 and 10 g/L. Excessive blood transfusion is contraindicated, as a postoperative hemoglobin of < 10 g/L reduces the risk of hepatic artery thrombosis.[81] Venesection is recommended for any patient with hemoglobin > 11 g/L during the first 2 postoperative weeks (Table 21.4).

Immunosuppression

There have been many recent advances in immunosuppressive drugs, but current protocols consist of the calcineurin inhibitors (CNI) with or without anti–interleukin-2 receptor antibodies (IL-2 antibodies; basiliximab or daclizumab),[82,83] for induction and renal-sparing drugs (such as mycophenolate mofetil[84] or sirolimus)[85] for maintenance. There is also a move to introduce steroid-free immunosuppression both at induction and for maintenance. Protocols (Table 21.5) consist of:

- Cyclosporine microemulsion (Neoral), prednisolone, and azathioprine
- Tacrolimus with prednisolone
- Basiliximab or daclizumab with either of the above
- Basiliximab or daclizumab with tacrolimus and mycophenolate mofetil

Table 21.4 Postoperative management of liver transplantation.

Fluid management Maintain: CVP > 6 cmH_2O Urine output > 1 mL/kg/h with 4.5% or 20% albumin or 5–10% dextrose Hb < 11 g/L *Prophylactic antibiotics* 1 Cefuroxime 25 mg/kg/dose t.d.s. for 48 h 2 Amoxicillin 25 mg/kg/dose t.d.s. for 48 h 3 Metronidazole 8 mg/kg/dose t.d.s. over 1 h for 48 h (or rectally) 4 Nystatin: 50 000 units orally q.d.s. if < 10 kg 100 000 units orally q.d.s. if > 10 kg 5 Amphotericin 1 mL/day orally 6 If CMV-positive donor, acyclovir 500 mg/m^2/i.v. dose t.d.s. over 1 h 7 Co-trimoxazole < 5 years 240 mg/day p.o.; > 5 years 480 mg/day p.o., for 6 months	*Antiplatelet therapy* 1 Aspirin 3 mg/kg/day per rectum or via nasogastric tube (maximum 75 mg) 2 Dipyridamole: If < 10 kg, 25 mg t.d.s. orally for 3 months If > 10 kg, 50 mg t.d.s. orally Anticoagulation (if necessary) Heparin (60–120 units/kg/day) to maintain PT 20–30 s *Antacids* Ranitidine 3 mg/kg/dose t.d.s. If gastric pH < 5, omeprazole 10–20 mg i.v. b.i.d. *Antihypertensives* Acute: 1 Labetalol 1–3 mg/kg/h 2 Nifedipine 5–10 mg/dose sublingually as needed Chronic: 1 Nifedipine 5–10 mg t.i.d. 2 Atenolol 25–50 mg/day

CVP, central venous pressure; Hb, hemoglobin; CMV, cytomegalovirus; PT, prothrombin time.

Table 21.5 Immunosuppression.

Trough levels	Cyclosporine (ME) 5 mg/kg b.i.d.		Tacrolimus 0.075 mg/kg b.i.d.		Tacrolimus with IL-2 antibodies* ± MMF† 0.1 mg/kg b.i.d.
		or		*or*	
0–1 month	200–250 ng/mL		8–12 ng/mL		7–11 ng/mL
1–3 months	180–200 ng/mL		5–8 ng/mL		4–7 ng/mL
3–12 months	150–200 ng/mL		3–8 ng/mL		2–4 ng/mL
> 12 months	70–100 ng/mL		3–5 ng/mL		2–4 ng/mL
	Prednisolone 2 mg/kg (↓) 3 months		Prednisolone 2 mg/kg (↓) 3 months		
	Azathioprine 1–2 mg/kg 12 months				

IL-2, interleukin-2; ME, microemulsion.
* Daclizumab (1 mg/kg): intraoperatively and days 4 and 18; basiliximab (10–20 mg/kg): intraoperatively and day 4.
† MMF: mycophenolate mofetil 10–40 mg/kg.

The majority of units use steroids at induction, gradually reducing them over the first 2 weeks. Some units withdraw or reduce to alternate-day therapy after 3 months to improve growth. Azathioprine is usually discontinued after 1 year. Cyclosporine or tacrolimus are continued for life. Although most immunosuppressant drug monitoring is based on trough levels, it is possible that peak cyclosporine levels (C2 levels) may be more effective in preventing rejection and reducing side effects.[86]

A European multicenter study that directly compared tacrolimus with cyclosporine after transplantation demonstrated a significant reduction in the incidence of acute and steroid-resistant rejection in the tacrolimus group in comparison with the cyclosporine group, without significant differences in adverse side effects[87] and with a better long-term outcome.

Mycophenolate mofetil (MMF) 10–40 mg/kg has recently been developed as an adjuvant immunosuppressive agent. It is an antiproliferative agent that is similar in action to azathioprine and may depress the bone marrow. It is effective induction when combined with a CNI drug and an IL-2 antibody[82] and can be used as monotherapy for maintenance if renal dysfunction is an issue.[88] Its long-term safety is undetermined, and there are significant gastrointestinal and hematological side effects in adults, although these are less severe in children. It has no cosmetic side effects, is renal-sparing and it does not require drug monitoring. Although it is possible to measure mycophenolic acid (MPA) pharmacokinetics, there are few data on effective therapeutic levels.[84]

Anti–interleukin-2 receptor antibodies (IL-2 antibodies) are monoclonal antibodies that selectively target the IL-2 receptors on activated T-cells, which is a key step in the development of cell-mediated immunity. Two antibodies are available, basiliximab and daclizumab, both of which are renal-sparing and provide effective induction immunosuppression after transplantation in combination with a calcineurin inhibitor in children.[89,90]

Sirolimus is a macrocyclic triene antibiotic that prevents T-cell proliferation by inhibiting cytokine production and does not inhibit calcineurin. In adults, sirolimus has been evaluated as both primary and rescue immunosuppression for liver transplant recipients, and it has the advantage of being both renal-sparing and reducing the need for high-dose steroids.[91] Significant side effects include delayed wound healing, hyperlipidemia, and an increase in the rate of hepatic artery thrombosis; it should not be used immediately after transplantation, but may be useful for chronic rejection. There are few studies of sirolimus in pediatric liver transplantation; it appears to be a potent immunosuppressant, but with a significant incidence of infectious side effects.[85]

Prophylactic antibiotics

Broad-spectrum antibiotics are prescribed for 48 h unless there is continuing infection (Table 21.4). Systemic antifungals, fluconazole, or liposomal amphotericin should be continued for 14 days in children with acute liver failure or those undergoing a second laparotomy for complications. Whilst patients are on steroids, it is advisable to give low-dose co-trimoxazole or trimethoprim as prophylaxis against *Pneumocystis carinii* infection. Oral nystatin and amphotericin to prevent oral and esophageal candidiasis may be continued for 6–12 months.

Prophylaxis for CMV infection is required for CMV-negative recipients of a CMV-positive donor. Acyclovir (1500 mg/m^2/day i.v. or 200–400 mg/dose q.d.s. orally) or ganciclovir (5 mg/kg) prevents infection in the short term when immunosuppression is intense.[92] There is no satisfactory prophylaxis for EBV, although some units use acyclovir or ganciclovir.

Other medications

The incidence of stress ulcers and excess gastric secretion is high in children recovering from liver transplantation, particularly those receiving high doses of steroids.[93,94] It is therefore important to prevent steroid-induced peptic ulceration with ranitidine, which unlike cimetidine does not interact with cyclosporine, sucralfate (2–4 g q.d.s.), and/or omeprazole (10–20 mg i.v. b.i.d.).

Antiplatelet drugs, aspirin, and dipyridamole are prescribed to prevent vascular thrombosis and discontinued at 3 months. Intravenous heparin and/or warfarin may be indicated for children with a high risk of thrombosis. Antihypertensive medication is usually required because of the effects of the immunosuppressive therapy. Nifedipine (5–10 mg/dose) and/or atenolol (25–50 mg/dose) are usually adequate for immediate use.

Postoperative complications

Early postoperative complications

Complications in the early postoperative period may be due to:

- The recipient's preoperative condition (e.g., malnutrition, sepsis, renal failure)
- The quality of the graft (e.g., primary nonfunction, acidosis, coagulopathy)
- Surgical complications (e.g., intra-abdominal hemorrhage, vascular thrombosis, venous outflow obstruction)
- Side effects of drugs (e.g., cyclosporine-induced renal failure; hyperglycemia from either tacrolimus or cyclosporine).

A number of factors may predispose to postoperative renal failure. Some patients have impaired renal function preoperatively that may have been aggravated by intraoperative cardiovascular instability requiring inotrope support. In such patients, induction therapy with IL-2 antibodies allows the use of low-dose CNI or a delay in their introduction. Alternatively, renal-sparing drugs such as MMF or sirolimus should be administered once the initial postoperative period is past. Oliguria is common and should be managed by ensuring adequate fluid replacement or furosemide challenge (1–2 mg/kg i.v., or infusion 0.25 mg/kg/h). Anuria with rising urea, creatinine, or potassium levels requires renal hemodialysis or filtration and may be associated with graft dysfunction.

The main causes of graft loss in the first week include:

- Primary nonfunction (PNF) secondary to hyperacute rejection, which occurs on day 4–5
- Hepatic artery or portal vein thrombosis
- Systemic sepsis

Primary nonfunction is a serious complication that requires immediate retransplantation. It may be suspected if there is persistent coagulopathy, acidosis, a high potassium level and transaminases > 10 000 IU/L. If nonfunction is secondary to hyperacute rejection, the diagnosis can only be made by liver biopsy (which may be impractical) or by identification of raised immunoglobulins.[95] Treatment consists of retransplantation or an increase in immunosuppression.

Hepatic artery thrombosis occurs in 10% of children. The incidence has fallen following the introduction of reduction hepatectomy and split-liver grafts, with the use of larger donor blood vessels.[57,96] Medical prevention of hepatic artery

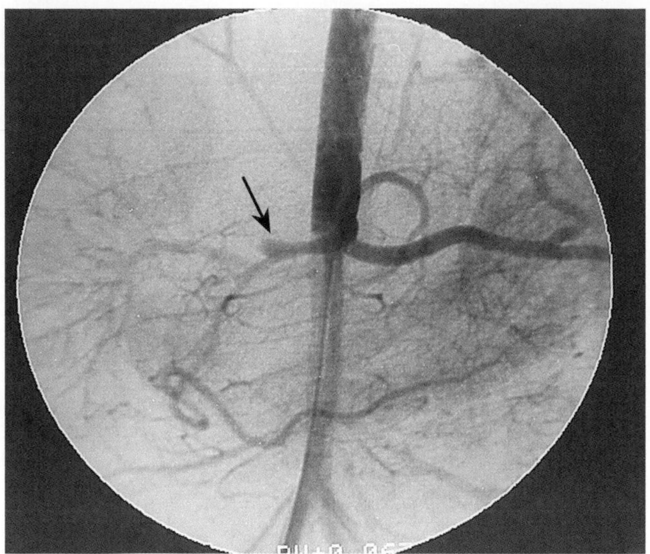

Figure 21.3 Hepatic angiogram showing a patent celiac axis but absent hepatic artery secondary to hepatic artery thrombosis. The patient underwent successful re-transplantation.

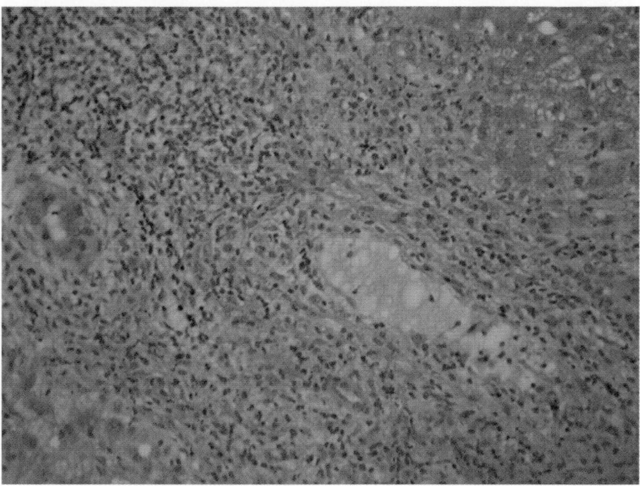

Figure 21.4 Liver histology, showing acute rejection. There is a mixed inflammatory infiltrate in the portal tract, with eosinophils, endotheliitis, lymphoid infiltration, and inflammation of bile ducts. There is some hepatocyte loss (hematoxylin–eosin, original magnification × 200).

thrombosis is by maintaining a low hematocrit (< 10 g/hemoglobin) and using antiplatelet agents such as aspirin (3 mg/kg/day) and dipyridamole (25–50 mg t.d.s.).[81] Portal vein thrombosis is less common. The diagnosis of hepatic artery or portal vein thrombosis is made by Doppler ultrasound and confirmed by angiography or MRI angiography (Figure 21.3). Treatment includes:

- Immediate laparotomy with thrombectomy or thrombolysis[97]
- Anticoagulation: intravenous heparin initially, followed by oral warfarin
- Retransplantation

Retransplantation is not always required, as collateral blood vessels may develop. Late complications of hepatic artery thrombosis include biliary leaks and strictures or hepatic abscesses.[70]

Systemic sepsis is treated as indicated, with broad-spectrum antibiotics and antifungals. Retransplantation is not indicated if sepsis leads to multiorgan failure and graft nonfunction.

Hemorrhage from the cut surface of the liver is a rare complication and is managed conservatively unless there is confirmed bleeding or hemodynamic instability. Abdominal tamponade may decrease renal blood flow, causing renal failure.

Complications after the first postoperative week

Complications arising after the first postoperative week include:

- Acute rejection
- Biliary leaks/strictures
- Persistent wound drainage or ascites
- sepsis
- Neurological side effects

Acute rejection is less common in infants (20%), but increases to 50–60% in older children.[98] The clinical signs and symptoms include fever, irritability, and abdominal discomfort. The diagnosis is confirmed by detecting a rise in bilirubin, alkaline phosphatase, aspartate and alanine transaminases, and γ-glutamyltransferase (GGT). It is always necessary to have histological confirmation. Acute rejection is indicated by a mixed inflammatory infiltrate in the portal tracts, with subendothelial lymphoid infiltration (endothelialitis) and inflammatory infiltration of the bile ducts (Figure 21.4).[99] Treatment is with pulse methylprednisolone (20–40 mg/kg/day) intravenously over 2 or 3 days. If there is inadequate histological or biochemical response, treatment with methylprednisolone may be repeated, but conversion to a more potent immunosuppressive drug such as sirolimus may be required.[85]

Chronic rejection occurs in < 10% of children at any time after transplantation.[98] The diagnosis is suggested by the gradual onset of jaundice, pruritus, and pale stools, which indicate biliary obstruction. Biochemical changes include a higher rise in bilirubin, alkaline phosphatase, and GGT than in transaminases. Histology may demonstrate extensive damage and loss of bile ducts (vanishing bile duct syndrome), with arterial obliteration and fibrosis (Figure 21.5). Most children respond to an increase in immunosuppression, such as the addition of MMF or conversion to tacrolimus or sirolimus, but some require retransplantation. Newer therapies such as alemtuzumab (Campath) have yet to be evaluated.[100]

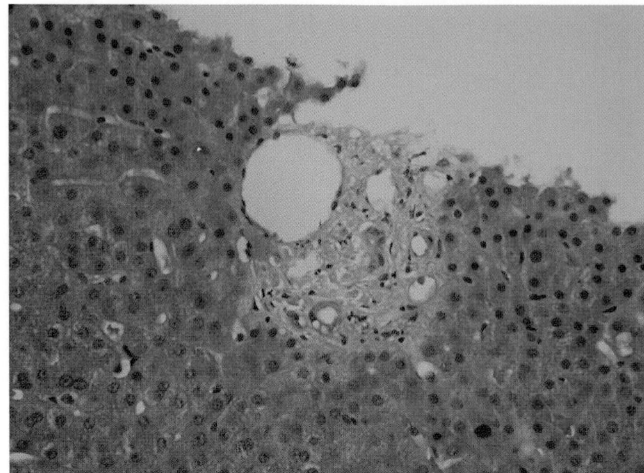

A

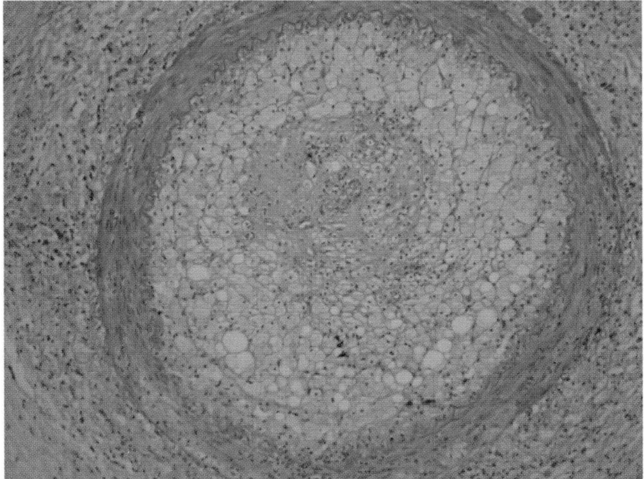

B

Figure 21.5 Liver histology, showing chronic rejection. **A** There is an inflammatory infiltrate in the portal tract, with loss of bile ducts—vanishing bile duct syndrome (hematoxylin–eosin, original magnification × 200). **B** In the later stages, there is foam-cell arteriopathy (hematoxylin–eosin, original magnification × 100).

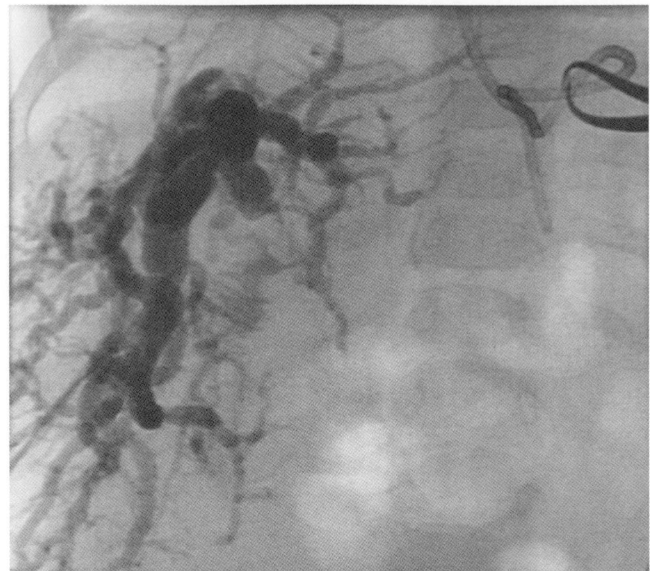

A

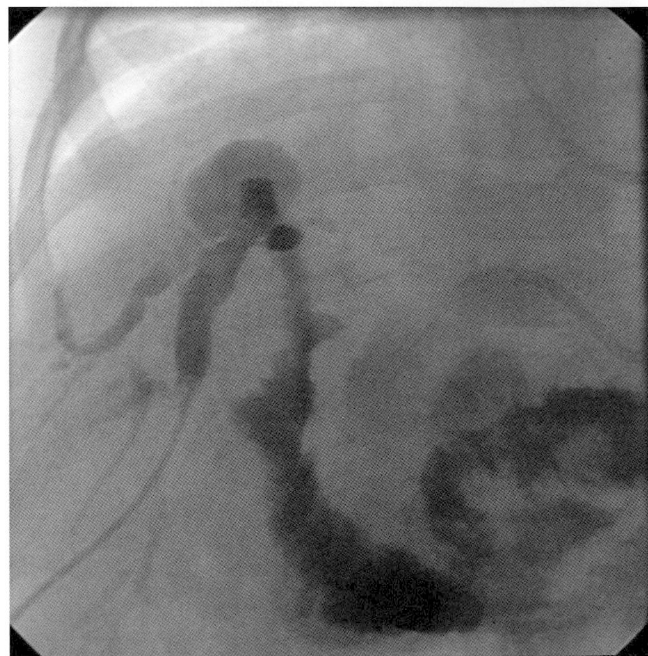

B

Figure 21.6 **A** Biliary obstruction occurs in 20% of children after liver transplantation, due to hepatic artery ischemia or a biliary anastomotic stricture). **B** Following balloon dilation of the stricture using a percutaneous transhepatic approach, there is good drainage of contrast from the intrahepatic bile ducts across the biliary anastomosis into the jejunal Roux loop.

The incidence of biliary complications has increased with the use of reduction hepatectomies and split-liver grafts.[57,70] Biliary strictures may be secondary to an anastomotic stricture, edema of the bile ducts, or hepatic artery ischemia. Biliary leaks may be secondary to leakage from the cut surface of the liver or from hepatic artery ischemia. Most biliary leaks will settle with conservative management. Large leaks causing biliary peritonitis, biliary abscesses, or sepsis will require surgical drainage and reconstruction. The majority of intrahepatic biliary strictures are now managed medically with ursodeoxycholic acid, or radiologically using percutaneous transhepatic cholangiography. The dilated biliary tree is cannulated and external biliary drainage is established (Figure 21.6). Biliary dilation can be carried out using balloons and biliary stents. Surgical reconstruction is required for the management of extrahepatic biliary strictures, or if interventional radiology fails.

Persistent drain losses may be due to preoperative ascites or secondary to rejection, sepsis, hepatic vein obstruction, or peritonitis. They may lead to acidosis and coagulopathy or an enhanced coagulable state due to loss of bicarbonate and coagulation factors. Treatment is of the primary cause, fluid restriction, and diuretics. Hepatic vein outflow obstruction may be related to the use of the "piggy-back" technique for anastomosis. It may be difficult to detect on ultrasound alone and may require venography and stenting.[101]

Sepsis is still the commonest complication following liver transplantation (60–70%).[3] The majority of infections are bacterial infections related to central line insertion (*Streptococcus faecalis* and *S. viridans*, *Pseudomonas aeruginosa*, and *Staphylococcus aureus*). Fungal infections with *Candida albicans* and *Aspergillus* spp. are documented in approximately 20% of patients and are particularly common in patients with fulminant hepatitis with acute hepatic necrosis before transplantation. Vancomycin-resistant enterococcus (VRE) is a common gut pathogen, but systemic infection requires treatment with quinupristin/dalfopristin (Synercid) or linezolid.[102]

Neurological side effects such as convulsions were common following the use of intravenous cyclosporine or high-dose tacrolimus. The development of convulsions is still reported, as is the development of a reversible leukoencephalopathy, which may be related to toxic CNI levels.[103]

Late complications after liver transplantation

Late complications (after 3 weeks) may occur at any time after transplantation. They include:

- Side effects of immunosuppression
- CMV or EBV infection
- Post-transplant lymphoproliferative disease (PTLD)
- Late biliary stricture
- Late hepatic artery or portal vein thrombosis
- Chronic rejection

There are numerous side effects of immunosuppressive therapy (Table 21.6). Some are short-term, such as stunting and hypertension secondary to steroids, while nephrotoxicity and increased risk of viral infection are lifelong. Hirsutism and gingival hyperplasia are side effects of cyclosporine which, although cosmetic, have an important effect on quality of life. With careful monitoring of immunosuppression to ensure adequate trough levels, nephrotoxicity should be minimized.[104]

Table 21.6 Immunosuppressive complications after transplantation.

Drug	Complications
Steroids	Stunting Hypertension Cushingoid facies
Cyclosporine	Hirsutism Gingival hyperplasia Hyperlipidemia
Cyclosporine/tacrolimus	Renal dysfunction Hypertension Neurotoxicity Hyperglycemia ? Lymphoproliferative disease
Tacrolimus	? Cardiomyopathy

CMV infection occurs 5–6 weeks after transplantation despite prophylaxis with acyclovir or ganciclovir.[92,105,106] It is more common in children than adults, reflecting the number of CMV-negative children undergoing liver transplantation. The risk of CMV disease, as opposed to CMV infection, is indirectly related to receiving a transplant from a CMV-positive donor, but the condition is usually treated effectively with high-dose ganciclovir 5 mg/kg and a hyperimmune CMV globulin dose.

The development of primary EBV is a significant long-term problem. Approximately 65% of children undergoing liver transplantation will be EBV-negative before the operation, and 75% of this group will have a primary EBV infection within 6 months of transplantation.[92] It is important to diagnose primary EBV infection and reduce immunosuppression, if possible, in order to prevent further progression to lymphoproliferative disease.[107]

There is a close relationship between primary EBV infection and the development of lymphoproliferative disease.[108] The spectrum of B-lymphocyte proliferation ranges from benign hyperplasia to malignant lymphoma. The clinical features may represent infectious mononucleosis, isolated lymphoid involvement, or malignant lymphoma EBV. Polymerase chain reaction (PCR) is usually positive, but is not diagnostic of PLTD. The diagnosis is based on identifying the characteristic histology from the affected tissue, which may demonstrate polymorphic B-cell proliferation or lymphomatous features of nuclear atypia and necrosis. Epstein–Barr encoded RNA (EBER) staining for EBV is positive (Figure 21.7). Immunofluorescent staining of heavy-chain and light-chain immunoglobulins may differentiate monoclonal from polyclonal infiltrates. Almost any organ in the body can be affected, although the liver and gut are most commonly involved. There is no difference in incidence between tacrolimus and cyclosporine.[109]

Treatment includes:

- Reduction of immunosuppression.
- Intravenous acyclovir (3 mg/m^2) or ganciclovir (6–10 mg/kg) may be effective.
- Infusion of autologous T cells directed against EBV cells[110] is an effective technique, but is very labor-intensive and costly.
- Chemotherapy, tailored to the type of lymphoma, is necessary if the lymphoproliferative disease becomes overtly malignant.
- If the reduction in immunosuppression leads to rejection, then balancing therapy, as above, is difficult.

Late biliary strictures are usually due to hepatic artery thrombosis and lead to cholangitis and biliary cirrhosis. They are treated radiologically as above (Figure 21.6) or by surgery.

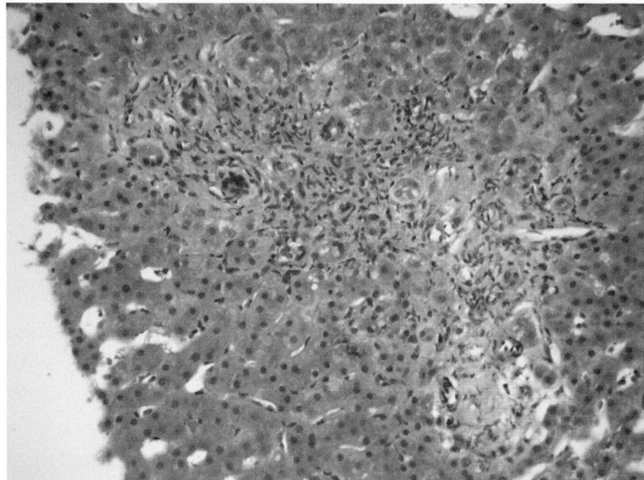

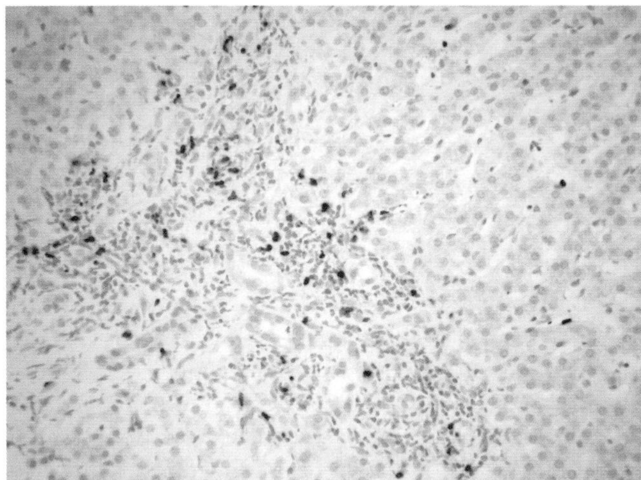

Figure 21.7 Children are more likely to develop a primary Epstein–Barr virus (EBV) infection after transplantation because they are negative before transplantation and receive a donor from an older (EBV-positive) donor. **A** Histologically, there is an inflammatory infiltrate, mainly with B cells (hematoxylin–eosin, original magnification × 200). **B** Immunocytochemistry demonstrates positive EBV cells in the affected tissue (Epstein–Barr encoded RNA, original magnification × 200).

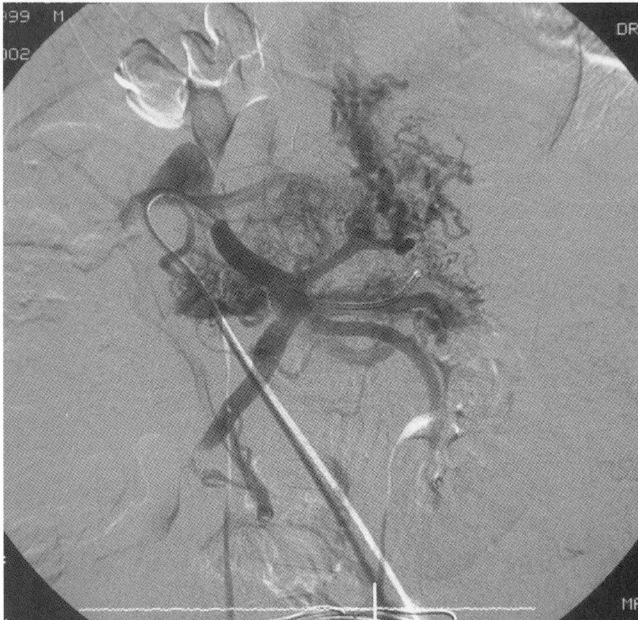

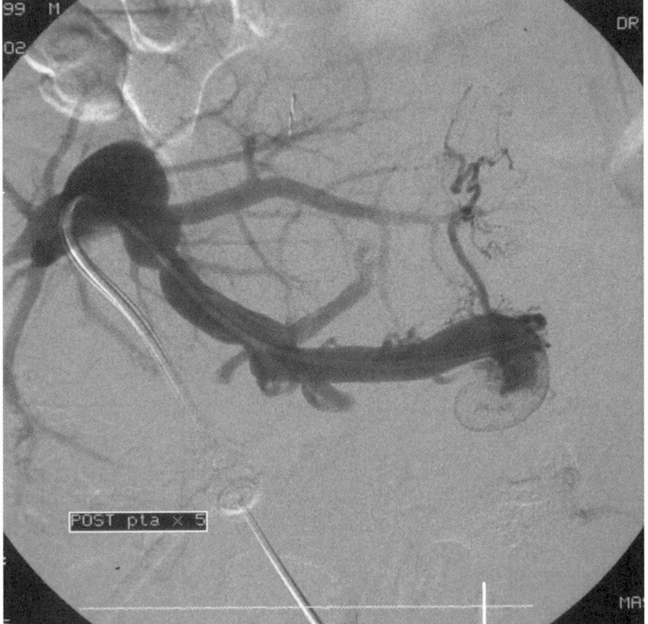

Figure 21.8 **A** The percutaneous transhepatic portogram shows a critical stenosis of the portal vein anastomosis after transplantation, with numerous varices in the upper abdomen. **B** This was successfully treated with balloon dilation, reducing the pressure gradient across the portal vein anastomosis and a reduction in variceal filling.

Late hepatic thrombosis does not usually require treatment, as a collateral blood supply becomes established. Portal vein stenosis due to an anastomotic stricture may lead to portal hypertension and varices. It should be treated radiologically by venoplasty or surgical reconstruction or a meso-rex shunt (Figure 21.8).

Chronic rejection can occur at any time, especially if there is noncompliance. Treatment is as above.

Survival following liver transplantation

Current results from international units indicate that 1-year survival after elective pediatric liver transplantation is 90%.[1,3] Long-term survival (10–15 years) ranges from 60% to 80%.[111–113] Patients who receive elective living related liver transplantation may have a higher 1-year survival (94%) in comparison with those receiving cadaveric grafts (78%) (Figure 21.9).[114]

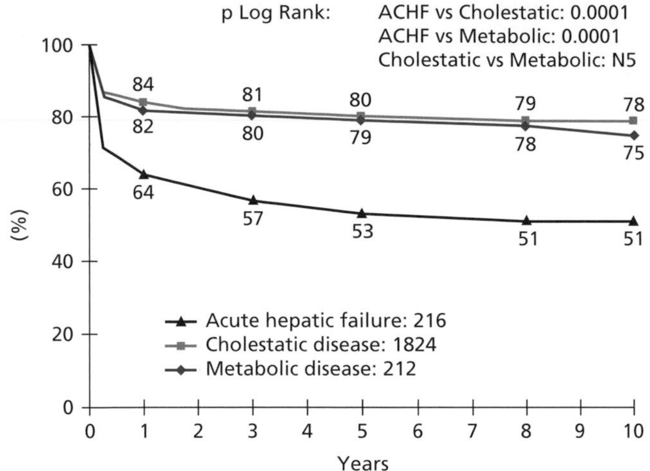

Figure 21.9 Survival after liver transplantation according to recipient age, 1988–2005. (European Liver Transplant Registry.)

Factors affecting survival

There are a number of factors that may influence survival. Age at transplantation has previously been considered a significant risk factor, and transplantation was originally contraindicated in infants under 1 year old.[115] Technical developments, which have included reduction hepatectomy, split-liver transplantation, and living related donor transplantation, have reduced waiting-list mortality[116] and extended liver transplantation to this young age group,[3,58] even in infants weighing less than 5 kg.[69,117]

Many studies have indicated that the inevitable protein malnutrition that affects children with end-stage liver disease had a significant influence on morbidity and mortality after liver transplantation. Chin *et al.*[118] found a significant difference in the 2-year actuarial survival for children with standard deviation scores (SDS for weight) of less than −1 (57%) compared with those greater than −1 (95%). This was confirmed using height standard deviation scores, in which children who are less stunted at the time of their operation had an improved outcome, indicating the necessity for preoperative nutritional support (Chapter 15).[119]

The severity of liver disease has a significant effect on short-term survival, as children transplanted electively have an improved survival in comparison with those transplanted for acute liver failure or fulminant hepatitis.[120–122]

Recurrent disease after transplantation

In some instances, survival may be affected by recurrence of the original disease. Recurrence of hepatitis B virus (HBV infection) is almost 100% likely in those children who are positive for HBV DNA or hepatitis B e antigen at the time of their operation.[123] Recurrent HBV disease is associated with chronic hepatitis or cirrhosis (79%), submassive necrosis (9%), or fibrosing cholestatic hepatitis, which is a fatal form of fulminant hepatic failure (25%).[124] Prophylaxis with anti-HBV human immunoglobulin (HBIg) has been replaced with the nucleoside analogues lamivudine and adefovir, which effectively prevent recurrence, but at the expense of the emergence of viral mutants.[23] Recurrence of hepatitis B infection in children who have undergone transplantation for fulminant hepatitis B is unusual.

Although chronic hepatitis C is an unusual indication for liver transplantation in childhood, a number of children were infected preoperatively before screening became available (Chapter 6).[125,126] Reinfection of the graft is inevitable, but treatment outcomes have improved following treatment with the combination of pegylated interferon and ribavirin.[127]

Recent studies have indicated that autoimmune hepatitis may recur both immunologically and histologically and may be more severe than the original disease.[128] Giant-cell hepatitis in association with autoimmune hemolytic anemia is a rare disease that has been shown to recur after transplantation.[129] The outcome for children who undergo transplantation for malignant hepatic tumors is related to the rate of recurrence, and if no extrahepatic metastases were present at the time of surgery, the long-term outcome may be excellent.[130,131]

De novo autoimmune hepatitis

A number of recent studies have documented the development of autoantibodies—antinuclear antibody (ANA), smooth muscle antibody (SMA), and rarely liver-kidney microsomal (LKM) antibody—after transplantation in both children and adults, in recipients who had not had autoimmune disease before transplantation.[132,133] The incidence varies from 2–3% to 50% with time, and is associated with a graft hepatitis and progressive fibrosis.[134] Although the etiology is unknown, the hepatitis resolves with steroid therapy or with azathioprine (Figure 21.10; see also Chapter 8).[135]

Long-term renal function

The development of nephrotoxicity with both cyclosporine and tacrolimus was considered inevitable. There is a 30% reduction in renal function after transplantation, which stabilizes or improves with low-dose maintenance immunosuppression or a transfer to renal-sparing drugs such as mycophenolate mofetil or sirolimus.[88,104,136] Only 4–5% of patients develop severe chronic renal failure in the longer term, requiring renal transplantation. Acute postoperative hypertension is seen in 65% of children, but only persists in 28%.[137] Treatment with Losartan, an angiotensin II antagonist (2 mg/kg/day; usually 25–50 mg/day) is effective for chronic hypertension and may be more effective than nifedipine (5–10 mg/dose) and/or atenolol (25–50 mg/dose).

Hyperlipidemia

Cyclosporine and sirolimus both increase serum lipids, particularly cholesterol, which resolves on transfer to tacrolimus or mycophenolate mofetil.[138]

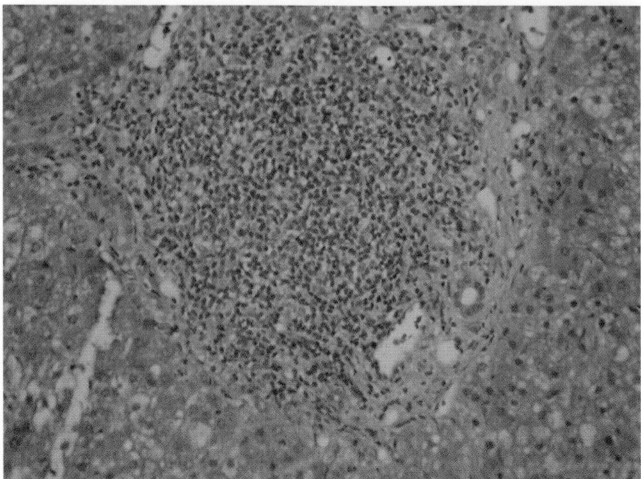

Figure 21.10 Chronic graft hepatitis develops 5–10 years after transplantation and may be related to chronic rejection or de-novo hepatitis. In this section, there is a mixed inflammatory infiltrate confined to the portal tract (hematoxylin–eosin, original magnification × 200).

Hematological complications

Graft-versus-host disease is rare after liver transplantation, but may respond to increased immunosuppression.[139] Both autoimmune hemolytic anemia and idiopathic thrombocytopenia are reported and may be immunological or drug-related, particularly with tacrolimus.[140] Both respond to high-dose steroids or intravenous immunoglobulin.

Transplant tolerance

There is considerable interest in the development of transplant tolerance, and adult studies have demonstrated that approximately 20% of patients can be withdrawn from immunosuppression.[141] Complete withdrawal of immunosuppression in children is anecdotal and related to case reports of anergy following post-transplantation lymphoproliferative disease. Children may be more likely to become tolerant after transplantation, as they require less immunosuppression and are less likely to develop rejection than older children and adults, perhaps because neonates have a greater T-helper response than adults, which is more likely to lead to graft acceptance.[142]

Quality of life after transplantation

Children who survive the initial 3 months after transplantation without major complications should achieve a normal lifestyle, despite the necessity for continuous monitoring of immunosuppressive treatment. Children who undergo transplantation for metabolic liver disease have both phenotypic and functional recovery (α_1-antitrypsin deficiency, Wilson's disease, and tyrosinemia type I). Children with organic acidemias will only have palliation of their defect if the enzyme defect is not restricted to the liver (propionic acidemia or methylmalonic acidemia).[143–145]

Growth after transplantation

Early studies evaluating growth in children after liver transplantation indicated that up to 59% of children did not achieve catch-up growth.[146] In contrast, more recent studies have indicated that approximately 80% of survivors achieve normal growth patterns and body habitus.[118,146,147]

In the majority of children who have had a successful liver transplant, there is a rapid return to normal in the mid-arm muscle area and mid-arm fat area within 6–12 months after transplantation.[29] Weight gain may initially be excessive due to the effects of steroids, appetite, and salt and water retention. Most children will regain normal weight within 12 months. Linear growth may be delayed for between 6 and 24 months, which is directly related to steroid dosage and preoperative stunting.[148,149] Newer regimens that avoid or reduce steroids will benefit growth in the longer term.[150]

Growth failure after transplantation

The most important factors inhibiting growth after transplantation are:

- Excessive use of steroids
- Preoperative stunting
- Genetic disorders
- Behavioral feeding problems

Children who are particularly stunted before transplantation (height SDS <–1) initially have rapid catch-up growth, but do not achieve their genetic potential, while children who are less stunted (height SDS >–1) have slower catch-up growth, but will eventually achieve normal height.[151]

The growth-suppressant effects of corticosteroids in liver transplantation have been documented by many units. Catch-up growth will be observed either when alternate-day steroids are instituted or steroids are discontinued after transplantation, as is routine in some units.[146,152] Steroid avoidance, if successful, may alleviate this problem.

Failure to thrive and stunting are intrinsic features of certain genetic disorders, such as Alagille's syndrome. Linear growth may improve after transplantation for Alagille's syndrome, but approximately half of these children do not achieve normal height.[153]

Behavioral feeding problems

Children with end-stage liver disease have associated anorexia and vomiting. They often receive unpalatable feeds, sometimes by nasogastric tube. Many of these infants may never have fed normally before transplantation and thus will have missed their developmental milestones for chewing, swallowing, and normal feeding behavior. The perioperative emphasis on nutritional support often creates parental anxiety about feeding, which further exacerbates these difficult behavioral problems. A review of data from our unit in Birmingham shows that up to 60% of patients who were tube-fed before liver transplantation develop significant feeding problems postoperatively. The management of these disorders includes a multidisciplinary approach with a dietitian and food psychologist, and with a strict behavioral feeding regimen. In the minority of patients, however, nocturnal enteral feeding may be required for 1–2 years to maintain normal growth.[154]

Psychosocial development

There is an initial deterioration in psychosocial development after transplantation, as noted by deteriorations in social skills, language development, and eye/hand coordination for up to 1 year postoperatively.[30,46]

The majority of children will achieve normal psychosocial development after transplantation, but the rate of improvement is related to the age of onset of liver disease and age at the time of transplantation.[155] Children who do not undergo transplantation until significant motor or psychological developmental delay has taken place are unlikely to catch up adequately and achieve normal developmental scores after transplantation. In contrast, children who have undergone transplantation earlier have been shown to have complete nutritional and developmental catch-up within 1–4 years postoperatively and to be capable of attending a normal school (see also Chapter 24).[30,156] Long-term studies have indicated that although within the normal range, transplant recipients fall in the lower intelligence quotient (IQ) range, although it is not clear whether this is due to pretransplantation factors or post-transplantation immunosuppression.[157]

Noncompliance with therapy

Nonadherence is the major cause of graft loss or rejection in adolescent transplant recipients, accounting for 17% of liver grafts.[80,158] It is the main cause of late graft loss in adolescence after liver transplantation (see Chapter 25).[80] Additional risk factors for nonadherence are the age at which transplantation takes place, social and economic factors, and the process of transition to adult care.[159] There is good evidence that nonadherence to medication, clinic visits, and medical advice increases after transfer to adult care, indicating the need for an appropriate transition policy.[160] The management of nonadherence is difficult and relies on a nonjudgmental approach and efforts to improve education, social functioning, and behavioral strategies to encourage self-motivation (see also Chapter 25).[161]

Endocrine development

Long-term studies in France have shown that children surviving liver transplantation will enter puberty normally, girls will develop menarche, and both boys and girls will have pubertal growth spurts.[149] Successful pregnancies have been reported.[162,163] It is important that appropriate advice about fertility, contraception, and immunosuppressive therapy should be provided (see Chapter 25).[164]

Family functioning

Recent data on family functioning indicate that the extreme stress experienced by families may lead to marital breakup and dysfunctional family behavior.[165] Health-related quality-of-life scores are less than for normal families, as expected, but within the normal range.[166–168]

Outpatient monitoring

Initial post-transplantation management includes frequent follow-up by the transplant center, usually at weekly intervals, extending with time to monthly, 3-monthly, and then 6-monthly intervals. Monitoring should include:

- Assessment of nutritional status by measuring height, weight, triceps skinfold, mid-arm circumference, and mid-arm muscle area.
- Detection of potential complications (e.g., rejection, infection, hepatic artery thrombosis, biliary complications, development of de-novo autoimmune hepatitis) by performing regular liver function tests, serology (hepatitis B, C, CMV) screening for autoantibodies (ANA, SMA, LKM) annually and 6-monthly, or annual abdominal ultrasound examinations.
- Monitoring of immunosuppression to maintain adequate peak or trough levels of cyclosporine and trough levels of tacrolimus or sirolimus to prevent rejection and reduce toxicity (Table 21.5).
- Monitoring for PTLD by EBV PCR 3–6-monthly; and measuring serum albumin, as a falling albumin level may be an early sign of gut PTLD.
- Protocol liver biopsies. Although annual liver biopsies produce little additional information unless other investigations are abnormal,[169] 5- and 10-year biopsies may detect chronic hepatitis and fibrosis in 25–50% of children that is not related to hepatitis C or G, but may be autoimmune in origin.[134,170]
- Renal function. Regular monitoring of the calculated glomerular filtration rate (cGFR) using the Schwartz formula—40 × height (cm)/creatinine (μmol/L)—as a screen for renal function is of value. If the cGFR falls below 65 mL/min/1.73 m^2, chromium ethylenediamine tetraacetic acid (EDTA) estimation should be performed, as it is a more accurate measurement. Transfer to a renal-sparing drug or a reduction in CNI drugs should be considered if the chromium EDTA values fall below 65 mL/min/1.73 m^2, as transfer to a renal-sparing agent is effective if started before there is irreversible renal dysfunction.[171] New data suggesting that Cystatin C is a good screening test for renal dysfunction may be valuable and reduce dependency on chromium EDTA.[172]
- Regular measurement of blood pressure and/or ambulatory blood pressure monitoring may be required.
- As children become adolescents, appropriate advice about adolescent issues is required (Chapter 25).

It is essential to encourage both the child and family to return to a normal life by reducing outpatient visits and encouraging a return to school, nursery, and playgroup, and discouraging the parents from continuing to maintain their child in a sick role. Many families may find the transition from intensive management in specialist units to the more relaxed outpatient follow-up difficult to cope with and may need additional support and encouragement to regain a normal life. Outreach clinics held in the referring hospital are a good way of ensuing a return to normality.

Promising lines of research

For the moment, liver transplantation is here to stay, although the rapid development of techniques to improve hepatocyte transplantation for acute liver failure or metabolic liver disease is encouraging.[39] The continued advance in targeted less toxic immunosuppressive drugs can only improve the outcome for children undergoing liver transplantation.

Case study

A.M. was a 5-year-old boy who initially had a successful Kasai portoenterostomy for biliary atresia. He developed recurrent cholangitis, cirrhosis, and portal hypertension and was on a variceal banding program for hematemesis. Abdominal examination revealed distended veins, ascites, and hepatosplenomegaly. He was receiving supplemental feeding with Nutrini Extra 70 mL/h for 6 hours overnight and 400 mL in the daytime, with a small amount of solid food.

Indications for transplantation included: decompensated cirrhosis with poor nutrition, a falling albumin level, ascites, and increasing coagulopathy.

He received a segment II/III orthotopic liver; the donor was O rhesus-positive and CMV-negative. At transplantation, due to severe fibrous tissue at the porta hepatis, it was impossible to dissect out the venous and arterial vessels, and both venous and arterial conduits were formed. A Roux loop was formed for the biliary anastomosis. There were many varices around the porta hepatis. He had a straightforward postoperative course and was discharged 3 weeks postoperatively on tacrolimus 0.2 mg twice daily and prednisolone 10 mg daily.

He returned after 12 months with a history of recurrent fever, abdominal pain, and loose watery stools without blood or mucus. He complained of mild abdominal pain, not associated with food. His blood culture showed *Streptococcus pneumoniae,* and he was treated with a 10-day course of intravenous antibiotics. Abdominal examination revealed ascites and splenomegaly.

Investigations: hemoglobin 9.2 g/L; white count 5.0×10^9 g/L; platelets 173×10^9 g/L; mean corpuscular volume (MCV) 63; film: microcytic hypochromic picture; prothrombin time (PT) 15 s (normal 12–15 s); activated partial thromboplastin time (APTT) 32 s (normal 33–37 s); bilirubin 13 mmol/L (normal < 20 mmol/L); alkaline phosphatase 432 IU/L (normal < 600 IU/L); alanine aminotransferase (ALT) 21 IU/L (normal < 40 IU/L); aspartate aminotransferase (AST) 3 IU/L (normal < 40 IU/L); GGT 56 IU/L (normal 35–40 IU/L); albumin 24 g/L (normal 35–52 g/L); total protein 44 (normal 52–82 g/L); lactate dehydrogenase (LDH) 354 IU/L (normal 375–700 IU/L); EBV PCR 20 000 copies/mL (slightly elevated); tacrolimus level 3.4 ng/L.

Immunology. Antinuclear antibodies negative; liver/kidney microsomal antibodies negative; mitochondrial antibodies negative; smooth muscle antibodies weakly positive; IgG 5.56 (normal); IgA 0.97 (normal); IgM 1.22 (normal).

Upper gastrointestinal endoscopy. Mild gastropathy was noted. No ulcers or erosions were seen. The duodenal and jejunal mucosa was normal. Duodenal aspirate: no *Cryptosporidia* or *Giardia* seen. Jejunal biopsies showed dilated lymphatics (Figure 21.11).

Abdominal ultrasonography. The liver parenchyma was normal, but the spleen was enlarged. The hepatic and portal veins were patent. There was a clot in the retrohepatic inferior vena cava (IVC). Both kidneys appeared grossly normal. There was a moderate amount of ascites.

Computed tomography. The renal veins were patent and drained into collateral vessels, as the IVC appeared thrombosed throughout its length. Prominent azygous vein was noted. There was a significant amount of ascites within the abdomen and edema within the mesenteric fat. There was thickening of the wall and valvulae conniventes in the small bowel. The spleen was enlarged, measuring 14 cm in length. The kidneys and pancreas were normal. No pelvic or intra-abdominal lymphadenopathy was identified.

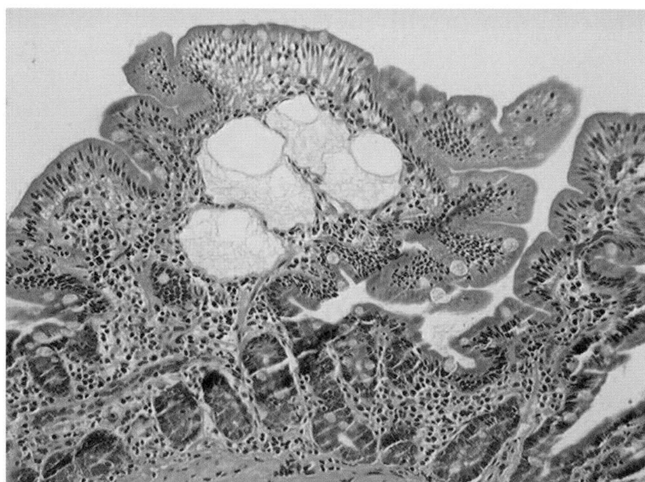

Figure 21.11 A jejunal biopsy, showing dilated lymphatics suggestive of intestinal lymphangiectasia. This is due to obstruction of the inferior vena cava and hepatic veins after transplantation. It leads to protein-losing enteropathy and loss of albumin, immunoglobulins, and lymphocytes. In immunosuppressed patients after transplantation, it may lead to significant infections unless managed with immunoglobulins and correction of the block.

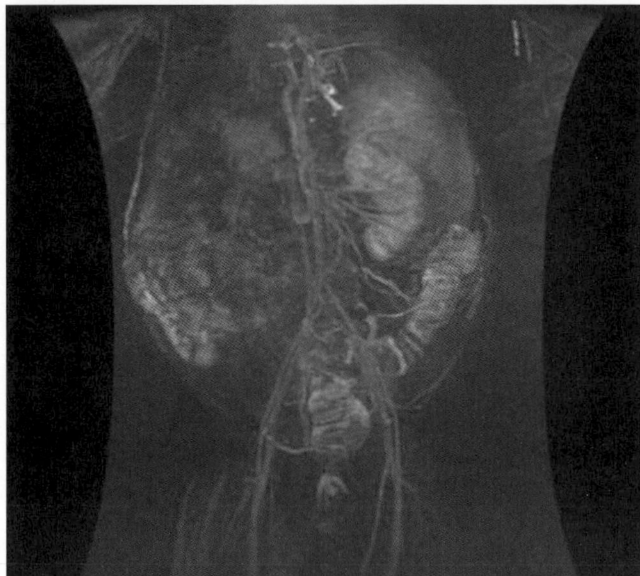

Figure 21.12 Magnetic resonance angiogram, showing obstruction of inferior vena cava and collateral blood vessels, which return the venous drainage to the heart.

Hematology: fibrinogen 3.7; prothrombin 20210A; gene mutation, normal Hind 3 restriction pattern; Factor V Leiden, normal.

Treatment. He was started on an medium-chain triglyceride (MCT)-based diet, intravenous albumin and immunoglobulin infusions, warfarin, spironolactone 10 mg twice daily, penicillin V 250 mg twice daily, and continued on tacrolimus 0.3 mg twice daily, omeprazole 10 mg daily, prednisolone 2.5 mg daily. He continued to lose weight and have troublesome ascites and recurrent infections. He was admitted electively for angiography and dilation of the IVC and hepatic vein after his albumin levels, which had been monitored locally, had dropped despite twice-weekly infusions.

Angiogram. The IVC was occluded, with probable stenosis of hepatic vein except to the IVC. The IVC was occluded just to level of the renal vein entrance (Figure 21.12). Hepatic vein dilation was carried out via the right internal jugular and left femoral vein with a 12-mm balloon, and full inflation was achieved twice, with good flow after balloon dilation. Final pressures were hepatic vein 9 mm and right atrium 7 mm. He recovered well and no longer requires albumin or immunoglobulin infusions or courses of antibiotics, but continues on warfarin.

Comment. The patient developed obstruction of the retrograde IVC following transplantation, due to technical difficulties during the operation. There was no evidence of a primary coagulation defect. This obstruction may affect hepatic vein outflow and is often difficult to diagnose on ultrasound. In this case, the extensive thrombosis was easy to see in the IVC, but the hepatic veins appeared patent until visualized at angiography. He developed intestinal lymphangiectasia with a protein-losing enteropathy, losing lymphocytes, albumin, and immunoglobulins through the intestine. This acquired immunodeficiency led to repeated infections, requiring recurrent courses of antibiotics and intravenous immunoglobulins. There was no resolution of the thrombosis on warfarin, and he required 2–3-weekly albumin and immunoglobulin infusions to control his ascites and infections and was receiving an MCT diet to reduce protein loss. His symptoms finally resolved after successful dilation of the hepatic vein outflow using interventional radiology.[173]

References

1 European Liver Transplant Registry 2006: www.eltr.org.

2 McDiarmid SV, Anand R, Lindblad AS. The Principal Investigators and Institutions of the Studies of Pediatric Liver Transplantation (SPLIT) Research Group. Development of a pediatric end-stage liver disease score to predict poor outcome of children awaiting liver transplantation. *Transplantation* 2002; **74**:173–81.

3 Beath SV, Brook GD, Kelly DA, *et al.* Successful liver transplantation in babies under 1 year. *BMJ* 1993;**307**:825–8.

4 Metzelder ML, Bottländer M, Melter M, Petersen C, Ure BM. Laparoscopic partial external biliary diversion procedure in progressive familial intrahepatic cholestasis: a new approach. *Surg Endosc* 2005;**19**:1641–3.

5 Hadzic N, Francavilla R, Chambers SM, Castellaneta S, Portmann B, Mieli-Vergani G. Outcome of PiSS and PiSZ alpha-1-antitrypsin deficiency presenting with liver involvement. *Eur J Pediatr* 2005;**164**:250–2.

6 Francavilla R, Castellaneta SP, Hadzic N, *et al.* Prognosis of alpha-1-antitrypsin deficiency-related liver disease in the era of paediatric liver transplantation. *J Hepatol* 2000;**32**:986–92.

7 Kayler LK, Rasmussen CS, Dykstra DM, *et al.* Liver transplantation in children with metabolic disorders in the United States. *Am J Transplant* 2003;**3**:334–9.

8 Lindstedt S, Holme E, Lock E, *et al.* Treatment of hereditary tyrosinaemia type I by inhibition of 4-hydroxphenyl pyruvate dioxygenase. *Lancet* 1992;**340**:813–7.

9 Mohan N, McKiernan P, Preece MA, Green A, Kelly DA. Indications and outcome of liver transplantation in tyrosinaemia type I. *Eur J Pediatr* 1999;**158**(Suppl 2): S49–54.

10 van Spronsen FJ, Bijleveld CM, van Maldegem BT, Wijburg FA. Hepatocellular carcinoma in hereditary tyrosinemia type I despite 2-(2 nitro-4-3 trifluoro- methylbenzoyl)-1, 3-cyclohexanedione treatment. *J Pediatr Gastroenterol Nutr* 2005;**40**: 90–3.

11 Baumann U, Duhme V, Auth MK, McKiernan PJ, Holme E. Lectin-reactive alpha-fetoprotein in patients with tyrosinemia type I and hepatocellular carcinoma. *J Pediatr Gastroenterol Nutr* 2006;**43**:77–82.

12 Macvicar D, Dicks-Mireaux C, Leonard JV, Wight DG. Hepatic imaging with computed tomography of chronic tyrosinaemia type I. *Br J Radiol* 1990;**63**:605–8.

13 Manowski Z, Silver, MM, Roberts EA, Superina RA, Philips MJ. Liver cell dysplasia and early liver transplantation in hereditary tyrosinaemia. *Mod Pathol* 1990;**36**:694–701.

14 Dhawan A, Taylor RM, Cheeseman P, De Silva P, Katsiyiannakis L, Mieli-Vergani G. Wilson's disease in children: 37-year experience and revised King's score for liver transplantation. *Liver Transpl* 2005;**11**:441–8.

15 Rela M, Heaton ND, Vougas V, *et al.* Orthotopic liver transplantation for hepatic complications of Wilson's disease. *Br J Surg* 1993;**80**:909–11.

16 Debray D, Lykavieris P, Gauthier F, *et al.* Outcome of cystic fibrosis-associated liver cirrhosis: management of portal hypertension. *J Hepatol* 1999;**31**:77–83.

17 Melzi ML, Kelly DA, Colombo C, *et al.* Liver transplant in cystic fibrosis: a poll among European centers. A study from the European Liver Transplant Registry. *Transpl Int* 2006;**19**:726–31.

18 Couetil JP, Soubrane O, Houssain, DP, *et al.* Combined heart–lung–liver, double lung–liver, and isolated liver transplantation for cystic fibrosis in children. *Transpl Int* 1997;**10**:33–9.

19 Milkiewicz P, Skiba G, Kelly D, *et al.* Transplantation for cystic fibrosis. Outcome following early liver transplantation. *J Pediatr Gastroenterol Nutr* 2002;**17**:208–13.

20 Sokal EM, Van Hoof F, Alberti D, de Ville de Goyet J, de Barsy T, Otte JB. Progressive cardiac failure following orthotopic liver transplantation for type IV glycogenosis. *Eur J Pediatr* 1992;**151**: 200–3.

21 Labrune P. Glycogen storage disease type I: indications for liver and/or kidney transplantation. *Eur J Pediatr* 2002;**161** (Suppl 1):S53–5.

22 Gregorio GV, Portmann B, Reid F, *et al.* Autoimmune hepatitis in childhood: a 20 year experience. *Hepatology* 1997;**25**:541–7.

23 Mutimer D. Review article: hepatitis B and liver transplantation. *Aliment Pharmacol Ther* 2006;**23**:1031–41.

24 Hadzic N. Paediatric sclerosing cholangitis associated with primary immunodeficiency. *J Pediatr Gastroenterol Nutr* 1999; **28**:579.

25 Oellerich M, Burdelski M, Lautz HU, Schulz M, Schmidt FW, Herrmann H. Lidocaine metabolite formation as a measure of liver function in patients with cirrhosis. *Ther Drug Monit* 1990;**12**:219–26.

26 Malatack JJ, Schaid DJ, Urbach AH, *et al.* Choosing a pediatric recipient for orthotopic liver transplantation. *J Pediatr* 1987; **111**:479–89.

27 McDiarmid SV, Merion RM, Dykstra DM, Harper AM. Selection of pediatric candidates under the PELD system. *Liver Transpl* 2004;**10**(10 Suppl 2):S23–30.

28 Shneider BL, Suchy FJ, Emre S. National and regional analysis of exceptions to the Pediatric End-Stage Liver Disease scoring system (2003–2004). *Liver Transpl* 2006;**12**:40–5.

29 Beath S, Kelly DA, Booth I. Nutritional support in children with liver disease. *Arch Dis Child* 1993;**69**:545–9.

30 van Mourik ID, Beath SV, Brook GA, *et al.* Long-term nutritional and neurodevelopmental outcome of liver transplantation in infants aged less than 12 months. *J Pediatr Gastroenterol Nutr* 2000;**30**:269–75.

31 O'Grady J, Alexander G, Hayllar KM, Williams R. Early indicators of prognosis in fulminant hepatic failure. *Gastroenterology* 1989;**97**:439–45.

32 Lee WS, McKiernan P, Kelly DA. Etiology, outcome and prognostic indicators of childhood fulminant hepatic failure in the United Kingdom. *J Pediatr Gastroenterol Nutr* 2005;**40**:575–81.

33 Bonatti H, Muiesan P, Connolly S, *et al.* Liver transplantation for acute liver failure in children under 1 year of age. *Transplant Proc* 1997;**29**:434–5.

34 Liver Advisory Group UK: http://www.ultransplant.org.uk.

35 Lauterberg BH, Vaishnar Y, Stillwell WB, Mitchell JR. The effects of age and glutathione depletion on hepatic glutathione turnover in vivo determined by acetaminophen probe analysis. *J Pharmacol Exp Ther* 1980;**213**:54–8.

36 Mahadevan SB, McKiernan PJ, Davies P, Kelly DA. Paracetamol induced hepatotoxicity. *Arch Dis Child* 2006;**91**:598–603.

37 Flynn D, Mohan N, McKiernan PJ, *et al.* Progress in therapy and outcome for children with neonatal haemochromatosis. *Arch Dis Child* 2003;**88**:F124–F127.

38 Rela M, Muiesan P, Andreani P, *et al.* Auxiliary liver transplantation for metabolic diseases. *Transplant Proc* 1997;**29**:444–5.

39 Dhawan A, Mitry RR, Hughes RD. Hepatocyte transplantation for liver-based metabolic disorders. *J Inherit Metab Dis* 2006; **29**:431–5.

40 Raper SE, Grossman M, Rader DJ, *et al.* Safety and feasibility of liver-directed ex vivo gene therapy for homozygous familial hypercholesterolaemia. *Ann Surg* 1996;**223**:116–26.

41 Ellis SR, Hulton SA, McKiernan PJ, de Ville de Goyet J, Kelly DA. Combined liver–kidney transplantation for primary hyperoxaluria type 1 in young children. *Nephrol Dial Transplant* 2001;**16**:348–54.

42 Pimpalwar AP, Sharif K, Ramani P, *et al.* Strategy for hepatoblastoma management: transplant versus non-transplant surgery. *J Pediatr Surg* 2002;**37**:240–5.

43 Lilly JR, Starzl TE. Liver transplantation in children with biliary atresia and vascular anomalies. *J Pediatr Surg* 1974;**9**:707–14.

44 Hobeika J, Houssain D, Bernard O, DeVictor D, Grimon J, Chapui Y. Orthotopic liver transplantation in children with chronic liver disease and severe hypoxaemia. *Transplantation* 1995;**57**:224–8.

45 Uemoto S, Vinomarta Y, Tanarka A, *et al.* Living related liver transplantation in children with hypoxaemia related to intrapulmonary shunting. *Transpl Int* 1996;**9**(Suppl 1):S157–9.

46 Wayman KI, Cox KL, Esquivel CO. Neurodevelopmental outcome of young children with extrahepatic biliary atresia 1 year after liver transplantation. *J Pediatr* 1997;**131**:894–8.

47 Hosey MT, Gordon G, Kelly DA, Shaw L. Oral findings in children with liver transplants. *Int J Paediatr Dent* 1995;**5**:29–34.

48 Thomson M, McKiernan P, Buckels J, Mayer D, Kelly D. Generalised mitochondrial cytopathy is an absolute contraindication to orthotopic liver transplantation in childhood. *J Pediatr Gastroenterol Nutr* 1998;**26**:478–81.

49 Roland ME, Stock PG. Liver transplantation in HIV-infected recipients. *Semin Liver Dis* 2006;**26**:273–84.

50 Wali MH, Heydtmann M, Harrison RF, Gunson BK, Mutimer DJ. Outcome of liver transplantation for patients infected by hepatitis C, including those infected by genotype 4. *Liver Transpl* 2003;**9**:796–804.

51 Kano H, Mizuta K, Sakakihara Y, *et al.* Efficacy and safety of immunization for pre- and post-liver transplant children. *Transplantation* 2002;**74**:543–50.

52 Reinoso MA, Sharp HL, Rank J. Endoscopic variceal ligation in pediatric patients with portal hypertension secondary to liver cirrhosis. *Gastrointest Endosc* 1997;**46**:244–6.

53 Johnson SP, Leyendecker JR, Joseph FB, *et al.* Transjugular portosystemic shunts in paediatric patients awaiting liver transplantation. *Transplantation* 1996;**62**:1178–81.

54 Heyman MB, LaBerge JM. Role of transjugular portosystemic shunt in the treatment of portal hypertension in pediatric patients. *J Pediatr Gastroenterol Nutr* 1999;**29**:240–9.

55 Sen S, Mookerjee RP, Davies NA, Williams R, Jalan R. Review article: the Molecular Adsorbents Recirculating System (MARS) in liver failure. *Aliment Pharmacol Ther* 2002;16(Suppl 5):32–8.

56 De Ville de Goyet J, Hausleithner V, Reding R, Lerut J, Janssen M, Otte JB. Impact of innovative techniques on the waiting list and results in paediatric liver transplantation. *Transplantation* 1993;**56**:1130–6.

57 Mirza DF, Achilleos O, Pirrenne J, Buckels JA, McMaster P, Mayer AD. Encouraging results of split-liver transplantation. *Br J Surg* 1998;**85**:494–7.

58 Millis JM, Cronin, DC, Brady LM, *et al.* Primary living-donor liver transplantation at the University of Chicago: technical aspects of the first 104 recipients. *Ann Surg* 2000;**232**:104–11.

59 Broelsch CE, Emond JC, Whitington PF, *et al.* Application of reduced-size liver transplants as split grafts, auxiliary orthotopic grafts and living related segmental transplants. *Ann Surg* 1990; **212**:368–75.

60 Couinaud C. *Le Foie: études anatomiques et chirurgicales.* Paris: Masson, 1957.

61 Bismuth H. Surgical anatomy and anatomical surgery of the liver. *World J Surg* 1982;**6**:3–9.

62 Strong R, Lynch S, Yamanaka J, *et al.* Monosegment liver transplantation. *Surgery* 1995;**118**:904–6.

63 Bismuth H, Houssain D. Reduced size orthotopic liver grafts in hepatic transplantation in children. *Surgery* 1984;**95**:367–70.

64 Kalayoglu M, Stratta RJ, Hoffmann RN, *et al.* Extended preservation of the liver for clinical transplantation. *Lancet* 1988;**i**:617–9.

65 Busuttil RW, Goss JA. Split liver transplantation. *Ann Surg* 1999;**229**:313–21.

66 Feng S, Si M, Taranto S, *et al.* Trends over a decade of pediatric transplantation in the United States. *Liver Transpl* 2006;**12**: 578–84.

67 Pichlmayr R, Ringe B, Gubernatis G, Hauss J, Bunzendahl H. [Transplantation of a donor liver to 2 recipients (splitting transplantation)—a new method in the further development of segmental liver transplantation; in German.] *Langenbecks Arch Chir* 1988;**373**:127–30 .

68 Noujaim HM, Gunson B, Mayer D, *et al.* Ex-situ split liver transplantation. Impact of a new protocol. *Transplantation* 2002;**74**: 1386–90.

69 Noujaim HM, Mayer AD, Buckels JAC, *et al.* Techniques for and outcome of liver transplantation in neonates and infants up to 5 kg of body weight. *J Pediatr Surg* 2000;**37**:159–64.

70 Chardot C, Candinas D, Mirza D, *et al.* Biliary complications after paediatric liver transplantation: Birmingham's experience. *Transpl Int* 1995;**8**:133–40.

71 De Ville de Goyet J, Struye de Swielande Y, Reding R, *et al.* Delayed primary closure of the abdominal wall after cadaveric and living related donor liver graft transplantation in children: a safe and useful technique. *Transpl Int* 1998;**11**:117–22.

72 Broelsch CE, Whitington PF, Emond JC, *et al.* Liver transplantation in children from living related donors. *Ann Surg* 1991; **214**:428–37.

73 Florman S, Miller CM. Liver donor liver transplantation. *Liver Transpl* 2006;**12**:499–510.

74 Renz JF, Kin CJ, Saggi BH, Emond JC. Outcomes of living donor transplantation. In: Busuttil RW, Klintmalm GB, eds. *Transplantation of the Liver*. Philadelphia: Elsevier, 2005: 713–24.

75 Nanashima A, Yamaguchi H, Shibasaki S, *et al.* Comparative analysis of postoperative morbidity according to type and extent of hepatectomy. *Hepatogastroenterology* 2005;**52**:844–8.

76 Emond JC, Renz JF, Ferrel LD, *et al.* Functional analysis of grafts from living donors. Implications for the treatment of older recipients. *Ann Surg* 1996;**224**:544–54.

77 Tanaka K, Uemoto S, Tokunaga Y, *et al.* Liver transplantation in children from living-related donors. *Transplant Proc* 1993;**25**: 1084–6.

78 Roberts J, Hulbert-Shearon TE, Merion RM, *et al.* Influence of graft type on outcomes after pediatric liver transplantation. *Am J Transplant* 2004;**4**:373–7.

79 Boudjema K, Bachellier P, Wolf P, Tempe JD, Jaeck D. Auxiliary liver transplantation and bioartificial bridging procedures in treatment of acute liver failure. *World J Surg* 2002;**26**:264–74.

80 Sudan DL, Langnas AN, Shaw BW Jr. Long-term follow-up of auxiliary liver transplantation for fulminant hepatic failure. *Transplant Proc* 1997;**29**:485–6.

81 Buckels JAC, Tisone G, Gunsen BK, McMaster P. Low haematocrit reduces hepatic artery thrombosis after liver transplantation. *Transplant Proc* 1989;**21**:2460–1.

82 Schuller S, Wiederkehr JC, Coelho-Lemos IM, Avilla SG, Schultz C. Daclizumab induction therapy associated with tacrolimus-MMF has better outcome compared with tacrolimus-MMF alone in pediatric living donor liver transplantation. *Transplant Proc* 2005;**37**:1151–2.

83 Spada M, Petz W, Bertani A, *et al.* Randomized trial of basiliximab induction versus steroid therapy in pediatric liver allograft recipients under tacrolimus immunosuppression. *Am J Transplant* 2006;**6**:1913–21.

84 Aw MM, Brown NW, Itsuka T, *et al.* Mycophenolic acid pharmacokinetics in pediatric liver transplant recipients. *Liver Transpl* 2003;**9**:383–8.

85 Sindhi R, Seward J, Mazariegos G, *et al.* Replacing calcineurin inhibitors with mTOR inhibitors in children. *Pediatr Transplant* 2005;**9**:391–7.

86 Ganschow R, Richter A, Grabhorn E, *et al.* C2 blood concentrations of orally administered cyclosporine in pediatric liver graft recipients with a body weight below 10 kg. *Pediatr Transplant* 2004;**8**:185–8.

87 Kelly D, Jara P, Rodeck B, *et al.* Tacrolimus and steroids versus ciclosporin microemulsion, steroids and azathioprine in children undergoing liver transplantation: randomized multicentre trial. *Lancet* 2004;**364**:1054–61.

88 Evans HM, McKiernan PJ, Kelly DA. Mycophenolate mofetil for renal dysfunction after pediatric liver transplantation. *Transplantation* 2005;**79**:1575–80.

89 Ganschow R, Grabhorn E, Schulz A, Von Hugo A, Rogiers X, Burdelski M. Long-term results of basiliximab induction immunosuppression in pediatric liver transplant recipients. *Pediatr Transplant* 2005;**9**:741–74.

90 Kelly DA. The use of anti-interlukin-2 receptor antibodies in pediatric liver transplantation. *Pediatr Transplant* 2001;**5**:386–9.
91 McAlister VC, Peltekian KM, Malatjalian DA, *et al.* Orthotopic liver transplantation using low-dose tacrolimus and sirolimus. *Liver Transplant* 2001;**7**:401–8.
92 Davison SM, Murphy MS, Adeodu OO, Kelly DA. Impact of cytomegalovirus and Epstein–Barr virus infection in children following liver transplantation. *Gut* 1993;**34**:S32.
93 Dimand EJ, Burchkart G, Concepcion W, Hall RH, Starzl TE. Pharmacodynamics of continuous infusion ranitidine in post-operative pediatric liver transplant patients: intragastric pH, bleeding and metabolic alkalosis. *Gastroenterology* 1989;**96**:A125.
94 Kelly DA. Do H2 receptor antagonists have a therapeutic role in childhood? *J Pediatr Gastroenterol Nutr* 1994;**19**:270–6.
95 Adams DH, Hubscher SG, Burnett D, Elias E. Immunoglobulins in liver allograft rejection: evidence for deposition and secretion within the liver. *Transplant Proc* 1990;**22**:1834–5.
96 Rela M, Muiesan P, Bajtnagar V, *et al.* Hepatic artery thrombosis after liver transplantation in children under 5 years of age. *Transplantation* 1996;**61**:1355–7.
97 Perkins JD. Thrombolysis for early hepatic artery thrombosis: Definitive therapy or diagnostic aid? *Liver Transpl* 2007;**13**:927–31.
98 Murphy MS, Harrison R, Davies P, *et al.* Risk factors for liver rejection: evidence to suggest enhanced allograft tolerance in infancy. *Arch Dis Child* 1996;**75**:502–6.
99 Hubscher S. Diagnosis and grading of liver allograft rejection: a European perspective. *Transplant Proc* 1996;**28**:504–7.
100 Kato T, Selvaggi G, Panagiotis T, *et al.* Pediatric liver transplant with Campath 1H induction—preliminary report. *Transplant Proc* 2006;**38**:3609–11.
101 Lorenz JM, Van Ha T, Funaki B, *et al.* Percutaneous treatment of venous outflow obstruction in pediatric liver transplants. *J Vasc Interv Radiol* 2006;**17**:1753–61.
102 Gray J, Darbyshire PJ, Beath SV, Kelly D, Mann JR. Experience with quinupristin/dalfopristin in treating infections with vancomycin-resistant *Enterococcus faecium* in children. *Pediatr Infect Dis J* 2000;**19**:234–8.
103 Hinchley J, Chaves C, Appingnani B, *et al.* A reversible posterior leukoencephalopathy syndrome. *N Engl J Med* 1996;**334**:494–500.
104 Arora-Gupta N, Davies P, McKiernan P, Kelly DA. The effect of long-term calcineurin inhibitor therapy on renal function in children after liver transplantation. *Pediatr Transplantation* 2004;**8**:145–50.
105 Mellon A, Shepherd RW, Faoagali JL, *et al.* Cytomegalovirus infection after liver transplantation in children. *J Gastroenterol Hepatol* 1993:**8**:540–4.
106 Gane E, Saliba F, Valdecasas GJC, *et al.* Randomised trial of efficacy and safety of oral ganciclovir in the prevention of cytomegalovirus disease in liver-transplant recipients. *Lancet* 1997;**350**:1729–33.
107 Newell KA, Alonso EM, Whitington PF, *et al.* Posttransplant lymphoproliferative disease in paediatric liver transplantation. Interplay between primary Epstein–Barr virus infection and immunosuppression. *Transplantation* 1996;**62**:370–5.
108 Ho M, Jaffe R, Miller G, *et al.* The frequency of Epstein–Barr virus infection and associated lymphoproliferative syndrome after transplantation and its manifestations in children. *Transplantation* 1988;**45**:719–27.
109 Kelly DA, Lloyd C, Jara P, *et al.* Long term follow up of children receiving tacrolimus (tac) or cyclosporin A microemulsion (cya) post liver transplantation. *Pediatr Transplant* 2007;**11**(Suppl 1): 110.
110 Haque T, Wilkie GM, Jones MM, *et al.* Allogeneic cytotoxic T-cell therapy for EBV-positive posttransplantation lymphoproliferative disease: results of a phase 2 multicenter clinical trial. *Blood* 2007;**110**:1123–31.
111 Andrews W, Sommerauer J, Roden J, Andersen J, Conlin C, Moore P. 10 years of pediatric liver transplantation. *J Pediatr Surg* 1996;**31**:619–24.
112 Sudan DL, Shaw BW Jr, Langnas AN. Causes of late mortality in pediatric liver transplant recipients. *Ann Surg* 1998;**227**:289–95.
113 Busuttil RW, Farmer DG, Yersiz H, *et al.* Analysis of long-term outcomes of 3200 liver transplantations over two decades: a single-center experience. *Ann Surg* 2005;**241**:905–16.
114 Hashikura Y, Kawasaki S, Terada M, *et al.* Long-term results of living-related donor liver graft transplantation: a single-center analysis of 110 transplants. *Transplantation* 2001;**72**:95–9.
115 Zitelli BJ, Gartner B, Malatack JJ, *et al.* Pediatric liver transplantation: patient evaluation and selection, infectious complications, and life-style after transplantation. *Transplant Proc* 1987;**19**:3309–16.
116 Ryckman FC, Flake AW, Fisher RA, *et al.* Segmental orthotopic hepatic transplantation as a means to improve patient survival and waiting-list mortality. *J Pediatr Surg* 1991;**26**:422–7.
117 Mekeel KL, Langham MR, Gonzalez-Peralta RP, Hemming AW. Liver transplantation in very small infants. *Pediatr Transplant* 2007;**11**:66–72.
118 Chin SE, Shepherd RW, Cleghorn GJ, *et al.* Survival, growth and quality of life in children after orthotopic liver transplantation: a 5 year experience. *J Paediatr Child Health* 1991;**27**:380–5.
119 Moukarzel AA, Najm I, Vargas J, McDiarmid SV, Busuttil RW, Ament ME. Effect of nutritional status on outcome of orthotopic liver transplantation in paediatric patients. *Transplant Proc* 1990;**22**:1560–3.
120 Rodeck B, Melter M, Kardorff R, *et al.* Liver transplantation in children with chronic end stage liver disease: factors influencing survival after transplantation. *Transplantation* 1996;**62**:1071–6.
121 Martin SR, Atkison P, Anand R, Lindblad AS; SPLIT Research Group. Studies of Pediatric Liver Transplantation 2002: patient and graft survival and rejection in pediatric recipients of a first liver transplant in the United States and Canada. *Pediatr Transplant* 2004;**8**:273–83.
122 Rhee C, Narsinh K, Venick RS, *et al.* Predictors of clinical outcome in children undergoing orthotopic liver transplantation for acute and chronic liver disease. *Liver Transpl* 2006;**12**:1347–56.
123 O'Grady JG, Smith HM, Davies SE, *et al.* Hepatitis B virus reinfection after orthotopic liver transplantation. *J Hepatol* 1992;**14**:104–11.
124 Davies SE, Portman BC, O'Grady JG, *et al.* Hepatic histological findings after transplantation for chronic hepatitis B virus infection, including a unique pattern of fibrosing cholestatic hepatitis. *Hepatology* 1991;**13**:150–7.
125 Nowicki MJ, Ahmad N, Heubi JE, Kuramoto IK, Baroudy BM, Balistreri WF. The prevalence of hepatitis C virus (HCV)

in infants and children after liver transplantation. *Dig Dis Sci* 1994;**39**:2250–4.
126 Pastore M, Willems M, Cornu C, *et al.* Role of hepatitis C virus in chronic liver disease occurring after orthotopic liver transplantation. *Arch Dis Child* 1995;**72**:403–7.
127 Belli LS, Burroughs AK, Burra P, *et al.* Liver transplantation for HCV cirrhosis: improved survival in recent years and increased severity of recurrent disease in female recipients: results of a long term retrospective study. *Liver Transpl* 2007;**13**:733–40.
128 Birnbaum AH, Benkov KJ, Pittman NS, McFarlane-Ferreira Y, Rosh JR, LeLeiko NS. Recurrence of autoimmune hepatitis in children after liver transplantation. *J Pediatr Gastroenterol Nutr* 1997;**25**:20–5.
129 Horsmans Y, Galant C, Nicholas ML, Lamy M, Geubel AP. Failure of ribavirin or immunosuppressive therapy to alter the course of post-infantile giant-cell hepatitis. *J Hepatol* 1995;**22**: 382.
130 Achilleos QA, Buist LJ, Kelly DA, *et al.* Unresectable hepatic tumors in childhood and the role of liver transplantation. *J Pediatr Surg* 1996;**31**:1563–7.
131 Austin MT, Leys CM, Feurer ID, *et al.* Liver transplantation for childhood hepatic malignancy: a review of the United Network for Organ Sharing (UNOS) database. *Pediatr Surg* 2006;**41**: 182–6.
132 Kerkar N, Hadzi N, Davies ET, *et al.* De-novo autoimmune hepatitis after liver transplantation. *Lancet* 1998;**351**:409–13.
133 Andries S, Casamayou L, Sempoux C, *et al.* Posttransplant immune hepatitis in pediatric liver transplant recipients: incidence and maintenance therapy with azathioprine. *Transplantation* 2001;**72**:267–72.
134 Evans HM, Kelly DA, McKiernan PJ, Hubscher S. Progressive histological damage in liver allografts following pediatric liver transplantation. *Hepatology* 2006;**43**:1109–17.
135 Salcedo M, Vaquero J, Banares R, *et al.* Response to steroids in de novo autoimmune hepatitis after liver transplantation. *Hepatology* 2002;**35**:349–56.
136 Berg UB, Ericzon BG, Nemeth A. Renal function before and long after liver transplantation in children. *Transplantation* 2001; **27**:561–2.
137 Bartosh SM, Alonso EM, Whitington PF. Renal outcomes in pediatric liver transplantation. *Clin Transplant* 1997;**11**:354–60.
138 Reyes J, Jain A, Mazariegos G, *et al.* Long-term results after conversion from cyclosporine to tacrolimus in pediatric liver transplantation for acute and chronic rejection. *Transplantation* 2000;**69**:2578–80.
139 Ghali MP, Talwalkar JA, Moore SB, Hogan WJ, Menon KV, Rosen CB. Acute graft-versus-host disease after liver transplantation. *Transplantation* 2007;**83**:365–6.
140 Taylor RM, Bockenstedt P, Su GL, Marrero JA, Pellitier SM, Fontana RJ. Immune thrombocytopenic purpura following liver transplantation: a case series and review of the literature. *Liver Transpl* 2006;**12**:781–91.
141 Riordan SM, Williams R. Tolerance after liver transplantation: does it exist and can immunosuppression be withdrawn. *J Hepatol* 1999;**31**:1106–19.
142 Ganschow R, Broering DC, Nolkempter D, *et al.* Th2 cytokine profile in infants predisposes to improved graft acceptance after liver transplantation. *Transplantation* 2001;**72**:929–34.
143 Kelly DA. Organ transplantation for inherited metabolic disease. *Arch Dis Child* 1994;**71**:181–3.
144 Gissen P, Chakrapani A, Wraith JE, *et al.* Long-term survival post early liver transplantation in organic acidemias. *Hepatology* 2001:**34**:503A.
145 Chakrapani A, Sivakumar P, McKiernan PJ, Leonard JV. Metabolic stroke in methylmalonic acidemia five years after liver transplantation. *J Pediatr* 2002;**140**:261–3.
146 Rodeck B, Melter M, Hoyer PF, Ringe B, Brodehi J. Growth in long-term survivors after orthotopic liver transplantation in childhood. *Transplant Proc* 1994;**26**:165–6.
147 Holt RI, Broide E, Buchanan CR, *et al.* Orthotopic liver transplantation reverses the adverse nutritional changes of end-stage liver disease in children. *Am J Clin Nutr* 1997;**65**:534–42.
148 Viner RM, Forton JTM, Cole TJ, Clark IH, Nobel-Jamieson G, Barnes ND. Growth of long term survivors of liver transplantation. *Arch Dis Child* 1999;**80**:235–40.
149 Codoner-Franch P, Bernard O, Alvarez F. Long-term follow-up of growth in height after successful liver transplantation. *J Pediatr* 1994;**124**:368–73.
150 Reding R, Webber SA, Fine R. Getting rid of steroids in pediatric solid-organ transplantation? *Pediatr Transplant* 2004;**8**: 526–30.
151 Sarna S, Siplia I, Vihervuori E, Koistinen R, Holmberg C. Growth delay after liver transplantation in childhood: studies of underlying mechanisms. *Pediatr Res* 1995;**38**:366–72.
152 Dunn SP, Falkenstein K, Lawrence JP, *et al.* Monotherapy with cyclosporine for chronic immunosuppression in pediatric liver transplant recipients. *Transplantation* 1994;**57**:544–7.
153 Cardona A, Houssin D, Gauthier F, *et al.* Liver transplantation in children with Alagille's syndrome—a study of 12 cases. *Transplantation* 1995;**60**:339–42.
154 Kelly DA. Posttransplant growth failure in children. *Liver Transplant Surg* 1997;**3**:1–9.
155 Stewart SM, Uauy R, Waller D, Kennard BD, Benser M, Andrews WS. Mental and motor development, social competence, and growth one year after successful pediatric liver transplantation. *J Pediatr* 1989;**114**:574–81.
156 Stone RD, Beasley PJ, Treacy SJ, Twente AW, Vacanti JP. Children and families can achieve normal psychological adjustment and a good quality of life following pediatric liver transplantation: a long-term study. *Transplant Proc* 1997;**29**:1571–2.
157 Krull K, Fuchs C, Yurk H, Boone P, Alonso E. Neurocognitive outcome in pediatric liver transplant recipients. *Pediatr Transplant* 2003;**7**:111–8.
158 Molmenti E, Mazariegos G, Bueno J, *et al.* Noncompliance after pediatric liver transplantation. *Transplant Proc* 1999;**31**:408.
159 McDonagh JE, Kelly DA. Transitioning care of the pediatric recipient to adult caregivers. *Pediatr Clin North Am* 2003;**50**: 1561–83, xi–xii.
160 Fredericks EM, Lopez MJ, Magee JC, Shieck V, Opipari-Arrigan L. Psychological functioning, nonadherence and health outcomes after pediatric liver transplantation. *Am J Transplant* 2007;**7**: 1974–83.
161 Dobbels F, van Damme-Lombaert R, Vanhaecke J, De Geest S. Growing pains: non-adherence with the immunosuppressive regimen in adolescent transplant recipients. *Pediatr Transplant* 2005;**9**:381–90.

162 Armenti VT. Pregnancy after liver transplantation. *Liver Transpl* 2006;**12**:1037–9.

163 Laifer SA, Guido RS. Reproductive function and outcome of pregnancy after liver transplantation in women. *Mayo Clin Proc* 1995;**70**:388–94.

164 Sucato GS, Murray PJ. Developmental and reproductive health issues in adolescent solid organ transplant recipients. *Semin Pediatr Surg* 2006;**15**:170–8.

165 Rodrigue JR, MacNaughton K, Hoffman RG III, *et al.* Perceptions of parenting stress and family relations by fathers of children evaluated for organ transplantation. *Psychol Rep* 1996;**79**:723–7.

166 Sundaram SS, Landgraf JM, Neighbors K, Cohn RA, Alonso EM. Adolescent health-related quality of life following liver and kidney transplantation. *Am J Transplant* 2007;**7**:982–9.

167 Bucuvalas JC, Alonso E. Outcome after liver transplantation: more than just survival rates. *Liver Transpl* 2005;**11**:7–9.

168 Avitzur Y, De Luca E, Cantos M, *et al.* Health status ten years after pediatric liver transplantation-looking beyond the graft. *Transplantation* 2004;**78**:566–73.

169 Rosenthal P, Emond JC, Heyman MB, *et al.* Pathological changes in yearly protocol liver biopsy specimens from healthy pediatric liver recipients. *Liver Transplant Surg* 1997;**6**:559–62.

170 Davison SE, Skidmore SJ, Collingham KE, Irving WL, Hubscher SG, Kelly DA. Chronic hepatitis in children after liver transplantation: role of hepatitis C virus and hepatitis G virus infections. *J Hepatol* 1998;**28**:764–70.

171 Kelly DA. Current issues in pediatric transplantation. *Pediatr Transplant* 2006;**10**:712–20.

172 Samyn M, Cheeseman P, Bevis L, *et al.* Cystatin C, an easy and reliable marker for assessment of renal dysfunction in children with liver disease and after liver transplantation. *Liver Transpl* 2005;**11**:344–9.

173 Lee WS, John P, McKiernan P, de Ville de Goyet J, Kelly DA. Inferior vena cava occlusion and protein-losing enteropathy after liver transplantation in children. *J Pediatr Gastroenterol Nutr* 2002;**34**:413–6.

22 Small-Bowel Transplantation in Children

Jorge Reyes

Introduction

Organ transplantation in children has been successful and clinically applicable for over 50 years in organs such as the liver, kidney, and heart. Successful transplantation of the intestine, however, remained difficult because of the need to provide sufficient immunosuppression to prevent rejection without creating untreatable clinical circumstances such as overwhelming infection and disabling drug toxicity. The intestinal allograft did not fit the paradigm that had been defined for other organs and experimentally tested in dogs by Lillehei *et al.* in 1959[1] and Starzl and Kaupp in 1960.[2] Although these studies served as technical centerpieces for intra-abdominal transplant procedures that involved more than one organ, the predicted cellular events of rejection and also potentially graft-versus-host disease (GVHD) were poorly understood.

Early experience with cyclosporine immunosuppression was largely unsuccessful,[3–7] although it was notable that transplantation of the intestine in combination with a liver allograft appeared to reduce rejection.[3,8,9] Until 1990, only the isolated intestine recipient reported by Goulet *et al.* and a living related donor intestinal segment transplanted by Deltz *et al.* had survived.[10,11] The introduction of the immunosuppressant tacrolimus (previously FK-506) into clinical transplantation significantly improved survival,[12] although the postoperative course remains complex and the long-term outcomes are still unraveling (Figure 22.1).

Advances in clinical surgery and immunosuppressive management over the last 17 years have made human intestinal transplantation a clinical reality. In this chapter, we will examine the basis of successful clinical pediatric intestinal and liver transplantations, which are a result of advances in the following principles:

- Indications for transplantation
- Surgical technique
- Advances in immunosuppression
- Induction of donor-specific nonreactivity

Diseases of the Liver and Biliary System in Children, 3rd edition. Edited by Deirdre Kelly. © 2008 Blackwell Publishing, ISBN: 978-1-4051-6334-7.

Indications

Successful intestinal transplantation has changed the outcome for many children who develop complications from total parenteral nutrition (TPN). Table 22.1 summarizes the diagnoses by cause that distribute patients by age, risk for early or late mortality, and outcome after transplantation. A multidisciplinary approach to intestinal failure in the setting of an intestinal transplant program can facilitate the identification and management of serious medical and surgical problems which allows appropriate selection of candidates and the optimum transplant procedure. Most large pediatric gastrointestinal units which manage 10–15 home parenteral nutrition patients per year can expect that up to five patients will develop a serious complication meriting assessment for small-bowel transplantation, one or two of whom may then be listed for small-bowel transplantation.[13] Optimization of TPN and enteral management may stabilize patients' clinical syndromes and in some patients may lead to resolution of cholestasis and independence from TPN, thus avoiding transplantation. Optimization strategies in children are best guided by the ability to achieve growth and development.

Indications for intestinal transplantation

The introduction of TPN in 1969 dramatically improved the outcome for children with short-bowel syndrome,[14] but long-term outcome is related to the rate of intestinal adaptation and the development of TPN complications. Intestinal transplantation, either alone or as a composite graft with other intra-abdominal organs, is indicated for children with irreversible intestinal failure who develop life-threatening complications related to direct toxicity of TPN or the catheters needed to infuse it.

Causes of intestinal failure (Table 22.1)

Intestinal failure is defined as gastrointestinal disease that leads to failure to maintain a sufficient fluid, electrolyte, and nutritional status that leads to dependency on TPN.

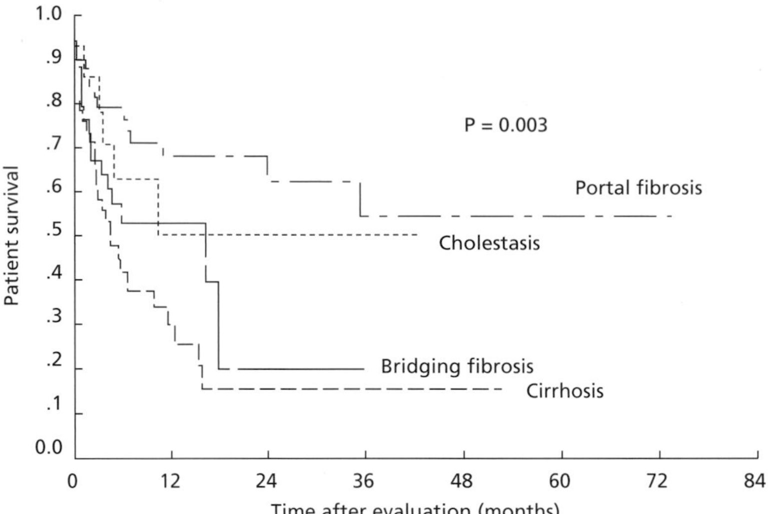

Figure 22.1 Kaplan–Meier survival curve according to histopathology on liver biopsies from 161 patients referred for intestinal transplant evaluation. Bridging fibrosis (n = 37) and cirrhosis (n = 48) had similar clinical behavior and warrant liver replacement in the face of persistent jaundice and coagulopathy. (Reproduced with permission from Bueno *et al.*[39])

Table 22.1 Causes of intestinal failure requiring intestinal transplantation in children.

Surgical short gut, as a consequence of:
Congenital malformations
Necrotizing enterocolitis (NEC)
Trauma
Volvulus
Intestinal atresia
Gastroschisis*
Intestinal dysmotility
Intestinal pseudo-obstruction
Intestinal aganglionosis (Hirschsprung disease)
Enterocyte absorptive impairment
Microvillus inclusion disease
Autoimmune or idiopathic enteropathy
Tumors
Familial polyposis
Inflammatory pseudotumor

*Gastroschisis may be associated with intestinal atresia, volvulus, NEC, or vascular occlusion.

Surgical causes. The commonest cause of intestinal failure in childhood is the short-bowel syndrome, due to surgical correction of congenital defects such as gastroschisis, midgut volvulus, intestinal atresia, or surgery for necrotizing enterocolitis (Table 22.1). Patients with gastroschisis may have intestinal dysmotility in association with their abdominal wall defect.

The capacity for intestinal adaptation is influenced by the length and type of residual small bowel (whether it is ileum or jejunum), the site of intestinal resection, the presence or absence of the ileocecal valve, the length of remaining colon, and the age of the patient. In clinical practice, the minimum length of intestine necessary for adaptation is difficult to establish because of inadequacies in assessing bowel length following resection and the subsequent development of dysmotility, inflammation, and shortening of the remaining bowel. The presence of an ileocecal valve is crucial for adaptation, as it may reduce bacterial overgrowth and improve function.[15,16] In general, ileum adapts better than jejunum. Adaptation may be improved by enteral supplementation, utilization of oral glutamine,[17–20] and growth hormone.[21]

Functional causes. Functional causes for intestinal failure include disorders of motility—e.g., chronic intestinal pseudo-obstruction (CIP), Hirschsprung disease and aganglionosis; or mucosal disorders such as microvillous inclusion disease and protracted diarrhea of unknown cause.

In CIP, patients present at birth or in the first year of life with signs and symptoms of intestinal obstruction without an anatomical cause. The disorder may be secondary to neuropathic or myopathic dysfunction.[22] Abdominal distension and constipation are common symptoms. Many patients with the neuropathic form have severe abdominal pain and become narcotic-dependent. Patients with the myopathic form are at risk of spontaneous intestinal perforation, megacystis/megaureter with consequent repeated urinary tract infections, and eventual renal dysfunction. Hirschsprung disease may rarely present with extensive jejunoileal involvement; since surgical procedures for this extensive form are generally unsuccessful, intestine transplantation may be the only treatment.[23]

Microvillus inclusion disease is an autosomal-recessive disorder characterized by the combination of hypoplastic villous atrophy, in which the apical surface enterocytes contain vesicles with microvilli and secretory granules.[24] Eighty per cent of children die in infancy from malabsorption and malnutrition without TPN. Long-term survivors are dependent on TPN.

Intestinal tumors. Unlike adult practice, malignancy is an unusual cause of intestinal failure. Diffuse intestinal polyposis requiring extensive surgery is occasionally encountered.

Complications of TPN

Parenteral nutrition permits children with intestinal failure to survive for many years, but is associated with a number of life-threatening complications. These include catheter sepsis, metabolic disorders, loss of venous access from extensive venous thrombosis (Figure 22.2), pulmonary embolism, and the development of TPN-induced liver dysfunction,[25–27] now termed "intestinal failure–associated liver disease" (IFALD).

By far the most severe complication induced by TPN is cholestatic liver disease, IFALD, which varies in frequency depending on age, the etiology of intestinal failure, the duration of TPN use, and associated complications such as infection.[28] This complication is more common in children than in adults on TPN, especially in neonates who have suffered extensive loss of their intestine due to necrotizing enterocolitis or intestinal atresias. Many studies have noted that IFALD is more common in premature or low-birth-weight infants, which may be related to the immaturity of the neonatal liver.[29] There is both diminished hepatic uptake and synthesis of bile salts and a reduced enterohepatic circulation.[30] Inability to establish enteral feeding is common in children requiring parenteral nutrition, and TPN liver disease is more likely to develop in those children who are unable to tolerate any enteral feeding.[31] Prolonged fasting leads to a reduction in the secretion of gastric inhibitory polypeptide (GIP) and vasoactive intestinal polypeptide (VIP), which when combined with reduced gastrin catabolism results in increased serum gastrin and gastric hypersecretion, leading to intestinal stasis, reduction in gallbladder contractility, and decreased exocrine pancreatic secretion.[32] Intestinal stasis may lead to bacterial overgrowth, bacterial translocation, and sepsis. The reduction in cholecystokinin release may influence gallbladder size and contractility and cause the development of biliary sludge and gallstones.[33] TPN liver disease is more common in neonates with recurrent episodes of sepsis, which may be related to either central line infections or bacterial translocation, with release of endotoxin into the portal vein circulation.[34]

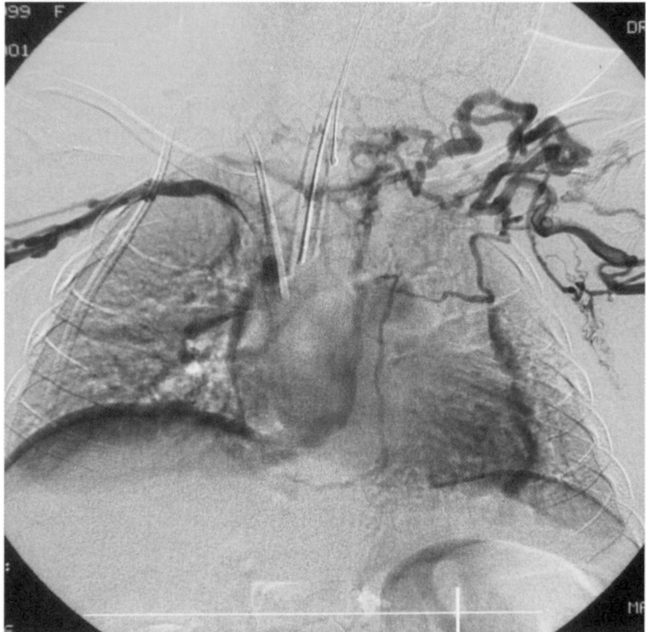

Figure 22.2 Chronic venous occlusion secondary to central venous lines is a common complication of total parental nutrition (TPN). This bilateral arm venogram shows occlusion of the left axillary, left subclavian, and left innominate veins, with a stenosis of the right subclavian vein. There is a right internal jugular vein tunneled central line, with its tip in the superior vena cava. Lack of venous access for TPN is an indication for small-intestinal transplantation.

It is possible that hepatotoxicity may be related to the components of TPN, and a variety of precipitating factors have been suggested, such as the excessive provision of protein and carbohydrates, glycine, alanine, tryptophan, and flavonoids, associated with relative deficiencies in selenium, tocopherol, and taurine.[35,36] Hypermagnesemia has been reported in children with TPN cholestasis related to excessive manganese supplementation,[37] suggesting that manganese toxicity exacerbates cholestasis in children with established liver disease. The end result is a disruption of bile flow and bile acid metabolism, sequestration of bile in the gallbladder, and tenacious bile in the biliary system.[38]

Histology. The early histological changes are related to centrilobular cholestasis without inflammation, necrosis, or fatty infiltration. Steatosis is relatively uncommon in infants, but is secondary to hepatic accumulation of lipid or glycogen. More advanced liver disease includes portal fibrosis, pericellular fibrosis, and bile ductular proliferation. Patients with more severe pathological damage to the liver will have a higher mortality rate (Figure 22.3).[39]

Clinical features of IFALD. Clinical jaundice is a sensitive indicator of ongoing liver damage, although bilirubin may improve with treatment of sepsis or intestinal adaptation. Persistently elevated bilirubin (> 100 μmol/L) carries a high 1-year mortality and is an indication for transplantation.[40] Splenomegaly may develop early and is helpful in staging hepatic fibrosis. Clinical evidence of portal hypertension (history of bleeding esophageal varices, hepatosplenomegaly and ascites) suggests irreversible liver disease. The use of endoscopic ultrasound, which detects submucosal esophageal and gastric varices, may be helpful in staging the disease and in making the choice between isolated intestinal and combined liver and bowel disease (see Chapter 2).

Management of TPN and liver disease. The loss of different sections of the gastrointestinal tract leads to differing clinical

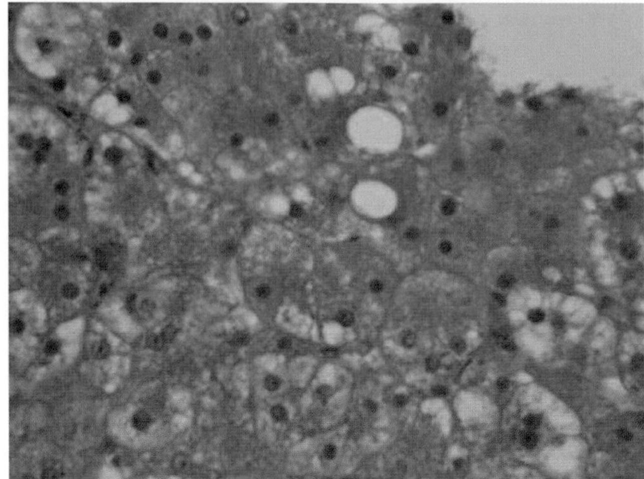

A

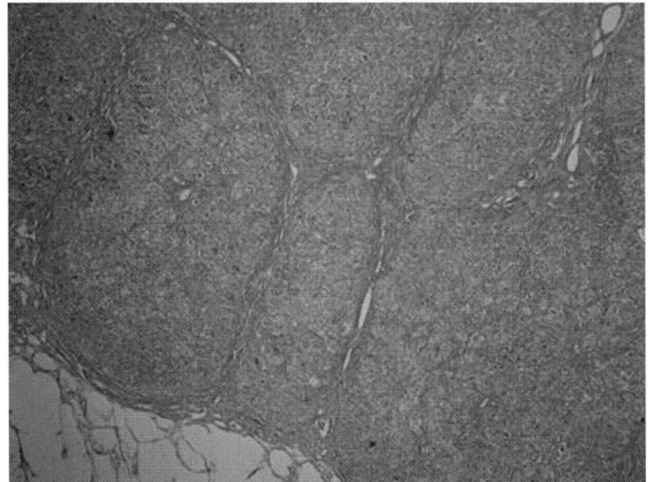

B

Figure 22.3 Severe total parenteral nutrition cholestasis is an indication for a liver or combined liver and intestinal transplant. The early histological changes are related to centrilobular cholestasis without inflammation, necrosis or fatty infiltration (**A**), but the development of perivenular fibrosis and cirrhosis indicates advanced intestinal failure–associated liver disease (IFALD) (**B**).

syndromes and management problems. Malabsorption of minerals and folic acid is common with duodenal resections, while protein and carbohydrate malabsorption are major problems with jejunal resections. Disruption of the enterohepatic circulation of bile salts with malabsorption of vitamin B_{12} occurs with ileal resection. The reduction in intestinal transit time, in association with malabsorption of carbohydrate, may precipitate fermentation and small-bowel bacterial overgrowth syndrome[41–44] and may cause steatorrhea with saponification of luminal ionized calcium and excessive free oxalate absorption by the colon, leading to hyperoxaluria and the development of oxalate urolithiasis.

IFALD is potentially reversible if TPN is discontinued before the development of severe fibrosis of cirrhosis,[45] although this is not an option for children with irreversible intestinal failure, from mucosal causes (e.g., microvillous atrophy) or functional causes (e.g., pseudo-obstruction). In children with a short gut from neonatal surgery, the aim is to reduce cholestasis by encouraging intestinal adaptation, thus achieving independence from TPN and avoiding transplantation. It is critical to begin early use of the remaining gut, and also to consider surgical procedures aimed at improving surface area.[46] Procedures such as longitudinal intestinal lengthening[47] and serial transverse enteroplasty[48] may be indicated in some patients with remaining small bowel, if they have not developed significant liver disease.[49]

Hepatic dysfunction may be reduced by the introduction of enteral feeding, which may encourage normal biliary dynamics, improve bile flow, and reduce intestinal stasis and bacterial overgrowth. The use of modular feeds given continuously initially, in increasing volumes, is useful for bowel adaptation in patients with the short-bowel syndrome, and may be used in association with codeine and/or loperamide to increase transit times. Bile flow and the formation of biliary sludge may be improved using oral ursodeoxycholic acid (10–20 mg/kg).[50,51]

It is important to prevent sepsis, particularly catheter sepsis, and bacterial overgrowth using oral decontamination therapy.[52] The addition of glutamine to TPN solutions may improve gut immunity and intestinal adaptation. Other strategies used include cycling of TPN,[53] selective bowel decontamination,[54] and the use of intravenous cholecystokinin.[55] Innovative bowel tapering and lengthening surgery has successfully improved the motility of previously dilated segments of bowel.[49] This improvement in function together with an increase in the surface area of the intestine may allow sufficient adaptation for TPN to be discontinued.[56,57]

In children with an adequate length of small bowel and/or an ileocecal valve in whom there is potential for further intestinal adaptation, an isolated liver transplant may be preferred to a combined liver and intestinal transplant.[57,58]

Vascular access. Vascular access and infectious problems are the next TPN-induced complications, and are a consequence of the need for lifelong venous catheterization. In practical terms, venous accessibility is limited to six sites—the pairs of internal jugular, subclavian, and iliac veins. The loss of 50% of these sites warrants consideration for intestinal transplantation. Likewise, patients presenting life-threatening catheter sepsis with metastatic infections, unusual pathogens, or multisystem organ failure should be referred for intestinal transplantation.[59]

Evaluation for transplantation (Table 22.2)

Children referred for intestinal transplantation generally have complex medical, surgical, and social histories. A thorough multidisciplinary evaluation is required, including:

Table 22.2 Evaluation of pediatric small-bowel transplantation candidates.

Intestinal assessment
Anatomy of remaining bowel
Upper and lower gastrointestinal barium studies
Motility studies
Histology of bowel
Hepatic assessment
Bilirubin, alkaline phosphatase, aspartate aminotransferase (AST)
Albumin
α-Fetoprotein
Prothrombin time, partial thromboplastin time
Liver ultrasound for hepatic vessels
Liver histology (when indicated)
Vascular access
Doppler ultrasound for patency of central veins
Nutritional evaluation
Weight, height, triceps, skinfold, mid-arm circumference
Transferrin, albumin, prealbumin, serum amino acid analysis
Vitamins A, D, E, B_{12}, thiamine
Triglycerides
General
Full blood count
Blood type (ABO), tissue typing, cross-matching
Blood urea nitrogen (BUN), serum creatinine
Chest radiograph
Echocardiogram, electrocardiogram
Ventilation/perfusion scan (if indicated)
Investigations for infection
Blood, urine, throat, feces, ascites culture: bacterial, fungal, viral, hepatitis screen, cytomegalovirus, Epstein–Barr virus
Quantitative stool cultures

- Confirmation of the cause and extent of intestinal failure
- Potential for intestinal adaptation and medical or surgical intervention
- identification of other organ dysfunction, such as cardiac, pulmonary, or central nervous system

Intestinal assessment

Confirmation of diagnosis

It is essential to confirm the diagnosis in patients with motility disorders or mucosal lesions by reviewing the patient's history and radiographic and histological findings. There may be considerable variation in the extent of gastrointestinal tract involvement and manometric findings in patients with CIP. Thus, functional assessment of the entire gastrointestinal tract (including the esophagus) is critical in the selection of the appropriate intestinal graft.[60]

Patients with extensive long-segment Hirschsprung disease require a thorough review of all pathological material prior to transplantation to establish the extent of the disease, with further examination of intraoperative frozen-section samples of residual intestine at the time of transplantation.

Intestinal tract anatomy is assessed by barium studies to ascertain continuity, deformities, or gross functional abnormalities.

The length of bowel in patients with short-bowel syndrome is estimated as far as possible, identifying the length of ileum and jejunum, the presence or absence of the ileocecal valve, and any evidence of dysmotility.

Intestinal function

The best test of intestinal function is tolerance to enteral feeds, and it is therefore important to obtain a good feeding history in order to establish whether there is any potential for adaptation or medical therapy.

Assessment of motility can be carried out by:

- Carmine red marker transit time (normal > 6 h).
- Technetium-labeled gastric emptying (normal < 4 h).
- Intestinal manometry.
- In patients with dysmotility syndromes, it may be useful to measure the response to prokinetic drugs such as domperidone, metoclopramide, cisapride, or erythromycin. Children with significant dysmotility are unlikely to adapt easily.

Absorption studies that include xylose absorption are rarely performed, but measurement of stool electrolytes, reducing substances, and steatocrit may be helpful in assessing the severity of mucosal disease.

It is essential to assess the potential for adaptation in patients with short-gut syndrome by:

- Encouraging either continuous or bolus enteral feeds.
- Treating bacterial overgrowth with antibiotics (amoxicillin and metronidazole).
- Addition of glutamine to TPN or enteral feeds.[20]
- Consideration of growth hormone therapy.[21]
- Consideration of corrective surgery in children with short gut; reestablishing continuity of bowel or bowel lengthening may improve intestinal function. Patients with "extreme short gut," defined as resection of more than 80% of the small bowel, including the ileocecal valve, are unlikely to adapt and should be considered early for transplantation.

Hepatic function

Most children who are referred for intestinal transplantation will have some hepatic dysfunction. The assessment of hepatic function is critical in establishing whether the patient requires an isolated intestinal transplant or a combined liver/intestinal transplant, as well as determining preoperative and postoperative morbidity.

Persistently elevated bilirubin (> 100 μmol/L) carries a high 1-year mortality and is an indication for transplantation if persistent.[40] Splenomegaly may develop early and is helpful in staging hepatic fibrosis. Clinical evidence of portal hypertension (history of bleeding esophageal varices, hepatosplenomegaly, and ascites) suggests irreversible liver disease and the need for liver transplantation with or without intestinal transplantation. The emerging use of endoscopic ultrasound may detect submucosal varices and aid in this decision (see Chapter 2).

The assessment should include:

- Biochemical liver function tests.
- Coagulation profile.
- Serum albumin.
- Liver histology, to establish the severity and extent of hepatic fibrosis or cirrhosis and also to exclude other potential liver diseases such as viral hepatitis (Figure 22.3).
- Upper gastrointestinal endoscopy, to establish the presence of varices or portal gastropathy.
- Doppler ultrasound studies of splanchnic venous anatomy, including the portal vein, splenic vein, hepatic veins, and inferior vena cava, are performed routinely, since the patency of these vessels may modify the operative procedure.
- The presence of gallstones and common duct stones can be established by ultrasound, magnetic resonance cholangiography (MRC), or endoscopic retrograde cholangiography.

Vascular access

Vascular access should be assessed by ultrasound to confirm patency of the internal jugular, subclavian, and iliac veins, with venography as required (Figure 22.2).

General assessment

Nutritional and developmental status is established as for liver transplantation (Chapter 21).

All patients are screened for active bacterial or fungal infection and previous exposure to cytomegalovirus (CMV) and Epstein–Barr virus (EBV). Immunological deficiencies are assessed when clinically indicated.

Cardiac assessment includes electrocardiography and echocardiography to exclude cardiomyopathy or evidence of previous pulmonary embolism. A ventilation/perfusion scan is occasionally required.

Psychological assessment

Small-bowel transplantation remains a complex procedure with an unknown long-term prognosis, and it is important that both child and family are appraised of the risks and complications of this procedure in order to make an informed decision. Psychological preparation of the child is paramount and should include preparation for a stoma and ileostomy (see Chapter 24).

On completion of the assessment, the decision will be made whether the child requires an isolated small-bowel transplant or combined liver and small-bowel transplantation, or in rare cases an isolated liver transplant only. The indications for isolated small-bowel transplantation include:

- Irreversible intestinal failure with expected long-term dependence on parenteral nutrition
- Loss of vascular access, with normal liver function and histology
- Mild to moderate hepatic fibrosis (grade 1–3) with normal hepatic synthesis
- Intractable gastrointestinal fluid loss

The current indications for combined small-bowel/liver transplantation are:

- Irreversible liver disease secondary to IFALD
- Loss of vascular access, with evidence of significant hepatic disease
- Inborn errors of liver metabolism leading to small-bowel failure (e.g., protein C or S deficiency)

Liver-only transplantation in children with intestinal failure is only indicated in children with surgical short gut who are considered to have the potential for intestinal adaptation, but have irreversible liver failure.[61] These patients are usually premature infants with surgical short bowel and are at a high risk of developing liver disease as a consequence of early bacterial overgrowth and sepsis, and metabolic disorders.[62]

Contraindications for small-bowel transplantation

The current contraindications include:

- Uncontrolled sepsis or malignancy elsewhere in the body
- Severe cerebral, cardiac or respiratory disease.

Human immunodeficiency virus (HIV) infection is no longer a contraindication for transplantation, with the development of effective antiviral drugs. There are no age or size limitations, although in practice infants weighing < 5 kg rarely undergo transplantation because of the lack of similar-sized small donors.

Timing of transplantation

As quality of life may be acceptable for many children maintained on parenteral nutrition, the timing of this operation may be difficult. Furthermore, the difficulty in obtaining suitable age-matched and size-matched donors for small children means a lengthy wait for a suitable organ in Europe (although this is not so in the United States). Between 37% and 50% of patients have died while awaiting small-bowel transplantation,[13,63] although newer techniques, such as the use of reduced grafts, have significantly reduced the waiting time and the mortality (from 60% to 14%).[64] Children with surgical short-gut syndrome and those with a high plasma bilirubin at the time of evaluation have the shortest duration of survival,[13,39] and this high risk has been substantiated by the high mortality on the organ transplant waiting list with the United Network for Organ Sharing (UNOS).[65] Children with a falling platelet count and increasing splenomegaly also have a poor prognosis.[60] Referral should therefore proceed whenever there is the development of persistent jaundice, a falling platelet count, or significant vascular access complications.

Preoperative management

Management of patients awaiting small-bowel transplantation requires careful attention to the prevention of sepsis, maintenance of nutrition, and prevention and management of vascular and hepatic complications.

Sepsis rates may be reduced by aseptic catheter techniques and by the use of selective bowel contamination (polymyxin B, gentamicin, and amphotericin administered orally). TPN protocols may need modification to ensure adequate nutrition for growth and to overcome hepatic catabolism. Tolerance to oral intake is crucial, since this can affect post-transplantation nutritional management. Children should be stimulated to eat before transplantation, even if no nutritional benefit is gained, as this encourages developmental progress for eating and swallowing. Prevention of vascular thrombosis is difficult and the use of anticoagulation is not universally accepted.

Liver failure in the setting of intestinal failure has an ominous prognosis and a significant 1-year mortality secondary to infection, bleeding, and encephalopathy.[39] Because such children have a high mortality rate, it is essential that intestinal failure patients should be referred for assessment once identified.

Hepatic complications should be managed as described in Chapters 15, 19, and 21. Cholestatic patients should be treated with ursodeoxycholic acid (10–20 mg/kg) and supplemented with adequate fat-soluble vitamins parenterally. Bleeding esophageal varices are treated with sclerotherapy or banding, but the majority of these patients will bleed from portal gastropathy, which can be controlled with continuous infusion of somatostatin (octreotide) or oral losartan, an angiotensin II receptor antagonist (2 mg/kg/day; usually 25–50 mg/day), may be effective in reducing portal pressure and bleeding (see Chapters 15 and 19). The use of transjugular intrahepatic portosystemic shunts (TIPS) is rarely indicated. Hypersplenism with severe thrombocytopenia may have a transient response to splenic artery embolization.

The transplant procedure

Selection of donors

Grafts for intestinal transplantation are obtained for ABO-identical brain-dead donors from neonates to age 55 years. Donors with a history of prolonged cardiopulmonary arrest or significant inotrope requirement should be avoided, as this may result in significant bowel ischemia. Donors with malignancy are excluded, but those with systemic viral or bacterial infection in the absence of an identifiable thoracic or abdominal source are acceptable. Matching with human leukocyte antigen (HLA) is unnecessary. CMV-positive donors are only considered for transplantation into CMV-positive recipients unless the patient is dying from liver failure. CMV-negative patients awaiting isolated intestinal grafts should only receive organs from CMV-negative donors. Graft pretreatment to deplete the lymphoid population of the intestinal allograft with either irradiation or a monoclonal antibody—such as OKT3 (muromonab-CD3) or antithymocyte globulin—as prophylaxis for GVHD is performed in some centers.[66]

Ideally, donors should be of similar size to the recipient. However, reductions of intestinal and liver/intestine allografts may be necessary because of the prolonged wait for age-matched and size-matched donors.

Donor operation

The procurement of abdominal visceral organs, either *en bloc* or as separate components, is similar to a large cluster of grapes with a double central stem consisting of the celiac axis and superior mesenteric arteries (Figure 22.4).[67] The separate grape clusters represent the different abdominal organs, which include the liver, stomach, duodenum, pancreas, small intestine, and colon. These can be removed or retained according to the clinical needs of the recipient, with preservation of the double arterial stem structures in the larger composite grafts, which include the complete multivisceral, modified multivisceral, liver/small-bowel, and modified liver/small-bowel allografts. In the isolated small-bowel allograft, only the superior mesenteric artery stem is retained.

The procurement technique focuses on simple isolation and cooling of the organs to be transplanted, with preservation of the vascular and parenchymal anatomy.[68] This procedure has been simplified using a limited hilar dissection by preserving the duodenal loop and pancreas with the liver/small-bowel allograft, thus avoiding transection of the common bile duct. Procurement is limited then to simple isolation of the stomach and division at the pylorus, and transection of the ileum at the ileocecal valve with mobilization of the colon.[69] The pancreas, when it is not required, is removed as a back-table dissection to the right of the superior mesenteric vein. These grafts are ideally suited to very small donors (neonates), thus avoiding manipulation of the hepatic hilum, and larger donors in whom graft reduction is necessary (Figure 22.5). Both situations have allowed for reductions of the liver and intestine component of the graft, thus allowing for increased donor utilization.[64,70,71]

The isolated small-bowel graft can be procured as a composite graft with the other organs and then separated as a back-table procedure into separate intestine, pancreas, and liver allografts. The entire multivisceral procurement will take 3–4 h.[72]

These composite grafts are removed with minimal contamination, since the hollow viscera are sealed off by stapling and transection. The succus entericus is left undisturbed and transplanted with the graft.

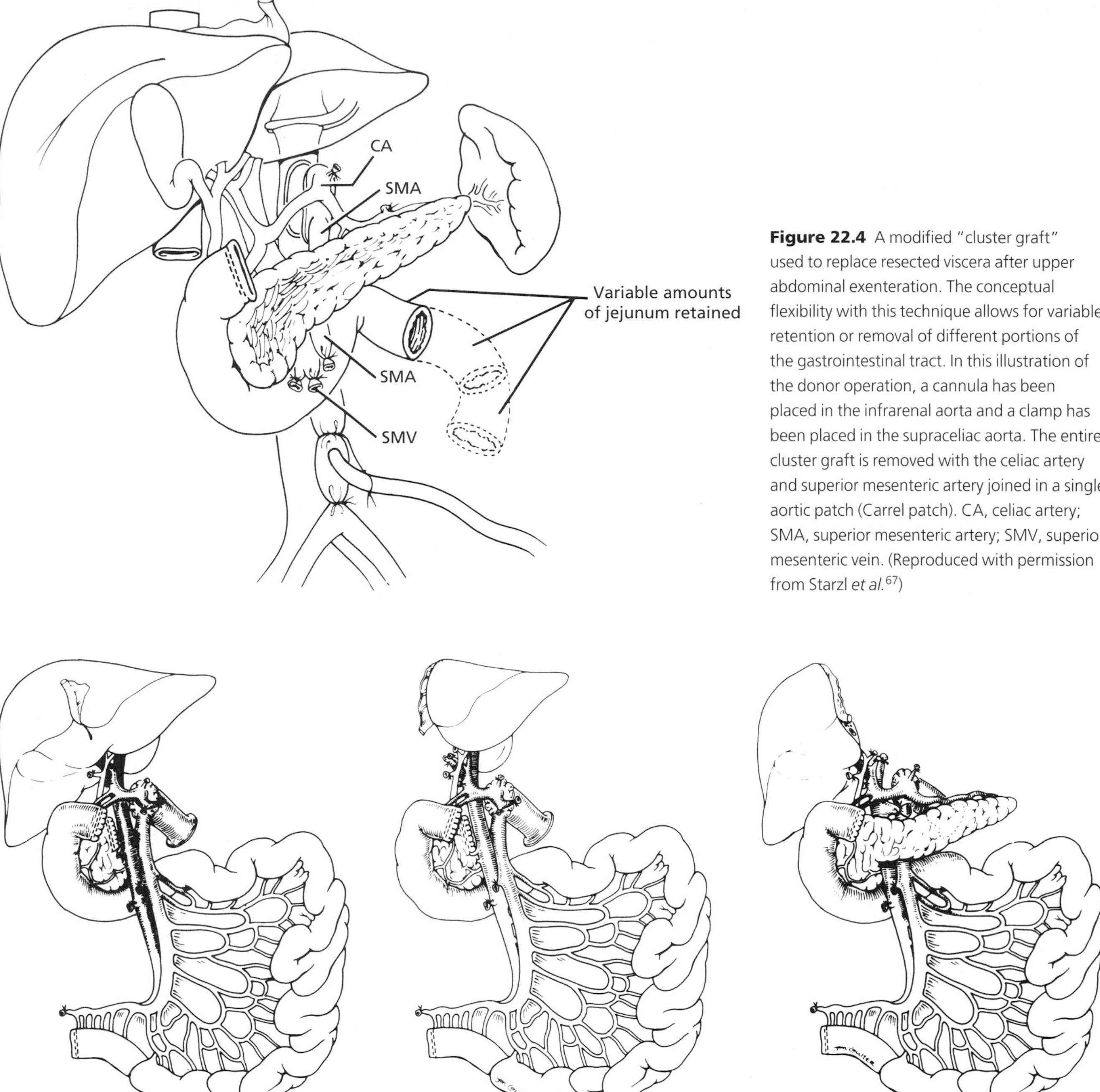

Figure 22.4 A modified "cluster graft" used to replace resected viscera after upper abdominal exenteration. The conceptual flexibility with this technique allows for variable retention or removal of different portions of the gastrointestinal tract. In this illustration of the donor operation, a cannula has been placed in the infrarenal aorta and a clamp has been placed in the supraceliac aorta. The entire cluster graft is removed with the celiac artery and superior mesenteric artery joined in a single aortic patch (Carrel patch). CA, celiac artery; SMA, superior mesenteric artery; SMV, superior mesenteric vein. (Reproduced with permission from Starzl *et al.*[67])

Figure 22.5 The composite liver/small-bowel allograft with preservation of the duodenum in continuity with the graft jejunum and hepatic biliary system is a practical variation of the original cluster graft. The pancreas is transected to the right of the portal vein, but in patients suffering total parenteral nutrition–induced pancreatic disease (with endocrine or exocrine deficiencies), it may be preserved. The aortic patch containing the celiac trunk and superior mesenteric arteries is anastomosed to a conduit of donor thoracic aorta. This technique allows reductions of the liver and/or intestinal components of the allograft, thus permitting the use of larger donor organs for smaller recipients. (Reproduced with permission from Bueno *et al.*[70])

Graft preservation

After completion of the donor dissection, systemic heparinization is performed and the proximal aorta is cross-clamped. In-situ perfusion using cold University of Wisconsin (UW) solution, with venous bed decompression via a venotomy in the intrapericardial suprahepatic vena cava,[73,74] is performed. Separation of organs is performed on the back table, and the graft is stored in ice for transport. Preservation time can vary from 2.8 to 14.8 h, with a mean of 7.83 h without significant evidence of preservation injury.

Recipient operations

Most children who need an intestinal or multiorgan transplant have had multiple previous abdominal explorations for intestinal resection, lengthening procedures, or treatment of complications. The combination of severe adhesions and portal hypertension presents a significant surgical challenge. The volume contraction of the abdominal cavity resulting from previous resections has required the use of Silastic silos, closure using only skin and subcutaneous tissue, and recently, graft reductions of the intestinal and liver allograft by extended right hepatic resection or left lateral segmentectomy (Figure 22.5).[70] Tissue expanders, applied either before or after transplantation, have been used. The use of abdominal wall from the donor as a composite tissue graft to facilitate abdominal closure after intestinal transplantation has recently been described.[75]

Once the donor organs are found to be satisfactory, the recipient operation begins in order to avoid prolonged cold ischemia times. The recipient operation involves removal of the failed organs, with exposure of the vascular anatomy for arterialization and venous drainage, identification of proximal and distal recipient bowel remnants, and finally allograft implantation.

Composite grafts

Composite grafts include multivisceral grafts and liver/small bowel. For these composite procedures, the native liver is removed, with preservation of the recipient inferior vena cava. It is necessary to ensure that the axial stem of the portal vein between the donor organs remains intact. In recipients of a liver/small-bowel graft, the portal vein of the remaining foregut is attached to the intact portal stem of the donor.

Arterialization of these grafts is accomplished with the double arterial stem of the celiac and superior mesenteric arteries (as a Carrel patch), anastomosed to the infrarenal or supraceliac aorta, with an interposed aortic conduit or iliac artery homograft. The composite graft is connected first to a common conduit of recipient hepatic veins ("piggy-back" to the skeletonized recipient vena cava), and then to the arterio-aortic anastomosis. In the multivisceral operation, the recipient's portal vein and gastrointestinal tract, pancreas, and liver are removed with the enterectomy and replaced with the donor portal vein in continuity via the liver, which prevents the need for a portal vein anastomosis. In the modified multivisceral operation, the liver is excluded and only the gastropancreatic-intestinal tract is transplanted. In this operation, the portal venous return is directed into the recipient's portal vein.

Restoration of intestinal continuity requires an anastomosis with native proximal gut (an esophagogastric anastomosis in the multivisceral procedure) and distal native gut, usually a coloenteric anastomosis with the distal ileum allograft. Because the duodenum- preserving composite liver/intestine allograft leaves the hepatic hilum undisturbed, biliary anastomosis is not necessary (Figure 22.5).

A "chimney" or "loop" allograft ileostomy is performed for routine surveillance of the intestinal allograft. This ileostomy can be taken down after several months when a stable immunosuppressive regimen has been achieved and there has been freedom from rejection without the need for frequent endoscopic surveillance.

Isolated intestinal grafts

Many patients with functional intestinal failure will not have had abdominal operations or resections. In patients with Crohn's disease with multiple abdominal fistulas, enterectomy may be performed before the transplant procedure in order to have a well-healed abdominal cavity. In patients with surgical short gut, the proximal and distal remnants of the intestine are identified. Arterialization of the graft will be from the donor superior mesenteric artery to the infrarenal aorta. Venous drainage through the superior mesenteric vein may be to the recipient portal vein, superior mesenteric vein, splenic vein, or inferior vena cava. An interposition donor venous graft can be applied to any of the aforementioned native veins in order to avoid a difficult surgical exposure and tension on the vascular anastomosis. Intestinal continuity is provided with anastomoses to previously identified native proximal and distal bowel, with a "chimney" ileostomy for endoscopic surveillance.

The time between procurement and implantation of the allograft (cold ischemia time) ranges from 2 to 17 h, while the warm ischemia time (the time that it takes to sew the graft in) is approximately 30 min. Both of these intervals are important determinants of preservation injury to the intestine.

In order to reduce postoperative fluid loss, a segment of large intestine was included in 32 patients,[76] but this led to an increased rate of infection and graft failure. In order to improve postoperative motility, donor celiac ganglia preservation of the intestinal allograft was also studied, but with no apparent benefit.

Living donor grafts

A small number of living-donor intestinal transplants have been performed, and the recipient outcomes appear to be similar to those with deceased-donor grafts, though in theory living donors may provide a survival advantage due to decreased waiting times, cold ischemia time, and better HLA matching. These living-donor grafts have been performed as an isolated intestine graft using ileum, and also as a sequential combined (but not composite) liver plus intestine graft, using the ileum and the left lateral segment of the liver.[77,78]

Postoperative management

The key to successful postoperative management is effective teamwork between anesthetists, surgeons, pediatricians, and nursing and paramedical staff. Recipients of composite grafts (multivisceral, liver/small bowel, or cluster grafts) suffer from end-stage liver/disease and may require a longer intensive-care stay to manage pulmonary, cardiac, and hepatic function. Recipients of isolated small-bowel transplants are less likely to require intensive care, but still present similar infectious risks and the potential to develop hepatic or pancreatic complications. Recipients of isolated intestinal transplants have a median intensive-care unit and hospital stay of 5 days and 9 weeks, respectively, vs. 17 days and 12.4 weeks, respectively, for larger composite grafts.[79] Recipients of isolated liver transplant in the context of intestinal failure have a prolonged postoperative course because of the need to encourage intestinal adaptation.

The prolonged intensive-care stay is related to the potential for graft malfunction, infection, and preoperative liver failure, as well as difficulties with early extubation, which may be exacerbated by the significantly longer operative times for the composite grafts (median time 13 h) in comparison with isolated small-bowel transplants (median time 9 h).

Discrepancies in donor/recipient size may prevent initial closure of the abdominal wall at the time of transplant, requiring the use of Silastic or collagen patches until appropriate fluid and electrolyte management can permit definitive closure. The increase in intra-abdominal volume with compression of the thoracic cavity may be an additional factor responsible for respiratory impairment. Unusually severe rejection of an isolated small-intestine allograft with systemic venous drainage into the inferior vena cava can produce respiratory insufficiency and an acute respiratory distress syndrome (ARDS) picture.

The main principles of postoperative management are:

- Immunosuppression and prevention of rejection
- Prevention and treatment of infection
- Fluid balance and maintenance of nutritional status
- Assessment of graft function
- Long-term rehabilitation

Immunosuppression

The same postoperative immunosuppression is used in both isolated and composite intestinal allograft recipients. This is based on a combination of tacrolimus (previously FK-506) with or without steroids. Some units begin immunosuppression in the operating room and others immediately afterwards.

The introduction of tacrolimus (previously known as FK-506) in 1987 brought intestinal transplantation to the forefront. It was initially used with intravenous methylprednisolone (10 mg/kg), followed by a steroid taper of methylprednisolone (5 mg/kg/day), reduced over 5 days to 1 mg/kg/day. Tacrolimus (0.1 mg/kg/day) was given by continuous intravenous infusion and maintained at a steady-state whole-blood level of 20–25 ng/mL (microparticle enzyme immunoassay, MEIA), and oral tacrolimus was started (0.15 mg/kg/day) once gastrointestinal motility was observed, although some units start oral tacrolimus immediately postoperatively. Trough levels were run at 20–25 ng/mL initially, reducing to 8–12 ng/mL after 6–12 months. This combination had significant toxicities and facilitated opportunistic infections. Consequently, the addition of "third agents" to the maintenance regimen began after 1995, using azathioprine, cyclophosphamide, mycophenolate mofetil (MMF), and most recently rapamycin. There was no benefit with cyclophosphamide or MMF, and their use was therefore abandoned. Rapamycin administration has allowed for good graft function and freedom of rejection under lower levels of tacrolimus.[80,81]

Induction therapy using humanized IgG1 monoclonal antibodies directed at the subunit of the human interleukin-2 receptor (daclizumab or basilimax) has significantly increased rejection-free survival.[82] Protocols are presently under study using pretreatment (before allograft implantation) and induction protocols with other antilymphocyte antibodies such as Thymoglobulin and Campath (alemtuzumab).[83] Indeed, monotherapy with tacrolimus after perioperative lymphoid depletion using rabbit antithymocyte globulin (Thymoglobulin) has allowed for improved rejection-free survival, early minimization of tacrolimus exposure, and a decreased incidence of opportunistic infections, and has resulted in a higher rate of patient and graft survival.[84] With such protocols, tacrolimus trough levels can be run at 10–15 mg/mL.

These strategies alter the lymphocyte population of donor and recipient, and have been used principally to avoid GVHD.[4,66] The paradigm of donor and recipient lymphocyte populations forming "genetic composites"[85] is known as "microchimerism." It is believed that the engagement of these two immunocyte populations leads to mutually canceling immune reactions, with the eventual development of varying disease of nonreactivity.[86] Interestingly, however, the augmentation of microchimerism using the infusion of donor bone-marrow cells recovered from donor vertebral bodies at the time of intestinal allograft procurement has not resulted in enhanced intestinal allograft acceptance.[87] Although none of the aforementioned protocols is tolerogenic, the lymphocyte-depleting agents have allowed for minimization strategies, thus decreasing the development of complications.

Prevention of infection

Prophylactic antibiotics are given for 14 days after transplantation. They include ciprofloxacin 5 mg/kg/dose b.i.d.; amoxyl 25 mg/kg/dose t.d.s.; or vancomycin if the patient has been colonized with methicillin-resistant *Staphylococcus aureus* or resistant fecal streptococci; metronidazole 8 mg/kg/dose t.d.s. Co-trimoxazole (240 mg orally if less than

5 years; 480 mg orally over 5 years) is used as prophylaxis against *Pneumocystis carinii*.

Oral nonabsorbable selective bacterial and fungal decontamination is given every 6 h for 2 weeks.[88] Surveillance stool cultures are performed weekly. Quantitative cultures with colonies of > 10^8 organisms are considered significant only in the presence of systemic sepsis or ongoing acute cellular rejection of the intestinal allograft, and are treated appropriately. It is important to note that bacterial translocation can occur with intestinal allograft rejection or other opportunistic infections such as EBV enteritis. It is necessary to treat both the disease causing the immunological damage of the mucosal barrier and the infection.[89]

Antiviral prophylactic strategy is directed towards prevention of infection with CMV and EBV, and includes:

- A 2-week course of intravenous ganciclovir (10 mg/kg/day) with concomitant CMV-specific hyperimmune globulin (CytoGam/super R).[90]
- Oral acyclovir (200 mg q.d.s. < 5 years; 500 mg q.d.s. > 5 years) or oral ganciclovir may be continued for 3 or 6 months.

Management of fluid balance

Fluid balance in this group of patients may be difficult to manage because of previous liver disease and the requirement for intraoperative coagulation or colloid support. In the first 2–3 days after transplantation, fluid shifts between graft, lungs, and peripheral tissues can result in overall fluid retention, but intravascular volume depletion. This is exacerbated by high-dose steroids, tacrolimus, nephrotoxic antibiotics, and antifungals. Fluid balance must take into account fluid losses from abdominal drains, nasogastric and stoma output, and urine output. Fluids should be restricted to two-thirds maintenance and provided as dextrose/saline with colloid as required to maintain central venous pressure (6–10 cmH_2O), urine output 0.5–1.5 mL/kg/h.

Nutrition

Total parenteral nutrition is provided with standard TPN formulas and tapered gradually as oral or enteral nutrition is advanced. Enteral feeds by continuous infusion may start as soon as bowel sounds are obvious. In general, it is best to start with simple feeds such as isotonic dipeptide formulas containing medium-chain triglycerides, glutamine, and glucose polymers. This is later converted to a lactose-free and gluten-free diet that contains dietary fiber such as pectin to promote normalization of intestinal motility and function. Long-chain triglyceride is added later when lymphatics are established. Many children will not voluntarily eat after transplantation, as this may be the first time many of them will have experienced normal feeding. Management requires a multidisciplinary approach involving psychological support. Enteral supplementation may be required on a long-term basis. Independence from TPN is achieved in all functioning grafts within 4–6 weeks.[91]

Assessment of the graft

Monitoring of liver and pancreatic components of composite intestinal allografts is performed as for isolated transplantation of these solid organs. Regular assessment of liver function tests, amylase, and insulin requirements is routine; abdominal ultrasound and biopsies from transplanted organs are performed as required.

Intestinal grafts

Assessment of the anatomical and functional viability of an intestinal allograft begins in the operating room immediately after graft reperfusion. Venous outflow disturbances may result in congestion and ecchymosis, which must be differentiated from hyperacute rejection and ischemic damage. Similar changes may be seen in the ileal stoma postoperatively.

As intestinal allografts may be composed of varying lengths of the gastrointestinal tract with functionally and anatomically differing segments (stomach, duodenum, small intestine, colon), the assessment of these grafts must be flexible, aggressive, and multidisciplinary. There are no good functional or biochemical markers to assess injury or rejection of intestinal allografts, although a rise in the gentamicin levels in children receiving oral decontamination may be an early indicator.[92] There has been recent interest in the use of fecal calprotectin to screen for rejection.[93]

Radiological evaluation using barium usually reveals a normal mucosal pattern, with intestinal transit times of 2–4 h. Serum nutritional markers (transferrin, albumin, retinoic acid) and absorption studies (D-xylose, tacrolimus, quantification of fat in the stool) provide long-term measures of function in a stable graft, but little useful information about clinical disease.

The most effective methods of assessing graft status and diagnosing rejection are:

- Assessment of stomal output for volume, consistency, reducing substances, and bacterial overgrowth. An increase in stomal output suggests either infection or rejection, but does not differentiate between the two. The presence of blood in the stool is always an ominous sign, requiring an urgent endoscopy, since this may be due to rejection or infection.
- Routine enteroscopic surveillance performed twice a week through the allograft ileostomy provides adequate information in the majority of cases. Occasionally, upper gastrointestinal endoscopy with visualization and biopsy of the proximal allograft is necessary.
- The use of magnification or zoom endoscopy[94] has enhanced clinical assessment, although histopathology remains the gold standard.
- Formal motility testing is occasionally required for long-term functional assessment.[95]

Complications after transplantation

Clinical/surgical factors

Complications related to the surgical procedure or the postoperative clinical management of the recipient are common (47%). The major technical complications are biliary or intestinal anastomotic leaks, intestinal perforation, and thrombosis of the hepatic artery in the larger composite grafts, which may be complicated by severe intra-abdominal infections with polymicrobial and fungal organisms. The most serious clinical management issues are rejection, infection, fluid and electrolyte disturbances, renal dysfunction, and hypertension, which are exacerbated by high levels of tacrolimus and steroids.[96]

Rejection

Historically, the incidence of intestinal allograft rejection has been reported to be as high as 90%, and it is more frequent and severe in recipients of isolated intestinal grafts in comparison with liver/small bowel or multivisceral allografts. Most episodes occur within the first 90 days. The use of OKT3 (muromonab-CD3) for the treatment of severe steroid-resistant rejection is also more common in isolated small-bowel transplantation. The rate of rejection of the liver when it is part of a composite graft is 43%, suggesting that the liver graft may protect the intestinal component. In composite grafts that included other organs, the rejection rates were as follows: colon 34%, stomach 12%, and pancreas 12%.[69]

Acute intestinal rejection presents with nonspecific symptoms such as:

- Fever, abdominal pain, and distension.
- Nausea, vomiting.
- Increase in stomal output.
- The stoma may become edematous, erythematous and friable.
- Gastrointestinal bleeding can occur in severe rejection, with ulceration and sloughing of the intestinal mucosa.

Sepsis due to bacterial or fungal translocation occurs as a result of disruption of the intestinal mucosal barrier from rejection. Paradoxically, such severe infections can only be treated by stabilizing the allograft mucosal barrier with augmented immunosuppression.

Endoscopically, the transplanted intestinal mucosa loses its velvety appearance and becomes hyperemic or dusky, as well as hypoperistaltic. Erythema may be focal or diffuse; the mucosa becomes friable, and diffuse ulceration appears (Figure 22.6).[97]

Histologically, there is variable presence of lamina propria, edema, and villous blunting. The diagnosis rests on the presence of a mononuclear cell infiltrate, cryptitis with apoptosis, and regeneration. Neutrophils, eosinophils, and macrophages may be seen traversing the muscularis mucosa.[98–100] The degree of epithelial and crypt cell damage varies (Figure 22.7A). The histologic assessment of endoscopic biopsies can be hampered by viral infections and the presence of "patchy" changes; however, a recent grading system has addressed these difficulties.[101]

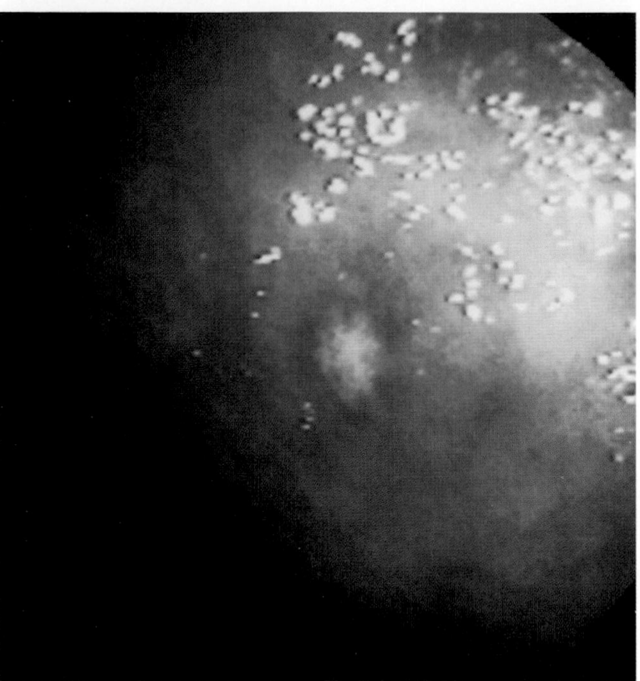

Figure 22.6 Endoscopic appearance of severe intestinal allograft rejection. There has been sloughing of the mucosa and ulceration.

It is unclear whether, in the most severe form of rejection, the progressively worsening apoptosis or a vascular response to rejection leading to ischemia results in the severe mucosal sloughing and crypt destruction. The mucosal surface becomes replaced by inflammatory pseudomembranes and granulation tissue, which precipitate continuous blood loss, as well as intermittent septic episodes from bacterial and fungal translocation (Figure 22.6).

Chronic rejection has been observed in patients with persistent intractable rejection episodes. These patients present with:

- Progressive weight loss, chronic diarrhea, intermittent fever and gastrointestinal bleeding.
- Endoscopic mucosal biopsies reveal a scant cellular infiltrate, with villous blunting, focal ulceration, and epithelial metaplasia (Figure 22.7B). Full-thickness intestinal biopsies may reveal obliterative arteriopathy, which is uncommon in children.
- Radiographically, it may present areas of strictures and dilations, with areas of arteriopathy on angiography.

The most important factor responsible for improvement in clinical outcomes has been a decrease in the frequency and severity of rejection. This has been achieved by increasing experience, use of antilymphocyte globulin immunosuppression, and early diagnosis of opportunistic infections.[84]

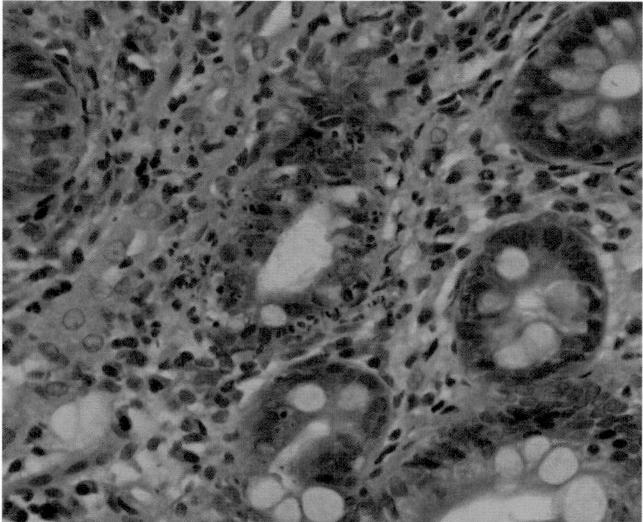

A

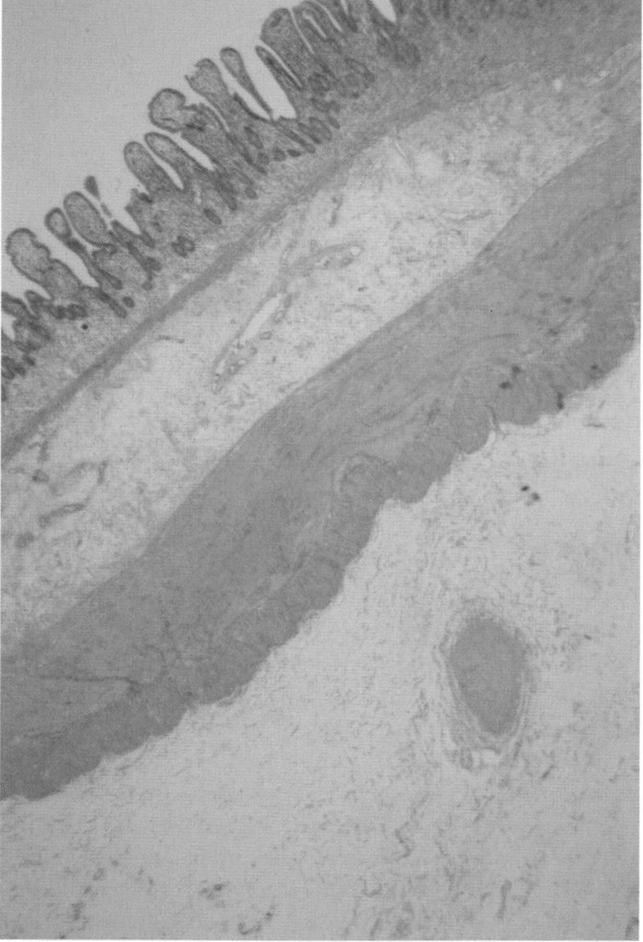

B

Figure 22.7 A Histological appearance of severe intestinal allograft rejection, with loss of villi and crypts and multiple apoptosis in the crypt (hematoxylin–eosin, original magnification × 400). **B** Chronic rejection demonstrates thickening and fibrosis of the mucosa, which is best appreciated in the resected bowel (hematoxylin–eosin, original magnification × 40).

Therapy

Graft rejection is treated with high doses of intravenous methylprednisolone (10 mg/kg) as bolus therapy in cases of mild rejection, and with a taper in cases of moderate to severe rejection. The tacrolimus trough levels in whole blood are maintained at around 15 ng/mL. OKT3 or Thymoglobulin is reserved for steroid-resistant rejection, or in cases of severe mucosal injury and crypt damage.[87] Addition of sirolimus (rapamycin) or mycophenolate mofetil may also be useful in the treatment of resistant rejection.[81]

Infections

Infectious complications are frequent due to several predisposing factors, which include:

- The severity of preoperative liver failure
- The presence of intra-abdominal, pulmonary, or catheter sepsis prior to transplantation
- The higher level of immunosuppression required to prevent rejection in intestinal grafts

There is a higher incidence of infectious complications in recipients of large composite intestinal allografts, perhaps because of the technically challenging transplant procedures, with increased operative time, transfusion requirements, and intestinal cold ischemia times.

Bacterial pathogens include staphylococci (intravenous line–induced), enterococci, and Gram-negative rods. Recently, the hospital-acquired vancomycin-resistant enterococcus (VRE) has been a problem in the United Kingdom.[102] Enteric organisms are usually associated with abdominal wound infections, deep abdominal abscesses, peritonitis, pneumonia, and bacterial translocation from grafts damaged by rejection. Multiple sources of infection can occur simultaneously, or there may be mixed infections from the same source. The multiple antibiotic regimens required to treat these infections may precipitate the development of resistant organisms such as the nascent strain of panresistant enterococci, and fungal infections.

Fungal infections are usually the result of intravenous line contamination, translocation due to rejection, massive antibiotic usage, and intestinal leaks. Aggressive medical and surgical therapy is required in patients with this complication. It is not usually wise to reduce immunosuppression, as the coexistence of cellular rejection warrants maintaining an intact mucosal barrier by appropriate augmentation of immunosuppression. Complete withdrawal of immunosuppression is impossible in this recipient population, due to a high incidence of rebound rejection.

CMV infection develops in 22% of pediatric intestinal graft recipients and often involves the allograft intestine (91%). Children have comparable morbidity to adults, but a lower mortality. CMV disease is highest in CMV-negative recipients of CMV-positive grafts;[90,103] these recipients have more aggressive disease, manifested by a higher incidence of recurrence, persistence of disease, involvement of native intestine,

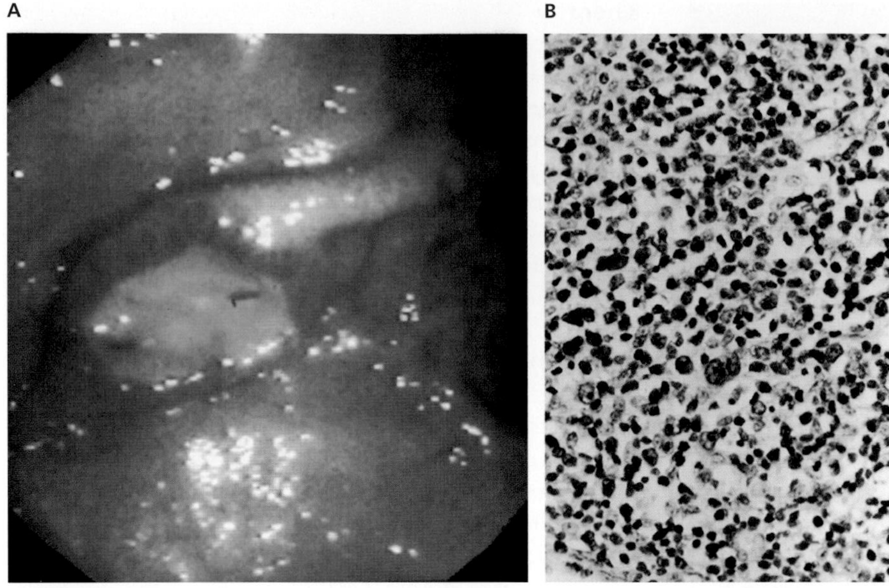

Figure 22.8 A Typical endoscopic appearance of "shallow" ulcer surrounded by normal mucosa. **B** Histopathology shows typical cytomegalovirus inclusion bodies. The number of inclusion bodies has been associated with more severe clinical disease, with gradual disappearance as the disease resolves.

hepatitis, central nervous disease, and retinal involvement. Diagnosis is usually made after nonspecific symptoms have prompted measurement of CMV RNA,[104] CMV antigenemia in the peripheral blood, and/or an endoscopy (Figure 22.8). Endoscopic images usually reveal superficial ulcers against a background of normal mucosa. Histopathology shows typical CMV inclusion bodies, although care must be taken not to associate occasional crypt epithelium apoptosis with rejection. Successful clinical management has been accomplished in over 95% of episodes using ganciclovir, alone or in combination with CMV-specific hyperimmunoglobulin. It is essential to avoid rejection by maintaining immunosuppression at baseline and reducing it only in the face of deteriorating clinical disease.[89]

EBV-associated post-transplant lymphoproliferative disease (PTLD) has occurred in 31% of children, which puts them at a significantly higher risk than adult intestinal recipients (11%). Recipients of multivisceral grafts have a higher incidence of infection (50%) in comparison with recipients of isolated small bowel (29%) or liver/small bowel (27%).

The clinical presentation includes nonspecific intestinal and systemic symptoms, hypoalbuminemia, bleeding, lymphadenopathy, and tumors found on physical examination, endoscopy, or histology (Figure 22.9). Risk factors include recipient age, history of previous splenectomy, and the use of OKT3. Therapy includes the reduction and withdrawal of immunosuppression, antivirals (ganciclovir, acyclovir, hyperimmunoglobulin), cytokines (interferon-α) and chemotherapy. More recently, rituximab (a monoclonal antibody) and infusion of HLA-matched T cells have had some success in treating this difficult disorder.[105,106] The disease may be fatal in up to 45% of patients, in whom rebound rejection was a significant contributor to mortality.[107] It is important to prevent and diagnosis PTLD early using in-situ hybridization staining for EBV early RNA in all suspicious histology, and establishing "viremia" by EBV-PCR.[108] This strategy of preemptive antiviral therapy using ganciclovir and CMV-IVIg (and when possible reduction of immunosuppression) was utilized when increasing viral loads were detected in the peripheral blood of recipients, and has resulted in decreased incidence of PTLD, as well as improved outcomes.[109]

Although viral infections are less common, respiratory syncytial virus, rotavirus, adenovirus, and parainfluenza virus lead to significant morbidity and severe mortality in this population.

Chimerism and GVHD

The phenomenon of donor and recipient cell migration observed in all solid-organ recipients has been described as "chimerism." This hypothesis forms the basis of the two-way paradigm of transplantation immunology, in which donor and recipient cell populations interact with mutually canceling effects, producing eventual allograft acceptance.[86] Using bone-marrow augmentation with adjuvant donor bone-marrow cells, the presence of donor cell chimerism was documented in 100% of the study population and 80% of the control patients.[69]

GVHD is unusual in this population unless there is preexisting immunodeficiency and may be asymptomatic or associated with rejection. Skin changes consistent with GVHD were diagnosed by histopathological criteria in only seven children (8%), and in only two patients who had received adjunct bone marrow, with onset ranging from 6 days to 8 years following transplantation. Histological criteria for GVHD include keratinocyte necrosis, epithelial apoptosis of native gastrointestinal tract, or epithelial cell necrosis of oral mucosa (see Figure 17.16, p. 416). Spontaneous resolution occurred in all but one patient, who had

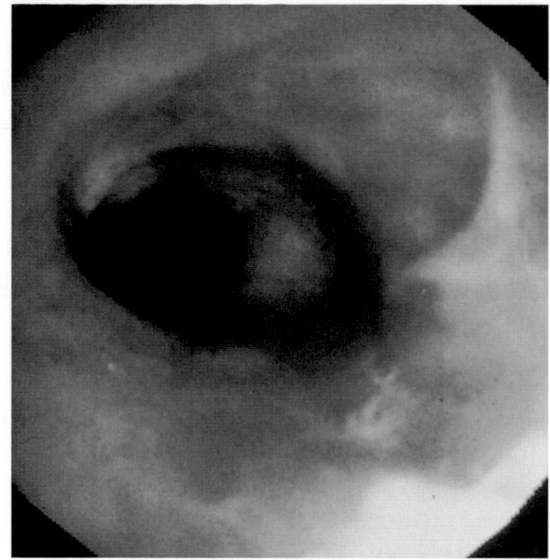
A

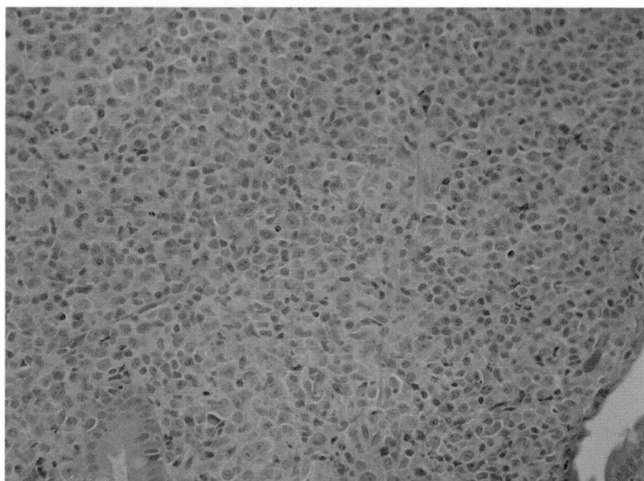
B

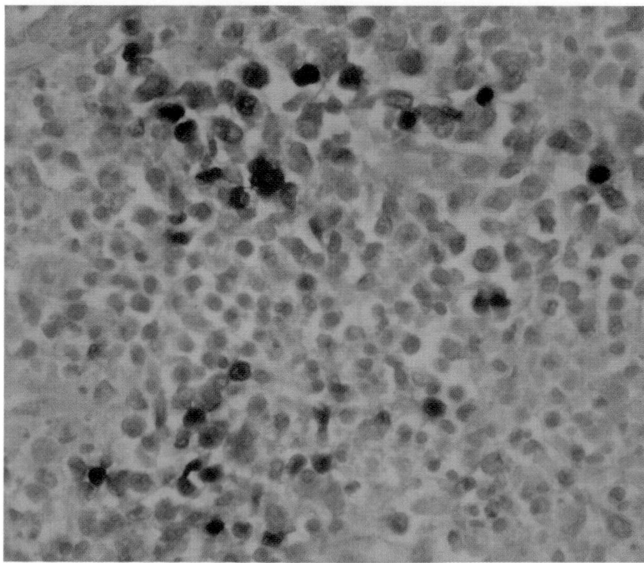
C

hereditary IgG and IgM deficiency and died from septicemia. GVHD was diagnosed 4 days after immunosuppression stopped and was confirmed by immunohistochemical studies visualizing donor cell infiltration into the lesions.[110]

Consequently, the impact of GVHD in clinical transplantation is not significant.[69,84] Also, it is presently unclear whether graft irradiation or donor pretreatment can alter the incidence of clinical GVHD.[111,112]

Causes of graft loss

The main cause of intestinal graft loss is infection, which may be associated with rejection or PTLD in 48% of grafts lost. Twenty-eight percent of grafts are lost due to surgical technical/clinical complications. The decision for graft enterectomy should be based on significant intestinal graft dysfunction and the need to withdraw immunosuppression, prior to the development of infectious complications, which may persist after removal of the graft.

Retransplantation of the intestine is required for acute and chronic rejection and hepatic artery thrombosis, and has a high failure rate due to the precarious clinical status of the patient when the retransplant is performed. Retransplantation should be restricted to highly selected cases, such as early vascular thrombosis or primary nonfunction of the graft prior to significant manifestations of other organ failure.[79]

Survival

Survival has improved with the use of tacrolimus, and international experience has confirmed the feasibility and lifesaving potential of this therapeutic modality.[94,113]

Survival after intestinal transplantation has seen dramatic improvements in the last 5 years, with centers reporting 1-year survival rates varying from 30% to 100%.[84,100,114] Data from the International Intestine Transplant Registry indicate a 1-year graft survival rate of 70%;[115] however, there was a superior survival of 81% in patients induced with antilymphocyte globulin.

The inclusion of allograft colon did not affect survival, but increased patient and graft loss from infection in the recipients of this intestinal segment. There was no benefit in weaning TPN or intravenous fluids in comparison with patients who did not receive allograft colon. Thus, the only

Figure 22.9 (**A**) Endoscopic appearance of a post-transplant lymphoproliferative disease (PTLD) lesion, with a raised, "tumorous," ulcerated lesion surrounded by normal-appearing mucosa. Histopathology shows a polymorphic infiltrate (**B**) (hematoxylin–eosin, original magnification × 40), which demonstrates "transformed" PTLD lymphocytes staining positive for Epstein–Barr early RNA (EBER) (**C**; in-situ hybridization for Epstein–Barr virus early RNA, original magnification × 600).

indication for inclusion of allograft colon should be as a reconstructive segment in selected cases of Hirschsprung disease or CIP, where a pull-through procedure through the rectum may be functionally beneficial.[116]

Use of bone marrow augmentation did not improve actuarial patient or graft survival, although there was no morbidity associated with the infusions.

Indeed, an analysis of survival statistics after intestinal transplantation shows that the 1-year survival figures reflect surgical experience and appropriate perioperative clinical management, which should result in an approximately 70% rate of patient survival. However, because of the high incidence of rejection and the need for higher long-term immunosuppression, survival continues to decrease, with a 3-year patient survival of 55%. Most of the deaths are from opportunistic infections such as CMV and PTLD-associated EBV infection, which may be prevented by early diagnosis and preemptive therapy. Further improvement in survival, however, rests on decreasing the incidence of rejection and providing long-term rehabilitation and graft acceptance without the need for high baseline immunosuppression.[115]

Nutritional status and long-term rehabilitation

Independence from TPN has been accomplished in most children within the first 4–6 weeks. Although all children tolerate a regular oral diet, 87% of these receive their complete nutritional requirements solely from this route. The remainder (17%) require enteral supplementation because of behavioral feeding problems or inadequate calorie intake. Food allergies to lactose and gluten have been common.[117]

Linear growth occurs to a greater degree in older children than in recipients aged 1–5 years, and it progresses after weaning from TPN as calories are provided via oral and/or enteral routes. Deficiencies in red blood cell folate, zinc, and copper levels have been documented postoperatively in some patients.

The intensity of home medical services, however, decreases over a 1–3-year period after transplantation as the patient recovers and is reintegrated into the home and school environment. Children are able to make physical and developmental progress. All school-aged children participate in a school program. Older children and adolescents are often upset about the alterations to their bodies, with protruding lines, tubes, and an ileostomy. Thus, removal of medical appliances may be psychologically and developmentally beneficial, helping the child adapt more easily to life after intestinal transplantation.[118,119]

There is now evidence that although small-bowel transplantation is expensive, the improvement in outcome and the reduction in the costs of home parenteral nutrition make it economically viable.[120,121]

Present and future status

Rapidly accumulating international experience has allowed the development of clinical and surgical strategies demonstrating the feasibility, reliability, and lifesaving potential of intestinal transplant procedures.[113,115] This reserved optimism must be weighed against the poor outlook for patients with intestinal failure, many of whom will die without transplantation. The most significant preoperative risk factors reflect liver failure and include: clinical jaundice, coagulopathy, fibrosis/cirrhosis on liver biopsy, and hypersplenism.[39] Thus, early referral for management of intestinal failure and consideration for intestinal transplantation should occur before the development of significant liver dysfunction, particularly in infants with short-gut syndrome.

The improved survival of both patient and graft with the isolated intestinal transplant in comparison with composite grafts is mainly due to the absence of these critical risk factors and simpler surgical and clinical post-transplant management. However, it also reflects the ability to remove a failed intestinal graft and resume TPN if the clinical circumstances permit. This advantage is such that it is not justified to remove a normal liver as part of the transplant procedure, nor to allow a patient to develop liver failure prior to consideration for intestinal transplantation.

From these data, it is evident that the balance between the need for high levels of immunosuppression to prevent rejection, and the incidence of opportunistic infection as a consequence of immunosuppression remains the major obstacle to the further development of intestinal transplantation. The improvements in technical and clinical skills, such as the early diagnosis and prevention of infection with the use of pp65 CMV antigenemia, EBV-PCR in peripheral blood, and Epstein–Barr early RNA (EBER) in tissue sampling, have enhanced our ability to reduce post-transplant complications and improve survival. However, strategies aimed at decreasing the immunogenicity of the intestinal allograft, thereby reducing the incidence and intensity of rejection and the need for augmentation of immunosuppression, are required to make survival rates for intestinal transplantation comparable to those with other forms of solid-organ transplantation.

It is possible that the development of an immunomodulation strategy that changes the immunogenicity of the intestinal allograft while permitting the phenomenon of bidirectional cell migration and chimerism could reduce the incidence and severity of rejection. Although much progress has been made with modifications in immunosuppression and clinical management, it is still a work in progress. Intestinal failure management must evolve to a better understanding of the physiologic and immunologic changes inherent in losing the intestine, as well as a better sense of the drug toxicity produced by TPN. Organ availability for children awaiting transplantation must improve in order to decrease the mortality while waiting. Most importantly, increased clinical and bench research must develop a better understanding of the complex immunologic events occurring with intestinal transplantation, thus facilitating improved outcomes.

Case study

A previously healthy 5-year-old boy developed an acute abdomen, which at laparotomy was found to be due to a midgut volvulus. He had extensive resection of infarcted bowel, leaving him with an ultrashort-bowel syndrome (around 5 cm of bowel). The third part of the duodenum was made into an end stoma. He was managed with parenteral nutrition, but rapidly developed liver disease induced by intestinal failure. He had a poor quality of life because of excessive stomal output, and he missed eating.

At assessment, liver function tests were: bilirubin 231 mmol/L (normal < 20); alanine aminotransferase (ALT) 497 IU/L (normal > 40), albumin 29 g/L (normal 35–45). Coagulation and full blood count were normal.

Ultrasound of the abdomen demonstrated that the liver echotexture was normal, but the spleen size was 11 cm (enlarged for his age). Liver vasculature was normal and he had patent internal jugular, brachiocephalic, and subclavian veins. He was listed for a combined liver and intestinal transplant.

He received an en-bloc full-size liver and a whole small-intestine graft from a 14-kg, O-negative blood group CMV-positive donor. He had hepatic vein–hepatic vein anastomosis and inferior vena cava–inferior vena cava anastomosis. The cuff of the donor aorta and the superior mesenteric and celiac arteries were sutured to an aortic conduit. There were no portal or biliary anastomoses. The intestine was joined by jejunojejunal anastomosis and ileocolic anastomosis. The total ischemic time was 7 h. His abdomen was left opened with a Silastic patch, which was subsequently closed along with creation of a loop ileostomy 15 cm proximal to the ileocolic anastomosis.

He made a rapid recovery and was started on standard immunosuppression. This included tacrolimus, methylprednisolone for the first 14 days, oral prednisolone after the second week, and basiliximab during transplant and day 4 postoperatively. On day 6 after transplantation, his γ-glutamyltransferase (GGT) and liver enzymes were raised, although a liver biopsy showed no evidence of graft rejection, but perfusion injury. His surveillance stoma allograft biopsy demonstrated mild acute rejection, which was not treated.

On day 5, enteral feeds via a nasojejunal tube were introduced based on a medium-chain triglyceride modular feed. His stoma output was around 600 mL/day and controlled with loperamide. He was discharged 4 weeks after transplantation on full enteral feeds.

At outpatient follow-up he has remained well and has been maintained on sirolimus and prednisolone.

Comment. This young boy developed a devastating mid-gut volvulus which infarcted all of his intestine, leaving him with an ultrashort bowel. He would have died without expert surgery and parenteral nutrition. However, the extremely short bowel meant that he rapidly developed liver disease associated with intestinal failure, and due to the poor quality of life he received a combined liver and intestinal transplant. He received an en-bloc full-size graft, and this may have reduced his post-transplant complications. He only developed mild rejection and was rapidly weaned off PN. He has remained well, without significant episodes of sepsis.

References

1 Lillehei RC, Goott B, Miller FA. The physiological response of the small bowel of the dog to ischemia including prolonged in vitro preservation of the bowel with successful replacement and survival. *Ann Surg* 1959;**150**:543–60.

2 Starzl TE, Kaupp HA Jr. Mass homotransplantation of abdominal organs in dogs. *Surg Forum* 1960;**11**:28–30.

3 Grant D. Intestinal transplantation: current status. *Transplant Proc* 1989;**21**(1 Pt 3):2869–71.

4 Starzl TE, Rowe MI, Todo S, *et al.* Transplantation of multiple abdominal viscera. *JAMA* 1989;**261**:1449–57.

5 Grant D, Wall W, Mimeault R, *et al.* Successful small-bowel/liver transplantation. *Lancet* 1990;**335**:181–4.

6 Margreiter R, Konigsrainer A, Schmidt T, *et al.* Successful multivisceral transplantation. *Transplant Proc* 1992;**24**:1226–7.

7 McAlister V, Wall W, Ghent C, *et al.* Successful small intestine transplantation. *Transplant Proc* 1992;**24**:1236–7.

8 Calne RY, Sells RA, Pena JR, *et al.* Introduction of immunologic tolerance by porcine liver allograft. *Nature* 1969;**223**: 472–4.

9 Kamada N, Davies HS, Wight D, *et al.* Liver transplantation in the rat: biochemical and histological evidence of complete tolerance induction in nonrejector strains. *Transplantation* 1983;**35**: 304–11.

10 Deltz E, Schroeder PH Gebhardt H, *et al.* Successful clinical small bowel transplantation: report of a case. *Clin Transplant* 1989;**3**: 89–91.

11 Goulet O, Revillon Y, Brousse N, *et al.* Successful small bowel transplantation in an infant. *Transplantation* 1992;**53**:940–3.

12 Todo S, Tzakis AG, Abu-Elmagd K, *et al.* Cadaveric small bowel and small bowel-liver transplantation in humans. *Transplantation* 1992;**53**:369–7.

13 Beath SV, Needham SJ, Kelly DA, *et al.* Clinical features and prognosis of children assessed for isolated small bowel (ISBTx) or combined small bowel and liver transplantation (CSBLTx). *J Paediatr Surg* 1997;**32**:459–61.

14 Wilmore DW, Groff DB, Bishop HB, *et al.* Total parenteral nutrition in infants with catastrophic gastrointestinal anomalies. *J Paediatr Surg* 1969;**4**:181–9.

15 Wilmore DW. Factors correlating with a successful outcome following extensive intestinal resection in newborn infants. *J Pediatr* 1972;**80**:88–95.

16 Grosfeld JL, Rescorla FJ, West KW. Short bowel syndrome in infancy and childhood: analysis of survival of 60 patients. *Am J Surg* 1986;**151**:41–6.

17 Windmueller HG, Spaeth AE. Identification of ketone bodies and glutamine as the major respiratory fuels in vivo for post absorptive rat small intestine. *J Biol Chem* 1978;**253**:69–76.

18 O'Dwyer ST, Smith RJ, Hwang TL, Wilmore DW. Maintenance of small bowel mucosa with glutamine-enriched parenteral nutrition. *J Parenter Enteral Nutr* 1989;**13**:579–85.

19 Wilmore DW, Smith RJ, O'Dwyer ST, *et al.* The gut: a central organ after surgical stress. *Surgery* 1988;**104**:917–23.

20 Vanderhoof JA, Blackwood DJ, Mohammadpour H, Park JH. Effects of oral supplementation of glutamine on small intestinal mucosal mass following resection. *J Am Coll Nutr* 1992;**11**: 223–7.

21 Byrne TA, Morrissey TB, Nattakom TV, *et al.* Growth hormone, glutamine, and a modified diet enhance nutrient absorption in patients with severe short bowel syndrome. *J Parenter Enteral Nutr* 1995;**19**:296–302.

22 Hyman PA, DiLorenzo C. Chronic intestinal pseudoobstruction. In: Willie R, Hyams JS, eds. *Pediatric Gastrointestinal Disease.* Philadelphia: Saunders, 1993: 641–51.

23 Fortuna RS, Weber TR, Tracy TF Jr, Silen ML, Cradock TV. Critical analysis of the operative treatment of Hirschsprung's disease. *Arch Surg* 1996;**131**:520–4.

24 Davidson GP, Cutz E, Hamilton JR, Gall DG. Familial enteropathy: a syndrome of protracted diarrhea from birth, failure to thrive, and hypoplastic villous atrophy. *Gastroenterology* 1978; **75**:783–90.

25 Steiger E, Srp F. Morbidity and mortality related to home parenteral nutrition in patients with gut failure. *Am J Surg* 1983;**145**:102–5.

26 Ricour C, Gorski AM, Goulet O, *et al.* Home parenteral nutrition in children. Eight years experience with 112 patients. *Clin Nutr* 1990;**9**:65–71.

27 Pollard AJ, Sreeram N, Wright JG, *et al.* Pulmonary embolism in children/endlash another hazard of parenteral feeding. *Gut* 1994;**35**:S33.

28 Kelly DA. Intestinal failure associated liver disease—what do we know today? *Gastroenterology* 2006;**130**(2 Suppl):S70–7.

29 Beale EF, Nelson RM, Bucciarelli RL, *et al.* Intrahepatic cholestasis associated with parenteral nutrition in premature infants. *Pediatrics* 1979;**64**:342–7.

30 Tzakis AJ, Todo S, Reyes J. Clinical intestinal transplantation: focus on complications. *Transplant Proc* 1992;**24**:1238–40.

31 Colomb V, Goulet O, Rambaud C, *et al.* Long-term parenteral nutrition in children: liver and gallbladder disease. *Transplant Proc* 1992;**24**:1054–5.

32 Rombeau JL, Rolandelli RH. Enteral and parenteral nutrition in patients with enteric fistulas and short bowel syndrome. *Surg Clin North Am* 1987;**67**:551–71.

33 Barbier J, Gineste D, Kraimps JL, *et al.* [Hepatobiliary complications of total parenteral nutrition; in French.] *Chirurgie* 1992;**118**:47–53.

34 Balisteri WF, Bove KE. Hepatobiliary consequences of parenteral alimentation. *Prog Liver Dis* 1990;**9**:567–601.

35 Manginello FP, Javitt NB. Parenteral nutrition and neonatal cholestasis. *J Pediatr* 1981;**99**:445–9.

36 Das JB, Cosentino CM, Levy MF, *et al.* Early hepatobiliary dysfunction during total parenteral nutrition: an experimental study. *J Pediatr Surg* 1993;**28**:14–8.

37 Fell JM, Reynolds AP, Meadows N, *et al.* Manganese toxicity in children receiving long-term parenteral nutrition. *Lancet* 1996;**347**:1218–21.

38 Hofmann AF. Defective biliary secretion during total parenteral nutrition: probable mechanisms and possible solutions. *J Pediatr Gastroenterol Nutr* 1995;**4**:376–90.

39 Bueno J, Ohwada S, Kochosis S, *et al.* Factors impacting on the survival of children with intestinal failure referred for intestinal transplantation. *J Pediatr Surg* 1999;**34**:27–33.

40 Beath SV, Booth IW, Murphy MS, *et al.* Nutritional care in candidates for small bowel transplantation. *Arch Dis Child* 1995;**73**:348–50.

41 Gorgstrom B, Dahlquist A, Lundh G, *et al.* Studies of intestinal digestion and absorption in the human. *J Clin Invest* 1957; **36**:1521–36.

42 Dudrick SJ, Latifi R, Fosnocht DE. Management of the short-bowel syndrome. *Surg Clin North Am* 1991;**71**:625–43.

43 Edes TE. Clinical management of short-bowel syndrome: enhancing the patient's quality of life. *Short-Bowel Syndrome* 1990;**88**:91–5.

44 Bond JH, Currier BE, Buchwals H, *et al.* Colonic conservation of malabsorbed carbohydrates. *Gastroenterology* 1980;**78**:444–7.

45 Dahms BB, Halpin TC Jr. Serial liver biopsies in parenteral nutrition–associated cholestasis of early infancy. *Gastroenterology* 1981;**81**:136–44.

46 Vanderhoof JA, Young RJ. Enteral and parenteral nutrition in the care of patients with short-bowel syndrome. *Best Pract Res Clin Gastroenterol* 2003;**17**:997–1015.

47 Bianchi A. Intestinal loop lengthening—a technique for increasing small intestinal length. *J Pediatr Surg* 1980;**15**:145–51.

48 Kim HB, Lee PW, Garza J, *et al.* Serial transverse enteroplasty for short bowel syndrome: a case report. *J Pediatr Surg* 2003;**38**: 881–5.

49 Sudan D, DiBaise J, Torres C, *et al.* A multidisciplinary approach to the treatment of intestinal failure. *J Gastrointest Surg* 2005; **9**:165–76.

50 Spagnuolo MI, Iorio R, Vegnente A, Guarino A. Ursodeoxycholic acid for treatment of cholestasis in children on long-term total parenteral nutrition: a pilot study. *Gastroenterology* 1996; **111**:716–9.

51 Heubi JE, Wiechmann DA, Creutzinger V, *et al.* Tauroursodeoxycholic acid (TUDCA) in the prevention of total parenteral nutritional associated liver disease. *J Pediatr Gastroenterol Nutr* 2003;**36**:422–3.

52 Spaeth G, Berg RD, Specian RD, Deitch EA. Food without fiber promotes bacterial translocation from the gut. *Surgery* 1990; **108**:240–6.

53 Hwang TL, Lue MC, Chen LL. Early use of cyclic TPN prevents further deterioration of liver functions for the TPN patients with impaired liver function. *Hepatogastroenterology* 2000;**47**:1347–50.

54 Kubota A, Okada A, Imura K, *et al.* The effect of metronidazole on TPN-associated liver dysfunction in neonates. *J Pediatr Surg* 1990;**25**:618–21.

55 Teitelbaum DH, Han-Markey T, Schumacher RE. Treatment of parenteral nutrition-associated cholestasis with cholecystokinin-octapeptide. *J Pediatr Surg* 1995;**30**:1082–5.

56 Hassan KO, Beath SV, McKiernan PJ. Difficult management choices for infants with short bowel syndrome and liver failure. *J Pediatr Gastroenterol Nutr* 2002;**35**:216–9.

57 Kumar N, Beath S, van Mourik I, *et al.* New strategies to improve outcome of children awaiting small bowel transplantation. *Am J Transplant* 2002;**2**:939.

58 Gupte GL, Kumar N, Kelly DA, *et al.* 11 years' experience of evaluating children with intestinal failure (if) referred for possible intestinal transplantation. *J Pediatr Gastroenterol Nutr* 2002; **34**:449.

59 Kaufman SS, Atkinson JB, Bianchi A, *et al.* Indications for pediatric intestinal transplantation. *Pediatr Transpl* 2001;**5**:80–7.

60 Gupte GL, Beath SV, Protheroe S, *et al.* Improved outcome of referrals for intestinal transplantation in the UK. *Arch Dis Child* 2007;**92**:147–52.

61 Botha JF, Grant WJ, Torres C, *et al.* Isolated liver transplantation in infants with end-stage liver disease due to short bowel syndrome. *Liver Transpl* 2006;**12**:1062–6.

62 Wolf A, Pohlandt F. Bacterial infection: the main cause of acute cholestasis in newborn infants receiving short-term parenteral nutrition. *Pediatr Gastroenterol Nutr* 1989;**8**:297–303.

63 Reyes J, Tzakis A, Todo S, *et al.* Candidates for small bowel transplantation and possible indicators of outcome. *Transplant Proc* 1994;**26**:1445.

64 Deville D, Goyet J, Mitchell A, *et al.* En block combined reduced liver and small bowel transplants: from large donors to small children. *Transplantation* 2000;**69**:555–9.

65 Fryer J, Pellar S, Ormond D, *et al.* Mortality in candidates waiting for combined liver-intestine transplants exceeds that for other candidates waiting for liver transplants. *Liver Transpl* 2003;**9**:748–53.

66 Langnas AN, Shaw BW Jr, Antonson DL, *et al.* Preliminary experience with intestinal transplantation in infants and children. *Pediatrics* 1996;**97**:443–8.

67 Starzl TE, Todo S, Tzakis A, *et al.* The many faces of multivisceral transplantation. *Surg Gynecol Obstet* 1991;**172**:335–44.

68 Starzl TE, Hakala TR, Shaw BW Jr, *et al.* A flexible procedure for multiple cadaveric organ procurement. *Surg Gynecol Obstet* 1984;**158**:223–30.

69 Abu-Elmagd K, Reyes J, Todo S, *et al.* Clinical intestinal transplantation: new perspectives and immunologic considerations. *J Am Coll Surg* 1998;**186**:512–27.

70 Bueno J, Abu-Elmagd K, Mazariegos G, *et al.* Composite liver-small bowel allografts with preservation of donor duodenum and hepatic biliary system in children. *J Pediatr Surg* 2000; **35**:291–5.

71 Sudan DL, Iyer KR, Deroover A, *et al.* A new technique for combined liver-small intestinal transplantation. *Transplantation* 2001;**72**:1846–8.

72 Abu-Elmagd K, Fung J, Bueno J, *et al.* Logistics and technique for procurement of intestinal, pancreatic, and hepatic grafts from the same donor. *Ann Surg* 2000;**323**:680–97.

73 Kalayoglu M, Sollinger WH, Stratta RJ, *et al.* Extended preservation of the liver for clinical transplantation. *Lancet* 1988;**i**: 617–9.

74 Todo S, Nery J, Yanaga K, *et al.* Extended preservation of human liver grafts with UW solution. *JAMA* 1989;**261**:711–4.

75 Levi DM, Tzakis AG, Kato T, *et al.* Transplantation of the abdominal wall. *Lancet* 2003;**361**:2173–6.

76 Todo S, Reyes J, Furukawa H, *et al.* Outcome analysis of 71 clinical intestinal transplantations. *Ann Surg* 1995;**333**:270–82.

77 Gruessner RW, Sharp HL. Living-related intestinal transplantation: first report of a standardized surgical technique. *Transplantation* 1997;**15**:1605–7.

78 Testa G, Holterman M, John E, *et al.* Combined living donor liver/small bowel transplantation. *Transplantation* 2005;**27**: 1401–4.

79 Reyes J, Bueno J, Kocoshis S, *et al.* Current status of intestinal transplantation in children. *J Pediatr Surg* 1998;**33**:243–54.

80 Lauro A, Dazzi A, Ercolani G, *et al.* Rejection episodes and 3-year graft survival under sirolimus and tacrolimus treatment after adult intestinal transplantation. *Transplant Proc* 2007;**39**: 1629–31.

81 Sindhi R, Seward J, Mazariegos G, *et al.* Replacing calcineurin inhibitors with mTOR inhibitors in children. *Pediatr Transpl* 2005;**9**:391–7.

82 Bond GJ, Mazariegos GV, Sindhi R, Abu-Elmagd KM, Reyes J. Evolutionary experience with immunosuppression in pediatric intestinal transplantation. *J Pediatr Surg* 2005;**40**:274–9.

83 Nishida S, Levi DM, Moon JI, *et al.* Intestinal transplantation with alemtuzumab (Campath-1H) induction for adult patients. *Transplant Proc* 2006;**38**:1747–9.

84 Reyes J, Mazariegos GV, Abu-Elmagd K, *et al.* Intestinal transplantation under tacrolimus monotherapy after perioperative lymphoid depletion with rabbit anti-thymocyte globulin (Thymoglobulin). *Am J Transpl* 2005;**5**:1430–6.

85 Murase N, Demetris AJ, Metasuaki T, *et al.* Long survival in rats after multivisceral versus isolated small bowel allotransplantation under FK506. *Surgery* 1991;**110**:87–8.

86 Starzl TE, Demetris AJ, Trucco M, *et al.* Cell migration and chimerism after whole-organ transplantation: the basis of graft acceptance. *Hepatology* 1993;**17**:1127–56.

87 Reyes J, McGhee W, Mazariegos G, *et al.* Thymoglobulin in the management of steroid resistant acute cellular rejection in children. *Transplantation* 2002;**74**:419.

88 Green M, Reyes J, Nour B, *et al.* Early infectious complications of liver-intestinal transplantation in children: preliminary analysis. *Transplant Proc* 1994;**26**:1420–1.

89 Sigurdsson L, Green M, Putnam P, *et al.* Bacteremia frequently accompanies rejection following pediatric small bowel transplantation. *J Pediatr Gastroenterol Nutr* 1995;**21**:356.

90 Bueno J, Green M, Kocoshis S, *et al.* Cytomegalovirus infection after intestinal transplantation in children. *Clin Infect Dis* 1997; **25**:1078–83.

91 Janes S, Beath SV, Jones R, *et al.* Enteral feeding after intestinal transplantation: the Birmingham experience. *Transplant Proc* 1997;**29**:1855–6.

92 Haghighi KS, Sharif K, Gupte G, *et al.* Is serum gentamicin level a good predictor of graft injury in intestinal transplantation? *Transplant Proc* 2006;**38**:1733–4.

93 Sudan D, Vargas L, Sun Y, Bok L, Dijkstra G, Langnas A. Calprotectin: a novel noninvasive marker for intestinal allograft monitoring. *Ann Surg* 2007;**246**:311–5.

94 Kato T, Gaynor JJ, Nishida S, *et al.* Zoom endoscopic monitoring of small bowel allograft rejection. *Surg Endosc* 2006;**20**:773–82.

95 Mousa H, Bueno J, Griffiths J, *et al.* Intestinal motility after small bowel transplantation. *Transplant Proc* 1998;**30**:2535–6.

96 Kato T, Gaynor JJ, Selvaggi G, *et al.* Intestinal transplantation in children: a summary of clinical outcomes and prognostic factors in 108 patients from a single center. *J Gastrointest Surg* 2005;**9**:75–89.

97 Sigurdsson L, Reyes J, Todo S, *et al.* Anatomic variability of rejection in intestinal allografts after pediatric intestinal transplantation. *J Pediatr Gastroenterol Nutr* 1998;**27**:403–6.

98 White FV, Reyes J, Jaffe R, *et al.* Pathology of intestinal transplantation in children. *Am J Surg Path* 1995;**19**:687–98.

99 Lee RG, Nakamura K, Tsamauda ACM, *et al.* Pathology of human intestinal transplantation. *Gastroenterology* 1996;**110**: 1820–34.

100 Sudan DL, Kauffman SS, Shaw BW, *et al.* Isolated intestinal transplantation for intestinal failure. *Am J Gastroenterol* 2000;**95**: 1506–15.

101 Wu T, Abu-Elmagd K, Bond G, *et al.* A schema for histologic grading of small intestine allograft acute rejection. *Transplantation* 2003;**27**:1241–8.

102 Gray J, Darbyshire PJ, Beath SV, *et al.* Experience with quinupristin/dalfopristin in treatment of infections with vancomycin-resistant *Enterococcus faecium* in children. *J Pediatr Infect Dis* 2000;**19**:234–8.

103 Green M, Bueno J, Sigurdsson L, *et al.* Unique aspects of the infectious complications of intestinal transplantation. *Curr Opin Org Transpl* 1999;**4**:361–7.

104 Hebert H, Muller C, Loffler J, *et al.* Monitoring of CMV infection: a comparison of PCR from whole blood, plasma-PCR, pp65-antigenaemia and virus culture in patients after bone marrow transplantation. *Bone Marrow Transplant* 1996;**17**:861–8.

105 Haque T, Wilkie GM, Jones MM, *et al.* Allogeneic cytotoxic T-cell therapy for EBV-positive posttransplantation lymphoproliferative disease: results of a phase 2 multicenter clinical trial. *Blood* 2007;**110**:1123–31.

106 Choquet S, Oertel S, Leblond V, *et al.* Rituximab in the management of post-transplantation lymphoproliferative disorder after solid organ transplantation: proceed with caution. *Ann Hematol* 2007;**86**:599–607.

107 Reyes J, Green M, Bueno J, *et al.* Epstein–Barr virus associated posttransplant lymphoproliferative disease after intestinal transplantation. *Transplant Proc* 1996;**28**:2768–9.

108 Green M, Reyes J, Jabbour N, *et al.* Use of quantitative PCR to predict onset of Epstein–Barr viral infection and post-transplant lymphoproliferative disease after intestinal transplantation in children. *Transplant Proc* 1996:**28**:2759–60.

109 Green M, Reyes J, Webber S, Rowe D. The role of antiviral and immunoglobulin therapy in the prevention of Epstein–Barr virus infection and post-transplant lymphoproliferative disease following solid organ transplantation. *Transpl Infect Dis* 2001;**3**: 97–103.

110 Reyes J, Todo S, Green M, *et al.* Graft-versus-host disease after liver and small bowel transplantation in a child. *Clin Transplant* 1997;**11**:345–8.

111 Murase N, Ye Q, Nalesnik MA, *et al.* Immunomodulation for intestinal transplantation by allograft irradiation, adjunct donor bone marrow infusion, or both. *Transplantation* 2000;**15**:1632–41.

112 Bakonyi A, Berho M, Ruiz P, *et al.* Donor and recipient pretransplant conditioning with nonlethal radiation and antilymphocyte serum improves the graft survival in a rat small bowel transplant model. *Transplantation* 2001;**27**:983–8.

113 Reyes JD. Intestinal transplantation. *Semin Pediatr Surg* 2006;**15**: 228–34.

114 Pinna AD, Weppler D, Nery JR, *et al.* Intestinal transplantation at the University of Miami-five years of experience. *Transplant Proc* 2000;**32**:1226–7.

115 Grant D, Abu-Elmagd K, Reyes J, *et al.* Intestine Transplant Registry. 2003 report of the intestine transplant registry: a new era has dawned. *Ann Surg* 2005;**241**:607–13.

116 Tzakis A, Nour B, Reyes J, *et al.* Endorectal pull-through of transplanted colon as part of intestinal transplantation. *Surgery* 1995;**117**:451–3.

117 Strohm S, Koehler A, Reyes J. Management in pediatric small bowel transplant. *Nutr Clin Prac* 1999;**14**:58–63.

118 Kosmach B. Care routines following pediatric intestinal transplantation. [Paper presented at the 5th International Symposium on Intestinal Transplantation, Cambridge, UK, 1998.]

119 Sudan D, Horslen S, Botha J, *et al.* Quality of life after pediatric intestinal transplantation: the perception of pediatric recipients and their parents. *Am J Transplant* 2004;**4**:407–13.

120 Sudan D. Cost and quality of life after intestinal transplantation. *Gastroenterology* 2006;**130**(2 Suppl 1):S158–62.

121 Longworth L, Young T, Beath SV, *et al.* An economic evaluation of pediatric small bowel transplantation in the United Kingdom. *Transplantation* 2006;**82**:508–15.

12 The Developing World

23 Liver Disease in the Developing World

Seng-Hock Quak, Anupam Sibal, and Mei-Hwei Chang

Liver disease in children is a common problem in the developing world. The most important etiology is infection, which includes viral hepatitis, dengue fever, typhoid, malaria, and tuberculosis.

As a result of improved environmental sanitation and socio-economic conditions, there has been a change in the pattern of disease in the developing world. International programs such as the universal hepatitis B vaccination program in hyperendemic areas have changed the natural history of hepatitis B and have implications for the control of infectious liver diseases in other parts of the world.

As modern medicine and sanitation control reduce the incidence of infectious diseases, it has become apparent that both genetic and metabolic liver diseases are as important a cause of liver disease in children in the developing world as in developed countries. Unfortunately, lack of resources, training, and specialized laboratory support makes the diagnosis and management of these rare diseases a problem in many areas.

The success of liver transplantation internationally has led to its development in many countries. As the organization of an effective cadaveric donor program is difficult for many reasons, the most effective form of transplantation for treatment of children with end-stage liver disease is a living related donation program.

Much needs to be done to improve child health in many developing countries. It is important to continue to control the remaining infectious causes of liver diseases and to develop better ways to diagnose and treat genetic and metabolic liver diseases.

Neonatal liver disease

Neonatal liver disease includes many clinical conditions. Although these are addressed in detail elsewhere in this book (see Chapter 4), the spectrum of neonatal liver disease and cholestasis in developing countries differs significantly from that in developed nations with regard to both etiology and management (Table 23.1).

Etiology

Neonatal cholestasis (NC) constitutes around one-third of hepatobiliary disorders in India, Malaysia, and Taiwan. In Delhi, data collected over 9 years showed that NC constituted 21% (427/1998) of all pediatric hepatobiliary referrals. Biliary atresia was responsible for about 21% of these (90/427).

Table 23.1 Spectrum of neonatal cholestasis syndrome in India (n = 1008).

	Subgroups		Total NCS	
	n	%	n	%
Hepatocellular			533	53
Neonatal hepatitis	468			
Idiopathic giant-cell hepatitis		64%		
TORCHES infections		22%		
Sepsis		8%		
Others (malaria, UTI, etc.)		6%		
Metabolic	43			
Galactosemia		35%		
α_1-Antitrypsin deficiency		33%		
TPN-related		19%		
Others		13%		
Others	22			
Obstructive			385	38
Biliary atresia		89%		(34)
Choledochal cyst		11%		(3)
Ductal paucity			29	3
Non-syndromic		83%		
Syndromic		17%		
Idiopathic			61	6
Total			1008	

NCS, neonatal cholestasis syndrome; TORCHES, toxoplasmosis, rubella, cytomegalovirus, herpes, syphilis; TPN, total parenteral nutrition; UTI, urinary tract infection.

Diseases of the Liver and Biliary System in Children, 3rd edition. Edited by Deirdre Kelly. © 2008 Blackwell Publishing, ISBN: 978-1-4051-6334-7.

Idiopathic giant-cell hepatitis (29%) and cholestasis due to multiple factors (19%) were the other major causes (Sibal, personal communication). The relative incidence of conditions leading to NC, as reported from a countrywide analysis in India, is shown in Table 23.1.[1] Metabolic conditions constituted only 4% of these cases, which reflects the lack of diagnostic facilities in India.

In a series of 50 consecutive cases of obstructive jaundice seen at a tertiary center in Singapore, 66% were due to idiopathic hepatitis, 28% due to biliary atresia, 4% to choledochal cysts, and 2% to galactosemia.[2] In Taiwan, about 49% of cases of neonatal hepatitis were due to cytomegalovirus (CMV) infection.[3] Neither α_1-antitrypsin deficiency nor cystic fibrosis was documented in either the Singapore or Taiwan series. Metabolic diseases such as abnormal bile salt metabolism were not excluded because of a lack of laboratory support.

Over 50% of children with NC are referred to hospital later than in the developed countries. This may be due to a lack of appreciation of jaundice and because initially they appear well. Other reasons for delay are a lack of awareness at the primary and secondary levels of health care and the absence of a standardized approach to diagnosis.[4] Furthermore, parents may delay seeking medical advice due to the complex social set-up (with decisions being made by the extended family), or because alternative medicine systems are consulted before appropriate medical attention is sought. The average age at presentation to a specialized center with NC is usually 3.5 months.

Diagnosis

Diagnosis is as described in Chapter 4, but many of the specialized investigations are not available in developing countries and accurate diagnosis depends on collaboration with specialized units in the developed world.

Treatment and outcome

The final outcome in a significant proportion of cases is dependent on the age at diagnosis and the availability of appropriate management. The delay in diagnosis and referral is reflected in the reported prevalence of cirrhosis, at 75–100% of patients undergoing laparotomy for NC. The importance of early detection and operative management is evident through collective results, showing that the success of a portoenterostomy is related to the age at the time of procedure and reduces significantly with every month of delay. While 70–80% of children who undergo surgery before 2 months of age achieve adequate bile drainage, the number drops to 40–50% with surgery at 2–3 months, and the average success rate further falls from 25% to 10% for children operated beyond 3 or 4 months of age. Many of the children are referred too late with advanced liver disease and cannot benefit from the Kasai portoenterostomy (Chapters 4 and 19), leaving transplantation as the only option. However, the high cost and the lack of available donor organs make this an unrealistic option for many children. Of 44 children who underwent the Kasai procedure in India,[5] only 20% became jaundice-free, which was attributable to their advanced age at presentation (> 90 days) in 60% of cases, in comparison with Singapore, where biliary atretic patients are regularly operated on and 37% of the patients have successful portoenterostomy, as defined by clearance of jaundice.[6] In a long-term follow-up of patients in India with successful biliary drainage, a 15-year survival rate of 87% has been reported, which is comparable with European or Japanese results.[4]

Of 215 children considered for liver transplantation in Delhi, 142 had NC (biliary atresia constituted 62% of these). Ninety-one children were found to be unfit for transplantation, of whom 64 had NC along with severe malnutrition (Sibal, personal communication). As specific commercial liver feeds are not available in many developing countries, most units rely on modular feeds incorporating medium-chain triglycerides.

A greater awareness regarding diagnosis and referral of patients, a uniform approach to investigation and treatment, and strengthening/improvement of laboratory and surgical facilities at referral centers will hopefully improve the outcome for these infants in developing countries in the near future. There are already signs of hope in India, with public awareness campaigns and education programs showing positive results. A comparison of numbers prior to the national consensus and initiation of the continued awareness campaign in 1999 with those thereafter showed an increase in patients presenting with NC per month from 1.5 to 3.2 during the corresponding periods. The mean age of patients with extrahepatic biliary atresia at presentation also showed a trend to earlier referral, with the average age decreasing from 132 days to 97 days and the delay in referral falling from 121 days to 78 days after the awareness measures.[4,7]

Chronic liver disease

Most chronic liver disease is due to chronic viral hepatitis (Table 23.2). The accuracy of the diagnosis depends on local expertise and the degree of specialization of laboratory support. The etiological profile of chronic liver disease (CLD), as determined in a nationwide survey of teaching medical institutions in India from 1988 to 1997, is shown in Table 23.2. Category I centers are those with specialist pediatric gastroenterology and hepatology units and category II centers are those without such units. It is likely that metabolic and autoimmune liver disease is underrepresented because of a lack of diagnostic facilities.

While treatment for each of these conditions is no different from that in the West, a lack of specialized metabolic feeds and the high cost of drugs such as interferon are serious limitations.

Table 23.2 Etiological profile of chronic liver disease in India.

Etiology	Category I centers (n = 6)	Category II centers (n = 5)
Total patients	809	175
Viral hepatitis	147 (18.2%)	32 (18.3%)
Autoimmune	49 (6.0%)	3 (1.7%)
Metabolic	170 (21.0%)	24 (13.7%)
Others*	83 (10.3%)	65 (37.1%)
Unknown	360 (44.5%)	51 (29.1%)

*Others: galactosemia, hereditary fructose intolerance, glycogen storage disease, tyrosinemia type I, Niemann–Pick disease, Gaucher disease.

Table 23.3 Specialized formulas available in Malaysia.

Disorders	Formula
Galactosemia	Soy formulas: Isomil,* Prosobee,† Formula-S,‡ Nursoy,§ Alsoy#
Maple syrup urine disease	MSUD diet powder†
Tyrosinemia	Low Phe/Tyr diet powder¶
Nutritional supplement for end-stage liver disease	Neocate¶

* Abbott.
† Mead-Johnson.
‡ Nutricia.
§ Wyeth.
\# Nestle.
¶ Scientific Hospital Supplies (SHS).

Metabolic liver disease

In the developing world, the diagnosis and management of metabolic liver disease pose several challenges. As the clinical presentation may be nonspecific, accurate diagnosis requires specific and reliable diagnostic facilities, which only exist in a few centers in developing countries. Even in centers where these facilities exist, social, cultural, and economic factors may reduce the number of families willing to allow their child to undergo invasive tests or to consider prenatal testing.

In a nationwide survey involving 11 teaching medical institutions in India (six with specialized pediatric gastroenterology and hepatology services and five without such services), metabolic liver diseases (MLDs) constituted up to 46% (8–43% in specialized centers) of the reported cases of chronic liver disease over a period of 1–9 years. Wilson's disease was the most frequently diagnosed MLD, and Indian childhood cirrhosis (ICC) was infrequently reported.[8] Other frequently diagnosed MLDs were α_1-antitrypsin deficiency, galactosemia, hereditary fructose intolerance, glycogen storage diseases, tyrosinemia type l, Niemann–Pick disease, and Gaucher disease. Most metabolic defects were diagnosed on the basis of clinical features and liver histology, as specific enzyme assays were rarely available. Isolated metabolic diseases such as tyrosinemia have been reported from Singapore.[9]

The treatment of metabolic liver disease is a challenge in developing countries, as therapeutic options are limited. Dietary management involves unpalatable diets and the use of nasogastric feeding, which is difficult to support in the community without the appropriate infrastructure. Specialized feeding formulas are not freely available. Although many nutritional companies have agents in developing countries, the process of importing the required formula is slow, expensive, and may be impossible (Table 23.3).

Liver transplantation is limited to a few centers and is rarely an option (see below).

Indian childhood cirrhosis (see also Chapter 14)

Indian childhood cirrhosis (ICC) was formerly one of the commonest causes of chronic liver disease in children in India and responsible for a large number of childhood deaths, but has now become practically nonexistent. In the 1980s, the incidence was one in 4000 rural live births, but recently it has accounted for less than 2% of cases of metabolic liver disease treated at large teaching hospitals.[10]

Etiology

The etiology of ICC was thought to be related to copper toxicosis[11] due to ingestion of animal milk that had been contaminated by copper in brass cooking pots.[12,13]

Clinical features

The mean age at presentation was 18 months (range 6 months to 5 years). It was more common in males than in females (3 : 1) and had an insidious onset, with abdominal distension and malaise, with rapid progression to liver failure and death. Physical features included hepatomegaly, ascites, and portal hypertension.

The diagnosis was based on liver histology, which included: hepatocyte necrosis with ballooning and Mallory hyaline; pericellular interlobular fibrosis; inflammatory infiltration; and grossly elevated liver copper (> 250 mg/g dry weight).

Treatment and prognosis

Although untreated ICC has a high mortality rate (86% within 6 months of hospital attendance), treatment early in the course of the disease (at the preicteric stage) has recently been shown to allow long-term disease-free survival.

All 29 patients treated with D-penicillamine were found to be growing well, with normal liver function tests, 5–12 years after diagnosis. Only four had residual hepatosplenomegaly, which showed inactive micronodular cirrhosis on biopsy. No major side effects of penicillamine therapy were reported.[14]

The disappearance of ICC remains enigmatic, but it may have been related to a change in feeding practices and a reduction in the use of brass cookware (see Chapter 14).[15]

Sporadic cases of an ICC-like disorder in infants have been reported from other countries (idiopathic copper toxicosis). It is possible that different mechanisms (environmental, genetic, or a combination of the two) may give rise to copper-associated childhood toxicosis. Further developments in the mapping of genes involved in copper metabolism may shed more light on the etiopathogenesis of this disorder, which is fortunately now rare.

Infectious diseases

For yellow fever, Lassa fever, schistosomiasis, hydatid disease, Marburg and Ebola viruses, see Chapter 6.

Typhoid

Enteric fever is an acute systemic bacterial illness caused by the *Salmonella* group of organisms and is a major health problem in developing countries. Typhoid bacilli are filtered by the liver and Kupffer cells and excreted in the bile. Hepatic enlargement is a common occurrence in enteric fever and has been recognized since a report by Osler in 1899.

Clinical features and diagnosis

Between 23% and 90% of children with typhoid fever are reported to have mild to moderate hepatomegaly, and approximately 1–16% are jaundiced. Moderately elevated hepatic transaminases are common. Hepatic manifestations are more severe in relapses and in infections by multidrug-resistant *Salmonella typhi*.[16] A study in New Delhi showed that of 93 children with culture proven *Salmonella typhi* infection, hepatomegaly was seen in 88% and splenomegaly in 46%. Fever was the presenting symptom in all children, with 75.8% having high-grade fever and 72.6% presenting with history of more than 7 days of fever at the time of admission. Seventy-four percent of the children were toxic at admission, and a total of 30.6% developed complications (hepatitis 14.5%, intestinal bleeding 4.8%, pleural effusion 1.6%). Further manifestations were diarrhea (74.2%), abdominal pain (62.9%), vomiting (61.2%), malaise (48.3%), anorexia (33.8%), nausea (32.2%), cough (32.2%), constipation (14.5%), and gastrointestinal bleeding (12.9%).[17]

Salmonella endotoxin may induce consumptive coagulopathy, depletion of complement, and arteritis, all of which may damage hepatocytes. Direct invasion of the hepatocyte by the organism may also contribute to the hepatic insult.

The differential diagnosis includes:

- Hemolysis (in patients with glucose-6-phosphate dehydrogenase (G6PD) deficiency or thalassemia)
- Ascending cholangitis
- *Salmonella* liver abscess
- Cholecystitis
- Amebic liver disease
- Malaria with jaundice
- Viral hepatitis

An important differentiating clinical feature is that the jaundice associated with typhoid fever tends to occur at the peak of fever, whereas in viral hepatitis, jaundice is usually followed by a decrease in fever. Furthermore, an alanine aminotransferase (ALT)/lactate dehydrogenase (LDH) ratio of < 4 is seen in typhoid hepatitis and > 4 in viral hepatitis.[18] Hepatic encephalopathy has been rarely reported.[19] Acute typhoid cholecystitis is rare.

Liver histology

The liver biopsy may demonstrate mild hepatitis, parenchymatous degeneration, peripheral infiltration by mononuclear cells, and central necrosis, with characteristic granulomatous collections of mononuclear cells called typhoid/Mallory nodules.

Treatment and outcome

In view of the high proportion of multidrug-resistant strains (50% in China, 50–88% in Vietnam, 16–25% in Singapore, 40–92% in India) the treatment of typhoid in developing countries is with third-generation cephalosporins (i.v. ceftriaxone or cefotaxime 100 mg/kg/day, oral cefuroxime 10 mg/kg/day) or quinolones (ciprofloxacin or ofloxacin i.v. 10 mg/kg/day or oral 20 mg/kg/day). Maintenance of adequate hydration and dietary intake is essential. Treatment is continued for 5 days after fever settles. Hospital admission is required for complications, toxicity, and for hydration/nutrition. Recent published data in Delhi showed that 66.6% of children had multidrug-resistant typhoid fever, of which the maximum numbers of patients were seen in the 2–5-year-old age group (30.6%). Ofloxacin (20 mg/kg/day) showed comparable efficiency to ceftriaxone (100 mg/kg/day), with a defervescence time of 5.0 days versus 4.3 days, respectively.[17]

If hepatitis is associated, other causes of jaundice need to be excluded. Hepatomegaly and jaundice usually resolve within the first 7–10 days with appropriate therapy, whereas the transaminases resolve within 2–3 weeks.

Dengue fever

Dengue infection—also known as dengue fever, dengue hemorrhagic fever (DHF), and dengue shock syndrome—caused by mosquito-borne flavivirus, is endemic in many areas of the tropics and subtropics, including South-East Asia, India, the Pacific islands, and the Caribbean.

DHF is a severe, often fatal, febrile disease caused by dengue viruses and characterized by capillary permeability and abnormalities of hemostasis.

Clinical features

Dengue fever is usually characterized by:

• Biphasic fever (saddle-backed).
• Myalgia.
• Arthralgia.
• Severe headache and retro-orbital pain.
• Rash, which may be petechial.
• Leukopenia and lymphadenopathy.
• Hepatomegaly in almost all patients (79–100%).
• A protein-losing shock syndrome may develop—dengue shock syndrome (DSS).
• Bleeding complications may be present, ranging from gingival bleeding and epistaxis to hematuria.
• Fulminant hepatitis with encephalopathy and Reye syndrome has been reported from Thailand (Nimmannitya *et al.* 1987).[20]
• Myocarditis with a congested liver and ascites.
• Pleural effusion.

According to the World Health Organization, Dengue hemorrhagic fever (DHF) is characterized by:
• High-grade fever
• Thrombocytopenia
• Hemorrhagic phenomena
• Increased vascular leakage

Dengue shock syndrome (DSS) additionally shows:
• Weak rapid pulse
• Narrow pulse pressure (less than 20 mmHg)
• Hypotension for age
• Cold, clammy skin and restlessness

Hepatic transaminases—aspartate aminotransferase (AST) and ALT—often rise in dengue patients and may be elevated up to fivefold.[21] They usually peak in the second week of illness, with gradual normalization by the third to fourth week of illness. Clinically, patients can have hepatomegaly, with complaints of hepatic tenderness. Jaundice is a less common symptom (15–62%), except in those with DHF or DSS.[22]

DHF is graded from I to IV depending on clinical parameters, with DSS showing typical signs of circulatory failure. Hypoxia/ischemia resulting from the prolonged shock and metabolic acidosis may be responsible for the severity of hepatic dysfunction. The differential diagnosis includes acute hepatitis, while the clinical features of DSS may be confused with acute liver failure, in view of the changes in sensorium, bleeding tendency, and hepatomegaly.

A study conducted at the University of Colombia documented 168 out of 913 children with DHF grade III/IV who had atypical clinical manifestations, including hepatitis (27%), neurological alterations (25%), acute abdominal pain (11%), pulmonary alterations (9%), acalculous cholecystitis (9%), cardiac involvement (8%), and renal impairment (7%).[23] In addition, a pediatric study in Thailand, which included 35 children with acute liver failure, showed that dengue virus was present in 34.3% of cases. There were no cases of hepatitis A or B-induced liver failure in this study, due to the enforcement of vaccination.[24] This suggests that the dengue virus could become a more serious contributor in acute liver disease than initially assumed, requiring fast establishment of the diagnosis (dengue IgM, IgG enzyme-linked immunosorbent assay) and appropriate management.

The liver histology demonstrates centrilobular necrosis, fatty change, Kupffer cell hyperplasia, acidophilic bodies and monocyte infiltration of the portal tract.

Outcome

Treatment is supportive. Hepatic involvement is self-limited, although a few patients may develop hepatic failure. Recovery is usual within 48 hours, except for DHF or DSS.

The case-fatality rate of DHF is 5%, but can decline to 1% with appropriate treatment. The fatality rates of DSS can reach above 10% and a secondary antibody response (especially to type 2/DEN-2 virus) in patients with DHF or DSS is associated with a very high risk of mortality, with some sources mentioning even up to 100%.

Malaria

The liver is intimately related to *Plasmodium falciparum* and *P. vivax,* as it has a key role both in the life cycle of the organism and also in protective immunity against it.

Clinical features

Jaundice and hepatomegaly are more common in pediatric malarial infections (68%) in comparison with adult infections (6%). Jaundice is usually unconjugated, but may also be conjugated, which is more common with *P. falciparum* malaria than with *P. vivax.* Mild elevation of hepatic aminotransferases is common. Severe infection may occur in neonates, who present with clinical features suggestive of cholestasis.

Liver histology usually reveals fatty change, liver cell necrosis, nuclear vacuolation, Kupffer cell hyperplasia, and mononuclear cell infiltration. Kupffer cells contain malarial pigment in the form of dark brown granules, and in acute malaria due to *P. falciparum* numerous parasitized red blood cells and iron. Immunofluorescence staining in liver biopsy sections reveals intense deposition within the reticuloendothelial elements.[25]

In hyperendemic regions, an aberrant immunological response to *Plasmodium* results in hyperreactive malarial splenomegaly (tropical splenomegaly). This condition is characterized by massive splenomegaly and an elevated malarial antibody (polyclonal IgM). Significant hepatomegaly is a common associated finding, but liver histology demonstrates normal hepatocytes, with numerous lymphocytes in dilated sinusoids and enlarged Kupffer cells. Malarial pigment is usually absent.

Sudden massive intravascular hemolysis occurring in a previously infected individual, followed by fever and hemoglobinuria, is known as blackwater fever. Now fortunately rare, it is observed in nonimmune individuals residing in endemic areas and taking quinine irregularly for prophylaxis or presumptive treatment. It is associated with *P. falciparum* and scanty or absent parasitemia and carries a poor prognosis. The attack consists of fever with or without rigors, pain in the loins, hemoglobinuria, icterus, bilious vomiting, circulatory collapse, and acute renal failure. Fulminant hepatic failure has also been reported. Treatment is with antimalarial chemotherapy and measures to maintain circulatory volume. Cholestasis may occur, but hepatotoxicity may also be due to the toxic effects of antimalarial agents, such as amodiaquine, pyrimethamine, and sulfadoxine.

Outcome

Jaundice and hepatomegaly usually improve quickly after treatment of malaria, within 4–6 days. Treatment varies from region to region, depending on resistance. Chloroquine, sulfadoxine/pyrimethamine, and quinine may be used. *P. falciparum* malaria is more severe in jaundiced patients[26] and is associated with higher mortality,[27] perhaps because of the increased numbers of parasites causing severe intravascular hemolysis, rather than hepatitis. The aims of treatment are to reduce parasitemia and manage associated complications such as hypoglycemia and lactic acidosis. In severe and complicated *P. falciparum* malaria, treatment is quinine salt 10 mg/kg 8-hourly i.v. in 5% dextrose, irrespective of the chloroquine resistance status of the area. Quinine therapy should be for a minimum duration of 7 days, including both parenteral and oral doses. Alternative treatment includes artemisinin derivatives, such as:

- Artemisinin 10 mg/kg once a day i.v. for 5 days, with a double divided dose administered on the first day
- Artesunate 1 mg/kg (two doses) i.m./i.v. at an interval of 4–6 h on the first day, followed by 1 mg/kg once daily for 5 days
- Artemether 1.6 mg/kg (two doses) i.m. at an interval of 4–6 h on the first day, followed by 1.6 mg/kg once daily for 5 days

In children with G6PD deficiency, certain antimalarial agents (sulfadoxine/pyrimethamine) may provoke severe intravascular hemolysis.

Neither chronic hepatitis nor cirrhosis are reported in the longer term, but there may be residual reticuloendothelial cell changes due to hyperreactive malarial splenomegaly.

Hepatic tuberculosis

Liver involvement is seen in miliary and congenital tuberculosis (TB), or as a result of the hepatotoxicity of antitubercular drugs.

Clinical features

Primary hepatobiliary TB is associated with fever, abdominal pain, and hepatomegaly. Hepatomegaly is found in 60% of children with abdominal or disseminated TB.[28] Other presentations include:[29]

- Recurrent obstructive jaundice (30%)
- Hepatic calcification
- Tuberculous cholangitis
- Bile duct strictures and lymph nodes at the porta hepatis
- Liver abscess, particularly in endemic areas

Diagnosis and outcome

Elevation of hepatic aminotransferases is usual. The diagnosis is based on finding caseating granulomas on liver biopsy with evidence of TB elsewhere in the body. In children with a liver abscess, liver function tests may be normal. A diagnostic tap of the abscess is rarely helpful, but a biopsy from the wall of the abscess may show caseating granulomas or acid-fast bacilli. Alternatively, the diagnosis should be suspected if the diagnostic tap reveals sterile yellowish fluid, the immunodiagnostic tests for amebiasis are negative, and there is no response to combined therapy with antibiotics and antiprotozoal agents.

Treatment of hepatic TB requires balancing the hepatotoxic effect of the anti-TB therapy with its beneficial effects. Use of streptomycin may be needed along with ethambutol and ciprofloxacin, which are safe for the liver (Table 23.4). If the patient is compliant, treatment is usually successful.

Hepatotoxicity associated with anti-TB therapy

(see also Chapter 9)

Hepatotoxicity is a significant problem with antitubercular therapy (ATT). The reported rates of hepatotoxicity with ATT are 4.28% in Western countries[30] and 11.5% in Indian studies.[31] ATT-induced hepatitis causes a mortality of 6–12% if the drugs are continued after the onset of symptoms. Evidence of hepatitis in a patient receiving ATT presents a particularly difficult dilemma, as it is necessary to decide whether the hepatotoxicity is part of the disease or is a potentially severe hepatotoxic reaction that warrants discontinuation of therapy.

Although the mechanism of hepatotoxicity and the risk factors predisposing to it are still not clearly defined, advanced age, female sex, poor nutritional status, high alcohol intake, underlying liver disease (hepatitis B and hepatitis C) and human immunodeficiency virus (HIV) infection have been reported as risk factors for ATT-induced hepatotoxicity in adults. Acetylator status, previously considered a factor

Table 23.4 Recommended doses of antitubercular drugs in children.

Drug	Dose (mg/kg/day)
Isoniazid	5
Rifampicin	10
Pyrazinamide	25
Ethambutol	20
Streptomycin	20
Ciprofloxacin	10

in hepatotoxicity, does not appear to be an important determinant of hepatotoxicity due to isoniazid (isonicotinohydrazide, INH), particularly in children.[32] The risk factors for ATT-induced hepatitis in children are not clear, but it is more likely if there is underlying liver disease, severe malnutrition, or extensive TB (tuberculous meningitis or miliary TB).

The rate of INH-induced hepatotoxicity in children is 3–10%, with fulminant hepatitis in 0.6% of cases. Hepatotoxicity is more likely in adolescents, but there is no difference between slow and rapid acetylators. Rifampicin was initially thought to potentiate isoniazid-induced hepatotoxicity, but subsequent studies showed similar rates of hepatotoxicity when INH was used alone or in combination with rifampicin. Only 0.6% of patients receiving rifampicin may develop jaundice. Pyrazinamide at recommended dosages (20–35 mg/kg/day) does not potentiate INH-induced hepatitis, although it may give rise to an increase in transaminases.[32] Hepatitis is more likely with combination therapy.

Diagnosis and management

Although clear-cut guidelines about monitoring liver function are not agreed, it would seem prudent to measure AST and ALT every 2–3 weeks for the first 8 weeks. The development of jaundice or hepatomegaly would warrant immediate action.

ALT or AST more than twice the upper limit of normal, or visible jaundice, or serum bilirubin > 2 mg/dL (> 40 μmol/L) in the presence of ATT indicates hepatotoxicity secondary to ATT. The differential diagnosis should include other causes of infectious hepatitis.[33] Absence of fever, a prodromal illness, or tender hepatomegaly are important clues to the presence of drug-induced hepatitis.

If jaundice develops or if transaminases rise to more than four times normal, INH, rifampicin and pyrazinamide should be stopped and streptomycin (20 mg/kg) and ethambutol (20 mg/kg) should be started. Continuing unmodified ATT in the presence of liver dysfunction can result in liver failure. Weekly transaminase levels should be assessed until AST and ALT return to less than twice normal (usually 2–4 weeks), and INH can then be restarted 1 week later. Pyrazinamide may be added a further 1 week later if it has been stopped during the intensive phase of therapy.[32,34] Streptomycin and ethambutol may be stopped when two of the drugs have been reintroduced. Weekly monitoring of live enzymes should continue until all hepatotoxic drugs have been reintroduced and continued for 2 weeks. The last drug to be introduced should be stopped if transaminases rise again to more than twice normal.

Hepatobiliary and pancreatic ascariasis

Ascariasis is caused by the nematode *Ascaris lumbricoides,* which is the largest and most prevalent of the human helminths. *Ascaris* infections are usually asymptomatic, unless there is a heavy infection. In the Indian subcontinent, ascariasis is highly endemic in Kashmir, central and southwest India, and Bangladesh. Hepatobiliary and pancreatic ascariasis (HPA) is a well-described entity in which the helminth enters the ampullary orifice from the duodenum and either blocks the duct or advances into the common bile duct, the hepatic ducts, or the cystic duct. Occasionally, the worms enter the gallbladder or the pancreatic duct. Worm invasion of the hepatobiliary tree is less common in children than in adults, possibly due to the smaller size of the ductal system, which makes it difficult for the worms to enter.[35]

The clinical spectrum includes acute cholecystitis, pancreatitis, cholangitis, or a hepatic abscess. The worms either move from the ducts or die there, forming a nidus for bile duct calculi. The diagnosis is suggested by finding adult worms or eggs in stool.[36] The worms may also be detected on computed tomography (CT) of the liver.[37] Treatment of biliary ascariasis includes conservative management for cholangitis and pancreatitis and oral anthelmintics to paralyze the worms, which are then expelled by the peristaltic activity of the intestine. Endoscopic intervention (removal by basket) can be used when patients do not respond to the initial symptomatic treatment or when the worm has not moved out of the ducts within 3 weeks of treatment. Pyrantel pamoate (10 mg/kg, single dose) and mebendazole (100 mg b.i.d. for 3 days) are effective against the worm and safe to use. Albendazole (200 mg orally < 2 years; 400 mg orally ≥ 2 years) has the advantage of requiring a single dose when used for *A. lumbricoides.* A second course may be given if the patient is not cured by 3 weeks after treatment.

Portal hypertension

Extrahepatic portal hypertension

Portal hypertension is an important cause of morbidity and mortality in children with liver disease, with high risk related to variceal bleeding, mainly from esophageal varices. The causes are categorized into cirrhotic and noncirrhotic etiology. More than three-quarters of Indian children with portal hypertension were found to have extrahepatic portal hypertension,[38] and Indian studies have shown extrahepatic portal venous obstruction (EHPVO) to be the commonest noncirrhotic cause for portal hypertension. The etiology of EHPVO is difficult to assess in most cases, but case reviews suggest congenital malformation of the portal vein or acquired thrombosis following umbilical sepsis, intraluminal trauma following exchange transfusion for neonatal hyperbilirubinemia, and pyelophlebitis following intestinal infection as possible causes. Many of these cases are commonly seen in children from the poorer sections of society.[39] In a prospective study, Yaccha *et al.* provided support for the hypothesis that the etiology of upper gastrointestinal bleeding in children may differ between developed and developing countries. They showed that 95% of children had upper gastrointestinal variceal bleeding, 92% of whom had bleeding due to EHPVO, a figure significantly higher than that seen in the West.[40]

Hepatoportal sclerosis

Hepatoportal sclerosis (also known as noncirrhotic portal fibrosis or idiopathic portal hypertension) is a common cause of portal hypertension among adults in India.[41] Although there have been few studies in children, hepatoportal sclerosis was present in 1.7% of 115 pediatric patients with portal hypertension,[42] and in another study in 3.25% of 338 children with portal hypertension seen over 6.5 years.[43]

Liver disease

Portal hypertension secondary to cirrhosis is mostly due to biliary atresia. Most of these children are too old at presentation for a portoenterostomy, because of a delay in referral.

Clinical features

Children may present with asymptomatic splenomegaly, failure to thrive, or gastrointestinal hemorrhage. Ascites is a rare feature. Most pediatric patients with EHPVO in developing countries present later than their counterparts in the West. They are likely to have had two or more previous episodes of variceal hemorrhage and usually have massive splenomegaly and moderate iron-deficiency anemia.

The median age at presentation of children with hepatoportal sclerosis is 11 years (range 5–14 years), and in contrast to adults, children rarely present with a variceal bleed. The clinical features of children with liver disease are as described elsewhere (Chapter 15).

Differential diagnosis

Isolated splenomegaly without upper gastrointestinal hemorrhage or evidence of hepatic decompensation has to be differentiated from other causes of splenomegaly such as lymphoma, leukemia, and Epstein–Barr virus infection, among others. In India, congestive splenomegaly (hyperreactive malarial splenomegaly), sickle-cell disease, thalassemia, and kala azar (which may also present with pancytopenia and upper gastrointestinal hemorrhage) need to be considered, and schistosomiasis should be excluded in endemic areas.

Treatment and outcome

Treatment options are the same as in the West and include endoscopic sclerotherapy, variceal banding, and shunt surgery.[44,45] Banding is now the preferred treatment option, as it requires fewer sessions, has fewer side effects, and compliance is better. The latter is of particular relevance for patients on low incomes who have long journeys to hospital.[44]

Patients with portal hypertension due to hepatoportal sclerosis have an excellent prognosis, as the histological changes are rarely progressive and the development of spontaneous shunts tends to protect these patients from variceal bleeding. Four of six patients with variceal bleeding were managed with endoscopic sclerotherapy and two with shunt surgery. All were alive and well after a median follow-up of 5.7 months.[43]

Although liver transplantation is the treatment of choice for those with cirrhotic portal hypertension, it remains unrealistic for most patients due to nonavailability of organs, prohibitive cost, and lack of specialized centers.

Viral hepatitis

Viral hepatitis is a worldwide health problem and is most prevalent in children in the developing world. Hepatitis A to E viruses are the main causes of viral hepatitis. Hepatitis A and E viruses are enterally transmitted and do not lead to chronic liver disease, while hepatitis B, C, and D viruses are parenterally transmitted and lead to chronic viral hepatitis, liver cirrhosis, and hepatocellular carcinoma (HCC).

Hepatitis D and E are rare in children even in the developing world, and this section will therefore discuss the relevance of hepatitis A, B, and C virus infection to child health in these countries.

Hepatitis A virus infection (see also Chapter 6)

Hepatitis A virus (HAV) is a nonenveloped, single-stranded RNA virus. It has four genotypes, with a single serotype. It belongs to a new genus, *Hepatovirus,* within the family *Picornaviridae*. It has been the most common viral hepatitis in the developing world.

The main route of transmission is through the fecal–oral route by contaminated food, water, or household contact. Uncooked or partially cooked shellfish is an important source of HAV infection, while transmission from food handlers and infected children to medical personnel has been reported. Travelers to endemic areas are at high risk and may transmit HAV after infection. After 10–12 days, HAV is detectable in the blood and feces, but becomes undetectable after the appearance of jaundice.

Epidemiology

HAV infection is prevalent in Asia, southern Europe, South America, and many other parts of the world. The epidemiological status of hepatitis A is divided into high, intermediate and low endemicity. The prevalence has declined gradually in the past 20 years[46–48] as a result of improved sanitation and socio-economic conditions, and many developing countries have moved from high to intermediate endemicity. However, even within the same developing country, low and intermediate areas may be mixed with high-endemicity areas, with a series of local epidemics. With these changes in epidemiology, there has been a decrease in immunity against hepatitis A,[49] increasing the number of children and adolescents who are now susceptible to HAV.

The Shanghai hepatitis A epidemic in 1988 demonstrated the impact of a large epidemic in the context of reduced immunity and exposure. More of the population was susceptible to hepatitis A in the Shanghai epidemic because it was a low to intermediate endemic area, while the surrounding areas were of high endemicity. Almost 300 000 people developed clinical hepatitis A, and 47 (15 of whom were hepatitis B surface antigen carriers) died.[50]

HAV infection is still a health problem in developing countries. For example, in a recent study of Mongolian children from 2005 to 2006, total antibody against HAV was detected in 19.5% (17/87) of those in the 1–3-year-old age group, 50.0% (69/138) of those in the 4–6-year-old age group, and 81.4% (105/129) of those in the 7–9-year-old age group. Notably, 97.2% of children in the 16–20-year-old year age group had anti-HAV antibody.[51] With increasing travel and international communication, prevention of HAV infection is now an important worldwide problem, particularly for travelers or food handlers.

A study conducted in Delhi on patients attending the outpatient department of a private hospital for almost a year until 2004 showed an overall seroprevalence for hepatitis A of 49% in the 2–12-year-old age group (Sibal *et al.*, personal communication), while the overall seroprevalence in other major Indian cities has been reported to average 65.9% (varying from 26.2% to 85.3%). Cochin, a city in South India with a higher literacy rate, showed the lowest prevalence at 26.2%. Seropositivity increased with age from 52.2% in the 1–5-year-old age group to 80.8% in those aged 16 or over.[52] These percentages demonstrate the shifting epidemiology in some pockets of the country, while many studies conducted across India still show results for high endemicity, with more than 90–95% of children being anti-HAV-positive by the age of 10 years. An association between rising seroprevalence and increasing age is common to many studies.[53,54]

Clinical features

Hepatitis A remains an important cause of morbidity in the developing world. The incubation period ranges from 15 to 50 days. The prodrome is abrupt, with general malaise, fever, anorexia, nausea, vomiting, and abdominal pain or discomfort. Jaundice appears within 1 week and lasts for < 2 weeks in the majority of cases. Hepatomegaly and elevation of aminotransferases are usual during the prodromal period. Serum bilirubin and aminotransferases return to normal within 2–3 months. HAV infection is often asymptomatic in young children, in contrast to infection in adults. It is more severe in those with chronic liver diseases, such as chronic hepatitis B or C.[55,56]

Extrahepatic manifestations are rare and may range from neurological, renal, and hematological manifestations to acute pancreatitis (see Chapter 6). Data from Delhi on hepatobiliary referrals (n = 1998) showed that of 961 children presenting with acute liver disease, 79% had typical hepatitis A and 15% had atypical manifestations of hepatitis A (Sibal *et al.*, personal communication).

Both the relapsing and cholestatic forms of hepatitis A are seen in children, with an increased incidence in older age. Prolonged cholestasis is seen as a protracted period of jaundice for more than 3 months, which resolves without intervention. The cholestatic course may present with pruritus, fever, diarrhea, weight loss, and serum bilirubin more than 10 mg/dL.[57] Relapsing acute viral hepatitis can be seen in 3–20% of patients with hepatitis A, with the patient initially showing partial or complete resolution of clinical and biochemical manifestations, but relapsing within a period of 3 weeks with a clinically milder presentation. Multiple relapses are uncommon and a tendency to increased cholestasis in patients may be noticed.[58]

The severity of the hepatitis and the numbers of symptomatic cases depend on age. The case-fatality rate has been reported to be 0.1% in children < 14 years old, 0.4% in adolescents and young adults (15–39 years), and 1.1% in patients 40 years of age or over. Although hepatitis A is mostly a self-limited acute disease, it can lead to fulminant hepatic failure on rare occasions, mainly in South America and South-East Asia. Among 5529 children in Pakistan with symptoms of acute hepatitis between 1991 and 1998, 2735 children had positive IgM antibody to HAV. Thirty children (1%) showed progressive hepatic dysfunction and liver failure.[59] In children with viral hepatitis A, particularly fulminant hepatitis A, who present with anemia and very high bilirubin levels, an association with G6PD should be considered (Sibal *et al.*, personal communication).

Prevention

Improvements in sanitation and water supply and the introduction of HAV vaccine are important factors contributing to the control of HAV. Seroepidemiological studies conducted in Taipei showed intermediate endemicity in 1975–1976.[60] When the study was repeated in 1984, anti-HAV was undetectable in children < 5 years of age, and only in 5% of children 5–10 years old.[61] When the study was repeated again in the same area in 1989, no children < 10 years were anti-HAV-positive.[62] In 2000, hardly any children or young adults < 20 years of age had immunity to HAV.[63] In contrast, 50% of those in the 20–30-year-old age group were anti-HAV positive and 90% of those over 30 were positive.

Before the introduction of hepatitis A vaccine, immunoglobulin was used to control local epidemics or prevent infection in travelers, but only provided immunity for 3–6 months. The development of effective hepatitis A vaccine has produced long-term immunity. Formalin-inactivated HAV vaccines are currently in clinical use and are highly immunogenic and safe, with mild side effects in both children and adults. Live attenuated vaccines are still under clinical investigation. A recent study in children in Taiwan demonstrated that inactivated HAV vaccine administered on a schedule of 0, 1, and 6 months provided protection for > 5 years and by mathematical calculation for > 25 years.[64,65]

The seroprevalence rate of anti-HAV was 95% at 1 month after the first dose of HAV vaccine and 100% at 6 and 7 months and 1–5 years after the first dose of vaccine.

A large double-blind, community-based control trial of an inactivated hepatitis A vaccine was conducted in a total of 40 119 children aged 1–16 years in Thailand. During the trial, there were 40 cases of hepatitis A, 38 of which were in the control group. The protective efficacy was 94% after two doses of hepatitis A vaccine, suggesting that two doses of HAV vaccine are as effective as three. Two double doses of HAV vaccine are more convenient for those traveling to endemic areas, and this is now the recommended schedule.

In Israel, a two-dose universal hepatitis A immunization program aimed at children aged 18 and 24 months (without a catch-up campaign) was started in 1999. Before this program, the mean annual incidence of hepatitis A disease was 50.4 per 100 000 in 1993–1998. The annual incidence of 2.2 to 2.5 per 100 000 in 2002–2004 represents a 95% or greater reduction for each year relative to the mean incidence in 1993–1998. This universal toddlers-only HAV immunization program in Israel demonstrated not only the high effectiveness of hepatitis A vaccination but also marked herd protection.[66] A combined hepatitis A and B vaccine (Twinrix) has been successfully developed for children or young adults to prevent hepatitis A and hepatitis B, with good immunogenicity to both viruses.[67]

The administration of two doses of hepatitis A virus vaccine on a 0- and 6-month schedule starting at 11–18 months of age was as immunogenic and as well tolerated as the administration of two doses in children 2 years of age. Immune responses to diphtheria–tetanus–acellular pertussis and *Haemophilus influenzae* type b, either given alone or coadministered with hepatitis A virus vaccine, were similar except for the antipertussis toxoid response.[68]

Hepatitis A infection is considered to be a mild disease in the majority of cases and the hepatitis A vaccine is optional in India. However, in children with G6PD deficiency, the virus can cause hemolytic anemia, severe hyperbilirubinemia, renal failure, and fulminant hepatic failure.[69] Personal experience showed that nine patients with hepatitis A also had G6PD deficiency, five of whom developed fulminant hepatic failure (55.6%). All of them were anemic and their G6PD levels were less than 100 mU/10^9 red blood cells. The mean peak serum bilirubin was 56.8 mg/dL (range 24.7–87.0 mg/dL) and the rate of rise was more than 10 mg/dL in 24 hours. Three patients were ventilated electively because of worsening encephalopathy. Four developed renal dysfunction, two of whom required hemodialysis. One child underwent a living related donor liver transplant. There were four children with concomitant hepatitis A and G6PD deficiency who did not develop fulminant hepatic failure. The mean serum bilirubin level in this group was 28.1 mg/dL (range 18–42 mg/dL). Although the rise was not as much as in the patients who developed fulminant hepatic failure, it was higher than that found in patients with hepatitis A virus infection (16 mg/dL; range 6–20 mg/dL) without an associated G6PD deficiency. Looking at this risk, recommending hepatitis A vaccine to children with G6PD deficiency should be justified.[70]

Table 23.5 Problems in the control of hepatitis A virus (HAV) infection.

- Frequent, rapid international travel
- Increasing susceptibility of the population, due to improved sanitation
- High cost of the HAV vaccine
- Inadequate resources for immunization

A vaccine of Chinese origin (a live attenuated H2 strain) against hepatitis A has been a focus of interest, and studies have been carried out since 1999. Given in a single dose, it is showing good immunogenicity and appears to be safe for use in children.[71]

The problems with control of hepatitis A are listed in Table 23.5.

Hepatitis B virus infection (see also Chapters 6 and 7)

Epidemiology

Hepatitis B virus (HBV) infection is a worldwide health problem. It is prevalent in Asia, Africa, southern Europe, and Latin America, where the hepatitis B surface antigen (HB_sAg)-seropositive rate ranges from 2% to 20%.[72,73] In most parts of Asia, the HB_sAg carrier rate in the general population is approximately 5–20% (Table 23.6) (Chen, personal communication).

In highly prevalent areas, primary HBV infections occur mainly during infancy and early childhood. The age of primary infection is an important factor affecting the outcome. Infection during infancy and early childhood leads to a high rate of chronicity. Before the implementation of the universal HBV vaccination program, the HBV infection rate

Table 23.6 Seroprevalence of hepatitis B surface antigenemia in the general population in Asian countries prior to the hepatitis B virus vaccination program.

Country	HB_sAg+ rate
Japan	–1%
Korea	3–15%
Malaysia	–5%
Singapore	5–7%
Thailand	8–10%
Indonesia	–10%
Philippines	–13%
Vietnam	–15%
China	10–20%
Hong Kong	–12%
Taiwan	15–20%

(i.e., the chronicity rate) in Taipei increased with age and was nearly 50% at age 14 years. The chronic infection rate was 5% in infants and remained stationary at 10% after the age of 2.[61,74] This suggested that most chronic HBV infection developed before 2 years of age in this hyperendemic population.[71] In parts of Africa such as rural Senegal, horizontal infection occurs very early. By the age of 2 years, 25% of children were infected, while at age 15 the infection rate was 80%.[75]

Perinatal transmission. Perinatal transmission from HB_sAg carrier mothers to their infants is a very important route of transmission leading to chronicity in hyperendemic areas. It accounts for the transmission route in 40–50% of HB_sAg carriers in Asia. Around 90% of the infants of seropositive mothers carrying hepatitis B e antigen (HB_eAg) became HB_sAg carriers,[76] irrespective of high or low HB_sAg and/or the HB_eAg carrier rate in the population. Studies in India have shown rates of vertical transmission from HB_eAg-positive mothers to their children of 58–90% (mean 73.76%) and from HB_sAg-positive mothers (HB_eAg/anti-HB_e-negative) of 5.5–20.0% (mean 15.36%).[77]

Horizontal and parenteral transmission. Horizontal transmission from highly infectious family members such as elder siblings is common, particularly in Africa. Parenteral transmission from improperly sterilized syringes or other contaminated instruments remains a problem in the developing world.[78,79] Other sources of infection include institutionalized children and multiple or large amounts of blood transfusions, etc. In Africa, HBV transmission occurs mainly horizontally during early childhood.

Clinical features and natural history

Acute or fulminant hepatitis B. HBV infects all ages. The normal incubation period is 2–6 months, and symptoms may occur as early as 2 months of age in infants of HB_sAg carrier mothers. Acute hepatitis B usually runs a self-limited course, and recovery follows anti-HB_s seroconversion. Acute or fulminant hepatitis B occurs mainly in infants of hepatitis B e antibody-seropositive mothers in areas of high prevalence.[80,81] There is a high mortality rate in children with fulminant hepatitis B, but those who survive do not develop chronic liver disease. The presence of the HBV precore mutant (from G to A at nucleotide 1896) has been described in fulminant hepatitis B in adults,[82] but was not confirmed by later studies.[83] A study in children in Taiwan revealed that although 33% (five of 14) of children with fulminant hepatitis B had the hepatitis B precore stop codon mutant, this was a similar proportion (30%, three of 10) to that in children with acute hepatitis B only.[84] The remaining nine of the 14 children with fulminant hepatitis had wild-type HBV, suggesting that the precore stop codon mutant did not cause the severe liver damage. Identical precore sequences were obtained from five mothers and their infants who developed fulminant hepatitis, suggesting maternal–infant transmission.

Chronic hepatitis B. Children with chronic HBV infection are usually asymptomatic. The liver histology findings are mild initially,[85] but may progress to severe liver damage in later life during the process of acute exacerbation and HB_eAg seroconversion.

Hepatitis B e antigen is an important marker reflecting active viral replication and infectivity, and its clearance is therefore used as a marker for seroconversion or the success of antiviral therapy.[86] With age, serum HB_eAg gradually clears, and HBV replication reduces over a period of 2–7 years,[87] although the mechanism remains unclear. HB_eAg clearance is usually preceded by an acute exacerbation, with elevated aminotransferase levels and active inflammation of the liver. The peak levels of aminotransferases range from ALT < 300 IU/L to > 800 IU/L in adolescents and young adults. It is occasionally accompanied by bridging necrosis on liver histology. Seroconversion takes place in 40% of children within 1 year of an acute exacerbation.

After HB_eAg clearance, aminotransferase levels gradually return to normal, and anti-HB_e develops spontaneously. An acute exacerbation with reactivation of HBV replication and reelevation of aminotransferases is unusual in children once anti-HB_e appears.[84] Unfortunately, it is likely that permanent liver damage and integration of the genome of HBV may have already taken place, despite the disappearance of HB_eAg.

Viral genetic factors and titers and host factors may affect the clinical course and outcome of HBV infection. Although HBV genotype B dominates in children with chronic HBV infection and HCC in Taiwan, genotype C delays HB_eAg seroconversion in pediatric chronic HBV infection.[88] Some types of human leukocyte antigen (HLA) have also been considered to affect the clinical courses of patients with HBV infection. Major histocompatibility complex (MHC) class II alleles HLA-DRB1*1301–2 were associated with protection against persistent HBV infection in Gambia, Germany, and Korea.[89–91] HLA class I antigen B61 and class II antigen DQB1*0503 were reported to be associated with earlier HB_eAg seroconversion in Taiwanese children with chronic HBV infection.[92]

Complications. The development of liver cirrhosis or HCC is rare but occasionally observed during childhood, particularly in areas hyperendemic for HBV infection.[93] Approximately 80% of children with HCC in Taiwan were anti-HB_e-seropositive.[94] It is estimated that the lifetime risk of HCC in HB_sAg carriers is around 25% and that it is higher in those with persistent HB_eAg positivity.[95]

Prevention of hepatitis B and related liver diseases

Immunoprophylaxis is the most cost-effective way of achieving global control of HBV infection and its related complications.[96,97] Passive immunization using hepatitis B immunoglobulin (HBIg) provides temporary immunity, but the cost of antenatal screening and HBIg is beyond most developing countries. The most important strategy has been the universal immunization program to prevent both perinatal and horizontal transmission of HBV infection (Table 23.6), which depends on the local epidemiological conditions—e.g., a high or low prevalence rate of HB_sAg carriage in children—and the government's budget.

The world's first universal hepatitis B immunization program was launched in Taiwan in July 1984. In this program, a combination of passive and active immunization effectively prevents HBV transmission from highly infectious mothers (HB_eAg-positive mothers). Routine prenatal screening of pregnant mothers for both HB_sAg and HB_eAg has been conducted. HBIg is given within 24 h after birth for infants of high-risk mothers with positive HB_eAg and HB_sAg. To all infants, the first dose of hepatitis B vaccine is given within the first week after birth, and the second and third doses 1 and 6 months later.[98] The efficacy of prevention for infants of high-risk mothers is approximately 85%.[99]

Table 23.7 Seroprevalence of hepatitis B surface antigen before (1984) and after (1989, 1994, 1999) universal vaccination against hepatitis B virus in Taiwan.

Age (years)	HB_sAg seropositive rates (%)			
	1984	1989	1994	1999
< 1	5.1	3.0	0.0	0.0
1–2	10.7	1.5	0.5	1.2
3–4	10.1	2.2	0.3	0.0
5–6	10.6	3.9	0.8	0.0
7–8	9.7	4.7	0.9	2.0
9–10	11.0	9.8	1.5	1.3
11–12	9.1	10.5	6.8	0.0
13–14	11.7	–	–	0.5

In areas in which the prevalence of HBV infection is low or financial resources are limited, immunization with three doses of HBV vaccine on a schedule of 0, 1, and 6 months without antenatal screening of the mothers or administration of HBIg is a reasonable strategy to save costs. Such programs have been successful in Thailand and many other countries in Asia.[100] To align with the National Immunization Program, some local governments in India, such as in Delhi, have commenced universal hepatitis B vaccination at birth, 6 weeks, 10 weeks, and 6 months. Long-term protection after HBV immunization in infancy has been a concern. In children who have not received a booster, the average decay of anti-HB_s from 7 to 16 years of age was approximately 20% of the geometric mean titer per year.[101]

Effect of universal hepatitis B immunization on the control of liver diseases in children. Universal hepatitis B vaccination has effectively reduced both perinatal and horizontal transmission of HBV[62] and thus the rate of chronic HBV infection worldwide.

The seroprevalence rates of HB_sAg in Taiwan children before and during the 15 years after the start of the vaccination program are shown in Table 23.7.[61,102,103] The HB_sAg carrier rate decreased significantly from around 10% before the vaccination program to < 1% afterward in children younger than 15 years.

In reports from many countries, such as Gambia and Korea,[104,105] universal vaccination programs have been equally successful. The hepatitis B carrier rate has fallen from 5–10% to < 1%, demonstrating that universal vaccination is more effective than selective immunization for high-risk groups (Table 23.8).[106]

The reduction in HBV infection after the launch of the universal hepatitis B vaccination program in July 1984 in Taiwan has had a dramatic effect on the incidence of HCC in children. The annual incidence of HCC in children aged 6–14 years was reduced to one-quarter, from 0.52–0.54 per 100 000 children born before July 1984 to 0.13–0.20 per 100 000 children born after July 1984.[107,108] This trend has

Table 23.8 Strategies for hepatitis B virus (HBV) immunization in regions with different HBV epidemiological conditions and resources.

Maternal screening HB_sAg/HB_eAg	HBV immunization HBIG*/HBV vaccine	Population HBV prevalence	Budget
Yes/yes	Yes/yes	High	High
Yes/no	Yes/yes	Low, but with high-risk groups	High
No/no	No/yes	High	Lower
No/no	No/yes	Low	Lower

* For infants of high-risk mothers (with positive HB_eAg or high reciprocal titer of HB_sAg (> 2560).

continued, and it is expected that there will be a subsequent decline in the incidence of HCC in adults in the future.

After the introduction of a universal vaccination program, HBV now rarely causes fulminant hepatic failure in older children, but remains a significant cause of fulminant hepatic failure in infants. HBV-positive fulminant hepatic failure develops in infants born to HB_eAg-negative, HB_sAg-carrier mothers who have not received hepatitis B immunoglobulin in accordance with the vaccination program in place.[109]

Long-term immunity after HBV immunization and booster doses

The levels of antibody against HB_sAg (anti-HB_s) wane gradually with time after primary HBV immunization in infancy. Hyporesponders who have lower initial antibody titers after vaccination lose detectable antibodies within a shorter period than the responders. The determination of serum levels of anti-HB_s after hepatitis B vaccination is currently the only simple test available to predict the decay of protection and to plan the administration of booster doses. Long-term protection against HBV infection is high, and booster vaccination at age 7 did not significantly increase this protection against HBV infection at age 16.[110] Even in the absence of detectable anti-HB_s, the maintenance of HB_sAg-specific cellular immune memory after primary HBV immunization confers protection against clinical breakthrough infection.[111]

It is not clear whether primary HBV vaccination in infancy can provide long-term protection against HBV transmission in adolescents who undertake high-risk behavior in HBV endemic areas. According to recent data in Taiwan, universal HBV vaccination in infancy provides long-term protection for up to 20 years, and a universal booster is not recommended for primary HBV vaccinees before adulthood.[112,113]

Future problems with HBV

In spite of the success of HBV immunization in preventing HBV infection and its complications, there remain significant problems with the eradication of HBV infection. Current problems include inadequate vaccination rates, vaccine failure, lack of response to the vaccine, and the development of viral mutants. The main causes of vaccine failure are high maternal viral load, HBV surface gene variants, and genetic nonresponsiveness or hyporesponsiveness, particularly in immune-compromised children. The prevalence of viral mutants in HBV-DNA–positive children was 7.8% before the HBV vaccination program and has increased to 19.6%, 28.1%, and 23.1% at 5, 10, and 15 years, respectively, after the launch of the program. There was a higher rate of mutants in children fully vaccinated in comparison with those not vaccinated (15/46 vs. 15/153). However, the overall number of children infected with mutant HBV has not increased after vaccination, due to the reduction in the HB_sAg carrier pool.[114]

Difficulties with therapy for hepatitis B

Treatment of chronic hepatitis B is unsatisfactory (see Chapter 6), particularly in Asian children, who have a lower seroconversion rate with interferon therapy compared with European children.[115] In addition, few developing countries have the resources to obtain therapy. The cost of either a 6-month course of interferon therapy or 12 months' lamivudine therapy is much higher than that of HBV immunoprophylaxis and cannot be justified on a large scale, given the low success rate of the therapy.

Although universal HBV immunization is more cost-effective in comparison with therapy, effective and cheaper antiviral therapy is needed for children who have not been vaccinated or who have failed to respond to HBV immunization. Currently, five antiviral drugs—interferon (conventional interferon alpha or pegylated interferon alpha), and nucleoside/nucleotide analogs (lamivudine, adefovir, entecavir, and telbivudine), have been approved by the Food and Drug Administration (FDA) in the United States for adult use. However, only conventional interferon alpha and lamivudine are approved for use in children. With immune tolerance to HBV, relatively high viral replication, and limited efficacy with the current antiviral therapy, further research to develop more effective therapies for children is needed.

Hepatitis C virus infection (see also Chapter 6)

Epidemiology

The seroprevalence of hepatitis C virus (HCV) infection is around 0.8–3.0% in the adult population and < 0.2% in children in most parts of the world, except for some hyperendemic areas.[116,117] HCV infection occurs mainly in high-risk children, such as those who have been exposed to blood products (children with hemophilia, thalassemia, blood transfusions, hemodialysis, malignancy, and organ transplantation) or in children of HCV-infected mothers. In hyperendemic areas, such as the Nile delta in Egypt, anti-HCV prevalence increases sharply with age, from 9.3% in those < 20 years of age to > 50% in those over 35. A history of antischistosomal injection therapy (reported by 19% of anti-HCV positive patients) was found to be a risk for anti-HCV.[118]

Perinatal transmission. In comparison with maternal transmission of HBV infection (maternal HBV titers 10^6–10^9 copies/mL, average 10^{7-8} copies/mL),[119] the level of HCV in maternal circulation is lower (10^5–10^7, mean $10^{6.4 \pm 0.5}$ copies/mL,[120] which may explain why perinatal infection is much lower than that in HBV.[121] Transmission is related to the level of maternal HCV RNA. The rate of maternal transmission in infants of mothers who were seropositive for HCV RNA and seronegative for HIV was between 0% and 15%, with a mean of 5%. HCV RNA can be detected in breast milk, but the titer (10 000 copies/mL) is much lower than that in maternal serum (10^5 to 2.5×10^7 copies/mL)[122] and breast-feeding is considered safe, which is of particular relevance for the developing world. In another cohort study, nine of 190 (4.7%) infants born to mothers who were HCV RNA–positive at delivery became infected, in comparison with none of 54 infants born to HCV RNA–negative mothers. The rate of transmission was 3.8% from the 182 who were HIV-negative, in comparison with 25.0% from the eight who were HIV-positive ($P < 0.05$). Membrane rupture > 6 h and internal fetal monitoring were associated with transmission of HCV to infants.[123] There was no protective effect of elective cesarean section delivery on vertical transmission of HCV.[124]

Parenteral exposure to HCV. Transfusion and injection using nonsterile needles were the most important causes of HCV transmission in the developing world. They continue to be important routes of HCV transmission in children in those areas of the developing world with limited resources, where mass blood screening for anti-HCV is not universally carried out even nowadays.

The HCV infection rate in thalassemic children in Taiwan ranged from 43% to 60%,[125] while approximately 15–20% of the pediatric hemodialysis populations and 3–4% of survivors of childhood malignancy were infected with HCV. Screening of anti-HCV in donated blood has reduced HCV infection to minimal levels in Taiwan, but it remains a source of infection in less developed countries.[126]

Sporadic cases. The proportion of cases without identifiable risk factors has consistently ranged from 35% to 40%. Intramuscular injection using nonsterile syringes or needles is the most likely route of transmission.

Clinical features

After primary infection with HCV, 60–80% of children have a chronic course, as in the West. HCV RNA is detectable in serum by 2 weeks after exposure, and anti-HCV is detectable in serum by 4–8 weeks. Most chronically infected children remain asymptomatic, with normal liver function profiles. However, transient or persistent elevation of aminotransferase levels is not uncommon, particularly in perinatally infected children. Chang *et al.* followed up 10 children with new HCV infection; four later lost HCV RNA, while six had a chronic course.[127] Fujisawa *et al.* followed up 53 children with chronic HCV infection. Hepatic transaminases remained abnormal for 1.5–13 years, but virological clearance of HCV RNA was only demonstrated in four of the 53.[128] Ten children had biochemical remission for more than 3 years, while 39 children remained abnormal biochemically.

Prevention

In contrast to hepatitis B, there is currently no approved effective vaccine for the prophylaxis of HCV infection. Screening of blood and blood products and use of disposable syringes and needles have reduced post-transfusion HCV infection and hepatitis effectively in those countries with sufficient resources and organization in the developing world. In Taiwan, the incidence of post-transfusion HCV infection in children after open-heart surgery has declined to zero after HCV screening of blood was instituted in 1992. However, infection through mother–infant transmission, parenteral exposure through invasive instruments, and organ transplantation are still sources of infection and can only be prevented by education of the public to avoid nonsterile invasive procedures such as injections, acupuncture, tattooing, etc. Recently, a recombinant protein-based HCV vaccine using viral envelope protein E1 and E2 has been undergoing phase II clinical trials in humans.[129]

Treatment

Treatment for hepatitis C with sustained viral clearance is more effective than that for hepatitis B, particularly since the development of combination therapy. Approximately 10–20% of adults achieve a sustained virologic response (SVR) after interferon alpha monotherapy.[130] A meta-analysis of interferon alpha therapy with at least 1.75 MU/m^2 three times weekly, administered for at least 6 months, included 366 treated and 105 untreated children. The average end-of-treatment response was 54% (0–91%) and the average sustained response was 36% (0–73%). The sustained response rate in children with genotype 1 was 27%, in comparison with 70% for non–genotype 1 ($P < 0.001$). Five of the 105 (5%) untreated control individuals had spontaneous viral clearance.[131]

The addition of ribavirin to interferon-based regimens markedly improves virological responses. Interferon alfa 2b 3 MU/m^2 in combination with ribavirin 15 mg/kg/day for a 48-week treatment period was found to be safe and effective in children with chronic hepatitis C in a multicenter study. A total of 46% of 118 optimally treated children achieved SVR (undetectable serum HCV RNA 24 weeks after completion of therapy). SVR was significantly more frequent in children with HCV genotypes 2 and 3 (84%) than in those with HCV genotype 1 (36%). Adverse events led to dose modification in 37 children (31%) and discontinuation in eight (7%).[132]

Peginterferon alfa 2a (40 kDa) improves antiviral efficacy in comparison with conventional interferon in both adults and children with chronic HCV infection.[133]

Other causes of viral hepatitis

Hepatitis D, hepatitis E, and other types of non-A–E hepatitis are uncommon forms of viral hepatitis in children. Hepatitis D is particularly rare in children in the developing world. Hepatitis G, transfusion-transmitted (TT) virus, and SEN virus (acronym from the original patient's initials) can be detected frequently in the serum of children with or without hepatitis and are not seen as causing viral hepatitis in children.

Hepatitis E virus (HEV) infection is endemic in south and central Asia and is transmitted enterically. Outbreaks of acute and fulminant hepatitis E have occurred in the Middle East, India, northern and western parts of Africa, and Mexico. Unlike hepatitis A in endemic areas, HEV infection rarely occurs in children younger than 10 years. In India, coinfection with hepatitis E and hepatitis A has been observed in children with fulminant hepatitis (Sibal *et al.*, personal communication). Hepatitis E appears to be changing the etiological spectrum of acute viral hepatitis, and increasing evidence is being found to make it the second most common cause of acute hepatitis in children in India.[134] A study to compare the pattern of HEV among urban and rural children in north India showed that HEV IgG was positive in 28.7% of urban children, in comparison with 23.8% of rural children, and that HEV IgM was positive in 42.8% of urban children and 47.3% of rural children. Seropositivity for HEV increased more than two times beyond 4 years of age in comparison with younger ages. Anti-HEV IgG appears to decline with increasing age.[135] Mixed infection with hepatitis A and E represented the largest etiological group in a study aiming to identify risk factors for fulminant hepatic failure.[136] In addition, HEV was associated with another hepatitis virus in 88% of cases of acute viral hepatitis, thus raising a high suspicion of multiple etiology in cases of HEV positivity. In multiple infections, however, the frequency of anicteric state, prolonged cholestasis, relapsing hepatitis, ascites, hemolysis, and mortality rates are similar in single and multiple infection groups for both acute viral hepatitis and fulminant hepatic failure. Coinfection with multiple viruses in one-quarter of patients with sporadic acute viral hepatitis does not produce a more severe disease.[137] A vaccine against hepatitis E might be the key for endemic areas, as previous infection with HEV does not confer protection as in the case of HAV.

In children with fulminant hepatitis, non-A–E hepatitis and dengue hemorrhagic fever are important etiological agents. Treatment is supportive (Chapter 7).

Orthotopic liver transplantation

Orthotopic liver transplantation (OLT) is an accepted treatment for children with end-stage liver disease (Chapter 21). Survivors lead high-quality normal lives and contribute actively to their family and society. As the 5-year actuarial survival rate is well over 85% for children in many international centers, many developing countries have set up liver transplantation programs in recent years. Many centers in developing countries have recently reported comparable outcomes.[138–140] Despite limited resources and support, many of these programs have been successfully established by hepatologists and transplant surgeons. This section attempts to discuss the many problems faced by OLT programs in the developing world and to highlight the differences from developed countries.

Organization of liver transplant program

In contrast to the rest of the world, many transplant programs in developing countries are initiated by the medical profession with or without institutional or government support, and consequently they may not have the full range of support needed to establish a successful program. This should be discouraged, as OLT is a lifelong commitment and only well-established institutions can offer meaningful long-term follow-up.

Not all developing countries have the resources and expertise to manage the complexities of an organ donation program, let alone the cultural and legal difficulties involved, and so for many countries it is best to begin with a living related donation program.

It is essential to obtain ethical support and approval before establishing a transplant program, particularly when a living related donor program is being considered. There may well be issues related to the sale of donor organs, even in developed countries, and both transplant surgeons and hepatologists in developing countries must be aware of this problem.

The transplant team includes many people (see Chapter 21)—such as anesthetists, immunologists, pathologists, psychiatrists, intensivists, microbiologists, radiologists, hematologists, pharmacists, dietitians, nurses, transplant coordinators, and biochemists. The team must be well organized and have good communication mechanisms, with regular meetings such as pretransplant assessment discussions and mortality and morbidity conferences. In many developing countries, not all team members have equal expertise, and this may compromise both the care of the recipient and the success of the program.

Before considering a transplant program, time and effort should be spent in training the supporting staff and the team to manage all aspects of liver transplantation. Pretransplantation care and assessment, immediate post-transplantation care, and long-term care are as important as surgical technique.[141] Liver transplantation is very much a team effort, and all the members of the team must be fully committed to the care of the patient.

Intensivists play a key role in the successful management of a transplant, particularly in the immediate postoperative period, when hemodynamic instability can adversely affect graft function. In developing countries, there are few well-trained intensivists, and many hepatologists may have to function as intensivists as well.

It is also essential to have appropriate support services, especially good laboratory and radiology support. The laboratory must be equipped with up-to-date facilities and able to perform the essential tests over 24 h. These tests include routine liver and kidney function tests, coagulation tests, and blood counts. This is not usually a significant problem in most developing countries, although there may be more difficulty with specialized tests such as drug monitoring (cyclosporine and tacrolimus), viral serology such as hepatitis B DNA, hepatitis C RNA, and CMV polymerase chain reaction or antigen detection.

Adequate radiological imaging of the vascular and hepatobiliary system is crucial for both pretransplantation and post-transplantation assessment (see Chapter 21). Interventional radiologists play an important role postoperatively in the management and treatment of many complications (see Chapter 2). Such expertise may not be available in the developing world, while Doppler ultrasonography, magnetic resonance imaging, and CT angiography are expensive. Transplant surgeons in developing countries often have to rely solely on their clinical judgment to manage these problems during the postoperative period.

A well-trained liver pathologist who is familiar with transplantation is important to help the clinician decide between rejection, ischemia, or infection in the graft. There is a shortage of pathologists worldwide, and this is particularly true in many developing countries. It is not uncommon for transplant centers to courier biopsy specimens to specialized centers in the West for opinions, which is far from ideal, as precious time is lost and this may adversely affect the outcome for the recipients.

Donor issues

Survival rates with liver transplantation have improved with experience and medical advances, thus creating more demand for such procedures. The increasing demand has caused a further shortage of cadaveric organs in the West and poses an even greater challenge in the developing world. Cadaveric organ donation is not widely accepted in many developing countries, due to lack of education and for religious and cultural reasons, and thus few national donor programs have been established. Apart from the delicate situation of approaching a family who are in mourning for donation, reasons include legal issues associated with brain death. When there are existing transplantation facilities, many families are not even aware of the option of cadaver organ donation. Furthermore, there are technical aspects of coordination, appropriate delivery, and timing, collaboration among different hospitals, and lack of a centralized cadaver organ donor program. There are only a few networks for sharing donor organs, as most developing countries function independently and many suitable organs are wasted. Lack of political agreement, poor communication, and variable standards of health care are major factors preventing the sharing of organs in the developing world.

In India, the Human Organ Transplantation Act was passed in 1994, and regulations were made in 1995 that recognize the concept of brain death and allow cadaver organs to be removed for transplantation. In spite of this, there is a lack of knowledge and reluctance on the part of the public to donate the organs of their brain-dead relatives. There may also be ignorance on the part of doctors, who do not approach the relatives of brain-dead patients with a request for donation. Infrastructure and organizational difficulties compound the problem. Thus, organs from only less than 1000 cadaver donors have been available in India for transplantation in the last 12 years (Mehta, personal communication).

Most children die during the long waiting period for a suitable cadaver organ, due to the severe shortage of grafts and long waiting lists for adults. In a center in New Delhi, of 30 families willing to accept liver transplantation, 17 opted for cadaveric transplantation but only one patient received the cadaveric organ, while the others died on the waiting list (Sibal *et al.*, personal communication).

In countries with a cadaveric donor program, the organ donation rate is lower than in the West. In Singapore, where there is a well-established organ donation program, cadaveric liver donation is only about 10 per million population, and overall there are fewer organ transplants per head of the population in developing countries in comparison with western Europe and North America.[142] This is partly because the medical community is neither aware nor fully convinced of the benefit of OLT, so that patients with brain death are not routinely referred to the transplant coordinators. In some countries, legislation is necessary before instigating a successful organ donation campaign. Ethical committees should be established to ensure that organ donation is within the ethical guidelines of the countries concerned, followed by public education and political support to promote organ donation.

Hepatitis B-positive donors

In many endemic areas in the developing world, there is a high incidence of donors positive for antibody to the hepatitis B core antigen (anti-HB_c). The exact incidence varies from country to country. In Singapore, anti-HB_c antibody is detected in about 30–40% of healthy adults and in 53% of organs donors, while in Taiwan anti-HB_c antibody is found in up to 80% of adults.[143] Due to the shortage of donor organs, it in not possible to reject these anti-HB_c antibody–positive donor organs, despite the risk of reactivating hepatitis B and infecting the immunosuppressed recipients, who have a high risk of fulminant hepatic failure. In Singapore, of the anti-HB_c–positive grafts that have been transplanted, 18% of the recipients subsequently developed hepatitis B de novo and are receiving long-term antiviral treatment.

It is essential to vaccinate the recipient against hepatitis B if this has not already been done. Liver recipients who have antibodies to hepatitis B core antigen (anti-HB_c) or who have received an anti-HB_c–positive liver graft are at risk of acquiring de novo hepatitis B infection without any further immunoprophylaxis. Studies have shown that lifelong treatment with lamivudine can prevent de novo infection, and hepatitis B immunoglobulin can be stopped in cases of post-transplant vaccinated patients.[144,145]

Fatty liver

In South-East Asia, many donor grafts are rejected because of severe fatty infiltration. In Singapore, out of 98 consecutive cadaveric liver donors, 16 (16%) were rejected because of severe fatty change. Among 61 healthy living donors who volunteered for liver donation, nine organs (15%) were rejected for the same reasons. This may be because of underlying obesity, the dietary pattern of Asians, and/or ingestion of native herbal medicine. Further research is necessary to solve this problem, but in the meantime it is a major limitation for the program.

Living related organ donation

In the light of the shortage of cadaver organs, living related donor liver transplantation is an essential option in pediatric transplantation in countries such as Japan, Korea, Taiwan, Hong Kong, and India. Studies show comparable patient and graft survival rates in both living related donor and cadaveric donor groups,[146] with a trend toward less initial graft malfunction in living related liver donor transplantation.[147] This modality has a number of advantages, as it can be performed in an elective manner, selecting the most appropriate time for surgery depending on the child's clinical status. Supportive measures, nutritional augmentation, and preoperative preparation can be completed, thus improving factors for the outcome. Other practical benefits include a very short cold ischemia time, which facilitates better graft quality and may reduce primary nonfunction of grafts. Theater staff and theater time can be planned in such a way that the transplant operation is not performed during the theater's busy hours. Toyoki *et al.* demonstrated that although the overall incidence of rejection and the graft survival rate were comparable in cadaver grafts and living related donor graft recipients, rejection episodes in living related donor liver transplantation diagnosed more than 1 year after transplantation were significantly fewer than in cadaver recipients. Living related recipients therefore appeared to show a partial immunological advantage in comparison with cadaver liver recipients.[148] A large cohort pediatric study by Bourdeaux *et al.* in Brussels in which the results of cadaver donors and living related donors were compared showed that the overall post-transplantation outcome at 5 years was better with living related donor liver transplantation.[149]

However, there are reservations regarding living related donation because of the risk for the healthy donor and the reported morbidity of 5% due to bile leakage, hemorrhage, infection, small-bowel obstruction, and incisional hernia. The donor mortality has been estimated at 0.5%, which is low enough to allow a parent or a close relative the option to donate a segment of their liver. Collective data worldwide, however, need to be assessed adequately to provide an accurate percentage of the donor mortality risk, as it varies from 0.2% to 2% across all centers, and there is as yet no living donor registry.[150]

Ethical debates on living related donor liver transplantation continue, with concerns about emotional pressure on a potential living related donor. In addition, in countries like India, most organ donors are women, partly because of social and family pressure, or because the husband is the wage-earner. A strict pre-assessment protocol has to be followed, including all diagnostic tests and psychological support as well as counseling of the whole family. The donor must be aware of potential risks, which range from bile leakage and hemorrhage to infection, gastritis, and peptic ulceration.

Pretransplant issues

Infections

Hepatitis B. Hepatitis B infection is endemic in eastern and South-East Asia, and although hepatitis B vaccination has been incorporated into many national vaccination programs, it is still not universally implemented. In places such as Taiwan, Malaysia, Hong Kong, and Singapore, where hepatitis B vaccination has been implemented since 1980s, chronic hepatitis B carriers are less common in the pediatric age group. However, even with hepatitis B vaccination in infancy, 5% of infants born to HB_eAg-positive mothers are chronic carriers. Thus, a number of pediatric patients with end-stage liver disease are chronic hepatitis B carriers. In Singapore, out of 33 pediatric liver recipients, two were hepatitis B carriers. They required oral lamivudine before transplantation, hepatitis B immunoglobulin during the perioperative period, and then long-term oral lamivudine with reduced levels of immunosuppression. An alternative strategy is high-dose hepatitis B revaccination after transplantation, which has shown conflicting results.[151]

Tuberculosis. TB is endemic in many developing countries, and childhood TB is not uncommon. Children with end-stage liver disease who are both malnourished and immunodeficient are more likely to be infected. It is well known that bacille Calmette–Guérin vaccination during early childhood does not fully protect against the infection. Thus, it is essential to exclude TB by chest radiography, sputum culture, and Mantoux test during the pretransplant assessment. Family members should be screened, as the child will be at high risk of infection during the immediate postoperative period, with a potentially fulminant course. TB may also be transmitted via the donor graft. Prophylactic isoniazid should be considered if there has been any contact with TB.

Nutritional status

Malnutrition in liver disease is a common problem and improved strategies for supporting and improving nutritional status prior to transplantation have shown a clear association with better post-transplantation outcomes. Severe malnutrition is a particular problem in the developing world and is compounded by late referral. Many primary health-care pediatricians still are unaware of the clinical course in children with end-stage liver disease and of the benefits and possibilities of liver transplantation in their own country. The implications of liver disease for nutritional status and the focus on nutritional management is often underestimated. Thus, many pediatric patients in the developing world present with protein malnutrition, gross nutritional rickets, iron-deficiency anemia, and coagulopathy. In an series in New Delhi, 70% of the children presented for liver transplantation were malnourished and required nutritional augmentation with nasojejunal tube feeding. Sixty-four of 142 babies with neonatal cholestasis were so severely malnourished that they were unsuitable for transplantation, as they would have required weeks of nutritional rehabilitation and their liver failure was too advanced to allow them that much time (Sibal, personal communication). This is particularly tragic, as appropriate management and vitamin supplementation can avoid many of the problems encountered.

Parental attitude

Liver transplantation is accepted as a treatment option in developing countries, but many parents in developing countries are unwilling to accept it. The emotional shock that parents suffer when hearing that their child needs a liver transplantation is undeniable, but many parents in the developing world are unwilling to accept liver transplantation as a life-saving modality. Poor education, lack of understanding, fear of long-term medications, religious objections, and cultural factors contribute to rejection of this treatment option. In India, more than half of the families refuse OLT, with a clear bias against transplantation in girls—with only two girls out of a total of 14 patients who underwent transplantation in a hospital in Delhi (Sibal, personal communication). In recent years, parental attitudes have changed and many parents have requested liver transplantation, particularly in countries in which the outcome of OLT is acceptable—leading to "transplant tourism," when the rich travel abroad for transplantation.

A great deal of public and professional education is required in order to highlight the success and benefits of transplantation and the need for adequate management and early referral. Obviously, the outcomes of OLT in developing countries should be publicized and made available to the public, so that parents can make an intelligent choice about OLT for their children.

Indications for transplantation

Chronic liver disease

The main indication for transplantation in the developing world is biliary atresia (Figure 23.1). The numbers of children reaching referral centers for Kasai portoenterostomy represent one-third of the estimated cases. Most are referred late in India and neighboring countries, and further delay is caused by the investigative work-up.[1] It is well established that early presentation is key.[152] Late referrals reduce the chances of survival, leaving only liver transplantation as an option, which not only has a much higher financial burden on the family but also involves higher risk and life-long immunosuppression.

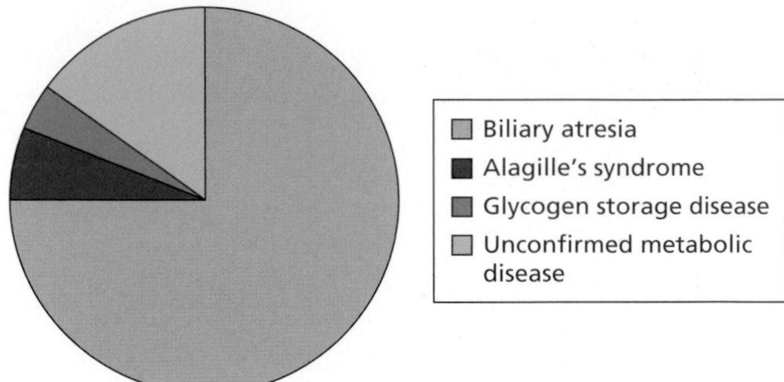

Figure 23.1 Indications for liver transplantation in Singapore. Biliary atresia is the commonest indication in Asia and in other countries such as India. The high proportion of unconfirmed liver disease, thought to represent metabolic liver disease, should be noted.

A "Yellow Alert" campaign was launched in 2000 in northern India to create awareness about the need for early referral of babies with neonatal cholestasis. This improved referrals, with the average age at presentation falling from 132 days to 97 days.[7]

Mehrotra *et al.*[153] reported that 79% of babies with extrahepatic biliary atresia in their center in north India required transplantation. Sixty-one percent of older children with cirrhosis and 67% of those with fulminant hepatic failure fulfilled the criteria for liver transplantation. Overall, 30% of children with liver diseases—consisting of cirrhosis (45%), biliary atresia (38%), and fulminant hepatic failure (11%)—were found to have an indication for liver transplantation. Many other diseases were undiagnosed and thought to represent metabolic liver disease. Liver transplantation for hepatitis B–related cirrhosis is not common in children, but liver transplantation may be indicated for HCC in hepatitis B carrier children if the tumor is located in the liver.

In a series in New Delhi, there was a total of 1998 hepatological referrals, in 215 of which the patient had an indication for liver transplantation in accordance with the international criteria. The commonest indications identified were neonatal cholestasis syndrome in 66% (n = 142), followed by fulminant hepatic failure (16%), cryptogenic cirrhosis (9%), Wilson's disease, progressive familial intrahepatic cholestasis, and others (Figure 23.2). The reasons for patients being considered unsuitable for transplantation, apart from advanced clinical pathology with gross clinical features, included severe ascites, protein calorie malnutrition, and multiple vitamin deficiencies with severe coagulopathy (Sibal, personal communication).

Acute liver failure

In children in the developing world, acute liver failure is mainly due to infection or to drugs. Hepatitis A is common in

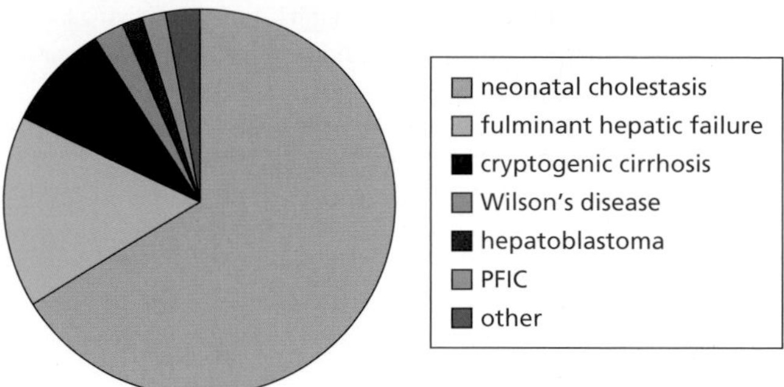

Figure 23.2 Indications for liver transplantation in a hospital in Delhi.

tropical countries, but only a small proportion of children develop fulminant liver failure. Studies in India have reported an association with acute viral hepatitis markers in up to 75% of patients with liver failure. Isolated viral markers for hepatitis A have been identified in more than 50% of cases of fulminant hepatic failure, followed by multiple infection with hepatitis A and E. Experience in a center in New Delhi showed that out of 81 children with fulminant hepatic failure, 41 were identified as having hepatitis A, of whom almost 44% had G6PD deficiency. Thirty-five children satisfied the criteria for liver transplantation, of whom 31 children died, however, mainly due to sepsis and multi-organ failure (Sibal *et al.*, personal communication).

The causes of drug-induced liver failure include accidental or nonaccidental acetaminophen overdose and the ingestion of native herbal medicines. Although a number of native herbal concoctions are known to cause hepatic injury, the exact mechanism and the hepatotoxic ingredients are not known.

Post-transplantation outcomes

The outcome of OLT in developing countries varies. Few patients survive long enough on the cadaveric waiting list to receive a donor, and thus only countries with living related donor programs are able to offer a viable procedure. However, in countries with relatively well-established programs, such as South Africa, Hong Kong, India, Singapore, and Taiwan, the graft and patient survival rates are acceptable, with actuarial survival ranging from 50% to 90%.[154]

There are a number of liver dialysis machines available on the market. However, they are very costly to use, and most developing countries are not able to afford such machines to treat patients with acute liver failure. In fact, it is futile to use such tools in centers that do not have an active liver transplantation program.[155]

Retransplantation is not available in developing countries, in view of the unavailability of cadaveric donors. The only option possible in such cases is living related donor transplantation, but sadly in most cases the child dies.

As in the West, cyclosporine and tacrolimus are the two main immunosuppressants used, but other agents such as mycophenolate mofetil, interleukin-2 receptor antagonists, and rapamycin have become available. The main problems with post-transplantation immunosuppressants are their cost and the difficulties in providing accurate and affordable therapeutic drug monitoring. Depending on the regimen used and the age of the patient, the cost of immunosuppressants can be as high as US$ 1000 per month, which is beyond the means of the vast majority of patients in the developing world. The availability of generic drugs has brought down the monthly cost to as low as US$ 250 in India.

Long-term survival depends on the availability of immunosuppression and the rate of intercurrent infection. Post-OLT tuberculosis is particularly difficult to manage, as a number of the anti-TB medicines are also hepatotoxic. Often, third-line medications and a combination of four or more drugs may be necessary. Although it is always mandatory to exclude active TB in the recipient, latent TB can be activated as a result of the immunosuppressive therapy. Infection with multidrug-resistant strains is common in many developing countries, and the sensitivity of the organism should be assessed.

Published data on the outcome of orthotopic liver transplantation in Asia and South America are presented in Tables 23.9 and 23.10.[156–174]

Table 23.9 Published reports and survival rates in pediatric liver transplantation in Asia, as well as Turkey and Saudi Arabia.

Country	Survival rates	References
China	1-year 93%	Wang *et al.* 2006[155]
	3-year 92%	Wang *et al.* 2006[155]
Hong Kong	3-year 79%	Saing *et al.* 2002[156]
	1-year 82%	Lo *et al.* 2002[157]
	5-year 74%	Lo *et al.* 2002[157]
India	First report in India	Poonacha *et al.* 2001[158]
Korea	1-year 80–92%	Annual Report 2005, Korea
	3-year 70–90%	Annual Report 2005, Korea
Malaysia	No published data yet	
Saudi Arabia	Reports on donor experience	Al-Shurafa *et al.* 2003[160]
		Al Sebayel *et al.* 2001[161]
Singapore	5-year 80%	Aw *et al.* 2006[159]
Taiwan	1 year 80–97%	Cheng *et al.* 2004[162]
		Ho *et al.* 2004[163]
Thailand	Report in adults only	Nivatvongs *et al.* 2003[164]
Turkey	1-year 80–86%	Aydogdu *et al.* 2005[165]
	4-year 65–67%	Aydogdu *et al.* 2005[165]
Vietnam	First pediatric report	Reading and Tran 2006[166]

Table 23.10 Published survival rates in pediatric liver transplantation in South America, along with Cuba and Mexico.

Country	Survival rates	References
Argentina	1-year 93%	Cuarterolo *et al.* 2005[167]
	1-year 78%	Williams *et al.* 1998[168]
	4-year 71%	Williams *et al.* 1998[168]
Brazil	5-year 70.2%	Tannuri *et al.* 2004[169]
Chile	1-year graft 81.3%	Uribe *et al.* 2005[170]
	5-year graft SR 72%	Uribe *et al.* 2005[170]
	1-year 82%	Buckel *et al.* 2003[171]
	5-year 74.8%	Buckel *et al.* 2003[171]
Cuba	1-year 92%	Gonzalez *et al.* 2006[172]
Mexico	Overall:	
	1-year 77.1%	Varela-Fascinetto *et al.* 2005[173]
	5-year 74.2%	Varela-Fascinetto *et al.* 2005[173]
	Period 1998–2000:	
	1-year 91.6%	Varela-Fascinetto *et al.* 2005[173]

Acknowledgment

Dr. Sheena Sharma's help and contribution in preparing this manuscript is acknowledged.

References

1 Indian Academy of Pediatrics, Pediatric Gastroenterology Subspecialty Chapter. Consensus report on neonatal cholestasis syndrome. Pediatric Gastroenterology Subspecialty Chapter of Indian Academy of Pediatrics. *Indian Pediatr* 2000;**37**:845–51.

2 Ramzan M, Quak SH. A clinical study of obstructive jaundice among Singapore infants. *J Singapore Paediatr Soc* 1992;**34**:205–8.

3 Chang MH, Lee CY, Chen DS, Hsu HC, Lai MY. Fulminant hepatitis in children in Taiwan: the important role of hepatitis B virus. *J Pediatr* 1987;**111**:34–9.

4 Yachha SK. Cholestatic jaundice during infancy. *Indian J Gastroenterol* 2005;**24**:47–8.

5 Narasimhan KL, Chowdhary SK, Vaiphei K, *et al.* Outcome of biliary atresia from Chandigarh: results of a prospective analysis. *Indian Pediatr* 2001;**38**:1144–8.

6 Marret MJ, Quak SH, Prabhakaran K. Biliary atresia: the NUH experience. *J Singapore Paediatr Soc* 1994;**36**:58–61.

7 Sharma A, Poddar U, Yachha SK. Positive impact of awareness campaign on referral of neonatal cholestasis syndrome in India. *J Gastroenterol Hepatol* 2004;**19**(Suppl):A800.

8 Pediatric Liver Study Group of India. Metabolic liver disease in childhood: Indian scenario. *Indian J Pediatr* 1999;**66**(1 Suppl):S97–103.

9 Goh DYT, Quak SH, Yap HK. Neonatal fulminant hepatic failure from tyrosinaemia in 2 Chinese infants. *J Singapore Paediatr Soc* 1993;**35**:186–90.

10 Arora NK, Lodha R, Gulati S, *et al.* Portal hypertension in north Indian children. *Indian J Pediatr* 1999;**28**:193–200.

11 Tanner MS, Portmann B, Mowat AP, *et al.* Increased hepatic copper concentration in Indian childhood cirrhosis. *Lancet* 1979;**i**:1203–5.

12 Tanner MS, Kantarjian AH, Bhave SA, Pandit AN. Early introduction of copper-contaminated animal milk feeds as a possible cause of Indian childhood cirrhosis. *Lancet* 1983;**ii**:992–5.

13 Bhave SA, Pandit AN, Tanner MS. Comparison of feeding history of children with Indian childhood cirrhosis and paired controls. *J Pediatr Gastroenterol Nutr* 1987;**6**:562–7.

14 Bavdekar AR, Bhave SA, Pradlan AM, Pandit AN, Tanner MS. Long term survival in Indian childhood cirrhosis treated with D-penicillamine. *Arch Dis Child* 1996;**74**:32–5.

15 Bhave SA, Pandit AN, Singh S, Walia BN, Tanner MS. The prevention of Indian childhood cirrhosis. *Ann Trop Paediatr* 1992;**12**:23–30.

16 Jagdish K, Patwari AK, Sarin SK, *et al.* Hepatic manifestations in typhoid fever. *Indian Pediatr* 1994;**31**:807–11.

17 Kumar R, Gupta N; Shalini. Multidrug-resistant typhoid fever. *Indian J Pediatr* 2007;**74**:39–42.

18 El Newihi HM, Alamy ME, Reynolds TB. *Salmonella* hepatitis: analysis of 27 cases and comparison with acute viral hepatitis. *Hepatology* 1996;**24**:516–9.

19 Olubodun JO, Kuti JA, Adefuye BO, Talabi AO. Typhoid fever associated with severe hepatitis. *Cent Afr J Med* 1994;**40**:262–4.

20 Nimmannitya S, Thisyakorn U, Hemsrichart V. Dengue haemorrhagic fever with unusual manifestations. *Southeast Asian J Trop Med Public Health* 1987;**18**:398–406.

21 Nguyen TL, Nguyen TH, Tieu NT. The impact of dengue haemorrhagic fever on liver function. *Res Virol* 1997;**148**:273–7.

22 Mohan B, Patwari AK, Anand VK. Hepatic dysfunction in childhood dengue infection. *J Trop Pediatr* 2000;**46**:40–3.

23 Mendez A, Gonzalez G. Dengue haemorrhagic fever in children: ten years of clinical experience. *Biomedica* 2003;**23**:180–93.

24 Poovorawan Y, Hutagalung Y, Chongrisawat V, *et al.* Dengue virus infection: a major cause of acute hepatic failure in Thai children. *Ann Trop Paediatr* 2006;**26**:17–23.

25 Cook GC. Liver in Malaria. *Postgrad Med J* 1994;70:780–4.

26 Wilairatana P, Looareesuwan S, Charoenlarp P. Liver profile changes and complications in jaundiced patients with falciparum malaria. *Trop Med Parasitol* 1994;**45**:298–302.

27 Murthy GC, Sahay RK, Sreeniwas DV, Sundram C, Shanker V. Hepatitis in falciparum malaria. *Trop Gastroenterol* 1998;**19**:152–4.

28 Thapa BR, Yachha SK, Mehta S. Abdominal tuberculosis. *Indian Pediatr* 1991;**28**:1093–1100.

29 Alvarez SZ, Carpio R. Hepatobiliary tuberculosis. *Dig Dis Sci* 1983;**28**:193–200.

30 Steele MA, Burk RF, Desprez RM. Toxic hepatitis with isoniazid and rifampicin. A Meta-analysis. *Chest* 1991;**19**:465–71.

31 Pande JN, Singh SN, Khilnani GC, Khilnani S, Tandon RK. Risk factors for hepatotoxicity from anti-tuberculosis drugs: a case-control study. *Thorax* 1996;**51**:132–6.

32 Seth V, Kabra SK, eds. *Essentials of Tuberculosis in Children,* 2nd ed. New Delhi: Jaypee Brothers, 2001.

33 Kumar A, Misra PK, Mehrotra R, Govil YC, Rama GS. Hepatotoxicity of rifampicin and isoniazid. Is it all drug-induced hepatitis? *Am Rev Respir Dis* 1991;**143**:1350–2.
34 Indian Academy of Pediatrics. Consensus statement and recommendations on treatment of childhood tuberculosis. *Indian Pediatr* 1997;**34**:1093–6.
35 Khurroo MS, Zargar SA, Mahajan R. Hepatobiliary and pancreatic ascariasis in India. *Lancet* 1990;**335**:1503–6.
36 Khurroo MS, Zargar SA, Mahajan R, Bhat RL, Javid G. Sonographic appearances in biliary ascariasis. *Gastroenterology* 1987;**93**:267–72.
37 Rocha MS, Costa NS, Angelo MT, *et al.* CT identification of ascaris in the biliary tract. *Abdom Imaging* 1995;**20**:317–9.
38 Arora NK, Lodha R, Gulati S, *et al.* Portal hypertension in north Indian children. *Indian J Pediatr* 1998;**65**:585–91.
39 Sharma AK, Rangam HK, Choubey RP. Splenectomy and lienorenal shunt for extra hepatic portal venous obstruction. *Indian Pediatr* 2000;**37**: 422–5.
40 Yaccha SK, Khanduri A, Sharma BC. Gastrointestinal bleeding in children. *J Gastroenterol Hepatol* 1996;**11**:903–7.
41 Dhiman RK, Chawla Y, Vasishta RK, *et al.* Non-cirrhotic portal fibrosis (idiopathic portal hypertension): experience with 151 patients and a review of the literature. *J Gastroenterol Hepatol* 2001;**17**:6–16.
42 Arora NK, Lodha R, Gulati S, *et al.* Portal hypertension in north Indian children. *Indian J Pediatr* 1999;**65**:585–91.
43 Poddar U, Thapa BR, Puri P, *et al.* Non-cirrhotic portal fibrosis in children. *Indian J Gastroenterol* 2000;**19**:12–3.
44 Mitra SK, Rao KL, Narasimham KL, *et al.* Side-to-side lienorenal shunt without splenectomy in noncirrhotic portal hypertension in children. *J Pediatr Surg* 1993;**28**:398–407.
45 Ganguly S, Dasgupta J, Das AS, Biswas K, Mazumdar DN. Study of hypertension in children with special reference to sclerotherapy. *Trop Gastroenterol* 1997;**18:**119–21.
46 Ikematsu H, Kashiwagi S, Hayashi J *et al.* A seroepidemiologic study of hepatitis A virus infections: statistical analysis of two independent cross-sectional surveys in Okinawa, Japan. *Am J Epidemiol* 1987;**126**:50–4.
47 Yap I, Guan R. Hepatitis A sero-epidemiology in Singapore: a changing pattern. *Trans R Soc Trop Med Hyg* 1993;**87**:22–3.
48 Poovorawan Y. Changing epidemiology and prevention of hepatitis A virus infection. *Zhonghua Min Guo Xiao Er Ke Yi Xue Hui Za Zhi* 1998;**39**:139–45.
49 Hadler SC. Global impact of hepatitis A infection: changing patterns. In: Hollinger FB, Lemon SM, Margolis H, eds. *Viral Hepatitis and Liver Disease.* Baltimore: Williams & Wilkins, 1991: 14–20.
50 Yao G. Clinical spectrum and natural history of viral hepatitis A in a 1988 Shanghai epidemic. In: Hollinger FB, Lemon SM, Margolis H, eds. *Viral Hepatitis and Liver Disease.* Baltimore: Williams & Wilkins, 1991: 76–8.
51 Tsatsralt-Od B, Takahashi M, Endo K, Agiimaa D, Buyankhuu O, Okamoto H. Comparison of hepatitis A and E virus infections among healthy children in Mongolia: evidence for infection with a subgenotype IA HAV in children. *J Med Virol* 2007;**79**: 18–25.
52 Mall ML, Rai RR, Philip M, *et al.* Seroepidemiology of hepatitis A infection in India: changing pattern. *Indian J Gastroenterol* 2001;**20**:132–5.
53 Aggarwal R, Naik S, Yachha SK, Naik SR. Seroprevalence of antibodies to hepatitis A virus among children in northern India. *Indian Pediatr* 1999;**36**:1248–50.
54 Mohanavalli B, Dhevahi E, Menon T, Malathi S, Thyagarajan SP. Prevalence of antibodies to hepatitis A and hepatitis E Virus in urban school children in Chennai. *Indian Pediatr* 2003;**40**: 328–31.
55 Keefe EB. Is hepatitis A more severe in patients with chronic hepatitis B and other chronic liver diseases? *Am J Gastroenterol* 1995;**90**:201–5.
56 Vento S, Garofano T, Renzini C, *et al.* Fulminant hepatitis associated with hepatitis A virus superinfection in patients with chronic hepatitis C. *N Engl J Med* 1998;**338**:286–90.
57 Gordon SC, Reddy KR, Schiff L, Schiff ER. Prolonged intrahepatic cholestasis secondary to acute hepatitis A. *Ann Intern Med* 1984;**101**:635–7.
58 Glikson M, Galun E, Oren R, Tur-Kaspa R, Shouval D. Relapsing hepatitis A. Review of 14 cases and literature survey. *Medicine (Baltimore)* 1992;**71**:14–23.
59 Shah U, Habib Z, Kleinman RE. Liver failure attributable to hepatitis A virus infection in a developing country. *Pediatrics* 2000;**105**:436–8.
60 Hwang LY, Beasley RP, Yang CS, Hsu LC, Chen KP. Incidence of hepatitis A virus infection in children in Taipei, Taiwan. *Intervirology* 1983;**20**:149–54.
61 Hsu HY, Chang MH, Chen DS, Lee CY Sung JL. Changing seroepidemiology of hepatitis A virus infection in Taiwan. *J Med Virol* 1985;**17**:297–301.
62 Tsen YI, Chang MH, Hsu HY, *et al.* Seroprevalence of hepatitis B virus infection in children in Taipei, 1989: five years after a mass hepatitis B vaccination program. *J Med Virol* 1991;**34**: 96–9.
63 Tseng HY, Lu CY, Lee CY *et al.* Hepatitis A virus infection in Taipei in 1999. *J Formos Med Assoc* 2001;**100**:604–7.
64 Horng YC, Chang MH, Lee CY, Safary A, Andre FE, Chen DS. Safety and immunogenicity of hepatitis A vaccine in healthy children. *Pediatr Infect Dis J* 1993;**12**:359–62.
65 Fan PC, Chang MH, Lee PI, Safary A, Lee CY. Follow-up immunogenicity of an inactivated hepatitis A vaccine in healthy children: results after five years. *Vaccine* 1998;**16**:232–5.
66 Dagan R, Leventhal A, Anis E, Slater P, Ashur Y, Shouval D. Incidence of hepatitis A in Israel following universal immunization of toddlers. *JAMA* 2005;**294**:202–10.
67 Tsai IJ, Chang MH, Chen HL, *et al.* Immunogenicity and reactogenicity of the combined hepatitis A and B vaccine in young adults. *Vaccine* 2001;**19**:437–41.
68 Nolan T, Bernstein H, Blatter MM, *et al.* Immunogenicity and safety of an inactivated hepatitis A vaccine administered concomitantly with diphtheria–tetanus–acellular pertussis and *Haemophilus influenzae* type B vaccines to children less than 2 years of age. *Pediatrics* 2006;**118**:e602–9.
69 Mishra D, Singh R, Sibal A. Liver transplantation for fulminant hepatitis A infection. *Indian Pediatr* 2002;**39**:189–92.
70 Sharma D, Sibal A. Making a case for hepatitis a vaccination in glucose-6 phosphate dehydrogenase deficient subjects. *Indian J Pediatr* 2005;**72**:640.
71 Bhave S, Bavdekar A, Madan Z, *et al.* Evaluation of immunogenicity and tolerability of a live attenuated hepatitis a vaccine in Indian children. *Indian Pediatr* 2006;**43**:983–7.

72 Maynard JE, Kane MA, Alter MJ, Hadler SC Control of hepatitis B by immunization: global perspective. In: Zuckerman AJ, ed. *Viral Hepatitis and Liver Diseases*. New York: Liss, 1998: 967–9.

73 Chen CJ, Wang LY, Yu MW. Epidemiology of hepatitis B virus infection in the Asia–Pacific region. *J Gastroenterol Hepatol* 2000;**15**(Suppl):E3–6.

74 Hsu HY, Chang MH, Chen DS *et al.* Baseline seroepidemiology of hepatitis B virus infection in children in Taipei, 1984: a study just before mass hepatitis B vaccination program in Taiwan. *J Med Virol* 1986;**18**:301–7.

75 Feret E, Larouze B, Diop B, *et al.* Epidemiology of hepatitis B virus infection in the rural community of Tip, Senegal. *Am J Epidemiol* 1987;**125**:140–9.

76 Stevens CE, Beasley RP, Tsui J, Lee WC. Vertical transmission of hepatitis B antigen in Taiwan. *N Engl J Med* 1975;**292**:771–4.

77 Nayak NC, Panda SK, Zuckerman AJ, *et al.* Dynamics and impact of perinatal transmission of hepatitis B virus in North India. *J Med Virol* 1984;**21**:137–45.

78 Beasley RP, Hwang LY, Lin CC *et al.* Incidence of hepatitis B virus infection in preschool children in Taiwan. *J Infect Dis* 1982;**146**:198–204.

79 Hsu SC, Chang MH, Ni YH, *et al.* Horizontal transmission of hepatitis B virus in children. *J Pediatr Gastroenterol Nutr* 1993; **292**:771–4.

80 Shiraki K, Yohihara N, Sakurai M, Eto T, Kawana T. Acute hepatitis B in infants born to carrier mothers with the antibody to hepatitis B e antigen. *J Pediatr* 1980;**97**:768–70.

81 Chang MH, Lee CY, Chen DS, Hsu HC, Lai MY. Fulminant hepatitis in children in Taiwan: the important role of hepatitis B virus. *J Pediatr* 1987;**111**:34–9.

82 Carman WF, Fagan EA, Hadziyannis S, *et al.* Association of a precore genome variant of hepatitis B virus with fulminant hepatitis. *Hepatology* 1991;**14**:219–22.

83 Feray C, Gigou M, Samuel D, Bernuau J, Bismuth H, Brechot C. Low prevalence of precore mutation in hepatitis B virus DNA in fulminant hepatitis type B in France. *J Hepatol* 1993;**18**: 119–22.

84 Hsu HY, Chang MH, Lee CY, *et al.* Precore mutant of hepatitis B virus in childhood fulminant hepatitis B: an infrequent association. *J Infect Dis* 1995;**171**:776–81.

85 Chang MH, Hwang LY, Hsu HC, Lee CY, Beasley RP. Prospective study of asymptomatic HB_sAg carrier children infected in the perinatal period: clinical and liver histologic studies. *Hepatology* 1988;**8**:374–7.

86 Nordenfelt E, Andrén-Sandberg M. Dane particle-associated DNA polymerase and e antigen: relation to chronic hepatitis among carriers of hepatitis B surface antigen. *J Infect Dis* 1976; **134**:85–9.

87 Chang MH, Hsu HY, Hsu HC, Ni YH, Chen JS, Chen DS. The significance of spontaneous HB_eAg seroconversion in childhood: with special emphasis on the clearance of HB_eAg before three years of age. *Hepatology* 1995;**22**:1387–92.

88 Ni YH, Chang MH, Wang KJ, *et al.* Clinical relevance of hepatitis B virus genotype in children with chronic infection and hepatocellular carcinoma. *Gastroenterology* 2004;**127**:1733–8.

89 Thursz MR, Kwiatkowski D, Allsopp CE, Greenwood BM, Thomas HC, Hill AV. Association between an MHC class II allele and clearance of hepatitis B virus in the Gambia. *N Engl J Med* 1995;**332**:1065–9.

90 Hohler T, Gerken G, Notghi A, *et al.* HLA-DRB1*1301 and *1302 protect against chronic hepatitis B. *J Hepatol* 1997;**26**:503–7.

91 Ahn SH, Han KH, Park JY, *et al.* Association between hepatitis B virus infection and HLA-DR type in Korea. *Hepatology* 2000; **31**:1371–3.

92 Wu JF, Chen CH, Hsieh RP, *et al.* HLA typing associated with hepatitis B e antigen seroconversion in children with chronic hepatitis B virus infection: a long term prospective sibling study in Taiwan. *J Pediatr* 2006;**148**:647–51.

93 Ni YH, Chang MH, Hsu HY *et al.* Hepatocellular carcinoma in childhood-the clinical manifestations and prognosis. *Cancer* 1991;68:1737–41.

94 Chang MH, Chen DS, Hsu HC, Hsu HY, Lee CY. Maternal transmission of hepatitis B virus in childhood hepatocellular carcinoma. *Cancer* 1989;**64**:2377–80.

95 Yang HI, Lu SN, Liaw YF, *et al.* Hepatitis B e antigen and the risk of hepatocellular carcinoma. *N Engl J Med* 2002;**347**:168–74.

96 Beasley RP, Hwang LY, Lee GCY, *et al.* Prevention of perinatally transmitted hepatitis B virus infections with hepatitis B immune globulin and hepatitis B vaccine. *Lancet* 1983;**ii**:1099–102.

97 Lee GCY, Hwang LY, Beasley RP, Chen SH, Lee TY. Immunogenicity of hepatitis B virus vaccine in healthy Chinese neonates. *J Infect Dis* 1983;**148**:526–9.

98 Chen DS, Hsu NHM, Sung JL, *et al.* A mass vaccination program in Taiwan against hepatitis B virus infection in infants of hepatitis B surface antigen carrier mothers. *JAMA* 1987;**257**:2597–603.

99 Hsu HM, Chen DS, Chuang CH, *et al.* Efficacy of a mass hepatitis B vaccination program in Taiwan: studies on 3464 infants of hepatitis B surface antigen-carrier mothers. *JAMA* 1988;**260**: 2231–5.

100 Poovorawan Y, Sanpavat S, Pongpunglert W, *et al.* Long term efficacy of hepatitis B vaccine in infants born to hepatitis B e antigen-positive mothers. *Pediatr Infect Dis J* 1992;**11**:816–21.

101 Wang CW, Wang LC, Chang MH, *et al.* Long-term follow-up of hepatitis B surface antibody levels in subjects receiving universal hepatitis B vaccination in infancy in an area of hyperendemicity: correlation between radioimmunoassay and enzyme immunoassay. *Clin Diagn Lab Immunol* 2005;**12**:1442–7.

102 Chen HL, Chang MH, Ni YH, *et al.* Seroepidemiology of hepatitis B virus infection in children—ten years of mass vaccination in Taiwan. *JAMA* 1996;**276**:906–8.

103 Ni YH, Chang MH, Huang LM, *et al.* Hepatitis B virus infection in children and adolescents in a hyperendemic area: 15 years after mass hepatitis B vaccination. *Ann Intern Med* 2001;**135**: 796–800.

104 Whittle HC, Maine N, Pilkington J, *et al.* Long-term efficacy of continuing hepatitis B vaccination in infancy in two Gambian villages. *Lancet* 1995;**345**:1089–92.

105 Choe YH, Seo JK, Yun JH, Lee HS. Recent changes in prevalence of hepatitis B viral markers in preschool children in Seoul,1995. *J Korean Pediatr Soc* 1996;**39**:1254–9.

106 Da Villa G, Picciottoc L, Elia S, Peluso F, Montanaro F, Maisto T. Hepatitis B vaccination: universal vaccination of newborn babies and children at 12 years of age versus high risk groups. A comparison in the field. *Vaccine* 1995;**13**:1240–3.

107 Chang MH, Chen CJ, Lai MS, *et al.* Universal hepatitis B vaccination in Taiwan and the incidence of hepatocellular carcinoma in children. *N Engl J Med* 1997;**336**:1855–9.

108 Chang MH, Chen T, Hsu HM, *et al.* Problems in the prevention of childhood hepatocellular carcinoma in the era of universal hepatitis B immunization. *Clin Cancer Res* 2005;**11**:7953–7.

109 Chen HL, Chang CJ, Kong MS, Huang FC, Lee HC, Lin CC. Pediatric fulminant hepatic failure in endemic areas of hepatitis B infection: 15 years after universal hepatitis B vaccination. *Hepatology* 2004;**39**:58–63.

110 Lin YC, Chang MH, Ni YH, Hsu HY, Chen DS. Long-term immunogenicity and efficacy of universal hepatitis B vaccination in Taiwan. *J Infect Dis* 2003;**187**:134–8.

111 Huang LM, Chiang BL, Lee CY, Lee PI, Chi WK, Chang MH. Long-term response to hepatitis B vaccination and response to booster in children born to mothers with hepatitis B e antigen. *Hepatology* 1999;**29**:954–9.

112 Beasley RP, Hwang LY, Lin CC, Ko YC, Twu SJ. Incidence of hepatitis among students at a university in Taiwan. *Am J Epidemiol* 1983;**117**:213–22.

113 Ni YH, Huang LM, Chang MH, *et al.* Two decades of universal hepatitis B vaccination in Taiwan: impact and implication for future strategies. *Gastroenterology* 2007;**132**:1287–93.

114 Hsu HY, Chang MH, Ni YH, Chen HL. Survey of hepatitis B surface variant infection in children 15 years after a nationwide vaccination program in Taiwan. *Gut* 2004;**53**:1499–503.

115 Lok ASF, Lai CL Wu PC, *et al.* Alpha-interferon treatment in Chinese patients with chronic hepatitis B. *J Hepatol* 1990;**11** (Suppl 1):S121–5.

116 Stevens CE, Taylor PE, Pindyck J, *et al.* Epidemiology of hepatitis C virus—a preliminary study in volunteer blood donors. *JAMA* 1990;**263**:49–53.

117 Chang MH, Lee CY, Chen DS. Minimal role of hepatitis C virus in childhood liver disease in an area hyperendemic for hepatitis B infection. *J Med Virol* 1993;**40**:322–5.

118 Abdel-Aziz F, Habib M, Mohamed MK, *et al.* Hepatitis C virus (HCV) infection in a community in the Nile delta: population description and HCV prevalence. *Hepatology* 2000;**32**:111–5.

119 Ngui SL, Andrews NJ, Underhill GS, Heptonstall J, Teo CG. Failed postnatal immunoprophylaxis for hepatitis B: characteristics of maternal hepatitis B virus as risk factors. *Clin Infect Dis* 1998;**27**:100–6.

120 Ohto H, Terazawa S, Sasaki N, *et al.* Transmission of hepatitis C virus from mothers to infants. *N Engl J Med* 1994;**330**:744–50.

121 Chang MH. Mother-to-infant transmission of hepatitis C virus. *Clin Invest Med* 1996;**19**:368–372.

122 Lin HH, Kao JH, Hsu HY, *et al.* Absence of infection in breast-fed infants born to hepatitis C virus-infected mothers. *J Pediatr* 1995;**126**:589–91.

123 Mast EE, Hwang LY, Seto DS, *et al.* Risk factors for perinatal transmission of hepatitis C virus (HCV) and the natural history of HCV infection acquired in infancy. *J Infect Dis* 2005;**192**: 1880–9.

124 European Paediatric Hepatitis C Virus Network. A significant sex—but not elective cesarean section—effect on mother-to-child transmission of hepatitis C virus infection. *J Infect Dis* 2005; **192**:1872–9.

125 Ni YH, Chang MH, Lin KS, *et al.* Hepatitis C viral infection in thalassemic children: clinical and molecular studies. *Pediatr Res* 1996;**39**:323–8.

126 Ni YH, Chang MH, Chang MH, *et al.* Post-transfusion hepatitis C virus infection in children. *J Pediatr* 1994;**24**:709–113.

127 Chang MH, Ni YH, Hwang LH, *et al.* Long-term clinical and virologic outcome of primary hepatitis C virus infection in children: a prospective study. *Pediatr Infect Dis* 1995;**13**:769–72.

128 Fujisawa T, Inui A, Komatsu H, Miyagawa Y, Onoue M. Interferon-alpha therapy for children with chronic hepatitis C. *Zhonghua Min Guo Xiao Er Ke Yi Xue Hui Za Zhi* 1998;**39**:146–9.

129 McNeil C. Hepatitis C vaccine approaches phase II trial. *J Natl Cancer Inst* 2006;**98**:301–2.

130 Davis GL. Treatment of acute and chronic hepatitis C. *Clin Liver Dis* 1997;**1**:615–30.

131 Jacobson KR, Murray K, Zellos A, *et al.* An analysis of published trials of interferon monotherapy in children with chronic hepatitis C. *J Pediatr Gastroenterol Nutr* 2002;**34**:52–8.

132 Gonzalez–Peralta RP, Kelly DA, *et al.* Interferon alfa-2b in combination with ribavirin for the treatment of chronic hepatitis C in children: efficacy, safety, and pharmacokinetics. *Hepatology* 2005;**42**:1010–8.

133 Schwarz KB, Mohan P, Narkewicz MR, *et al.* Safety, efficacy and pharmacokinetics of peginterferon alpha2a (40 kd) in children with chronic hepatitis C. *J Pediatr Gastroenterol Nutr* 2006;**43**: 499–505.

134 Poddar U, Thapa BR, Prasad A, Singh K. Changing spectrum of sporadic acute viral hepatitis in Indian children. *J Trop Pediatr* 2002;**48**:210–3.

135 Mathur P, Arora NK, Panda SK, Kapoor SK, Jailkhani BL, Irshad M. Seroepidemiology of hepatitis E virus (HEV) in urban and rural children of north India. *Indian Pediatr* 2001;**38**:461–75.

136 Arora NK, Nanda SK, Gulati S, *et al.* Acute viral hepatitis types E, A, and B singly and in combination in acute liver failure in children in north India. *J Med Virol* 1996;**48**:215–21.

137 Kumar A, Yachha SK, Poddar U, Singh U, Aggarwal R. Does co-infection with multiple viruses adversely influence the course and outcome of sporadic acute viral hepatitis in children? *J Gastroenterol Hepatol* 2006;**21**:1533–7.

138 Botha JF, Spearman CW, Millar AJ, *et al.* Ten years of liver transplantation at Groote Schuur Hospital. *S Afr Med J* 2000; **99**:880–3.

139 Klein FR, Klin PA. Status and perspectives of liver transplantation in Argentina. *Int Anesthesiol Clin* 2006;**44**:99–109.

140 Aw MM, Phua KB, Ooi BC, *et al.* Outcome of liver transplantation for children with liver disease. *Singapore Med J* 2006;**47**: 595–8.

141 Quak SH. Pre-liver transplantation management of children. *Ann Acad Med Singapore* 1991;**20**:534–9.

142 Takagi H. Organ transplants still too few in Japan and Asian countries. *Transplant Proc* 1997;**29**:1580–3.

143 Chen YS, Wang CC, de Villa VH, *et al.* Prevention of de novo hepatitis B virus infection in living donor liver transplantation using hepatitis B core antibody positive donors. *Clin Transplant* 2002;**16**:405–9.

144 Prakoso E, Strasser SI, Koorey DJ, *et al.* Long-term lamivudine monotherapy prevents development of hepatitis B virus infection in hepatitis B surface-antigen negative liver transplant recipients from hepatitis B core-antibody-positive donors. *Clin Transplant* 2006;**20**:369–73.

145 Kwon CH, Suh KS, Yi NJ, *et al.* Long-term protection against hepatitis B in pediatric liver recipients can be achieved effectively with vaccination after transplantation. *Pediatr Transplant* 2006;**10**:479–86.

146 Katz SM, Ozaki CF, Monsour HP Jr, *et al.* Pediatric living-related and cadaveric liver transplantation: a single center experience. *Transplant Proc* 1994;**26**:145–6.
147 Oliveros FH, Santamaria ML, Gamez M, *et al.* Comparative study between living and cadaveric donors in pediatric liver transplantation. *Transplant Proc* 2005;**37**:3936–8.
148 Toyoki Y, Renz JF, Mudge C, *et al.* Allograft rejection in pediatric liver transplantation: comparison between cadaveric and living related donors. *Pediatr Transplant* 2002;**6**:301–7.
149 Bourdeaux, C., Darwish, A., Jamart, J. *et al.* Living-related versus deceased donor pediatric liver transplantation: a multivariate analysis of technical and immunological complications in 235 recipients. *Am J Transplant* 2007;**7**:440–7.
150 Bramstedt KA. Living liver donor mortality: where do we stand? *Am J Gastroenterol* 2006;**101**:1–5.
151 Sanchez-Fueyo A, Rimola A, Grande L, *et al.* Hepatitis B immunoglobulin discontinuation followed by hepatitis B virus vaccination: a new strategy in the prophylaxis of hepatitis B virus recurrence after liver transplantation. *Hepatology* 2000;**31**: 496–501.
152 Mieli-Vergani G, Howard ER, Portman B, Mowat AP. Late referral for biliary atresia: missed opportunities for effective surgery. *Lancet* 1989;**i**:421–3.
153 Mehrotra P, Yachha SK. Living related liver transplantation in Indian Children. *Indian Pediatr* 1999;**36**:357–62.
154 Lee DK, Lo SK, Quak SH, Prabhakaran K, Tan KC. Liver transplant in Singapore: coming of age. *Singapore Med J* 1998;**139**: 49–52.
155 Wai CT, Lin SG, Aung MO, *et al.* MARS: a futile tool in centres without active liver transplant support. *Liver Int* 2007;**27**:69–75.
156 Wang XH, Yan LN, Zhang F, *et al.* Early experiences on living donor liver transplantation in China: multicenter report. *Chin Med J (Engl)* 2006;**119**:1003–9.
157 Saing H, Fan ST, Tam PK, *et al.* Surgical complications and outcome of pediatric liver transplantation in Hong Kong. *J Pediatr Surg* 2002;**37**:1673–7.
158 Lo CM, Fan ST, Liu CL, *et al.* Ten-year experience with liver transplantation at Queen Mary Hospital: retrospective study. *Hong Kong Med J* 2002;**8**:240–4.
159 Poonacha P, Sibal A, Soin AS, Rajasekar MR, Rajakumari DV. India's first successful pediatric liver transplant. *Indian Pediatr* 2001;**38**:287–91.
160 Aw MM, Phua KB, Ooi BC, *et al.* Outcome of liver transplantation for children with liver disease. *Singapore Med J* 2006;**47**:595–8.
161 Al-Shurafa H, Jawdat M, Wali S, *et al.* Donor experience and outcome of pediatric living-related liver transplantation in Saudi Arabia. *J Hepatobiliary Pancreat Surg* 2003;**10**:428–31.
162 Al Sebayel MS, Ramirez CB, Abou Ella K. The first 100 liver transplants in Saudi Arabia. *Transplant Proc* 2001;**33**:2709.
163 Cheng YF, Chen CL, Huang TL, *et al.* Risk factors for intraoperative portal vein thrombosis in pediatric living donor liver transplantation. *Clin Transplant* 2004;**18**:390–4.
164 Ho MC, Wu YM, Hu RH, *et al.* Surgical complications and outcome of living related liver transplantation. *Transplant Proc* 2004;**36**:2249–51.
165 Nivatvongs S, Sirichindakul B, Nontasuti B, *et al.* Result of orthotopic liver transplantation at King Chulalongkorn Memorial Hospital: the first series from Thailand. *J Med Assoc Thai* 2003;**86**(Suppl 2):S445–50.
166 Aydogdu S, Arikan C, Kilic M, *et al.* Outcome of pediatric liver transplant recipients in Turkey: single center experience. *Pediatr Transplant* 2005;**9**:723–8.
167 Reading R, Tran DA. First pediatric liver transplantation in Ho Chi Minh City, Vietnam. *Pediatr Transplant* 2006;**10**:402–4.
168 Cuarterolo M, Ciocca M, López S, *et al.* [Evolution of children one year post liver transplant; in Spanish.] *Medicina (B Aires)* 2005;**65**:402–8.
169 Williams E, Questa H, Wacholder V, *et al.* Development of a pediatric liver transplantation program in Argentina. *Pediatr Surg Int* 1998;**13**:319–22.
170 Tannuri U, Velhote MC, Santos MM, *et al.* Pediatric liver transplantation: fourteen years of experience at the children institute in São Paulo, Brazil. *Transplant Proc* 2004;**36**:941–2.
171 Uribe M, Buckel E, Ferrario M, *et al.* Pediatric liver transplantation: ten years of experience in a multicentric program in Chile. *Transplant Proc* 2005;**37**:3375–7.
172 Buckel E, Uribe M, Brahm J, *et al.* Outcomes of orthotopic liver transplantation in Chile. *Transplant Proc* 2003;**35**:2509–10.
173 Gonzalez I, Abdo AA, Lopez O, *et al.* First 100 liver transplants at the medico–surgical research center (CIMEQ). *Transplant Proc* 2006;**38**:2473–4.
174 Varela-Fascinetto G, Davila-Perez R, Nieto-Zermeno J, *et al.* Experience of a successful pediatric liver transplant program in Mexico. *Transplant Proc* 2005;**37**:1201–2.

13 Supporting the Child and Family

24 The Role of the Multidisciplinary Team

Graham Gordon, Julie Reed, Jacqueline Blyth, and Caroline Patchell

Living with liver disease

In an age and culture in which good health is taken for granted, parents expect their children to be well and to survive them. Diseases that threaten children's autonomy and compromise their life expectancy challenge our emotions and coping resources to the limit. Childhood disease can turn the world upside down.[1]

Most liver disease is life-limiting. Medical therapy may control symptoms and long-term complications and thus optimize the quality of life. However, for many children with liver disease, there is no absolute cure, and ongoing monitoring with regular hospital visits for blood tests or admission is required. Thus, from the time of diagnosis, both child and family have to adapt to a life that is different from their expectations in order that the "upside-down" world becomes the norm for them. The child (infant–adolescent) with a chronic illness is automatically different from children of a similar age, while parents have an additional workload in caring for their child. "Normalizing" processes within this context should be encouraged, using the knowledge, skills, and active support of the different health professionals within the multidisciplinary team.[2,3]

The child (depending on age) and family pass through numerous processes. Firstly, both parents and child need to come to terms with the shock of the diagnosis, as well as (for the parents) the grief of losing their child's good health. Parents have to take in much information relating to the diagnosis and prognosis, as well as learning new skills in caring for their child. Ideally, information should be shared with the parents and child at their own pace and in the context of their family and social setting.

Parents may find it difficult to accept the unpredictability of their child's disease and the effect on immediate life plans. If the child's condition deteriorates, with a reduction in physical mobility and increasing symptoms such as ascites and malnutrition, the intensity of the care required increases exponentially. As a result, the extra time and attention given to the child with liver disease may impact adversely on siblings and other members of the family.[1]

As the child's disease progresses, parents have to be careful to detect subtle changes in their child's condition in order to seek appropriate help. As liver disease is relatively uncommon in the child population, many parents, children, and young people become "experts" in disease management and often know more about specific aspects of their disease than their local health-care team. This may be an added concern to the family, and it is vital that efficient communication systems are established with local services. Ideally, the child and family should experience a "seamless web" of care, treatment, and support centered on the needs of the child and his or her siblings and carers.[4] Multidisciplinary working is an essential feature of this "seamless" care.[5]

Effective team working

The multidisciplinary team will work most effectively if they follow a shared vision for the service. The National Service Framework for Children, Young People and Maternity Services in England advocates child-centered hospital services.[6]

Child-centered services are services that:

- Consider the "whole child," not simply the illness being treated
- Treat children as children, and young people as young people
- Are concerned with the overall experience for the child and family
- Treat children, young people, and parents as partners in care
- Integrate and coordinate services around the child and family's particular needs
- Gradate smoothly into adult services at the right time
- Work in partnership with children, young people, and parents to plan and shape services and to develop the workforce

These principles are now used to guide the development of services in our unit. There is a climate in which the skills and judgment of all team members are valued. Communication channels are constantly appraised to ensure they are effective,

Diseases of the Liver and Biliary System in Children, 3rd edition. Edited by Deirdre Kelly. © 2008 Blackwell Publishing, ISBN: 978-1-4051-6334-7.

so that shared decisions can be made. Staff support is provided so that training issues can be addressed and debriefing can occur, as the nature of the work is stressful.[7] This is often provided by a counselor from within the clinical psychology team.

Consent to treatment

The United Nations Convention on the Rights of the Child states in Article 12 that governments should "assure to the child who is capable of forming his or her own views, the right to express those views freely, in all matters affecting the child, the views of the child being given weight in accordance with the age and maturity of the child."

For consent to be valid, it is expected that an individual is fully informed as to the alternatives, expected benefits, and the possible complications for a procedure or a research project and able to understand the implications of the decision. Consent may be given by a young person (in British law, this is usually 16 years of age) or by another on behalf of the child, such as parent or guardian. Emphasis should be placed on whether a child is competent to give consent. A child or young person who has the capacity to fully understand a decision affecting his or her life automatically has the capacity to make that decision, unless statute law states otherwise. This is the Gillick competence test after the Gillick case in 1985.[8] This set a precedent, because it allowed under-16-year-olds to consent to medical treatment provided they could show sufficient understanding and competence to make wise choices.[9]

Although it may be difficult to define when a child or young person is competent, this can be overcome by establishing a clear process of information-sharing and opportunities for shared decision-making, involving all members of the multidisciplinary team with the child and their parents.[10] In Birmingham, we have developed a framework to empower children and young people, with their parents, to make choices in their care and treatment.[10]

The objectives of the framework are, for the team:

- To gain information about the child's knowledge, understanding, and experience of illness and health care in the context of the child's life.

For the children and young people:

- To provide them with an opportunity to increase their knowledge and understanding of their disease and treatments and to express their feelings, fears, and expectations.
- To help them develop confidence in participating in decisions by providing opportunities for them to make choices in their care and treatment.

For the parents:

- To help them to gain knowledge and understanding of their child's disease and treatment in order to make informed decisions with their child and as individuals.
- To enable parents to impart information to their child and siblings.
- To facilitate sharing information between the child and parent in order to help them make decisions together.

Members of the multidisciplinary team

Multidisciplinary team working is the ideal way to assess and meet the needs of children with liver disease and their families within the hospital. The composition of these teams will vary slightly from setting to setting within one country, and could vary greatly from one country to another. Individuals involved in a child's care should meet regularly to share information and to formulate a treatment plan that best meets a child's needs with the resources that are available to them.

The multidisciplinary team usually consists of the following members:

- Medical and surgical teams, led respectively by a consultant pediatric hepatologist and pediatric hepatobiliary and transplant surgeon
- Ward nursing team, led by a senior nurse
- Specialist nurse
- Dietitian
- Physiotherapist
- Psychologist
- Play specialist
- Youth worker
- Pharmacist
- Family support worker
- Schoolteacher
- Chaplaincy
- Secretarial and administrative support

Similar teams will be found in the referring team, who will enter into a shared care agreement for the ongoing care of the child. All of these hospital-based teams will depend on the local primary health team for implementing parts of the treatment plan, such as prescribing medication, administering vaccinations, and support during normal childhood illness. This team will include:

- A general practitioner, or primary pediatrician
- Health visitor
- Practice nurse
- Children's community nursing team
- Community physiotherapist
- Social services
- Pharmacy
- Other services, such as home tuition available through the education department

Effective communication is the key to ensuring that children receive optimum care as they move between hospitals and the community.

Roles within the multidisciplinary team

Medical and surgical team

The medical and surgical teams should have sufficient consultant or specialist grades to provide 24-h cover for medical and surgical care for the child, support, advice, training, and teaching for the other medical staff involved in the care of the child. The consultants will provide the lead in developing the overall treatment plan for the child. Increasingly, this will involve asking advice from the hospital's wider team, such as:

- Microbiologist
- Virologist
- Radiologist
- Gastroenterologist
- Cardiologist
- Respiratory physician
- Neurologist
- Histopathologist
- Clinical scientists

Communication between the team is essential. We have found the following structure helpful:

- Daily consultant-led ward rounds at which the needs of the children currently in hospital are discussed and new plans for investigation, treatment, and monitoring are made.
- Twice-weekly ward round with the multidisciplinary team, at which a business-like structure will ensure that the treatment plans for discharged children are fully known and a plan of follow-up care implemented. It also allows for planning for future admissions to the hospital and for information to be shared about children with problems in other hospitals or in the home and a plan made.
- Microbiologist and gastroenterologist attend one ward round a week.
- Weekly radiology and histopathology conferences.
- A weekly meeting to discuss specific issues for children being considered for transplantation and the management of children currently on the waiting list.
- Consultant outpatient reviews, for medical staff to provide feedback about how children seen as outpatients are progressing. Preparation can be made for the following week's clinics.
- Meetings for particularly challenging problems that need a face-to-face discussion between a number of consultants.

Ward nursing team

This team needs to develop its own routines, which ensure that evidenced-based care is given to children. The senior nurses on the ward will take on development roles to ensure that nursing practice is continually changing to meet the needs of the children, such as:

- A teaching sister who coordinates the training needs of the nursing team in relation to new:
  —Equipment
  —Policy and procedure
  —Ways of working
- A student coordinator who coordinates the needs of nurses in various stages of training.
- A stoma nurse, who provides specific advice to children and develops the policies and provides training.
- An intravenous therapy nurse, who implements hospital policy and provides training.
- Other nurses may become link nurses with other groups in the hospital so that practice is kept up to date:
  —Tissue viability
  —Moving and handling
  —Nutritional care
  —Safeguarding children
  —Pain assessment and management

It is important that nurses are given time in order to carry out these roles that improve care for children. In the United Kingdom, this link between taking on added roles, remuneration, and being adequately supported has been managed through a joint Department of Health/staff-side scheme called Agenda for Change.[11] This scheme is designed to provide career and pay progression, with a link to a knowledge and skills framework,[12] and allows nurses the opportunity to publish their experience of nursing.[13] Increasingly due to changes in medical training and careers, nurses are taking on duties that were traditionally seen as being the role of the doctor. The role of the advanced nurse is developing to take on a job description that includes:[14]

- Clinical assessment
- Prescribing of medication
- Venipuncture
- Ordering of diagnostic investigations and monitoring tests

It is important to work with local universities and colleges to support advanced nursing. In Birmingham, we work with the Birmingham City University[15] and run courses twice a year on the principles of hepatology and transplant care. This collaboration between university and hospital has recently been acknowledged by the award of the status of "center for excellence in teaching and learning" by the Higher Education Funding Council for England.[16]

Specialist nurse

Specialist nurses have a wider role than solely being on the ward. This allows them to build up a caseload of children whom they can support while in hospital, but also in the outpatient clinic and the home. This gives them the opportunity to act as a key worker for children and families. Their roles in our team include the following.

Provision of information

The need of each child and family is assessed and a plan of implementation is agreed in the multidisciplinary team. This is achieved using a framework of practice called "Helping children with their families to be involved with decisions about treatment."[10] This information for the child is achieved by involving the schoolteacher and the play specialist. The teacher involves the child with activities about the body in line with the national educational curriculum. This involves educational computer network–based activities for the older child. For the younger child, the play specialist uses a range of play-based activities, including anatomical puppets, books, and board games. The specialist nurse will indicate the specific disease and possible treatment options relevant to each child. The parents will have their own program of education on:[17]

- The hospital and the ward
- Facilities, including accommodation and provision of interpreters
- Team members and roles
- Reasons for investigation and what they are
- Basic understanding of the liver and its functions
- Understanding the signs and symptoms of liver disease
- When you can expect results
- Treatments of liver disease
- Looking after the child in the home
- How to stay in contact

The literature for explaining about procedures and conditions has been streamlined. In Birmingham, we have a library of procedure leaflets that meet standards that are recognized by the Clinical Negligence Standards for Trusts (CNST).[18] The use of a questioning style will give a friendlier feel to the leaflet:[19]

- Introduction—why are we writing this leaflet?
- Overview of the procedure—what does it involve, where will it take place, how will it help me?
- What are the benefits?
- What are the risks?
- Are there any alternatives?
- What happens afterwards?
- What care will my child need at home?
- Where can I get further information?
- Frequently asked questions
- Space to write down questions

The leaflets are peer-reviewed, and feedback is obtained from the users of the leaflet. The leaflets should include a production date and should be regularly reviewed. The series should be reproduced for the younger and older child (Figure 24.1).[19,20]

Our leaflets include:

- Liver biopsy (percutaneous and transjugular)
- Endoscopy and endoscopic ultrasound
- Endoscopic variceal banding
- Abdominal ultrasound
- Radionucleotide scanning of the liver (technetium trimethyl 1-bromoiminodiacetic acid, TEBIDA)
- Endoscopic retrograde cholangiopancreatography (ERCP)
- Percutaneous transhepatic cholangiogram (PTC)
- Angiography
- Transjugular intrahepatic portosystemic shunt (TIPS)
- Magnetic resonance imaging (MRI)
- Computed tomography (CT)

Each center should build up a set that reflects the investigations and treatments that are offered locally.

Disease and general support literature is well developed in the United Kingdom. This has happened through collaborative working between the three national liver units and the Children's Liver Disease Foundation (CLDF). This has resulted in a set of nationally agreed pediatric liver disease leaflets for parents. Some are available online (www.childliverdisease.org) or by postal or personal application. The liver transplantation series is called "Stepping Stone to Transplantation."[21] A series is being developed for intestinal transplantation. Guidelines should be used in producing disease specific literature:[19]

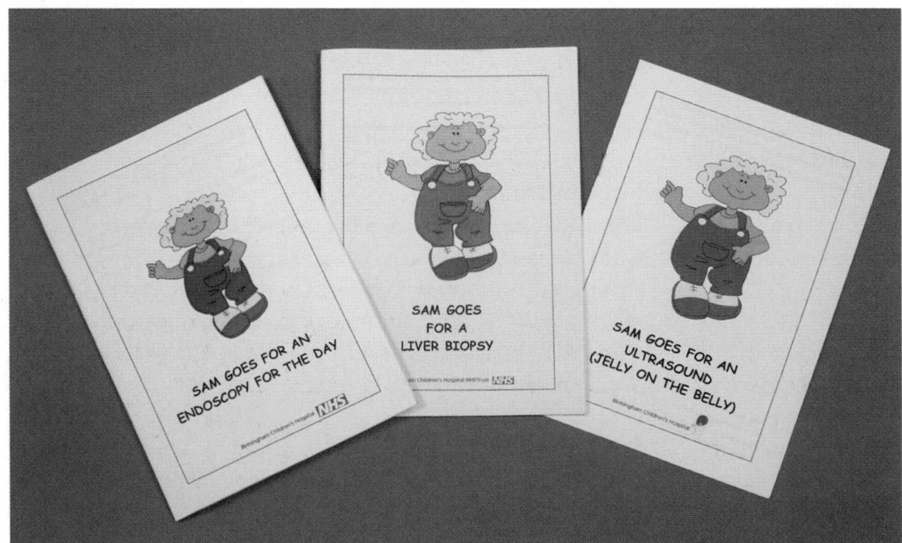

Figure 24.1 The Sam Series is an example of children's information leaflets used to prepare them for procedures. The leaflets can be read to the child by a parent or nurse, or used as a basis for explanation.

- Introduction—why are we writing this leaflet?
- What is the condition? What is it called and what are its characteristics?
- How is it diagnosed?
- What causes it?
- How common is it and whom does it affect?
- What treatments are available?
- What is the outlook?
- Is there a support group?
- Where can you get further information?

Skills training and discharge planning

This is achieved with the ward-based team and members of the multidisciplinary team. A plan is agreed with the child and family for the teaching of skills that will be needed in the home for the family to look after the child safely. This will include the safe administration of medicines, enteral feeding products by nasogastric or gastrostomy routes, stoma care, management of fluid balance, and problem-solving skills.[22] Discharge planning should begin early at the point of admission. With good planning and communication with the shared and primary health-care team, we have found that discharge can be facilitated at an early point. This planning can be done over the phone or by e-mail. For complex patients, we have found discharge meetings with local teams to be beneficial either in our hospital or local to the child's home. Recently with digital phone technology, we have achieved the same by telephone conference.

Providing continuing care

The specialist nurse is well placed to provide this rather than medical staff, who may move for training purposes. In Birmingham, we started a nurse-led telephone consultation service in 2001, called Liver Direct,[23] which proved very successful in managing the numerous calls that would come to the Liver Unit every day. Nurses were able to answer 90% of the calls. Voicemail, e-mail and improved hours have been added. The calls are logged on a database and become part of the patient record. The service is used by our shared and primary health teams, who appreciate being able to discuss patients with individuals who are knowledgeable about their present condition and understand how services are run and managed.

Coordination of immunosuppression

Specialist nurses are able to provide the skills and knowledge to do this very efficiently for 400 patients who are on immunosuppresion.[24] These children need follow-up of blood results, agreement on a new dosage, and a further review date. This is fed back to families, routinely by letter when no dose change is needed or by phone and confirming letter when a dose change is needed. Currently, the specialist nurses are managing over 2500 reviews a year. The letters are produced from the database.

Coordination of vaccination

In the past, general practitioners were advised by letter about the vaccination needs of children with liver disease and after transplantation. An audit of children with biliary atresia revealed that half of the children did not receive vaccinations on time or did not receive vaccines that might benefit them, such as pneumococcal vaccines. We became aware that vaccines were administered by practice nurses, who were unsure about the eligibility and timing. Our current practice is for the specialist nurse to send a recommended vaccination plan with timings for children with liver disease, for those being prepared for transplantation, and for those after transplant. The letter is copied to parents, who are able to see that the plan is implemented.[24]

Participation in outpatient and outreach clinics

The specialist nurse attends the outpatient clinic to see new children with the consultant and other members of the multidisciplinary team. They are ideally placed to develop these clinics to meet the needs of special groups. In our unit, we have listened to our young people and have developed the young people's clinic to meet their needs.[25] Children attend our unit from all over Britain. Increasingly, children with stable liver disease and after transplantation are managed in outreach clinics in other cities.[24] Children are seen by a consultant hepatologist, specialist nurse, and dietitian along with members of the local shared care team. The service is well received by families, as it reduces the travel burden. It is appreciated by the shared care teams, who have the benefit of discussion over specific and general management issues. For certain patient groups such as children with viral hepatitis, patients are being seen by a viral hepatitis specialist nurse alone along with the local team in these outreach clinics.

Participation in audit and research

Increasingly, specialist nurses are taking part in the audit and research activity of our unit. Specialist nurses lead specific audit projects and facilitate change and cost savings. A recent audit of serological results after transplantation has changed our practice and will save money. Specialist nurses run specific research projects and their skill in writing age-appropriate information leaflets is now an example of best practice in our hospital.[24]

Play specialist

Play specialists work with children of all ages.[26] Their work involves:

- Using play to enable children to have a positive image of hospital
- Preparing them to cope with admission, treatment, surgery, or other procedures
- Enabling them to manage fears and anxieties
- Offering coping strategies

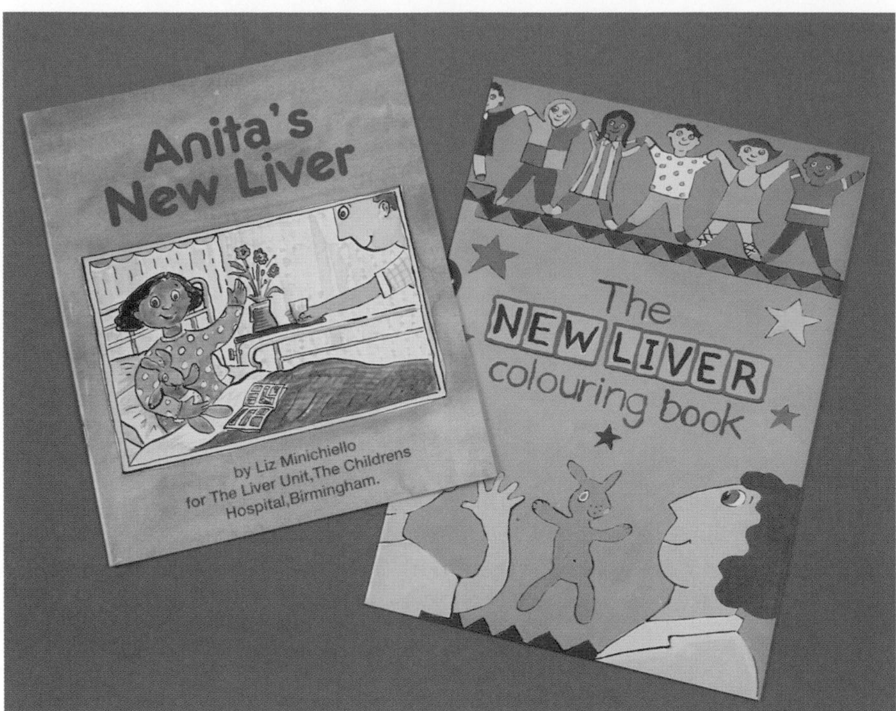

Figure 24.2 *Anita's New Liver* is a story-book for older children to prepare them for transplantation. It can be used in conjunction with the *New Liver Colouring Book*.

- Using specific play techniques to minimize stressful events by acting them out in advance or postprocedurally
- Assessing the child's level of cognitive understanding and development
- Education on condition and treatment
- Basic pain management

In our unit, the play specialists have a crucial role in:

- Preparing children for procedures and investigations
- Helping children cope with invasive and non invasive procedures
- Preparing children for transplantation, enabling them to make informed decisions regarding their treatment and admission, and to support the consent process (Figure 24.2)
- Normalizing the day for children who are hospitalized for long periods
- Using therapeutic play to help children express their fears and anxieties
- Issues in relation to chronic illness
- Supporting children postprocedurally, emotionally and psychologically

They work very closely with the specialist nurse, who highlights any particular disease issue; with the hospital schoolteacher, who may be able to use aspects of the national curriculum to teach the child normal body anatomy and physiology; and with the psychologist, who highlights particular aspects of psychological support that may be needed. They will also work with siblings, so that the whole family is informed about the treatment plan.

They will use a variety of different tools that will vary with each child. These will include:

- Various assessment tools that allow children to express what they already know and what they want us to know
- Hospital play to assess past experiences and anxieties
- Preparation books
- Real medical equipment (Figure 24.3)
- Body work
- Anatomical dolls, puppets, books, and body programs
- Handling of medical equipment, visits to other wards
- Developing the child's wish list about treatment
- Preparing children for lifestyle changes (Figure 24.4)
- Offering coping strategies

They will use the different skills of the adolescent play specialist and hospital youth worker when needed.

Family support worker

Our family support team includes a social worker. Issues of child safeguarding can thus be addressed promptly and with appropriate plans developed to keep children safe. The support worker's skills are in assessing the impact of the child's condition on social functioning, parenting capacity, assessing attachments, and facilitating help when needed. This may relate to help with claiming local and central government financial help, making applications to grant-awarding bodies, and liaising with local social services about ongoing practical support that may be available. Much of the time, support workers provide a listening ear. They facilitate a weekly parent support group within the ward.

Physiotherapist

The physiotherapist has a vital role in assessing the effects of

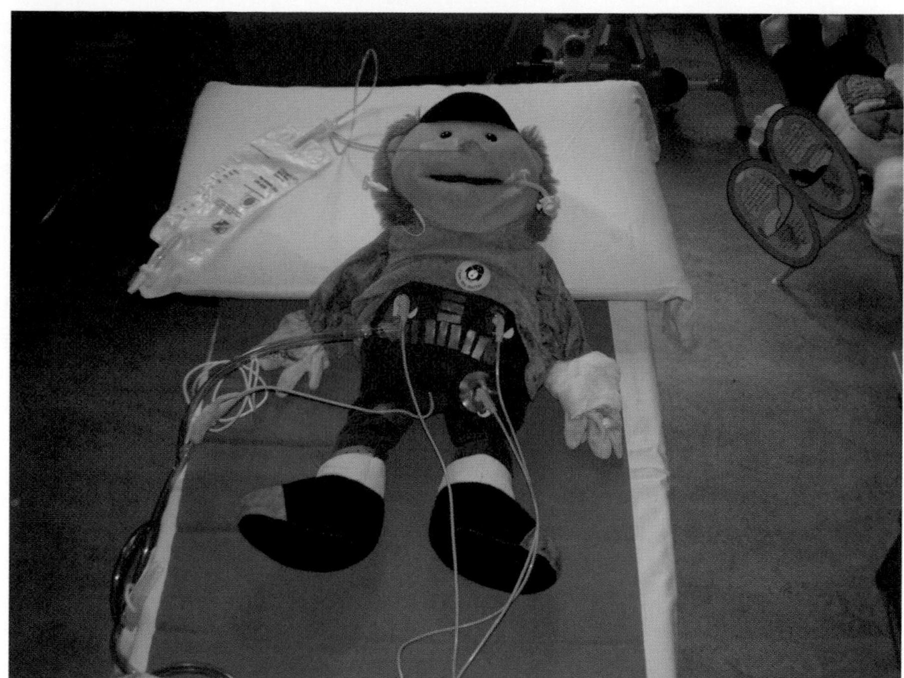

Figure 24.3 Children can be prepared for their postoperative experience using different play techniques. These puppets are very popular and allow the child to prepare for intensive care after surgery.

Stay Well
Your medicines stop your white blood cells looking after your body as well as they used to.
Therefore when a germ enters our body, like a germ which causes a cold, your white blood cells won't be able to get rid of it so easily, so you might become ill.
This is called Infection.
William
White Blood
Wendy
Cells
Colin
Cold germ
Claire
Cotrimoxazole
To help stop you getting ill, you have to take another special medicine for a short while called Cotrimoxazole

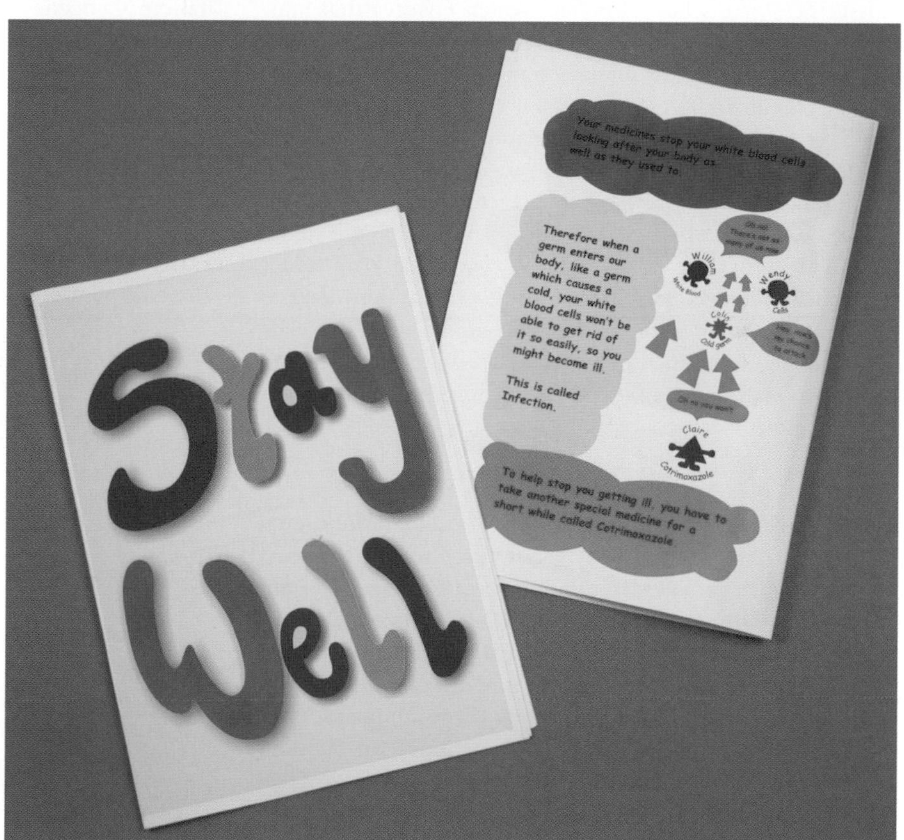

Figure 24.4 Life after transplantation may be different. It is helpful to encourage children to be independent and enjoy life using leaflets such as this one—"Stay Well".

liver disease and various treatments on movement. This is especially important in pediatrics, when developmental delay can occur quite readily. Once baseline assessments have been made, the physiotherapist will institute a treatment plan with the child and family, communicating this to the multidisciplinary team so that the plan can be supported. The role encompasses working on the ward, in the pediatric intensive-care unit, in outpatients, and facilitating continuing support either in other hospitals or in the community. The role increasingly involves health promotion and preventative health care, as obese children are seen in our clinics and ward with fatty liver disease. The effect of the organ donation crisis in the United Kingdom is causing children to wait longer on the active transplant list. These children are becoming less well as they reach transplant. The physiotherapist increasingly finds that respiratory and physical rehabilitation in children is longer and more challenging.

Pharmacist

Drug therapy in liver disease and after transplantation has become increasingly complex. The challenge in pediatrics is to have a preparation that can be taken by children and that ultimately is available in the local community. The ward-based pharmacy team has become a valuable part of the team in order to meet these challenges. We have pioneered ward-based pharmacy technicians, who keep ward-based drug stock levels constant and make sure that each child has his or her drugs dispensed in a form that can be taken by mouth. The technician is crucial to our "medicines for discharge" policy, which ensures that families have their take-home medication available for 5 days before discharge.[22] This enables training to be given in the complex medication regimens that are often needed in treating liver disease and after transplantation. The technician facilitates home delivery of certain medicines when general practitioners are not willing to prescribe major immunosuppressants, or when a medicine does not have a liquid formulation that a local pharmacist can access. The senior pharmacist reviews each child's drug prescription daily to identify any medication issues that need attention. The ward's policies that incorporate medicines are reviewed and amended so that there is good practice in the management of medicines.

Chaplain

The United Kingdom is now a multifaith society. The hospital chaplaincy has developed in recent years to reflect this.[27] The chaplaincy provides spiritual support for patients, staff, and relatives through chaplains and faith community representatives. Members of the chaplaincy team are seen around the ward and the hospital. They are mentioned in our ward literature and valued as team members. They offer religious and pastoral care, opportunity for children and families to continue their spiritual observances while in hospital, and support in times of crisis—in particular, when end-of-life decisions are to be made. They facilitate memorial services within and outside the hospital, which is appreciated by the wider hospital community and those in our service. They are part of the ethics advisory group in the hospital.

Shared-care protocols for patient management

Developing these documents is an important part of the multidisciplinary team role. Local teams need the support that these documents provide, enabling them to provide the continuity of care that children need. The scope of each of these documents should cover:

- An overview of the specific liver disease and its treatment
- Management of specific complications
- Specific information about the medication involved in treatment including dosage and side effects
- When to contact us and how

These should be available for primary and shared-care teams and will supplement discharge summaries and outpatient and other correspondence. Recently, the Department of Health in the United Kingdom has directed us to give copies of all outpatient correspondence to families who want them and to children above the age of 12 who would benefit from them.[28] This initiative, along with having copies of shared-care documents, is very empowering to families, particularly if there is a need to attend a health institution and records are not immediately available.

Case study

AB, aged 6 months, was admitted from his local hospital with cholangitis and deteriorating liver disease following a failed Kasai portoenterostomy at the age of 8 weeks. He was deeply jaundiced, with coagulopathy and deteriorating albumin levels. He had increasing signs of portal hypertension, ascites, pruritus, and failure to thrive. He was started on intravenous vitamin K, modified antibiotics, albumin infusions, and diuretics. His nutrition was modified to a medium-chain fat-based feed with increased calories and given via the nasogastric route.

His family were advised that he should be assessed for liver transplantation over the following days. A written timetable was given to the family for the next week, which included:

- Liver biopsy and endoscopy under general anesthesia
- Abdominal ultrasound
- Cardiac, neurological, renal assessment
- Developmental and psychosocial assessments
- Nutritional assessment
- Vaccination schedule
- An opportunity to meet senior members of the team, including hepatologist, anesthetist, surgeon, transplant coordinator, psychologist, support social worker, dietitian, physiotherapist and specialist nurse for information and counselling

The specialist nurse discussed with his family: ascites, portal hypertension, pruritus, liver biopsy, endoscopy, and the various assessments AB was to undergo. This was supported by the provision of literature. The process of assessment was explained and an opportunity was given to discuss indications, alternatives, logistics, organ donation, the call when a donor organ was found, the operation day, pediatric intensive care, recovery, surgical and medical complications such as infection and rejection, the long-term outcomes, medication, and lifestyle. The family were also taught how to carry out nasogastric feeding at home.

A recommendation was made to the family that AB should be placed on the waiting list for liver transplant following a vaccination program that would include varicella zoster, measles/mumps/rubella vaccine, influenza, and an accelerated program of hepatitis A and B.

AB was discharged 10 days after admission with community nursing support for home nasogastric feeding and home delivery of feed ingredients and disposable equipment from a community pharmacy company.

The support social worker had arranged support for father with work-related issues and ensured that the family were receiving all the available state benefits. The physiotherapist had taught the family fun-based activities to enable developmental progress.

After his admission, his family felt competent to deliver his nutrition, provide for his medication needs, and recognize signs of deterioration, and were confident about whom to contact both in the local and national unit if he became unwell.

Three months later, when he was fully vaccinated and in an improving nutritional state, and at a time when his family were ready for his operation psychologically, he received a suitable organ and had a successful liver transplant.

The Children's Liver Disease Foundation in Birmingham provides a useful web site (www.childliverdisease.org).

Psychological support

The psychologist will be involved in providing psychological support to the child and family, neuropsychological assessment, and evaluating psychosocial outcome.

Developmental, intellectual, and neuropsychological assessment

Developmental assessment involves the administration of standardized tests (e.g., Bayley Scales of Infant Development, Griffiths Mental Developmental Scales) to babies and preschool children in order to measure their developmental ability. Intellectual assessment involves the administration of norm-referenced tests (e.g., the Wechsler Preschool and Primary Scale of Intelligence III and Wechsler Intelligence Scale for Children IV) to preschool and school-aged children in order to measure their general intellectual ability. A neuropsychological assessment involves the administration of standardized tests of intellectual ability, learning, memory, and attention and the interpretation of these measures in the light of known brain functioning.

Neuropsychological impairment can arise as a direct result of liver disease, such as cirrhosis or Wilson's disease, or as a consequence of treatment—e.g., drug side effects. Assessment of a child's intellectual or neuropsychological functioning may be clinically indicated where there are concerns about low attainment relative to intellectual potential, specific learning difficulties, and problems with memory, attention, and concentration. Results of assessments may have important implications for a child's education, psychological and psychosocial adjustment, and professional–patient communication. Neuropsychological assessment may also be carried out as one component of a research protocol to investigate disease progression, effects of drug treatments, or outcome after liver transplantation.

Research on disease progression suggests that prior to overt signs of encephalopathy, children with chronic liver disease may have specific neuropsychological impairment (visual–spatial skills and attention/concentration), with intact verbal and memory skills. These impairments have been shown in adult patients with nonalcoholic cirrhosis,[29] and it is likely that these changes would be at least as significant in the pediatric population. In addition, some liver diseases, such as Wilson's disease, are associated with decrement in visual–spatial and visual scanning tasks prior to neurological impairment.[30]

Studies investigating outcome following liver transplantation have been hampered by small, heterogeneous samples; difficulties in making comparisons between psychometric tests measuring developmental ability and those measuring intellectual functioning; lack of baseline data prior to the onset of end-stage liver disease; absence of comparison groups; and a lack of research into specific components of neuropsychological functioning. Nevertheless, these studies suggest that post-transplant intellectual functioning is likely to be at least in the low average range.[31,32] Early studies suggested that children who were under 12 months at the onset of their liver disease may have global intellectual deficits at post-transplant assessment,[33] with poor growth being an important mediating factor. Modern management of pre-transplantation care and newer immunosuppression regimens have improved this outcome, but global difficulties may persist in some children. The results of a longitudinal study[34] suggest that there may be a dip in assessment scores following transplantation, with recovery to pretransplant intellectual level, or better, at 2 years after transplantation.[34] A child's growth may initially worsen after transplantation, with catch-up growth in height starting when the steroids are reduced or withdrawn.[35,36] This finding has important implications for supporting a child's return to education. In time, most children return to the normal range[34] and achieve a good quality of life and normal education.[37,38] In older children, clinical observations and two recent studies suggest that the effects of liver transplantation may adversely affect memory, learning processes, attention span, and vigilance.[39,40] Although the etiology is not known, it could be related to the severity of pretransplantation disease or to long-term immunosuppressant therapy.

In addition, both tacrolimus and cyclosporine, the most widely used immunosuppressant drugs, are both known to have neuropsychological effects—particularly cyclosporine[41] —and may affect neuropsychological functioning,[33] which has implications for the long-term educational prospects of survivors.

Treatment adherence

Children with liver disease before or after transplantation need to adhere to drug regimens with negative side effects, dietary restrictions, and undergo repeated invasive procedures. Adherence difficulties are among the most frustrating and perplexing problems for the multidisciplinary team, especially before and after transplantation. Adherence to a specific treatment is affected by a number of interrelated variables, including the child's developmental status, disease knowledge, health beliefs, and family support.[42] Nonadherence to medical therapy is a serious problem for adolescents and is one of the most common causes of chronic graft rejection in this population (see Chapter 25).

Although it is accepted that failure to take medication is important evidence of nonadherence, there are other measures such as attendance at clinic appointments and adherence with dietary and other medical advice that also need to be considered.[43] In order to determine whether or not a child is complying with treatment, an objective assessment method should be used, such as medication levels and nonattendance at clinics. There are electronic devices that record how many tablets are taken and when, but these are expensive and not always acceptable to young people.[44]

Interventions targeting adherence should be nonjudgmental and address the child's increasing role in self-care beginning in early adolescence.[45] Encouraging self-medication with the use of reminders (mobile phone alarms, etc.) at an early age may also be effective. In their study, Falkenstein *et al.*[46] found that noncompliance crosses all socio-economic and cultural groups. Improving flexibility of clinic hours, shortening the time between visits, and decreasing numbers and times of medication may increase adherence.

During the teenage years, parent support continues to be important, but peer support may have greater influence on a teenager's adherence. Involving healthy peers or slightly older patients as mentors[47] is a potentially promising area of research in treatment adherence. Nevertheless, treatment adherence remains a complex issue, and further research is needed to determine which intervention (or combination of interventions) is most suitable for an individual patient and their family.[48] Nonadherence is likely to increase following transfer to an adult unit and hence there is a need for a sound transition process (see Chapter 25).

Altered physical appearance

Most children with liver disease are likely to experience abnormal changes in their appearance at some stage during their treatment. These changes may be due to disease processes, e.g., jaundice, or as a consequence of medical or surgical treatment, such as cushingoid features, hirsutism, or abdominal scarring. Treatment adherence may be compromised by a patient's wish to avoid the negative side effects on physical appearance, especially steroids. Worries about altered appearance are likely to peak at adolescence, when many young people are concerned about how they look and the association with peer group acceptance.

There are a number of reasons why it is important to consider the psychological effects of growing up with a distinctive appearance. Firstly, children and adolescents describe themselves and their peers according to their physical appearance, and children as young as 3 years old are able to discriminate between attractive and unattractive peers.[49] Secondly, from adult studies there is evidence to suggest that individuals with an atypical appearance experience social avoidance.[50] Thirdly, if a child or young person experiences social avoidance by peers, then this may lead to decreased social competence, teasing, and low esteem.

Children with liver disease may also experience difficulty in establishing peer relationships because of their frequent hospital stays. Social competence in childhood is predictive of the formation of adult social relationships and may be seen as a component of an individual's quality of life. Lack of social competence is a risk factor for social isolation, low self-esteem, and depression.

There are a number of ways in which psychologists can help patients with abnormal physical appearance. Firstly, it is useful to enable patients to develop age-appropriate ways of explaining their altered appearance. Assistance with social skill development and coping strategies for teasing may also be indicated, and role-play with video feedback can be a useful adjunct. For preschool children, this work can be carried out with the child's parents, with the expectation that the child will imitate the parents' behavior. Secondly, patients can be involved in preparing photographs, video materials, and written text to send to their school prior to the child's return. Healthy peers will habituate to the patient's abnormal appearance and have an opportunity to ask questions and their desire to stare will be reduced. Thirdly, cognitive therapy may be useful for adolescents whose abnormal appearance is associated with depression, social anxiety, or poor treatment adherence.

Liver transplantation

Liver transplantation presents the child and family with ongoing medical and psychological challenges. As transplant survival rates have risen, transplant teams have become increasingly aware of the need to implement practices that enhance the child's and family's quality of life throughout the transplant process.[51,52]

Research in this area includes issues relating to health-related quality of life, family cohesion, global and general health, global mental health, physical abilities, and family functioning and cohesion.[53]

As a consequence, psychologists and other members of the psychosocial team have become involved in pretransplant evaluation of children and their families, and support through the transplant process. Psychological intervention can help ameliorate both the child's and parents' distress, reduce the need for drugs, increase adherence to medical regimens, decrease hospital stay, and facilitate adjustment to daily life.[54–56] Issues covered by the pretransplant assessment include the child's cognitive and developmental functioning, coping styles and mental health of the child and family, family functioning, assessment of adherence, and—in the case of live-related donation—evaluation of the donor.

Preparing children for surgery

Research has shown that children's experience of and recovery from medical intervention significantly improves when they are given age-appropriate information about the procedures.[57]

Consequently, transplant teams need to take into account both a child's cognitive and emotional development when making decisions about how much and in what way children should be informed about the disease, transplantation procedure, and medical regimen. Assessment can also reveal anxieties about medical procedures that affect the transplant process—for example, procedural anxiety and needle phobia. Certain times during the process of undergoing invasive procedures are particularly hard on children. These "stress points" include venipuncture, separation from parents at the time of transport to the operating room, and anesthesia induction.[58]

Psychological techniques that can help children cope with specific medical procedures include psycho-education, play therapy, distraction, relaxation, behavioral therapy, and cognitive behavioral therapy. In addition, guided by an understanding of the child's cognitive and developmental functioning, hospital play specialists have an important role in educating children about their transplant through innovative play activities and educational toys and books. Integrating therapeutic play and parental involvement is therefore an essential component in the provision of holistic and quality medical care in the preparation of children for surgery.[59]

In addition, in specific cases it can be useful to assess the cognitive functioning of the parents to determine whether they will require additional support in being able to comprehend and recall details of the child's medical regimen.

Coping styles

Assessment of family functioning and coping styles is integral to developing a transplant treatment plan, in order to minimize the impact of stressors on the family. Common stressors affecting the transplant process, identified by Meltzer and Rodrigue,[60] include waiting and competition for a suitable organ (7% of patients die waiting for a donor);[61] uncertainties of rejection and the child's future health and well-being; changes in role within the family—for example, siblings having to become more independent; social isolation; and financial burdens. Clinical experience suggests that families of children who require a second transplant find the process particularly stressful, and further research is required to understand the issues that face this patient group. Likewise, children may experience illness-related uncertainty, anxiety, depression, and problems with adherence.[62]

Mental health

Children may experience depressive and anxiety disorders during the transplant process due to psychological stressors, medications, physiological disturbances, and post-traumatic stress.[63,64] Adults tend to underestimate the child's post-transplantation emotional symptoms, possibly because they focus on the improved prognosis, whereas the children focus on the concrete experience of illness.[65] In addition, some children experience changes in mood related to death anxiety, guilt due to perceived and real burdens on the family, survival guilt when other transplant patients have died, changes in family dynamics, and body image concerns.[66]

Furthermore, according to Rothenhäusler *et al.*,[67] the duration of intensive-care treatment, the number of medical complications, and the occurrence of acute rejection are also positively correlated with the risk of post-traumatic stress symptoms in some children subsequent to liver transplantation. Consequently, it is important to monitor the child's mental state from pretransplant to post-transplant, enabling early psychological intervention if these symptoms reach clinically diagnostic levels.

Family functioning

Although not necessarily pathological, changes in the family system are inevitable when a child has a chronic illness such as liver disease and the family is subject to the transplant process—for example, parental role change, increase in the care-giving burden, and separation from siblings through hospital stays or resentment of the child by the siblings.[37,68] Following transplantation—particularly combined small-intestinal and liver transplantation—the impact of the illness may have a significant effect on parental time, emotions, and family activities.[69] Some parents also find it difficult to apply the same levels of discipline or become overprotective towards the child.

There are also issues due to difficulties in adjusting to a change in the level of dependence of the child on their parents and their increasing autonomy from the family unit. Therefore, families often require ongoing psychosocial intervention to facilitate adaptation to the different stages of the transplantation process.

Living related donor liver transplantation

Although cadaveric liver transplantation is the established procedure for children in need of liver transplantation, living related donor liver transplantation may be an option in some cases, because of donor shortages or lack of a cadaver donor program (see Chapter 24).

When a family decides to consider living related donor surgery, the potential donor must undergo extensive assessment. This process may add to the stress of the parents with a child who is seriously ill. Common concerns include possible organ failure, increased risk of two family members undergoing surgery, with an increased risk of mortality in both the donor and recipient, feelings of guilt from non-donating parents, and concern for other children.[70,71]

Whilst most parents approach living related donor liver transplantation with optimism, they should be advised that there is a high chance of unsuitability, as only 10–30% of parents are suitable donors. They may also be found to have significant pathology, both physical or psychosocial, which precludes donation.[72]

A parental decision to pursue living related donor liver transplantation should include evaluation of the possibility of coercion, the effect of culture, psychopathological factors, and parental guilt.[73] There is also the possibility that donors may lack self-awareness or may be disingenuous regarding their apparent altruism.[74]

The decision to undertake living related donor liver transplantation should be interdisciplinary and involve hepatologists, psychologists, social workers, and liaison nurses, to ensure that the donor is making a rational and voluntary decision based on a good understanding of all the relevant information. Of primary importance is that the living related donor program should include psychological evaluation, with particular reference to motivational factors as well as the quality of life of the family members (i.e., adult donor, partner of the donor, siblings of the recipient, and the recipient). There is an emerging evidence base to show that psychological input has a positive impact on health outcomes for children with liver disease.[74]

Journeying towards death—issues for palliative care

Hospital deaths are inevitable, and dying children have distinct needs.[75] An important aspect of caring for a dying child is to recognize that patients have changing medical, psychological, religious, and spiritual needs at every stage of end-of-life care and that family carers' needs are also significant. For example, some children have never lived outside the hospital, some have traumatic symptoms, and others have interventions delivered until they are too ill to travel home. Whilst hospices can provide support, they offer limited space and in some families there is a cultural expectation that death will happen in hospital. Such evidence that exists points to the need for the dying child and the family to be supported by a multidisciplinary team.[76,77] However, multidisciplinary pediatric practice for dying patients is an emerging discipline that is currently underresearched.[78,79]

Family-centered care is embedded in the philosophy of pediatric medicine. The World Health Organization[80] and Department of Health[81] highlight that the dying child and their family should receive psychological, spiritual, and religious support. However, death is a difficult subject to manage, and difficulties tend to be magnified when there is a whole-family dynamic. Issues of communication are fraught with difficulties, and parents may be reluctant to allow clinicians to talk openly about the end of life to their child. There is a clear need for multidisciplinary training in order to equip professionals with the skills to manage such a dynamic. Since psychological, religious, and spiritual needs are often culturally defined,[82] this imposes wider imperatives to understand the diverse needs this group of patients.

A dying child's right to holistic care is stated in National Health Service codes of practice in the United Kingdom,[81] and families' needs are made explicit. The Association for Children's Palliative Care (info@act.org.uk; www.act.org.uk) and the Child Bereavement Trust (www.childbereavement.org.uk) offer information for families and professionals.

Nutritional support

The need for dietetic support for a child with acute, chronic, or metabolic liver disease will depend on the severity of the disease and symptoms (Figure 24.5). Nutritional problems are multifactorial in origin and their treatments diverse (Table 24.1; see Chapter 15). Inability to provide satisfactory nourishment is distressing for both the families and the child, and requires much support from the dietitian and the team.

Chronic liver disease

All infants with liver disease should have regular growth monitoring. Anthropometric measurements such as height, weight, mid-arm circumference (MAC), and triceps skinfolds (TSF) are useful tools in assessing nutritional status.[83] Weight may be affected by ascites and organomegaly, and arm anthropometry may therefore give a more accurate assessment. Because of their rapid growth, infants are particularly at risk. The dietitian should be in regular contact with the family and health professionals caring for the child, so that growth failure can be identified early.

The aim of nutritional support is to provide adequate calories to prevent or treat malnutrition (Chapter 16). The

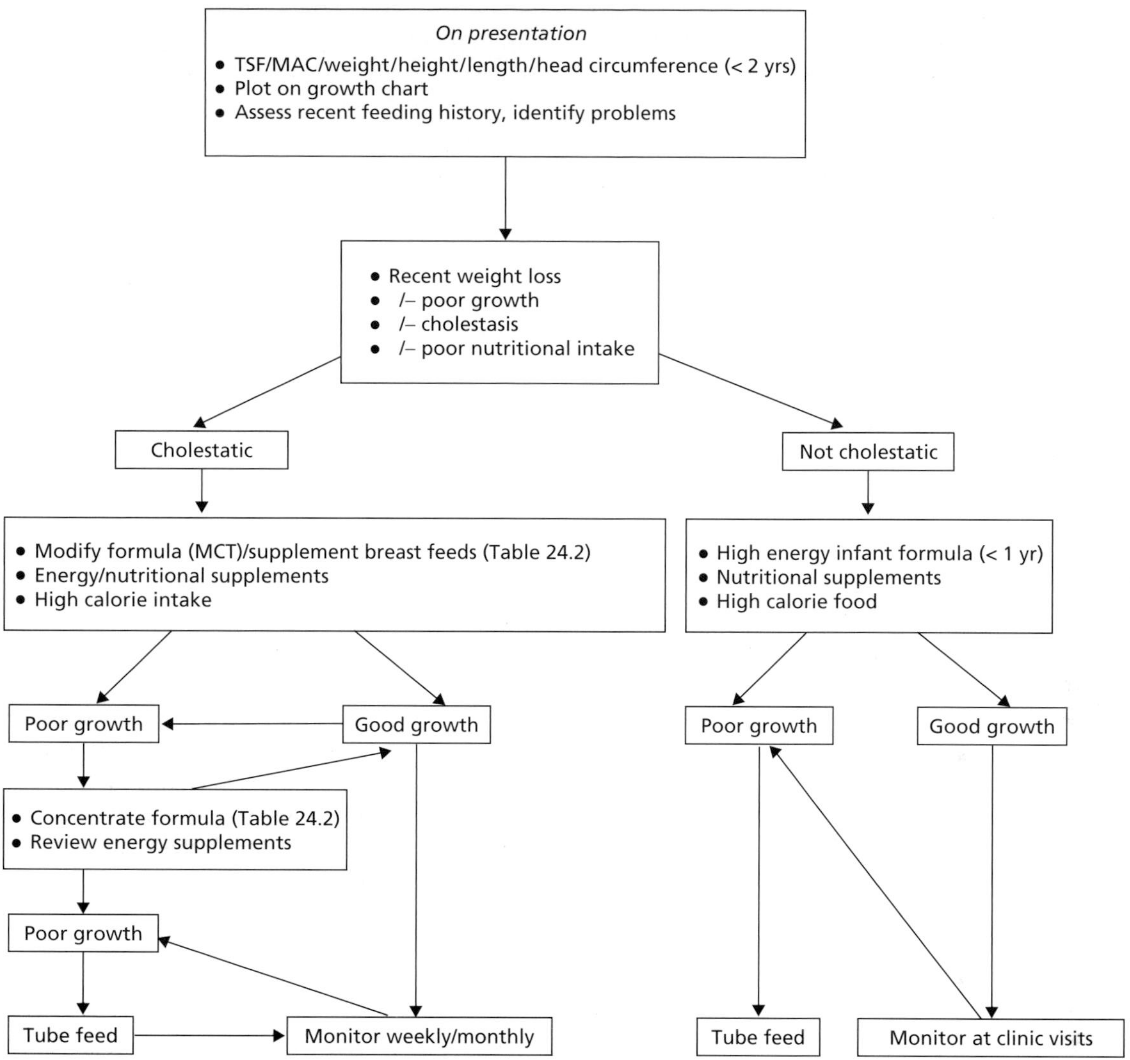

Figure 24.5 Algorithm for providing nutritional support to the child with liver disease.

Table 24.1 Causes of malnutrition in liver disease.

Inadequate intake
Anorexia, nausea, and vomiting
Early satiety due to organomegaly and ascites
Recurrent infections and hospitalization
Unpalatability of prescribed feeds and diet
Behavioral feeding difficulties
Taste changes caused by medications and biochemical disturbances
Impaired digestion and absorption of nutrients
Reduced bile flow causing fat and fat-soluble vitamin malabsorption, and essential fatty acid deficiency
Enteropathy due to portal hypertension
Disease-related pancreatic insufficiency
Increased nutritional requirements
Hypermetabolism due to infection or trauma
Insufficient protein synthesis and/or accelerated breakdown
Malabsorption

dietitian has a key role in designing and prescribing nutritional support.

Infants require adequate calories in their formula or breastfeeds to grow, but may be unable to consume adequate volumes of feed or be fluid-restricted because of ascites. It may be necessary either to offer a ready-to-use polymeric nutrient dense formula, or if specialized feeds are required, to concentrate formula milks to provide a more nutrient-dense feed (Table 24.2). This should be done under the supervision of an experienced pediatric dietitian to ensure that excessive amounts of protein and electrolytes are not consumed. Concentrating milk formulas maintains the optimal protein–energy ratio for growth and provides additional vitamins and minerals. If the infant is not cholestatic, a high-energy infant formula—e.g., Infatrini (Nutricia) or SMA High Energy (SMA Nutrition)—may be successful. Alternatively, extra carbohydrate in the form of glucose polymer—e.g., Maxijul powder or fat emulsions such as Calogen (long-chain triglyceride) or

Table 24.2 Example of how to concentrate infant formula: Peptijunior (Cow and Gate; nutrient density/100 mL).

Concentration (g/100 mL)	Energy (kcal, kJ)	Protein (g)	CHO (g)	Fat (g) 50% MCT	Na (mmol)	K (mmol)	Ca (mg)
Standard							
12.8%	67 (283)	1.8	6.9	3.6	0.9	1.7	53.8
15%	78 (335)	2.1	8.0	4.2	1.0	2.0	63
17%	89 (377)	2.4	9.1	4.8	1.1	2.2	71.4

MCT, medium-chain triglycerides.

Table 24.3 Treatment of disease-related symptoms.

Symptom	Possible dietetic treatment
Ascites	Sodium restriction Fluid restriction
Encephalopathy	Protein restriction < 1 g/kg[90] Use branched-chain amino acids[91,92]
Hypoglycemia	Continuous feeds, increased calorie density (maintain glucose > 4 mmol/L)
Malabsorption/feed intolerance	Continuous enteral feeds Manipulation of feed composition Parenteral nutrition

Liquigen (medium-chain triglyceride; all available from Scientific Hospital Supplies)—can be added, although this will adversely affect the nutrient profile of the feed.

Children with end-stage liver disease may develop portal hypertension and ascites and require salt and water restriction (Table 24.3). In some circumstances, a modular feed designed to meet the specific needs of the individual child may be required (Tables 24.4, 24.5). Cholestatic infants require specialized formula feeds (see below).

For most infants, solids should be introduced at 6 months of age, with no dietary restrictions. Some infants may be ready to commence solid food earlier. If this is the case, parents should be advised not to wean before 17 weeks of age. If additional calories are required, powdered foods can be mixed with infant formula, and/or energy supplements such as M.C.T. Duocal (Scientific Hospital Supplies, SHS) or glucose polymer can be added to increase calorie density. For some infants, this intervention can increase energy intake significantly (Tables 24.2, 24.6).

Older children will benefit from pediatric or adult nutritional supplements and from advice on increasing the energy and nutrient density of foods (Table 24.6).

Cholestatic liver disease

There are many causes of cholestatic liver disease, which can be divided into two groups: those presenting in infancy and those presenting in the older child (see also Chapters 4 and 15).

In infancy

- Neonatal infection/hepatitis
- Extrahepatic biliary atresia
- Intrahepatic biliary hypoplasia (progressive familial intrahepatic cholestasis, Alagille's syndrome)
- Liver disease induced by total parenteral nutrition (TPN).

Table 24.4 Modular feed ingredients.

Nutritional component	Product	Comments	Manufacturer
Protein	Protifar	Whole protein	Nutricia
Carbohydrate	Maxijul powder Polycal powder	Glucose polymer Glucose polymer	SHS Nutricia
Fat emulsions	Calogen Liquigen	Long-chain fat Medium-chain fat	SHS SHS
Vitamins and minerals	Pediatric Seravit	Contains carbohydrate	SHS
Electrolytes	Sodium chloride Potassium chloride	E.g., 1 mmol/mL E.g., 1 mmol/mL	

SHS, Scientific Hospital Supplies.

Table 24.5 Example of an 800-mL modular feed for an 8-kg 1-year-old child.

Product	Quantity	Energy (kcal)	Protein (g)	CHO (g)	Fat (g)	Na (mmol)	K (mmol)
Protifar	24 g	90	21.2	0.4	0.4	0.3	0.3
Maxijul	96 g	365	–	91.2	–	0.8	0.1
Pediatric Seravit	16 g	48	–	12.0	–	0.1	–
Calogen	34 mL	151	–	–	17	0.1	–
Liquigen	34 mL	151	–	–	17	0.4	–
Sodium chloride (1 mmol/mL)	12 mL	–	–	–	–	12	
Potassium chloride (1 mmol/mL)	16 mL	–	–	–	–	–	16
Per 100 mL		101	2.7	12.9	4.2	1.7	2.1
Per kg		101	2.7	12.9	4.2	1.7	2.1

Table 24.6 Suggestions on ways to add extra calories to food for infants and older children.

- Use breast milk/formula to make powdered baby foods
- Mix baby rice and breast milk/formula with pureed fruit, vegetables, or commercial baby foods
- Add a cheese-based sauce to potato or vegetables
- Add cream to soups, sauces, puddings
- Use full-fat products—e.g., yoghurts, milk, puddings
- Add margarine/butter/grated cheese to potato, sweet potato, vegetables, spaghetti, baked beans, omelettes
- Fry/roast foods where possible—e.g., sausages, bacon, fish fingers, potatoes
- Add lentils, beans, etc. to soups and casseroles
- Use sugar on hot drinks, cereals, and puddings
- Encourage sugary snacks—e.g., cakes, biscuits, sweets

These babies usually have increased energy and nutrient requirements—up to twice the estimated average requirement—as a result of malabsorption, higher energy expenditure, and infection (Chapter 4).

Most infants with cholestatic liver disease will require feed modification. If bile flow is limited from the liver into the gut, fat emulsification and digestion are reduced. This causes malabsorption of fat, fat-soluble vitamins, essential fatty acids, and some minerals, leading to steatorrhea, growth failure, and rickets.

Cholestatic babies often consume large volumes (200–300 mL/kg) of standard infant formula or breast milk, because of malabsorption of long-chain triglycerides (LCTs), which require bile for digestion and absorption. As fat is the major energy source at this age, the infants are not satisfied by their milk and consume large volumes to compensate. To promote growth, it is essential to improve fat absorption by manipulating dietary fat and substituting LCT with medium-chain triglycerides (MCTs). MCTs do not require emulsification with bile and are absorbed directly into the portal vein. The recommended practice is to change a cholestatic baby's feed to one containing a proportion (50–75%) of fat as MCT—e.g., Pregestimil (Mead Johnson), Peptijunior (Cow and Gate), Caprilon (SHS) or Generaid Plus (SHS) (Table 24.3). MCT is well tolerated, but in large quantities can cause abdominal pain, with or without diarrhea, and at high levels can cause vomiting (Table 24.7).

MCT does not contain essential fatty acids (EFAs), although the amount of EFAs required by cholestatic infants is unclear. Deficiencies may occur, but these are difficult to identify, as laboratory testing is difficult.[84] The infant formulas prescribed should meet the European Society for Pediatric Gastroenterology, Hepatology and Nutrition (ESPGHAN) guidelines for EFA (based on levels in breast milk), which recommend that 1–2% energy should come from linoleic acid (W6), with the linoleic acid–α-linolenic acid (W3) ratio being between 5 : 1 and 15 : 1. Walnut oil can be used as a natural source of EFAs, with 0.5 mL/100 kcal being prescribed to meet the recommended upper level.

Cholestatic breastfed babies will demand frequent feeds, which is exhausting for the mother. Mothers are encouraged to continue breastfeeding where possible, but the introduction of an MCT-containing formula as a top-up or supplementary feed will reduce the demand on the mother.

MCT-containing formula should continue until the infant's bilirubin level is within normal range or the child has undergone transplantation. Due to the strong flavor of these milks, the infant may reject them once solids are introduced, but an intake of around 600 mL daily should be encouraged. If growth is still failing despite resolution of cholestasis, the introduction of a high-energy infant formula—e.g., Infatrini (Nutricia) or SMA High Energy (SMA)—can be very successful in maintaining growth.

Table 24.7 Treatment of feeding problems.

Problem	Possible cause	Solutions
Diarrhea	MCT intolerance Medications Enteropathy/malabsorption	Change feed Review timing/type of medication Parenteral nutrition
Vomiting	Organomegaly Medication Reflux	Try continuous feeds Review medication Start feed thickener
Feed refusal	Taste of milk Disease state	Consider change of milk Tube-feed

MCT, medium-chain triglyceride.

Older children (> 2 years of age)

There are no specialized MCT-containing feeds available for this group of patients. Any pediatric energy supplements—e.g., Paediasure (1 kcal/mL; Abbott), Paediasure Plus (1.5 kcal/mL; Abbott), Fortini (1.5 kcal/mL; Nutricia)—or adult supplements such as Ensure Plus (1.5 kcal/mL; Abbott) or Fortisip (1.5 kcal/mL; Nutricia) can be used. Advice on fortifying foods with extra fat, carbohydrate, and energy supplements (Table 24.6) can have a huge impact on energy intake. Following "healthy eating" guidelines should be discouraged.

Nasogastric tube feeding

Supplementary nasogastric tube feeding should be considered at an early stage for any infant or child who is failing to thrive. The benefits are usually recognized and welcomed by all involved once commenced. These include:

- Reduction in pressure on parents and child
- Reduction in force-feeding
- Improved growth
- Happier mealtimes

Acceptance of tube feeding is enhanced by preparation, explanation, and support by the multidisciplinary team before and after it has been instigated. Parents and child (depending on age) should be taught to pass the tube and become familiar with the mechanics of the pump, particularly if enteral feeding is nocturnal. They should be conversant with the mode of feeding (bolus, nocturnal, or continuous). Parents should be expert in feed preparation and hygiene.

As up to 50–100% of energy requirements may be provided by tube feeding, this may impact on the oral feeding regimen. However, where possible the regimen should suit family life—i.e., overnight feeding with or without bolus feeds during the day while maintaining oral feeding to stimulate speech and swallowing. Often, continuous overnight feeding is better tolerated than bolus feeding for patients with organomegaly.

The use of gastrostomies in children with portal hypertension is controversial because of portal gastropathy and varices, but use of a soft nasogastric tube is safe.

Common problems

Intensive nutritional support in the ill infant or child may be problematic. A number of common problems are outlined in Table 24.7.

Parents of infants/children with liver disease feel immense pressure about feeding their child. They are aware of the importance of good nutrition and growth on prognosis and liver transplantation. They should not be burdened by unrealistic expectations, but should be reassured that the need for extra support and supplementary artificial feeding is often inevitable, particularly in end-stage disease.

Many children experience difficulty in feeding. This may be behavioral, usually as a result of long-term hospitalization, tube feeding when young, delayed weaning, or chronic illness, and will require different strategies (Table 24.8). Mealtimes can become a battleground, with both the child and carers using food as emotional manipulation. Often, the carer will feel guilty because the child has been ill for so long and that tackling feeding issues is cruel. Resolution of these feeding difficulties will need long-term input from speech therapists, clinical psychologists, dietitians, health visitors,

Table 24.8 Strategies for dealing with behavioral feeding difficulties.

- Never force/bribe/threaten a child to eat
- Try not to show anxiety or annoyance at mealtimes
- Reward good behavior at mealtimes with attention and positive feedback—e.g., smiling, talking to them, and ignore bad behavior (e.g., leaving the table before they should, throwing meals on the floor, etc.)
- Encourage family mealtimes, sitting at a table for social interaction
- Set a realistic time limit for the length of a meal—e.g., 30 min
- Encourage a regular meal pattern, which can include nutritious snacks
- Offer small portions and offer more when completed
- Discourage filling up on drinks between meals
- Allow infants to play with food and make a mess; this is part of normal development

pediatric community nurses, and specialist liaison nurses. Reassurance and practical support are invaluable.

Acute liver disease

Dietary treatment will depend on symptoms at presentation and on the speed of onset of disease. Initial assessment includes weight and height (length), and anthropometric measurements such as MAC and TSF. If the onset is rapid, the child is likely to be relatively well nourished at presentation, but may lose weight rapidly because of anorexia, vomiting, or fear of strange surroundings. Children require a high energy intake and sufficient carbohydrate to prevent hypoglycemia. If the child is encephalopathic, then protein reduction (1–2 g/kg) is required for a short period of time only (Table 24.3). Fluid volume should be restricted (50–75% maintenance) to prevent cerebral edema. Enteral feeding should be continued as long as possible using continuous nasogastric enteral feeding if the child is unable to feed because of drowsiness or the development of hepatic coma. Parenteral nutrition may be required if the child requires transplantation.

Liver transplantation

Children awaiting liver transplantation may need more intensive nutritional support, requiring extra nutritional supplements, enteral tube feeding, or in some circumstances parenteral feeding (Chapters 4 and 21; (Figure 24.5, Table 24.9). Modular enteral feeds may be helpful if the child requires electrolyte, fluid, or protein restriction (Tables 24.4, 24.5). Modular feeds must be prescribed and supervised by an experienced dietitian. Dietary and fluid restrictions should be kept to a minimum. Removing favorite foods from the diet may limit energy intake and is difficult for the child to accept, while prolonged dietary constraints can lead to nutritional deficiencies. Oral nutritional intake should be encouraged in order to maintain feeding skills, even if amounts are of little nutritional benefit.

Continuation of nutritional support after transplantation is vital, as it is important to maintain an adequate calorie intake (Chapter 22). If dietary restrictions have been implemented before transplantation, these should be lifted as soon as is practical unless there are complications such as chronic rejection. Many children will require tube feeding for some time, because of previous behavioral feeding problems.[85]

Parenteral nutrition

Parenteral nutrition has been used cautiously in children with liver disease, because of the well-recognized hepatobiliary complications that occur in premature infants with short-gut syndrome or intestinal failure.[86] There have been concerns about whether the potentially toxic components of parenteral nutrition could be exacerbated in children with established chronic liver disease or cholestasis. There is no evidence that amino acids, carbohydrates, or lipid emulsions are any more toxic in children with established liver disease, although amino acid levels and plasma lipids need careful monitoring. Standard amino acid and lipid solutions are well tolerated in stable patients, and lipids can be particularly beneficial in achieving adequate calorie intake. If encephalopathy develops, the amino acid content of the feed can be reduced to 1–2 g/kg/day; lipid administration requires careful monitoring in children with severe liver dysfunction,

Table 24.9 Feed composition commonly used in the treatment of cholestatic children (per 100 mL).

Feed	Manufacturer	Energy (kcal)	Protein (g)	Fat (g, % MCT)	Na (mmol)	EFAs W6 : W3
Pregestimil (13.5%)	MJ	68	1.9	3.8 (55%)	1.4	Yes 16.5 : 1
Peptijunior (12.8%)	C+G	67	1.8	3.6 (50%)	0.9	Yes 64 : 1
Caprilon (12.7%)	SHS	66	1.5	3.6 (75%)	0.9	Yes 7.5 : 1
Generaid Plus (17–34%)	SHS	79–157	1.9–3.7	3.2–6.5 (35%)	0.5–1.0	Yes 56 : 1
MCT Pepdite (15%)	SHS	68	2	2.7 (75%)	1.5	Yes 6.9 : 1
MCT Pepdite 1 + (20%)	SHS	91	2.8	3.6 (75%)	1.8	Yes 6.9 : 1
Modular feed	See individual products	70–200 50–65%	Flexible mmol/kg	Flexible	0–1.5	No

MJ, Mead Johnson; C+G, Cow and Gate; EFAs, essential fatty acids; MCT, medium-chain triglycerides; SHS, Scientific Hospital Supplies.

hepatic encephalopathy, or sepsis, and may need to be reduced in some children with sever disease, particularly if the plasma is lipemic.[87]

Although MCT emulsions have been suggested for adults with advanced liver failure, intravenous MCTs should be used with caution in children, because incomplete oxidation can occur, producing metabolic acidosis.[88] Parenteral structural lipid emulsions have not yet been evaluated in children. Special lipid emulsions (soya, MCT, olive oil, and fish oil, SMOF) may be beneficial.[89]

TPN may be necessary in children with liver disease if enteral nutrition has failed or there are complications such as feed intolerance or bleeding varices (Chapter 15), although the central venous catheters required are a potential source of infection.

The use of parenteral nutrition is particularly important for children with acute fulminant hepatitis who are awaiting liver transplantation because they are hypercatabolic. Standard formulas should be used, although the volume needs to be restricted to 75% of maintenance and the concentration should be increased to maintain glucose levels (> 4 mmol/L). There is no need to reduce protein content, particularly if the patient is electively ventilated (see Chapter 6).

Intestinal-failure liver disease

Parenteral nutrition is essential for children with intestinal failure and has transformed their outcome. The incidence of hepatic complications is associated with sepsis and prematurity[86] (see Chapter 22) and the parenteral nutrition may need to reflect the development of liver disease (see above). In this group of children, it is particularly important to encourage some enteral intake and to develop feeding and eating skills. Post-transplantation dietary regimens are focused on 24-h enteral feeding with a low-fat MCT diet initially, with a gradual increase in the concentration, volume, and fat content as enteral tolerance is achieved.

Conclusion

Intensive nutritional support may make a substantial difference to the quality of life of many children. Skilled intervention by the multidisciplinary team is vital.

References

1 Eiser C. The impact of chronic disease on sibling relationships. In: Eiser C, ed. *Growing Up with Chronic Disease: the Impact on Children and Their Families.* London: Kingsley, 1993: 175–95.

2 Krulik T. Successful normalisation tactics of parents of chronically ill children. *J Adv Nurs* 1980;**5**:573–8.

3 Knafl K, Deatrick J. How families manage chronic conditions—an analysis of the concepts of normalisation. *Res Nurs Health* 1986;**2**: 215–22.

4 Department of Health. *The NHS Plan.* London: Stationery Office, 2000.

5 Heywood J. Enhancing seamless care: a review. *Paediatr Nurs* 2002;**14**:18–20.

6 Department of Health. *Getting the Right Start: National Service Framework for Children.* London: Stationery Office, 2003.

7 Cook P. Supporting the staff. In: Cook P. *Supporting Sick Children and Their Families.* Edinburgh: Baillière Tindall, 1999: 239–55.

8 Gillick vs. West Norfolk and Wisbech Health Authority (1985) AC 112;(1985), 3 All ER 402;(1985), 3 WLR 830;(1986), 1FLR 224.

9 Coad J. *Oxford Handbook of Children and Young People's Nursing. Consent Issues.* Oxford: Oxford University Press, 2007.

10 Brook G. Children's competency to consent: a framework for practice. *Paediatr Nurs* 2000;**12**:31–5.

11 Department of Health. *Agenda for Change: Modernising the NHS Pay System.* London: Stationery Office, 1999.

12 Department of Health. *The NHS Knowledge and Skills Framework and the Development and Review Process.* London: Stationery Office, 2004.

13 Abel L, Press B, Hogg L, Hartt D, Gupte G. Intestinal transplantation in children: a new challenge for nursing. *Paediatr Nurs* 2007;**19**:20–4.

14 Department of Health. *The NHS Plan.* London: Stationery Office, 2004.

15 Whittle T, Thompson L. *Review of Learning Beyond Registration Provision in UCE Birmingham.* Birmingham: Faculty of Health, University of Central England, 2006.

16 Higher Education Funding Council for England (HEFCE). *Centres for Excellence in Teaching and Learning (CETL).* London: HEFCE, 2005.

17 Carter J, O'Reilly L, Stone E, Adams D, Hetherington J, Gordon G. Improving accessibility of information to children and families at the Liver Unit. *Pediatr Gastrenterol Nutr* 2004;**39**(Suppl 1):S149.

18 National Health Service Litigation Authority. *Clinical Negligence Scheme for Trusts.* http://www.nhsla.com, 2007.

19 Department of Health. *Toolkit for Producing Patient Information.* http://www.dh.gov.uk, 2003.

20 Carter J, Gordon G. Choices for children undergoing orthotopic liver transplant: how can we support them? *Pediatr Gastrenterol Nutr* 2004;**39**(Suppl 1):S152.

21 Gordon G, Brook G, Dudley L, *et al.* A multi-centre approach towards the development of national literature for families undergoing liver transplant in the United Kingdom. *Pediatr Gastrenterol Nutr* 2004;**39**(Suppl 1):S154.

22 Hogg L, Hartt D, Gordon G. Strategies used for managing families with challenging needs in the Liver Unit at Birmingham Children's Hospital. *Pediatr Gastrenterol Nutr* 2004;**39**(Suppl 1): S147.

23 Gordon G, Lloyd C, Gupte G, *et al.* Liver direct—a joined up way to manage long term care? *Arch Dis Child* 2002;**86**(Suppl 1):A46.

24 Gordon G. Nurse led services at the Liver Unit, Birmingham Children's Hospital. *Pediatr Gastrenterol Nutr* 2004;**39**(Suppl 1): S150.

25 Gordon G, Blythe J, Johnston A. Developing young people's clinics in a United Kingdom (UK) hepatology and transplantation unit. *Pediatr Transplant* 2007;**11**(Suppl 1):93.

26 Webster A. The facilitating role of the play specialist. *Paediatr Nurs* 2000;**12**:24–7.

27 Department of Health. *NHS Chaplaincy: Meeting the Religious and Spiritual Needs of Patients and Staff.* www.dh.gov.uk, 2003.

28 Department of Health. *Copying Letters to Patients: Good Practice Guidelines*. www.dh.gov.uk, 2003.

29 Tarter R, Gegedus A, Van Thiel D, Schade R, Gavaler J, Starzl T. Nonalcoholic cirrhosis associated with neuropsychological dysfunction in the absence of overt evidence of hepatic encephalopathy. *Gastroenterology* 1984;**86**:1421–7.

30 Tarter R, Switala J, Carra J, Edwards N, Van Thiel D. Neuropsychological impairment in patients with hepatolenticular degeneration (Wilson's disease) in the absence of overt encephalopathy. *Int J Neurosci* 1987;**37**:67–71.

31 Stewart SM, Uauy R, Waller DA, Kennard BD, Benser M, Andrews WS. Mental and motor development, social competence, and growth one year after successful paediatric liver transplantation. *J Pediatr* 1989;**114**:574–81.

32 Beath SV, Brook G, Kelly DA, *et al.* Successful liver transplantation in babies under 1 year. *BMJ* 1993;**307**:825–8.

33 Stewart SM, Kennard BD, Waller DA, Fixler D. Cognitive function in children who receive organ transplantation. *Health Psychol* 1994;**13**:3–13.

34 Van Mourik IDM, Beath SV, Brook GA, *et al.* Long-term nutritional and neurodevelopmental outcome of liver transplantation in infants aged less than 12 months. *J Pediatr Gastroenterol Nutr* 2000;**30**:269–75.

35 Fine RN, Alonson EM, Fischel JE, Bucuvalas JC, Enos RA, Gore-Langton RE. Pediatric transplantation of the kidney, liver and heart: summary report. *Pediatr Transplant* 2004;**8**:75–86.

36 Alonso EM, Neighbors K, Mattson C, *et al.* Functional outcomes of pediatric liver transplantation. *J Pediatr Gastroenterol Nutr* 2003;**37**:155–60.

37 Alonso EM, Neighbors K, Mattson C, *et al.* Functional outcomes of pediatric liver transplantation. *J Pediatr Gastroenterol Nutr* 2003;**37**:155–60.

38 Bucuvalas JC, Britto M, Krug S, *et al.* Health-related quality of life in pediatric liver transplant recipients: a single-center study. *Liver Transpl* 2003;**9**:62–71.

39 Krull K, Fuchs C, Uurk H. Neurocognitive outcome in pediatric liver transplant recipients. *Pediatr Transplant* 2003;**7**:111–8.

40 Qvist E, Pihko H, Fagerudd P, *et al.* Neurodevelopmental outcome in high-risk patients after renal transplantation in early childhood. *Pediatr Transplant* 2002;**6**:53–62.

41 Rubin AM, Kang H. Cerebral blindness and encephalopathy with cyclosporin A toxicity. *Neurology* 1987;**37**:1072–6.

42 Claude A, Brackis-Cott E, Dolezal CM, Abrams E. The role of psychosocial and family factors in adherence to antiretroviral treatment in human immunodeficiency virus-infected children. *Pediatr Infect Dis J* 2004;**23**:1035–41.

43 Cleemput I, Dobbels F. Measuring patient-reported outcomes in solid organ transplant recipients: an overview of instruments developed to date. *Pharmacoeconomics* 2007;**25**:269–86.

44 Dobbels F, Van Damme-Lombaert R, Vanhaecke J, De Geest S. Growing pains: non-adherence with the immunosuppressive regimen in adolescent transplant recipients. *Pediatr Transplant* 2005;**9**:381–90.

45 Shemesh E, Shneider BL, Savitzky JK, *et al.* Medication adherence in pediatric and adolescent liver transplant recipients. *Pediatrics* 2004;**113**:825–32.

46 Falkenstein K, Flynn L, Kirkpatrick B, Casa-Melley A, Dunn S. Non-compliance in children post-liver transplant. Who are the culprits? *Pediatr Transplant* 2004;**8**:233–6.

47 Pendley JS, Kasmen LJ, Miller DL, Donze J, Swenson C, Reeves G. Peer and family support in children and adolescents with type 1 diabetes. *J Pediatr Psychol* 2002;**27**:429–38.

48 La Greca AM, Schuman WB. Adherence to prescribed medical regimens. In: Roberts MC, ed. *Handbook of Pediatric Psychology*, 2nd ed. New York: Guilford Press, 1995: 55–83.

49 Langlois JH, Styczynski L. The effects of physical attractiveness on behavioural attributes and peer preferences of acquainted children. *Int J Behav Dev* 1979;**2**:325–41.

50 Rumsey N, Bull R, Gahagan D. The effect of facial disfigurement on the proxemic behaviour of the general public. *J Appl Psychol* 1982;**12**:137–50.

51 Maity S, Thomas AG. Quality of life in paediatric gastrointestinal and liver disease: a systematic review. *J Pediatr Gastroenterol Nutr* 2007;**44**:540–54.

52 Burra P, De Bona M. Quality of life following organ transplantation. *Transplant Int* 2007;**20**:397–409.

53 Cole C, Bucuvalas JC, Hornung RW, *et al.* Impact of liver transplantation on HRQOL in children less than 5 years old. *Pediatr Transplant* 2004;**8**:222–7.

54 Olbrisch ME, Benedict SM, Haller DL, Levenson JL. Psychosocial assessment of living organ donors: clinical and ethical considerations. *Progr Transplant* 2001;**11**:40–9.

55 Berquist RK, Berquist WE, Esquivel CO, Cox KL, Wayman KI, Litt IF. Adolescent non-adherence: prevalence and consequences in liver transplant recipients. *Pediatr Transplant* 2006;**10**:304–10.

56 Bucuvalas JC, Ryckman FC. Long-term outcome after liver transplantation in children. *Pediatr Transplant* 2002;**6**:30–6.

57 Brewer S, Gleditsch SL, Syblik D, Tietjens ME, Vacik HW. Pediatric anxiety: child life intervention in day surgery. *J Pediatr Nurs* 2006;**21**:13–22.

58 LeRoy S, Elixson EM, O'Brien P, Tong E, Turpin S, Uzark K. Recommendations for preparing children and adolescents for invasive cardiac procedures: a statement from the American Heart Association Pediatric Nursing Subcommittee of the Council on Cardiovascular Nursing in collaboration with the Council on Cardiovascular Diseases of the Young. *Circulation* 2003;**108**:2550–64.

59 Li HC, Lopez V, Lee TL. Psychoeducational preparation of children for surgery: the importance of parental involvement. *Patient Educ Couns* 2007;**65**:34–41.

60 Meltzer LJ, Rodrigue JR. Psychological distress in caregivers of liver and lung transplant candidates. *J Clin Psychol Med Settings* 2001;**8**:173–80.

61 McDiarmid SV, Davies D, Edwards EB. Improved graft survival of pediatric liver recipients transplanted with pediatric-aged liver donors. *Transplantation* 2000;**70**:1283–92.

62 Maikranz JM, Steele RG, Dreyer ML, Stratman AC, Bovaird JA. The relationship of hope and illness-related uncertainty to emotional adjustment and adherence among pediatric renal and liver transplant recipients. *J Pediatr Psychol* 2007;**32**:571–81.

63 Crone C, Gabriel G. Treatment of anxiety and depression in transplant patients: pharmacokinetic considerations. *Clin Pharmacokinet* 2004;**43**:361–94.

64 Walker AM, Harris G, Baker A, Kelly D, Houghton J. Post-traumatic stress responses following liver transplantation in older children. *J Child Psychol Psychiatry* 1999;**40**:363–74.

65 Shemesh E, Annunziato RA, Shneider B, *et al.* Parents and clinicians underestimate distress and depression in children who had a transplant. *Pediatr Transplant* 2005;**9**:673–9.

66 Fukunishi I, Sugawara Y, Takayama T, Makuuchi M, Kawarasaki H, Surman OS. Psychiatric disorders before and after living-related transplantation. *Psychosomatics* 2001;**42**:337–43.

67 Rothenhäusler HB, Ehrentraut S, Kapfhammer HP, *et al.* Psychiatric and psychosocial outcome of orthotopic liver transplantation. *Psychother Psychosomat* 2002;**71**:285–97.

68 Vilca-Melendez H, Heaton ND. Paediatric liver transplantation: the surgical view. *Postgrad Med J* 2004;**80**:571–6.

69 Sudan D, Horslen S, Botha J, *et al.* Quality of life after pediatric intestinal transplantation: the perception of pediatric recipients and their parents. *Am J Transplant* 2004;**4**:407–13.

70 Beavers KL, Sandler RS, Fair JH, Johnson MW, Shrestha R. The living donor experience: donor health assessment and outcomes after living donor liver transplantation. *Liver Transplant* 2003;**7**: 943–7.

71 Brown RS, Russo MW, Lai M, *et al.* A survey of liver transplantation from living adult donors in the United States. *N Engl J Med* 2003;**348**:818–25.

72 Baker A, Dhawan A, Devlin J, *et al.* Assessment of potential donors for living related liver transplantation. *Br J Surg* 2003;**86**: 200–5.

73 Surman OS, Fukunishi I, Allen T, Hertl M. Live organ donation: social context, clinical encounter, and the psychology of communication. *Psychosomatics* 2005;**46**:1–6.

74 Roberts MC. *Handbook of Pediatric Psychology*, 3rd ed. New York: Guilford, 2003.

75 Hyson J, Sutton D, Schwarz R, Devereux L, Sawyer S. *Paediatric Palliative Care: towards Best Practice at the Royal Children's Hospital, Melbourne*. Melbourne: Royal Children's Hospital, 2000.

76 Masera G, Spinetta JJ, Jankovic M, *et al.* Guidelines for assistance to terminally ill children with cancer: A report of the SIOP working committee on psychological issues in pediatric oncology. *Med Pediatr Oncol* 1999;**32**:44–8.

77 Contro N, Larson J, Scofield S, Sourkes B, Cohen H. Family perspectives on quality of pediatric palliative care. *Arch Pediatr Adolesc Med* 2002;**156**:14–9.

78 Donnelly JP, Huff SM, Lindsey ML, McMahon KA, Schumacher JD. The needs of children with life-limiting conditions: a healthcare-provider-based model. *Am J Hosp Palliat Care* 2005; **22**:259–67.

79 Davies R. The potential of integrated multi-agency care pathways for children. *Br J Nurs* 2006;**15**:764–8.

80 Sepúlveda C, Marlin A, Yoshida T, Ullrich A. Palliative care: the World Health Organization's global perspective. *J Pain Symptom Manage* 2002;**24**:91–6.

81 Craft A, Killen S. *Palliative Care Services for Children and Young People in England: an Independent Review for the Secretary of State for Health Crown.* London: Department of Health, 2007.

82 Taylor A, Box M. *Multicultural Palliative Care Guidelines.* Yarralumba, ACT: Palliative Care Australia, 1999.

83 Protheroe SM. Feeding the child with chronic liver disease. *Nutrition* 1998;**14**:796–800.

84 Socha P, Koletzko B, Jankowska I, *et al.* Long-chain PUFA supplementation improves PUFA profile in infants with cholestasis. *Lipids* 2002;**37**:953–7.

85 Kelly DA. Posttransplant growth failure in children. *Liver Transpl Surg* 1997;**3**:1–9.

86 Kelly DA. Intestinal failure associated liver disease—what do we know today? *Gastroenterology* 2006;**130**(2 Suppl):S70–7.

87 Kelly DA. Acute and chronic liver disease. In: Duggan C, Watkins JB, Walker WA, eds. *Nutrition in Pediatrics: Basic Science and Clinical Applications*, 4th ed. Hamilton, Ontario: Decker, 2008 [in press].

88 Glynn MJ, Powell-Tuck J, Reaveley DA, *et al.* High lipid parenteral nutrition improves port-systemic encephalopathy. *JPEN J Parenter Enteral Nutr* 1988;**12**:457–61.

89 Schlotzer E, Kanning U. Elimination and tolerance of a new parenteral lipid emulsion (SMOF)—a double-blind cross-over study in healthy male volunteers. *Ann Nutr Metab* 2004;**48**:263–8.

90 Gerber T, Schomerus H. Hepatic encephalopathy in liver cirrhosis. *Drugs* 2000;**60**:1353–70.

91 Teran JC. Nutrition and liver diseases. *Curr Gastroenterol Rep* 1999;**1**:335–40.

92 Chin SE, Shepherd RW, Thomas BJ, *et al.* Nutritional support in children with end-stage liver disease: a randomized crossover trial of a branched-chain amino acid supplement. *Am J Clin Nutr* 1992;**56**:158–63.

25 Adolescence and Transition to Adult Care

Janet E. McDonagh and Deirdre A. Kelly

Introduction

The addition of this chapter on transition in this latest edition of the present book reflects the increasing international recognition of the specific needs of young people and the importance of this area. Some 10–20% of all adolescents now have a significant ongoing health-care need related to a chronic health condition.[1–3] With advances in medical therapies and technologies, increasing numbers of young people with childhood-onset diseases—including those of the liver and biliary system—are surviving into adulthood, often with associated morbidities. The survival rate for child and adolescent recipients of liver transplantation is now 80% over 15 years. The challenge of developing transitional care for these young people is based on effective collaboration at the pediatric–adult interface and is a major challenge for pediatric and adult providers alike in the 21st century. Accompanying the improvements in survival is an increasing awareness of the need to consider the quality of life that these young people can expect into adulthood and in the longer term. Outcome research must not only consider the determinants of medical outcomes but also the psychosocial, educational, and vocational outcomes if the true picture is to be realized. One important area ripe for further study is that of the impact of the transition process itself on such outcomes.

Defining adolescence

Adolescence is best defined as the process of maturity in biological, psychological, and social terms. Adolescence starts around 10 years and may extend to 20 years.[4] Using such a wide age range definition highlights the importance of the diversity in individual development, especially in the adolescent phase of life; we may be dealing with a mature 10-year-old and a less mature 20-year-old. There is increasing evidence that key adolescent developmental milestones can be delayed in the context of chronic illness.[5,6]

Adolescence is a transitional stage in which the young person begins to move toward independence from parents and toward an increased reliance on peer-group acceptance. Adolescents have to learn to accept their developing sexuality and to make choices relating to education, employment, and a long-term career. These moves toward adulthood are challenging enough, but to a young person with chronic ill health they can be fraught with difficulties.[7] It may be more difficult for them to develop their own autonomy due to the dependence on their parents. Acceptance by peers may be more difficult due to social isolation, missing school or college due to ill health, and frequent hospital visits. Also, young people with liver disease may look "different" due to drug treatment (e.g., steroids) or the signs and symptoms of liver disease. Puberty may be delayed and growth stunted. The unpredictability of liver disease and treatment may make it difficult for young people and their families to plan realistically for the future.

Adolescents are a socially distinct group, not needing all the protection and security accorded to children but not yet ready for full independence. These young people and their parents require the support and guidance of the multidisciplinary team working within the specialist liver center to help them move into the adult world toward independence. The traditional pediatric model of care focusing on the parent may avoid the important issues of sexual and reproductive health care, substance misuse, risk behaviors, career counseling, and independent living.[8] Finally, the planning and development of adolescent-friendly services including the transition process must include the views of the young people themselves.[9]

Liver disease presenting in adolescence

Although most liver disease presents in infancy or early childhood, autoimmune liver disease, benign recurrent intrahepatic cholestasis (BRIC), and contraceptive-induced familial intrahepatic cholestasis (FIC) or adenomas present in adolescence. (see Chapters 3 and 8). Although autoimmune

Diseases of the Liver and Biliary System in Children, 3rd edition. Edited by Deirdre Kelly. © 2008 Blackwell Publishing, ISBN: 978-1-4051-6334-7.

liver disease responds to steroids and azathioprine, the increased weight gain, acne, striae, and facial disfigurement are difficult for both girls and boys, and careful counseling and support is required in order to ensure adherence. It is difficult for girls to regain their normal weight, often leading to increasing resentment and nonadherence.

BRIC and contraceptive-induced cholestasis are self-limiting but distressing conditions with jaundice and intense pruritus, but have major implications for future contraception and pregnancies. Genetic counseling may also be required because of the potential inheritance of these genetic defects (Chapter 3).

Transition

Transition is a multidimensional, active process that attends to the medical, psychosocial, and educational/vocational needs of adolescents as they move from child-centered to adult-centered services.[10] Transition, as with adolescent development itself, is therefore a time of change for the young person, the family, and the health-care team, in addition to the service configuration providing and the policies governing such care.

Confusion with respect to terminology has frustrated service and research development in this area to date, with professionals misinterpreting "transition" as meaning a single event of transfer of care to adult providers. Transition is a dynamic process with a beginning, middle, and end. The beginning is when the decision to begin or prepare for transition is made, usually within pediatric care and ideally by early adolescence. The middle phase is that of transition readiness, when the adolescent, family, and providers are prepared to begin, continue, and finish the process of transition. The final or end stage occurs when the adolescent or young adult not only transfers to adult care but is actively participating in adult care activities—e.g., of self-management and decision-making. It is important for clinicians, service providers, and policy-makers to distinguish the difference between the event of transfer and the process of transition, in order to ensure appropriate service development and not just the introduction of hand-over transfer procedures.

There is increasing agreement amongst practitioners and researchers in transitional care that there is more that unites young people with chronic conditions rather than divides them into distinct specialties. This chapter will therefore adopt a noncategorical approach to chronic illness and will refer to evidence from other specialties, acknowledging that young people with chronic illnesses face very similar issues during transition, although sometimes with different consequences.[7,11,12] In this era of financial restraint within health-care provision, such approaches are to be welcomed as enabling efficiencies of scale to be achieved in addition to an improved understanding of the common challenges facing all young people, their families, and clinicians during transition.[13]

Table 25.1 Key principles of transition.

- Active, dynamic process
- Future-focused
- Young person–centered
- Inclusive of parents/caregivers
- Early start
- Resilience framework
- Multidisciplinary, interagency
- Involves pediatric and adult services (health, social services, education, youth) in addition to primary care
- Coordinated, uninterrupted health care
  —Age-appropriate and developmentally appropriate
  —Culturally appropriate
  —Comprehensive, flexible, responsive
  —Holistic: medical, psychosocial, and educational/vocational aspects
- Skills training for the young person in communication, decision-making, assertiveness, self-management

The key principles of transition are summarized in Table 25.1 and quite clearly extend well beyond the remit of the event of transfer.

Transitions

Life in its entirety can be regarded as a series of transitions, with several major transitions congregating during adolescence—the transition from childhood to adulthood; from family relationships to those with peers; from platonic to intimate relationships; from dependent to interdependent living; and from school to further education, work, and/or further training. Interdependent with these transitions are those that are made between child-centered and adult-centered services. In today's world, these transitions are taking place at varying speeds—with some young people fast-tracking, such as teenage parents, and others on a much slower track, such as those remaining in further education well into their twenties and remaining financially dependent on their parents. Against this background, we therefore need to consider the added dimension that chronic illnesses or the post-transplantation condition bring to adolescent development. Such are the secular influences on adolescent development—so frequently ignored by health-care systems with rigid cut-off criteria—that young people are transferred to adult care in mid-adolescence with physical growth and puberty still incomplete and many of the other transitions yet to be embarked on.

Knowledge and skills in a resilience framework

The philosophy underpinning transitional care, as with the rest of adolescent health, is the concept of resilience.[14,15] Resilience has been defined as a "dynamic process involving an interaction of intrinsic and extrinsic processes of both risk and protection that act to modify the effects of an adverse life event such as illness."[16,17] Two major resources for the development of such resilience in the context of chronic illness and/or disability include knowledge and a range of skills or competencies. This knowledge-and-skills framework of transition will now be discussed further.

Knowledge

Salient information that is age-appropriate and developmentally appropriate is an integral part of transitional care for young people with chronic illnesses or long term conditions. The use of age-appropriate literature and a skilled play worker or teacher are invaluable to help young people understand and accept difficult issues such as having a dead person's organ, or facing a lifetime of medical monitoring and medication. Such information is requested by both young people and their parents, but is not always available or perceived as satisfactory by them.[18–21] Significant misunderstandings and inaccuracies have been reported among long-term clinic attendees,[22] raising the issue of education being primarily orientated toward parents during childhood and not revisited as the young person develops. Education was one of the most recommended services that young adults reported as an essential for an ideal diabetes center.[23]

Information regarding signs of disease relapse, graft rejection, and intercurrent infection whilst taking immunosuppressants are important if young people are going to take over the mantle of supervising their condition from their parent/caregivers. Similarly, information about drug therapy requested by young people includes rationale and risk–benefit discussions, and not just details of daily regimens and side effects.[19] Having a full understanding of the illness and being involved in medical decisions was rated as important by over two-thirds (69%) of young adult survivors of a pediatric dialysis and transplantation program and as the most helpful coping strategy overall by 36%.[24] Effective information has also been reported to improve quality of life, adherence to health regimens,[25] and coping with chronic disease.[26–29] For example, information regarding immunosuppressant therapies should include issues associated with preparation for travel abroad, as well as implications of practices such as tattooing and piercing and the necessity for prior hepatitis B vaccination. Other aspects of general health worthy of inclusion in education programs for young people with liver disease include dental care and the risks of sunbathing. The range of issues to address in an education program is detailed in Table 25.2.

Knowledge deficits in both adolescent and adult populations with childhood-onset disease have been reported by several authors, including knowledge about basic aspects of diagnosis and treatment.[30–32] Knowledge is important for various reasons, including disclosure. Disclosure to potential partners or employers is an unmet transitional need reported by adolescents themselves in several studies.[19,33] Accurate knowledge of diagnosis is also important for effective and appropriate information-seeking, particularly in the Internet era.

Table 25.2 The knowledge library for transition.

Condition, including effects on body, medical history, prognosis
- Therapy regimen including names, doses, side effects, rationale, risks of nonadherence
- Purposes of tests and procedures
- Relevant medical terminology
- Specific issues—e.g., antibiotic prophylaxis, immunizations

Role of individual health-care providers, what they do and how to access their services
- Meaning of transition
- Differences between pediatric and adult care
- Health insurance issues at transfer

Healthy lifestyles in terms of exercise, nutrition, dental care, emotional well-being, sun exposure, etc.
- Impact of drugs and alcohol on condition and therapy
- Impact of condition and therapy on sexual and reproductive health
- Impact of condition and therapy on education/vocation
- Advice on tattoos, body piercing

Confidentiality, consent and rights
- Social support groups and community organizations
- Reliable sources of information on: condition, therapy, general health, vocation, etc.

The range of information needs requested by young people is potentially wide and extends beyond the primary aspects of the disease and/or its therapy. Several authors have reported that young people with chronic illnesses perceive that health professionals fail to acknowledge the wider impact of the illness on the rest of their lives.[19,34] Disease education must resonate with the lives of the young people to be effective and acknowledge the realities of life as a young person today. Understanding the implications of the condition and its therapy for other aspects of health is an important component of education programs during transition.

A good working knowledge of what reliable resources are available to address these wider issues—in addition to issues such as education, vocation, leisure, financial support, disability legislation, and driving—is important for signposting. Finally, health professionals should always aim to provide up-to-date information—a significant challenge in itself.

In the delivery of any education program to young people, consideration must be given to the use of developmentally appropriate methods and the pacing and timing of delivery, in addition to assessment. Young people need to be able to access information when they need it and in a format that they prefer, and it has to be information that relates to them and addresses their own particular health needs—generic and disease-specific. Simple practices such as asking a young person to repeat the management plan to his or her parents when they return to the room after a one-to-one consultation are useful for assessing understanding. Checklists designed for self-completion in the waiting area are clinically useful, but must always be used in combination with an active assessment of understanding. Innovative approaches have been developed for this age group. The Division of Adolescent Medicine at the Hospital for Sick Children in Toronto hosts a web-based program called "My Health Passport," which produces an individualized, wallet-sized card for solid-organ transplant patients that contains important medical information. This program can be used interactively as well as independently. The practice of sending letters directly to the young person following consultations can further enhance the young person's knowledge[35] and can acknowledge the transition process as being patient-centered.

Parents and family remain a key resource of knowledge for young people, and any education program must address the informational needs of parents as well as young people, acknowledging that some of these needs will be similar but some will be different, reflecting their different perspectives. A core component of parental education during transition is developing an understanding of normal adolescent development itself and the impact of a chronic illness and/or disability on this.

Table 25.3 Skills for transition.

Health
• Feeling confident to see the health professional independent of parents when the young person so chooses
• Health information–seeking behaviors
• Accessing health care independently, including booking own appointments, contacting medical team for advice, refilling prescriptions, etc.
• Awareness of own health—taking temperatures
• Self-management of the condition
• Adherence to therapy, appointments
• Pain and fatigue management skills, including procedural pain management
• Emergency strategies
• Practical skills—e.g., urine/blood testing
Psychosocial
• Independent living skills
—Chores
—Meal preparation
—Self-care
—Mobility, including travel away from home
—Driving
—Hobbies and leisure activities
• Peer support, including independent social life
• Social competencies
Education/vocational
• Communication skills
• Work experience
• Part-time job
• Disclosure

Skills

Pediatrics is often criticized by adult counterparts as being too paternalistic and failing to recognize that young people are actually the "new users" of health services, the latter having been accessed previously by their parents/caregivers on their behalf. This concept is particularly useful when considering the skills training component of transition (Table 25.3). Skills training in self-advocacy for young people with chronic illness and/or disability reflects the resilience framework mentioned previously.[14] Such skills training has been reported to be associated with positive medical outcomes—e.g., diabetes self-management education and coping skills training programs have been shown to improve metabolic control, self-efficacy, and quality of life in adolescents.[36–39]

Independent consultations

One key skill in health is seeing the health professional independently of parents. This skill encompasses a range of other skills including confidence, communication skills, self-advocacy, negotiation, etc. Independent visits were reported to be one of the five main methods of "demonstrating transition" by providers of health care for adolescents with sickle cell disease in the United States,[40] along with encouraging patients to accept more responsibility, providing literature, making the patient more financially responsible, and having family conferences to discuss transition.[40] Independent visits have been shown to be important as one determinant of attendance at one adult congenital heart disease clinic appointment,[41] and as being a factor associated with improvement in health-related quality of life in adolescents with juvenile idiopathic arthritis (JIA).[42] However, although young people report valuing such opportunities,[19,43] not all services facilitate them.[44–46] Young people may be unaware of their rights to choose to be seen independently, and it is therefore important to proactively inform them, including such information in clinic literature and advertising it with posters in the waiting room, etc. In any discussion of such "independent" visits, consideration must be given to informed choice on the part of young people, their right to have a chaperone of their choice (not assuming that this will always be a parent), their awareness of their rights to confidentiality, and the circumstances in which this can be breached. An assessment by the health-care provider of the individual young person's skills with regard to the confidence and communication required to participate effectively in such dyadic consultations is also important.[34]

In addition to choosing to consult independently of their parents, young people need to know how to contact health-care providers independently—e.g., for advice (including in an emergency), making appointments, obtaining prescription refills, etc. Adolescence is the ideal time to start such skills training in anticipation of the time when young people will eventually leave home and live independently. The evidence suggests that such skills are not always fostered in pediatric settings.[45] Accessibility and publicity with specific reference to young people are key aspects in health services that are friendly to young people[9] and should be considered in the development of transitional care.

Practical skills

Integral to self-management is awareness of one's own health status. It is important to acquire practical skills such as taking temperatures, recognizing signs of intercurrent infection, measuring blood glucose, etc., as well as those involved with specific medications. Such detail is welcome in transitional programs, as exemplified by guidelines produced for young people with inflammatory bowel disease,[47] and it is of obvious relevance to all young people receiving immunosuppressant therapy.

Health information–seeking skills

There are now numerous sources of health information available to young people and their families that can be both empowering and unnerving. Knowing how and where to find reliable, accurate, and up-to-date information and how to distinguish such information from that which is inaccurate represents key knowledge and core skills for all young people with chronic illnesses. Health professionals can nurture such skills by providing young people with the relevant sources and assessing their awareness of these resources and the skills necessary in accessing them.

Pain and fatigue management skills

An important difference between child-centered and adult-centered services is procedural pain management, with many procedures in pediatric care being either performed by a limited number of professionals with continuity of care and/or under sedation or general anesthetic. Preparation for having such procedures performed by new people, and/or without sedation or anesthetic in accordance with adult practice, is vital to ensure successful and uneventful transfer.

Chronic pain and/or fatigue are common to many chronic conditions and can be associated with significant morbidity during adolescence in terms of schooling, social development, and physical activities. Psychological interventions have been reported to be beneficial in such situations.[48] Skills training in pain-coping strategies, pacing, and sleep hygiene is of relevance to many chronic conditions during adolescence and transition.

Communication skills

Young people have reported that their own communication skills influence their communication with doctors.[34] In addition, suboptimal communication by health-care providers with adolescents has also been reported, with health professionals frequently relying on unidirectional strategies rather than the preferable bidirectional strategies that nurture the young person's own skills and resilience.[49] Such skills are transferable to situations requiring disclosure, as well as to the world of work and other situations in which young people will have to communicate with other professionals.

Adherence and concordance

Finally, discussion of adolescents with chronic illnesses and/or disabilities would not be complete with considering the skills involved in adherence and concordance. Determinants of adherence incorporate many of the skills and much of the knowledge discussed here, in addition to a wide range of demographic and socio-economic factors, patient-related factors, condition-related factors, treatment-related factors, and factors related to the health-care setting and health-care provider (see below and also Chapter 25).

Generic health issues

In view of the recognized long-term morbidities of liver disease and transplantation—in terms of premature arteriosclerosis, hyperlipidemia, and osteoporosis—generic health issues such as substance use, alcohol, nutrition, and exercise should not be ignored. This is particularly pertinent during adolescence, which is the time when adult health-promoting behaviors often become established. Young people with chronic illnesses have been reported to have more age-related health concerns—e.g., in connection with weight and sexual health—in comparison with their healthy peers,[50] and have more serious and diverse concerns than perceived by their health-care providers.[51] Greater levels of exercise are associated with well-being and long-term functioning in patients with chronic conditions[52] and are to be encouraged when feasible, particularly in the light of concerns regarding the morbidity associated with inactivity among today's youth generally. A further issue is the importance of weight-bearing exercise for young people receiving steroid therapy, in view of the risk of premature osteoporosis after transplantation.[53] Mental health is another important component of transitional care, although psychosocial issues may vary with the primary diagnosis—e.g., adolescents with cystic fibrosis and transplants did not appear to have reduced self-esteem, unlike pediatric kidney transplant recipients.[54,55] Coping with teasing and/or bullying, side effects of drugs on body image, and disclosure issues are important issues to address with the young person during adolescence and transition.[19] Transplant recipients may be particularly vulnerable because of their altered appearance due to disease or medication, or because of time lost from school.

Sexual and reproductive health

Sexual health issues for young people with liver disease or after transplantation include all the usual concerns of their peers, which accompany the development of a sexual identity. In addition, they also have to deal with the reciprocal influences of puberty and chronic illness and/or transplantation, teratogenic drug therapy, effects on fertility, heredity issues, physical limitations, etc. Understanding the implications of a chronic illness for sexual and reproductive health was considered by physicians to be a key aspect of transitional care, although it was also the area in which there was the greatest gap between perceived importance and effectiveness.[56]

In any discussion regarding sensitive issues such as sexual health and substance use, it is important for health professionals to assess young people's understanding of what they have been told. One in 10 young men with cystic fibrosis confused infertility with impotence.[57] Reassurance about puberty and fertility is important, as both may be affected by chronic liver disease and transplantation.[58,59]

Both sexes need appropriate contraceptive advice, which should include the importance of barrier contraception for protection both against pregnancy and against sexually transmitted infections.

For young women, advice about safe and effective contraception and potential interactions with their medication is essential. The low-dose combined estrogen/progesterone pill, depot medroxyprogesterone contraception, and/or the "morning after" pill are safe for most young women before and after transplantation, unless they have other medical contraindications such as hypertension[60] (see also Chapter 21).

Likewise, advice about safe immunosuppressive medication during pregnancy is best given at an early stage. Most immunosuppressive medication is potentially teratogenic, but only mycophenolate mofetil has been consistently associated with fetal malformations. Young women planning a family should transfer to cyclosporine, tacrolimus, or prednisolone and azathioprine[61] either before or as soon as they become aware of their pregnancy (see also Chapter 21).

Many girls develop menorrhagia after transplantation, and specific advice from a specialist in adolescent medicine and/or gynecology trained in managing contraception and pregnancy in patients receiving immunosuppression is particularly useful.

Drugs and alcohol

Experimentation is part of "normal" adolescent psychosocial development, but becomes a matter of concern when it evolves into risk-taking behavior. A history of substance misuse has been reported in young people who are nonadherent with medication, and this is therefore an important (although at times difficult) aspect of history-taking.[62]

All recreational drugs affect the liver and should be strongly discouraged, as should smoking. Alcohol in moderate amounts is acceptable as long as it is well within national guidelines and unit limits, except for patients with severe liver disease. Coping strategies to deal with peer pressure with respect to alcohol intake and substance use are a further important component of transitional care.

Adherence issues

Nonadherence has been described as a risk-taking behavior[63] and is reported to be associated with other risk-taking behavior such as substance use, tattoos, and piercing,[64,65] highlighting the importance of taking a good psychosocial history. Screening tools such as the home, education, activities, drugs, sex activity, orientation, sexual abuse, and suicide (HEADSS) tool[66] are useful in this regard, both for determining risk as well as for providing information useful in the formulation of interventions to improve adherence and management. In any discussion regarding nonadherence in adolescence, it is important to reflect on what young people with chronic diseases have to face on a day-to-day basis. They often face long-term therapeutic regimens. They often have to continue medication even when they feel well. Many drug regimens also required regular monitoring in accordance with the course of the disease. All of these factors potentially lead to restrictions on leisure time, personal freedom, spontaneity, and peer interactions. Nonadherent behavior may be the only control mechanism open to the young person and/or be a simple wish to be heard and to take an active role in the decision-making process. Self-medication is an important aspect of becoming an independent young adult, but it must be seen in the context of shared decision-making, self-care, and self-management. Experimentation is a normal task of adolescent development and may be practiced by the self-medicating adolescent, but in the post-transplantation period nonadherence is the major cause of graft loss or rejection in adolescent transplant recipients, accounting for 17% of liver graft dysfunction. It is the main cause of late graft loss in adolescence after liver transplantation.[67] There is considerable evidence that nonadherence with clinic visits, medication, and compliance with medical advice increases after transfer to adult services, highlighting the importance of a good transfer process and sympathetic and skilled adult providers.[68] For further discussion regarding adherence during adolescence, several excellent reviews are available[69,70] (see also Chapter 25).

Key components of transitional care programs

In spite of the extensive literature on the evidence of a need for transition,[71,72] there are few detailed descriptions of actual transition programs in the literature other than models involving hand-over clinics involving pediatric and adult providers. The current literature on service evaluations

Table 25.4 Top 10 components of an effective transitional care program.

- Written policy
- Transitional care coordinator
- Transition program
- Involvement of interested adult service
- Multiagency involvement
- Primary care
- Involvement of young people
- Adequate administrative support
- Professional training
- Evaluation

is confusing with regard to what is meant by the term "transition" and whether it refers to the simple configuration of services and/or the content of the service provided—i.e., a transition program of care. There is, however, evidence available for individual components of the actual process of transition, which are discussed below and listed in Table 25.4.

Written policy

One of the most important aspects of transition is a written policy, developed and agreed with all the key players, to ensure consensus and a mutual understanding of the processes involved and to provide a structure for evaluation and audit (see below). There are now several excellent national policy statements advocating best practice in transition in the United Kingdom[73–77] and North America.[78–80] In practice, however, such policies are not developed[81] and/or not adhered to.[82]

An important component of such policies is a consideration of the transition timeline. An overriding principle of transition is that of flexibility, which acknowledges both the heterogeneity of adolescent developmental processes and also the potential impact of chronic illness on such processes. Developmental delay has been reported not only with regard to growth and puberty,[7] but also with regard to psychosexual, social, and vocational developmental milestones.[5,6,83] Many authors have discussed the need for consideration of the many determinants of the timing of transition and transfer in the development of transition policies,[79,84–86] albeit with a limited evidence base other than qualitative data from user accounts. Most policies advocate a start date by the age of 14 years.[76,78,79] Data from a British rheumatology study support an early start to transition. There was a maximum improvement in disease knowledge during early adolescence, with 11- and 14-year-olds reporting scores after 12 months' participation in a transitional care program that were significantly higher than those of 17-year-olds at baseline.[42] In agreement with the latter study, Hait *et al.* advocated a start at the age of 11–13 for young people with inflammatory bowel disease, with a timeline extending to 23 years.[47] In a study in the United States, transition planning was reported as having to be in place by the age of 12–14 to ensure vocational success.[87]

Coordinator and key worker role

Irrespective of whether a service can identify a key worker for every individual patient, a member of staff who is specifically designated as the transitional care program coordinator is vital to ensure both implementation as well as regular review, update, and evaluation. Such a role is identified as a core component in the majority of national policy statements to date.[73–80]

The role of a key worker and "case management" has similarly been advocated by many authors,[88–94] particularly in view of the frequently reported poor communication both between agencies and families as well as between agencies.[88] The role of such professionals is potentially diverse and wide-ranging—including clinical expert, consultant, change agent leader, researcher, and educator, to name but a few.[89] In a multicenter study of transitional care in rheumatology, the local coordinator role was considered better than paper-based resources by the adolescents themselves.[92] In the latter study, the role was undertaken by a range of personnel including occupational therapists, nurses, and physiotherapists.[92] Nurses are the profession most frequently advocated for this role in the literature.[76,89,95,96] Telfair *et al.* reported that nurse practitioners were more likely than other providers to demonstrate transition in their practice.[40] However, with the raised awareness of transition and increased opportunities for training, the potential for other professions should not be underestimated and should instead be recognized, encouraged and evaluated.

Program

The development of systematic transition programs has been supported by the majority of professionals in several major surveys.[40,92] Although there have been reported evaluations of "transitional programs," the specific details of the individual components of such programs, procedural factors, and logistics are only detailed in a few.[92] Furthermore, a weakness of the current evidence base is that research projects have tended to focus on a single aspect of transition—e.g., medical aspects, leaving home, transfer from pediatric to adult clinics—as opposed to taking a truly holistic view of transition.

In addition to meeting the transitional needs of young people, programs need to address the needs of their parents/caregivers and to remain inclusive, particularly as the young person gains more independence in the health-care setting. Health-care providers have been reported to consider a significantly earlier age than parents for young people to start being seen independently of their parents and to start teaching them self-management skills.[90] Parental difficulties and overprotectiveness have been reported to be a significant challenge during transition by several authors in a range of conditions.[20,97–99] Family support, including parental support without overprotectiveness, has been reported to be an important determinant of resilience for young people with chronic illnesses and/or disabilities.[100] Negotiating the appropriate level of protectiveness during the continuum of child and adolescent development is a key skill for *all* parents. An anticipatory approach supporting development of children and young people with chronic conditions assists families in this important task. Kieckhefer and Trahms eloquently describe the use of three theoretical models of practice for families in such an approach—developmental, leadership, and changing foci—thus enabling young people to grow up ready for adulthood.[101]

Planning and actively "envisioning a future" are integral to all transition programs.[102] Despite the widely advocated use of individualized transition plans, services have been slow to translate such policy into practice. In a 10-year audit of admissions of young adults aged 18 years and over to a major Australian pediatric hospital, 51% of surgical in-patients and 28% of medical in-patients had no documented plan for transition to adult care.[103] In addition to a lack of planning, disease complexity was reported to have contributed to the increased admissions.[103] Fiorentino also reported disease complexity as a negative predictor for transfer.[104] The American Academy of Pediatrics advocates the provision of a primary-care medical home for children and young people with chronic illnesses and/or disabilities, which specifically includes written care plans with regular review in addition to an emergency care plan.[105]

In various studies, young people have been very clear as to their desire to be involved in transition planning and/or goal-setting with their health-care team.[23,97] When individualized transition plans were implemented in a program of transitional care, they were successfully completed by 95% and 92% of adolescents and their parents respectively, efficiently identifying their needs.[92] Various other templates have been reported,[76] although not formally evaluated (Table 25.5).

Table 25.5 Transition web sites.

UK
- http://www.transitioninfonetwork.org.uk
- http://www.dh.gov.uk/transition
- http://www.dreamteam-uk.org

Australia
- http://www.rch.org.au/transition

Canada
- http://www.door2adulthood.com
- http://www.sickkids.ca/good2go

USA
- http://hctransitions.ichp.edu
- http://depts.washington.edu/healthtr/index.html
- http://chfs.ky.gov/ccshcn/ccshcntransition.htm

Interested adult service

To date, much of transition service development and research has been pediatrically driven. However, transition fundamentally involves both pediatric and adult providers, and engagement of the latter in service development is vital for success. Although there is no robust evidence to support one type of model over another, there is valuable evidence to support the key role of adult providers in transition. A "young adult team" in the United Kingdom has been reported to cost no more than ad hoc services and to be associated with significantly better participation in society.[106] In several studies of different chronic diseases, young people have reported a preference for meeting adult doctors prior to transfer.[19,23,107–112] In diabetes clinics, there was a higher rate of adherence to appointments in units where the young people had met the adult doctors before transfer.[108] Interestingly, providers treating both adolescent and adult populations have been reported to be more likely to demonstrate transition in practice in comparison with other professionals.[40]

Multidisciplinary and multiagency involvement

Due to the holistic nature of transition, care will, by definition, require a multidisciplinary and multiagency approach. The heterogeneity of these "virtual teams" has major implications for effective communication within and between services. Poor intra-agency and interagency coordination were reported by rheumatology professionals in a national survey of transitional care needs for young people with JIA.[20] Cross-boundary working has intrinsic challenges in itself, never mind in a relatively new area such as transitional care. Written communication between team members is vital and is discussed further under "Administrative support" below.

Primary-care models

The primary-care physician is an obvious candidate for the role of key worker, as he or she can potentially provide continuity of care for such young people and meet their broader health and social care needs. Primary-care teams may be particularly important for those patients who choose not to attend specialist adult services, by allowing some opportunity for monitoring and addressing physical health and psychosocial well-being. In spite of this, the majority of transitional care models are not focused on primary care.[113]

A Canadian study of young adults with diabetes reported that the family physician was the third most requested health-care professional they wanted as a member of the diabetes care team after the endocrinologist and the dietitian.[23] In contrast, in a national survey of professionals involved with adolescents with JIA, less than half perceived the primary-care practitioner (family practitioner) to be important in the planning of transitional care.[20] In their study in the United States, Telfair *et al.* reported that 81% of family practitioners reported no involvement in transitional care for adolescents with sickle cell disease.[40]

Addressing "broader health needs" is an obvious potential role for primary-care physicians. Chronically ill adolescents have been reported to be as likely or more likely to exhibit risky behaviors (e.g., substance misuse, sexual activity, etc.) than their healthy counterparts and should receive the same anticipatory guidance,[114] which may not always be available in specialty services.[115] Primary-care physicians are also the most likely to provide the patient with the only medical continuity during the period of transfer and are important in encouraging skills for appropriate health-care utilization. Learning to access health services independently has been shown to predict successful transfer.[41] However, discrepancies have been reported, with higher proportions of adolescents seeing the specialist independently in comparison with the proportion seeing their primary-care physician alone.[44] Primary-care physicians may also be unsure of their role with young people with chronic conditions, tending to leave issues to subspecialty providers.[104]

Training

In adolescent health care (including transitional care), the value of the therapeutic alliance between professionals and young people should never be underestimated. In a study of the determinants of adolescent satisfaction with a transitional care program, provider characteristics were significantly more important that the physical environment and process issues.[116] An important component of transitional care programs, therefore, is the availability of appropriately trained staff and in-service training to maintain their skills and knowledge in this area. In a Delphi study, the availability of professionals knowledgeable in transitional care was reported to be best practice, but was only feasible in a few hospitals in the United Kingdom,[117] reflecting the lack of formal training opportunities currently available in this area in Britain.[118] Transition has tremendous, although under-recognized, educational potential.[119] Topics such as the wider impact of chronic illness, adolescent development, dyadic vs. triadic consultations, ethics, confidentiality, multidisciplinary working, cultural competencies, and the differences in pediatric and adult service provision represent core knowledge for many health-care providers, not only those practicing in pediatric specialties.

Administrative support

Documentation of relevant information is important in view of the multidimensional and multidisciplinary nature of transitional care. Unfortunately, in a national audit of case notes of young people recently transferred to adult care, there was limited documentation of key transitional care issues in the case notes.[45] Interestingly, documentation significantly improved following participation in a research program evaluating an evidence-based transitional care program.[45] Similar problems with information exchange between pediatric and adult specialists were identified in a French study of the transfer arrangements for adolescents with diabetes.[120] The educational value of case notes and letters should not be underestimated as a tool for raising awareness of transition throughout the health service. The inclusion of a section addressing which transitional issues were discussed in that visit, and/or which stage transition planning has reached, is useful to ensure coordination between professionals involved with individual young people.

Effective communication both across disciplines and services and between pediatrics and adult services is imperative and yet challenging, in view of the number of professionals involved in addition to the need for the process to remain inclusive of the young person and family. The message represented by seeing a thin set of notes on arrival at the first clinic visit in the adult service can be disheartening for a young person who may have had several weighty volumes in the pediatric service, particularly if the onset of disease was in early childhood. Young people and their parents have expressed specific fears regarding the actual transfer of information.[19] Sawyer *et al.* also reported that summarizing such medical records in anticipation of transfer can take pediatric providers up to 4 h per record on average.[121] Despite participation in a multicenter transitional care research program, there was unfortunately no improvement in the number of patients for whom copy letters and/or medical and/or multidisciplinary team summaries were sent to the adult team prior to transfer.[45]

The importance of adequate administrative support is likely to be a determinant of successful transfer ultimately. The development of patient-held records, particularly for young people with complex needs, has been widely advocated[73,74]—although whether these records should be patient-held as opposed to parent-held is unclear. The practice of sending copies of clinic letters to families is likely to assist in this regard, although the implications of sending copy letters direct to the young people has not to date been specifically addressed, particularly with respect to confidentiality, comprehension, adolescent satisfaction, etc.[35] The evaluation of the use of web-based tools such as "My Health Passport" (www.sickkids.on.ca/myhealthpassport) and memory sticks in clinical practice is awaited with interest. Examples of the key areas of information to transfer to the adult health-care provider are listed in Table 25.6.

Involvement of young people in the development of services and policy

Actively involving young people in decision-making promotes citizenship and social inclusion, which are important for the health of the community. Moreover, strategies for enhancing participation will develop self-esteem, personal development, and a range of skills in young people. Such

Table 25.6 Information transfer.

- Date of diagnosis
- Diagnosis of primary condition
- Diagnosis of secondary conditions
- Diagnosis of other conditions
- Location and severity of disease
- Surgery and complications
- Medical therapies used: doses, duration, efficacy, adverse reactions, monitoring arrangements
- Role of other specialists
- Role of parents
- Primary-care involvement
- Plan for management if prior discussion with young person

Examples of templates available on the Internet:
- UK: http://www.dreamteam-uk.org
- Canada: http://www.sickkids.on.ca
- Australia: http://www.rch.org.au/transition

involvement should therefore be a fundamental component of any transitional care service. This is particularly pertinent in view of research that has identified differences between the views of young people and the views of the adults close to them, suggesting that adults cannot be used as reliable proxies for children's and young people's views.[122,123] Initiatives to involve young people's views in matters that concern them are therefore to be welcomed.[124–127]

Evaluation and audit

Finally, it is important to incorporate mechanisms of evaluation and audit into any interventional program, and this is particularly pertinent in an evolving area of health care such as adolescent health and transition.

Evidence to support transition

Benefits of effective transition have been reported by several authors, including improvements in follow-up,[128] satisfaction for young people,[42,111] disease control,[129] documentation of adolescent health issues,[45] and adherence to appointments after transfer.[130] The results of a large multicenter study of an evidence-based, coordinated transitional care program in rheumatology[92] showed significant improvements at 6 and 12 months for adolescents and their parents in comparison with the baseline with regard to health-related quality of life, knowledge, satisfaction with health care, and vocational readiness.[42] However, there remain more questions than answers, and more research is urgently needed. Do different models of transitional care produce equivalent medical and psychosocial outcomes? Which patient characteristics (medical, social, and psychosocial) identify those who need a transitional program? Are the majority of transitional issues truly noncategorical? What constitutes transition readiness? What defines "successful" transition? Can transitional care influence long-term outcomes? What are the most appropriate outcome measures for evaluative research?

Pediatric disease in an adult unit

Adult physicians may be inexperienced in handling adolescents or immature young people, but they also are unfamiliar with specific diseases historically confined to the pediatric age group in which there is little prospect of survival to adult life. These include metabolic liver disease, cholestatic diseases such as Alagille's syndrome and progressive familial intrahepatic cholestasis, biliary atresia, and post-transplant survivors.

There are now good long-term data on outcome for most of these diseases. There are two studies from Japan and France, respectively, which have demonstrated a 25% survival rate with native liver in children with biliary atresia for more than 20 years following initial Kasai portoenterostomy. Nearly all had developed cirrhosis and portal hypertension and some were being considered for transplantation. Nevertheless, they had all completed their education, both sexes had undergone puberty, and some had become parents of healthy children.[131–133]

There are similar data on Alagille's syndrome, which has a more variable outcome, with less requirement for transplantation. In a large French study, 70% of the children survived to adult life, 33% after successful transplantation. Most of the nontransplanted adults had persistent cholestasis and symptoms of liver disease, but little progression of cardiac disease or hypercholesterolemia.[134]

Children with metabolic disease such as the urea cycle defects, glycogen storage disease, and tyrosinemia type 1 are all new diseases for adult hepatologists, and are best managed by joint clinics with pediatric and adult specialists and dietitians indefinitely.[135]

Although adult hepatologists are well used to the management of patients who have undergone transplantation, they are less used to managing the long-term endocrine and emotional aspects of pretransplant chronic disease and the relative immaturity of these young people. Ensuring adequate psychosocial support in adult units is usually a difficult issue and is an important concern in planning transition (see above).

Conclusions

There are now approximately 10–20% of adolescents with chronic illnesses,[1–3] the majority of whom will survive into adult life and experience transition from child-centered to adult-centered care. In addition to this amazing improvement in survival rates, we need to ensure that the actual process of transition does not negatively influence such outcomes but rather enhances the improvement in the patients' social, vocational, and emotional outcomes. By adopting a resilience framework to transition rather than a purely medical model, health professionals can enrich the lives and maximize the potential of such young people. Above all, they are young people first and foremost. Transitional care is not just about addressing their condition, but about how they can live (and enjoy life) in spite of it.

Case study

AS was a 13-year-old girl who presented with autoimmune hepatitis type II (liver/kidney microsomal antibodies 1 : 1400 at diagnosis). She went into remission and was on maintenance immunosuppression with prednisolone 5 mg once daily and azathioprine 75 mg once daily for 2 years. She was assessed for liver transplantation at the age of 15 because of increasing portal hypertension, ascites, and peripheral edema. She complained of severe right hypochondrial pain, for which no cause was found. She underwent a successful transplant at the age of 16, with relief of the abdominal pain. She was maintained on cyclosporine and low-dose prednisolone. Twelve months after transplantation, she developed abnormal liver function tests and a recurrence of her abdominal pain. Histology and immunology demonstrated that she had a recurrence of the autoimmune hepatitis. She was restarted on high-dose immunosuppressive therapy. She became depressed and tearful about the recurrent disease, and pain management became more difficult. Despite tacrolimus, mycophenolate mofetil, and high-dose steroids, her disease progressed and she was once more considered for transplantation. In view of her age (nearly 18), it was felt best to transfer her to the adult unit for transplant assessment and future management. She was reluctant to transfer, but the transplant surgeon did not feel comfortable about operating on her in a children's hospital, and she was transferred to adult services at a series of clinics involving both pediatric and adult teams. There had been no formal, coordinated transition planning before her transfer.

She found the adjustment to the adult unit very difficult and struggled with the investigations needed for the transplant assessment. She missed being separated from her family on the ward and the multidisciplinary pediatric team. She became nonadherent with hospital visits and medication and was depressed and tearful. She often commented that she didn't wish to live. She received psychiatric support, but the psychiatrist was not experienced with young people, as he was used to counseling reformed alcoholics. She refused further psychological intervention.

She underwent her second transplantation, which went well. In the follow-up clinic 5 days later she seemed depressed and was told "to buck up and pull herself together." A review of her laboratory investigations showed that she had grossly abnormal renal and liver function tests due to a hepatic artery thrombosis. She was admitted to hospital and received an emergency transplant, but died immediately afterward from sepsis and multiorgan failure.

Comment. Transition can be particularly challenging for the young person and parents when disease presents during adolescence, when young people should be gaining in independence and finding their own personal identity. The evidence supports an early start to formal coordinated transition planning (see the section on "Written policy" above), and for AS this ideally should have started when she initially went into remission.

A key component of transition planning is the timing of transfer. It was not ideal to transfer AS at a time when her disease was uncontrolled and she was psychologically vulnerable and did not feel ready to transfer units. One solution would have been for her to have had the operation at the adult unit and return to the pediatric unit to recuperate and then transfer at a later date when her transition program was completed. It would also have been better if there had been a planned transition program prior to transfer, with a prolonged program to encourage independence, being seen on her own without her parents, starting self-medication. Although considerable discussion had taken place about transfer to the adult unit, she had not had a social visit to the adult unit and had not accepted the transfer psychologically.

Many young people become noncompliant following transfer to adult units and it is the main cause of graft loss in this age group. An integral component of transition programs prior to transfer to adult care is skills training in self-management (Table 25.3). However, transition is only completed when such skills are successfully undertaken in adult care, and adult teams should also embrace such practices. In addition, adult-trained physicians and surgeons may be impatient with young people who have been chronically unwell and find them difficult to handle and may not be sympathetic to their concerns. Parents who have been part of the decision-making process are often excluded, and in this case the patient's parents were not allowed to remain with her on the ward when she was an in-patient, which was a mutual cause of distress.

In addition, there may be little in the way of multidisciplinary support in the adult setting, which can be difficult for young people and parents to accept, particularly if they have not been prepared for such differences. Staff who are designated as transition coordinators (see the section on "Coordinator and key worker role" above) and work in both the pediatric and adult teams can facilitate transfer in such situations and gradually withdraw from active involvement when the young person has adapted to adult-centered care. They can also serve as a major resource for the training of adult team members in aspects of transitional care and adolescent health (see the section on "Training" above).

References

1 European Commission. *Report on the State of Young People's Health in the European Union.* Luxembourg: European Commission, 2000.

2 Newacheck PW, Strickland B, Shonkoff JP, *et al.* An epidemiologic profile of children with special health care needs. *Pediatrics* 1998;**102**:117–23.

3 Woodruffe C, Glickman M, Barker M, *et al. Children, Teenagers and Health: the Key Data.* Buckingham: Open University Press, 1993.

4 World Health Organization. *Young People's Health in Context.* Geneva: World Health Organization, 2004.

5 Lyon ME, Kuehl K, McCarter R. Transition to adulthood in congenital heart disease: missed adolescent milestones. *J Adolesc Health* 2006;**39**:121–4.

6 Stam H, Hartman EE, Deurloo JA, Groothoff J, Grootenhuis MA. Young adult patients with a history of pediatric disease: impact on course of life and transition into adulthood. *J Adolesc Health* 2006;**39**:4–13.

7 Suris JC, Michaud PA, Viner R. The adolescent with a chronic condition. Part 1: developmental issues. *Arch Dis Child* 2004;**89**: 938–42.

8 Payne D, Martin C, Viner R, Skinner R. Adolescent medicine in paediatric practice. *Arch Dis Child* 2005;**90**:1133–7.

9 Department of Health, United Kingdom. *You're Welcome Quality Criteria. Making Health Services Young People Friendly.* October, 2005 (www.dh.gov.uk).

10 Blum RW, Garell D, Hodgman CH, *et al.* Transition from child-centered to adult health-care systems for adolescents with chronic conditions. A position paper of the Society for Adolescent Medicine. *J Adolesc Health* 1993;**14**: 570–6.

11 Stein RE, Jessop DJ. A noncategorical approach to chronic childhood illness. *Public Health Rep* 1982;**97**:354–62.

12 Stein RE, Silver EJ. Operationalizing a conceptually based non-categorical definition: a first look at US children with chronic conditions. *Arch Pediatr Adolesc Med* 1999;**153**:68–74.

13 Sawyer SM, Drew S, Yeo MS, Britto MT. Adolescents with a chronic condition: challenges living, challenges treating. *Lancet* 2007;**369**:1481–9.

14 Olsson CA, Bond L, Burns JM, Vella-Brodrick DA, Sawyer SM. Adolescent resilience: a concept analysis. *J Adolesc* 2003;**26**: 1–11.

15 Ahern NR. Adolescent resilience: an evolutionary concept analysis. *J Pediatr Nurs* 2006;**21**:175–85.

16 Rutter M. Resilience in the face of adversity: Protective factors and resistance to psychiatric disorder. *Br J Psychiatry* 1985;**147**: 598–611.

17 Rutter M. Resilience concepts and findings: Implications for family therapy. *J Fam Ther* 1999;**21**:119–44.

18 Dovey-Pearce G, Hurrell R, May C, *et al.* Young adults' (16–25 years) suggestions for providing developmentally appropriate diabetes services: a qualitative study. *Health Soc Care Community* 2005;**13**:409–19.

19 Shaw KL, Southwood TR, McDonagh JE. Users' perspectives of transitional care for adolescents with juvenile idiopathic arthritis. *Rheumatology* 2004;**43**:770–8.

20 Shaw KL, Southwood TR, McDonagh JE. Developing a programme of transitional care for adolescents with juvenile idiopathic arthritis: results of a postal survey. *Rheumatology* 2004; **43**:211–9.

21 Ullrich G, Mattussek S, Dressler F, Thon A. How do adolescents with juvenile chronic arthritis consider their disease related knowledge, their unmet service needs and the attractiveness of various services? *Eur J Med Res* 2002;**7**:8–18.

22 Berry SL, Hayford JR, Ross CK, Pachman LM, Lavaigne JV. Conceptions of illness by children with juvenile rheumatoid arthritis: a cognitive developmental approach. *J Pediatr Psychol* 1993;**18**:83–97.

23 Scott L, Vallis M, Charette M, *et al.* Transition of care: researching the needs of young adults with type 1 diabetes. *Can J Diabetes* 2005;**29**:203–10.

24 Reynolds JM, Morton MJ, Garralda ME, *et al.* Psychosocial adjustment of adult survivors of a paediatric dialysis and transplant programme. *Arch Dis Child* 1993;**68**:104–10.

25 Klein JD, Allan MJ, Elster AB, *et al.* Improving adolescents preventive care in community health centers. *Pediatrics* 2001;**107**: 318–27.

26 Gage H, Hampson S, Skinner TC, Hart J, *et al.* Educational and psychosocial programmes for adolescents with diabetes: approaches, outcomes and cost effectiveness. *Patient Educ Couns* 2004;**53**:333–46.

27 Kyngas H. Patients education: perspective of adolescents with a chronic disease. *J Clin Nurs* 2003;**12**:744–51.

28 Guevara JP, Wolf FM, Grum CM, Clark NM. Effects of educational interventions for self management of asthma in children and adolescents: systematic review and meta-analysis. *BMJ* 2003;**326**:1308.

29 Last BF, Stam H, Onland-van Nieuwenhuizen AM, Grootenhuis MA. Positive effects of a psycho-educational group intervention for children with a chronic disease: first results. *Patient Educ Couns* 2007;**65**:101–12.

30 Shaw KL, Southwood TR, McDonagh JE. What's in a name? Disease knowledge in juvenile idiopathic arthritis (JIA). *Arch Dis Child* 2004;**89**(Suppl 1):A44.

31 Kadan-Lottick NS, Robison LL, Gurney JG, *et al.* Childhood cancer survivors' knowledge about their past diagnosis and treatment. Childhood Cancer Survivor Study. *JAMA* 2002;**287**: 1832–9.

32 Dore A, de Guise P, Merceir LA. Transition of care to adult congenital heart centers: what do patients know about their heart condition? *Can J Cardiol* 2002;**18**:141–6.

33 Telfair J, Myers J, Drezner S. Transfer as a component of the transition of adolescents with sickle cell disease to adult care: adolescent, adult and parent perspectives. *J Adolesc Health* 1994;**15**:558–65.

34 Beresford B, Sloper P. Chronically ill adolescents' experiences of communicating with doctors: a qualitative study. *J Adolesc Health* 2003;**33**:172–9.

35 James D, Yunas I, Jordan A, *et al.* Engaging young people in their healthcare: an audit of copy letters sent to adolescents in rheumatology. *Arch Dis Child* 2007;**92**(Suppl 1):A43.

36 Anderson BJ, Wolpert HA. A developmental perspective on the challenges of diabetes education and care during the young adult period. *Patient Educ Couns* 2004;**53**:347–52.

37 Grey M, Boland E, Davidson M, *et al.* Coping skills training for youth on intensive therapy has long-lasting effects on metabolic control and quality of life. *J Pediatr* 2000;**137**:107–13.

38 Grey M, Davidson M, Boland EA, *et al.* Clinical and psychosocial factors associated with achievement of treatment goals in adolescent with diabetes. *J Adolesc Health* 2001;**28**:377–85.

39 Anderson BJ, Wold FM, Burkhart MT, *et al.* Effects of peer group intervention on metabolic control of adolescent with IDDM. Randomised outpatient study. *Diabetes Care* 1989;**12**:179–83.

40 Telfair J, Alexander LR, Loosier PS, *et al.* Providers' perspectives and beliefs regarding transition to adult care for adolescents with sickle cell disease. *J Health Care Poor Underserved* 2004;**15**: 443–61.

41 Reid GJ, Irvine MJ, McCrindle BW, *et al.* Prevalence and correlates of successful transfer from pediatric to adult health care among a cohort of young adults with complex congenital heart defects. *Pediatrics* 2004;**113**:197–205.

42 McDonagh JE, Southwood TR, Shaw KL. The impact of a coordinated transitional care programme on adolescents with juvenile idiopathic arthritis. *Rheumatology* 2007;**46**:161–8.

43 Zack J, Jacobs CP, Keenan PM, *et al.* Perspectives of patients with cystic fibrosis on preventive counselling and transition to adult care. *Pediatr Pulmonol* 2003;**36**:376–83.

44 Shaw KL, Southwood TR, McDonagh JE. Growing up and moving on in rheumatology: a multicentre cohort of adolescents with juvenile idiopathic arthritis. *Rheumatology* 2005;**44**:806–12.

45 Robertson LP, McDonagh JE, Southwood TR, Shaw KL. Growing up and moving on. A multicentre UK audit of the transfer of adolescents with Juvenile Idiopathic Arthritis JIA from paediatric to adult centred care. *Ann Rheum Dis* 2006;**65**: 74–80.

46 Britto MT, Rosenthal SL, Taylor J, Passo MH. Improving rheumatologists' screening for alcohol use and sexual activity. *Arch Pediatr Adolesc Med* 2000;**154**:478–83.

47 Hait E, Arnold JH, Fishman LN. Educate, communicate, anticipate—practical recommendations for transitioning adolescents with IBD to adult health care. *Inflamm Bowel Dis* 2006;**12**: 70–3.

48 Eccleston C, Yorke L, Morley S, Williams AC, Mastroyannopoulou K. Psychological therapies for the management of chronic and recurrent pain in children and adolescents. *Cochrane Database Syst Rev* 2003;(**1**):CD003968.

49 Schubiner H, Eggly S. Strategies for health education for adolescent patients: a preliminary investigation. *J Adolesc Health* 1995;**17**:37–41.

50 Carroll G, Massarelli E, Opzoomer A, *et al.* Adolescents with chronic disease: are they receiving comprehensive health care? *J Adolesc Health Care* 1983;**4**:261–5.

51 Kowpak M. Adolescent health concerns: a comparison of adolescent and health care provider perceptions. *J Am Acad Nurse Pract* 1991;**3**:122–8.

52 Stewart AL, Hays RD, Wells KB, Rogers WH, Spritzer KL, Greenfield S. Long-term functioning and well-being outcomes associated with physical activity and exercise in patients with chronic conditions in the Medical Outcomes Study. *J Clin Epidemiol* 1994;**47**:719–30.

53 Rodino MA, Shane E. Osteoporosis after organ transplantation *Am J Med* 1998;**104**:459–69.

54 Burker EJ, Carels RA, Thompson LF, Rodgers L, Egan T. Quality of life in patients awaiting lung transplant: cystic fibrosis versus other end stage lung diseases. *Pediatr Pulmonol* 2000;**30**:453–60.

55 Baum M, Freier C, Freeman K, Chinnock RE. Developmental outcomes and cognitive functioning in infant and child heart transplant recipients. *Progr Pediatr Cardiol* 2000;**11**:159–63.

56 Scal P. Transition for youth with chronic conditions: primary care physicians' approaches. *Pediatrics* 2002;**110**:1315–21.

57 Sawyer SM, Farrant B, Cerritelli B, Wilson J. A survey of sexual and reproductive health in men with cystic fibrosis: new challenges for adolescent and adult services. *Thorax* 2005;**60**: 326–30.

58 Codoner-Franch P, Bernard O, Alvarez F. Long-term follow-up of growth in height after successful liver transplantation. *J Pediatr* 1994;**124**:368–73.

59 Cundy TF, O'Grady JG, Williams R. Recovery of menstruation and pregnancy after liver transplantation. *Gut* 1990;**31**: 337–8.

60 Sucato GS, Murray PJ. Developmental and reproductive health issues in adolescent solid organ transplant recipients. *Semin Pediatr Surg* 2006;**15**:170–8.

61 Armenti VT. Pregnancy after liver transplantation. *Liver Transpl* 2006;**12**:1037–9.

62 Millstein SG, Irwin CE, Adler NE, *et al.* Health risk behaviours and health concerns among young adolescents. *Pediatrics* 1992;**89**:422–8.

63 Penkower L, Dew MA, Ellis D, Sereika SM, Kitutu JM, Shapiro R. Psychological distress and adherence to the medical regimen among adolescent renal transplant recipients. *Am J Transplant* 2003;**3**:1418–25.

64 Lurie S, Shemesh E, Sheiner PA, *et al.* Nonadherence in pediatric liver transplant recipients—an assessment if risk factors and natural history. *Pediatr Transplant* 2000;**4**:200–6.

65 Stilley CS, Lawrence K, Bender A, Olshansky E, Webber SA, Dew MA. Maturity and adherence in adolescent and young adult heart recipients. *Pediatr Transplant* 2006;**10**:323–30.

66 Goldenring JM, Rosen DS. Getting into adolescent heads: an essential update. *Contemp Pediatr* 2004;**21**:64–90.

67 Sudan DL, Shaw BW Jr, Langnas AN. Causes of late mortality in pediatric liver transplant recipients. *Ann Surg* 1998;**227**:289–95.

68 Fredericks EM, Lopez MJ, Magee JC, Shieck V, Opipari-Arrigan L. Psychological functioning, nonadherence and health outcomes after pediatric liver transplantation. *Am J Transplant* 2007;**7**:1974–83.

69 Kyngas HA, Kroll T, Duffy ME. Compliance in adolescent with chronic diseases: a review. *J Adolesc Health* 2000;**26**:379–88.

70 Dobbels F, van Damme-Lombaert R, Vanhaecke J, De Geest S. Growing pains: non-adherence with the immunosuppressive regimen in adolescent transplant recipients. *Pediatr Transplant* 2005;**9**:381–90.

71 While A, Forbes A, Ullman R, Lewis S, Mathes L, Griffiths P. Good practices that address continuity during transition from child to adult care: syntheses of the evidence. *Child Care Health Dev* 2004;**30**:439–52.

72 Beresford B. On the road to nowhere? Young disabled people and transition. *Child Care Health Dev* 2004;**30**:581–7.

73 Department of Health, United Kingdom. *Getting the Right Start: National Service Framework for Children. Standard for Hospital Services.* London: Department of Health, 2003 (www.dh.gov.uk).

74 Department of Health, United Kingdom. *National Service Framework for Children, Young People and Maternity Services. Core Standard 4 Growing Up Into Adulthood.* London: Department of Health, 2004 (www.dh.gov.uk).

75 Department of Health, United Kingdom. *Transition. Getting it Right for Young People.* London: Department of Health, 2006 (www.dh.gov.uk/transition).

76 Royal College of Nursing. *Adolescent Transition Care: Guidance for Nursing Staff.* London: Royal College of Nursing, 2004 (www.rcn.org.uk).

77 Royal College of Paediatrics and Child Health. *Bridging the Gap: Health Care for Adolescents.* London: Royal College of Paediatrics and Child Health, 2003 (www.rcpch.ac.uk).

78 American Academy of Pediatrics, American Academy of Family Physicians, American College of Physicians-American Society of Internal Medicine. A consensus statement on health care transitions for young adults with special health care needs. *Pediatrics* 2002;**110**:1304–6.

79 Rosen DS, Blum RW, Britto M, Sawyer SM, Siegel DM; Society for Adolescent Medicine. Transition to adult health care for adolescents and young adults with chronic conditions. *J Adolesc Health* 2003;**33**:309–11.

80 Canadian Paediatric Society. Care of adolescents with chronic conditions. *Paediatr Child Health* 2006;**11**:43–8.

81 McDonagh JE, Shaw KL and Southwood TR. Translating policy into practice: development of a transitional care policy for adolescents with chronic illness. *Clin Exp Rheumatol* 2005;**23** (Suppl 37):S88.

82 Lotstein DS, McPherson M, Strickland B, Newacheck PW. Transition planning for youth with special health care needs: results from the national survey of children with special health care needs. *Pediatrics* 2005;**115**:1562–8.

83 Packham JC, Hall MA. Long-term follow-up of 246 adults with juvenile idiopathic arthritis: education and employment. *Rheumatology (Oxford)* 2002;**41:**1436–9.

84 Viner RM. Transition from paediatric to adult care. Bridging the gaps or passing the buck? *Arch Dis Child* 1999;**81**:271–5.

85 McDonagh JE. Growing up and moving on. transition from pediatric to adult care. *Pediatr Transplant* 2005;**9**:364–72.

86 Watson AR. Problems and pitfalls of transition from paediatric to adult renal care. *Pediatr Nephrol* 2005;**20**:113–7.

87 Wolf-Branigin M, Schuyler V, White P. Improving quality of life and career attitudes of youth with disabilities: experiences from the Adolescent Employment Readiness Centre. *Res Soc Work Pract* 2007;**17**:324–33.

88 Stevenson CJ, Pharoah POD, Stevenson R. Cerebral palsy—the transition from youth to adulthood. *Dev Med Child Neurol* 1997;**39**:336–42.

89 Betz CL, Redcay G. Dimensions of the transition service coordinator role. *J Spec Pediatr Nurs* 2005;**10**: 49–59.

90 Geenen SJ, Powers LE, Sells W. Understanding the role of health care providers during transition of adolescents with disabilities and special health care needs. *J Adolesc Health* 2003;**32**:225–33.

91 Garwick AW, Kohrman C, Wolman C, Blum RW. Families' recommendations for Improving Services with chronic conditions. *Arch Pediatr Adol Med* 1998;**152**:440–8.

92 McDonagh JE, Southwood TR, Shaw KL. Growing up and moving on in rheumatology: development and preliminary evaluation of a transitional care programme for a multicentre cohort of adolescents with juvenile idiopathic arthritis. *J Child Health Care* 2006;**10**:22–42.

93 Wojciechowski EA, Hurtig A, Dorn L. A natural history study of adolescent and young adults with sickle cell disease as they transfer to adult care: a need for case management services. *J Pediatr Nurs* 2002;**17**:18–27.

94 Joseph Rowntree Foundation. *Implementing Key Worker Services: a Case Study of Promoting Evidence-Based Practice.* 1999. York, England: Joseph Rowntree Foundation (www.jrf.org.uk).

95 Blomquist KB. Health, education, work and independence of young adults with disabilities. *Orthop Nurs* 2006;**25**:168–87.

96 Patterson D, Lanier C. Adolescent health transitions: focus group study of teens and young adults with special health care needs. *Fam Community Health* 1999;**22**:43–58.

97 Durst CL, Horn MV, MacLaughlin EF, *et al.* Psychosocial responses of adolescent cystic fibrosis patients to lung transplantation. *Pediatr Transplant* 2001;**5**:27–31.

98 Ehrich JHH, Rizzoni G, Broyer M, *et al.* Rehabilitation of young adults during renal replacement therapy in Europe 2. Schooling, employment and social situation. *Nephrol Dial Transplant* 1992;**7**:573–8.

99 Blum RW, Resnick MD, Nelson R, St Germaine A. Family and peer issues among adolescents with spina bifida and cerebral palsy. *Pediatrics* 1991;**88**:280–5.

100 Werner EE, Smith RS. *Overcoming the Odds: High Risk Children from Birth to Adulthood.* Ithaca, NY: Cornell University Press, 1992.

101 Kieckhefer GM, Trahms CM. Supporting development of children with chronic conditions: from compliance toward shared management. *Pediatr Nurs* 2000;**26**:354–63.

102 Reiss JG, Gibson RW, Walker LR. Health care transition: youth, family, and provider perspectives. *Pediatrics* 2005;**115**:112–20.

103 Lam PY, Fitzgerald BB, Sawyer SM. Young adults in children's hospitals: why are they there? *Med J Aust* 2005;**182**:381–4.

104 Fiorentino L, Datta D, Gentle S, *et al.* Transition from school to adult life for physically disabled young people. *Arch Dis Child* 1998;**79**:306–11.

105 Cooley WC, Committee on Children with Disabilities. Providing a primary care medical home for children and youth with cerebral palsy. *Pediatrics* 2004;**114**:1106–13.

106 Bent N, Tennant A, Swift T, Posnett J, *et al.* Team approach versus ad hoc health services for young people with physical disabilities: a retrospective cohort study. *Lancet* 2002;**360**: 1280–6.

107 Boyle MP, Farukhi Z, Nosky ML. Strategies for improving transition to adult cystic fibrosis care, based on patient and parent views. *Pediatr Pulmonol* 2001;**32**:428–36.

108 Kipps S, Bahu T, Ong K, *et al.* Current methods of transfer of young people with type 1 diabetes to adult services. *Diabet Med* 2002;**19**:649–54.

109 Miles K, Edwards S, Clapson M. Transition from paediatric to adult services: experiences of HIV-positive adolescents. *AIDS Care* 2004;**16**:305–14.

110 Nasr SZ, Campbell C, Howatt W. Transition program from paediatric to adult care for cystic fibrosis patients. *J Adolesc Health* 1992;**13**:682–5.

111 Steinkamp G, Ullrich G, Muller C, *et al.* Transition of adult patients with cystic fibrosis from paediatric to adult care—the patients' perspective before and after start-up of an adult clinic. *Eur J Med Res* 2001;**6**:85–92.

112 Landaw LI. Cystic fibrosis: transition from pediatric to adult physician's care. *Thorax* 1995;**50**:1031–2.

113 Scal P, Evans T, Blozis S, *et al.* Trends in transition from pediatric to adult health care services for young adults with chronic conditions. *J Adolesc Health* 1999;**24**:259–64.

114 Suris JC, Parera N. Sex, drugs and chronic illness: health behaviours among chronically ill youth. *Eur J Public Health* 2005;**15**:484–8.

115 Yeo MSM, Bond LM, Sawyer SM. Health risk screening in adolescents: room for improvement in a tertiary inpatient setting. *Med J Aust* 2005;**183**:427–9.

116 Shaw KL, Southwood TR, McDonagh JE. Young People's satisfaction of transitional care in adolescent rheumatology in the UK. *Child Care Health Dev* 2007;**33**:368–79.

117 Shaw KL, Southwood TR, McDonagh JE. Transitional care for adolescents with juvenile idiopathic arthritis: results of a Delphi study. *Rheumatology* 2004;**43**:1000–6.

118 McDonagh JE, Minnaar G, Kelly KM, O'Connor D, Shaw KL. Unmet education and training needs in adolescent health of health professionals in a UK Children's Hospital. *Acta Paediatr* 2006;**95**:715–9.

119 Hagood JS, Lenker CV, Thrasher S. A course on the transition to adult care of patients with childhood-onset chronic illness. *Acad Med* 2005;**80**:352–5.

120 Crosnier H, Tubiana-Rufi N. [Modalities of transition of diabetic adolescents from pediatrics to the adult care in the Paris-Ile-de-France region: an appeal to cooperative work for improving quality of care. Paris-Ile-de-France Section of DESG (Diabetes Education Study Group); in French.] *Arch Pediatr* 1998;**5**:1327–33.

121 Sawyer SM, Collins N, Bryan D, Brown D, Hope MA, Bowes G. Young people with spina bifida: transfer from pediatric to adult health care. *J Paediatr Child Health* 1998;**34**:414–7.

122 Shaw KL, Southwood TR, McDonagh JE. Growing up and moving on in rheumatology: parents as proxies of adolescents with Juvenile Idiopathic Arthritis. *Arthritis Care Res* 2006;**55**:189–98.

123 Waters E, Stewart-Brown S, Fitzpatrick R. Agreement between adolescent self-report and parent reports of health and well-being: results of an epidemiological study. *Child Care Health Dev* 2003;**29**:501–9.

124 Beresford B. *Personal Accounts: Involving Disabled Children in Research.* London: Stationery Office, 1997.

125 Department of Health, United Kingdom. Commission for Health Improvement. *Children's Voices.* London: Department of Health, 2004 (www.chi.nhs.uk).

126 Cutler D, Frost R. *Taking the Initiative: Promoting Young People's Involvement in Public Decision Making in the UK.* London: Carnegie Young People Initiative, 2001.

127 Royal College of Paediatrics and Child Health. *Coming out of the Shadows. A Strategy to Promote Participation of Children and Young People in RCPCH Activity.* London: Royal College of Paediatrics and Child Health, 2005 (www.rcpch.ac.uk).

128 Rettig P, Athreya BH. Adolescents with chronic disease: transition to adult health care. *Arthritis Care Res* 1991;**4**:174–80.

129 Salmi J, Huuponen T, Oksa H, Oksala H, Koivula T, Raita P. Metabolic control in adolescent insulin-dependent diabetics referred from pediatric to adult clinic. *Ann Clin Res* 1986;**4**: 174–80.

130 Vanelli M, Caronna S, Adinolfi B, *et al.* Effectiveness of an uninterrupted procedure to transfer adolescents with type 1 diabetes from the paediatric to the adult clinic held in the same hospital: eight-year experience with the Parma protocol. *Diabetes Nutr Metab* 2004;**17**:304–8.

131 Nio M, Ohi R, Hayashi Y, Endo N, Ibrahim M, Iwami D. Current status of 21 patients who have survived more than 20 years since undergoing surgery for biliary atresia. *J Pediatr Surg* 1996;**31**:381–4.

132 Lykaveris P, Chardot C, Sokhn M, Gauthier F, Valayer J, Bernard O. Outcome in adulthood of biliary atresia; a study of 63 patients who survived for over 20 years with their native liver. *Hepatology* 2005;**41**:366–72.

133 Kuroda T, Saeki M, Moikawa N, Fuchimoto Y. Biliary atresia and pregnancy; puberty may be an important point for predicting the outcome. *J Pediatr Surg* 2005;**40**:1852–5.

134 Lykavieris P, Hadchouel M, Chardot C, Bernard O. Outcome of liver disease in children with Alagille's syndrome: a study of 163 patients. *Gut* 2001;**49**:431–5.

135 Daublin G, Schwahn B, Wendel U. Type I glycogen storage disease: favourable outcome on a strict management regimen avoiding increased lactate production during childhood and adolescence. *Eur J Pediatr* 2002;**161**(Suppl 1):S40–5.

Index

Page numbers in *italics* represent figures and those in **bold** represent tables.

Index